D0946285

CLINICAL MANUAL OF ORIENTAL MEDICINE

AN INTEGRATIVE APPROACH

2

SECOND EDITION

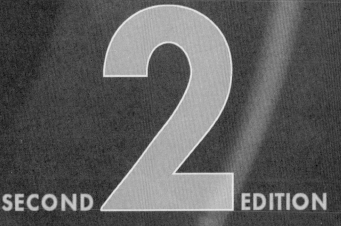
Lotus Institute Of Integrative Medicine

SYMPTOM/DISEASE INDEX

CHINESE DIAGNOSTIC INDEX

DRUG/HERB INDEX

EXEMPLAR FORMULAS

GENERAL INDEX

CLINICAL MANUAL OF ORIENTAL MEDICINE

An Integrative Approach

Second Edition

Lotus Institute of Integrative Medicine

PO Box 92493
City of Industry, CA 91715
Tel: (626) 780-7182
Fax: (626) 609-2929
Web: www.elotus.org
Email: info@elotus.org

中西醫結合臨床手冊

Copyright	Copyright © 1998, 2002, 2002, 2006 by the Lotus Institute of Integrative Medicine. 4th printing, 2nd Edition. All rights reserved. No part of this publication may be reproduced, stored in a retrieval system, or transmitted, in any form or by any means, electronic, mechanical, photocopying, recording, or otherwise, except for brief review, without the prior written permission of the Lotus Institute of Integrative Medicine.

Professional Use Only: This *Clinical Manual of Oriental Medicine* is intended as an educational guide for licensed health care practitioners only, as professional training and expertise are essential to the safe recommendation of and effective guidance for use of herbs. All herbal products discussed within this *Clinical Manual* must be used only through licensed health care practitioners.

The information in this *Clinical Manual* is presented in an accurate, truthful and non-misleading manner. The information is supported by modern research whenever possible and referenced accordingly throughout the entire *Clinical Manual*. Nonetheless, the FDA requires the following statements:

> *These statements have not been evaluated by the Food and Drug Administration. These products are not intended to diagnose, treat, cure or prevent any disease.*

General Disclaimer: Great care has been taken to maintain the accuracy of the information contained in this *Clinical Manual*. The information as presented in this *Clinical Manual* is for educational purposes only. We cannot anticipate all conditions under which this may be used. In view of ongoing research, changes in governmental regulation, and the constant flow of information relating to Chinese and western medicine, the reader is urged to check with other sources for all up-to-date information. The staff and authors of Lotus Institute of Integrative Medicine recognize that practitioners accessing this information will have varying levels of training and expertise; therefore, we accept no responsibility for the results obtained by the application of the information within this *Clinical Manual*. Nor are we liable for the safety and suitability of the products, either alone or in combination with others, with single herbs or with the products of other manufacturers. Neither the Lotus Institute of Integrative Medicine nor the authors of this *Clinical Manual* can be held responsible for errors of fact or omission, nor for any consequences arising from the use or misuse of the information herein.

Caution: Use of herbs during pregnancy or while nursing is *not* recommended.

Special Thanks: We would like to thank all the practitioners for submitting their case studies. We would also like to offer our appreciation to Jimmy Wei-Yen Chang, Alex Yuan-Da Chen, Laraine Crampton, Robert Doane, Li-Chun Huang, Jun-Qing Luo, Richard Tan, Hua-Long Zhang, Xiao-Ping Zhang and Victor Meng-Chau Jang for their expertise in bringing about this *Clinical Manual*.

ISBN: 0-9772270-0-6

Illustrator: Charles O. Funk

Publisher: **Lotus Institute of Integrative Medicine**
PO Box 92493 City of Industry, CA 91715
Tel: (626) 780-7182
Order: (866) 905-6887
Fax: (626) 609-2929
Web: www.elotus.org
Email: info@elotus.org

PREFACE

The cultural climate of contemporary healthcare is changing rapidly. As the North American public increasingly discovers the validity and efficacy of traditional Chinese medicine (TCM), both patients and practitioners here are catching glimpses of the potential for a comprehensive cooperation between the previously separate worlds of allopathic (that is, 'western' or 'modern') medicine and traditional Chinese medicine. This partnership has begun not only here but is also in progress in many of the nations in which modern and ancient medicines co-exist. There are notable examples of forward-looking hospitals and medical centers that are welcoming the assistance of TCM practitioners, and of TCM medical schools placing additional emphasis on the importance of graduates' having broad understanding of both medical worlds, and being able to speak effectively to and welcome partners within the allopathic model.

There are layers of action and potential throughout both worlds, but some are less 'integrated' than others. An acupuncturist need not know surgical techniques in order to appropriately address the presenting problems of a patient who desires assistance in recovering from surgery. A surgeon need not know how to do acupuncture in order to recommend that the surgical patient pursue a course of acupuncture to assist in resolving post-surgical pain and swelling. The partnership across this line is assisted by but not ultimately completely dependent upon communication between the two professionals.

However, when the TCM practitioner specializing in internal medicine, endocrinology, or gynecology (etc.) turns to prescribing herbal medicines, or the surgeon or internal medicine specialist or gynecologist (etc.) turn to prescribing pharmaceuticals, the potential for enhancing, exaggerating, undermining or complicating the other's efforts becomes much more apparent and potentially serious. When it comes to co-treating with medicines meant to be ingested, the need for communication becomes much clearer, and more urgent. The reasonable nexus of these two very different worlds would seem to be at the point of diagnosis, but even here it seems there could be for both parties a confounding welter of confusing terminology and approach creating a gulf between sincere professionals on either side.

While an M.D. neurologist would view and treat a headache sufferer from one angle, a TCM doctor would consider the same sufferer in light of a whole series of both similar and very different criterion. Neither is 'right' or 'wrong' for having a different approach than the other, and both have valuable healing service to offer. Although it is prohibitively expensive in terms of both time and life energy for all M.D.'s to learn TCM and all practitioners of Chinese medicine to earn medical degrees, there can and must increasingly be a shared vocabulary of understanding accessible to both medical traditions. This common ground can enhance the ability of both TCM and allopathic doctors to cooperate in providing the highest quality care to their patients while observing the utmost care to safeguard all patients from untoward reactions, interactions or complications resulting from co-treatment.

The following pages are certainly aimed primarily at TCM practitioners who are functioning either in independent or group practice, in complimentary care group practices or centers, or in hospitals incorporating both medical traditions. However, those nurses, M.D.'s, chiropractors, naturopaths, nutritionists and others who find themselves practicing alongside or in cooperation with TCM professionals will find the material in this text to be of help as they consider the purposes and actions of herbal medicines previously veiled by the mysteries of unfamiliarity, unique terminology and distinctive diagnostic strategies.

There is no disputing the superiority of combining individual skill, excellent training and longtime experience in selecting precisely the right combination of herbs for the particular patient and precise condition, given the surrounding climate, circumstances, unique patient constitution, previous patient responses to individual herbs or combinations. However, there is also a long-respected broader territory of reliable treatment using pre-processed combinations of herbs for very effective application to a specific range of action and symptomology. This middle ground, appropriately catalogued, documented and explained, can be very useful to the practitioner.

PREFACE

An M.D. debating whether a particular pharmaceutical product is appropriate for a patient who is already taking an herbal combination formula, need not return to TCM school to learn the individual characteristics of 5,000 herbal substances and the myriad applications of each substance and of combinations thereof, if appropriate information is available to her or him regarding the constituents and pharmaceutical actions of the herbal formula that the patient is taking.

Similarly, a doctor of Oriental medicine need not obtain a degree in pharmacology in an allopathic medical school in order to gain precise and adequate information as to the potential for enhanced or conflicting actions of the herbal medicines under consideration for a patient who has already begun taking pharmaceutical products to address symptoms. Having a clear and extensive resource for understanding the nature and TCM-context actions of commonly used pharmaceuticals is a key asset for this practitioner.

We have selected the Evergreen herbal formulas as the exemplars in this *Clinical Manual* because these formulas represent the most recent and innovative approach of TCM to address modern illnesses. For these new formulas, though their effectiveness have been documented by much clinical and laboratory research, there is not currently sufficient English-language explanation to ensure understanding and proper usage among practitioners. In other words, it is necessary to make sure contemporary practitioners understand how these newest formulas work, so they can make correct diagnoses and treat accordingly.

We choose to keep a simple focus in this volume, thus not to write about classic formulas, or formulas from multiple sources, in order to avoid repetition or unnecessary complication of the discussion. There is abundant documentation that exists for classic formulas from centuries of clinical application. There is no need to re-discuss those classics here, as we already know what they do and how they work. Naturally, a practitioner making careful note of the details of this volume will find that he or she can take general principles or specific information for use in considering other formulas, which is a positive by-product but not the central focus of this text.

The Lotus Institute of Integrative Medicine intends this *Clinical Manual* to provide not only a helpful resource for TCM practitioners and others, but also a bridge of communication precisely at the point of convergence of traditional Chinese medicine and other medical traditions. The thorough documentation and extensive discussion available for the products from Evergreen Herbs offer a broad and useful base from which to begin. It is our hope that the indexes, guidelines and supplementary material will make this volume even more accessible and helpful; we welcome your feedback and suggestions for future editions.

Sincere regards and best wishes for your endeavors in providing superlative health care,

Lotus Institute of Integrative Medicine
PO Box 92493 City of Industry, CA 91715
Tel: (626) 780-7182
Order: (866) 905-6887
Fax: (626) 609-2929
Web: www.elotus.org
Email: info@elotus.org

TABLE OF CONTENTS

TABLE OF CONTENTS

TABLE OF CONTENTS

Section 1

Introduction

介紹

Section 1

Introduction

STRATEGIC DOSING GUIDELINES

The standard dose of herbal extracts for an average adult is 6 to 10 grams per day. In treating acute or severe cases, the dosage may be increased up to 20 grams per day. Since not everybody is an "average adult," the fundamental concept in dosing is to realize that one size does not fit all. Every person is unique and must be treated individually.

The principle behind the *Age-To-Dose Dosing Guideline* is assessment of the maturity of the organs' ability to metabolize, utilize and eliminate herbs. This detailed chart is especially useful for adjusting dosages for infants and younger children. The recommendations are taken from *Herbology*, published by Nanjing College of Traditional Chinese Medicine.

The principle underlying the *Weight-To-Dose Dosing Guideline* is based on gauging the effective concentration of the herb after it is distributed throughout the body. This dosing strategy is especially useful for patients whose body weight falls outside of the normal range. All calculations are based on Clark's Rule in *Pharmaceutical Calculations*, by Mitchell Stoklosa and Howard Ansel.

These two charts provide the herbal practitioner with a handy reference for calculating dosages for those patients who fall outside the definition of an 'average adult.' It is still important to keep in mind, however, that these charts serve only as a guideline--not an absolute rule. Every person is unique and must be treated as such. One must always remember to treat each patient as an individual, not as a chart!

Table I. Age-to-Dose Dosing Guideline

Age	Recommended Daily Dosage	Fine Granules	Capsules
0 - 1 month	1/18 - 1/14 of adult dose	0.3 - 0.4 grams	N/R*
1 - 6 month	1/14 - 1/7 of adult dose	0.4 - 0.9 grams	N/R*
6 - 12 month	1/7 - 1/5 of adult dose	0.9 – 1.2 grams	N/R*
1 - 2 years	1/5 - 1/4 of adult dose	1.2 -1.5 grams	N/R*
2 - 4 years	1/4 - 1/3 of adult dose	1.5 - 2.0 grams	N/R*
4 - 6 years	1/3 - 2/5 of adult dose	2.0 - 2.4 grams	N/R*
6 - 9 years	2/5 - 1/2 of adult dose	2.4 - 3.0 grams	5 - 6 capsules**
9 - 14 years	1/2 - 2/3 of adult dose	3.0 - 4.0 grams	6 - 8 capsules**
14 - 18 years	2/3 - full adult dose	4.0 - 6.0 grams	8 - 12 capsules**
18 - 60 years	**adult dose**	**6.0 grams**	**12 capsules****
60 years and over	3/4 or less of adult dose	4.5 - 6.0 grams	9 - 12 capsules**

Table II. Weight-to-Dose Dosing Guideline

Weight	Recommended Daily Dosage	Fine Granules	Capsules
30 - 40 lbs	20% - 27% of adult dose	1.2 - 1.6 grams	N/R*
40 - 50 lbs	27% - 33% of adult dose	1.6 - 1.9 grams	N/R*
50 - 60 lbs	33% - 40% of adult dose	1.9 - 2.4 grams	N/R*
60 - 70 lbs	40% - 47% of adult dose	2.4 - 2.8 grams	N/R*
70 - 80 lbs	47% - 53% of adult dose	2.8 - 3.2 grams	5 - 6 capsules**
80 - 100 lbs	53% - 67% of adult dose	3.2 - 4.0 grams	6 - 8 capsules**
100 - 120 lbs	67% - 80% of adult dose	4.0 - 4.8 grams	8 - 10 capsules**
120 - 150 lbs	80% - 100% of adult dose	4.8 - 6.0 grams	10 - 12 capsules**
150 lbs	**adult dose**	**6.0 grams**	**12 capsules****
150 – 200 lbs	100% - 133% of adult dose	6.0 – 7.9 grams	12 - 16 capsules**
200 - 250 lbs	133% - 167% of adult dose	7.9 - 10.0 grams	16 - 20 capsules**
250 - 300 lbs	167% - 200% of adult dose	10.0 - 12.0 grams	20 - 24 capsules**

* N/R: Not Recommend for infants and young children since they may have difficulty swallowing.

** Each capsule weighs 500 mg or 0.5 gram.

LIST OF FORMULAS (Alphabetical Order)

NAME	CLINICAL APPLICATIONS	THERAPEUTIC FUNCTIONS
Adrenoplex	Adrenal support formula for individuals who are "burned out," with fatigue, no energy, lack of interest, lack of drive and satisfaction	Tonifies Kidney qi
Arm Support	Relieves shoulder, elbow and wrist pain	Dispels cold and damp, activates qi and blood circulation, relieves pain
Back Support (Acute)	Relieves acute low back pain	Disperses painful obstruction in the lower back
Back Support (Chronic)	Relieves chronic low back pain	Invigorates channel circulation, tonifies Kidney and Liver yin
Back Support (HD)	Relieves back pain from herniated disk	Activates blood circulation, eliminates blood stasis, reduces inflammation, relieves pain, strengthens the soft tissues
Back Support (Upper)	Relieves upper back pain (thoracic, chest, ribs, scapula)	Activates qi and blood circulation, dispels qi and blood stagnation, opens channels and collaterals, relieves pain
Balance (Cold)	Regulates menstruation in patients who are cold and weak	Nourishes Liver blood, dispels dampness and cold
Balance (Heat)	Treats menopause with manifestations of "heat" signs and symptoms (hot flashes, night sweats, emotional instability and irritability)	Clears deficiency heat
Blossom (Phase 1)	Female infertility: menstrual phase formula	Regulates menstruation, relieves pain
Blossom (Phase 2)	Female infertility: follicular phase formula	Tonifies qi and blood, nourishes Kidney *jing* (essence)
Blossom (Phase 3)	Female infertility: ovulatory phase formula	Tonifies *ming men* (life gate) fire and Kidney yang
Blossom (Phase 4)	Female infertility: luteal phase formula	Moves qi and blood
C/R Support	Strengthens the body and alleviates side effects associated with chemotherapy and/or radiation	Tonifies qi and yin, harmonizes the Stomach
CA Support	A support formula for individuals with cancer (may be late stage) who suffer extreme weakness and deficiency and cannot receive chemotherapy, radiation treatments or surgery	Clears heat, eliminates toxins, tonifies the underlying deficiencies (qi, blood, yin and yang)
Calm	Stress, anxiety, tension, nervousness, and restlessness; also a support formula for PMS (breast distention, irritability and/or mood swings)	Spreads Liver qi, relieves stagnation
Calm (ES)	Severe emotional and psychological disorders; also suppresses craving and withdrawal signs associated with addiction	Purges Liver fire, calms the *shen* (spirit)

LIST OF FORMULAS (Alphabetical Order)

NAME	CLINICAL APPLICATIONS	THERAPEUTIC FUNCTIONS
Calm (Jr)	ADD (attention deficit disorder), ADHD (attention deficit hyperactivity disorder), hyperactivity, restlessness, and difficulty concentrating	Extinguishes Liver wind, nourishes the *shen* (spirit)
Calm ZZZ	Treats stress, anxiety and restlessness with insomnia in patients with underlying weakness and deficiency	Calms the *shen* (spirit), regulates Liver qi, sedates liver fire, tonifies the deficiencies
Cholisma	Lowers cholesterol and triglyceride levels	Dispels dampness, invigorates blood circulation
Cholisma (ES)	Lowers the cholesterol and triglycerides levels in individuals with fatty liver and obesity	Dissolves damp, eliminates phlegm, invigorates blood circulation
Circulation	Treats cardiovascular disorders (such as coronary heart disease, angina pectoris, and arteriosclerosis)	Invigorates blood circulation in the upper *jiao*
Circulation (SJ)	Promotes blood circulation in the upper, middle and lower parts of the body (*San Jiao*); boosts treatment effect in patients who don't respond to standard treatments	Invigorates blood and qi circulation and eliminates blood and qi stagnations in *San Jiao*
Cordyceps 3	Provides general support to improve immune, respiratory and reproductive functions	Tonifies Lung and Kidney qi
Corydalin	Relieves acute headache	Invigorates qi and blood circulation in the head
Dermatrol (HZ)	Treats shingles (herpes zoster) with skin lesions and nerve pain	Drains damp-heat, purges fire, eliminates toxins, tonifies the underlying deficiencies
Dermatrol (PS)	Treats psoriasis and dermatological disorders with severe itching of the skin	Clears heat and detoxifies, nourishes blood
Dissolve (GS)	Dissolves gallstones (cholelithiasis) and relieves inflammation of the gallbladder and bile duct (cholecystitis)	Spreads Liver qi, clears damp-heat in the Gallbladder
Dissolve (KS)	Dissolves kidney and urinary bladder stones	Treats *shi lin* (stone dysuria)
Enhance Memory	Enhances memory, improves concentration, sharpens mental acuity	Tonifies Heart and Kidney *jing* (essence)
Equilibrium	Treats diabetes mellitus and normalizes blood glucose level	Nourishes yin, dispels dampness
Flex (CD)	Treats arthritis or joint pain that worsens with exposure to cold and damp	Warms the channels and relieves *bi zheng* (painful obstruction syndrome) with cold and deficiency
Flex (GT)	Treats gout, gouty arthritis	Drains damp-heat, opens the channels and collaterals, relieves pain
Flex (Heat)	Treats arthritis or joint pain characterized by heat (swelling, inflammation, redness and burning sensations of the affected joints)	Clears heat and relieves *bi zheng* (painful obstruction syndrome) with heat

LIST OF FORMULAS (Alphabetical Order)

NAME	CLINICAL APPLICATIONS	THERAPEUTIC FUNCTIONS
Flex (MLT)	Supports and rebuilds muscles, ligaments, tendons and cartilage	Tonifies qi and blood, nourishes yin, strengthens muscles, ligaments, tendons and cartilages.
Flex (NP)	Relieves nerve pain	Invigorates blood circulation in the extremities, relieves pain
Flex (SC)	Relieves muscle spasms and cramps	Nourishes Liver yin and blood, unblocks stagnation
Flex (Spur)	Relieves pain associated with bone spurs	Invigorates blood in the channels, disperses stagnation and relieves pain
Gardenia Complex	Purges excess fire in the body characterized by fever, high blood pressure and fast heart rate	Clears heat, purges fire, eliminates toxins
Gastrodia Complex	Treats deficient type of hypertension and vertigo	Reduces Liver yang rising, tonifies Liver and Kidney yin
Gentiana Complex	Treats excess type of hypertension. Also used for "damp-heat" affecting the Liver channel manifesting in genital herpes, genito-urinary infections	Dispels Liver channel damp-heat
Gentle Lax (Deficient)	Relieves chronic or habitual constipation	Moistens the intestines by nourishing yin and blood
Gentle Lax (Excess)	Relieves acute or severe constipation	Purges the intestines and unblocks stagnation
GI Care	Relieves general stomach disorders such as hyperacidity and treats stomach and duodenum ulcers	Clears Stomach fire and relieves pain
GI Care II	Relieves general intestinal disorders such as burning diarrhea due to infection, food poisoning or food sensitivities	Clears damp-heat, relieves diarrhea
GI Care (HMR)	Treats hemorrhoids, including internal or external hemorrhoids, with or without swelling, inflammation or bleeding	Clears damp-heat, eliminates toxic-heat from the intestines, regulates bowel movements
GI Care (UC)	Ulcerative colitis with chronic diarrhea with mucus, pus and blood, feeling of incomplete evacuation and abdominal cramps	Clears damp-heat, binds the intestines, stops bleeding
GI Harmony	Irritable bowel syndrome (IBS) with alternating diarrhea and constipation, abdominal bloating, pain or mucus, flatulence and rectal tenesmus	Spreads Liver qi, relieves diarrhea
GI Tonic	A gastrointestinal tonic formula to treat Spleen qi deficiency with loose stool, diarrhea, poor appetite, anorexia, and weakness	Tonifies Spleen qi, binds the intestines
Herbal ABX	An herbal antibiotic formula that treats bacterial, viral, and fungal infections; may be used individually or as an adjunct to another formula	Clears toxic-heat
Herbal Analgesic	An herbal analgesic formula that relieves pain and reduces inflammation; may be used individually or as an adjunct to another formula	Strongly unblocks stagnation and relieves pain

LIST OF FORMULAS (Alphabetical Order)

NAME	CLINICAL APPLICATIONS	THERAPEUTIC FUNCTIONS
Herbal DRX	An herbal diuretic formula that treats edema, generalized swelling, and water accumulation	Drains dampness, eliminates water accumulation
Herbal DTX	An herbal detox formula that cleanses the body and treats various poisoning conditions (chemicals, heavy metals, drugs, foods, and environmental or airborne toxins)	Clears heat, detoxifies, and nourishes yin
Herbal ENT	An herbal antibiotic formula that treats infections and inflammations of the ear, nose, throat and lung	Clears heat in the head and the upper *jiao*, eliminates toxins
Herbalite	An herbal formula that treats obesity by suppressing the appetite, increasing the metabolism, and elevating the energy level	Clears heat in the Stomach, dispels dampness
Immune +	Strengthens immune functions in individuals with normal or compromised immune system	Tonifies *wei* (defensive) *qi*
Imperial Tonic	A comprehensive herbal tonic formula that supplements qi, blood, yin and yang to promote optimal health and well-being	Tonifies qi, blood, yin and yang
Kidney DTX	A kidney detox formula that treats chronic nephritis, chronic nephrotic syndrome, proteinuria, and other chronic kidney diseases	Clears heat, detox the Kidneys, dispels dampness
Kidney Tonic (Yang)	A comprehensive Kidney yang tonic formula	Tonifies Kidney yang
Kidney Tonic (Yin)	A comprehensive Kidney yin tonic formula	Tonifies the Kidney yin
Knee & Ankle (Acute)	Treats acute knee and ankle disorders	Clears heat, activates blood circulation, eliminates blood stasis, drains fluids
Knee & Ankle (Chronic)	Treats chronic knee and ankle disorders	Tonifies qi, blood and yin; activates qi and blood circulation, opens channels and collaterals to relieve pain
Liver DTX	A liver detox formula that treats hepatitis, liver cirrhosis, elevated liver enzymes, and liver damages due to consumption of drugs or alcohol	Clears heat, detox the Liver
Lonicera Complex	An herbal formula that treats "wind-heat" conditions, such as common cold, influenza, oral herpes, cold sores, and fever blisters	Disperses wind-heat
LPS Support	Treats systemic lupus erythematosus (SLE) with inflammation in joints, tendons, and other connective tissues and organs	Clears heat, eliminates toxins, nourishes yin, tonifies blood, promotes generation of body fluids
Magnolia Clear Sinus	Treats sinusitis or rhinitis with clear or white nasal discharge	Disperses wind-cold, opens nasal orifices
Menotrol	Treats irregular or no menstruation due to cold and blood stagnation	Tonifies Kidney yang, invigorates blood
Mense-Ease	Eases painful menstruation	Invigorates blood circulation and removes stasis, relieves pain

LIST OF FORMULAS (Alphabetical Order)

NAME	CLINICAL APPLICATIONS	THERAPEUTIC FUNCTIONS
Migratrol	Relieves headache due to blood deficiency	Invigorates qi and blood circulation in the head, tonifies blood
Neck & Shoulder (Acute)	Relieves acute neck and shoulder pain	Disperses painful obstruction in the neck and shoulders
Neck & Shoulder (Chronic)	Relieves chronic neck and shoulder pain	Invigorates channel circulation, tonifies Kidney and Liver yin
Neuro Plus	Supports the nervous system and treats neuro-degenerative disorders such as Alzheimer's disease, Parkinson's disease, sequelae of stroke, and multiple sclerosis (MS)	Tonifies Kidney yang, opens channels and collaterals
Notoginseng 9	Stops bleeding	Cools the blood, disperses blood stasis, stops bleeding
Nourish	Nourishes Kidney yin, clears deficiency heat	Nourishes Liver and Kidney yin
Nourish (Fluids)	Nourishes yin and body fluids to treat dryness	Nourishes yin and replenishes body fluids, harmonizes the middle *jiao*
Osteo 8	Comprehensive bone support formula that increases bone density, maintains strong bones, and facilitates healing of bone injuries	Replenishes Kidney *jing* (essence)
Polygonum 14	An herbal hair tonic to promote healthy, shiny hair	Tonifies Liver blood and Kidney yin
Poria XPT	Relieves chest congestion and expels profuse yellow or green sputum	Clears Lung heat and phlegm
P-Statin	A prostate formula that addresses hypertrophy and enlargement with urinary difficulty	Disperses stagnation and relieves *lin zheng* (dysuria syndrome)
Pueraria Clear Sinus	Treats sinusitis or rhinitis with yellow nasal discharge	Disperses wind and heat, opens nasal orifices
Resolve (AI)	An herbal anti-inflammatory formula that resolves swelling and mass caused by inflammation	Disperse phlegm stagnation, clears heat and detoxifies
Resolve (Lower)	Resolves ovarian and uterine cysts, fibroids and mass	Disperses blood stasis and phlegm accumulation
Resolve (Upper)	Resolves breast lumps and cysts	Spreads Liver qi, disperses phlegm accumulation
Respitrol (CF)	Relieves cough	Releases exterior wind, eliminates phlegm, nourishes yin
Respitrol (Cold)	Relieves acute respiratory conditions with sneezing, dyspnea, chills, nasal congestion and clear nasal discharge	Warms the Lungs, dispels wind and cold

LIST OF FORMULAS (Alphabetical Order)

NAME	CLINICAL APPLICATIONS	THERAPEUTIC FUNCTIONS
Respitrol (Deficient)	Relieves chronic respiratory conditions with dyspnea, wheezing, shallow inhalation and general weakness	Tonifies and descends Lung qi
Respitrol (Heat)	Relieves acute respiratory conditions with dyspnea, wheezing, fever, dry mouth and thirst	Clears Lung heat, descends Lung qi
Saw Palmetto Complex	Treats enlarged prostrate gland (benign prostatic hypertrophy) with urinary urgency, painful urination with burning sensations	Clears heat in the lower *jiao*, relieves *lin zheng* (dysuria syndrome)
Schisandra ZZZ	Insomnia with difficulty falling and staying asleep; fragile mental state in individuals with excessive worries, insomnia, dizziness, constant fatigue and weakness	Tonifies Spleen and Heart blood, tranquilizes the *shen* (spirit)
Shine	Lifts depression, enhances mood, promotes positive outlook, increases energy and interest	Disperses phlegm and stagnation of qi, blood, food and damp
Silerex	Relieves general skin itching and irritation, such as rashes, eczema, dermatitis, and allergy	Clears heat and disperses wind; stops itching
Symmetry	Treats Bell's palsy, facial paralysis, TMJ (temporo-mandibular joint) pain, trigeminal neuralgia	Dispels wind attack, relieves pain
Thyrodex	Treats hyperthyroidism and its related symptoms	Drains Liver fire, softens hardness
Thyro-forte	Treats hypothyroidism and its related symptoms	Tonifies Kidney and Spleen yang
Traumanex	Treats trauma injuries with pain, swelling, inflammation, bruises, contusions, sprains, broken or fractured bones; also a post-surgical formula to facilitate recovery	Invigorates qi and blood circulation, relieves pain
Venus	An herbal formula for women to augment small or underdeveloped breasts, increase or maintain a healthy breast shape	Tonifies Kidney yang, invigorates blood circulation
Vibrant	A short-term tonic to boost energy and vitality, increase mental awareness and physical stamina, relieve tiredness, fatigue, and lack of energy	Tonifies qi
Vital Essence	Male reproductive disorders (infertility, low sperm count, poor sperm mobility, motility and morphology)	Tonifies Kidney yin, yang and *jing* (essence)
Vitality	Enhances male and female sexual awareness, increases sexual desire and libido, enhances sexual performance and pleasures, and treats sexual dysfunction	Tonifies Kidney yang and *jing* (essence)
V-Statin	Treats genito-urinary infections with itching and pain	Dispels damp-heat in the lower *jiao*

LIST OF FORMULAS (Body Systems)

MUSCULOSKELETAL DISORDERS

Arm Support	General musculoskeletal disorders of the arm (shoulders, elbows and wrists)	Dispels cold and damp, activates qi and blood circulation, relieves pain
Back Support (Acute)	Acute pain and inflammation of the lower back	Disperses painful obstruction in the lower back
Back Support (Chronic)	Chronic pain and inflammation of the lower back	Invigorates channel circulation, tonifies Kidney and Liver yin
Back Support (HD)	Herniated disk, lumbar radiculopathy, prolapsed or bulging disk, or slipped disk; localized or radiating pain from the spine	Activates blood circulation, eliminates blood stasis, reduces inflammation, relieves pain, strengthens the soft tissues
Back Support (Upper)	Stiffness and pain of the upper back, including chest, ribs, thoracic and scapula areas	Activates qi and blood circulation, dispels qi and blood stagnation, opens channels and collaterals, relieves pain
Corydalin	Acute headaches: vertex, occipital, frontal and temporal	Invigorates qi and blood circulation in the head
Flex (CD)	Joint pain that worsens with exposure to cold and dampness	Warms the channels and relieves *bi zheng* (painful obstruction syndrome) with cold and deficiency
Flex (GT)	Gout, gouty arthritis	Drains damp-heat, opens the channels and collaterals, relieves pain
Flex (Heat)	Joint pain with redness, swelling and inflammation	Clears heat and relieves *bi zheng* (painful obstruction syndrome) with heat
Flex (MLT)	Musculoskeletal disorders affecting the muscles, tendons and ligaments, including atrophy and wasting, damages from chronic wear and tear, and decreased range of motion and mobility	Tonifies qi and blood, activates qi and blood circulation, nourishes yin, strengthens muscles, ligaments, and tendons
Flex (NP)	Neuropathy and nerve-related pain and numbness	Invigorates blood circulation in the extremities, relieves pain
Flex (SC)	Muscle spasms and cramps	Nourishes Liver yin and blood, unblocks stagnation
Flex (Spur)	Bone spurs with swelling, inflammation and pain	Invigorates blood in the channels, disperses stagnation and relieves pain
Herbal Analgesic	For immediate and reliable relief of pain, an adjunct formula to relieve severe pain	Strongly unblocks stagnation and relieves pain
Knee & Ankle (Acute)	Acute injuries of knee and ankle with swelling, inflammation and pain	Clears heat, activates blood circulation, eliminates blood stasis, drains fluids

LIST OF FORMULAS (Body Systems)

MUSCULOSKELETAL DISORDERS (cont.)

Knee & Ankle (Chronic)	Chronic knee and ankle disorders, including atrophy and degeneration of the soft tissues, decreased range of motion and mobility, and generalized weakness and pain	Tonifies qi, blood and yin; activates qi and blood circulation, opens channels and collaterals to relieve pain
Migratrol	Chronic migraine and cluster headaches	Invigorates qi and blood circulation in the head, tonifies blood
Neck & Shoulder (Acute)	Acute neck and shoulder pain	Disperses painful obstruction in the neck and shoulders
Neck & Shoulder (Chronic)	Chronic neck and shoulder pain	Invigorates channel circulation, tonifies Kidney and Liver yin
Notoginseng 9	Bleeding disorders, including internal and external bleeding	Cools the blood, disperses blood stasis, stops bleeding
Osteo 8	Osteoporosis, bone fractures, and broken bones	Replenishes Kidney *jing* (essence)
Traumanex	Trauma injuries with bruises, swelling, inflammation; damages to soft tissues and bones	Invigorates qi and blood circulation, relieves pain

CARDIOVASCULAR/CIRCULATORY DISORDERS

Cholisma	Elevated cholesterol and triglycerides levels	Dispels dampness, invigorates blood circulation
Cholisma (ES)	High cholesterol and triglycerides levels in individuals with fatty liver and obesity	Dissolves damp, eliminates phlegm, invigorates blood circulation
Circulation	Coronary artery disease with decreased blood flow to the heart	Invigorates blood circulation in the upper *jiao*
Circulation (SJ)	Circulatory disorders with impaired blood circulation	Invigorates blood and qi circulation and eliminates blood and qi stagnations in the upper, middle and lower *jiaos*
Gastrodia Complex	Hypertension in individuals with "deficient" conditions	Reduces Liver yang rising, tonifies Liver and Kidney yin
Gentiana Complex	Hypertension in individuals with "excess" conditions	Dispels Liver channel damp-heat
Notoginseng 9	Bleeding disorders, including internal and external bleeding	Cools the blood, disperses blood stasis, stops bleeding

LIST OF FORMULAS (Body Systems)

RESPIRATORY DISORDERS

Herbal ABX	Herbal antibiotic formula for bacterial and viral infections	Clears fire, damp-heat and toxic heat, reduces swelling and redness
Herbal ENT	Herbal antibiotic formula for ear, nose, throat and lung infections and inflammations	Clears heat in the head and the upper *jiao*, eliminates toxins
Lonicera Complex	Initial stage of bacterial or viral infection with fever and sore throat	Disperses wind-heat
Magnolia Clear Sinus	Allergic sinusitis or rhinitis with nasal congestion and clear nasal discharge	Disperses wind-cold, opens nasal orifices
Notoginseng 9	Bleeding disorders, including internal and external bleeding	Cools the blood, disperses blood stasis, stops bleeding
Nourish (Fluids)	Chronic consumptive disorders characterized by dryness, such as thirst, dry mouth, post-infective cough, and non-productive cough	Nourishes yin and replenishes body fluids, harmonizes the middle *jiao*
Poria XPT	Lung infection with yellow phlegm, post-nasal drip, chest fullness and breathing difficulties	Clears Lung heat and phlegm
Pueraria Clear Sinus	Sinus infection with yellow, purulent nasal discharge and nasal congestion	Disperses wind and heat, opens nasal orifices
Respitrol (CF)	Cough from various causes (infection, drugs, smoking and others) with various complications (sputum, chest congestion, wheezing and dyspnea)	Releases exterior wind, eliminates phlegm, nourishes yin
Respitrol (Cold)	Acute respiratory conditions with dyspnea, chills, nasal congestion and clear nasal discharge	Warms the Lungs, dispels wind and cold
Respitrol (Deficient)	Chronic respiratory conditions with dyspnea, wheezing, shallow inhalation and general weakness	Tonifies and descends Lung qi
Respitrol (Heat)	Acute respiratory conditions with dyspnea, wheezing, fever, dry mouth, and thirst	Clears Lung heat, descends Lung qi

LIVER / GALLBLADDER DISORDERS

Dissolve (GS)	Gallstones and inflammation of the bile duct	Spreads Liver qi, clears damp-heat in the Gallbladder
Liver DTX	Herbal detox for liver diseases with elevated liver enzymes and compromised liver functions	Clears heat, detox the Liver

LIST OF FORMULAS (Body Systems)

GASTROINTESTINAL DISORDERS

Gentle Lax (Deficient)	Chronic constipation or habitual constipation with mild to moderate severity	Moistens the intestines by nourishing yin and blood
Gentle Lax (Excess)	Acute and severe constipation	Purges the intestines and unblocks stagnation
GI Care	Acid reflux, stomach ulcer, duodenal ulcer, stomach pain	Clears Stomach fire and relieves pain
GI Care II	Burning diarrhea due to infection or improper food intake, inflammatory bowel condition	Clears damp-heat, relieves diarrhea
GI Care (HMR)	Hemorrhoids, including internal or external hemorrhoids, with or without swelling, inflammation or bleeding	Clears damp-heat, eliminates toxic-heat from the intestines, regulates bowel movements
GI Care (UC)	Ulcerative colitis with diarrhea, mucus, blood and abdominal cramps	Clears damp-heat, binds the intestines, stops bleeding
GI Harmony	Irritable bowel syndrome with gas, pain, and alternating loose stools and constipation	Spreads Liver qi, relieves diarrhea
GI Tonic	General weakness and dysfunction of the gastrointestinal system, such as poor appetite, indigestion, and loose stools	Tonifies Spleen qi, binds the intestines
Herbal ABX	Herbal antibiotic formula to treat gastrointestinal infections	Clears fire, damp-heat and toxic heat, reduces swelling and redness
Herbal Analgesic	Herbal analgesic formula to relieve pain and reduce inflammation	Strongly unblocks stagnation and relieves pain
Notoginseng 9	Bleeding disorders, including internal and external bleeding	Cools the blood, disperses blood stasis, stops bleeding

GENITO-URINARY DISORDERS

Dissolve (KS)	Kidney and urinary stones	Treats *shi lin* (stone dysuria)
Gentiana Complex	Urinary tract infection, sexually transmitted diseases	Clears damp-heat in lower *jiao*
P-Statin	Enlarged prostate with urinary discomfort	Disperses stagnation and relieves *lin zheng* (dysuria syndrome)

LIST OF FORMULAS (Body Systems)

Saw Palmetto Complex	Enlarged prostate with pain and dysuria	Clears heat in the lower *jiao*, relieves *lin zheng* (dysuria syndrome)
V-Statin	General infection and inflammation of the genital area	Dispels damp-heat in the lower *jiao*

DERMATOLOGICAL DISORDERS

Dermatrol (HZ)	Shingles (herpes zoster) with skin lesions and nerve pain	Drains damp-heat, purges fire, eliminates toxins, tonifies the underlying deficiencies
Dermatrol (PS)	Psoriasis	Clears heat and detoxifies; nourishes blood
Herbal ABX	Herbal antibiotic formula to treat skin infections	Clears fire, damp-heat and toxic heat; reduces swelling and redness
Silerex	Itching from rashes, eczema, urticaria	Clears heat and disperses wind; stops itching

ENDOCRINE DISORDERS

Adrenoplex	Strengthens adrenal functions, for 'burned-out' individuals who have decreased mental and physical functions	Tonifies Kidney qi
Equilibrium	Diabetes mellitus	Nourishes yin, dispels dampness
Kidney Tonic (Yang)	A comprehensive Kidney yang tonic formula to address various conditions due to Kidney yang deficiency	Tonifies Kidney yang
Kidney Tonic (Yin)	A comprehensive Kidney yin tonic formula to address various conditions due to Kidney yin deficiency	Tonifies Kidney yin
Nourish	General endocrine imbalances	Nourishes Liver and Kidney yin
Thyrodex	Hyperthyroidism	Drains Liver fire, softens hardness
Thyro-forte	Hypothyroidism	Tonifies Kidney and Spleen yang
Please refer to "Formulas for Women" and "Formulas for Men" for other hormone-balancing formulas		

LIST OF FORMULAS (Body Systems)

STRESS / PSYCHOLOGICAL / SLEEP DISORDERS

Calm	Stress, frustration, irritability, anxiety, and emotional disturbance	Spreads Liver qi, relieves stagnation
Calm (ES)	Extra-strength formula to reduce severe restlessness, stress and anxiety	Purges Liver fire, calms the *shen* (spirit)
Calm (Jr)	ADD and ADHD, restlessness with difficulty focusing and concentrating	Extinguishes Liver wind, nourishes the *shen* (spirit)
Calm ZZZ	Stress, insomnia, and an overactive mind in individuals with underlying weakness and deficiencies	Calms the *shen* (spirit), regulates Liver qi, sedates Liver fire, tonifies the deficiencies
Schisandra ZZZ	Insomnia with excessive worries, pensiveness	Tonifies Spleen and Heart blood, tranquilizes the *shen* (spirit)
Shine	Depression	Disperses phlegm and stagnation of qi, blood, food and damp

INFECTIOUS DISORDERS

Gardenia Complex	Excess fire in the body characterized by fever, high blood pressure and fast heart rate	Purges fire in all three *jiaos*
Gentiana Complex	Genital herpes, genitourinary infections characterized by damp-heat affecting the Liver channel	Clears damp-heat and Liver fire
GI Care II	General intestinal disorders such as burning diarrhea due to infection, food poisoning or food sensitivities	Clears damp-heat in the intestines
Herbal ABX	An herbal antibiotic formula for bacterial, viral, and fungal infections	Clears toxic-heat
Herbal ENT	An herbal antibiotic formula for infections and inflammations of the ear, nose, throat and lung	Clears toxic-heat in the upper *jiao*
Lonicera Complex	Common cold, influenza, oral herpes, cold sores, and fever blisters characterized by wind-heat	Dispels wind-heat
Respitrol (Heat)	Acute respiratory conditions with dyspnea, wheezing, fever, dry mouth and thirst	Clears Lung heat
V-Statin	General infection and inflammation of the genital area	Dispels damp-heat in the lower *jiao*

LIST OF FORMULAS (Body Systems)

IMMUNE / ENERGY DISORDERS

CA Support	Cancer support formula for individuals who suffer extreme weakness and deficiency and cannot receive chemotherapy, radiation treatments or surgery	Clears heat, eliminates toxins, tonifies the underlying deficiencies (qi, blood, yin and yang)
C/R Support	Chemotherapy and radiation support formula for individuals receiving such treatments	Tonifies qi and yin, harmonizes the Stomach
Cordyceps 3	General support to improve immune and reproductive functions	Tonifies Lung and Kidney qi
GI Tonic	Gastrointestinal tonic formula to improve digestion of foods and absorption of nutrients	Tonifies Spleen qi, binds the intestines
Immune +	Promotes and strengthens immune function	Tonifies *wei* (defensive) *qi*
Imperial Tonic	A comprehensive and balanced tonic to improve mental and physical performances	Tonifies qi, blood, yin and yang
Vibrant	A quick and immediate tonic to boost energy and vitality	Tonifies qi

DETOX / CLEANSING FORMULAS

Circulation (SJ)	Chronic blood stagnation with multiple symptoms	Invigorates blood and qi circulation and eliminates blood and qi stagnations in the upper, middle and lower *jiaos*
Gardenia Complex	Any excess conditions characterized by heat, fire and toxins, including infectious diseases and inflammatory conditions	Clears heat, purges fire, eliminates toxins
Gentle Lax (Excess)	Herbal detox and cleanse for the digestive system	Purges the intestines and unblocks stagnation
Herbal DTX	Herbal detox to relieve adverse reactions to exposure to drugs, chemicals, heavy metals, environmental or airborne toxins	Clears heat, detoxifies, and nourishes yin
Kidney DTX	Herbal detox for chronic kidney disease with elevated creatinine and blood urea nitrogen	Clears heat, detox the Kidneys, dispels dampness
Liver DTX	Herbal detox for liver diseases with elevated liver enzymes and compromised liver functions	Clears heat, detox the Liver
Resolve (AI)	Herbal detox and cleanse for the lymphatic system	Disperse phlegm stagnation, clears heat and detoxifies

LIST OF FORMULAS (Body Systems)

FORMULAS FOR WOMEN

Balance (Cold)	Menstrual disorders with manifestations of cold (cold extremities, menstrual pain alleviated with warmth)	Nourishes Liver blood, dispels dampness and cold
Balance (Heat)	Menopause with manifestations of heat (hot flushes, irritability, insomnia and mood swings)	Clears deficiency heat
Blossom (Phase 1)	Female infertility (menstrual phase)	Regulates menstruation, relieves pain
Blossom (Phase 2)	Female infertility (follicular phase)	Tonifies qi and blood, nourishes Kidney *jing* (essence)
Blossom (Phase 3)	Female infertility (ovulatory phase)	Tonifies *ming men* (life gate) fire and Kidney yang
Blossom (Phase 4)	Female infertility (luteal phase)	Moves qi and blood
Calm	Premenstrual syndrome (PMS)	Spreads Liver qi, relieves stagnation
Menotrol	Amenorrhea, polycystic ovarian disease, and infertility	Tonifies Kidney yang, invigorates blood
Mense-Ease	Dysmenorrhea with pain and discomfort	Invigorates blood circulation and removes stasis, relieves pain
Nourish	Menopause with manifestations of yin-deficient heat (insomnia, mood swings, and dryness of the genito-urinary tissues)	Nourishes Liver and Kidney yin
Resolve (Lower)	Ovarian and uterine cysts and fibroids	Disperses blood stasis and phlegm accumulation
Resolve (Upper)	Breast lumps and cysts	Spreads Liver qi, disperses phlegm accumulation
Schisandra ZZZ	Pale complexion, anemia, insomnia, post-menstrual deficiencies	Tonifies Spleen and Heart blood, tranquilizes the *shen* (spirit)
Venus	Small and underdeveloped breasts	Tonifies Kidney yang, invigorates blood circulation
Vitality	Female sexual disorders, such as decreased libido, lack of interest and vitality	Tonifies Kidney yang and *jing* (essence)

LIST OF FORMULAS (Body Systems)

FORMULAS FOR MEN

Kidney Tonic (Yang)	Kidney yang deficiency	Warms and tonifies Kidney yang, replenishes *jing* (essence) and tonifies blood
Kidney Tonic (Yin)	Kidney yin deficiency	Tonifies the Kidney yin
P-Statin	Enlarged prostate with urinary discomfort	Disperses stagnation and relieves *lin zheng* (dysuria syndrome)
Polygonum 14	A general hair tonic to treat hair loss, premature grey hair, and unhealthy hair with split ends	Tonifies Liver blood and Kidney yin
Saw Palmetto Complex	Enlarged prostate with pain and dysuria	Clears heat in the lower *jiao*, relieves *lin zheng* (dysuria syndrome)
Vital Essence	Male reproductive disorders (infertility, low sperm count, poor sperm motility, mobility and morphology)	Tonifies Kidney yin, yang and *jing* (essence)
Vitality	Male sexual disorders (impotence, decreased libido, and premature ejaculation)	Tonifies Kidney yang and *jing* (essence)

HEATLTH / BEAUTY / ANTIAGING FORMULAS

Adrenoplex	Strengthens adrenal functions, for 'burned-out' individuals who have decreased mental and physical functions	Tonifies Kidney qi
Cordyceps 3	General support to improve immune and reproductive functions	Tonifies Lung and Kidney qi
Enhance Memory	Forgetfulness and poor memory	Tonifies Heart and Kidney *jing* (essence)
Herbalite	Obesity, promotes weight loss by suppressing appetite and increasing metabolic and energy levels	Clears heat in the Stomach, dispels dampness
Imperial Tonic	A comprehensive and balanced tonic to improve mental and physical performances	Tonifies qi, blood, yin and yang
Polygonum 14	A general hair tonic to treat hair loss, premature grey hair, and unhealthy hair with split ends	Tonifies Liver blood and Kidney yin
Venus	For breast augmentation, also increases libido in women	Tonifies Kidney yang, invigorates blood circulation

LIST OF FORMULAS (Body Systems)

SPECIALTY FORMULAS

Circulation (SJ)	Circulatory disorders with impaired blood circulation	Invigorates blood and qi circulation and eliminates blood and qi stagnations in the upper, middle and lower *jiaos*
Gardenia Complex	Any excess conditions characterized by heat, fire and toxins, including infectious diseases and inflammatory conditions	Clears heat, purges fire, eliminates toxins
Herbal DRX	An herbal diuretic formula for edema, swelling, and water accumulation	Drains dampness, eliminates water accumulation
Kidney Tonic (Yang)	A comprehensive Kidney yang tonic formula to address various conditions due to Kidney yang deficiency	Tonifies Kidney yang
Kidney Tonic (Yin)	A comprehensive Kidney yin tonic formula to address various conditions due to Kidney yin deficiency	Tonifies Kidney yin
LPS Support	Systemic lupus erythematosus (SLE)	Clears heat, eliminates toxins, nourishes yin, tonifies blood, promotes generation of body fluids
Neuro Plus	Neuro-degenerative disorders with impaired mental and/or physical functions, such as Alzheimer's disease, Parkinson's disease, and sequelae of stroke	Tonifies Kidney yang, opens channels and collaterals
Notoginseng 9	Bleeding disorders, including internal and external bleeding	Cools the blood, disperses blood stasis, stops bleeding
Nourish (Fluids)	Chronic consumptive disorders characterized by dryness, such as thirst, dry mouth, post-infective cough, and non-productive cough	Nourishes yin and replenishes body fluids, harmonizes the middle *jiao*
Resolve (AI)	Formation of hardness and nodules from general infectious or inflammatory disorders	Disperse phlegm stagnation, clears heat and detoxifies
Symmetry	Treats Bell's palsy, facial paralysis, TMJ (temporo-mandibular joint) pain, trigeminal neuralgia	Dispels wind attack, relieves pain

LIST OF FORMULAS (Body Systems)

SPECIALTY FORMULAS

Circulation (12)	Circulatory disorders with impaired blood circulation	Invigorates blood and qi circulation and eliminates blood and qi stagnations in the upper, middle and lower jiao
Gardenia Complex	Any excess conditions characterized by heat, fire and toxins, including infectious diseases and inflammatory conditions	Clears heat, purges fire, eliminates toxins
Herbal DRX	An herbal diuretic formula for edema, swelling and water accumulation	Drains dampness, eliminates water accumulation
Kidney Tonic (Yang)	A comprehensive Kidney yang tonic formula to address various conditions due to Kidney yang deficiency	Tonifies Kidney yang
Kidney Tonic (Yin)	A comprehensive Kidney yin tonic formula to address various conditions due to Kidney yin deficiency	Tonifies Kidney yin
LPS Support	Systemic lupus erythematosus (SLE)	Clears heat, eliminates toxins, nourishes yin, tonifies blood, promotes generation of body fluids
Neuro Plus	Neuro-degenerative disorders with impaired mental and/or physical functions, such as Alzheimer's disease, Parkinson's disease and sequelae of stroke	Tonifies Kidney yang, opens channels and collaterals
Notoginseng 9	Bleeding disorders, including internal and external bleeding	Cools the blood, disperses blood stasis, stops bleeding
Nourish (Yin)	Chronic consumptive disorders characterized by dryness, such as thirst, dry mouth, post-infectious cough and non-productive cough	Nourishes yin and replenishes body fluids, harmonizes the middle jiao
Resolve (AI)	Formation of hardness and nodules from general infectious or inflammatory disorders	Disperse phlegm stagnation, clears heat and detoxifies
Symmetry	Treats Bell's palsy, facial paralysis, TMJ (temporo-mandibular joint pain, trigeminal neuralgia	Dispels wind attack, relieves pain

Section 2

Symptom / Disease Index

病癥索引

Section 2

Symptom / Disease

Index

SYMPTOM / DISEASE INDEX

CONDITION	SYMPTON / DISEASE DESCRIPTION	TCM DIAGNOSIS	HERBAL FORMULAS
Abdominal Pain	Lower abdominal pain due to menstrual cramps	Blood stagnation in the uterus or lower *jiao*	*Mense-Ease*
	Lower abdominal pain with cold extremities	Cold and deficiency of blood	*Balance (Cold)*
	Lower abdominal pain due to endometriosis	Qi and blood stagnation in the lower *jiao*	*Resolve (Lower)*
	Lower abdominal pain due to pelvic inflammatory disease	Damp-heat in the lower *jiao*	*V-Statin*
	Intestinal spasms and cramps	Intestinal qi stagnation	*Flex (SC)*
	Due to gallstones	Damp-heat in the Liver and Gallbladder	*Dissolve (GS)*
	Due to food poisoning, traveler's diarrhea, or infection	Damp-heat in the Intestines	*GI Care II*
	Due to constipation	Heat in the Large Intestine	*Gentle Lax (Excess)*
	Due to irritable bowel syndrome (IBS)	Liver qi stagnation	*GI Harmony*
	Due to ulcerative colitis (UC), Crohn's disease	Damp-heat in the Large Intestine	*GI Care (UC)*
	With hypochondriac pain, fidgeting, restlessness, and irritability	Liver qi stagnation	*Calm*
	With acid regurgitation, belching	Stomach heat	*GI Care*
	Dull pain with fatigue and diarrhea	Spleen qi deficiency	*GI Tonic*
	Due to Kidney stone	Qi stagnation with dampness accumulation	*Dissolve (KS)*
	Severe abdominal pain	Severe qi and blood stagnation	*Add Herbal Analgesic*
	With severe blood stagnation	Blood stasis	*Add Circulation (SJ)*
Abscess	Lung abscess, profuse yellow phlegm	Phlegm and heat in the Lung	*Poria XPT*
	Breast abscess	Phlegm stagnation in the upper *jiao*	*Resolve (Upper)*
	Ulcerative colitis with mucus and blood in the stool	Damp-heat in the Large Intestine	*GI Care (UC)*
	All swelling and inflammation of the lymph nodes and glands	Phlegm accumulation	*Resolve (AI)*
	Irritable bowel syndrome with mucus and pus in the stool	Damp-heat in the Small and Large Intestine	*GI Harmony*
	With infection	Accumulation of toxic heat	*GI Harmony* and *Herbal ABX*
Abuse (Substance)	*See Addiction*		
AC Separation	Shoulder pain from injury	Qi and blood stagnation	*Arm Support* and *Traumanex*
	With severe pain	Severe qi and blood stagnation	*Add Herbal Analgesic*
Acid Reflux	Heartburn, belching, indigestion, gastritis, ulcers, foul breath	Stomach heat	*GI Care*
	Caused by stress	Liver qi stagnation	*GI Care* and *Calm*
	With excess heat, constipation, sweating, thirst, possible fever	Excess fire	*GI Care* and *Gardenia Complex*
	With bleeding	Excess heat	*Notoginseng 9*
Acne	With pus and redness	Toxic and damp heat accumulation	*Dermatrol (PS)* and *Herbal ENT*
ADD/ADHD	Inability to focus and concentrate	Liver qi stagnation	*Calm (Jr)*
(Children/Adults)...	Inability to focus and concentrate with hyperactivity	Liver wind with *shen* (spirit) disturbance	*Calm (Jr)*

Lotus Institute of Integrative Medicine

SYMPTOM / DISEASE INDEX

CONDITION	SYMPTOM / DISEASE DESCRIPTION	TCM DIAGNOSIS	HERBAL FORMULAS
	Inability to focus and concentrate with poor memory	Liver qi stagnation with Heart deficiency	*Calm (Jr)* and *Enhance Memory*
	Inability to focus due to deficiency	Heart and Kidney deficiencies	*Enhance Memory*
	With excess heat in all three *jiaos* manifesting in red face, constipation, hyperactivity and short-temper	Excess heat	*Calm (Jr)* and *Gardenia Complex*
	With blood stagnation manifesting in signs of purplish tongue, possible distended sublingual veins	Blood stagnation	*Calm (Jr)* and *Circulation (SJ)*
Addiction	Withdrawal symptoms associated with smoking, drugs or alcohol addiction	Toxic heat in the Liver and *shen* (spirit) disturbance	*Calm (ES)* and *Liver DTX*
Addison's Disease	Liver damage with elevated liver enzymes	Toxic heat in the Liver	*Liver DTX*
	Symptoms of adrenal insufficiency	Kidney yang deficiency	*Adrenoplex*
Adrenal Insufficiency	Diminished function of the adrenal glands and endocrine system	Deficiencies of Kidney yin, yang and *jing* (essence)	*Adrenoplex*
Aging	Early signs of aging with weakness, fatigue, forgetfulness, dizziness, etc.	Deficiencies of qi, blood, yin and yang	*Imperial Tonic*
	Neurodegeneration with early signs of dementia and Alzheimer's disease	Deficiencies of Kidney yin, yang and *jing* (essence)	*Neuro Plus*
	Poor memory and forgetfulness	Heart and Kidney deficiencies	*Enhance Memory*
	Premature aging with chronic fatigue	Kidney and Lung deficiencies	*Cordyceps 3*
	Premature aging with decreased mental and physical performances	Deficiencies of Kidney yin, yang and *jing* (essence)	*Adrenoplex*
	Degeneration of soft tissue (muscles, ligaments, tendons, cartilage)	Kidney and Liver yin deficiencies	*Flex (MLT)*
	Decrease in bone density	Kidney *jing* (essence) deficiency	*Osteo 8*
	Gray hair	Kidney *jing* (essence) deficiency and Liver blood deficiency	*Polygonum 14*
	Thirst with dry skin	Stomach and Lung yin deficiencies	*Nourish (Fluids)*
	General Kidney yin deficiency signs such as blurry vision, weakness of the back and knees, tinnitus, dryness, flushed cheeks, possible low-grade fever, etc.	Kidney yin deficiency	*Kidney Tonic (Yin)*
	General Kidney yang deficiency signs such as coldness, low libido, premature ejaculation, weakness and soreness of the back and knees, pale complexion, polyuria, etc.	Kidney yang deficiency	*Kidney Tonic (Yang)*
Agitation	Short temper, flushed face, possible constipation	Liver qi stagnation or Liver yang rising	*Calm* or *Calm (ES)*
AIDS...	Compromised immune system; frequent viral and bacterial infections	*Wei* (defensive) *qi* deficiency	*Immune +*

SYMPTOM / DISEASE INDEX

CONDITION	SYMPTOM / DISEASE DESCRIPTION	TCM DIAGNOSIS	HERBAL FORMULAS
	For complications, see appropriate disease and symptoms		
Alcohol Abuse	See Addiction		
Allergy	Allergic rhinitis or sinusitis, clear, watery nasal discharge, stuffy nose, sneezing	Wind-cold with fluid congestion	*Magnolia Clear Sinus*
	Allergic rhinitis or sinus infection, yellow nasal discharge, stuffy nose	Damp-heat with fluid congestion	*Pueraria Clear Sinus*
	Skin allergy, rash, itching, eczema, and other dermatological disorders	Wind-heat at the skin level, heat in the blood	*Silerex* or *Dermatrol (PS)*
	Adverse reactions from exposure to drugs, chemicals, heavy metals, environmental and airborne toxins	Toxic heat	*Herbal DTX*
	Asthma due to allergy with heat symptoms such as redness of the face, yellow phlegm and red tongue	Lung heat	*Respitrol (Heat)*
	Asthma due to allergy with cold symptoms such as clear or white sputum	Cold in the Lung	*Respitrol (Cold)*
	Profuse post-nasal drip and sputum in the throat	Phlegm accumulation	*Poria XPT*
	Ears plugged, nose and throat with yellow nasal discharge and ticklish sore throat	Toxic heat accumulation in the upper *jiao*	*Herbal ENT*
	Allergy with cough	Lung qi reversal	*Respitrol (CF)*
	Food allergy with underlying digestive weakness and loose stool	Spleen qi deficiency	*GI Tonic*
Alopecia	Hair loss, premature gray hair, split ends, dry and dull hair	Blood deficiency with dryness	*Polygonum 14*
	Stress related hair disorders	Blood deficiency with Liver qi stagnation	*Polygonum 14* and *Calm*
Alzheimer's Disease	Forgetfulness, poor concentration, compromised mental and physical functions	Deficiencies of Kidney yin, yang and *jing* (essence) with phlegm obstruction	*Neuro Plus*
	With constipation	Kidney deficiency with phlegm obstruction, and heat and dryness in the Large Intestine	*Neuro Plus* and *Gentle Lax (Deficient)*
Amenorrhea	Dull lower abdominal pain, cold extremities, edema, generalized weakness	Coldness of the uterus with underlying qi and blood deficiencies	*Balance (Cold)*
	Sharp lower abdominal pain in a fixed location due to fibroids with cold extremities, edema, generalized weakness	Coldness of the uterus with blood stagnation.	*Balance (Cold)* and *Resolve (Lower)*
	Amenorrhea with irregular or delayed menstruation with scanty discharge, cold extremities	Kidney yang deficiency and blood stagnation	*Menotrol*
	Caused by stress or change of environment	Liver qi stagnation	*Calm*
	With severe blood stagnation, purplish tongue, dark complexion, or past history of surgery	Severe blood stasis	*Circulation (SJ)*

SYMPTOM / DISEASE INDEX

CONDITION	SYMPTON / DISEASE DESCRIPTION	TCM DIAGNOSIS	HERBAL FORMULAS
Anemia	With fatigue, lack of energy, poor appetite	Blood and qi deficiencies	*Imperial Tonic*
	With insomnia, excessive worries, disturbed sleep	Spleen and Heart blood deficiencies	*Schisandra ZZZ*
	With irregular menstruation, cold extremities, dizziness, lumbago	Coldness of the uterus	*Balance (Cold)*
	With chronic headache	Blood deficiency	*Migratrol*
	With excessive stress, anxiety and insomnia	Liver qi stagnation with underlying deficiency	*Calm ZZZ*
Ankle	Acute ankle pain	Qi and blood stagnation	*Knee & Ankle (Acute)*
	Chronic ankle pain	Qi and blood stagnation	*Knee & Ankle (Chronic)*
	Ligament or connective tissue injury	Qi and blood stagnation	*Knee & Ankle (Acute)* and *Flex (MLT)*
	Acute sprain and strain with bruises and swelling	Qi and blood stagnation	*Knee & Ankle (Acute)* and *Traumanex*
Anorexia	Poor to no appetite, weight loss, sallow complexion	Spleen deficiency	*GI Tonic*
	Anorexia with fatigue, thirst, dryness, dizziness and general deficiencies	Qi, yin, yang and blood deficiencies	*GI Tonic* and *Imperial Tonic*
Antibiotics (Side Effects)	Dry mouth, thirst	Stomach yin deficiency	*Nourish (Fluids)*
Anxiety	Stress, irritability, restlessness, nervousness	Liver qi stagnation	*Calm*
	With pronounced anger, neurosis or insomnia	Liver fire with *shen* (spirit) disturbance	*Calm (ES)*
	With excessive worrying, pensiveness and indecisiveness	Liver qi stagnation with Spleen and Heart deficiencies	*Calm* and *Schisandra ZZZ*
	Anxiety and stress with inability to calm down, "overactive mind" in patients with deficiency	Liver qi stagnation with qi deficiency	*Calm ZZZ*
	ADD or ADHD in children	Liver wind with *shen* (spirit) disturbance	*Calm (Jr)*
	Anxiety caused by forgetfulness	Heart and Kidney deficiencies	*Enhance Memory*
	With hypertension	Liver and Kidney yin deficiency with Liver yang rising	*Gastrodia Complex*
Appendicitis (Chronic)	Chronic, dull pain in the lower right quadrant of the abdomen	Damp-heat	*Resolve (AI)*
	Moderate to severe infection	Toxic heat	*Resolve (AI)* and *Herbal ABX*
	With severe pain	Severe qi and blood stagnation	*Resolve (AI)* and *Herbal Analgesic*
	With fever	Toxic heat accumulation	*Add Gardenia Complex*
Appetite...	Loss of appetite due to excessive worrying	Spleen and Heart deficiencies	*Schisandra ZZZ*
	Loss of appetite because of generalized weakness and chronic illness	Spleen qi deficiency	*GI Tonic*
	Loss of appetite from stress and nervousness	Liver overacting on the Spleen	*Calm*

SYMPTOM / DISEASE INDEX

CONDITION	SYMPTOM / DISEASE DESCRIPTION	TCM DIAGNOSIS	HERBAL FORMULAS
	Excessive appetite with weight gain	Stomach heat	*Herbalite*
Apprehension	*See* Anxiety		
Arm	Arm pain from injury	Qi and blood stagnation	*Arm Support* and *Traumanex*
	Shooting pain with numbness originating from dysfunction of the cervical spine	Qi and blood stagnation	*Arm Support* and *Neck & Shoulder (Acute)*
Arrhythmia	With shortness of breath, general weakness	Kidney and Heart deficiencies	*Cordyceps 3*
	In angina pectoris	Chest *bi zheng* (painful obstruction syndrome)	*Circulation*
Arteries (blockage)	With high cholesterol/triglycerides	Damp accumulation	*Cholisma*
	With high cholesterol, fatty liver and obesity	Excessive damp accumulation	*Cholisma (ES)*
	In peripheral vascular disease	Qi and blood stagnation	*Flex (NP)*
	With deficient type of hypertension	Liver yang rising with Liver and Kidney yin deficiencies	*Gastrodia Complex*
	With excess type of hypertension	Liver fire	*Gentiana Complex*
	With excessive blood stagnation manifesting in purplish tongue, dark complexion	Blood stasis	*Circulation (SJ)*
Arteriosclerosis	*See* Cholesterol		
Arthralgia	*See* Arthritis		
Arthritis…	Pain, swelling, inflammation, redness with heat sensations	*Bi zheng* (painful obstruction syndrome) due to heat	*Flex (Heat)*
	Chronic arthritis with weakness, soreness, pain; worsens during cold and rainy seasons	*Bi zheng* (painful obstruction syndrome) due to cold and damp	*Flex (CD)*
	With severe pain	*Bi zheng* (painful obstruction syndrome) with severe qi and blood stagnation	*Add Herbal Analgesic*
	Of the neck and shoulder	*Bi zheng* (painful obstruction syndrome) with qi and blood stagnation	*Neck & Shoulder (Chronic)* with a *Flex* formula
	Of the arm	*Bi zheng* (painful obstruction syndrome) with qi and blood stagnation	*Arm Support* with a *Flex* formula
	Of the back	*Bi zheng* (painful obstruction syndrome) with qi and blood stagnation	*Back Support (Chronic)* with a *Flex* formula
	Of the knee and ankle	*Bi zheng* (painful obstruction syndrome) with qi and blood stagnation	*Knee & Ankle (Chronic)* with a *Flex* formula
	Osteoarthritis	Qi and blood stagnation with Kidney *jing* (essence) deficiency	*Osteo 8* with a *Flex* formula

SYMPTOM / DISEASE INDEX

CONDITION	SYMPTON / DISEASE DESCRIPTION	TCM DIAGNOSIS	HERBAL FORMULAS
	Gouty arthritis	*Re bi* (heat painful obstruction)	*Flex (GT)*
	With degeneration of soft tissue (muscles, ligaments, tendon, cartilage)	Liver and Kidney yin deficiencies	*Flex (MLT)*
	With blood stagnation manifesting in purplish tongue, previous trauma or history of surgery, dark complexion, etc.	Blood stasis	*Circulation (SJ)*
AST, ALT	Elevated levels of liver enzymes, AST and ALT (SGPT and SGOT)	Toxic-heat in the Liver	*Liver DTX*
	Elevated liver enzymes due to exposure to drugs, chemicals, heavy metals, environmental and airborne toxins	Toxic heat	*Liver DTX* and *Herbal DTX*
Asthma	Wheezing, dyspnea, yellow sputum, heat sensations	Lung heat	*Respitrol (Heat)*
	Wheezing, dyspnea, white sputum, chills	Lung cold	*Respitrol (Cold)*
	Chronic asthma with wheezing, shortness of breath, shallow inhalation	Deficiencies of the Lung and the Kidney	*Respitrol (Deficient)*
	Maintenance formula for asthma triggered by over-exertion	Lung and Kidney deficiencies	*Cordyceps 3*
	Maintenance formula for asthma triggered by allergies	Lung qi deficiency	*Immune +*
	Maintenance formula for asthma triggered by exposure to chemicals, heavy metals, environmental and airborne toxins	Toxic heat	*Herbal DTX*
	With cough	Lung qi reversal	*Respitrol (CF)* with a *Respitrol* formula
	With excessive phlegm or sputum that may or may not be easy to cough out	Excessive phlegm accumulation	*Poria XPT* with a *Respitrol* formula
	With allergy, sinusitis or rhinitis manifesting in yellow nasal discharge	Lung heat	*Pueraria Clear Sinus* with a *Respitrol* formula
	With allergy, sinusitis or rhinitis manifesting in clear or white nasal discharge	Lung cold	*Magnolia Clear Sinus* with a *Respitrol* formula
	With severe dry throat, mouth and skin	Stomach and Lung yin deficiencies	*Nourish (Fluids)* with a *Respitrol* formula
Atherosclerosis	*See Cholesterol*		
Attention deficit	*See ADD*		
Atrophy…	Muscle atrophy due to stroke	*Wei* (atrophy) syndrome	*Neuro Plus* and *Imperial Tonic*
	Muscle atrophy with weakness, poor appetite	Spleen qi deficiency	*GI Tonic*
	Congenital deficiency with weakness of the bones	Kidney *jing* (essence) deficiency	*Osteo 8*
	Degeneration and atrophy of soft tissue (muscles, ligaments, tendons, cartilage)	Kidney *jing* (essence) deficiency and Liver yin deficiency	*Flex (MLT)*

SYMPTOM / DISEASE INDEX

CONDITION	SYMPTON / DISEASE DESCRIPTION	TCM DIAGNOSIS	HERBAL FORMULAS
	Of the arm	Wei (atrophy) syndrome	Add Arm Support
	Of the neck and shoulder area	Wei (atrophy) syndrome	Add Neck & Shoulder (Chronic)
	Of the back area	Wei (atrophy) syndrome	Add Back Support (Chronic)
	Of the knee and ankle area	Wei (atrophy) syndrome	Add Knee & Ankle (Chronic)
	Muscle atrophy with weakness, dizziness, blurry vision, listlessness, palpitation, shortness of breath, spontaneous sweating	Qi, blood, yin and yang deficiency	Imperial Tonic
	With blood stagnation manifesting in numbness	Blood stagnation	Add Flex (NP)
Autism	Developmental delays and learning disabilities	Shen (spirit) disturbance	Calm (Jr)
Autoimmune Diseases	Grave's disease	Excess Liver yang	Thyrodex
	Multiple sclerosis	Qi and blood stagnation	Neuro Plus
	Rheumatoid arthritis	Bi zheng (painful obstruction syndrome) due to heat	Flex (Heat)
	Hashimoto's thyroiditis, chronic thyroiditis	Kidney yang deficiency	Thyro-forte
	Type I diabetes	Stomach, Lung and Kidney yin deficiencies	Equilibrium
	Sjogren's syndrome	Lung yin deficiency with heat	Nourish (Fluids) and Herbal ENT
	Myasthenia gravis	Zhong (central) qi deficiency	C/R Support
	Reiter's syndrome	Excess heat in all three jiaos	Gardenia Complex and Gentiana Complex
Aversion to Cold/Wind	Weak immune system with increased susceptibility to catching colds	Wei (defensive) qi deficiency	Immune + or Cordyceps 3
Back Pain...	Acute low back pain	Qi and blood stagnation	Back Support (Acute)
	Chronic aches, weakness and soreness of the lower back	Qi and blood stagnation with Liver and Kidney deficiencies	Back Support (Chronic)
	With spasms and cramps	Qi and blood stagnation with Liver yin and body fluid deficiencies	Back Support (Acute) and Flex (SC)
	Upper back pain in the chest, ribs, thoracic area	Qi and blood stagnation	Back Support (Upper)
	Due to slipped disk	Qi and blood stagnation	Back Support (HD)
	Due to bone spurs	Qi and blood stagnation	Flex (Spur)
	Due to osteoporosis	Kidney yin, yang and jing (essence) deficiencies	Osteo 8 and Back Support (Chronic)
	Due to recent traumatic injury	Qi and blood stagnation	Traumanex with Back Support (Acute)

SYMPTOM / DISEASE INDEX

CONDITION	SYMPTON / DISEASE DESCRIPTION	TCM DIAGNOSIS	HERBAL FORMULAS
	Due to kidney stones	Qi and blood stagnation	Dissolve (KS)
	Due to kidney infection	Heat in the lower jiao	V-Statin
	Due to dysmenorrhea	Qi and blood stagnation	Mense-Ease and Back Support (Chronic)
	And soreness due to chronic nephritis or nephritic syndrome	Toxic heat in the Kidney	Kidney DTX
	With severe blood stagnation from previous injury	Qi and blood stagnation	Add Circulation (SJ)
	Due to Kidney yin deficiency with symptoms of blurry vision, flushed cheeks, soreness and weakness of the back and knees, low-grade fever, night sweats, etc	Kidney yin deficiency	Kidney Tonic (Yin)
	Due to Kidney yang deficiency with symptoms of coldness, low libido, polyuria, weakness of the back and knees, etc.	Kidney yang deficiency	Kidney Tonic (Yang)
	Severe back pain	Severe qi and blood stagnation	Add Herbal Analgesic
Bacterial Infection	See Infection		
Bad Breath	Foul breath with excessive hunger	Stomach heat	Herbalite
	Excess heat in the body	Heat in all three jiaos	Gardenia Complex
	With bitter taste in the mouth, short temper	Liver fire	Gentiana Complex
	With dry mouth	Lung and Stomach yin deficiencies	Nourish (Fluids)
	With throat infection	Toxic heat accumulation	Herbal ENT
Balance	Poor balance with dizziness and vertigo	Liver wind rising	Gastrodia Complex
Baldness	See Hair Loss		
Bed-wetting	Bed-wetting, frequent urination, terminal dripping of urine	Kidney yang deficiency	Kidney Tonic (Yang)
Behavior	Disruptive, rude or aggressive behavior	Liver yang rising with shen (spirit) disturbance	Calm (ES)
	ADD or ADHD	Liver wind with shen (spirit) disturbance	Calm (Jr)
Belching	Acid reflux, heartburn, foul breath, indigestion	Stomach heat	GI Care
	Poor appetite, loose stool, fatigue	Spleen qi deficiency	GI Tonic
	Dry throat, thirst	Stomach yin deficiency	Nourish (Fluids)
	Chronic, stubborn belching with blood stagnation (purplish tongue) or for unknown reasons	Blood stasis	Circulation (SJ)
Bell's Palsy	Facial paralysis	Wind attack with qi and blood stagnation	Symmetry
Benign Prostatic Hyperplasia (BPH)...	With difficult, painful and burning urination	Damp-heat in the lower jiao	P-Statin or Saw Palmetto Complex
	With back soreness, terminal dripping of urine, coldness	Kidney yang deficiency	P-Statin or Saw Palmetto Complex and Kidney Tonic (Yang)

SYMPTOM / DISEASE INDEX

CONDITION	SYMPTON / DISEASE DESCRIPTION	TCM DIAGNOSIS	HERBAL FORMULAS
	Moderate to severe cases of infection and inflammation	Accumulation of toxic heat	*Saw Palmetto Complex* and *Resolve (AI)*
Bile Duct	Inflammation or obstruction of the bile duct	Damp-heat in the Liver and Gallbladder	*Dissolve (GS)*
	With severe pain due to bile duct obstruction	Severe qi and blood stagnation	*Dissolve (GS)* and *Herbal Analgesic*
Binge Eating	Excessive appetite	Stomach heat	*Herbalite*
Bipolar Disorder	Manic behavior	Liver yang rising with *shen* (spirit) disturbance	*Calm (ES)*
	Depression	Stagnation of phlegm, qi, blood and food with deficiencies of the Spleen and the Heart	*Shine*
Bladder	*See* Urinary Tract Infection, Urinary Stone, and Urination (Frequent)		
Bladder Stone	Kidney or urinary stones	*Shi lin* (stone dysuria)	*Dissolve (KS)*
	With severe pain due to kidney stone	Severe qi and blood stagnation	*Dissolve (KS)* and *Herbal Analgesic*
	With bleeding	Qi and blood stagnation with heat pushing blood out of the vessels	*Dissolve (KS)* and *Notoginseng 9*
	With fever or heat sensation	Qi and blood stagnation with heat or fire accumulation	*Dissolve (KS)* and *Herbal ABX*
Bleeding	General bleeding	All causes	*Notoginseng 9*
	Abnormal uterine bleeding due to heat	Heat in the lower *jiao*	*Notoginseng 9* with *V-Statin*
	Abnormal uterine bleeding due to cold	Coldness and deficiency of the uterus	*Notoginseng 9* with *Balance (Cold)*
	Bleeding from peptic and duodenal ulcers	Stomach heat	*Notoginseng 9* with *GI Care*
	Intestinal bleeding with diarrhea due to food poisoning	Toxic heat in the Large Intestine	*Notoginseng 9* with *GI Care II*
	Rectal bleeding due to hemorrhoids	Heat in the Large Intestine	*Notoginseng 9* with *GI Care (HMR)*
	Lower gastrointestinal bleeding due to ulcerative colitis	Damp-heat in the Large Intestine	*Notoginseng 9* with *GI Care (UC)*
	Subcutaneous bleeding, purpura	Spleen qi deficiency with inability to keep blood in the vessels	*Notoginseng 9* with *Schisandra ZZZ*
	Bleeding and bruises from traumas	Qi and blood stagnation	*Notoginseng 9* with *Traumanex*
	Excessive bleeding leading to anemia or fatigue and weakness	Qi and blood deficiency	*Notoginseng 9* with *Imperial Tonic*
	Oral herpes	Toxic heat	*Lonicera Complex* with *Gardenia Complex*
Blister(s) …	Genital herpes	Damp-heat in the lower *jiao* and Liver channel	*Gentiana Complex*

SYMPTOM / DISEASE INDEX

CONDITION	SYMPTON / DISEASE DESCRIPTION	TCM DIAGNOSIS	HERBAL FORMULAS
	Nerve pain, shingles due to herpes zoster	Qi and blood stagnation	*Dermatrol (HZ)* with *Herbal Analgesic*
	Chicken pox	Wind-heat invasion with toxic heat accumulation in the Lung	*Lonicera Complex* and *Silerex*
	Dermatitis	Toxic and damp-heat accumulation	*Dermatrol (PS)* or *Silerex* and *Gardenia Complex*
Bloating	With epigastric fullness, heartburn	Stomach heat with qi stagnation	*GI Care*
	With PMS, mood swings, breast distention, stress	Liver qi stagnation	*Calm*
	With dysmenorrhea	Liver qi stagnation with blood stasis	*Mense-Ease*
	Due to endometriosis	Qi and blood stagnation in the lower *jiao*	*Resolve (Lower)*
	Due to irritable bowel syndrome (IBS)	Liver qi stagnation	*GI Harmony*
	Due to ulcerative colitis	Damp-heat in the Large Intestine	*GI Care (UC)*
	Due to weakness of the digestive system	Spleen qi deficiency	*GI Tonic*
	Severe bloating and pain	Qi stagnation	*Add Herbal Analgesic*
	Hypochondriac distention with stress	Liver qi stagnation	*Calm*
Blood Clot	Severe blood stagnation in the extremities	Blood stagnation	*Flex (NP)*
	Coronary heart condition	Blood stagnation	*Circulation*
	Severe blood stagnation in the body	Blood stagnation	*Circulation (SJ)*
Blood Pressure	*See* Hypertension or Hypotension		
Blood Sugar Level	*See* Diabetes or Hyperglycemia		
Boils	With infection	Toxic heat accumulation	*Resolve (AI)* and *Herbal ABX*
Bone Disorder	Osteoporosis	Kidney yin and *jing* (essence) deficiencies	*Osteo 8*
	Acute phase of traumatic injuries with severe pain, inflammation and bruises	Qi and blood stagnation	*Traumanex*
	Moderate to severe cases of infection and inflammation with bone fracture	Accumulation of toxic heat	*Traumanex* with *Herbal ABX*
	Delayed healing of bone fracture	Deficiency of Kidney *jing* (essence)	*Osteo 8*
	Recovery phase of external injuries in all parts of the body; strengthens the bones, tendons and ligaments	Liver and Kidney deficiencies	*Flex (MLT)*
	Bone spur	Qi and blood stagnation	*Flex (Spur)*
	Bone spur with severe pain	Severe qi and blood stagnation	*Flex (Spur)* plus *Herbal Analgesic*
Bone Spur...	Bone spur	Qi and blood stagnation	*Flex (Spur)*
	Accompanied by severe pain	Severe qi and blood stagnation	*Flex (Spur)* plus *Herbal Analgesic*

SYMPTOM / DISEASE INDEX

CONDITION	SYMPTON / DISEASE DESCRIPTION	TCM DIAGNOSIS	HERBAL FORMULAS
	Neck and shoulder pain	Qi and blood stagnation in the upper *jiao*	*Flex (Spur)* plus *Neck & Shoulder (Acute)*
	Low back pain	Qi and blood stagnation in the lower *jiao*	*Flex (Spur)* plus *Back Support (Acute)*
	Upper back pain	Qi and blood stagnation in the upper *jiao*	*Flex (Spur)* plus *Back Support (Upper)*
	Arm (shoulder, elbow, wrist) pain	Qi and blood stagnation in the upper *jiao*	*Flex (Spur)* plus *Arm Support*
	Knee and ankle pain	Qi and blood stagnation in the lower *jiao*	*Flex (Spur)* plus *Knee & Ankle (Acute)*
Borborygmi	Due to food poisoning or gastrointestinal infection	Damp-heat in the Intestines	*GI Care II*
	Due to stress and anxiety	Liver qi stagnation	*Calm*
	Due to irritable bowel syndrome (IBS)	Liver qi stagnation	*GI Harmony*
	Due to weakness of the digestive system	Spleen qi deficiency	*GI Tonic*
Bowel Movement	*See* Constipation, Diarrhea, Ulcerative Colitis, Irritable Bowel Syndrome (IBS), Hemorrhoid, Crohn's disease		
BPH	*See* Benign Prostatic Hypertrophy		
Brain	Alzheimer's, dementia, Parkinson's, post-stroke complications and other neurodegenerative disorders with compromised mental and physical functions	Kidney yin, yang and *jing* (essence) deficiencies	*Neuro Plus*
	Poor memory, forgetfulness	Heart and Kidney deficiencies	*Enhance Memory*
	Under-developed breasts	Kidney yang and *jing* (essence) deficiencies	*Venus*
Breast	Breast distention, PMS, irritability	Liver qi stagnation	*Calm*
	Breast lumps, benign breast disorder, fibrocystic disorders	Liver qi stagnation with phlegm and heat	*Resolve (Upper)*
	Breast cancer patients receiving chemotherapy or radiation	*Wei* (defensive) *qi* and *zhong* (central) *qi* deficiencies	*C/R Support*
	End stage breast cancer	*Yuan* (source) *qi* deficiency	*CA Support*
Breathing	*See* Asthma, Cough, Dyspnea, or Common Cold		
Bronchitis / Bronchiectasis…	Cough	Lung qi reversal	*Respitrol (CF)*
	Cough, dyspnea, fever, yellow sputum	Lung heat	*Respitrol (Heat)*
	Cough, dyspnea, clear white sputum, intolerance to cold, chills	Lung cold	*Respitrol (Cold)*
	Cough, profuse yellow sputum, chest congestion	Lung heat with phlegm	*Poria XPT*
	Chronic bronchitis with dryness and scanty sputum	Lung qi and yin deficiency	*Respitrol (Deficient)* and *Nourish (Fluids)*

SYMPTOM / DISEASE INDEX

CONDITION	SYMPTON / DISEASE DESCRIPTION	TCM DIAGNOSIS	HERBAL FORMULAS
	Moderate to severe cases of chronic bronchitis with infection and inflammation	Accumulation of toxic heat	*Respirol (Deficient) and Herbal ABX*
	Coughing of blood	Lung heat	*Notoginseng 9* with one of the *Respirol* formula
	To enhance the antibiotic effect	Toxic heat in the Lung	*Add Herbal ABX*
Bruises	*See Trauma*		
Bruxism (Teeth Grinding)	With stress	Liver qi stagnation	*Calm*
	With severe stress and insomnia	Liver qi stagnation with *shen* (spirit) disturbance	*Calm (ES)*
Bulimia	Binge eating followed by abdominal pain or self-induced vomiting	*Shen* (spirit) disturbance	*Calm (ES)*
	Obesity, excess appetite with mental disorder	*Shen* (spirit) disturbance with Stomach heat	*Calm (ES)* with *Herbalite*
"Burned Out"	Fatigue, over-exhaustion, lack of interest, and decreased vitality	Kidney yang deficiency	*Adrenoplex*
	Chronic fatigue	Lung and Kidney deficiencies	*Cordyceps 3*
	Overall weakness and deficiency	Qi, blood, yin and yang deficiencies	*Imperial Tonic*
	Burned out with Kidney yin deficiency signs of night sweats, low-grade fever, blurry vision, tinnitus, weakness and soreness of the back and knees, etc.	Kidney yin deficiency	*Kidney Tonic (Yin)*
Bursitis	Inflammation and redness of the joints	*Bi zheng* (painful obstruction syndrome) due to heat	*Flex (Heat)*
	With severe pain	Severe qi and blood stagnation	*Flex (Heat)* and *Herbal Analgesic*
	Of the shoulder	Qi and blood stagnation	*Neck & Shoulder (Acute)*
	Of the elbow	Qi and blood stagnation	*Arm Support*
	Of the hip	Qi and blood stagnation	*Back Support (Acute)*
	Of the knee	Qi and blood stagnation	*Knee & Ankle (Acute)*
	With degeneration of the soft tissue (muscle, ligaments, tendons, cartilage)	Liver and Kidney yin deficiencies	*Flex (MLT)*
Calcification	Calcification of joints	Phlegm accumulation	*Flex (Spur)*
Calcium	Calcium deficiency seen in osteoporosis or decreased bone density	Deficiency of Kidney yin and *jing* (essence)	*Osteo 8*
Calculi	*See Stones*		
Calf	Spasm and cramps	Qi and blood stagnation	*Flex (SC)*
	With severe pain	Severe qi and blood stagnation	*Flex (SC)* with *Herbal Analgesic*
	Chronic stiffness from old injuries with blood stagnation	Blood stasis	*Flex (SC)* with *Circulation (SJ)*
	With knee or ankle pain	Qi and blood stagnation	*Flex (SC)* with *Knee & Ankle (Acute)*

SYMPTOM / DISEASE INDEX

CONDITION	SYMPTON / DISEASE DESCRIPTION	TCM DIAGNOSIS	HERBAL FORMULAS
Cancer / Carcinoma	Nausea, vomiting, compromised immune system, generalized weakness, and other side effects of chemotherapy and radiation	Deficiencies of yin, *yuan* (source) *qi*, and *wei* (defensive) *qi*	*C/R Support*
	Weakened or compromised immune system	*Wei* (defensive) *qi* deficiency	*Immune +*
	Compromised respiratory and reproductive systems	Lung and Kidney deficiencies	*Cordyceps 3*
	Dry mouth and thirst	Stomach yin deficiency	*Nourish (Fluids)*
	End stage cancer in patients who are too weak to receive chemotherapy or radiation	*Yuan* (source) *qi* deficiency	*CA Support*
Candidiasis	Genital itching and yellow discharge	Damp-heat in the lower *jiao* and Liver channel	*V-Statin*
Canker Sore	Ulcers in the mouth	Stomach heat	*Gardenia Complex*
Capsulitis	Frozen shoulder with pain	Qi and blood stagnation	*Arm Support* and *Neck & Shoulder (Acute)*
Carbuncle	Painful inflammation	Toxic heat with phlegm accumulation	*Resolve (AI)*
Carpal Tunnel Syndrome	Wrist pain	Qi and blood stagnation	*Arm Support*
	With severe pain	Severe qi and blood stagnation	*Arm Support* and *Herbal Analgesic*
Cartilage	Enhancing the growth of muscles, tendons, ligaments and cartilages	Liver blood and Kidney yin deficiencies	*Flex (MLT)*
Cataract	With blurry vision, dry eyes, weakness of the lower back and knees, tinnitus	Liver and Kidney yin deficiencies	*Nourish*
	With hypertension, flushed face, possible constipation	Liver yang rising	*Gentiana Complex*
Cellulite	Accumulation of cellulite with excessive hunger	Stomach heat	*Herbalite*
Cellulitis	Cellulitis due to infection	Toxic heat accumulation	*Herbal ABX* and *Herbal ENT*
	Swelling, inflammation and enlarged glands	Phlegm stagnation	*Resolve (AI)*
Cerebral Circulation Insufficiency	Forgetfulness, poor concentration associated with dementia or Alzheimer's Disease	Poor circulation with deficiencies of Kidney yin, yang and *jing* (essence)	*Neuro Plus*
	Poor memory and forgetfulness	Heart and Kidney deficiencies	*Enhance Memory*
	Severe blood stagnation	Blood stagnation	*Circulation (SJ)*
Chancre	Chancre of mouth	Toxic heat accumulation	*Herbal ABX* and *Herbal ENT*
	Chancre in the genital region	Damp-heat in the lower *jiao* and Liver channel	*Herbal ABX* with *Gentiana Complex* or *V-Statin*
Change of Life	See Menopause		
Chemical	See Poisoning		
Chemotherapy	See Cancer		
Chest Pain...	Cardiovascular/coronary heart disorders, chest pain, dyspnea with physical exertion	Blood stagnation in the chest	*Circulation*

SYMPTOM / DISEASE INDEX

CONDITION	SYMPTOM / DISEASE DESCRIPTION	TCM DIAGNOSIS	HERBAL FORMULAS
	Cardiovascular/coronary heart disorders with severe pain	Qi and blood stagnation	Circulation with Herbal Analgesic
	Asthma with fever, yellow phlegm	Heat in the Lung	Respitrol (Heat)
	Asthma with chills, white or clear phlegm	Cold in the Lung	Respitrol (Cold)
	Chest pain due to cough	Lung qi reversal	Respitrol (CF)
	Chronic respiratory condition	Lung qi deficiency	Respitrol (Deficient)
	Chest congestion, pain with coughing, yellow sputum	Heat and phlegm in the Lung	Poria XPT
	Severe blood stagnation or past history of injury or surgery in the chest area	Blood stagnation	Circulation (SJ)
	With stomach ulcer	Stomach fire	GI Care
Chicken Pox	Blisters with itching	Toxic heat invading the Lung	Lonicera Complex
	With severe itching	Wind-heat invasion	Lonicera Complex and Silerex
Chills	Common cold/flu with ticklish throat, fever	Wind-heat invasion	Lonicera Complex
	Common cold/flu with clear or white nasal discharge, sneezing	Wind-cold invasion	Respitrol (Cold)
	Fever and chills from stomach flu or food poisoning with diarrhea	Damp-heat in the intestine	GI Care II
	With fever, sore throat, ear pain	Toxic heat accumulation	Herbal ENT
Chinese Restaurant Syndrome	Hypersensitivity to MSG with headache, thirst and abdominal discomfort	Toxic, damp-heat	GI Care II with Liver DTX
Chlamydia	Burning sensation with urination, discharge and pain	Damp-heat in the lower jiao and Liver channel	V-Statin
Cholecystitis	Inflammation of the gallbladder with or without gallstones	Damp-heat in the Gallbladder	Dissolve (GS)
	With elevated liver enzymes, possibly with liver impairment	Damp-heat in the Liver and the Gallbladder	Dissolve (GS) with Liver DTX
	With fatty liver and high cholesterol	Damp-heat in the Liver and the Gallbladder	Dissolve (GS) with Cholisma (ES)
Cholelithiasis	Gallstones with or without cholecystitis	Damp-heat in the Gallbladder drying up the fluid	Dissolve (GS)
	Gallstones with elevated liver enzymes, possibly with liver impairment	Damp-heat in the Liver and the Gallbladder	Dissolve (GS) with Liver DTX
	With severe pain due to gallstones	With qi and blood stagnation	Dissolve (GS) with Herbal Analgesic
	With fatty liver and high cholesterol	Damp-heat in the Liver and the Gallbladder	Dissolve (GS) with Cholisma (ES)
	With fever	Liver fire	Dissolve (GS) with Gardenia Complex
Cholestasis	See Cholecystitis, Cholelithiasis		
Cholesterol / Triglycerides...	Elevated levels	Accumulation of damp and phlegm	Cholisma
	With excess type hypertension	Damp and phlegm with Liver fire	Cholisma with Gentiana Complex

SYMPTOM / DISEASE INDEX

CONDITION	SYMPTOM / DISEASE DESCRIPTION	TCM DIAGNOSIS	HERBAL FORMULAS
	With deficient type hypertension	Damp and phlegm with Liver yang rising	*Cholisma* with *Gastrodia Complex*
	With coronary heart disease	Damp and phlegm with blood stagnation	*Cholisma* and *Circulation*
	With obesity and excessive appetite	Damp and phlegm with Stomach heat	*Cholisma* and *Herbalite*
	With fatigue	Damp and phlegm with Lung and Kidney deficiencies	*Cholisma* with *Cordyceps 3*
	With fatty liver	Damp and phlegm in the Liver	*Cholisma (ES)*
	Short-term tiredness and lack of energy	Qi deficiency	*Vibrant*
Chronic Fatigue Syndrome	Chronic fatigue with generalized weakness	Qi, blood, yin and yang deficiencies	*Vibrant* plus *Imperial Tonic*
	Chronic fatigue with reproductive and respiratory deficiencies	Lung and Kidney qi deficiencies	*Vibrant* with *Cordyceps 3*
	Adrenal insufficiency	Kidney qi deficiency	*Adrenoplex*
	Inability to concentrate	Heart and Kidney deficiencies	*Enhance Memory*
Cigarette Smoking	*See* Addiction		
Circulation, Poor	Poor peripheral circulation with numbness and pain of the extremities	Qi and blood stagnation	*Flex (NP)*
	Poor circulation due to blood stagnation from previous injuries or surgery	Severe blood stasis	*Circulation (SJ)*
	Coronary heart condition	Qi and blood stagnation in the upper *jiao*	*Circulation*
	Acute or chronic cluster headache with blood deficiency	Qi and blood stagnation with blood deficiency	*Migratrol*
Cluster Headache	Acute cluster headache	Qi and blood stagnation	*Corydalin*
	Severe cluster headache	Severe qi and blood stagnation	*Migratrol* or *Corydalin* plus *Herbal Analgesic*
	Caused by stress	Liver qi stagnation or Liver yang rising	*Corydalin* with *Calm* or *Calm (ES)*
	With short-temper, irritability, red face, red eyes and possible constipation	Liver fire	*Corydalin* with *Gentiana Complex*
Cognitive Impairment	Memory impairment due to neurodegenerative disorders	Deficiencies of Kidney yin, yang and *jing* (essence) with phlegm	*Neuro Plus*
	Poor memory and forgetfulness	Heart and Kidney deficiencies	*Enhance Memory*
Cold...	*See* Common Cold		
	Cold extremities with weakness of the lower back and knees, clear polyuria	Kidney yang deficiency	*Kidney Tonic (Yang)*
	Cold extremities due to poor blood circulation	Blood stagnation	*Flex (NP)*
	In females with weakness and irregular menstruation	Cold in the uterus with qi and blood deficiencies	*Balance (Cold)* and *Kidney Tonic (Yang)*

SYMPTOM / DISEASE INDEX

CONDITION	SYMPTOM / DISEASE DESCRIPTION	TCM DIAGNOSIS	HERBAL FORMULAS
	Female infertility with no ovulation	Kidney yang deficiency	*Blossom (Phase 3)* and *Kidney Tonic (Yang)*
	Coldness and pain of the joints	Cold *bi zheng* (painful obstruction syndrome)	*Flex (CD)*
Cold Sores	Fever blisters with pain and inflammation	Wind-heat	*Lonicera Complex*
	Moderate to severe cases of infection and inflammation	Accumulation of toxic heat	*Lonicera Complex* and *Herbal ABX*
Colic Pain	*See* Gallstones, Kidney Stones or Bladder Stones		
Colitis	Ulcerative colitis or Crohn's disease	Damp-heat in the Large Intestine	*GI Care (UC)*
	Colitis with diarrhea due to infection	Damp-heat in the Large Intestine	*GI Care II*
	Moderate to severe cases of infection and inflammation	Accumulation of toxic heat	*GI Care II* plus *Herbal ABX*
	Irritable bowel syndrome (IBS)	Liver qi stagnation	*GI Harmony*
	With bleeding	Heat accumulation pushing blood out of the vessels	*Add Notoginseng 9*
Colon	*See* Constipation, Diarrhea, Colitis, Colitis, Diverticulosis, Irritable Bowel Syndrome (IBS), Crohn's Disease, Ulcerative Colitis, etc.		
	Cleansing	Toxic heat accumulation in the colon	*Gentle Lax (Excess)*
Common Cold	Sore throat, headache	Wind-heat	*Lonicera Complex*
	Fever, dyspnea, chest congestion	Lung heat	*Respitrol (Heat)*
	Runny nose with clear watery discharge, sneezing, nasal congestion	Lung cold	*Respitrol (Cold)*
	Chest congestion, profuse yellow sputum, cough	Lung heat with phlegm	*Poria XPT*
	Moderate to severe cases of infection and inflammation	Accumulation of toxic heat	*Poria XPT* and *Herbal ABX*
	Prevention of common cold and flu	*Wei* (defensive) *qi* deficiency	*Immune +*
	With severe sore throat and possible ear ache	Toxic heat in the Lung	*Herbal ENT*
Complexion	Pale with fatigue and weakness	Qi deficiency	*Imperial Tonic*
	Pale with dizziness and anemia	Blood deficiency	*Schisandra ZZZ* or *Balance (Cold)*
	Dark circles under the eyes, soreness and weakness of the lower back and knees, dizziness, tinnitus, possible spermatorrhea, hair loss and dryness	Kidney yin deficiency	*Nourish* or *Kidney Tonic (Yin)*
	Dark complexion with purplish tongue, dry hair, coldness; menstrual cramps and blood clots in women	Blood stagnation	*Menotrol*
	Dark complexion from chronic blood stagnation resulting from surgery or old injuries	Blood stasis	*Circulation (SJ)*
	Red complexion with high blood pressure and fast heart rate	Heat in all three *jiaos*	*Gardenia Complex*

SYMPTOM / DISEASE INDEX

CONDITION	SYMPTOM / DISEASE DESCRIPTION	TCM DIAGNOSIS	HERBAL FORMULAS
Conception	*See Infertility*		
Conjunctivitis	Redness and swelling of the eyes, "red eyes"	Liver fire rising	*Gentiana Complex*
	Inflammation and swelling of the eyes	Heat in all three *jiaos*	*Gardenia Complex*
	Moderate to severe cases of infection and inflammation	Accumulation of toxic heat	*Gardenia Complex* and *Herbal ABX*
Constipation	Excess type constipation with yellow tongue coat and red face	Excess heat in the Large Intestine	*Gentle Lax (Excess)*
	Deficient type constipation with dryness	Heat in the Large Intestine with yin deficiency	*Gentle Lax (Deficient)*
	Irritable bowel syndrome (IBS)	Liver qi stagnation	*Gentle Lax (Deficient)* and *GI Harmony*
	With cold extremities, pale complexion, preference for warmth, polyuria and excessive urinary urges at night	Kidney yang deficiency	*Gentle Lax (Deficient)* and *Kidney Tonic (Yang)*
	With thirst, dryness, dizziness; in postpartum or convalescing patients	Blood deficiency	*Gentle Lax (Deficient)* and *Schisandra ZZZ*
	With hemorrhoid	Blood stagnation	*GI Care (HMR)*
	With dryness and thirst	Stomach yin deficiency	*Nourish (Fluids)*
	With bleeding	Heat in the intestines	*Add Notoginseng 9*
	Post-surgical constipation	Qi and blood stagnation	*Traumanex* and *Gentle Lax (Deficient)*
Contagious Disease	*See Infection*		
Convulsion	Childhood convulsion	Liver wind	*Calm (Jr)*
	High blood pressure, redness of the face and eyes, tremors	Liver wind with Liver yang rising	*Symmetry* with *Gastrodia Complex*
	Dryness of the eyes, soreness of the back and knees, tinnitus	Liver and Kidney yin deficiency	*Symmetry* with *Nourish*
Coronary Heart Disease	Chest pain with numbness due to poor blood circulation	Blood stagnation	*Circulation*
	Chest pain with high cholesterol/triglycerides	Blood stagnation with damp and phlegm	*Circulation* and *Cholisma*
	Chest pain with high cholesterol/triglycerides, fatty liver and obesity	Blood stagnation with damp and phlegm	*Circulation* and *Cholisma (ES)*
	Chest pain with deficient type hypertension, dizziness, tinnitus	Blood stagnation with Liver yang rising	*Circulation* and *Gastrodia Complex*
	Chest pain with excess type hypertension, headache, flushed face, red eyes, anger	Blood stagnation with Liver fire	*Circulation* with *Gentiana Complex*
	Chest pain with generalized weakness	Blood stagnation with qi deficiency	*Circulation* with *Imperial Tonic*
	Severe chest pain	Qi and blood stagnation	*Circulation* and *Herbal Analgesic*
	Severe blood stasis manifesting in dark, purplish complexion, purplish tongue, possible distended sublingual veins	Blood stasis	*Circulation (SJ)*

SYMPTOM / DISEASE INDEX

CONDITION	SYMPTON / DISEASE DESCRIPTION	TCM DIAGNOSIS	HERBAL FORMULAS
Cough	General cough	Any cause	*Respitrol (CF)*
	Dyspnea, yellow nasal discharge or sputum, fever	Lung heat	*Respitrol (Heat)*
	Dyspnea, white nasal discharge or sputum, chills	Lung cold	*Respitrol (Cold)*
	Early stage of infection, cough with pronounced sore throat	Wind-heat	*Respitrol (CF)* and *Herbal ENT*
	Mid-to-late stage of infection, cough with chest congestion and yellow sputum	Lung heat with phlegm	*Respitrol (Heat)* and *Poria XPT*
	Chronic dry and non-productive cough, chest pain	Lung yin deficiency	*Respitrol (Deficient) and Nourish (Fluids)*
	Moderate to severe cases of infection and inflammation	Accumulation of toxic heat	*Respitrol (Deficient)* and *Herbal ABX*
	Cough due to exposure to drugs, chemicals, heavy metals, environmental and airborne toxins	Toxic heat	*Respitrol (CF)* and *Herbal DTX*
	Chronic respiratory disease with weakness	Lung and Kidney deficiencies	*Respitrol (Deficient)* and *Cordyceps 3*
	With phlegm or feeling of plum-pit syndrome, hypochondriac distension, short temper	Liver qi stagnation or Liver fire	*Respitrol (CF)* and *Calm (ES)*
	Dry cough, thirst, dryness	Lung and Stomach yin deficiencies	*Respitrol (CF)* and *Nourish (Fluids)*
Cramps	Muscle spasms or intestinal cramping	Liver yin and body fluid deficiencies	*Flex (SC)*
	Menstrual cramps	Blood stagnation	*Mense-Ease*
	Stomach cramp with acid reflux or ulcer	Stomach heat	*GI Care with Flex (SC)*
	Intestinal cramps from irritable bowel syndrome (IBS)	Liver qi stagnation	*Flex (SC)* with *GI Harmony*
	Intestinal cramps from ulcerative colitis	Damp-heat in the intestine	*Flex (SC)* with *GI Care (UC)*
	With severe pain	Severe qi and blood stagnation	*Flex (SC)* with *Herbal Analgesic*
Crohn's Disease	Diarrhea, rectal bleeding, poor appetite, fever, night sweats, weight loss	Toxic heat accumulation in the intestines with yin-deficient heat	*GI Care (UC)*
	With pronounced poor appetite and weakness	Spleen qi deficiency	*GI Tonic*
	With severe bleeding	Heat pushing blood out of the vessels	*Add Notoginseng 9*
Crying	Emotional disturbance during menopause	Kidney yin deficiency with *shen* (spirit) disturbance	*Balance (Heat)*
	From stress	Liver qi stagnation	*Calm* or *Calm (ES)*
	With stress, fatigue, insomnia	Liver qi stagnation with qi deficiency	*Calm ZZZ*
Cyst...	Cysts in the breast	Liver qi stagnation with phlegm accumulation	*Resolve (Upper)*

SYMPTOM / DISEASE INDEX

CONDITION	SYMPTON / DISEASE DESCRIPTION	TCM DIAGNOSIS	HERBAL FORMULAS
	Ovarian or uterine cysts	Qi and blood stagnation in the lower *jiao*	*Resolve (Lower)*
	Cysts elsewhere in the body	Qi and phlegm stagnation	*Resolve (AI)*
Cystitis	Acute stage with urinary urgency, burning and painful urination	Damp-heat in the Urinary Bladder	*V-Statin*
	Chronic stage with urinary urgency, frequent re-infection	Damp-heat in the Urinary Bladder with yin deficiency	*Gentiana Complex* with *Nourish*
	Moderate to severe cases of infection and inflammation	Accumulation of toxic heat	*Gentiana Complex* and *Herbal ABX*
	Interstitial cystitis	Damp-heat accumulation and blood stagnation in the lower *jiao*	*V-Statin* with *Circulation (SJ)*
	With bleeding	Heat pushing blood out of the vessels	*V-Statin* with *Notoginseng 9*
	With fever	Fire accumulation in the lower *jiao*	*V-Statin* with *Gardenia Complex*
Dairy Product Intolerance	Diarrhea and bloating	Spleen qi deficiency	*GI Tonic*
Degeneration	Of the nervous system	Kidney yin, yang and *jing* (essence) deficiencies	*Neuro Plus*
	Of bone density	Kidney yin and *jing* (essence) deficiencies	*Osteo 8*
	Decrease in function of adrenal glands and the endocrine system	Kidney qi deficiency	*Adrenoplex*
	Pre-mature aging with gray hair and hair loss	Liver blood deficiency with Kidney yin deficiency	*Polygonum 14*
	Hypothyroidism	Kidney yang deficiency	*Thyro-forte*
	Degenerative arthritis of the upper body	Liver yin and Kidney yin deficiencies	*Neck & Shoulder (Chronic)*
	Degenerative arthritis of the lower body	Liver yin and Kidney yin deficiencies	*Back Support (Chronic)*
	Poor memory and forgetfulness	Heart and Kidney deficiencies	*Enhance Memory*
	Of soft tissue (muscle, tendon, ligament, cartilage)	Liver and Kidney yin deficiencies	*Flex (MLT)*
	Decreased or absence of libido	Kidney yang deficiency	*Vitality*
	Causing cramps	Blood deficiency with qi and blood stagnation	*Flex (SC)*
Dehydration	From diarrhea due to food poisoning	Damp-heat in the Intestines	*Nourish (Fluids)* with *GI Care II*
	Due to chronic diarrhea with weak digestion and poor appetite	Spleen qi deficiency	*Nourish (Fluids)* with *GI Tonic*
	Due to excess fire, fever, inflammation or infection	Fire in the *qi* (energy) level	*Gardenia Complex*
	Resulting in excessive thirst and dryness	Yin and fluid deficiency	*Nourish (Fluids)*
Delirium…	With anxiety, irritability, restlessness and insomnia	Liver fire	*Calm (ES)*
	With constipation	Qi stagnation and excess fire	*Calm (ES)* with *Gentle Lax (Excess)*
	With heat sensation	Excess fire	*Gardenia Complex*

SYMPTOM / DISEASE INDEX

CONDITION	SYMPTON / DISEASE DESCRIPTION	TCM DIAGNOSIS	HERBAL FORMULAS
	With severe blood stagnation manifesting in purplish tongue, dark complexion or in cases where other herbs don't seem to work	Severe blood stasis	*Circulation (SJ)*
Dementia	Memory impairment due to neurodegenerative disorders	Deficiencies of Kidney yin, yang and *jing* (essence) with phlegm	*Neuro Plus*
	Poor memory and forgetfulness	Heart and Kidney deficiencies	*Enhance Memory*
Dependence	*See Addiction*		
Depression	With fatigue, lack of interest	Stagnation of phlegm, qi, blood and food	*Shine*
	With signs of vegetative state	Severe stagnation of phlegm, qi, blood and food	*Shine* with *Vibrant*
	With restlessness, irritability, anger (manic depressives)	Stagnation of phlegm, qi, blood and food with Liver and Heart fire	*Shine* with *Calm (ES)*
	With increased appetite and weight gain	Stagnation of phlegm, qi, blood and food with Stomach heat	*Shine* with *Herbalite*
	With poor appetite	Stagnation of phlegm, qi, blood and food with Spleen qi deficiency	*Shine* with *GI Tonic*
	With sexual dysfunction or lack of libido	Stagnation of phlegm, qi, blood and food with Kidney yang deficiency	*Shine* with *Vitality*
	With low energy	Stagnation of phlegm, qi, blood and food with qi deficiency	*Shine* with *Cordyceps 3*
	With insomnia or too little sleep	Stagnation of phlegm, qi, blood and food with lack of nourishment to the *shen* (spirit)	*Shine* with *Schisandra ZZZ*
	Post-partum depression	Stagnation of phlegm, qi, blood and food with blood deficiency	*Shine* with *Imperial Tonic*
	Pre-menopausal and menopausal depression	Stagnation of phlegm, qi, blood and food with yin-deficient heat	*Shine* with *Balance (Heat)*
	With inability to concentrate	Stagnation of phlegm, qi, blood and food with Heart and Kidney deficiencies	*Shine* with *Enhance Memory*
	With headache	Stagnation of phlegm, qi, blood and food	*Shine* with *Corydalin*
Dermatitis	Rash, itching, redness	Wind-heat or damp-heat at the skin level	*Silerex*
	Moderate to severe cases of infection and inflammation	Accumulation of toxic heat	*Silerex* with *Herbal ABX*
	Severe itching	Toxic heat	*Dermatrol (PS)*
	With redness and heat sensation	Excess heat accumulation	*Add Gardenia Complex*
Detox…	Accumulation of toxic substances in the body leading to compromised liver function (alcohol, drugs, medication, smoking, etc.)	Toxic heat in the Liver	*Liver DTX*

SYMPTOM / DISEASE INDEX

CONDITION	SYMPTON / DISEASE DESCRIPTION	TCM DIAGNOSIS	HERBAL FORMULAS
	Accumulation of toxic substances in the body leading to compromised kidney function	Toxic heat in the Kidney	*Kidney DTX*
	Adverse reactions from exposure to drugs, chemicals, heavy metals, hormones in meat, environmental and airborne toxins	Toxic heat accumulation	*Herbal DTX*
	Accumulation of toxic substances in the gastrointestinal tract	Toxic heat accumulation	*Gentle Lax (Excess)*
	To cleanse the blood	Blood stagnation	*Circulation (SJ)*
	To cleanse the lymphatic system	Damp and phlegm accumulation	*Resolve (AI)*
	For weight loss	Stomach fire	*Herbalite*
Diabetes	High blood glucose	Yin deficiencies of the Lung, the Stomach and the Kidney	*Equilibrium*
	With impotence	Yin deficiencies of the Lung, the Stomach and the Kidney with yang deficiency of the Kidney	*Equilibrium* with *Vitality*
	With urinary tract infection	Yin deficiencies of the Lung, the Stomach and the Kidney with damp-heat in the Urinary Bladder	*Equilibrium* and *Gentiana Complex*
	With blurry vision	Yin deficiencies of the Lung, the Stomach and the Kidney with false heat	*Equilibrium* and *Nourish*
	With high cholesterol	Yin deficiencies of the Lung, the Stomach and the Kidney with damp and phlegm accumulation	*Equilibrium* and *Cholisma*
	With peripheral neuropathy	Yin deficiencies of the Lung, the Stomach and the Kidney with qi and blood stagnation	*Equilibrium* and *Flex (NP)*
	With excessive thirst	Stomach and Lung yin and fluid deficiency	*Equilibrium* and *Nourish (Fluids)*
Diarrhea	Loose stool or diarrhea with poor appetite and weakness	Spleen deficiency	*GI Tonic*
	With foul-smelling stool, burning sensation of anus, abdominal discomfort and pain, nausea and vomiting, traveler's diarrhea	Damp-heat in the Intestines	*GI Care II*
	Due to ulcerative colitis, Crohn's disease, diarrhea with pus and blood	Toxic heat in the intestines	*GI Care (UC)*
	Due to irritable bowel syndrome (IBS)	Liver qi stagnation	*GI Harmony*
	Moderate to severe cases of infection and inflammation	Accumulation of toxic heat	*GI Harmony* and *Herbal ABX*
	With bleeding	Heat pushing blood out of the vessels	*Add Notoginseng 9*
	Extreme thirst and dryness from diarrhea	Yin and fluid deficiency	*Add Nourish (Fluids)*
	Poor appetite, fatigue, loose stool	Spleen qi deficiency	*GI Tonic*
Diet...	Excess appetite, overweight	Dampness accumulation with Stomach heat	*Herbalite*

SYMPTOM / DISEASE INDEX

CONDITION	SYMPTON / DISEASE DESCRIPTION	TCM DIAGNOSIS	HERBAL FORMULAS
	Food poisoning or traveler's diarrhea	Damp-heat in the intestine	*GI Care II*
	Excessive appetite with high cholesterol	Damp accumulation	*Cholisma*
	Excessive appetite with high cholesterol, fatty liver and obesity	Damp phlegm accumulation	*Cholisma (ES)*
	Excessive appetite with gallstone	Damp-heat in the Gallbladder	*Dissolve (GS)*
	Excessive appetite with hepatitis	Toxic heat in the Liver	*Liver DTX*
Discharge	Clear and watery nasal discharge	Wind-cold at the exterior	*Magnolia Clear Sinus*
	Thick and yellow nasal discharge	Damp-heat at the nose	*Pueraria Clear Sinus*
	Yellow vaginal discharge	Damp-heat in the lower *jiao*	*V-Statin*
	Clear vaginal discharge	Kidney yang deficiency	*Balance (Cold)*
	Moderate to severe cases of infection and inflammation	Accumulation of toxic heat	*V-Statin* and *Herbal ABX*
	Ear discharge from infection	Toxic heat invasion	*Herbal ENT*
	Nipple discharge from fibrocystic disorder	Phlegm accumulation and Liver qi stagnation	*Resolve (Upper)*
Distention	Head	Qi and blood stagnation	*Corydalin*
	Head: due to deficient type of hypertension	Liver yang rising with yin deficiency	*Gastrodia Complex*
	Head: due to excess type of hypertension	Liver fire	*Gentiana Complex*
	Chest: coronary heart disease	*Xiong bi* (painful obstruction of the chest)	*Circulation*
	Chest: wheezing or dyspnea with fever, yellow sputum	Lung heat	*Respitrol (Heat)* with *Poria XPT*
	Chest: wheezing or dyspnea with white sputum	Lung cold	*Respitrol (Cold)*
	Chest: chronic respiratory disorder with dyspnea	Lung qi deficiency	*Respitrol (Deficient)*
	Hypochondriac area	Liver qi stagnation	*Calm*
	Abdomen: due to irritable bowel syndrome (IBS)	Liver qi stagnation	*GI Harmony*
	Abdomen: due to ulcerative colitis (UC) or Crohn's disease	Damp-heat in the intestine	*GI Care (UC)*
	Abdomen: with weakness of digestion	Spleen qi deficiency	*GI Tonic*
	Lower abdomen: due to fibroids	Qi, blood and phlegm stagnation	*Resolve (Lower)*
	Lower abdomen: due to endometriosis	Qi and blood stagnation	*Resolve (Lower)*
	Breast distention	Liver qi stagnation	*Calm*
	Severe breast distention	Liver qi stagnation	*Calm* and *Resolve (Upper)*
	Swelling and edema	Fluid and damp accumulation	*Herbal DRX*
Dizziness...	Due to anemia	Spleen and Heart deficiencies	*Schisandra ZZZ*
	Due to hypertension	Liver yang rising or Liver fire	*Gastrodia Complex* or *Gentiana Complex*

SYMPTOM / DISEASE INDEX

CONDITION	SYMPTOM / DISEASE DESCRIPTION	TCM DIAGNOSIS	HERBAL FORMULAS
	From exposure to drugs, chemicals, heavy metals, environmental and airborne toxins	Toxic heat	*Herbal DTX*
	With migraine or headache from blood deficiency	Blood deficiency	*Migratrol*
	With ear, nose or throat infection	Wind-heat and toxic heat invasion	*Herbal ENT*
	With blurry vision, tinnitus, hot flashes, low-grade fever or night sweats	Kidney yin-deficient heat	*Balance (Heat)* or *Kidney Tonic (Yin)*
	With flu or common cold	Wind-heat or wind-cold invasion	*Lonicera Complex* or *Respitrol (Cold)*
Diverticulitis	Diverticulitis with inflammation	Damp-heat in the intestine	*Resolve (AI)* with *GI Harmony*
	With acute constipation	Qi stagnation with heat	*Resolve (AI)* with *Gentle Lax (Excess)*
	With chronic constipation or dry stool	Yin deficiency with stagnation	*Resolve (AI)* and *Gentle Lax (Deficient)*
	With severe pain	Severe qi and blood stagnation	*Resolve (AI)* and *Herbal Analgesic*
Dreams	Increased dreams, difficulty falling and staying asleep, poor appetite, epigastric fullness and distension, fatigue	Spleen and Heart deficiencies	*Schisandra ZZZ*
	Nervousness, forgetfulness, restlessness, weakness	Heart and Kidney deficiencies	*Enhance Memory*
	Anger, short temper, hypochondriac discomfort	Liver fire	*Calm (ES)*
	Difficulty falling or staying asleep, stress, anxiety, restlessness with deficiency	Liver qi stagnation with qi deficiency	*Calm ZZZ*
Drooling of Saliva	With paralysis, bell's palsy	Liver wind	*Symmetry*
	With profuse saliva, poor appetite, pale complexion, loose stool	Spleen qi deficiency	*GI Tonic*
	With ulceration in the tongue, bitter taste, constipation, irritability	Stomach heat	*Herbal ENT* and *Gentle Lax (Excess)*
Drugs	*See Addiction, Detox, Poisoning*		
Dryness	Dry eyes	Liver and Kidney yin deficiencies	*Nourish*
	Dry skin, hair, nails	Liver blood and Kidney yin deficiencies	*Polygonum 14*
	General dryness with thirst	Lung and Stomach yin deficiency	*Nourish (Fluids)*
	Severe dryness with tinnitus, hair loss, blurry vision, weakness and soreness of back and knees, hot flashes, low-grade fever, malar flush, night sweats, etc.	Kidney yin deficiency	*Kidney Tonic (Yin)* and *Balance (Heat)*
Duodenum	Ulcer with abdominal pain	Stomach heat	*GI Care*

Lotus Institute of Integrative Medicine

SYMPTOM / DISEASE INDEX

CONDITION	SYMPTOM / DISEASE DESCRIPTION	TCM DIAGNOSIS	HERBAL FORMULAS
Dysentery	Diarrhea with foul-smelling stool, burning sensation of anus, abdominal discomfort and pain, nausea and vomiting	Damp-heat in the Intestines	*GI Care II*
	Moderate to severe cases of infection and inflammation	Accumulation of toxic heat	*GI Care II* with *Herbal ABX*
	With bleeding	Heat pushing blood out of the vessels	Add *Notoginseng 9*
	With fever	Excess heat accumulation	Add *Gardenia Complex*
Dysmenorrhea	With bloating and blood clots	Qi and blood stagnation	*Mense-Ease*
	Due to endometriosis or uterine fibroids	Qi and blood stagnation	*Mense-Ease* with *Resolve (Lower)*
	With pelvic infection or inflammation	Toxic heat accumulation and blood stagnation	*Mense-Ease* with *V-Statin*
	With severe pain	Severe qi and blood stagnation	*Mense-Ease* with *Herbal Analgesic*
Dyspnea	Cough, dyspnea, chest congestion, yellow sputum, with or without fever	Lung heat	*Respitrol (Heat)*
	Cough, white sputum or nasal discharge, chills	Lung cold	*Respitrol (Cold)*
	Chronic respiratory disorder; dyspnea with light physical exertion	Deficiencies of the Lung and the Kidney	*Respitrol (Deficient)*
	Cough with no other significant signs	Lung qi reversal	*Respitrol (CF)*
	Chronic respiratory disorder with underlying Lung and Kidney deficiency	Lung and Kidney qi deficiency	*Cordyceps 3*
Dysuria	Painful urination due to heat	Damp-heat in the Urinary Bladder	*V-Statin*
	Kidney or urinary stones	Dysuria due to stone; *shi lin* (stone dysuria)	*Dissolve (KS)*
	Moderate to severe cases of kidney stone with infection and inflammation	Accumulation of toxic heat	*Dissolve (KS)* with *Herbal ABX*
	Chronic nephritis	Toxic heat with dampness and Kidney deficiency	*Kidney DTX*
	Due to prostatitis	Damp-heat accumulation in the lower *jiao*	*Saw Palmetto Complex*
	Due to prostate enlargement	Damp accumulation and qi stagnation	*P-Statin*
	With bleeding	Heat pushing blood out of the vessels	Add *Notoginseng 9*
	With fever	Excess heat accumulation	Add *Gardenia Complex*
	With severe pain	Severe qi and blood stagnation	Add *Herbal Analgesic*
Ear Infection	Ear infection with fever, pain	Damp-heat in the Liver and Gallbladder channels	*Herbal ENT*
	Moderate to severe cases of infection and inflammation	Accumulation of toxic heat	*Herbal ENT* and *Gentiana Complex*
	With swelling	Damp-heat accumulation	*Herbal ENT* and *Resolve (AI)*
	With fever	Excess heat accumulation	*Herbal ENT* and *Gardenia Complex*
Eating Disorder	*See Anorexia, Bulimia*		

SYMPTOM / DISEASE INDEX

CONDITION	SYMPTON / DISEASE DESCRIPTION	TCM DIAGNOSIS	HERBAL FORMULAS
Eczema	Skin allergy, rash, eczema, itching, general dermatological disorders	Wind-heat at the skin level, heat in the blood	*Silerex*
	Of the genital area	Damp-heat in the lower *jiao*	*V-Statin*
	Chronic itching	Toxic heat accumulation	*Add Dermatrol (PS)*
	Skin reaction due to exposure to drugs, chemicals, heavy metals, environmental and airborne toxins	Toxic heat accumulation	*Silerex or Dermatrol (PS)* and *Herbal DTX*
	Chronic eczema with underlying blood deficiency or anemia	Toxic heat accumulation with blood deficiency	*Silerex with Schisandra ZZZ*
	With redness, burning or fever	Excess heat accumulation	*Silerex and Gardenia Complex*
	Stubborn eczema due to blood stagnation with dark appearance and purplish tongue	Blood stagnation	*Silerex and Circulation (SJ)*
Edema	General edema with swelling	Water accumulation	*Herbal DRX*
	With coldness of extremities, dizziness, irregular menstruation	Spleen deficiency with damp and cold	*Balance (Cold)*
	Edema in hypothyroid patients	Kidney yang deficiency with damp accumulation	*Thyro-forte* and *Herbal DRX*
	Due to hypertension	Liver yin deficiency with Liver yang rising	*Gastrodia Complex*
	Due to obesity and excess appetite	Stomach heat with damp	*Herbalite*
	With coldness and weakness	Kidney yang deficiency	*Kidney Tonic (Yang)*
	Due to chronic kidney disease	Kidney deficiency	*Kidney DTX*
	With weak digestive system and diarrhea	Spleen deficiency	*GI Tonic*
	With lymphedema	Damp and phlegm accumulation	*Resolve (AI)*
	Due to diabetes	Yin deficiency with damp	*Equilibrium*
Elbow	Tennis elbow, golfer's elbow, pain	Qi and blood stagnation	*Arm Support*
	With severe pain	Severe qi and blood stagnation	*Add Herbal Analgesic*
	Soft tissue degeneration (muscles, tendons, ligaments and cartilage)	Liver and Kidney yin deficiencies	*Add Flex (MLT)*
Emaciation	Weight loss, fatigue, over-all deficiency	Qi, blood, yin and yang deficiencies	*Imperial Tonic*
	Chronic fatigue with compromised lung and kidney functions	Lung and Kidney deficiencies	*Cordyceps 3*
	Weight loss, loose stool, poor appetite, fatigue with weak digestive system	Spleen deficiency	*GI Tonic*
	General Kidney yin deficiency signs such as blurry vision, weakness of the back and knees, tinnitus, dryness, flushed cheeks, possible low-grade fever, etc.	Kidney yin deficiency	*Kidney Tonic (Yin)*
	General Kidney yang deficiency signs such as coldness, low libido, premature ejaculation, weakness and soreness of the back and knees, pale complexion, polyuria, etc.	Kidney yang deficiency	*Kidney Tonic (Yang)*
Emotion...	Instability with stress, PMS, nervousness	Liver qi stagnation	*Calm*

SYMPTOM / DISEASE INDEX

CONDITION	SYMPTOM / DISEASE DESCRIPTION	TCM DIAGNOSIS	HERBAL FORMULAS
	Instability with Heart fire manifesting in restlessness, insomnia and anger	Liver and Heart fire	*Calm (ES)*
	Instability with mood swings in menopause patients	Kidney and Liver yin deficiencies	*Balance (Heat)*
	Instability, over-active mind, stress and insomnia in patients with deficiency	Liver qi stagnation with qi deficiency	*Calm ZZZ*
	Excessive worrying, pensiveness, anemia	Spleen and Heart blood deficiencies	*Schisandra ZZZ*
	Depression	Qi, blood, phlegm, food, fire and damp accumulation	*Shine*
	Pent-up emotion with red face, constipation, excess fire	Excess accumulation of fire	*Add Gardenia Complex*
	Chronic, stubborn emotional imbalance that doesn't seem to respond to any treatment	Blood stagnation	*Add Circulation (SJ)*
Emphysema	Dyspnea, wheezing, scanty or no sputum, weakness	Deficiencies of the Lung and the Kidney	*Respirol (Deficient)*
	Dyspnea, wheezing, white sputum	Lung cold	*Respirol (Cold)*
	Dyspnea, wheezing, fever	Lung heat	*Respirol (Heat)*
	Maintenance formula to improve breathing	Lung and Kidney deficiencies	*Cordyceps 3*
	Cough with no other pronounced symptoms	Lung qi reversal	*Respirol (CF)*
Endocrine Disorder	Diminished function of the adrenal glands and endocrine system	Deficiencies of Kidney yin, yang and *jing* (essence)	*Adrenoplex*
	Diabetes mellitus	Yin deficiency with dampness and heat	*Equilibrium*
	Hyperthyroidism	Excess heat	*Thyrodex*
	Hypothyroidism	Kidney yang deficiency	*Thyro-forte*
	Addison's disease	Kidney deficiency	*Adrenoplex*
Endometriosis	Cramps and pain with or without menstruation	Blood stagnation in the lower *jiao*	*Resolve (Lower)*
	Severe menstrual cramps	Blood stagnation in the lower *jiao*	*Resolve (Lower)* and *Mense-Ease*
	With back pain	Blood stagnation in the lower *jiao*	*Resolve (Lower)* and *Back Support (Acute)*
	Causing infertility	Blood stagnation in the lower *jiao*	*Resolve (Lower)* and *Blossom (Phase 1-4)*
Energy…	Short-term tiredness and lack of energy	Qi deficiency	*Vibrant*
	Chronic fatigue with generalized weakness and deficiency in qi, blood, yin and yang	Qi, blood, yin and yang deficiencies	*Vibrant* and *Imperial Tonic*
	Chronic fatigue with Lung and Kidney weakness	Lung and Kidney deficiencies	*Cordyceps 3*
	Low energy and weak immune system	*Wei* (defensive) *qi* deficiency	*Immune +*

Lotus Institute of Integrative Medicine

SYMPTOM / DISEASE INDEX

CONDITION	SYMPTON / DISEASE DESCRIPTION	TCM DIAGNOSIS	HERBAL FORMULAS
	Low energy and weak digestive function	Spleen qi deficiency	GI Tonic
	Chronic sluggishness with blood stagnation signs of purplish tongue, dark complexion, past history of trauma or surgery	Blood stagnation	Circulation (SJ)
Enhancement (Breast)	To enhance the size and the shape of the breasts	Kidney yang and jing (essence) deficiencies	Venus
Enteritis	Diarrhea with foul-smelling stool, burning sensation of anus, abdominal discomfort and pain, nausea and vomiting	Damp-heat in the Intestines	GI Care II
	Ulcerative colitis, Crohn's disease	Damp-heat in the Large Intestine	GI Care (UC)
	Moderate to severe cases of ulcerative colitis and Crohn's disease	Accumulation of toxic heat	GI Care (UC) and Herbal ABX
	Chronic enteritis with weakness, poor appetite, and diarrhea	Spleen qi deficiency	GI Care II and GI Tonic
	Due to chemotherapy	Qi deficiency and heat accumulation	C/R Support
	With excess heat and inflammation	Excess heat	GI Care II and Gardenia Complex
	Enteritis with pain	Qi and blood stagnation	GI Care II and Herbal Analgesic
	Enteritis with bleeding	Heat pushing blood out of the vessels	GI Care II and Notoginseng 9
Epicondylitis (Lateral or Medial)	Tennis elbow	Qi and blood stagnation	Arm Support
	For degeneration of the joint and related soft tissue (muscle, ligaments, tendons, cartilages)	Wei (atrophy) syndrome	Flex (MLT)
	For severe pain		Add Herbal Analgesic
Epigastric Pain	Epigastric fullness and pain, stomach ulcer, gastritis, acid reflux	Stomach heat	GI Care
	Irritable bowel syndrome (IBS), Crohn's disease, gas with indigestion	Liver qi stagnation	GI Harmony
	Pain due to gallstones	Damp-heat in the Liver and Gallbladder	Dissolve (GS)
	With severe pain	Severe qi and blood stagnation	Herbal Analgesic
	With obesity and excessive appetite	Stomach fire	Herbalite
Epilepsy	Childhood convulsions, epilepsy, seizures and twitching of muscles	Liver wind	Calm (Jr)
	Convulsion, epilepsy, seizure or twitching in adults	Liver wind	Symmetry
Erection Difficulty	See Impotence		
Erysipelas	Skin and lymph infection	Toxic heat accumulation with phlegm	Herbal ENT and Herbal ABX
Esophageal Reflux	See Acid Reflux		
Estrogen...	Breast discomfort with PMS	Liver qi stagnation	Calm
	Breast discomfort with lumps, possible fibroids	Liver qi stagnation with phlegm stagnation	Resolve (Upper)
	Infertility	Depends on each phase	Blossom (Phase 1-4)

SYMPTOM / DISEASE INDEX

CONDITION	SYMPTON / DISEASE DESCRIPTION	TCM DIAGNOSIS	HERBAL FORMULAS
	Menopause	Kidney yin deficiency	Balance (Heat) and/or Nourish
	Osteoporosis	Kidney jing (essence) deficiency	Osteo 8
	Dryness of the eyes with blurred vision	Liver and Kidney yin deficiencies	Nourish
Eyes	Hypertensive patients with red eyes, blurred vision, dizziness or vertigo	Liver yang rising	Gastrodia Complex
	Hypertensive patients with red eyes, flushed face, short temper	Liver fire rising	Gentiana Complex
	Red eyes due to infection	Accumulation of toxic heat	Herbal ABX
	Dry eyes with blurred vision	Liver and Kidney yin deficiencies	Nourish
Eye (With Dark Circles)	With generalized weakness, possible tinnitus, blurry vision, night sweating, low-grade fever	Kidney yin deficiency	Kidney Tonic (Yin)
	With coldness, soreness and weakness of the low back and knees, spermatorrhea, low libido, polyuria, hair loss, etc.	Kidney yang deficiency	Kidney Tonic (Yang)
Facial Paralysis	Bell's Palsy	Wind attack with qi and blood stagnation	Symmetry
Fainting	See Hypoglycemia, Hypotension		
Fallopian Tubes	Infertility due to obstruction	Qi and blood stagnation of the lower jiao	Resolve (Lower) with Blossom (Phase 1-4)
	Inflammation of the fallopian tubes	Damp-heat in the lower jiao	V-Statin
	Abscess and inflammation	Phlegm obstruction	Resolve (AI) and V-Statin
	Infertility due to scarring, coldness and weakness	Blood stagnation with Kidney yang deficiency	Menotrol
Fat	Obesity with excess appetite	Damp-heat accumulation with heat	Herbalite
	High cholesterol and triglycerides levels	Damp-heat accumulation	Cholisma
	Fatty tissue deposit, such as lipomas	Phlegm stagnation	Resolve (AI)
	Short-term tiredness and lack of energy	Qi deficiency	Vibrant
Fatigue...	Chronic fatigue with generalized weakness	Qi, blood, yin and yang deficiencies	Vibrant with Imperial Tonic
	Weakness, insomnia, excess worries	Spleen and Heart qi deficiencies	Schisandra ZZZ
	Patients who are burned out with fatigue, lack of energy and drive	Deficiency of Spleen and Stomach	Adrenoplex
	Chronic fatigue with lung and kidney weakness	Lung and Kidney deficiencies	Cordyceps 3
	Low energy and weak immune system	Wei (defensive) qi deficiency	Immune +
	Low energy and weak digestive function, poor appetite, loose stool	Spleen qi deficiency	GI Tonic
	Due to coronary artery disease	Chest pain; chest bi zheng (painful obstruction syndrome)	Circulation
	Due to chronic nephritis	Toxic heat in the Kidney	Kidney DTX

Lotus Institute of Integrative Medicine

SYMPTOM / DISEASE INDEX

CONDITION	SYMPTON / DISEASE DESCRIPTION	TCM DIAGNOSIS	HERBAL FORMULAS
	In cancer patients	*Yuan* (source) *qi* and *wei* (defensive) *qi* deficiencies	*C/R Support* or *CA Support*
	In chronic patients with severe blood stagnation manifesting in purplish tongue	Blood stasis	*Circulation (SJ)*
Fatty Liver	Fatty liver with high cholesterol and obesity	Damp and phlegm accumulation	*Cholisma (ES)*
	With hepatitis	Toxic heat in the Liver	*Cholisma (ES)* and *Liver DTX*
Fear	Fear, restlessness, anxiety	*Shen* (spirit) disturbance with fire	*Calm (ES)*
	Easily frightened, poor sleep, excessive dreams	Spleen and Heart blood deficiency with *shen* (spirit) disturbance	*Schisandra ZZZ*
Fertility	*See Infertility*		
Fever	General fever	Heat in all three *jiaos*	*Gardenia Complex*
	Fever in viral infections, common cold and flu	Wind-heat	*Lonicera Complex*
	Fever in bacterial infections, pneumonia, or bronchitis, cough, dyspnea	Lung heat	*Respitrol (Heat)*
	Fever, chest congestion, yellow sputum	Damp-heat in the Lung	*Poria XPT*
	Low-grade fever in the evening with perspiration	Yin deficiency with false heat	*Nourish* with *Balance (Heat)*
	Various types of infection	Heat at various parts of body	*Herbal ABX*
	Fever due to hyperthyroidism	Liver fire excess	*Thyrodex*
	Fever due to exposure to drugs, chemicals, heavy metals, environmental and airborne toxins	Toxic heat	*Herbal DTX*
	Fever with swelling and inflammation	Heat with phlegm stagnation	*Gardenia Complex* with *Resolve (AI)*
	Unremitting fever due to blood stagnation manifesting in purplish tongue	Blood stasis	*Circulation (SJ)* with *Gardenia Complex*
Fever Blister	Cold sores with pain and inflammation	Wind-heat	*Lonicera Complex*
	Moderate to severe cases of infection and inflammation	Accumulation of toxic heat	*Herbal ENT* and *Herbal ABX*
	Fever blister with severe pain	Qi and blood stagnation	*Herbal ENT* and *Herbal Analgesic*
Fibrocystic Disease	Fibrocystic breast masses	Liver qi stagnation with phlegm	*Resolve (Upper)*
	Fibroids in the uterus and ovaries	Blood stagnation in the lower *jiao*	*Resolve (Lower)*
Fibromyalgia…	With coldness and/or numbness	*Bi zheng* (painful obstruction syndrome) with cold and deficiency	*Flex (CD)*
	With heat sensations	*Bi zheng* (painful obstruction syndrome) with heat	*Flex (Heat)*

SYMPTOM / DISEASE INDEX

CONDITION	SYMPTON / DISEASE DESCRIPTION	TCM DIAGNOSIS	HERBAL FORMULAS
	With spasms and cramps	*Bi zheng* (painful obstruction syndrome) with Liver yin and body fluid deficiencies	*Flex (SC)*
	Due to stress	*Bi zheng* (painful obstruction syndrome) with Liver qi stagnation	*Calm* or *Calm (ES)*
	With extreme fatigue due to deficiency	*Bi zheng* (painful obstruction syndrome) with qi deficiency	*Calm* or *Calm (ES)* and *Imperial Tonic*
	Due to bone spurs	Qi and blood stagnation	*Flex (Spur)*
	With severe pain	Severe qi and blood stagnation	*Flex (Spur)* and *Herbal Analgesic*
	Due to blood stagnation manifesting in purplish tongue	Blood stasis	*Circulation (SJ)*
Fidgeting	*See Irritability*		
Filatov's Disease	Fever, pharyngitis, enlarged lymph	Toxic heat accumulation with dampness	*Resolve (AI)* and *Herbal ENT*
Fire	Excess fire and heat signs	Excess fire in all three *jiaos*	*Gardenia Complex*
	Fissures with dryness	Yin deficiency	*Nourish*
Fissures	With ulceration or from hemorrhoids	Damp-heat in the lower *jiao*	*V-Statin* and *GI Care (HMR)*
	With acute constipation	Qi and blood stagnation	*Gentle Lax (Excess)*
	With chronic constipation or dry stool	Yin deficiency	*Gentle Lax (Deficient)*
	With infection	Toxic heat	*Gentle Lax (Deficient)* and *Herbal ABX*
	With sweating, irritability	Yin deficiency with heat	*Balance (Heat)*
Five-Center Heat	With thirst, dryness	Yin deficiency	*Balance (Heat)* and *Nourish (Fluids)*
	With extreme Kidney yin deficiency	Kidney yin deficiency	*Kidney Tonic (Yin)*
	Due to irritable bowel syndrome	Liver qi stagnation	*GI Harmony*
Flatulence	With burning diarrhea or infection	Damp-heat in the intestine	*GI Care II*
	With weakness, poor appetite with diarrhea	Spleen qi deficiency	*GI Tonic*
	With ulcerative colitis, Crohn's disease	Damp-heat accumulation	*GI Care (UC)*
	Stress related bloating and distension	Liver qi stagnation	*Calm*
	With gallstones	Damp-heat in the Liver	*Dissolve (GS)*
Flu	*See Common Cold, Influenza*		
	Intestinal Flu	Toxic, damp-heat in the Intestines	*GI Care II*
	ADD, ADHD	Liver wind with *shen* (spirit) disturbance	*Calm (Jr)*
Focus…	Inability to focus, poor memory, forgetfulness	Heart and Kidney deficiencies	*Enhance Memory*

SYMPTOM / DISEASE INDEX

CONDITION	SYMPTOM / DISEASE DESCRIPTION	TCM DIAGNOSIS	HERBAL FORMULAS
	Alzheimer's disease	Kidney yang deficiency	*Neuro +*
Follicular Phase	Infertility; follicular phase	Qi and blood deficiency, Kidney *jing* (essence) deficiency	*Blossom (Phase 2)*
Food Poisoning	Diarrhea, abdominal pain, nausea, vomiting	Damp-heat in the Intestines	*GI Care II*
	Moderate to severe cases of infection and inflammation	Accumulation of toxic heat	*GI Care II* and *Herbal ABX*
	With fever	Accumulation of toxic heat	*GI Care II* and *Gardenia Complex*
Forgetfulness	Poor memory, forgetfulness	Heart and Kidney deficiencies	*Enhance Memory*
	Poor memory, poor concentration associated with Alzheimer's disease	Deficiencies of Kidney yin, yang and *jing* (essence)	*Neuro Plus*
	With dizziness, weakness, difficulty sleeping, anemia, excessive thinking and worrying	Spleen and Heart deficiency	*Schisandra ZZZ*
	ADD or ADHD in children	Liver wind with *shen* (spirit) disturbance	*Calm (Jr)*
	Diminished mental and physical functions	Deficiencies of Kidney yin, yang and *jing* (essence)	*Adrenoplex*
	With Kidney yin deficient signs of blurry vision, weakness of the back and knees, tinnitus, dryness, flushed cheeks, possible low-grade fever, etc.	Kidney yin deficiency	*Kidney Tonic (Yin)*
	With Kidney yang deficient signs of coldness, low libido, premature ejaculation, weakness and soreness of the back and knees, pale complexion, polyuria, etc.	Kidney yang deficiency	*Kidney Tonic (Yang)*
Fracture	*See Bone Disorders*		
Frozen Shoulder	Acute pain and immobility	Qi and blood stagnation	*Neck & Shoulder (Acute)* and *Arm Support*
	Chronic, dull pain, immobility, numbness	Qi and blood stagnation with Liver yin deficiency	*Neck & Shoulder (Chronic)* and *Arm Support*
	Pain due to bone spur	Qi and blood stagnation	*Neck & Shoulder (Acute)* and *Flex (Spur)*
	With severe pain	Severe qi and blood stagnation	*Neck & Shoulder (Acute)* and *Herbal Analgesic*
Fullness...	Due to peptic ulcers	Stomach heat	*GI Care*
	With irritability and stress	Liver overacting on the Spleen and Stomach	*Calm*
	With constipation	Qi stagnation of the Large Intestine	*Gentle Lax (Excess)* or *Gentle Lax (Deficient)*
	Before or during menstruation	Liver qi stagnation	*Calm*

SYMPTOM / DISEASE INDEX

CONDITION	SYMPTON / DISEASE DESCRIPTION	TCM DIAGNOSIS	HERBAL FORMULAS
	Due to endometriosis, uterine or ovarian fibroids	Blood stagnation in the lower *jiao*	*Resolve (Lower)*
	Due to gallstone	Damp-heat in the Gallbladder	*Dissolve (GS)*
	Due to irritable bowel syndrome (IBS), Crohn's disease	Liver qi stagnation	*GI Harmony*
	Due to ulcerative colitis	Damp-heat accumulation	*GI Care (UC)*
	With weakness, poor appetite and loose stool	Spleen qi deficiency	*GI Tonic*
	In those undergoing chemotherapy/radiotherapy	Stomach yin and qi deficiencies	*C/R Support*
Fungal Infection	*See Infection*		
Furuncle	Swelling with redness and pain	Damp-heat	*Resolve (AI)*
	Moderate to severe infection	Toxic heat	*Resolve (AI)* and *Herbal ABX*
	With severe pain	Severe qi and blood stagnation	*Resolve (AI)* and *Herbal Analgesic*
	Chronic, non-healing cases with blood stagnation manifesting in purplish tongue	Blood stasis	*Circulation (SJ)*
Gallbladder	*See Cholecystitis, Cholelithiasis*		
Gallstones	*See Stones*		
Gas	*See Flatulence*		
Gastritis	Heartburn, acid reflux, stomach pain	Stomach fire	*GI Care*
	Stress related gastritis with heartburn, acid reflux, stomach pain	Stomach fire with Liver qi stagnation	*GI Care* and *Calm*
	Gastritis with weakness, poor appetite and loose stool	Spleen qi deficiency	*GI Tonic*
	With bleeding	Heat pushing blood out of the vessels	*Add Notoginseng 9*
	With dryness and thirst	Stomach yin deficiency	*Nourish (Fluids)*
Gastroenteritis	Diarrhea with foul-smelling stool, burning sensation of anus, abdominal discomfort and pain, nausea and vomiting	Damp-heat in the Intestines	*GI Care II*
	Moderate to severe cases of infection and inflammation	Accumulation of toxic heat	*GI Care II* and *Herbal ABX*
	Ulcerative colitis, Crohn's disease or symptoms like such	Damp-heat accumulation	*GI Care (UC)*
	Gastrointestinal symptoms associated with exposure to drugs, chemicals, heavy metals, environmental and airborne toxins	Toxic heat	*Herbal DTX*
	With bleeding	Heat in the blood	*Notoginseng 9*
	With fever or excess heat	Excess accumulation of heat	*Gardenia Complex*
Gastroesophageal Reflux Disease (GERD)	Acid reflux, heartburn, stomach pain and discomfort	Stomach fire with rising Stomach qi	*GI Care*
	Stress related	Liver qi stagnation	*GI Care* and *Calm*
Gastroptosis	Downward displacement of the stomach	Qi and yang deficiency	*C/R Support* and *GI Tonic*

SYMPTOM / DISEASE INDEX

CONDITION	SYMPTOM / DISEASE DESCRIPTION	TCM DIAGNOSIS	HERBAL FORMULAS
Genital Herpes	*See Herpes*		
Genital Itching	Itching and discomfort in the genital area	Damp-heat in the lower *jiao*	*V-Statin* or *Gentiana Complex*
	Moderate to severe cases of infection and inflammation	Accumulation of toxic heat	Use either above with *Herbal ABX*
	Chancre, sore, warts	Damp and toxic heat in the lower *jiao*	*V-Statin* and *Herbal ABX*
Germs	*See Infection*		
Glandular Fever	Fever, pharyngitis, enlarged lymph	Toxic heat accumulation with dampness	*Resolve (AI)* and *Herbal ABX*
Glomerulonephritis	Compromised kidney function with proteinuria and edema	Toxic heat accumulation	*Kidney DTX*
	Drug related	Toxic heat accumulation	*Kidney DTX* and *Herbal DTX*
Glucose	*See Diabetes, Hypoglycemia*		
Goiter	Enlargement of the thyroid gland due to hyperthyroidism	Liver qi and phlegm stagnation with *shen* (spirit) disturbance	*Thyrodex*
	Enlargement of the thyroid gland due to hypothyroidism	Spleen and Kidney yang deficiencies	*Thyro-forte*
Gonorrhea	Discharge, dysuria with burning sensation and pain	Damp-heat in the lower *jiao*	*Gentiana Complex* or *V-Statin*
Gout	Pain, redness and swelling	Hot *bi zheng* (painful obstruction syndrome)	*Flex (GT)*
	With severe pain	Severe qi and blood stagnation	*Flex (GT)* and *Herbal Analgesic*
Grave's Disease	*See Hyperthyroidism*		
Growth	Growth retardation	Kidney yin, yang and *jing* (essence) deficiencies	*Osteo 8*
Gums	Bleeding or swollen gums	Stomach heat	*Gardenia Complex*
Hair	Premature gray hair, dry scalp, hair, nails	Liver yin and blood deficiencies	*Polygonum 14*
	Stress-related hair disorders	Liver qi stagnation with yin and blood deficiencies	*Polygonum 14* and *Calm*
Halitosis	*See Bad Breath*		
Hands	Cold hands with weakness or anemia	Liver blood deficiency	*Balance (Cold)*
	Cold hands due to poor circulation	Qi and blood stagnation	*Flex (NP)*
	Feeling of heat in the palms and feet	Yin deficiency with heat	*Balance (Heat)* or *Nourish*
	Pain or numbness of the arm	Qi and blood stagnation	*Arm Support*
	Tingling, pain or numbness of the hands originating from cervical disorder	Qi and blood stagnation	*Neck & Shoulder (Acute)*
Hangover...	Excessive consumption of alcohol	Toxic heat in the Liver	*Liver DTX*
	Hangover with headache	Toxic heat in the Liver with qi and blood stagnation	*Liver DTX* and *Corydalin*
	Hangover with stomach pain, nausea and vomiting	Heat in the Liver and the Stomach	*Liver DTX* and *GI Care*

SYMPTOM / DISEASE INDEX

CONDITION	SYMPTON / DISEASE DESCRIPTION	TCM DIAGNOSIS	HERBAL FORMULAS
	With excessive thirst	Yin and fluid deficiencies	*Nourish (Fluids)*
	With excess heat and fire signs	Excess fire accumulation	*Liver DTX* and *Gardenia Complex*
Hardness	*See Nodules*		
Hashimoto's Thyroiditis	*See Hypothyroidism*		
Hay Fever	*See Allergy*		
Headache	Immediate relief for a variety of headache or migraine	Qi and blood stagnation	*Corydalin*
	Due to hypertension with dizziness	Liver yin deficiency with Liver yang rising	*Corydalin* and *Gastrodia Complex*
	Due to stress	Liver qi stagnation	*Corydalin* and *Calm*
	Temporal or vertex headache with flushed face, anger	Damp-heat in the Liver channel	*Corydalin* and *Gentiana Complex*
	Due to common cold, fever, sore throat	Wind-heat	*Corydalin* and *Lonicera Complex*
	Sinus headache with white watery nasal discharge	Wind-cold with fluid congestion	*Corydalin* and *Magnolia Clear Sinus*
	Sinus headache with yellow thick nasal discharge	Damp-heat with fluid congestion	*Corydalin* and *Pueraria Clear Sinus*
	With ear, nose or throat infection	Toxic heat invasion	*Corydalin* and *Herbal ENT*
	Blood deficient type of hollow headache	Blood deficiency with qi and blood stagnation	*Migratrol*
	Stubborn, stabbing headache due to previous trauma to the head or blood stagnation	Blood stasis	*Corydalin* and *Circulation (SJ)*
	Headache with excess heat signs manifesting in red face, fast heartbeat and possible constipation	Excess heat	*Corydalin* and *Gardenia Complex*
	With facial paralysis, Bell's palsy, TMJ or trigeminal neuralgia	Qi and blood stagnation	*Corydalin* and *Symmetry*
Hearing Loss	Diminished hearing or ringing of the ear	Kidney yin deficiency	*Nourish*
	Tinnitus	Lung and Kidney qi deficiencies	*Cordyceps 3* and *Nourish*
Heart	*See Angina Pectoris, Cholesterol, Hypertension, Hypotension, Coronary Heart Disease*		
Heart Attack (Prevention)	Coronary heart disease	Blood stagnation in the upper *jiao*	*Circulation*
Heartbeat	Fast with high blood pressure	Excess fire	*Gardenia Complex*
Heartburn	Acid reflux with stomach pain and discomfort	Stomach fire	*GI Care*
Heaviness	Heaviness and/or sluggish feeling	Damp accumulation	*Herbal DRX*
	Obesity with excessive appetite	Stomach heat	*Herbalite*
Heavy Metal	*See Poisoning, Detox*		

SYMPTOM / DISEASE INDEX

CONDITION	SYMPTON / DISEASE DESCRIPTION	TCM DIAGNOSIS	HERBAL FORMULAS
Helicobacter pylori Infection	Stomach or duodenal ulcer due to *H. Pylori* infection	Stomach heat	*GI Care*
Hematemesis	Vomiting of blood	Stomach heat	*Notoginseng 9*
	Blood in the stool	Heat in the Intestines	*Notoginseng 9*
Hematochezia	In ulcerative colitis, Crohn's disease	Damp-heat and toxic heat in the Intestines	*Notoginseng 9* with *GI Care (UC)*
	With hemorrhoid	Heat and blood stagnation in the lower *jiao*	*Notoginseng 9* with *GI Care (HMR)*
Hematuria	Blood in the urine with infection	Heat in the bladder or lower *jiao*	*Notoginseng 9* with *V-Statin*
Hemiplegia	Muscle stiffness, paralysis, difficult movement	Qi and blood stagnation	*Neuro Plus*
	With muscle cramps and spasms	Qi and blood stagnation with Liver yin and body fluid deficiencies	*Neuro Plus* with *Flex (SC)*
	Facial paralysis, Bell's Palsy	Qi and blood stagnation	*Symmetry*
Hemoptysis	Coughing of blood	Heat in the Lung or deficiency	*Respitrol (CF)* and *Notoginseng 9*
Hemorrhage	*See Bleeding*		
Hemorrhoids	Excess type constipation with hemorrhoids	Heat in the Large Intestine	*Gentle Lax (Excess)* with *GI Care (HMR)*
	Deficient type constipation with hemorrhoids	Heat in the Large Intestine with yin deficiency	*Gentle Lax (Deficient)* with *GI Care (HMR)*
	With severe pain	Severe qi and blood stagnation	*GI Care (HMR)* with *Herbal Analgesic*
	With bleeding	Heat pushing blood out of the vessels	*GI Care (HMR)* with *Notoginseng 9*
Hepatitis	With elevated liver enzymes	Toxic heat in the Liver	*Liver DTX*
	With gallstones or cholecystitis	Toxic heat in the Liver, damp-heat in the Gallbladder	*Liver DTX* with *Dissolve (GS)*
	Due to exposure to drugs, chemicals, heavy metals, environmental and airborne toxins	Toxic heat	*Liver DTX* with *Herbal DTX*
	With fatigue and weakness	Qi, yin, yang and blood deficiency	*Liver DTX* with *Imperial Tonic*
	Moderate to severe cases of infection and inflammation	Accumulation of toxic heat	*Liver DTX* with *Herbal ABX*
Herbicide Poisoning	Adverse reactions from exposure to insecticide, pesticide, herbicide and other toxins	Toxic heat in the Liver	*Herbal DTX*
	Compromised liver function due to exposure to toxins	Toxic heat in the Liver	*Liver DTX*
	Compromised kidney function due to exposure to toxins	Toxic heat in the Kidney	*Kidney DTX*

SYMPTOM / DISEASE INDEX

CONDITION	SYMPTOM / DISEASE DESCRIPTION	TCM DIAGNOSIS	HERBAL FORMULAS
Herniated Disk	Slipped disk with pain	Qi and blood stagnation	*Back Support (HD)*
	With back sprain and strain	Qi and blood stagnation	*Back Support (HD)* and *Back Support (Acute)*
	With severe pain	Severe qi and blood stagnation	*Back Support (HD)* and *Herbal Analgesic*
Herpes (Genital)	Genital herpes outbreak with lesions and pain	Damp-heat in the Liver and Gallbladder channels	*Gentiana Complex* or *V-Statin*
	Frequent genital herpes outbreaks	Damp-heat in the Liver and Gallbladder channels with underlying yin deficiency	*Gentiana Complex* with *Nourish*
	Moderate to severe cases of infection and inflammation	Accumulation of toxic heat	*Gentiana Complex* and *Herbal ABX*
	With severe pain	Severe qi and blood stagnation with heat	*Gentiana Complex* and *Herbal Analgesic*
Herpes (Oral)	Fever blisters with pain and inflammation	Wind-heat	*Lonicera Complex* and *Herbal ABX*
	Moderate to severe cases of infection and inflammation	Accumulation of toxic heat	*Lonicera Complex* and *Herbal ENT*
Herpes Zoster	Acute pain and inflammation of herpes zoster	Damp-heat	*Dermatrol (HZ)*
	Moderate to severe cases of infection and inflammation	Accumulation of toxic heat	*Dermatrol (HZ)* and *Gentiana Complex*
	With severe pain	Severe qi and blood stagnation with heat	*Dermatrol (HZ)* and *Herbal Analgesic*
Hiccup	With foul breath, hunger, redness of the face	Stomach heat	*Herbalite*
	With poor appetite, loose stool or diarrhea, generalized weakness	Spleen qi deficiency	*GI Tonic*
	Chronic and unknown in cause	Blood stagnation	*Circulation (SJ)*
High Blood Pressure	*See* Hypertension		
Hip Fracture	Post-traumatic care	Qi and blood stagnation	*Traumanex*
	To strengthen and rebuild the bones and connective tissues (muscles, ligaments, tendons, cartilage)	Kidney *jing* (essence) deficiency	*Osteo 8* and *Flex (MLT)*
	For pain associated with hip fractures	Qi and blood stagnation	*Add Back Support (Acute)*
	With severe pain	Severe qi and blood stagnation with heat	*Add Herbal Analgesic*
HIV	Immune deficiency with frequent infections	*Wei* (defensive) *qi* deficiency	*Immune +* with *Herbal ABX*
	Chronic fatigue with immune deficiency	Lung and Kidney deficiencies	*Immune +* with *Cordyceps 3*

Lotus Institute of Integrative Medicine

SYMPTOM / DISEASE INDEX

CONDITION	SYMPTOM / DISEASE DESCRIPTION	TCM DIAGNOSIS	HERBAL FORMULAS
Hives	See Itching		
Hordeolum (Sty)	Localized infection of one or more sebaceous glands	Toxic heat accumulation	*Herbal ABX* and *Resolve (AI)*
Hormones	Estrogen deficiency	Kidney yin deficiency	*Kidney Tonic (Yin)*
	Testosterone deficiency	Kidney yang deficiency	*Vitality and Kidney Tonic (Yang)*
	Low libido in men or women	Kidney yang deficiency	*Vitality*
	Hypothyroidism	Kidney yang deficiency	*Thyro-forte*
	Hyperthyroidism	Liver fire	*Thyrodex*
	Diabetes Mellitus	Yin deficiency	*Equilibrium*
	To detox hormones present in milk and meat	Toxic heat	*Herbal DTX*
Hospital-acquired Infection	See Infection		
Hot Flashes	With menopause signs	Yin deficiency with deficient heat	*Balance (Heat)*
	With thirst, dryness, and sweating	Yin deficiency with deficient heat and dryness	*Balance (Heat)* with *Nourish*
	With irritability and restlessness	Yin deficiency with Liver qi stagnation	*Balance (Heat)* with *Calm ZZZ*
	With insomnia due to deficiency	Yin deficiency with Spleen and Heart deficiencies	*Balance (Heat)* and *Schisandra ZZZ*
	With insomnia due to excess	Yin deficiency with *shen* (spirit) disturbances	*Balance (Heat)* and *Calm (ES)*
	See Menopause		
Hyperactivity	ADD, ADHD	Liver wind with *shen* (spirit) disturbance	*Calm (Jr)*
Hyperglycemia	See Diabetes		
Hyperhydrosis	Excessive sweating with a weak immune system	Lung qi deficiency and *wei* (defensive) *qi* deficiency	*Immune* +
Hyperlipidemia	See Cholesterol		
Hypertension...	Due to excess heat manifesting in red face, fast heartbeat, possible high blood pressure and constipation	Excess heat accumulation	*Gardenia Complex*
	Excess type with flushed face, anger, redness of eyes	Damp-heat in the Liver	*Gentiana Complex*
	Deficient type with dizziness, vertigo, tinnitus, and blurry vision	Liver yang rising with Liver and Kidney yin deficiencies	*Gastrodia Complex*
	Hypertension in patients with chronic kidney disorder	Toxic heat in the Kidney	*Gastrodia Complex* and *Kidney DTX*
	With excess fire manifesting in red face, red eyes, heat sensation, fast heart rate, high blood pressure and possible constipation	Excess fire in all three *jiaos*	*Add Gardenia Complex*
	With high cholesterol	Damp and phlegm accumulation	*Add Cholisma* or *Cholisma (ES)*

SYMPTOM / DISEASE INDEX

CONDITION	SYMPTON / DISEASE DESCRIPTION	TCM DIAGNOSIS	HERBAL FORMULAS
	With coronary heart disease	Blood stagnation	*Add Circulation*
	With headache	Qi and blood stagnation	*Add Corydalin*
	With blood stagnation manifesting in purplish tongue	Blood stasis	*Add Circulation (SJ)*
Hyperthermia	Hyperthermia due to hyperthyroidism	Liver qi stagnation with heat	*Thyrodex*
Hyperthyroidism	With elevated T3 and T4 levels and enlarged thyroid gland	Qi and phlegm stagnation with *shen* (spirit) disturbance	*Thyrodex*
	With irritability	Qi and phlegm stagnation with *shen* (spirit) disturbance and Liver qi stagnation	*Thyrodex* and *Calm*
	With hypertension	Qi and phlegm stagnation with *shen* (spirit) disturbance and rising Liver yang	*Thyrodex* and *Gastrodia Complex*
	With excess heat or fever	Excess fire	*Thyrodex* and *Gardenia Complex*
Hyper-triglyceridemia	*See* Cholesterol		
Hypochondriac Pain	With fidgeting, restlessness, irritability	Liver qi stagnation	*Calm*
	With anger, neurosis	Liver fire	*Calm (ES)*
	Due to hepatitis	Toxic heat in the Liver	*Liver DTX*
	With cholecystitis or gallstones	Damp-heat in the gallbladder	*Dissolve (GS)*
	In patients with irritable bowel syndrome (IBS)	Liver qi stagnation	*GI Harmony*
	With severe pain	Severe qi and blood stagnation	*Add Herbal Analgesic*
	Chronic pain with blood stagnation	Blood stagnation	*Calm and Circulation (SJ)*
Hypoglycemia	Low blood sugar level, dizziness	Spleen and Heart blood deficiencies	*Schisandra ZZZ*
	With overall weakness and deficiencies of yin, yang, qi and blood	Qi, blood, yin and yang deficiencies	*Imperial Tonic*
Hypotension	Low blood pressure with dizziness, fatigue	Deficiencies of qi and yang	*Imperial Tonic*
Hypothermia	Coldness of the body and extremities	Cold accumulation with Kidney yang deficiency	*Kidney Tonic (Yang)*
Hypothyroidism	With fatigue, aversion to cold, decreased heart rate and blood pressure, muscle weakness or sluggishness, and other related symptoms	Yang deficiency of Heart, Spleen, and Kidney	*Thyro-forte*
	With low energy	Qi deficiency	*Thyro-forte* with *Imperial Tonic*
	With depression	Qi, blood, food and phlegm stagnation	*Thyro-forte* with *Shine*
	With coldness or slow metabolism	Yang deficiency	*Thyro-forte* with *Adrenoplex*
	Post-operative healing	Blood stagnation	*Traumanex*
Hysterectomy...	Decrease in bone density following the operation	Kidney yin and *jing* (essence) deficiencies	*Osteo 8*
	Hot flashes, irritabilities, mood swings, night sweating	Kidney yin deficiency with deficient fire	*Balance (Heat)* with *Nourish*

CONDITION	SYMPTOM / DISEASE DESCRIPTION	TCM DIAGNOSIS	HERBAL FORMULAS
	With dryness and thirst	Yin and body fluids deficiencies	Nourish (Fluids)
	With dry hair or graying of hair	Kidney jing (essence) and Liver blood deficiencies	Polygonum 14
Hysteria	Mild to moderate cases of irritability and stress	Liver qi stagnation	Calm
	Moderate to severe cases of mood swings, anger, restlessness, irritability	Liver fire with shen (spirit) disturbance	Calm (ES)
	Disorientation, crying spells, inability to control oneself, restless sleep	Yin deficiency with false heat	Calm (ES) with Balance (Heat)
	Stress, anxiety, restlessness, insomnia in patients with deficiency	Liver qi stagnation with qi deficiency	Calm ZZZ
	Excessive worrying, pensiveness, dreams, anemia, mostly in women	Spleen and Heart blood deficiencies with shen (spirit) disturbance	Schisandra ZZZ
IBS (Irritable Bowel Syndrome)	See irritable bowel syndrome		
Immuno-deficiency	With frequent viral or bacterial infections	Wei (defensive) qi deficiency	Immune +
	With weak constitution	Qi, blood, yin and yang deficiencies	Immune + with Imperial Tonic
	Due to chemotherapy and radiation	Qi and yin deficiencies	Immune + with C/R Support
	With respiratory and reproductive weakness	Lung and Kidney deficiencies	Immune + with Cordyceps 3
	End-stage cancer patients who cannot receive chemotherapy or radiation	Yuan (source) qi deficiency	CA Support
Impotence	Generalized male sexual dysfunction	Kidney yang deficiency	Vitality
	Due to complications of diabetes	Kidney yin and yang deficiencies	Vitality with Equilibrium
	Decreased sexual desire and stamina due to adrenal depletion	Kidney yang deficiency	Adrenoplex
	Due to nervousness and anxiety	Liver fire with shen (spirit) disturbance	Calm (ES)
	With poor appetite, weakness, loose stool or diarrhea	Spleen qi deficiency with Kidney yang deficiency	Vitality with GI Tonic
	With palpitation, shortness of breath, spontaneous sweating, sallow complexion, emaciation, listlessness, poor appetite, loose stool	Spleen and Heart deficiencies	Schisandra ZZZ
Incomplete Evacuation	Due to irritable bowel syndrome (IBS) or stress	Liver qi stagnation	GI Harmony
	Due to ulcerative colitis, Crohn's disease	Toxic heat in the Intestines	GI Care (UC)
	Due to food poisoning, improper food intake, traveler's diarrhea or colitis	Damp-heat in the Intestines	GI Care II
Incomplete Emptying	Urinary symptoms due to benign prostatic hypertrophy	Stagnation or damp-heat in the lower jiao	P-Statin or Saw Palmetto Complex

SYMPTOM / DISEASE INDEX

CONDITION	SYMPTOM / DISEASE DESCRIPTION	TCM DIAGNOSIS	HERBAL FORMULAS
Incontinence	With coldness symptoms such as cold extremities, weakness and coldness of the lower back and knees, light-colored urine	Kidney yang deficiency	*Kidney Tonic (Yang)*
Indigestion	Indigestion and burning diarrhea with stomach pain, fullness and discomfort due to improper food intake	Damp-heat in the intestines	*GI Care II*
	Loose stool, poor appetite, weak digestion and generalized weakness	Spleen qi deficiency	*GI Tonic*
	Food stagnation	Food stagnation	*Shine*
	Slow digestion, or due to irritable bowel syndrome (IBS)	Liver qi stagnation	*GI Harmony*
Infection	Generalized: Various types of infection	Heat at various parts of body	*Herbal ABX*
	Sinus: infection with clear and watery discharge	Wind-cold at exterior	*Magnolia Clear Sinus*
	Sinus: infection with sticky and yellowish discharge	Damp-heat in the interior	*Pueraria Clear Sinus*
	Lung: Fever, dyspnea, chest congestion	Lung heat	*Respitrol (Heat)*
	Lung: Runny nose with clear watery discharge, sneezing, nasal congestion	Lung cold	*Respitrol (Cold)*
	Lung: Chest congestion, profuse yellow sputum, cough	Lung heat with phlegm	*Poria XPT*
	Lung: Common cold and influenza	Wind-heat or wind-cold at the exterior	*Lonicera Complex*
	Severe sore throat, strep throat, or tonsillitis	Toxic heat invasion	*Herbal ENT*
	Oral herpes with blisters	Wind-heat or Stomach heat	*Lonicera Complex*
	Gastrointestinal infection with abdominal pain and diarrhea	Damp-heat in the Intestines	*GI Care II*
	Genital: Infection of the genital area, such as herpes, gonorrhea, and other sexually transmitted diseases; bacterial or fungal infections	Damp-heat in lower *jiao*	*Gentiana Complex* or *V-Statin*
	Genito-urinary infection in both women and men	Damp-heat in the lower *jiao*	*V-Statin*
	Infection with inflammation and swelling	Damp-heat	*Herbal ABX with Resolve (AI)*
	Infection with pain	Toxic heat accumulation	*Herbal ABX with Herbal Analgesic*
	Shingles	Toxic heat invasion	*Dermatrol (HZ)*
Infectious Mononucleosis	Fever, pharyngitis, enlarged lymph	Toxic heat accumulation with dampness	*Herbal ENT*
Infertility…	Male infertility, low sperm count, poor sperm motility, morphology and mobility of the sperm, generalized male sexual dysfunction	Kidney yang deficiency	*Vitality*
	Female infertility (Menstrual Phase)	Qi and blood stagnation	*Blossom (Phase 1)*
	Female infertility (Follicular Phase)	Qi and blood deficiency, Kidney *jing* (essence) deficiency	*Blossom (Phase 2)*
	Female infertility (Ovulatory Phase)	Kidney yang deficiency	*Blossom (Phase 3)*

SYMPTOM / DISEASE INDEX

CONDITION	SYMPTON / DISEASE DESCRIPTION	TCM DIAGNOSIS	HERBAL FORMULAS
	Female infertility (Luteal Phase)	Liver qi stagnation	*Blossom (Phase 4)*
	Female infertility due to weakness and cold	Coldness in the uterus	*Blossom (Phase 1-4)* with *Balance (Cold)*
	Female infertility due to obstruction (cysts, endometriosis, tubal obstruction, fibroids, etc.)	Blood stagnation in the lower *jiao*	*Blossom (Phase 1-4)* with *Resolve (Lower)*
	Female infertility with coldness, irregular or delayed menstruation with scanty discharge	Kidney yang deficiency and blood stagnation	*Blossom (Phase 1-4)* with *Menotrol*
	With extreme stress	Liver qi stagnation	*Blossom (Phase 1-4)* with *Calm*
	With inflammation or infection of the pelvis (ovaries, uterus, fallopian tubes)	Heat accumulation in the lower *jiao*	*Blossom (Phase 1-4)* with *V-Statin*
	Women past 35 years of age with more prominent signs of yin deficiency and heat signs	Kidney yin deficiency	*Blossom (Phase 1-4)* with *Kidney Tonic (Yin)*
	Women past 35 years of age with more prominent signs of yang deficiency and cold signs	Kidney yang deficiency	*Blossom (Phase 1-4)* with *Kidney Tonic (Yang)*
Inflammation	Soft tissue or joint inflammation with pain and redness	Hot *bi zheng* (painful obstruction syndrome)	*Flex (Heat)*
	Joint pain that worsens with cold and dampness	Cold *bi zheng* (painful obstruction syndrome)	*Flex (CD)*
	Inflammation with severe pain	Qi and blood stagnation	Add *Herbal Analgesic*
	Muscle spasm and cramps	Liver yin and body fluid deficiencies	*Flex (SC)*
	Inflammation and pain due to external injuries	Qi and blood stagnation	*Traumanex*
	Tonsillitis	Wind-heat	*Lonicera Complex* or *Herbal ENT*
	Pelvic inflammatory disease	Damp-heat in the lower *jiao*	*V-Statin*
	With swelling and redness	Damp-heat	*Resolve (AI)*
	Inflammation in ulcerative colitis	Damp-heat in the Intestines	*GI Care (UC)*
	Inflammation due to intestinal flu or traveler's diarrhea	Damp-heat in the Intestines	*GI Care II*
	Chronic nephritis or nephrotic syndrome	Toxic heat in the Kidney	*Kidney DTX*
	Hepatitis	Toxic heat in the Liver	*Liver DTX*
	Ear infection and inflammation	Heat in the Liver channel	*Herbal ENT*
	Moderate to severe cases of infection and inflammation	Accumulation of toxic heat	Add *Herbal ABX*
	With fever and other heat signs of red face, fast heartbeat, high blood pressure or constipation	Excess heat	Add *Gardenia Complex*
	Inflammation of soft tissue (muscle, ligaments, tendon, cartilage)	Qi and blood stagnation	*Flex (MLT)*
	Herniated disk	Qi and blood stagnation	*Back Support (HD)*
	Gout	*Re bi* (heat painful obstruction)	*Flex (GT)*

SYMPTOM / DISEASE INDEX

CONDITION	SYMPTON / DISEASE DESCRIPTION	TCM DIAGNOSIS	HERBAL FORMULAS
Influenza	See Common Cold		
Injury	Bone fracture, severe pain, bruises	Blood stagnation	Traumanex
	Of the neck and shoulder area	Qi and blood stagnation	Add Neck & Shoulder (Acute)
	Of the upper back	Qi and blood stagnation	Add Back Support (Upper)
	Of the low back	Qi and blood stagnation	Add Back Support (Acute)
	Of the arm	Qi and blood stagnation	Add Arm Support
	Of the leg, knee or ankle	Qi and blood stagnation	Add Knee & Ankle (Acute)
	With severe pain	Severe qi and blood stagnation	Add Herbal Analgesic
	Chronic history of injury/trauma with residual pain	Qi and blood stagnation	Add Circulation (SJ)
	Sprain and strain of muscles	Qi and blood stagnation	Flex (SC) or Flex (MLT)
Inner Ear Disorder	Inner ear infection and pain	Toxic fire accumulation	Herbal ENT
	Dizziness, vertigo and poor balance	Liver wind rising	Gastrodia Complex
	With severe pain	Severe qi and blood stagnation	Gastrodia Complex and Herbal Analgesic
	Swelling and feeling of pressure	Dampness accumulation	Gastrodia Complex and Resolve (AI)
	Tinnitus	Kidney yin deficiency	Nourish or Kidney Tonic (Yin)
Insecticide Poisoning	Adverse reactions from exposure to insecticide, pesticide, herbicide and other toxins	Toxic heat	Herbal DTX
	Compromised liver function due to exposure to toxins	Toxic heat in the Liver	Liver DTX
	Compromised kidney function due to exposure to toxins	Toxic heat in the Kidney	Kidney DTX
Insomnia	Due to restlessness, stress, anxiety	Shen (spirit) disturbance with Liver fire	Calm (ES)
	Due to excessive worries and dreams, fatigue, pensiveness, poor appetite	Shen (spirit) disturbance due to Spleen and Heart deficiencies	Schisandra ZZZ
	Due to hyperthyroidism	Shen (spirit) disturbance with qi and phlegm stagnation	Thyrodex
	Due to depression	Stagnation of phlegm, qi, blood and food	Shine
	Fatigue with stress and an overactive mind with difficulty falling or staying asleep	Liver qi stagnation and qi deficiency	Calm ZZZ
	Chronic insomnia with blood stagnation manifesting in dark complexion, purplish tongue	Blood stagnation	Add Circulation (SJ)
Insulin	Diabetes Mellitus	Yin deficiency	Equilibrium
Intercourse...	Causing bladder infection	Damp-heat in the lower jiao	V-Statin

Lotus Institute of Integrative Medicine

SYMPTOM / DISEASE INDEX

CONDITION	SYMPTOM / DISEASE DESCRIPTION	TCM DIAGNOSIS	HERBAL FORMULAS
	Painful intercourse due to endometriosis	Qi and blood stagnation	*Resolve (Lower)* and *Mense-Ease*
	Difficult intercourse with yeast infection	Damp-heat in the lower *jiao*	*V-Statin*
	See also Infertility, Impotence, Libido		
Intermittent Claudication	With pain in the calf	Qi and blood stagnation	*Flex (NP)*
	With spasms and cramps	Liver yin deficiency with qi and blood stagnation	*Flex (NP)* and *Flex (SC)*
	With severe pain	Severe qi and blood stagnation	*Flex (NP)* and *Herbal Analgesic*
Intestinal Flu	Nausea, vomiting, diarrhea and abdominal discomfort	Damp-heat in the Intestines	*GI Care II*
	Moderate to severe cases of infection and inflammation	Accumulation of toxic heat	*Add Herbal ABX*
	With bleeding	Heat forcing blood out of the vessels	*Add Notoginseng 9*
Intestines	*See* Constipation, Diarrhea, or specific disorders		
Irritability	Stress, anxiety, restlessness, insomnia, nervousness, poor appetite	Liver qi stagnation	*Calm*
	Above symptoms, but more severe, with or without neurosis	Liver fire	*Calm (ES)*
	With crying spells and melancholy attacks during menopause	Liver yin deficiency with false heat	*Balance (Heat)*
	With Fidgeting, restlessness, short temper, high blood pressure	Liver fire	*Gentiana Complex*
	Irritability due to hyperthyroidism	*Shen* (spirit) disturbance with qi and phlegm stagnation	*Thyrodex*
	ADD, ADHD	Liver wind and *shen* (spirit) disturbance	*Calm (Jr)*
	With anxiety, stress, insomnia and an over-active mind in patients with deficiency	Liver qi stagnation with qi deficiency	*Calm ZZZ*
	With high blood pressure, excess heat, red face, fast heartbeat and possible constipation	Excess heat accumulation	*Add Gardenia Complex*
Irritable Bowel Syndrome (IBS)	IBS	Damp-heat in the Intestines	*GI Harmony*
	IBS due to stress	Damp-heat in the Intestines with Liver qi stagnation	*GI Harmony* and *Calm*
Itching	General skin itching	Wind-heat at the skin level, heat in the blood	*Silerex*
	Genital itching	Damp-heat in the lower *jiao*	*V-Statin*
	Genital itching with hypertension	Damp-heat in the Liver channel	*Gentiana Complex*
	Severe itching	Toxic heat	*Silerex* and *Dermatrol (PS)*
	Psoriasis	Toxic heat	*Dermatrol (PS)*
	Moderate to severe cases of infection and inflammation	Accumulation of toxic heat,	*Dermatrol (PS)* and *Herbal ABX*
	With fever	Toxic heat	*Add Gardenia Complex*
IVF	To increase the success of *in vitro* fertilization	Kidney *jing* (essence) deficiency	*Blossom (Phase 1–4)*

SYMPTOM / DISEASE INDEX

CONDITION	SYMPTON / DISEASE DESCRIPTION	TCM DIAGNOSIS	HERBAL FORMULAS
Jaundice	Yellow skin and sclera with hepatitis	Damp-heat in the Liver	*Liver DTX*
	Yellow skin and sclera with cholecystitis or gallstones	Damp-heat in the Gallbladder	*Dissolve (GS)*
	Infectious jaundice	Toxic heat	*Liver DTX* and *Herbal ABX*
	With fatty liver and obesity	Damp-heat accumulation	*Add Cholisma (ES)*
Jock Itch	Genital itching	Damp-heat in the lower *jiao* and Liver channel	*V-Statin*
Joint	See Neck Pain, Shoulder Pain, Back Pain, Arthritis and other related disorders		
	Degeneration of joint and surrounding tissue (muscle, ligaments, tendons, cartilages)	*Wei* (atrophy) syndrome	*Flex (MLT)*
	Spurs or stiffness or calcification	Qi and blood stagnation	*Flex (Spur)*
Kidney	Kidney or urinary stones	Dysuria due to stone; *shi lin* (stone dysuria)	*Dissolve (KS)*
	Moderate to severe cases of infection and inflammation	Accumulation of toxic heat	*Dissolve (KS)* and *Herbal ABX*
	Chronic nephritis or nephritic syndrome	Toxic heat	*Kidney DTX*
	Compromised kidney functions	Kidney deficiency	*Cordyceps 3*
	With bleeding	Heat forcing blood out of the vessels	*Add Notoginseng 9*
	With back pain	Qi and blood stagnation	*Add Back Support (Acute)*
Kissing Disease	Fever, pharyngitis, enlarged lymph glands	Toxic heat accumulation with dampness	*Herbal ENT*
Klebsiella Infection	Urinary, pulmonary, wound infections	Toxic heat	*Herbal ABX*
Knee	Acute knee pain	Qi and blood stagnation	*Knee & Ankle (Acute)*
	Chronic knee pain	Qi and blood stagnation	*Knee & Ankle (Chronic)*
	Ligament injury	Qi and blood stagnation	*Knee & Ankle (Acute)* and *Flex (MLT)*
	Acute sprain and strain	Qi and blood stagnation	*Knee & Ankle (Acute)* and *Traumanex*
	Gout	Toxic heat accumulation with qi and blood stagnation	*Flex (GT)*
	With fracture	Qi and blood stagnation	*Traumanex* and *Osteo 8*
	With severe pain	Severe qi and blood stagnation	*Knee & Ankle (Acute)* and *Herbal Analgesic*
Lactation	Lack of lactation during nursing period	Blockage	*Venus*
	Due to deficiency	Qi, blood, yin and yang deficiency	*Add Imperial Tonic*
Lactose Intolerance	Weakness of the digestive function, loose stool or diarrhea	Spleen qi deficiency	*GI Tonic*

SYMPTOM / DISEASE INDEX

CONDITION	SYMPTOM / DISEASE DESCRIPTION	TCM DIAGNOSIS	HERBAL FORMULAS
Large Intestine	*See* Diarrhea, Constipation, Ulcerative Colitis, Colitis, Crohn's Disease, Enteritis, or the specific disorder		
Lateral Epicondylitis	Tennis elbow	Qi and blood stagnation	*Arm Support*
	For degeneration of the joint and related soft tissue (muscle, ligaments, tendons, cartilage)	*Wei* (atrophy) syndrome	*Flex (MLT)*
	For severe pain		*Add Herbal Analgesic*
LDL Cholesterol	Elevated levels	Damp accumulation	*Cholisma*
	With hypertension due to deficiency	Liver yang rising with yin deficiency	*Cholisma* and *Gastrodia Complex*
	With hypertension due to excess	Liver fire with dampness	*Cholisma* and *Gentiana Complex*
	With hepatitis	Toxic heat in the Liver	*Cholisma* and *Liver DTX*
	With fatty liver and obesity	Damp heat accumulation	*Cholisma (ES)*
Leg	*See* Circulation (Poor), Pain, Osteoporosis, Restless Leg, Cramps, Knee, Ankle		
Libido	Decreased libido	Kidney yang deficiency	*Vitality*
	Excess libido	Kidney yin deficiency with rising fire	*Gardenia Complex* with *Balance (Heat)*
Ligament	Enhancing the growth of muscles, tendons, ligaments and cartilages	Liver blood and Kidney yin deficiencies	*Flex (MLT)*
Lin (Dysuria) Syndrome	Burning sensations during urination due to infection	Damp-heat in the lower *jiao*	*V-Statin*
	Kidney stone	Phlegm accumulation in the lower *jiao*	*Dissolve (KS)*
	Frequent urination profuse in amount, coldness	Kidney yang deficiency	*Kidney Tonic (Yang)*
	Chronic nephritis or nephritic syndrome	Toxic heat in the Kidney	*Kidney DTX*
	Moderate to severe infection	Toxic heat	*Kidney DTX* and *Herbal ABX*
	With severe pain	Severe qi and blood stagnation	*Kidney DTX* and *Herbal Analgesic*
	With fever, painful urination and dark yellow urine	Excess heat	*Add Gardenia Complex*
	With edema and water accumulation	Damp accumulation	*Add Herbal DRX*
Lipid	*See* Cholesterol		
Lipoprotein	*See* Cholesterol		
Lithiasis	*See* Stones		
Liver	*See* Hepatitis, Detoxification, Gallstones, Cholecystitis, Fatty Liver and Cancer		
Low Back Pain	*See* Back Pain		
Lumbago	*See* Back Pain		

SYMPTOM / DISEASE INDEX

CONDITION	SYMPTON / DISEASE DESCRIPTION	TCM DIAGNOSIS	HERBAL FORMULAS
Lumbar Radiculopathy	Herniated disk with pain	Qi and blood stagnation	Back Support (HD)
	With recent trauma	Qi and blood stagnation	Add Traumanex
	With severe back pain	Qi and blood stagnation	Add Back Support (Acute) or Herbal Analgesic
Lump	Hard swelling with redness and pain	Dampness accumulation	Resolve (AI)
Lung	See Asthma, Cough, Dyspnea, Bronchitis and Pneumonia, etc.		
Lupus	Lupus	Toxic heat accumulation with yin deficiency	LPS Support
Luteal Phase	Female infertility, Luteal Phase	Qi and blood stagnation	Blossom (Phase 4)
Lyme Disease	Early symptoms of rash, fever, malaise, body ache	Toxic heat invasion	Dermatrol (PS) with Gardenia Complex and Herbal ABX
Lymph Nodes	Swelling	Damp accumulation	Resolve (AI)
Lymphadenitis	Swelling and pain	Dampness with toxic heat	Resolve (AI) with Herbal ABX or Herbal ENT
Lymphedema	Accumulation of lymphatic fluids causing swelling	Dampness and phlegm accumulation	Resolve (AI)
	All types of inflammation and swelling with heat sensation	Damp accumulation	Resolve (AI)
Lymphadenopathy	Moderate to severe cases of infection and inflammation	Accumulation of toxic heat	Resolve (AI) with Herbal ABX
	Swelling and enlarged lymph nodes with possible nodules or fibroids in the breasts	Liver qi and phlegm stagnation	Resolve (AI) with Resolve (Upper)
	Swelling and enlarged lymph nodes with possible nodules or fibroids in the female reproductive organs	Blood and phlegm stagnation in the lower jiao	Resolve (AI) with Resolve (Lower)
	Lymphadenopathy with immune deficiency	Wei (defensive) qi deficiency	Resolve (AI) with Immune +
	With edema	Damp and water accumulation	Resolve (AI) with Herbal DRX
Macula	Degeneration of macula and diminished vision	Liver and Kidney yin deficiencies	Nourish
Malabsorption Syndrome	Malabsorption, diarrhea, fatigue, poor appetite	Spleen qi deficiency	GI Tonic
Malignancy	See Cancer		
	Malnutrition in children with fatigue, poor energy, lack of appetite	Spleen qi deficiency	GI Tonic
Malnutrition	Malnutrition with generalized deficiency and over-all constitutional weakness	Qi, blood, yin and yang deficiencies	Imperial Tonic
Mammary Gland	See Breast		
Mania	Mild cases of hyperactivity with anger and irritability	Liver heat with shen (spirit) disturbance	Calm (ES)
	In severe cases with blood stagnation signs of dark complexion, purplish tongue	Blood stagnation	Add Circulation (SJ)

SYMPTOM / DISEASE INDEX

CONDITION	SYMPTON / DISEASE DESCRIPTION	TCM DIAGNOSIS	HERBAL FORMULAS
Manic Depressive Illness	See Bipolar		
Mastitis	See Breast		
Mass	Mass, swelling or nodules	Phlegm and damp accumulation	Resolve (AI)
	In the breast	Liver qi stagnation with phlegm accumulation	Resolve (Upper)
	In the female reproductive organs (ovarian cysts, uterine fibroids, myomas, etc)	Qi and blood stagnation with phlegm accumulation	Resolve (Lower)
Medial Epicondylitis	Golfer's elbow	Qi and blood stagnation	Arm Support
	With severe pain	Qi and blood stagnation	Add Herbal Analgesic
Memory	Forgetfulness, poor memory	Heart and Kidney deficiencies	Enhance Memory
	Decreased mental function due to injury and/or degeneration	Deficiency of Kidney yin and jing (essence)	Neuro Plus
	Decreased mental function due to excessive stress and exhaustion	Deficiency of qi and Kidney	Adrenoplex
Meniere's Disease	Dizziness, vertigo, and loss of balance	Liver wind rising	Gastrodia Complex
Menopausal Syndrome	Mood swings, emotional instability, hot flushes, night sweating	Yin deficiency with deficient heat	Balance (Heat)
	With thirst and dryness with yin deficient signs listed above	Yin deficiency with deficient heat and dryness	Balance (Heat) with Nourish
	With pronounced irritability and mood swings	Yin deficiency with Liver qi stagnation	Balance (Heat) with Calm
	With pronounced anger, restlessness	Yin deficiency with shen (spirit) disturbance	Balance (Heat) with Calm (ES)
	With tiredness, insomnia and excessive worrying	Yin deficiency with Spleen and Heart blood deficiencies	Balance (Heat) and Schisandra ZZZ
	With qi deficiency, insomnia, irritability, restlessness, stress, restless mind	Liver qi stagnation with qi deficiency	Balance (Heat) with Calm ZZZ
Menstruation (Disorders During Period) ...	Diarrhea: Loose stool or diarrhea with lower abdominal fullness, profuse menstrual amount, sallow complexion, edema, bland taste in the mouth, poor appetite	Spleen qi deficiency	GI Tonic
	Diarrhea: Watery stool, lower abdominal coldness and feeling of prolapse, coldness of limbs, delayed menstruation	Spleen and Kidney yang deficiencies	GI Tonic and Kidney Tonic (Yang)
	Diarrhea: Abdominal pain followed by loose stool, abdominal pain lessens with defecation, hypochondriac distension and pain, nausea, breast tenderness	Liver qi stagnation	Calm
	Edema: Edema of the face and limbs, loose stool, scanty urine, light in color	Spleen qi deficiency with deficiency cold	GI Tonic and Herbal DRX

SYMPTOM / DISEASE INDEX

CONDITION	SYMPTON / DISEASE DESCRIPTION	TCM DIAGNOSIS	HERBAL FORMULAS
	Fever: Low-grade fever during the period and subsides after each cycle, period usually comes early, profuse in amount, purplish in color and thick in texture, chest and hypochondriac distension, irritability, dizziness, redness of the face and eyes, bitter taste in the mouth, dry throat	Liver fire	*Gentiana Complex*
	Fever: Low-grade fever or heat sensation which is exacerbated before each cycle, early periods, dark in color and scanty in amount, irritability, dry mouth, throat, emaciation	Kidney yin deficiency with deficient heat	*Balance (Heat)* and *Nourish*
	Headache: Usually occurs before or during each cycle, fixed in location and stabbing in nature, blood clots with lower abdominal pain	Blood stagnation	*Resolve (Lower)*
	Headache: Dizziness, distension and pain before the period, irritability, short temper, restless sleep, tinnitus, hypochondriac pain, bitter taste in the mouth, bright red menstrual color, yellow vaginal discharge	Liver yang rising	*Gentiana Complex*
	Headache: Feeling of emptiness and pain after cycles, dizziness, fear of light and prefers quiet environments, palpitation, insomnia, dry mouth, poor appetite, sallow complexion, light menstrual amount	Blood deficiency	*Schisandra ZZZ* with *Migratrol*
	Low back pain: Acute pain, lower abdominal bloating, possible blood clots	Qi and blood stagnation	*Back Support (Acute)*
	Low back pain: Soreness and weakness sensation with fatigue	Kidney deficiency	*Back Support (Chronic)*
	Nose bleeding: Bleeding occurs usually during or before periods, bitter taste in the mouth, dry throat, redness of the face, eyes, dizziness, irritability, short temper, insomnia, breast tenderness or hypochondriac pain	Liver fire	*Gentiana Complex*
	Nose bleeding: Bleeding occurs usually during or after periods, dizziness, tinnitus, dry mouth, throat, afternoon fever	Yin deficiency	*Nourish*
	Nose bleeding: Bleeding usually occurs during or after periods, light colored menstrual blood, fatigue, loose stool, poor appetite	Spleen qi deficiency with inability to keep blood within the vessels	*Schisandra ZZZ*
	See also amenorrhea		
Menstrual Amount…	**Profuse:** Early and profuse in amount or incessant bleeding, bright red in color, emaciation, flushed cheeks, *wu xin re* (five-center heat), dizziness, tinnitus, tidal fever, night sweating, insomnia, soreness of the lower back and knees, dry eyes, dry stool	Kidney and Liver yin deficiency	*Nourish* with *Balance (Heat)* and *Notoginseng 9*

SYMPTOM / DISEASE INDEX

CONDITION	SYMPTON / DISEASE DESCRIPTION	TCM DIAGNOSIS	HERBAL FORMULAS
	Profuse: Early, profuse in amount or prolonged in length, bright red or dark and black in color, thick in texture with clots, redness of the face, irritability, short temper, stifling sensation in the chest, breast tenderness, dizziness, headache, bitter taste in the mouth	Liver fire	*Gentiana Complex* and *Notoginseng 9*
	Profuse: Prolonged duration, light in color, sensations of emptiness in the lower abdomen, preference for pressure, pale complexion, listlessness, shortness of breath, spontaneous sweating, poor appetite, loose stool, edema	Spleen qi deficiency	*GI Tonic* and *Notoginseng 9*
	Profuse: Delayed, profuse in amount or incessant in bleeding, dark in color with clots, lower abdominal coldness and pain with preference for warmth and pressure, possible infertility	Deficiency and coldness of the *chong* (thoroughfare) channel	*Balance (Cold)* and *Notoginseng 9*
	Profuse: Profuse yellow vaginal discharge before and after cycles, fetid in smell and thick in texture, genital itching, epigastric fullness, heaviness sensation	Damp-heat in the lower *jiao*	*V-Statin* and *Notoginseng 9*
	Scanty: As little as a few drops, light in color, delayed onset, dull abdominal pain, preference for pressure, pale complexion, dizziness, blurry vision, palpitation, forgetfulness, insomnia, dry skin and hair	Blood deficiency	*Schisandra ZZZ*
	Scanty: Dark purple with clots, delayed onset, thick in texture, stabbing or needling pain in the lower abdomen, dark complexion, breast distension	Blood stagnation	*Resolve (Lower)*
	Scanty: Light red or dark red in color, scanty in amount, lower abdominal pain after each cycle, irregular menstruation, dizziness, tinnitus, weakness of the back and extremities	Kidney yin deficiency	*Kidney Tonic (Yin)*
	Scanty: Light or dark in color, possible clots, lower abdominal coldness and pain that lessens with warmth, cold extremities, clear vaginal discharge	Deficiency and coldness of the *chong* (thoroughfare) channel	*Balance (Cold)* and *Imperial Tonic*
	Scanty: Thick yellow in texture, turbid vaginal discharge, overweight, epigastric fullness, nausea, heaviness sensation	Damp-heat in the lower *jiao*	*V-Statin*
Menstrual Color...	**Light red:** Scanty in amount, delayed, lower abdominal dull pain, lusterless complexion, dizziness, palpitation, insomnia, dry skin, hair and nails	Blood deficiency	*Schisandra ZZZ*
	Light red: Scanty, early and profuse in amount, lochia, pale complexion, fatigue, spontaneous sweating, aversion to wind, feeling of emptiness in the lower abdomen	Qi deficiency	*Imperial Tonic*

SYMPTOM / DISEASE INDEX

CONDITION	SYMPTON / DISEASE DESCRIPTION	TCM DIAGNOSIS	HERBAL FORMULAS
	Light red: Clots, coldness of the limbs, lower abdominal pain that is alleviated by warmth, soreness and weakness of the lower back, clear leukorrhea, loose stool	Kidney and Spleen yang deficiency	*GI Tonic* and *Kidney Tonic (Yang)*
	Dark purple: Thick with clots, lower abdominal pain, irritability, thirst, low grade fever before menstrual cycles, yellow thick vaginal discharge	Damp-heat accumulation	*V-Statin*
	Dark purple: Clots, lower abdominal fullness, distension and pain that worsens with pressure, emotional instability, breast distension and tenderness	Liver qi stagnation	*Calm*
	Dark purple: Blood clots with coldness in the lower abdominal and legs, purplish tongue, symptoms alleviated with warmth	Cold accumulation	*Balance (Cold)* with *Menotrol*
Menstrual Cramps/Pain	Severe menstrual pain with bloating and blood clots	Blood and qi stagnation in the lower *jiao*	*Mense-Ease*
	Dull menstrual pain, coldness of extremities, fatigue	Coldness and blood deficiency with blood stagnation	*Balance (Cold)* and *Mense-Ease*
	With severe pain and cramps due to endometriosis	Severe qi and blood stagnation	*Resolve (Lower)* and *Mense –Ease*
	Pain with water retention	Qi and blood stagnation with damp accumulation	*Herbal DRX* and *Mense-Ease*
Menstrual Duration	**Prolonged:** Bright red or purplish red in color, thick in texture with blood clots, soreness and weakness of low back and extremities, dizziness, five-heart heat, thirst	Kidney yin deficiency with heat	*Nourish*
	Prolonged: Light in color, coldness of extremities, low back pain, slightly overweight	Kidney yang deficiency	*Kidney Tonic (Yang)*
	Prolonged: Light in color, edema, listlessness, poor appetite, lower abdominal fullness and distension, loose stool	Spleen qi deficiency	*GI Tonic* and *Balance (Cold)*
	Prolonged: Dark purple with clots, lower abdominal pain which worsens with pressure, pain lessens with passage of clots	Blood stagnation	*Resolve (Lower)*
	Shortened: Light in color, low-grade fever, night sweats, flushed cheeks, tinnitus	Kidney yin deficiency	*Kidney Tonic (Yin)*
	During menopause	Yin deficiency with false heat	*Balance (Heat)* or *Nourish*
Menstrual Irregularity…	**Early:** Profuse in amount, dark red or purplish in color, thick with fetid odor, irritability, dry mouth, preference for coldness, constipation, yellow urine	Damp-heat in the lower *jiao*	*V-Statin*
	Early: Scanty in amount, red in color with no clots, dizziness, palpitation, insomnia, soreness of the lower back, *wu xin re* (five-center heat), flushed cheeks	Yin deficiency	*Balance (Heat)* and *Nourish*

SYMPTOM / DISEASE INDEX

CONDITION	SYMPTON / DISEASE DESCRIPTION	TCM DIAGNOSIS	HERBAL FORMULAS
	Early: Amount may be profuse or scanty, color may be red or purplish with clots, breast distension and tenderness, chest, hypochondriac and lower abdominal fullness and pain, emotional instability with possible short temper, bitter taste in the mouth or dryness	Liver qi stagnation	*Calm*
	Early: Light in color, scanty in amount, feeling of emptiness in the lower abdomen, listlessness, palpitation, shortness of breath, poor appetite, loose stool	Qi deficiency	*Imperial Tonic*
	Early: Profuse during the first day and dramatically decreases later or incessant bleeding that is purple with clots, lower abdominal fullness, distension and pain	Blood stagnation	*Resolve (Lower)*
	Delayed: Scanty in amount, light in color, dizziness, palpitation absence of abdominal pain	Blood deficiency	*Schisandra ZZZ*
	Delayed: Scanty in amount, dark in color with clots, lower abdominal dull pain, preference for pressure, pain lessens with warmth, cold extremities, dark complexion	Deficiency and coldness of the *chong* (thoroughfare) channel	*Balance (Cold)* and *Kidney Tonic (Yang)*
	Delayed: Scanty in amount, purplish in color, lower abdominal pain which worsens with pressure and lessens with warmth, purplish complexion	Excess cold	*Menotrol*
	Delayed: Purplish red blood with lower abdominal distension and pain, chest and hypochondriac pain, breast tenderness	Liver qi stagnation	*Calm*
	Irregular: May be twice a month or once in two months, may be profuse or scanty in amount, breast tenderness, lower abdominal distension and pain, hypochondriac distension, lower back soreness	Liver qi stagnation with Kidney yin deficiency	*Calm* and *Kidney Tonic (Yin)*
	Irregular: Pale in color and scanty in amount, dizziness, palpitation, fatigue, listlessness, loose stool	Heart and Spleen deficiency	*Schisandra ZZZ*
Mental Health Disorders...	Anxiety	Liver qi stagnation	*Calm*
	Delusion	*Shen* (spirit) disturbance	*Calm (ES)*
	Depression	Qi stagnation	*Shine*
	With high blood pressure, fast heart rate, high temperature	Excess heat accumulation	*Add Gardenia Complex*
	Chronic case with blood stasis signs of dark complexion, purplish tongue with distended sublingual veins	Blood stagnation	*Add Circulation (SJ)*
	Developmental delays	Kidney *jing* (essence) deficiency	*Enhance Memory*
	See Addiction for substance dependence		

Lotus Institute of Integrative Medicine

SYMPTOM / DISEASE INDEX

CONDITION	SYMPTON / DISEASE DESCRIPTION	TCM DIAGNOSIS	HERBAL FORMULAS
	See Bulimia, Anorexia, Sexual Dysfunction for eating and sexual disorders		
Metabolic Disorder	Hyperlipidemia	Dampness accumulation	*Cholisma*
	Obesity with excessive appetite	Dampness accumulation	*Herbalite*
	Slow metabolism with low energy	Qi deficiency	*Vibrant*
	Slow metabolism in chronic fatigue syndrome	Severe qi deficiency	*Cordyceps 3*
	Slow metabolism with overall weakness and deficiency	Qi and blood deficiencies	*Imperial Tonic*
	Slow metabolism with adrenal insufficiency	Kidney qi deficiency	*Adrenoplex*
	Slow metabolism due to hypothyroidism	Kidney yang deficiency	*Thyro-forte*
	Rapid metabolism due to hyperthyroidism	Excess heat	*Thyrodex*
Metastasis	*See* Cancer		
Migraine	*See* Headache		
Miscarriage	Weakness, fatigue, and coldness after miscarriage	Coldness in the uterus with qi, blood, yin and yang deficiencies	*Balance (Cold)* and *Imperial Tonic*
	Habitual miscarriage with yin deficient signs of low-grade fever, night sweats, flushed cheeks, dizziness, tinnitus, etc.	Kidney yin deficiency	*Kidney Tonic (Yin)*
	Habitual miscarriage with yang deficient signs of coldness, low libido, soreness and weakness of the back and knees, polyuria	Kidney yang deficiency	*Kidney Tonic (Yang)*
Molds	*See* Allergy		
Mononucleosis	Infection causing swelling of lymph glands with fatigue	Toxic heat with dampness	*Herbal ENT with Resolve (AI)*
Mood Swing	Mood swings, irritability	Liver qi stagnation	*Calm*
	Insomnia, restlessness and anger in excess patients	Liver fire	*Calm (ES)*
	During menopause	Kidney yin deficiency with Liver qi stagnation	*Balance (Heat)*
	In depression	Food, phlegm, qi and blood stagnation	*Shine*
	Insomnia, stress, overactive mind, anxiety with weakness in patients with deficiency	Liver qi stagnation with qi deficiency	*Calm ZZZ*
	Excessive worrying, pensiveness, dream-disturbed sleep	Spleen and Heart blood deficiencies	*Schisandra ZZZ*
	In chronic cases with blood stagnation signs of dark complexion, purplish tongue, distended sublingual veins	Blood stagnation	*Add Circulation (SJ)*
Mouth	Dry mouth	Stomach yin deficiency	*Nourish (Fluids)*
	Ulcers	Stomach fire	*Gardenia Complex*
Mucus...	Profuse yellow phlegm, chest congestion, cough and possible fever	Phlegm and heat in the Lung	*Poria XPT*
	Cough, dyspnea, chest congestion, yellow sputum	Lung heat	*Respirol (Heat)*

Lotus Institute of Integrative Medicine

SYMPTOM / DISEASE INDEX

CONDITION	SYMPTON / DISEASE DESCRIPTION	TCM DIAGNOSIS	HERBAL FORMULAS
	Clear or white phlegm, nasal congestion, sneezing	Lung cold	*Respitrol (Cold)*
	Moderate to severe cases of infection and inflammation	Accumulation of toxic heat	*Add Herbal ABX*
	Irritable bowel syndrome with mucus in stool	Liver qi stagnation	*GI Harmony*
	Ulcerative colitis or Crohn's disease with mucus in stool	Damp-heat in the intestine	*GI Care (UC)*
	Mucus in stool due to food poisoning or traveler's diarrhea	Damp-heat in the intestine	*GI Care II*
	With bleeding	Heat forcing blood out of the vessels	*Add Notoginseng 9*
Mumps	Swollen, painful glands with infection and inflammation	Toxic heat with phlegm accumulation	*Herbal ENT with Resolve (AI)*
Muscle Tension	Muscle tightness and tension	Liver yin and body fluid deficiencies	*Flex (SC)*
	Muscle tension in the neck and shoulders	Qi and blood stagnation	*Neck & Shoulder (Acute)*
	Tension due to stress	Liver qi stagnation	*Flex (SC) with Calm*
	Tightness or degeneration of soft tissues: muscles, tendons, ligaments and cartilages	Liver blood and Kidney yin deficiencies	*Flex (MLT)*
Myasthenia Gravis	General weakness and fatigability after exercise	*Yuan* (source) *qi* deficiency	*C/R Support*
Nasal Congestion	Thick yellow nasal discharge, nasal obstruction, sinus infection	Damp-heat with fluid congestion	*Pueraria Clear Sinus*
	Clear watery nasal discharge, nasal obstruction, allergy	Wind-cold with fluid congestion	*Magnolia Clear Sinus*
	Moderate to severe cases of infection and inflammation	Accumulation of toxic heat	*Add Herbal ABX*
Nausea	With stomach pain, acid regurgitation	Stomach heat	*GI Care*
	With vomiting due to chemotherapy	Stomach yin deficiency	*C/R Support*
	With vomiting, abdominal pain and diarrhea due to food poisoning	Damp-heat in the lower *jiao*	*GI Care II*
	With vomiting and abdominal pain due to gallstones	Damp-heat in the Liver and Gallbladder	*Dissolve (GS)*
	With poor appetite and weakness	Spleen qi deficiency	*GI Tonic*
	With dryness and thirst	Stomach yin deficiency	*Nourish (Fluids)*
	Unexplained cause, exhibiting dark complexion, purplish tongue	Blood stagnation	*Circulation (SJ)*
Neck Pain	Acute neck and shoulder pain	Qi and blood stagnation	*Neck & Shoulder (Acute)*
	Chronic neck and shoulder pain	Qi and blood stagnation with Liver yin deficiency	*Neck & Shoulder (Chronic)*
	Chronic neck pain due to osteoporosis	Kidney yin and *jing* (essence) deficiencies	*Osteo 8 with Neck & Shoulder (Chronic)*
	Pain due to bone spurs	Qi and blood stagnation	*Neck & Shoulder (Acute) with Flex (Spur)*
	With severe pain	Severe qi and blood stagnation	*Neck & Shoulder (Acute) with Herbal Analgesic*

SYMPTOM / DISEASE INDEX

CONDITION	SYMPTON / DISEASE DESCRIPTION	TCM DIAGNOSIS	HERBAL FORMULAS
Nephritis	Compromised kidney function with edema and proteinuria	Kidney deficiency with dampness	*Kidney DTX*
	Compromised kidney and liver function	Kidney deficiency with damp-heat in the Liver	*Kidney DTX and Liver DTX*
	Compromised kidney function due to exposure to drugs, chemicals and other toxins	Kidney deficiency with toxic heat	*Kidney DTX and Herbal DTX*
	To improve kidney function for recovery	Kidney deficiency	*Kidney DTX and Cordyceps 3*
	With edema	Water accumulation	*Add Herbal DRX*
	With high blood pressure	Kidney and Liver yin deficiency with Liver yang rising	*Add Gastrodia Complex*
	With lupus	Toxic heat accumulation	*Add LPS Support*
Nephrotic Syndrome	*See* Nephritis		
Nerves	Oral herpes	Stomach fire flaring upward	*Lonicera Complex and Herbal ENT*
	Genital herpes	Damp-heat in the lower *jiao* and Liver channel	*Gentiana Complex*
	Neuropathy with numbness and pain of extremities	Qi and blood stagnation	*Flex (NP)*
	Pain due to multiple sclerosis with generalized weakness and deficiency	Qi and blood stagnation with Kidney deficiency	*Neuro Plus*
	Shingles	Toxic and damp heat accumulation	*Dermatrol (HZ)*
	Temporo-mandibular joint pain	Wind attack with qi and blood stagnation	*Symmetry*
	See Stress, Anxiety		
Nervousness	*See* Stress, Anxiety		
Neuralgia	Peripheral neuralgia with pain, numbness, tingling and swelling	Qi and blood stagnation	*Flex (NP)*
	Pain due to bone spurs	Qi and blood stagnation	*Flex (Spur)*
	With severe pain	Severe qi and blood stagnation	*Add Herbal Analgesic*
Neuropathy	*See* Neuralgia		
Neurosis	Stress, irritability, restlessness, insomnia, nervousness	Liver qi stagnation	*Calm*
	Above symptoms, more severe	Liver fire	*Calm (ES)*
	Excessive worrying, pensiveness, over thinking, poor appetite	Spleen and Heart deficiencies	*Schisandra ZZZ*
	Insomnia, nervousness, anxiety, overactive mind, stress and weakness	Liver qi stagnation with qi deficiency	*Calm ZZZ*
	Severe or chronic condition with blood stagnation signs of dark complexion, purplish tongue, distended sublingual veins	Blood stagnation	*Circulation (SJ)*
Night Sweat	Perspiration at night	Yin deficiency with false heat	*Nourish and Balance (Heat)*

Lotus Institute of Integrative Medicine

SYMPTOM / DISEASE INDEX

CONDITION	SYMPTOM / DISEASE DESCRIPTION	TCM DIAGNOSIS	HERBAL FORMULAS
Nocturnal Emission	Nocturnal emission	Kidney yin deficiency	*Nourish* or *Kidney Tonic (Yin)*
Nodules	Anywhere in the body due to infection and inflammation	Phlegm stagnation	*Resolve (AI)*
	In the breast area	Phlegm stagnation	*Resolve (Upper)*
	In the lower abdominal area	Phlegm and blood stagnation	*Resolve (Lower)*
	In the neck due to hyperthyroidism	Liver fire with phlegm stagnation	*Thyrodex*
	In the neck due to hypothyroidism	Yang deficiency with phlegm stagnation	*Thyro-forte*
	In the lymphatic system	Phlegm stagnation	*Resolve (AI)*
Nose	Profuse white or clear nasal discharge, sneezing	Lung cold	*Respitrol (Cold)*
	Allergy with clear or white nasal discharge	Wind-cold attacking the Lung	*Magnolia Clear Sinus*
	Allergy with yellow nasal discharge	Wind-heat attacking the Lung	*Pueraria Clear Sinus*
	Nose bleeding	Heat pushing blood out of the vessels	*Notoginseng 9*
	Dry nose, throat, thirst	Lung and Stomach yin deficiencies	*Nourish (Fluids)*
Nutrition	*See* Malnutrition		
Obesity	With excessive hunger	Stomach fire	*Herbalite*
	With high cholesterol	Stomach fire with phlegm and damp	*Herbalite* and *Cholisma*
	With diabetes	Stomach fire with yin deficiency	*Herbalite* and *Equilibrium*
	With excess type hypertension	Stomach fire with damp-heat	*Herbalite* and *Gentiana Complex*
	With deficient type hypertension	Stomach fire with Liver yin deficiency	*Herbalite* and *Gastrodia Complex*
	With coronary artery disease	Stomach fire with phlegm stagnation	*Herbalite* and *Circulation*
	With fatty liver and high cholesterol	Damp-phlegm accumulation	*Cholisma (ES)*
Obsessive-Compulsive Disorder (OCD)	Presence of recurrent, unwanted and intrusive physical and mental activities	*Shen* (spirit) disturbance	*Calm (ES)*
Olecranon Bursitis	Painful elbow	Qi and blood stagnation	*Arm Support*
	With severe pain	Severe qi and blood stagnation	*Add Herbal Analgesic*
Operation (Post-Op Care)	Enhances recovery and prevents adhesions and complications	Qi and blood stagnation	*Traumanex*
	To treat or reduce the risk of infection in post-operative patients	Toxic heat	*Add Herbal ABX*
	To enhance growth of bones	Kidney *jing* (essence) deficiency	*Add Osteo 8*
	To enhance the recovery and growth of soft tissue (muscles, tendons, ligaments and cartilage)	Kidney yin and Liver blood deficiencies	*Add Flex (MLT)*
	Post-operative recovery in deficient and weak patients	Qi and blood deficiency	*Add Imperial Tonic*
	Post-operative pain: *See* pain or the affected parts of the body		

SYMPTOM / DISEASE INDEX

CONDITION	SYMPTON / DISEASE DESCRIPTION	TCM DIAGNOSIS	HERBAL FORMULAS
Osteoarthritis	Joint pain	Qi and blood stagnation with Kidney jing (essence) deficiency	Osteo 8 and a Flex formula
Osteoporosis	Decreased density of bones	Deficiency of Kidney jing (essence)	Osteo 8
	Osteoporosis with bone fracture or broken bone	Deficiency of Kidney jing (essence) with blood stagnation	Osteo 8 and Traumanex
	With low libido	Kidney jing (essence) deficiency	Osteo 8 and Vitality
	With menopause symptoms such as hot flashes, irritability and night sweating	Kidney jing (essence) deficiency and deficient heat flaring	Osteo 8 and Balance (Heat)
Otitis Media	Inflammation of the ear with pain, fever or hearing impairment	Toxic heat accumulation	Herbal ENT
	With flu or common cold symptoms of sore throat, etc.	Wind-heat invasion	Add Lonicera Complex
	With severe pain	Toxic heat accumulation	Add Herbal Analgesic
Otolaryngological Disorders	Disorders of the ear, nose and throat	Toxic heat accumulation	Herbal ENT
Ovaries	See Fibrocystic Disease, Endometriosis, Infertility, Menstrual Irregularities		
Overdose	Overdose of drugs or other toxic materials	Toxic heat	Herbal DTX or Liver DTX
Overeating	Excessive appetite	Stomach heat	Herbalite
Overweight	See Obesity		
Ovulation	Ovulation difficulties due to coldness, weakness and blood clots during menstruation	Blood stagnation with Kidney yang deficiency	Menotrol
	Coldness, soreness and weakness of the lower back and knees with constitutional weakness	Kidney yang deficiency	Kidney Tonic (Yang) or Balance (Cold)
	Stress related	Liver qi stagnation	Calm
	Due to endometriosis or fibroids	Qi and blood stagnation	Resolve (Lower)
	Infertility	Varies	Blossom (Phase 1-4)
Pain	A general formula to relieve pain	Qi and blood stagnation	Herbal Analgesic
	See specific condition, disease, or body part		
Palpitation	Increased heart rate with insomnia, fatigue, and over-thinking	Heart and Spleen blood deficiencies	Schisandra ZZZ
	Increased heart rate with chest pain, coronary heart disorder	Blood stagnation	Circulation
	Increased heart rate and blood pressure due to hyperthyroidism	Qi and phlegm stagnation	Thyrodex
	Increased heart rate in menopausal women	Deficient heat	Balance (Heat)
Pancreas	See Diabetes		
Paralysis ...	Impaired function of the extremities or the face in post-stroke	Qi and blood stagnation	Neuro Plus

SYMPTOM / DISEASE INDEX

CONDITION	SYMPTOM / DISEASE DESCRIPTION	TCM DIAGNOSIS	HERBAL FORMULAS
Paranoia	Facial paralysis	Qi and blood stagnation	*Symmetry*
	Personality disorder	*Shen* (spirit) disturbance	*Calm (ES)*
Parkinson's Disease	Tremor, muscle rigidity, poor balance, impaired mental and physical functions	Deficiencies of Kidney yin, yang and *jing* (essence) with Liver yang rising	*Neuro Plus*
Parotitis	Inflammation or infection of the parotid salivary gland	Toxic heat with phlegm accumulation	*Herbal ENT* with *Resolve (AI)*
Patella	Acute knee pain	Qi and blood stagnation	*Knee & Ankle (Acute)*
	Chronic knee pain	Qi and blood stagnation	*Knee & Ankle (Chronic)*
	With severe pain	Severe qi and blood stagnation	*Add Herbal Analgesic*
	Yellow discharge with foul odor	Damp-heat in the lower *jiao*	*V-Statin*
Pelvic Inflammatory Disease (PID)	Foul smelling yellow discharge, pelvic pain in hypertensive patients	Damp-heat in the lower *jiao*	*Gentiana Complex*
	Endometriosis	Qi and blood stagnation	*V-Statin* and *Resolve (Lower)*
	Chronic pelvic inflammatory disease with weakness and thirst	Damp-heat accumulation in the lower *jiao* with Kidney yin deficiency	*V-Statin* and *Nourish*
	Moderate to severe cases of infection and inflammation	Accumulation of toxic heat	*V-Statin* and *Herbal ABX*
	With severe pain	Severe qi and blood stagnation	*V-Statin* and *Herbal Analgesic*
Pelvic Pain	Due to pelvic inflammatory disease	Damp-heat in the lower *jiao*	*V-Statin*
	Due to dysmenorrhea	Blood stagnation in the lower *jiao*	*Mense-Ease*
	Due to fibroids or endometriosis	Blood and phlegm stagnation in the lower *jiao*	*Resolve (Lower)*
	Due to genito-urinary infection	Damp-heat in the lower *jiao*	*Gentiana Complex* or *V-Statin*
	Post-surgical pelvic pain or scar tissues	Qi and blood stagnation	*Traumanex*
	With severe pain	Severe qi and blood stagnation	*Add Herbal Analgesic*
	Moderate to severe cases of infection and inflammation	Accumulation of toxic heat	*Add Herbal ABX*
	With high fever	Excess heat accumulation	*Add Gardenia Complex*
Penis	*See* Impotence, Premature Ejaculation, Sexual Dysfunction, Sexually Transmitted Disease, Infection		
Peptic Ulcer	Gastric and duodenal ulcer	Stomach heat	*GI Care*
	Stress-induced gastric and duodenal ulcers	Stomach heat with Liver qi stagnation	*GI Care* with *Calm*
	Peptic ulcer with poor appetite, fatigue, loose stool	Stomach heat with Spleen qi deficiency	*GI Care* with *GI Tonic*
	With severe pain	Severe qi and blood stagnation	*GI Care* with *Herbal Analgesic*
	With bleeding	Heat forcing blood out of the vessels	*Add Notoginseng 9*
Period	*See* Menstrual Irregularity, Menstrual Cramp, Amenorrhea, Menopausal Syndrome		

SYMPTOM / DISEASE INDEX

CONDITION	SYMPTON / DISEASE DESCRIPTION	TCM DIAGNOSIS	HERBAL FORMULAS
Peripheral Neuropathy	Neuropathy with pain, numbness, tingling and swelling	Qi and blood stagnation	*Flex (NP)*
	Diabetic neuropathy	Yin deficiency with stagnation	*Flex (NP)* with *Equilibrium*
Personality Disorder	*See* Mental Health Disorder		
Pesticide Poisoning	Adverse reactions from exposure to insecticide, pesticide, herbicide and other toxins	Toxic heat	*Herbal DTX*
	Compromised liver function due to exposure to toxins	Toxic heat in the Liver	*Liver DTX*
	Compromised kidney function due to exposure to toxins	Toxic heat in the Kidney	*Kidney DTX*
Pfeiffer's Disease	Fever, pharyngitis, enlarged lymph	Toxic heat accumulation with dampness	*Resolve (AI)* and *Herbal ABX*
	With sore throat	Wind-heat invasion	*Lonicera Complex*
Pharyngitis	With fever, cough, dyspnea	Lung heat	*Respirol (Heat)* and *Herbal ENT*
	Moderate to severe cases of infection and inflammation	Accumulation of toxic heat	*Herbal ENT* and *Herbal ABX*
	With severe pain	Toxic heat with severe qi and blood stagnation	*Herbal ENT* and *Herbal Analgesic*
Phlegm	Profuse yellow phlegm, chest congestion, cough and possible fever	Phlegm and heat in the Lung	*Poria XPT*
	Cough, dyspnea, chest congestion, yellow sputum	Lung heat	*Respirol (Heat)*
	Clear or white phlegm, nasal congestion, sneezing	Lung cold	*Respirol (Cold)*
	Moderate to severe cases of infection and inflammation	Accumulation of toxic heat	Add *Herbal ABX*
	Nodules or swellings	Phlegm accumulation	*Resolve (AI)*
	Nodules or swellings with redness and pain	Toxic heat with phlegm	*Resolve (AI)* and *Herbal ABX*
	With cough	Lung qi reversal	*Respirol (CF)*
	With bleeding	Heat pushing blood out of the vessels	Add *Notoginseng 9*
Pituitary Gland	Diminished function of the adrenal glands and endocrine system	Deficiencies of Kidney yin, yang and *jing* (essence)	*Adrenoplex*
	Diabetes mellitus	Yin deficiency with dampness and heat	*Equilibrium*
	Hyperthyroidism	Excess heat	*Thyrodex*
	Hypothyroidism	Kidney yang deficiency	*Thyro-forte*
Plaque	*See* Cholesterol		
Plasma	*See* Blood		
	Breast distention, bloating, mood swings	Liver qi stagnation	*Calm*
PMS (Premenstrual Syndrome) ...	Insomnia, restlessness and anger	Liver fire	*Calm (ES)*
	With lower abdominal pain and dysmenorrhea	Liver qi stagnation with blood stagnation	*Calm* and *Mense-Ease*

SYMPTOM / DISEASE INDEX

CONDITION	SYMPTON / DISEASE DESCRIPTION	TCM DIAGNOSIS	HERBAL FORMULAS
	With edema and coldness	Liver qi stagnation with coldness	*Calm* and *Balance (Cold)* or *Herbal DRX*
	With insomnia, anxiety, stress, irritability, overactive mind and weakness in patients with deficiency	Liver qi stagnation with qi deficiency	*Calm ZZZ*
Pneumonia	Cough, dyspnea, fever	Lung heat	*Respitrol (Heat)*
	Chest congestion, fever, cough with yellow sputum	Phlegm and heat in the Lung	*Poria XPT*
	Moderate to severe cases of infection and inflammation	Accumulation of toxic heat	*Poria XPT* and *Herbal ABX*
	With high fever	Excess heat accumulation	*Add Gardenia Complex*
Poison Oak/Ivy	Itching of the skin	Toxic heat	*Silerex* or *Dermatrol (PS)*
	With infection	Toxic heat	*Silerex* and *Herbal ABX*
Poisoning	Food poisoning with abdominal pain and diarrhea	Damp-heat in the Intestines	*GI Care II*
	Adverse reactions from exposure to insecticide, pesticide, herbicide, heavy metal, and other toxins	Toxic heat	*Herbal DTX*
	Compromised liver function due to exposure to toxins	Toxic heat in the Liver	*Liver DTX*
	Compromised kidney function due to exposure to toxins	Toxic heat in the Kidney	*Kidney DTX*
	With fever	Excess heat accumulation	*Add Gardenia Complex*
	Chronic cases with blood stagnation signs of dark complexion, purplish tongue with distended sublingual veins	Blood stagnation	*Add Circulation (SJ)*
	Itching of skin	Wind-heat attacking the exterior	*Silerex*
	Moderate to severe cases of infection and inflammation of the skin	Accumulation of toxic heat	*Silerex* and *Herbal ABX*
	To strengthen the immune system	*Wei* (defensive) *qi* deficiency	*Immune +*
Pollution	*See* Detox, Poisoning		
Polycystic Ovary Syndrome	*See* Fibrocystic Disease, Endometriosis, Infertility, Menstrual Irregularities		
	Irregular menstruation with severe pain and coldness	Blood stagnation with cold accumulation	*Menotrol*
	Irregular menstruation with pain but no coldness	Qi, blood and phlegm stagnation	*Resolve (Lower)*
	Infertility	Varies	*Blossom (Phase 1-4)*
Polydypsia	Increased intake of fluid, thirst	Lung yin deficiency with heat	*Nourish (Fluids)*
Polydypsia	Increased intake of fluid, thirst in diabetes	Lung yin deficiency with heat	*Equilibrium* and *Nourish (Fluids)*
Polyneuropathy	Neuropathy with pain, numbness, tingling and swelling	Qi and blood stagnation	*Flex (NP)*
Polyps	Intestinal polyps	Damp accumulation	*Resolve (AI)*
Polyphagia...	Increased intake of food in diabetic patients	Stomach yin deficiency with heat	*Equilibrium*

SYMPTOM / DISEASE INDEX

CONDITION	SYMPTON / DISEASE DESCRIPTION	TCM DIAGNOSIS	HERBAL FORMULAS
	Increased hunger	Stomach heat	*Herbalite*
Polyuria	With coldness and weakness	Kidney yang deficiency	*Adrenoplex*
	Due to infection with dark urine and pain	Damp-heat in the lower *jiao*	*V-Statin*
	In diabetic patients	Kidney yin deficiency	*Equilibrium*
	Due to enlarged prostate	Damp-heat in the lower *jiao*	*Saw Palmetto Complex* or *P-Statin*
	Due to chronic nephritis or nephritic syndrome	Toxic heat in the Kidney	*Kidney DTX*
	Moderate to severe cases of infection and inflammation	Accumulation of toxic heat	*Add Herbal ABX*
Poor Memory	*See Forgetfulness*		
Post-Menstrual Care	Dizziness with signs of anemia, poor sleep, excessive dreams and worrying	Blood deficiency	*Schisandra ZZZ*
	Fatigue and generalized weakness	Qi and blood deficiencies	*Imperial Tonic*
	Soreness and weakness of the back and knees, feeling of emptiness in the lower abdomen	Kidney yin deficiency	*Kidney Tonic (Yin)*
Post-Nasal Drip	Post-nasal drip that is yellow in color, possible inflammation	Damp-heat with fluid congestion	*Pueraria Clear Sinus*
	Post-nasal drip that is white in color, nasal obstruction	Wind-cold with fluid congestion	*Magnolia Clear Sinus*
	Moderate to severe cases of infection and inflammation	Accumulation of toxic heat	*Add Herbal ABX*
	Plum-pit syndrome with feeling of foreign object obstructed in the throat	Liver qi stagnation with phlegm accumulation	*Poria XPT* and *Calm*
Postpartum Care	Residual blood stagnation with pain	Blood stagnation	*Traumanex*
	To treat or reduce the risk of infection	Toxic heat	*Herbal ABX*
	Generalized weakness, dizziness, post-partum tonic	Blood, qi, yin and yang deficiencies	*Imperial Tonic*
	Pale face, insomnia with anemia	Blood deficiency	*Schisandra ZZZ*
	With severe pain	Severe qi and blood stagnation	*Add Herbal Analgesic*
	Post-partum depression	Qi, blood, phlegm and food stagnation	*Schisandra ZZZ* and *Shine*
	With bleeding	Qi deficiency	*Add Notoginseng 9*
	Insufficient lactation due to blockage or deficiency	Qi and blood deficiencies with qi stagnation	*Venus* and *Imperial Tonic*
	Constipation	Qi and blood stagnation and deficiencies	*Imperial Tonic* and *Gentle Lax (Deficient)*
Premature Aging…	Prematurely gray hair, hair loss, brittle hair with split ends	Liver blood deficiency	*Polygonum 14*
	Prematurely gray hair, hair loss due to stress	Liver blood deficiency with Liver qi stagnation	*Polygonum 14* and *Calm*
	With decreased mental and physical functions	Deficiency of qi, blood, yin and yang	*Imperial Tonic*
	With poor memory and forgetfulness	Kidney yin and *jing* (essence) deficiency	*Neuro Plus* or *Enhance Memory*

SYMPTOM / DISEASE INDEX

CONDITION	SYMPTOM / DISEASE DESCRIPTION	TCM DIAGNOSIS	HERBAL FORMULAS
	With decreased libido in men and women	Kidney yang deficiency	*Vitality*
	To prevent osteoporosis	Kidney *jing* (essence) deficiency	*Osteo 8*
	General Kidney yin deficiency signs such as blurry vision, weakness of the back and knees, tinnitus, dryness, flushed cheeks, possible low-grade fever, etc.	Kidney yin deficiency	*Kidney Tonic (Yin)*
	General Kidney yang deficiency signs such as coldness, low libido, premature ejaculation, weakness and soreness of the back and knees, pale complexion, polyuria, etc.	Kidney yang deficiency	*Kidney Tonic (Yang)*
Premature Ejaculation	With soreness and weakness of the low back and knees, hair loss, coldness, polyuria, or loose stool	Kidney yang deficiency	*Kidney Tonic (Yang)*
	With *wu xin re* (five-center heat), night sweating, dry mouth, dizziness, tinnitus, dry stool	Kidney yin deficiency	*Nourish*
	With irritability, bitter taste in the mouth, yellow urine, possible genital itching	Damp-heat in the lower *jiao*	*V-Statin*
	With emaciation, fatigue, weakness of limbs, poor appetite, loose stool	Spleen qi deficiency	*GI Tonic*
	Generalized male sexual dysfunction with low libido	Kidney yang deficiency	*Vitality*
Premenstrual Syndrome (PMS)	Breast distention, bloating, mood swings	Liver qi stagnation	*Calm*
	Insomnia, restlessness and anger	Liver fire	*Calm (ES)*
	PMS with lower abdominal pain and dysmenorrhea	Liver qi stagnation with blood stagnation	*Calm* and *Mense-Ease*
	PMS with edema and coldness	Liver qi stagnation with coldness	*Calm* and *Balance (Cold)* or *Herbal DRX*
	With insomnia, anxiety, stress, irritability, overactive mind and weakness in patients with deficiency	Liver qi stagnation with qi deficiency	*Calm ZZZ*
Prolapse	Organ prolapse	Spleen qi deficiency with inability to hold the organs in place	*C/R Support*
Prostate	Hemorrhoid	Damp-heat accumulation with blood stagnation	*GI Care (HMR)*
	Enlarged prostate with difficult, painful and burning urination	Damp-heat in the lower *jiao*	*Saw Palmetto Complex*
	Enlarged prostate with back soreness, terminal dripping of urine, overall coldness	Kidney yang deficiency	*P-Statin* or *Saw Palmetto Complex* and *Kidney Tonic (Yang)*
	Moderate to severe cases of infection and inflammation	Accumulation of toxic heat	*Add V-Statin*
	Excessive swelling with thick tongue coating	Phlegm accumulation	*Add Resolve (AI)*
Proteinuria...	Proteinuria due to nephritis	Kidney deficiency with dampness	*Kidney DTX*

SYMPTOM / DISEASE INDEX

CONDITION	SYMPTOM / DISEASE DESCRIPTION	TCM DIAGNOSIS	HERBAL FORMULAS
	With edema	Damp accumulation	Add Herbal DRX
Psoriasis	Itching, silvery, scaling papules and plaques on the skin	Toxic heat	Dermatrol (PS)
	With heat sensation, red discoloration of the skin, possible burning sensation	Excess heat accumulation	Add Gardenia Complex
Psychosis	Mental impairment and confusion	Shen (spirit) disturbance with Liver fire	Calm (ES)
Psychological Disorder	See Mental Health Disorder		
Pulmonary Disorders	See Asthma, Cough, Dyspnea, Pneumonia, Bronchitis, Common Cold, Flu or other specific disorders		
Purple Tongue	Severe blood stagnation manifesting in chronic symptoms	Severe blood stagnation	Circulation (SJ)
	Purpura due to fatigue, weakness and Spleen qi deficiency	Spleen qi deficiency	Schisandra ZZZ
Purpura	Subcutaneous bleeding	Heat pushing blood out of the vessels	Add Notoginseng 9
	Excess heat with feverish sensation, red face, red tongue, rapid pulse	Excess heat accumulation	Notoginseng 9 and Gardenia Complex
	Lung abscess, profuse yellow phlegm	Phlegm and heat in the Lung	Poria XPT
	Breast abscess	Phlegm stagnation in the upper jiao	Resolve (Upper)
Pus	General formation of abscess due to infection and inflammation	Accumulation of toxic heat	Add Herbal ABX
	With hard mass	Phlegm and damp accumulation	Resolve (AI)
	Infection of the kidneys	Damp-heat in the lower jiao	V-Statin
Pyelonephritis	Chronic nephritis or nephritic syndrome	Toxic heat in the Kidney	Kidney DTX
	Moderate to severe cases of infection and inflammation	Accumulation of toxic heat	Kidney DTX and Herbal ABX
Radiation Therapy	See Cancer		
	Itching, redness and swelling of skin	Wind-heat at the skin level, heat in the blood	Silerex
Rash	Genital rash and itching	Damp-heat in the lower jiao	V-Statin
	Severe itching	Toxic heat	Dermatrol (PS)
	Rash due to exposure to drugs, chemicals, heavy metals, environmental and airborne toxins	Toxic heat	Dermatrol (PS) and Herbal DTX
Raynaud's Syndrome	Coldness of the extremities	Yang deficiency	Kidney Tonic (Yang)
	To increase peripheral blood circulation	Qi and blood stagnation	Add Flex (NP)
Red Blood Cells	Deficiency of red blood cells in anemia	Blood deficiency	Schisandra ZZZ
Regurgitation	See Nausea, Vomiting, Acid Reflux		
Rehabilitation	See Detoxification, Addiction		

SYMPTOM / DISEASE INDEX

CONDITION	SYMPTOM / DISEASE DESCRIPTION	TCM DIAGNOSIS	HERBAL FORMULAS
Reiter's Syndrome	Urinary urgency, burning urination, redness and painful eyes, ulcers, pain, etc.	Toxic heat accumulation	*Gardenia Complex* and *Gentiana Complex*
Renal Colic	With severe pain in the flank due to kidney stones	Dysuria due to stone; *shi lin* (stone dysuria)	*Dissolve (KS)*
	With severe pain	Severe qi and blood stagnation	Add *Herbal Analgesic*
	With edema	Damp accumulation	Add *Herbal DRX*
Reproductive System	*See* Sexual Dysfunction, Infertility, Infection, and other related organs		
Respiratory Disorders	*See* Asthma, Cough, Dyspnea, Pneumonia, Bronchitis, Common Cold, Flu		
Restless Leg Syndrome	Constant movement of the leg	Liver wind rising with lack of nourishment to the tendons and muscles	*Flex (SC)*
Restlessness	*See* Stress, ADD/ADHD		
Rheumatism	*See* Arthritis		
Rheumatoid Arthritis	*See* Arthritis		
Rhinitis	*See* Sinusitis		
Rib Pain	Pain in the chest, ribs, thoracic area	Qi and blood stagnation in the upper *jiao*	*Back Support (Upper)*
	With spasms	Liver blood deficiency	Add *Flex (SC)*
	With severe pain	Severe qi and blood stagnation	Add *Herbal Analgesic*
Ringing of Ears	*See* Tinnitus		
Rotator Cuff Tear / Tendonitis	Acute pain and immobility	Qi and blood stagnation	*Neck & Shoulder (Acute)* and *Arm Support*
	Chronic, dull pain, immobility, numbness	Qi and blood stagnation with Liver yin deficiency	*Neck & Shoulder (Chronic)* and *Arm Support*
	With neck pain	Qi and blood stagnation	*Neck & Shoulder (Acute)*
	With severe pain	Severe qi and blood stagnation	Add *Herbal Analgesic*
	With degeneration of soft tissue (muscle, ligaments, tendons, cartilage)	Liver blood deficiency and Kidney yin deficiency	*Flex (MLT)*
Runny Nose	*See* Common Cold		
Sadness	*See* Depression		
Salpingitis	Inflammation of the fallopian tube	Damp-heat in the lower *jiao*	*V-Statin*
	To reduce adhesions and scar tissue	Blood stagnation	Add *Resolve (Lower)*
	With fever	Excess heat accumulation	Add *Gardenia Complex*

SYMPTOM / DISEASE INDEX

CONDITION	SYMPTOM / DISEASE DESCRIPTION	TCM DIAGNOSIS	HERBAL FORMULAS
Scabies	Dermatitis with eruptions	Wind-heat or toxic heat	*Silerex* and *Herbal ABX*
Scapular Pain	Pain in the scapula or in between the scapulas	Qi and blood stagnation	*Back Support (Upper)*
	With severe pain	Severe qi and blood stagnation	*Add Herbal Analgesic*
Schizophrenia	Disturbed thoughts, delusion, hallucination, bizarre behavior	*Shen* (spirit) disturbance with Liver fire	*Calm (ES)*
Sciatica	Sciatica with back pain	Qi and blood stagnation	*Back Support (HD)*
	Sciatic pain with arthritis that worsens during cold and rainy seasons	Coldness and deficiency of the lower back	*Add Flex (CD)*
	Pain due to bone spurs	Qi and blood stagnation with phlegm formation	*Add Flex (Spur)*
	With severe pain	Severe qi and blood stagnation	*Add Herbal Analgesic*
Scrofula	Scrofula	Dampness accumulation	*Resolve (AI)*
	With redness and heat sensation	Heat accumulation	*Resolve (AI)* and *Herbal ABX*
Scrotum	Itching of the scrotum	Damp-heat in the lower *jiao*	*V-Statin*
	Infection of the scrotum, swelling with pain with possible eczema or oozing of fluids, yellow urine, constipation	Damp-heat in the lower *jiao* and Liver channel	*V-Statin* and *Herbal ABX*
Seizure	For prevention and treatment of seizure	Liver wind rising	*Gastrodia Complex* or *Symmetry*
Semen	*See Sexual Dysfunction*		
Sexual Dysfunction	Diminished sexual and physical performances	Kidney yin, yang and *jing* (essence) deficiencies	*Vitality*
	Impotence, premature ejaculation, inability to sustain erection	Kidney yang deficiency	*Vitality*
	Sexual dysfunction due to complications of diabetes	Kidney yin and yang deficiencies	*Vitality* and *Equilibrium*
	Decreased libido in men and women	Kidney yang deficiency	*Vitality*
	Sexual dysfunction with chronic fatigue	Kidney and Lung deficiencies	*Vitality* and *Cordyceps 3*
	Excess libido in men and women with emaciation, dry stool or constipation, dry mouth, yellow urine	Kidney yin deficiency with deficient fire	*Balance (Heat)* and *Nourish*
	Excess libido in men and women with dysuria, thirst, decreased appetite	Damp-heat in the lower *jiao*	*Gentiana Complex* with *Gardenia Complex*
	Male infertility due to sperm disorder (morphology, motility and mobility)	Kidney *jing* (essence) deficiency	*Vital Essence*
	Female infertility	Varies	*Blossom (Phase 1-4)*
Sexually Transmitted Disease (STD)	Infection in the genital area with itching, pus, discharge, and pain	Damp-heat in the lower *jiao*	*V-Statin* and *Herbal ABX*
SGPT, SGOT ...	Elevated levels of liver enzymes SGPT and SGOT (AST and ALT)	Toxic heat in the Liver	*Liver DTX*
	Moderate to severe cases of infection and inflammation	Accumulation of toxic heat	*Liver DTX* and *Herbal ABX*

SYMPTOM / DISEASE INDEX

CONDITION	SYMPTON / DISEASE DESCRIPTION	TCM DIAGNOSIS	HERBAL FORMULAS
	Elevated liver enzymes due to exposure to drugs, chemicals and other toxins	Toxic heat	*Liver DTX* and *Herbal DTX*
Shin Splints	Muscle spasms and cramps	Liver yin or blood deficiency	*Flex (SC)*
Shingles	Pain of the affected area with or without lesions	Damp-heat in the Liver channel	*Dermatrol (HZ)*
	With severe pain	Severe qi and blood stagnation	*Dermatrol (HZ)* and *Herbal Analgesic*
Shortness of Breath	*See* Asthma, Cough, Dyspnea		
Shoulder Pain	Frozen shoulder, acute pain and immobility	Qi and blood stagnation	*Neck & Shoulder (Acute)*
	Frozen shoulder, chronic dull pain	Qi and blood stagnation with Liver yin deficiency	*Neck & Shoulder (Chronic)*
	Bone spurs	Qi and blood stagnation	*Flex (Spur)*
	With severe pain	Severe qi and blood stagnation	*Add Herbal Analgesic*
	Shoulder pain radiating down the arm	Qi and blood stagnation	*Add Arm Support*
	With degeneration or for maintenance of soft tissue (muscle, tendons, cartilage, ligaments)	Liver blood deficiency and Kidney yin deficiency	*Add Flex (MLT)*
	Radiating to the right shoulder blade or the back due to gallstones	Damp-heat in the Liver and Gallbladder	*Dissolve (GS)*
Sigh	Frequent sighing with chest or hypochondriac distension, poor appetite	Liver qi stagnation	*Calm*
	Due to depression	Qi, blood, food, phlegm stagnation	*Shine*
	With shortness of breath, spontaneous sweating, fatigue	Lung qi deficiency	*Immune +*
	With anxiety, stress, restlessness, overactive mind, insomnia and weakness	Liver qi stagnation with qi deficiency	*Calm ZZZ*
Sinusitis	Thick yellow nasal discharge, nasal obstruction, sinus infection	Damp-heat with fluid congestion	*Pueraria Clear Sinus*
	Clear watery nasal discharge, nasal obstruction, allergy	Wind-cold with fluid congestion	*Magnolia Clear Sinus*
	Moderate to severe cases of infection and inflammation	Accumulation of toxic heat	*Add Herbal ABX*
	With headache	Qi and blood stagnation	*Add Corydalin*
Sjogren's Syndrome	Dry mouth, itchy eyes, swollen glands, dental cavity, fatigue	Lung and Stomach yin deficiency	*Nourish (Fluids)* and *Herbal ENT*
	Yellow discoloration of the skin in jaundice patients	Damp-heat in the Liver and Gallbladder	*Liver DTX*
Skin...	Dry skin and hair	Blood deficiency	*Polygonum 14*
	Itching, redness and swelling of skin, dermatitis	Wind-heat at the skin level, heat in the blood	*Silerex*
	Dermatitis with moderate to severe cases of infection and inflammation	Accumulation of toxic heat	*Add Herbal ABX*

SYMPTOM / DISEASE INDEX

CONDITION	SYMPTOM / DISEASE DESCRIPTION	TCM DIAGNOSIS	HERBAL FORMULAS
	Psoriasis or severe itching	Toxic heat	*Dermatrol (PS)* and *Gardenia Complex*
	Rash in the lower body and genital region	Damp-heat in the lower *jiao*	*Gentiana Complex*
	Nodules, swellings and redness	Phlegm heat accumulation	*Resolve (AI)*
	Adverse reactions on the skin from exposure to drugs, chemicals, heavy metals, environmental and airborne toxins	Toxic heat	*Herbal DTX*
	Redness and burning sensation affecting the upper body	Toxic heat invading the upper *jiao*	*Herbal ENT*
	With fever, redness and burning sensation all over the body	Excess heat accumulation	*Add Gardenia Complex*
	Shingles	Toxic heat	*Dermatrol (HZ)*
Sleep	Insomnia in weak or deficient patients with excessive worrying, pensiveness and poor or dream-disturbed sleep	Deficiency of blood in the Heart and Spleen	*Schisandra ZZZ*
	Insomnia with stress, anxiety, irritability, overactive mind and restlessness in patients with overall weakness and deficiency	Liver qi stagnation with qi deficiency	*Calm ZZZ*
	Insomnia due to stress and anxiety in excess patients	*Shen* (spirit) disturbance	*Calm (ES)*
	Hypersomnia, constant sleepiness, poor appetite, loose stool, weakness	Spleen qi deficiency	*GI Tonic*
	Generalized coldness, tinnitus, polyuria, edema	Kidney yang deficiency	*Kidney Tonic (Yang)*
Slipped Disk	Herniated disk with pain	Qi and blood stagnation	*Back Support (HD)*
Sluggishness	Sluggishness or heavy sensation in the body	Damp accumulation	*Herbal DRX*
	Sluggishness or heaviness with poor appetite, loose stool and edema	Spleen qi deficiency with water accumulation	*Herbal DRX* and *GI Tonic*
	Sluggishness due to deficiency	Qi deficiency	*Vibrant*
Small Intestine	*See Diarrhea, Constipation, Enteritis, Crohn's Disease*		
Smoking	*See Addiction, Detoxification*		
	Dryness	Yin deficiency	*Nourish (Fluids)*
	Chronic chest tightness, dyspnea or wheezing	Lung qi deficiency	*Respitrol (Deficient)*
Social Diseases	*See Sexually Transmitted Diseases*		
Soft Tissue	Enhancing the growth of muscles, tendons, ligaments and cartilages	Liver blood and Kidney yin deficiencies	*Flex (MLT)*
Sore Throat	Redness and swelling of the throat from common cold or influenza	Wind-heat invasion	*Lonicera Complex*
	Moderate to severe cases of infection and inflammation	Accumulation of toxic heat	*Herbal ENT*
	With swollen tonsils	Toxic heat accumulation	*Add Resolve (AI)*
	With fever	Excess heat accumulation	*Add Gardenia Complex*
	With yellow or greenish phlegm	Toxic heat with phlegm accumulation	*Add Poria XPT*

SYMPTOM / DISEASE INDEX

CONDITION	SYMPTOM / DISEASE DESCRIPTION	TCM DIAGNOSIS	HERBAL FORMULAS
Spasm	Spasms and cramps of the skeletal or intestinal muscles	Liver yin and body fluid deficiencies	*Flex (SC)*
	Spastic colon or irritable bowel syndrome (IBS)	Liver qi stagnation	*GI Harmony*
Sperm Count (Low)	Infertility, generalized male sexual dysfunction	Kidney yang deficiency	*Vital Essence*
	Infertility, generalized male sexual dysfunction with chronic fatigue	Lung and Kidney deficiencies	*Vital Essence* and *Cordyceps 3*
	Infertility with impotence	Kidney yang deficiency	*Vital Essence* and *Vitality*
Spermatorrhea	With emaciation, fatigue, listlessness, pale complexion, shortness of breath, spontaneous sweating, poor appetite, forgetfulness	Qi, blood, yin and yang deficiencies	*Imperial Tonic* with *Vitality*
	Easily aroused, bitter taste in the mouth, yellow urine, low grade fever	Kidney yin deficiency	*Nourish* with *Balance (Heat)*
	Irritability, genital itching or feeling of dampness	Damp-heat in the lower *jiao*	*V-Statin*
Spider bite	Toxic reactions	Toxic heat	*Herbal ABX* and *Gardenia Complex*
Spleen	*See Anemia, Immunodeficiency*		
Sports Formulas	Desire for added energy, improved athletic performance	Qi deficiency	*Vibrant*
	Lack of energy, history of low energy	Qi, blood, yin and yang deficiencies	*Imperial Tonic*
	Sports injuries, trauma	Blood stagnation	*Traumanex*
	Spasms, muscle cramps, sprain and strains	Liver yin and body fluid deficiencies	*Flex (SC)*
	Severe muscle pain	Qi and blood stagnation	*Flex (SC)* and *Herbal Analgesic*
	For maintainance of healthy soft tissue (muscles, tendons, ligaments and cartilage)	Liver blood deficiency and Kidney *jing* (essence) deficiency	*Flex (MLT)*
Sprain and Strain	Acute muscle and tendon or ligaments sprain and strain	Qi and blood stagnation	*Traumanex*
Spur (Bone)	Bone spurs	Qi and blood stagnation	*Flex (Spur)*
	Bone spur with severe pain	Severe qi and blood stagnation	*Add Herbal Analgesic*
	Pain of the neck and shoulder	Qi and blood stagnation in the upper *jiao*	*Add Neck & Shoulder (Acute)*
	Low back pain	Qi and blood stagnation in the lower *jiao*	*Add Back Support (Acute)*
	Arm pain	Qi and blood stagnation in the upper *jiao*	*Add Arm Support*
	Knee or ankle pain	Qi and blood stagnation in the lower *jiao*	*Add Knee & Ankle (Acute)*
Sputum...	Yellow, profuse, purulent sputum, chest congestion	Phlegm and heat in the Lung	*Poria XPT*
	Yellow sputum, fever, dyspnea, cough or asthma	Lung heat	*Respitrol (Heat)*
	White sputum, nasal obstruction or discharge, sneezing	Lung cold	*Respitrol (Cold)*
	Moderate to severe cases of infection and inflammation	Accumulation of toxic heat	*Add Herbal ABX*

SYMPTOM / DISEASE INDEX

CONDITION	SYMPTOM / DISEASE DESCRIPTION	TCM DIAGNOSIS	HERBAL FORMULAS
	Profuse white or clear sputum with poor appetite, fatigue, loose stool	Spleen qi deficiency	GI Tonic
Staphylococcal Infection	Infection	Toxic heat accumulation	Herbal ABX
Stiffness	See Neck, Shoulder, Back, Arthritis, Bone Spurs, Spasms		
Stomach	Heartburn, acid reflux, stomach pain, ulcers, gastritis	Stomach fire	GI Care
	Stomach pain due to stress	Stomach fire with Liver qi stagnation	GI Care and Calm
	Stomach pain due to gallstones	Damp-heat in the Liver and Gallbladder	Dissolve (GS)
	Dull stomach pain with poor appetite, fatigue and loose stool	Spleen qi deficiency	GI Tonic
	Severe stomach pain	Qi and blood stagnation	Add Herbal Analgesic
	General stomach problem with thirst and dryness	Stomach yin deficiency	Nourish (Fluids)
	Chronic, stubborn stomach pain with manifestations of blood stagnation such as dark complexion, purplish tongue with distended sublingual veins	Blood stagnation	Add Circulation (SJ)
Stones	Kidney or urinary stones	Shi lin (stone dysuria)	Dissolve (KS)
	Gallstones	Damp-heat in the Liver and Gallbladder	Dissolve (GS)
	Moderate to severe cases of infection and inflammation	Accumulation of toxic heat	Add Herbal ABX
	With severe pain	Severe qi and blood stagnation	Add Herbal Analgesic
	With bleeding	Heat in the blood	Add Notoginseng 9
Stool	See Diarrhea, Constipation		
Strep Throat	See Sore Throat, Infection		
Stress...	Moderate cases of stress, anxiety, irritability, restlessness, nervousness	Liver qi stagnation	Calm
	Moderate cases of stress with excess type hypertension	Liver qi stagnation with damp-heat	Calm and Gentiana Complex
	Stress with acute headache	Liver qi stagnation with qi and blood stagnation	Calm and Corydalin
	Stress with chronic headache	Liver qi stagnation with qi and blood stagnation	Calm and Migratrol
	Moderate cases of stress with stomach or duodenal ulcer	Liver overacting on the Stomach	Calm and GI Care
	Severe cases of stress, anxiety, irritability, restlessness, nervousness	Liver fire with shen (spirit) disturbance	Calm (ES)
	Severe cases of stress with excess type hypertension	Liver fire with damp-heat	Calm (ES) and Gentiana Complex
	Severe cases of stress with headache	Liver fire with qi and blood stagnation	Calm (ES) and Corydalin
	ADD or ADHD	Liver wind with shen (spirit) disturbance	Calm (Jr)
	Stress causing weakness of the digestive system with loose stool	Spleen qi deficiency with Liver qi stagnation	Calm and GI Tonic

SYMPTOM / DISEASE INDEX

CONDITION	SYMPTOM / DISEASE DESCRIPTION	TCM DIAGNOSIS	HERBAL FORMULAS
	Stress, anxiety, restlessness, insomnia in patients with deficiency	Liver qi stagnation with qi deficiency	*Calm ZZZ*
	Irritable bowel syndrome (IBS) due to stress	Liver qi stagnation	*Calm* and *GI Harmony*
	Ulcerative colitis (UC) or Crohn's disease due to stress	Liver qi stagnation with damp-heat accumulation	*Calm* and *GI Care (UC)*
Stroke	Patients with increased risk of stroke due to excess type hypertension	Liver fire rising	*Gentiana Complex*
	Patients with increased risk of stroke due to deficient type hypertension	Liver yang rising with Liver and Kidney yin deficiencies	*Gastrodia Complex*
	Patients with increased risk of stroke due to high cholesterol levels	Phlegm and damp	*Cholisma* or *Cholisma (ES)*
	Patients with increased risk of stroke due to coronary heart disease	Blood stagnation	*Circulation*
	Treats the complications of stroke; to be used only after hemorrhage stops	Deficiencies of Kidney yin, yang and *jing* (essence) with qi and blood stagnation	*Neuro Plus*
	Facial paralysis	Qi and blood stagnation	*Symmetry*
Subluxation	Neck, cervical vertebrae	Qi and blood stagnation	*Neck & Shoulder (Acute)*
	Upper back, thoracic vertebrae	Qi and blood stagnation	*Back Support (Upper)*
	Low back, lumbar vertebrae	Qi and blood stagnation	*Back Support (Acute)*
	Herniated disk	Qi and blood stagnation	*Back Support (HD)*
	With severe pain	Severe qi and blood stagnation	*Add Herbal Analgesic*
Sugar	*See Diabetes, Hypoglycemia*		
Surgery	Post-surgical weakness	Qi, blood, yin and yang deficiencies	*Imperial Tonic*
	Enhances post-surgical recovery, reduces adhesions	Qi and blood stagnation	*Traumanex*
	With severe pain during post-surgical recovery	Severe qi and blood stagnation	*Traumanex* and *Herbal Analgesic*
	Enhances bone growth	Kidney *jing* (essence) deficiencies	*Add Osteo 8*
	Enhances soft tissue growth (muscles, tendons, ligaments, cartilage)	Liver blood and Kidney *jing* (essence) deficiencies	*Add Flex (MLT)*
	Post-surgical constipation	Qi and blood stagnation	*Traumanex* and *Gentle Lax (Deficient)*
Sweat…	Night sweating, irritability, hot flushes	Yin deficiency with deficiency heat	*Balance (Heat)*
	Spontaneous sweating with impaired immune system	*Wei* (defensive) *qi* deficiency	*Immune +*
	Sticky, yellowish sweating	Damp-heat accumulation	*Gentiana Complex*
	Sweating due to hyperthyroidism	Qi and phlegm stagnation with *shen* (spirit) disturbance	*Thyrodex*
	Profuse sweating due to excess heat, red face, possible constipation, rapid heart rate, high blood pressure	Excess heat	*Gardenia Complex*

SYMPTOM / DISEASE INDEX

CONDITION	SYMPTOM / DISEASE DESCRIPTION	TCM DIAGNOSIS	HERBAL FORMULAS
	With thirst, dryness	Stomach and Lung yin deficiencies	*Nourish (Fluids)*
	With common cold, *See* Common Cold		
Swelling	Swelling with edema	Water accumulation	*Herbal DRX*
	Swelling with pain and inflammation	Damp-heat accumulation	*Resolve (AI)*
	Moderate to severe infection	Toxic heat accumulation	*Resolve (AI)* and *Herbal ABX*
	With severe pain	Severe qi and blood stagnation	*Resolve (AI)* and *Herbal Analgesic*
	Edema of the lower body with coldness	Kidney yang deficiency	*Kidney Tonic (Yang)*
	Swelling and inflammation of the upper body with heat sensation and redness	Toxic heat invasion	*Herbal ENT*
Swimmer's Ear	Infection with pain	Toxic heat invasion	*Herbal ENT*
	With severe pain	Severe qi and blood stagnation with toxic heat	*Herbal ENT* and *Herbal Analgesic*
Systemic Lupus Erythematosus (SLE)	Lupus with inflammation in joints, tendons, and other connective tissues and organs	Toxic heat accumulation with yin deficiency	*LPS Support*
Tachycardia	*See* Palpitation		
Tan yin (Phlegm Retention)	Swelling with edema	Phlegm, damp and water retention	*Herbal DRX*
	Yellow phlegm and sputum in the chest	Phlegm and damp retention in the chest	*Poria XPT*
Taste	Bitter taste, short temper, headache, hypochondriac pain, possible stickiness sensation in the mouth	Liver fire	*Gentiana Complex*
	Above symptoms with constipation	Excess heat with stagnation	*Add Gentle Lax (Excess)*
	Sweet taste, fatigue, poor appetite, epigastric distension, irregular bowel movement, possible stickiness sensation in the mouth	Spleen qi deficiency	*GI Tonic*
	Sour taste	Qi, blood, phlegm and food stagnation	*Shine*
Tendonitis	*See* Neck, Shoulder, Arm, Wrist, Elbow, Ankle, Knee, Back		
Tendon	Enhancing the growth of muscles, tendons, ligaments and cartilages	Liver blood and Kidney yin deficiencies	*Flex (MLT)*
	Due to food poisoning or traveler's diarrhea	Damp-heat in the Intestines	*GI Care II*
Tenesmus	With feeling of incomplete evacuation, hypochondriac pain, bloating, pain which lessens with defecation	Liver qi stagnation	*Calm* and *GI Harmony*
	With pain, feeling of rectal prolapse, fatigue	Spleen qi deficiency	*GI Tonic*
Tension	Stress, irritability, anxiety	Liver qi stagnation	*Calm*
	Severe restlessness with insomnia, redness of the face, anger	Liver fire	*Calm (ES)*
Tension Headache	Headache with stress and anxiety	Liver qi stagnation	*Corydalin* and *Calm*
Headache...	Headache with excessive emotional distress, insomnia	Liver qi stagnation with *shen* (spirit) disturbance	*Corydalin* and *Calm (ES)*

SYMPTOM / DISEASE INDEX

CONDITION	SYMPTON / DISEASE DESCRIPTION	TCM DIAGNOSIS	HERBAL FORMULAS
	With severe pain	Severe qi and blood stagnation	*Corydalin* and *Herbal Analgesic*
	Maintenance formula for chronic pain or in cases of deficient type of headaches with dull and hollow pain	Blood deficiency	*Migratrol*
	Chronic headache with possible previous head injuries manifesting in dark complexion, purplish tongue and distended sublingual vein	Blood stagnation	*Corydalin* and *Circulation (SJ)*
Terminal Cancer	Terminal, end-stage cancer patients with extreme weakness	*Yuan* (source) *qi* deficiency	*CA Support*
Terminal Dribbling	Urinary symptoms, painful urination that is dark in color due to benign prostatic hypertrophy and heat	Damp-heat in the lower *jiao*	*P-Statin* or *Saw Palmetto Complex*
	With polyuria, coldness and frequent urinary urges at night and coldness	Kidney yang deficiency	*Kidney Tonic (Yang)*
Testicles	*See* Impotence, Premature Ejaculation, Infection		
Testosterone	Impotence due to lack of testosterone	Kidney yang deficiency	*Vitality*
	Lack of libido in women	Kidney yang deficiency	*Vitality*
Thirst	General thirst and dryness	Lung and Stomach yin deficiency	*Nourish (Fluids)*
	Increased desire and intake of water in diabetic patients	Lung yin deficiency with heat	*Equilibrium*
Thoracic Pain	Pain in the chest, ribs, thoracic area	Qi and blood stagnation	*Back Support (Upper)*
	For severe pain	Severe qi and blood stagnation	*Add Herbal Analgesic*
	For stabbing pain with previous trauma history, purplish tongue, dark distended sublingual vein, dark complexion	Blood stagnation	*Add Circulation (SJ)*
Throat	*See* Sore Throat		
Thrombocytopenia	Decrease in number of blood platelets	Blood deficiency	*Schisandra ZZZ* or *Imperial Tonic*
Thrombosis	Obstruction in the vessels	Blood stagnation	*Circulation* or *Traumanex*
Throwing Up	*See* Vomiting		
Thyroid Gland	Hyperthyroidism	Liver fire rising	*Thyrodex*
	Hypothyroidism	Kidney, Heart and Spleen yang deficiencies	*Thyro-forte*
Tidal Fever	Afternoon fever with sweating, irritability	Yin deficiency with heat	*Balance (Heat)*
	With thirst, dryness	Yin deficiency	*Balance (Heat)* and *Nourish (Fluids)*
Tinnitus ...	Dizziness and vertigo in hypertensive patients	Liver yin deficiency with Liver yang rising	*Gastrodia Complex*
	Dizziness, night sweats, and generalized weakness	Liver and Kidney yin deficiencies	*Nourish*
	Tinnitus due to compromised Kidney and ear functions	Kidney deficiency	*Cordyceps 3*
	Tinnitus due to exposure to drugs, chemical, and other toxins	Toxic heat	*Kidney DTX*

SYMPTOM / DISEASE INDEX

CONDITION	SYMPTOM / DISEASE DESCRIPTION	TCM DIAGNOSIS	HERBAL FORMULAS
	General Kidney yin deficiency signs such as blurry vision, weakness of the back and knees, tinnitus, dryness, flushed cheeks, possible low-grade fever, etc.	Kidney yin deficiency	Kidney Tonic (Yin)
TMJ	Temporo-mandibular joint pain	Wind attack with qi and blood stagnation	Symmetry
Tonic	Generalized fatigue, lack of energy, dizziness, and weakness	Qi, blood, yin and yang deficiencies	Imperial Tonic
	Short-term tiredness and lack of energy	Qi deficiency	Vibrant
	Weakened immune system with frequent viral or bacterial infections	Wei (defensive) qi deficiency	Immune +
	Respiratory and reproductive weakness	Lung and Kidney qi deficiencies	Cordyceps 3
	Weak digestion, fatigue, loose stool	Spleen qi deficiency	GI Tonic
	Forgetfulness and poor memory	Heart and Kidney deficiencies	Enhance Memory
	Female infertility due to deficiency	Kidney jing (essence) deficiency	Blossom (Phase 1-4)
	Thirst and dryness	Body fluids deficiency	Nourish (Fluids)
	General Kidney yin deficiency signs such as blurry vision, weakness of the back and knees, tinnitus, dryness, flushed cheeks, possible low-grade fever, etc.	Kidney yin deficiency	Kidney Tonic (Yin)
	General Kidney yang deficiency signs such as coldness, low libido, premature ejaculation, weakness and soreness of the back and knees, pale complexion, polyuria, etc.	Kidney yang deficiency	Kidney Tonic (Yang)
Tonsillitis	Sore throat with redness and swelling	Wind-heat invasion	Lonicera Complex
	Moderate to severe cases of infection and inflammation	Accumulation of toxic heat	Herbal ENT and Herbal ABX
	With severe pain and swelling	Toxic heat with phlegm stagnation	Herbal ENT and Resolve (AI)
Toothache	With swelling and pain, worsens with intake of spicy food and lessens with coldness	Wind-heat invasion	Lonicera Complex
	Pain with stomach ulcer	Stomach heat	GI Care
	Toothache especially at the root, dry throat, palpitation, dizziness, irritability, insomnia	Kidney yin deficiency	Nourish or Balance (Heat)
	With bleeding	Heat forcing blood out of the vessels	Add Notoginseng 9
	With inflamed gums, bad breath, thirst and excess hunger	Stomach heat	Gardenia Complex
Toxins...	Compromised liver function due to exposure to toxins	Toxic heat in the Liver	Liver DTX
	Compromised kidney function due to exposure to toxins	Toxic heat in the Kidney	Kidney DTX
	Adverse reactions from exposure to drugs, chemicals, heavy metals, environmental and airborne toxins	Toxic heat	Herbal DTX
	Headache from exposure to toxic substances	Toxic heat with qi and blood stagnation	Herbal DTX and Corydalin

SYMPTOM / DISEASE INDEX

CONDITION	SYMPTOM / DISEASE DESCRIPTION	TCM DIAGNOSIS	HERBAL FORMULAS
	Respiratory symptoms from exposure to toxic substances	Toxic heat in the Lung	*Herbal DTX* and *Respirol (Heat)*
	Dermatological reactions from exposure to toxic substances	Toxic heat in the exterior	*Herbal DTX* and *Silerex*
	Moderate to severe cases of infection and inflammation	Accumulation of toxic heat	*Herbal DTX* and *Herbal ABX*
	For chronic exposure to toxins with blood stagnation signs of dark complexion, purplish tongue and distended sublingual veins	Blood stagnation	*Herbal DTX* and *Circulation (SJ)*
	To strengthen the immune system to guard against toxic invasion	*Wei* (defensive) *qi* deficiency	*Immune +*
Traumatic Injuries	With severe pain, inflammation, bruises, broken bones	Blood stagnation	*Traumanex*
	To facilitate recovery following traumatic injuries to the bones	Kidney yin and *jing* (essence) deficiencies	*Osteo 8*
	Broken bone or bone fracture in patients with osteoporosis	Blood stagnation with Kidney yin and *jing* (essence) deficiencies	*Traumanex* and *Osteo 8*
	To enhance recovery of connective tissue (muscles, tendons, ligaments, cartilage)	Liver blood and Kidney yin deficiencies	*Flex (MLT)*
	Moderate to severe cases of infection and inflammation	Accumulation of toxic heat	*Add Herbal ABX*
	With severe pain	Severe qi and blood stagnation	*Add Herbal Analgesic*
	Chronic, old injury with recurrent pain	Chronic blood stagnation	*Add Circulation (SJ)*
	Injury to the head	Qi and blood stagnation	*Add Corydalin*
	Injury to the neck and shoulder area	Qi and blood stagnation	*Add Neck & Shoulder (Acute)*
	Injury to the arm	Qi and blood stagnation	*Add Arm Support*
	Injury to the back	Qi and blood stagnation	*Add Back Support (Acute)*
	Injury to the upper back	Qi and blood stagnation	*Add Back Support (Upper)*
	Herniated disk	Qi and blood stagnation	*Add Back Support (HD)*
	Injury to the knees or ankles	Qi and blood stagnation	*Add Knee & Ankle (Acute)*
Traveler's Diarrhea	Diarrhea with foul-smelling stool, burning sensation of anus, abdominal discomfort and pain, nausea and vomiting	Damp-heat in the Intestines	*GI Care II*
	Moderate to severe cases of infection and inflammation	Accumulation of toxic heat	*GI Care II* and *Herbal ABX*
	For severe pain	Qi and blood stagnation and toxic heat	*GI Care II* and *Herbal Analgesic*
	With bleeding	Toxic heat	*GI Care II* and *Notoginseng 9*
Trichomoniasis	Infection in the genital region	Damp-heat in the lower *jiao* and Liver channel	*V-Statin*
	Moderate to severe cases of infection and inflammation	Accumulation of toxic heat	*V-Statin* and *Herbal ABX*
Trigeminal Neuralgia	Facial nerve pain	Wind attack with qi and blood stagnation	*Symmetry*
Triglycerides	*See Cholesterol*		

SYMPTOM / DISEASE INDEX

CONDITION	SYMPTOM / DISEASE DESCRIPTION	TCM DIAGNOSIS	HERBAL FORMULAS
Tuberculosis	Cough, yellow-greenish sputum, dyspnea	Phlegm and heat in the Lung	*Respitrol (CF)* and *Poria XPT*
	Dry cough with scanty sputum, dyspnea	Yin and qi deficiencies of the Lung	*Respitrol (Deficient)*
	Moderate to severe cases of infection and inflammation	Accumulation of toxic heat	*Respitrol (Deficient)* and *Herbal ABX*
Tumor	*See* Cancer		
Twitching	Of the face, dizziness, tinnitus, short temper	Liver yang rising	*Gastrodia Complex* or *Calm*
	Of the face, intermittent in nature, dizziness, wiry, possible stiffness and cramping of other parts of the body	Liver blood deficiency	*Symmetry*
Type "A" Personality	Excessive competitive drive, impatience, overactive mind, stress but with deficient constitution	Liver qi stagnation with qi deficiency	*Calm ZZZ*
	All the above symptoms but excess in body constitution also manifesting in possible red face, eyes, constipation, high blood pressure, fast heart rate	Liver and Heart fire	*Calm (ES)*
Ulcer	Gastric and duodenal ulcer	Stomach heat with yin deficiency	*GI Care*
	Stress-induced gastric and duodenal ulcers	Stomach heat with Liver qi stagnation	*GI Care* and *Calm*
	Ulcerative colitis, Crohn's disease	Toxic heat in the intestine	*GI Care (UC)*
	Ulcer in the oral cavity	Stomach heat	*Gardenia Complex*
	With severe pain	Severe qi and blood stagnation	*Add Herbal Analgesic*
	Moderate to severe cases of infection and inflammation	Accumulation of toxic heat	*Add Herbal ABX*
	With dry mouth and thirst	Stomach yin deficiency	*Add Nourish (Fluids)*
Ulcerative Colitis (UC)	Ulcerative colitis with mucus, pus and blood in the stools with feeling of incomplete evacuation and abdominal cramps	Damp-heat in the Intestines	*GI Care (UC)*
Upper Back Pain	Pain in the upper back, chest, ribs, thoracic area	Qi and blood stagnation	*Back Support (Upper)*
Upper Respiratory Infection	Initial stage of infection with slight sore throat, feverish sensation, cough, yellow phlegm	Wind-heat invasion	*Lonicera Complex*
	Severe sore throat, ear infection and yellow nasal discharge	Toxic heat	*Herbal ENT*
	Fever, cough, dyspnea	Lung heat	*Respitrol (Heat)*
	Sneezing, white or clear nasal discharge	Wind-cold invasion	*Respitrol (Cold)*
	Cough	Lung qi reversal	*Respitrol (CF)*
	Recurrent infection or to enhance the antibiotic function of any of the formulas above	Toxic heat	*Add Herbal ABX*
Urinary Stones...	Kidney or urinary stones	*Shi lin* (stone dysuria)	*Dissolve (KS)*
	Moderate to severe cases of infection and inflammation	Accumulation of toxic heat	*Add Herbal ABX*

SYMPTOM / DISEASE INDEX

CONDITION	SYMPTON / DISEASE DESCRIPTION	TCM DIAGNOSIS	HERBAL FORMULAS
	With severe pain	Severe qi and blood stagnation	*Add Herbal Analgesic*
	With bleeding	Heat pushing blood out of the vessels	*Add Notoginseng 9*
Urinary Tract Infection (UTI)	Painful and difficult urination with itching and discharge	Damp-heat in the lower *jiao*	*Gentiana Complex* or *V-Statin*
	Frequent recurrences of urinary tract infection due to diabetes	Damp-heat in the lower *jiao* with yin deficiency	*Equilibrium* with *V-Statin*
	Moderate to severe cases of infection and inflammation	Accumulation of toxic heat	*Add Herbal ABX*
	With severe pain	Severe qi and blood stagnation	*Add Herbal Analgesic*
	With bleeding	Heat pushing blood out of the vessels	*Add Notoginseng 9*
	With high fever	Excess heat accumulation	*Add Gardenia Complex*
	Recurrent infection with yin-deficient heat signs of thirst, dryness, flushed cheeks, low-grade fever	Yin-deficient heat	*Nourish*
	In diabetic patients	Kidney yang deficiency	*Equilibrium*
Urination (Frequent)	Frequent urination with burning sensations, cystitis, urinary tract infection (UTI)	Damp-heat in the lower *jiao*	*V-Statin*
	Moderate to severe cases of infection and inflammation	Accumulation of toxic heat	*V-Statin* with *Herbal ABX*
	Due to prostate enlargement	Damp-heat in the lower *jiao*	*P-Statin* or *Saw Palmetto Complex*
	Frequent urinary urges, especially at night, coldness, clear urination	Kidney yang deficiency	*Kidney Tonic (Yang)*
	Chronic nephritis or nephritic syndrome	Toxic heat in the Kidney	*Kidney DTX*
	Interstitial cystitis	Blood stagnation	*V-Statin* and *Resolve (Lower)*
Urination (Incontinent)	With coldness, weakness and soreness of the lower back and knees, clear urination	Kidney yang deficiency	*Kidney Tonic (Yang)*
Urine	Clear, profuse, frequent urges especially at night, coldness	Kidney yang deficiency	*Kidney Tonic (Yang)*
	Dark, yellow, painful urination	Damp-heat in the lower *jiao*	*V-Statin*
	High urine ketone level or high blood glucose level	Deficient fire with damp accumulation	*Equilibrium*
Urolithiasis	Kidney or urinary stones	Dysuria due to stone; *shi lin* (stone dysuria)	*Dissolve (KS)*
	With severe pain	Severe qi and blood stagnation	*Dissolve (KS)* with *Herbal Analgesic*
Urticaria	Rash, itching of the body	Wind-heat at the skin level, heat in the blood	*Silerex*
	Rash of the lower body and genital region	Damp-heat in the lower *jiao*	*Gentiana Complex* or *V-Statin*
	Severe itching	Toxic heat	*Dermatrol (PS)* and *Gardenia Complex*
Uterus	*See* Fibroids, Infertility, Menopause, Dysmenorrhea, Endometriosis, Pelvic Inflammatory Disease, Irregular Menstruation		
Vaginal Infection…	Foul smelling-yellow discharge, pelvic pain, itching due to infection	Damp-heat in the lower *jiao*	*V-Statin*

SYMPTOM / DISEASE INDEX

CONDITION	SYMPTON / DISEASE DESCRIPTION	TCM DIAGNOSIS	HERBAL FORMULAS
	Vaginal infection due to complications of diabetes	Damp-heat in the lower *jiao* with yin deficiency	*V-Statin* with *Equilibrium*
	Moderate to severe cases of infection and inflammation	Accumulation of toxic heat	*V-Statin* with *Herbal ABX*
	Vaginal infection leading to lower abdominal pain	Qi and blood stagnation	*V-Statin* with *Herbal Analgesic*
Vaginitis	Vaginitis with yellow discharge and foul odor	Damp-heat in the lower *jiao*	*V-Statin*
	Moderate to severe cases of infection and inflammation	Accumulation of toxic heat	*V-Statin* with *Herbal ABX*
	Vaginal infection leading to lower abdominal pain	Qi and blood stagnation	*V-Statin* with *Herbal Analgesic*
Varicocele	Causing male infertility	Blood stagnation	*Resolve (Lower)*
Varicose Veins	Distended purplish black veins mostly on the legs	Blood stagnation	*Circulation (SJ)*
	With water retention	Blood stagnation with water accumulation	*Circulation (SJ)* with *Herbal DRX*
Vein	Distended sublingual vein	Blood stagnation	*Circulation (SJ)*
Venereal Diseases	*See* Sexually Transmitted Diseases		
Vertigo	Dizziness and vertigo with headache, flushed face and anger	Liver fire rising	*Gentiana Complex*
	Dizziness and vertigo with or without nausea and vomiting and yin deficiency	Liver yin deficiency with Liver yang or Liver wind rising	*Gastrodia Complex*
Viral Infection	*See* Infection, Common Cold, Gastritis, Gastroenteritis, Hepatitis, Herpes, HIV, Influenza, Pneumonia, Sore Throat, Urinary Tract Infection		
	Blurry vision due to deficient type hypertension	Liver yin deficiency with Liver yang rising	*Gastrodia Complex*
Vision	Blurry vision due to excess type hypertension	Liver fire	*Gentiana Complex*
	Vision impairment due to diabetes	Yin deficiency	*Equilibrium*
	Dry, blurry vision	Kidney deficiency with false heat	*Nourish*
Voice	Hoarseness due to a common cold/flu with itching, painful throat	Wind-heat invasion	*Lonicera Complex*
	Hoarseness due to overuse, dry throat, scanty sputum	Yin deficiency	*Nourish*
	Nausea and vomiting due to chemotherapy	Stomach yin deficiency	*C/R Support*
	Nausea, vomiting, abdominal pain and diarrhea due to food poisoning	Damp-heat in the Intestines	*GI Care II*
Vomiting	Nausea, vomiting, epigastric, chest and hypochondriac distension and pain, emotional instability, stress related	Liver qi stagnation	*Calm*
	With dryness and thirst	Stomach yin deficiency	*Nourish (Fluids)*
	From exposure to toxic materials or smell	Toxic heat invasion	*Liver DTX* or *Herbal DTX*
	Caused by gallstones	Damp-heat in the Liver and Gallbladder	*Dissolve (GS)*
Vulvitis...	Inflammation of the vulva	Damp-heat in the lower *jiao*	*V-Statin*

SYMPTOM / DISEASE INDEX

CONDITION	SYMPTON / DISEASE DESCRIPTION	TCM DIAGNOSIS	HERBAL FORMULAS
	Moderate to severe cases of infection and inflammation	Accumulation of toxic heat	*V-Statin* with *Herbal ABX*
	Severe itching	Toxic heat	Add *Dermatrol (PS)*
	Due to immune deficiency	*Wei* (defensive) *qi* deficiency	*Immune +*
Wasting Syndrome	Due to cancer with chemotherapy and radiation treatments	*Yuan* (source) *qi* and yin deficiencies	*C/R Support*
	End-stage cancer	*Yuan* (source) *qi* deficiency	*CA Support*
	Weight loss, decreased energy, overall weakness	Qi, blood, yin and yang deficiencies	*Imperial Tonic*
	Digestive weakness, loose stool, fatigue	Spleen qi deficiency	*GI Tonic*
	Degeneration of soft tissue (muscles, ligaments, tendons, cartilage)	Liver blood and Kidney *jing* (essence) deficiencies	*Flex (MLT)*
	Degeneration of bones	Kidney *jing* (essence) deficiency	*Osteo 8*
Water Retention	*See* Edema		
Weak Muscle	Low energy and fatigue, weakness and soreness especially of the back and knees	Qi, blood, yin and yang deficiencies	*Imperial Tonic* with *Back Support (Chronic)*
	Weakness of muscle due to adrenal gland under-activity	Kidney yang deficiency	*Adrenoplex*
	Lack of muscle tone, digestive weakness, loose stool, fatigue	Spleen qi deficiency	*GI Tonic*
	Post-stroke complications	Qi and blood stagnation	*Neuro Plus*
	Degeneration of soft tissue (muscles, ligaments, tendons, cartilage)	Liver blood and Kidney *jing* (essence) deficiencies	*Flex (MLT)*
	For immediate boost of energy	Qi deficiency	*Vibrant*
Weakness...	Decreased energy, overall weakness of constitution	Qi, yin, yang and blood deficiencies	*Imperial Tonic*
	Poor appetite, loose stool	Spleen qi deficiency	*GI Tonic*
	Respiratory and reproductive weakness	Lung and Kidney deficiencies	*Cordyceps 3*
	Anemia, restless sleep, pale complexion	Blood deficiency	*Schisandra ZZZ*
	Adreno-insufficiency in patients who are "burned-out" with decreased mental and physical functions	Kidney deficiency	*Adrenoplex*
	Weakness of the immune system	*Wei* (defensive) *qi* deficiency	*Immune +*
	End stage cancer patients who cannot receive chemotherapy or radiation	*Yuan* (source) *qi* deficiency	*CA Support*
	Weakness in cancer patients receiving chemotherapy or radiation	*Yuan* (source) *qi* deficiency	*C/R Support*

Lotus Institute of Integrative Medicine

SYMPTOM / DISEASE INDEX

CONDITION	SYMPTON / DISEASE DESCRIPTION	TCM DIAGNOSIS	HERBAL FORMULAS
	Weakness of the bones	Kidney *jing* (essence) deficiency	Osteo 8
	Degeneration of soft tissue (muscles, ligaments, tendons, cartilage)	Liver blood and Kidney *jing* (essence) deficiencies	Flex (MLT)
	Weakness of the back and knees	Kidney deficiency	Back Support (Chronic)
	Weakness of the legs, knees and ankles	Kidney deficiency	Knee & Ankle (Chronic)
	Weakness of the neck and shoulders	Liver blood deficiency	Neck & Shoulder (Chronic)
	General Kidney yin deficiency signs such as blurry vision, weakness of the back and knees, tinnitus, dryness, flushed cheeks, low-grade fever, etc.	Kidney yin deficiency	Kidney Tonic (Yin)
	General Kidney yang deficiency signs such as coldness, low libido, premature ejaculation, weakness and soreness of the back and knees, pale complexion, polyuria, etc.	Kidney yang deficiency	Kidney Tonic (Yang)
Weight Control	See Obesity		
Wheezing	See Asthma		
Whiplash	See Neck Pain		
White Blood Cells	Low white blood cells count in immuno-compromised patients	Qi deficiency	Immune +
	Compromised respiratory and reproductive functions	Lung and Kidney qi deficiencies	Cordyceps 3
Withdrawal	See Addiction		
Wrist	Wrist pain	Qi and blood stagnation	Arm Support
	Degeneration of soft tissue (muscles, ligaments, tendons, cartilage)	Liver blood & Kidney *jing* (essence) deficiencies	Add Flex (MLT)
	With severe pain	Severe qi and blood stagnation	Add Herbal Analgesic
Worrying	With insomnia, weakness, poor appetite	Spleen and Heart deficiency	Schisandra ZZZ
	Short-term fatigue and lack of energy	Qi deficiency	Vibrant
Yawning	Fatigue, coldness, decreased dietary intake, loose stool, frequent urinary urges especially at night, decreased libido	Kidney yang deficiency	Vitality
	Overall weakness of the constitution	Qi, blood, yin and yang deficiencies	Imperial Tonic
	With listlessness, stifling sensation in the chest, sighing, abdominal distension, plum-pit sensation, emotional instability	Liver qi stagnation	Calm
	With chest congestion and stabbing pain in a fixed location, palpitation, shortness of breath, dizziness, intermittent pulse	Chest *bi zheng* (painful obstruction syndrome)	Circulation
Yeast Infection (Vaginal)	Itching and pain in the genital region	Damp-heat in the lower *jiao*	Gentiana Complex or V-Statin
	Frequent yeast infection due to complications of diabetes	Damp-heat in the lower *jiao* with yin deficiency	Add Equilibrium
	Moderate to severe cases of infection and inflammation	Accumulation of toxic heat	Add Herbal ABX

Section 3

Chinese Diagnostic Index

中醫診斷索引

Section 3

Chinese Diagnostic

Index

CHINESE DIAGNOSTIC INDEX

I.   ***Ba Gang Bian Zheng* (Eight Principle Differentiation)**
1. Exterior
2. Interior
3. Cold
4. Heat
5. Deficiency
6. Excess
7. Yin
8. Yang

II.   ***Zang Fu Bian Zheng* (Organ Pattern Differentiation)**
1. Liver (Wood Element)
2. Gall Bladder (Wood Element)
3. Heart (Fire Element)
4. Small Intestine (Fire Element)
5. Spleen (Earth Element)
6. Stomach (Earth Element)
7. Lung (Metal Element)
8. Large Intestine (Metal Element)
9. Kidney (Water Element)
10. Urinary Bladder (Water Element)

III.   ***Wei Qi Ying Xue Bian Zheng* (Defensive, Qi, Nutritive, Blood Differentiation)**
1. *Wei* (defense) level
2. *Qi* (energy) level
3. *Ying* (nutritive) level
4. *Xue* (blood) level

IV.   ***Liu Jing Bian Zheng* (Six Stages Differentiation)**
1. *Taiyang*
2. *Yangming*
3. *Shaoyang*
4. *Taiyin*
5. *Shaoyin*
6. *Jueyin*

V.   ***San Jiao Bian Zheng* (Triple Burner Differentiation)**
1. Upper *jiao*
2. Middle *jiao*
3. Lower *jiao*

VI.   **Qi, Blood, Body Fluids and *Jing* (Essence)**
1. Qi deficiency
2. Reversed flow of qi
3. Qi stagnation
4. Qi and blood stagnation
5. Blood deficiency
6. Blood stagnation
7. Bleeding
8. Body fluids
9. *Jing* (essence)

CHINESE DIAGNOSTIC INDEX

VII. *Liu Yin* (Six Exogenous Factors)
1. Wind
2. Cold
3. Summer-heat
4. Damp
5. Dryness
6. Heat

VIII. *Qi Qing* (Seven Emotions)
1. Joy
2. Anger
3. Melancholy
4. Meditation (Over-Thinking)
5. Grief
6. Fear
7. Fright

IX. **Other Factors**
1. Food (diet)
2. Traumatic injuries
3. Phlegm
4. *Bi zheng* (painful obstruction syndrome)
5. *Shen* (spirit)

CHINESE DIAGNOSTIC INDEX

I. *BA GANG BIAN ZHENG* (EIGHT PRINCIPLE DIFFERENTIATION)

1. EXTERIOR

- *Corydalin* – <u>headache</u> from invasion of wind
- *Dermatrol (PS)* – <u>psoriasis</u> caused by toxic heat
- *Herbal ABX* – all types of <u>infection</u> or <u>inflammation</u> with or without fever, inflammation, redness and swelling
- *Herbal DTX* – pathogenic accumulation from chronic exposure to <u>chemical</u> <u>compounds</u> and <u>environmental</u> <u>toxins</u>
- *Herbal ENT* – ear, nose, throat and lung <u>infection</u>
- *Lonicera Complex* – <u>common</u> <u>cold</u>, <u>flu</u>, <u>sore</u> <u>throat</u> caused by wind–heat
- *Magnolia Clear Sinus* – <u>allergy</u>, <u>stuffy</u> <u>nose</u> and other <u>nasal</u> <u>disorders</u> from invasion of wind–cold
- *Migratrol* – prevention and treatment of <u>migraine</u> <u>headache</u>
- *Neck & Shoulder (Acute)* – <u>neck</u> and <u>shoulder</u> <u>pain</u> from wind–cold
- *Pueraria Clear Sinus* – <u>sinusitis</u>, <u>rhinitis</u> and other <u>nasal</u> <u>disorders</u> caused by wind–heat
- *Respitrol (Cold)* – <u>flu</u>, <u>runny</u> <u>nose</u> and other <u>respiratory</u> <u>disorders</u> from wind–cold
- *Respitrol (CF)* – cough
- *Respitrol (Heat)* – <u>cough</u>, dyspnea, and other <u>respiratory</u> <u>disorders</u> caused by wind–heat
- *Silerex* – <u>rash</u>, <u>itching</u>, and other <u>dermatological</u> <u>disorders</u> because of wind–heat
- *Symmetry* – <u>Bell's</u> <u>palsy</u>, <u>TMJ</u> (temporo-mandibular joint pain), <u>trigeminal</u> <u>neuralgia</u> due to wind

2. INTERIOR – Refer to the specific diagnostic criteria below for additional information

3. COLD

- *Adrenoplex* – fatigue, lack of interest, lack of drive and satisfaction, 'burned <u>out</u>,' with diminished mental and physical performance
- *Arm Support* – <u>shoulder</u>, <u>elbow</u> and <u>wrist</u> pain
- *Balance (Cold)* – women's <u>disorders</u> characterized by cold and deficiency
- *Cordyceps 3* – <u>lung</u>, <u>kidney</u>, <u>immune</u>, <u>reproductive</u>, and <u>chronic</u> <u>fatigue</u> disorders remedied by tonifying the <u>Lung</u> and <u>Kidney</u> to strengthen the body and relieve underlying coldness and deficiency
- *Corydalin* – <u>headache</u> arising from cold
- *Flex (CD)* – <u>bi</u> <u>zheng</u> (<u>painful</u> <u>obstruction</u> <u>syndrome</u>) because of cold and damp
- *Flex (NP)* – <u>peripheral</u> <u>neuropathy</u> with pain, numbness, tingling, swelling and muscle wasting especially at the extremities
- *GI Tonic* – strengthens <u>Spleen</u> and <u>Stomach</u> to stop <u>diarrhea</u>, <u>indigestion</u>, <u>lethargy</u>, and addresses general disorders of the gastrointestinal tract
- *Herbal Analgesic* – <u>pain</u> in various parts of the body caused by qi and <u>blood</u> <u>stagnation</u>
- *Magnolia Clear Sinus* – <u>allergy</u>, <u>stuffy</u> <u>nose</u> and other <u>nasal</u> <u>disorders</u> caused by cold and fluid congestion in the Lungs
- *Mense–Ease* – <u>dysmenorrhea</u> with cold and blood stagnation
- *Menotrol* – <u>amenorrhea</u>, <u>infertility</u>, <u>irregular</u>, and <u>delayed</u> or <u>scanty</u> <u>menstruation</u>
- *Neck & Shoulder (Acute)* – <u>acute</u> <u>neck</u> and <u>shoulder</u> <u>pain</u>
- *Neck & Shoulder (Chronic)* – <u>chronic</u> <u>neck</u> and <u>shoulder</u> <u>pain</u>
- *Neuro Plus* – <u>Alzheimer's</u>, <u>Parkinson's</u>, or <u>stroke</u> <u>complications</u> with deteriorating mental and physical functions (<u>neurodegenerative</u> <u>disorders</u>) arising from Kidney deficiency with phlegm and blood stagnation
- *Resolve (Lower)* – <u>fibroids</u>, <u>endometriosis</u>, or <u>infertility</u> because of blood and phlegm stagnation with cold in the lower *jiao*

❧ *Respitrol (Cold)* – <u>common</u> <u>cold</u>, <u>flu</u>, <u>runny</u> <u>nose</u>, and other respiratory disorders accompanying Lung cold
❧ *Thyro–forte* – <u>hypothyroidism</u> with fatigue, lack of energy, coldness of the body
❧ *Venus* – increases the <u>size</u> and improves the <u>shape</u> of <u>breasts</u>

4. HEAT

4.1 Deficiency Heat

❧ *Balance (Heat)* – <u>menopause</u> and other <u>women's</u> <u>disorders</u> with yin deficiency and deficiency heat
❧ *CA Support* – <u>cancer</u> <u>support</u> for weak patients who cannot tolerate chemotherapy or radiation
❧ *Calm (Jr)* – attention deficit disorder (<u>ADD</u>) or attention deficit hyperactivity disorder (<u>ADHD</u>)
❧ *Equilibrium* – <u>diabetes</u> with yin deficiency and deficiency heat
❧ *Gentle Lax (Deficient)* – deficient type <u>constipation</u> with heat and dryness in the Large Intestine
❧ *Gastrodia Complex* – <u>hypertension</u> with Liver yang rising and underlying Liver and Kidney yin deficiencies
❧ *GI Care* – <u>stomach</u> <u>pain</u>, gastritis, and <u>ulcers</u> with Stomach fire and Stomach yin deficiencies
❧ *Herbal DTX* – accumulation of <u>chemical</u> <u>compounds</u> and <u>environmental</u> <u>toxins</u> from chronic exposure
❧ *Kidney DTX* – <u>nephritis</u> and <u>nephrotic</u> <u>syndrome</u> by increasing its ability to <u>excrete</u> and <u>eliminate</u> <u>toxins</u>
❧ *LPS Support* – <u>systemic</u> <u>lupus</u> <u>erythematosus</u> (<u>SLE</u>)
❧ *Nourish* – various signs and symptoms of Liver and Kidney yin deficiencies
❧ *Nourish (Fluids)* – yin and <u>body</u> <u>fluid</u> <u>deficiency</u> with <u>dryness</u>
❧ *Neck & Shoulder (Acute)* – <u>acute</u> <u>neck</u> and <u>shoulder</u> <u>pain</u>
❧ *Resolve (Lower)* – <u>endometriosis</u> with pain and cramps

4.2 Excess Heat

❧ *Calm* – <u>stress</u>, <u>irritability</u> and other <u>emotional</u> <u>imbalances</u> of Liver qi stagnation and heat
❧ *Calm (ES)* – <u>restlessness</u>, <u>anger</u>, <u>insomnia</u> and <u>severe</u> <u>emotional</u> <u>imbalance</u> arising from Liver fire with *shen* (spirit) disturbance
❧ *Dermatrol (HZ)* – <u>shingles</u> caused by damp–heat
❧ *Dissolve (GS)* – <u>gallstones</u> or <u>cholecystitis</u> caused by damp–heat in the Liver and Gallbladder
❧ *Dissolve (KS)* – <u>kidney</u> or <u>urinary</u> <u>stones</u> with difficult urination
❧ *Flex (Heat)* – <u>bi zheng</u> (<u>painful</u> <u>obstruction</u> <u>syndrome</u>) arising from heat
❧ *Flex (Spur)* – resolves <u>bone</u> <u>spurs</u> to alleviate pain and inflammation
❧ *Gardenia Complex* – excess <u>fire</u> in all three *jiaos*
❧ *Gentiana Complex* – <u>hypertension</u> and <u>lower</u> *jiao* <u>disorders</u> arising from damp–heat and fire in the Liver and Gallbladder channels
❧ *Gentle Lax (Excess)* – excess type <u>constipation</u> with heat in the Large Intestine
❧ *GI Care* – <u>stomach</u> pain, <u>gastritis</u>, and <u>ulcers</u> with Stomach fire and Stomach yin deficiencies
❧ *GI Care II* – <u>diarrhea</u>, foul–smelling stools with burning sensations of the anus, mucus, abdominal discomfort, pain, borborygmus, possible nausea, vomiting and feelings of incomplete defecation
❧ *GI Care (HMR)* – <u>hemorrhoids</u>
❧ *GI Care (UC)* – prevents and treats <u>ulcerative</u> <u>colitis</u> (<u>UC</u>) characterized by diarrhea with mucus, pus and blood
❧ *GI Harmony* – prevents and treats <u>irritable</u> <u>bowel</u> <u>syndrome</u> (<u>IBS</u>) by harmonizing the gastrointestinal tract

CHINESE DIAGNOSTIC INDEX

- *Herbal ABX* – all types of <u>infection</u> or <u>inflammation</u> with or without fever, inflammation, redness and swelling
- *Herbal Analgesic* – <u>pain</u> in various parts of the body caused by qi and <u>blood stagnation</u>
- *Herbal DTX* – pathogenic accumulation of <u>chemical compounds</u> and <u>environmental toxins</u> arising from chronic exposure
- *Herbal ENT* – ear, nose, throat and lung <u>infection</u>
- *Herbalite* – <u>obesity</u> <u>with</u> <u>excessive hunger</u> and <u>appetite</u> because of Stomach heat
- *Liver DTX* – <u>liver damage with elevated liver enzymes</u> from toxic damp–heat in the Liver and Gallbladder
- *Lonicera Complex* – <u>common cold</u>, <u>flu</u>, <u>sore throat</u> arising from wind–heat
- *Notoginseng 9* – bleeding
- *Poria XPT* – <u>cough with yellow sputum</u> because of heat and phlegm in the Lungs
- *P–Statin* – <u>benign prostatic hyperplasia</u> (<u>BPH</u>) with dysuria and incontinence
- *Pueraria Clear Sinus* – <u>sinusitis</u>, <u>rhinitis</u>, and other <u>nasal disorders</u> with yellow discharge caused by heat
- *Resolve (AI)* – resolves <u>hardness</u> and <u>nodules</u> arising from <u>swelling</u> and <u>inflammation</u>
- *Resolve (Upper)* – <u>benign breast disorders</u> caused by stagnation of Liver qi, phlegm, blood, heat
- *Respitrol (Heat)* – <u>cough</u>, <u>dyspnea</u>, and other <u>respiratory disorders</u> because of Lung heat
- *Saw Palmetto Complex* – <u>prostatic enlargement</u> caused by damp–heat in the lower *jiao*
- *Shine* – <u>depression</u> arising from stagnation of blood, phlegm, food, and Liver qi with heat
- *Silerex* – <u>rash</u>, <u>itching</u>, and other <u>dermatological disorders</u> caused by heat in the blood
- *Symmetry* – <u>Bell's palsy</u>, <u>TMJ</u> (temporo-mandibular joint pain), <u>trigeminal neuralgia</u> due to wind
- *Thyrodex* – <u>hyperthyroidism</u> arising from Liver fire and phlegm stagnation with underlying qi and yin deficiencies
- *V–Statin* – <u>vaginitis</u>, <u>pelvic inflammatory disease</u> and <u>urogenital infections</u>

4.3 Toxic Heat

- *Dermatrol (HZ)* – <u>shingles</u> caused by damp–heat and toxicity
- *Herbal ABX* – all types of <u>infection</u> or <u>inflammation</u> with or without fever, inflammation, redness and swelling
- *Herbal ENT* – ear, nose, throat and lung <u>infection</u>

5. DEFICIENCY

5.1 Yin Deficiency

- *Balance (Heat)* – <u>menopause</u> and other <u>women's disorders</u> with yin deficiency and deficiency heat
- *Blossom (Phase 2)* – female infertility: follicular phase
- *CA Support* – <u>cancer support</u> for weak patients who cannot tolerate chemotherapy or radiation
- *Calm* – <u>stress</u>, <u>irritability</u> and other <u>emotional imbalances</u> because of Liver qi stagnation with underlying deficiency
- *Calm (Jr)* – attention deficit disorder (<u>ADD</u>) or attention deficit hyperactivity disorder (<u>ADHD</u>)
- *Equilibrium* – <u>diabetes</u> with yin deficiency and deficiency heat
- *Flex (CD)* – <u>bi zheng</u> (<u>painful obstruction syndrome</u>) because of deficiency, cold and damp
- *Flex (MLT)* – <u>degeneration</u> of muscle, ligament, tendons and cartilage
- *Flex (SC)* – <u>spasms</u> and <u>cramps</u> caused by Liver yin and blood deficiencies
- *Gastrodia Complex* – <u>hypertension</u> with Liver and Kidney yin deficiencies and Liver yang rising
- *Gentle Lax (Deficient)* – deficient type <u>constipation</u> with heat and dryness in the Large Intestine
- *GI Care* – <u>stomach pain</u>, <u>gastritis</u>, and <u>ulcers</u> with Stomach fire and Stomach yin deficiencies

- *Imperial Tonic* – <u>weak</u> <u>constitution</u> with qi, blood, yin and yang deficiencies
- *Knee & Ankle (Chronic)* – Chronic knee and ankle pain
- *LPS Support* – <u>systemic</u> <u>lupus</u> <u>erythematosus</u> (<u>SLE</u>)
- *Neck & Shoulder (Chronic)* – <u>chronic</u> <u>neck</u> and <u>shoulder</u> <u>pain</u>
- *Nourish* – various signs and symptoms of Liver and Kidney yin deficiencies
- *Osteo 8* – <u>decreased</u> <u>bone</u> <u>density</u> with soreness, weakness and pain
- *Respitrol (CF)* – cough
- *Respitrol (Deficient)* – <u>asthma</u>, <u>dyspnea</u>, <u>cough</u> and other <u>chronic</u> <u>respiratory</u> <u>disorders</u> arising from Lung and Kidney deficiency
- *Thyrodex* – <u>hyperthyroidism</u> because of Liver fire and phlegm stagnation with underlying qi and yin deficiencies
- *Venus* – increases the <u>size</u> and improves the <u>shape</u> of <u>breasts</u>
- *Vital Essence* – <u>male</u> <u>infertility</u>

5.2 Yang Deficiency

- *Adrenoplex* – fatigue, lack of interest, lack of drive and satisfaction, '<u>burned</u> <u>out</u>,' with diminished mental and physical performance
- *Blossom (Phase 3)* – female infertility: ovulatory phase
- *Circulation* – <u>cardiovascular</u> <u>disorders</u> from phlegm and blood stagnation in the chest, with Heart yang deficiency
- *Cordyceps 3* – <u>lung</u>, <u>kidney</u>, <u>immune</u>, <u>reproductive</u>, and <u>chronic</u> <u>fatigue</u> disorders, remedied by tonifying the <u>Lung</u> and <u>Kidney</u> to strengthen the body and relieve underlying coldness and deficiency
- *Imperial Tonic* – <u>weak</u> <u>constitution</u> with qi, blood, yin and yang deficiencies
- *Menotrol* – <u>amenorrhea</u>, <u>infertility</u>, <u>irregular</u>, and <u>delayed</u> <u>or</u> <u>scanty</u> <u>menstruation</u>
- *Neuro Plus* – <u>Alzheimer's</u>, <u>Parkinson's</u>, or <u>stroke</u> <u>complications</u> with deteriorating mental and physical functions (neurodegenerative disorders) because of Kidney deficiency with phlegm and blood stagnation
- *Osteo 8* – <u>decreased</u> <u>bone</u> <u>density</u> with soreness, weakness and pain
- *Thyro–forte* – <u>hypothyroidism</u> with fatigue, lack of energy, coldness of the body
- *Venus* – increases the <u>size</u> and improves the <u>shape</u> of <u>breasts</u>
- *Vitality* – <u>male</u> <u>sexual</u> <u>disorders</u> from deficiencies of Kidney yang and Kidney *jing* (essence)
- *Vital Essence* – <u>male</u> <u>infertility</u>

5.3 Qi Deficiency

- *CA Support* – <u>cancer</u> <u>support</u> for weak patients who cannot tolerate chemotherapy or radiation
- *C/R Support* – <u>generalized</u> <u>deficiency</u> in patients receiving <u>chemotherapy</u> and <u>radiation</u>
- *Cordyceps 3* – <u>lung</u>, <u>kidney</u>, <u>immune</u>, <u>reproductive</u>, and <u>chronic</u> <u>fatigue</u> disorders remedied by tonifying the <u>Lung</u> and <u>Kidney</u> to strengthen the body and relieve underlying coldness and deficiency
- *Flex (MLT)* – <u>degeneration</u> of muscle, ligament, tendons and cartilage
- *GI Tonic* – strengthens <u>Spleen</u> and <u>Stomach</u> to stop <u>diarrhea</u>, <u>indigestion</u>, <u>lethargy</u>, and addresses general disorders of the gastrointestinal tract
- *Immune +* – <u>weakened</u> <u>immune</u> <u>system</u> because of *wei* (defensive) *qi* deficiency
- *Imperial Tonic* – <u>weak</u> <u>constitution</u> with qi, blood, yin and yang deficiencies
- *Respitrol (CF)* – cough
- *Schisandra ZZZ* – <u>fatigue</u> and *shen* (spirit) <u>disturbance</u> with <u>Spleen</u> and Heart deficiencies
- *Vibrant* –<u>fatigue</u> and <u>lack</u> <u>of</u> <u>energy</u> caused by qi deficiency
- *Vital Essence* – <u>male</u> <u>infertility</u>

5.4 Blood Deficiency

- ☯ *Balance (Cold)* – <u>women's</u> <u>disorders</u> characterized by cold and blood deficiency
- ☯ *Blossom (Phase 2)* – female infertility: follicular phase
- ☯ *Enhance Memory* – improves <u>memory</u> and <u>mental</u> <u>functions</u>
- ☯ *Imperial Tonic* – <u>weak</u> <u>constitution</u> with qi, blood, yin and yang deficiencies
- ☯ *Menotrol* – <u>amenorrhea</u>, <u>infertility</u>, <u>irregular</u>, and <u>delayed</u> or <u>scanty</u> <u>menstruation</u>
- ☯ *Osteo 8* – <u>decreased</u> <u>bone</u> <u>density</u> with soreness, weakness and pain
- ☯ *Polygonum 14* – <u>gray</u> <u>hair</u>, <u>hair</u> <u>loss</u>, and other <u>hair</u> <u>disorders</u> because of deficiencies of Liver blood and Kidney *jing* (essence)
- ☯ *Venus* – increases the <u>size</u> and improves the <u>shape</u> of <u>breasts</u>
- ☯ *Vital Essence* – <u>male</u> <u>infertility</u>

6. EXCESS

6.1 Excess Heat

- ☯ *Calm* – <u>stress</u>, <u>irritability</u> and other <u>emotional</u> <u>imbalances</u> from Liver qi stagnation with heat
- ☯ *Calm (ES)* – <u>restlessness</u>, <u>anger</u>, <u>insomnia</u> and <u>severe</u> <u>emotional</u> <u>imbalance</u> because of Liver fire with *shen* (spirit) disturbance
- ☯ *Calm (Jr)* – attention deficit disorder (<u>ADD</u>) or attention deficit hyperactivity disorder (<u>ADHD</u>)
- ☯ *Dermatrol (HZ)* – <u>shingles</u> caused by damp–heat
- ☯ *Dissolve (GS)* – <u>gallstones</u> or <u>cholecystitis</u> arising from damp–heat in the Liver and Gallbladder
- ☯ *Dissolve (KS)* – <u>kidney</u> or <u>urinary</u> <u>stones</u> with difficult urination
- ☯ *Flex (Heat)* – <u>bi</u> <u>zheng</u> (<u>painful</u> <u>obstruction</u> <u>syndrome</u>) because of heat
- ☯ *Flex (Spur)* – resolves <u>bone</u> <u>spurs</u> to alleviate pain and inflammation
- ☯ *Gastrodia Complex* – <u>hypertension</u> with Liver yang rising and underlying Liver and Kidney yin deficiencies
- ☯ *Gentiana Complex* – <u>hypertension</u> and <u>lower</u> <u>jiao</u> <u>disorders</u> from damp–heat and fire in the Liver and Gallbladder channels
- ☯ *Gentle Lax (Excess)* – excess type <u>constipation</u> with heat in the Large Intestine
- ☯ *GI Care* – <u>stomach</u> <u>pain</u>, <u>gastritis</u>, and <u>ulcers</u> with Stomach fire and Stomach yin deficiencies
- ☯ *GI Care II* – <u>diarrhea</u>, foul–smelling stools with burning sensations of the anus, mucus, abdominal discomfort, pain, borborygmus, possible nausea, vomiting and feelings of incomplete defecation
- ☯ *GI Care (UC)* – prevents and treats <u>ulcerative</u> <u>colitis</u> (<u>UC</u>) characterized by diarrhea with mucus, pus and blood
- ☯ *GI Harmony* – prevents and treats <u>irritable</u> <u>bowel</u> <u>syndrome</u> (<u>IBS</u>) by harmonizing the gastrointestinal tract
- ☯ *Herbal ABX* – all types of <u>infection</u> or <u>inflammation</u> with or without fever, inflammation, redness and swelling
- ☯ *Herbal DTX* – pathogenic accumulation of <u>chemical</u> <u>compounds</u> and <u>environmental</u> <u>toxins</u> arising from chronic exposure
- ☯ *Herbal ENT* – ear, nose, throat and lung <u>infection</u>
- ☯ *Herbalite* – <u>obesity</u> <u>with</u> <u>excessive</u> <u>hunger</u> and <u>appetite</u> caused by Stomach heat
- ☯ *Kidney DTX* – <u>nephritis</u> and <u>nephrotic</u> <u>syndrome</u>: increases Kidney ability to <u>excrete</u> and <u>eliminate</u> <u>toxins</u>
- ☯ *Liver DTX* – <u>liver</u> <u>damage</u> <u>with</u> <u>elevated</u> <u>liver</u> <u>enzymes</u> because of toxic damp–heat in the Liver and Gallbladder
- ☯ *LPS Support* – <u>systemic</u> <u>lupus</u> <u>erythematosus</u> (<u>SLE</u>)
- ☯ *Poria XPT* – <u>cough</u> with yellow sputum, arising from heat and phlegm in the Lungs
- ☯ *P–Statin* – <u>benign</u> <u>prostatic</u> <u>hyperplasia</u> (<u>BPH</u>) with dysuria and incontinence

CHINESE DIAGNOSTIC INDEX

- ☙ *Pueraria Clear Sinus* – <u>sinusitis</u>, <u>rhinitis</u>, and other <u>nasal</u> <u>disorders</u> with yellow discharge caused by heat
- ☙ *Resolve (AI)* – resolves hardness and <u>nodules</u> caused by <u>swelling</u> and <u>inflammation</u>
- ☙ *Respitrol (Heat)* – <u>cough</u>, <u>dyspnea</u>, and other <u>respiratory</u> <u>disorders</u> arising from Lung heat
- ☙ *Saw Palmetto Complex* – <u>prostatic</u> <u>enlargement</u> because of damp–heat in the lower *jiao*
- ☙ *Silerex* – <u>rash</u>, <u>itching</u>, and other <u>dermatological</u> <u>disorders</u> caused by heat in the blood
- ☙ *Thyrodex* – <u>hyperthyroidism</u> from Liver fire and phlegm stagnation with underlying qi and yin deficiencies
- ☙ *V–Statin* – <u>vaginitis</u>, <u>pelvic</u> <u>inflammatory</u> <u>disease</u> and <u>urogenital</u> <u>infections</u>

6.2 Excess Cold

- ☙ *Adrenoplex* – fatigue, lack of interest, lack of drive and satisfaction, '<u>burned</u> <u>out</u>,' with diminished mental and physical performance
- ☙ *Circulation* – <u>cardiovascular</u> disorders of phlegm and blood stagnation in the chest, with Heart yang deficiency
- ☙ *Flex (NP)* – <u>peripheral</u> <u>neuropathy</u> with pain, numbness, tingling, swelling and muscle wasting, especially at the extremities
- ☙ *Magnolia Clear Sinus* – <u>allergy</u>, <u>nasal</u> <u>congestion</u> and other <u>nasal</u> <u>disorders</u> from cold and fluid congestion in the Lungs
- ☙ *Menotrol* – <u>amenorrhea</u>, <u>infertility</u>, <u>irregular</u>, and <u>delayed</u> <u>or</u> <u>scanty</u> <u>menstruation</u>
- ☙ *Mense–Ease* – <u>dysmenorrhea</u> with cold and blood stagnation
- ☙ *Respitrol (Cold)* – <u>common</u> <u>cold</u>, <u>flu</u>, <u>runny</u> <u>nose</u>, and other <u>respiratory</u> <u>disorders</u> from Lung cold and phlegm
- ☙ *Venus* – increases the <u>size</u> and improves the <u>shape</u> of <u>breasts</u>

6.3 Stagnation

- ☙ *Back Support (Acute)* – <u>acute</u> <u>lower</u> <u>back</u> <u>pain</u>
- ☙ *Cholisma* – <u>high</u> <u>cholesterol</u> because of accumulation of damp and phlegm
- ☙ *Circulation (SJ)* – moves blood in all three *jiaos*
- ☙ *Corydalin* – <u>headache</u> caused by qi and blood stagnation
- ☙ *Dissolve (KS)* – <u>kidney</u> or <u>urinary</u> <u>stones</u> with difficult urination
- ☙ *Flex (NP)* – <u>peripheral</u> <u>neuropathy</u> with pain, numbness, tingling, swelling and muscle wasting, especially at the extremities
- ☙ *Flex (Spur)* – resolves <u>bone</u> <u>spurs</u> to alleviate pain and inflammation
- ☙ *Herbal Analgesic* – <u>pain</u> in various parts of the body caused by qi and <u>blood</u> <u>stagnation</u>
- ☙ *Menotrol* – <u>amenorrhea</u>, <u>infertility</u>, <u>irregular</u>, and <u>delayed</u> <u>or</u> <u>scanty</u> <u>menstruation</u>
- ☙ *Migratrol* – prevention and treatment of <u>migraine</u> <u>headache</u>
- ☙ *Neck & Shoulder (Acute)* – <u>acute</u> <u>neck</u> and <u>shoulder</u> <u>pain</u>
- ☙ *Neuro Plus* – <u>Alzheimer's</u>, <u>Parkinson's</u>, or <u>stroke</u> <u>complications</u> with deteriorating mental and physical functions (neurodegenerative disorders) because of Kidney deficiency with phlegm and blood stagnation
- ☙ *P–Statin* – for <u>benign</u> <u>prostatic</u> <u>hyperplasia</u> (<u>BPH</u>) with dysuria and incontinence
- ☙ *Resolve (AI)* – resolves <u>hardness</u> and <u>nodules</u> caused by <u>swelling</u> and <u>inflammation</u>
- ☙ *Resolve (Lower)* – <u>fibroids</u>, <u>endometriosis</u>, or <u>infertility</u> because of blood and phlegm stagnation with cold in the lower *jiao*
- ☙ *Resolve (Upper)* – <u>benign</u> <u>breast</u> <u>disorders</u> from stagnation of Liver qi, phlegm, blood and heat
- ☙ *Shine* – <u>depression</u> arising from stagnation of blood, phlegm, food, and Liver qi with heat
- ☙ *Traumanex* – injuries with qi and blood stagnation

CHINESE DIAGNOSTIC INDEX

7. YIN

- ☯ *Back Support (Chronic)* – weakness and pain of the lower back and knees with Kidney deficiency
- ☯ *Balance (Heat)* – menopause and other women's disorders with yin deficiency and deficiency heat
- ☯ *C/R Support* – nausea and vomiting caused by Stomach yin deficiency from chemotherapy and radiation
- ☯ *Calm* – stress, irritability because of Liver qi stagnation with underlying yin deficiency
- ☯ *Calm (Jr)* – attention deficit disorder (ADD) or attention deficit hyperactivity disorder (ADHD)
- ☯ *Equilibrium* – diabetes with yin deficiency and deficiency heat
- ☯ *Enhance Memory* – improves memory and mental functions
- ☯ *Flex (SC)* – spasms and cramps caused by Liver yin and blood deficiencies
- ☯ *Gastrodia Complex* – hypertension with Liver yang rising and underlying Liver and Kidney yin deficiencies
- ☯ *Gentle Lax (Deficient)* – deficient type constipation with heat and dryness in the Large Intestine
- ☯ *GI Care* – stomach pain, gastritis, and ulcers with Stomach fire and Stomach yin deficiencies
- ☯ *Imperial Tonic* – weak constitution with qi, blood, yin and yang deficiencies
- ☯ *Neuro Plus* – Alzheimer's, Parkinson's, or stroke complications with deteriorating mental and physical functions (neurodegenerative disorders) arising from Kidney yin, yang and *jing* (essence) deficiencies with phlegm and blood stagnation
- ☯ *Nourish* – Various signs and symptoms of Liver and Kidney yin deficiencies
- ☯ *Osteo 8* – decreased bone density with soreness, weakness and pain
- ☯ *Polygonum 14* – gray hair, hair loss, and other hair disorders from deficiencies of Liver blood and Kidney *jing* (essence)
- ☯ *Thyrodex* – hyperthyroidism because of Liver fire and phlegm stagnation with underlying qi and yin deficiencies
- ☯ *Venus* – increases the size and improves the shape of breasts

8. YANG

8.1 Excess Yang

- ☯ *Calm* – stress, irritability and other emotional imbalances arising from Liver qi stagnation with heat
- ☯ *Calm (ES)* – restlessness, anger, insomnia and severe emotional imbalance because of Liver fire with *shen* (spirit) disturbance
- ☯ *Calm (Jr)* – attention deficit disorder (ADD) or attention deficit hyperactivity disorder (ADHD)
- ☯ *Dermatrol (HZ)* – shingles caused by damp–heat
- ☯ *Dissolve (GS)* – gallstones or cholecystitis from damp–heat in the Liver and Gallbladder
- ☯ *Dissolve (KS)* – kidney or urinary stones with difficult urination
- ☯ *Gardenia Complex* – excess fire in all three *jiaos*
- ☯ *Gastrodia Complex* – hypertension with Liver yang rising and underlying Liver and Kidney yin deficiencies
- ☯ *Gentiana Complex* – hypertension and lower *jiao* disorders because of damp–heat and fire in the Liver and Gallbladder channels
- ☯ *Gentle Lax (Excess)* – excess type constipation with heat in the Large Intestine
- ☯ *GI Care* – stomach pain, gastritis, and ulcers with Stomach fire and Stomach yin deficiencies
- ☯ *GI Care II* – diarrhea, foul–smelling stools with burning sensations of the anus, mucus, abdominal discomfort, pain, borborygmus, possible nausea, vomiting and feelings of incomplete defecation
- ☯ *Herbal ABX* – all types of infection or inflammation with or without fever, inflammation, redness and swelling

- *Herbal DTX* – pathogenic accumulation of <u>chemical</u> <u>compounds</u> and <u>environmental</u> <u>toxins</u> following chronic exposure
- *Herbal ENT* – ear, nose, throat and lung <u>infection</u>
- *Kidney DTX* – strengthens the <u>kidney</u> and improves its ability to <u>excrete</u> and <u>eliminate</u> <u>toxins</u>
- *Liver DTX* – <u>liver</u> <u>damage</u> <u>with</u> <u>elevated</u> <u>liver</u> <u>enzymes</u> from toxic damp–heat in the Liver and Gallbladder
- *Respitrol (Deficient)* – <u>asthma</u>, <u>dyspnea</u>, <u>cough</u>, and other <u>chronic</u> <u>respiratory</u> <u>disorders</u> caused by deficiencies of the Lung and the Kidney yang
- *Thyrodex* – <u>hyperthyroidism</u> arising from Liver fire and phlegm stagnation with underlying qi and yin deficiencies
- *V–Statin* – <u>vaginitis</u>, <u>pelvic</u> <u>inflammatory</u> <u>disease</u> and <u>urogenital</u> <u>infections</u>

8.2 Deficient Yang

- *Adrenoplex* – fatigue, lack of interest, lack of drive and satisfaction, '<u>burned</u> <u>out</u>,' with diminished mental and physical performance
- *Back Support (Chronic)* – <u>soreness</u> and <u>pain</u> <u>of</u> <u>the</u> <u>lower</u> <u>back</u> and <u>knees</u> with Kidney yang deficiency
- *Circulation* – <u>cardiovascular</u> disorders of phlegm and blood stagnation in the chest with Heart yang deficiency
- *Cordyceps 3* – <u>lung</u>, <u>kidney</u>, <u>immune</u>, <u>reproductive</u>, and <u>chronic</u> <u>fatigue</u> disorders remedied by tonifying the <u>Lung</u> and <u>Kidney</u> to strengthen the body and relieve underlying coldness and deficiency
- *GI Tonic* – strengthens <u>Spleen</u> and <u>Stomach</u> to stop <u>diarrhea</u>, <u>indigestion</u>, <u>lethargy</u>, and addresses general disorders of the gastrointestinal tract
- *Imperial Tonic* – <u>weak</u> <u>constitution</u> with qi, blood, yin and yang deficiencies
- *Menotrol* – <u>amenorrhea</u>, <u>infertility</u>, <u>irregular</u>, and <u>delayed</u> <u>or</u> <u>scanty</u> <u>menstruation</u>
- *Mense–Ease* – <u>dysmenorrhea</u> with cold and blood stagnation and yang deficiency
- *Neuro Plus* – <u>Alzheimer's</u>, <u>Parkinson's</u>, or <u>stroke</u> <u>complications</u> with deteriorating mental and physical functions arising from Kidney yin, yang and *jing* (essence) deficiencies with phlegm and blood stagnation
- *Osteo 8* – <u>decreased</u> <u>bone</u> <u>density</u> with soreness, weakness and pain
- *P–Statin* – <u>benign</u> <u>prostatic</u> <u>hyperplasia</u> (<u>BPH</u>) with dysuria and incontinence
- *Thyro–forte* – <u>hypothyroidism</u> with fatigue, lack of energy, coldness of the body
- *Venus* – increases the <u>size</u> and improves the <u>shape</u> of <u>breasts</u>
- *Vitality* – <u>male</u> <u>sexual</u> <u>disorders</u> from deficiencies of Kidney yang and Kidney *jing* (essence)

II.   *ZANG FU BIAN ZHENG (ORGAN PATTERN DIFFERENTIATION)*

1.   LIVER (WOOD ELEMENT)

- *Balance (Cold)* – <u>women's</u> <u>disorders</u> with deficiencies of the <u>Liver</u> and the <u>Spleen</u>
- *Balance (Heat)* – <u>menopause</u> and other <u>women's</u> <u>disorders</u> with yin deficiency and deficiency heat
- *Calm* – <u>stress</u>, <u>irritability</u> and other <u>emotional</u> <u>imbalances</u> because of Liver qi stagnation with heat
- *Calm (ES)* – <u>restlessness</u>, <u>anger</u>, <u>insomnia</u> and <u>severe</u> <u>emotional</u> <u>imbalance</u> from Liver fire with *shen* (spirit) disturbance
- *Calm (Jr)* – attention deficit disorder (<u>ADD</u>) or attention deficit hyperactivity disorder (<u>ADHD</u>)
- *Calm ZZZ* – <u>insomnia</u> due to stress and deficiency
- *Cholisma (ES)* – <u>high</u> <u>cholesterol</u> with <u>fatty</u> <u>liver</u> and <u>obesity</u>
- *Dermatrol (HZ)* – <u>shingles</u> caused by damp–heat

CHINESE DIAGNOSTIC INDEX

- ❧ *Dissolve (GS)* – gallstones or cholecystitis caused by Liver qi stagnation and damp–heat in the Liver and Gallbladder
- ❧ *Flex (CD)* – *bi zheng* (painful obstruction syndrome) from Liver and Kidney deficiencies
- ❧ *Flex (NP)* – peripheral neuropathy with pain, numbness, tingling, swelling and muscle wasting, especially at the extremities
- ❧ *Flex (SC)* – spasms and cramps caused by Liver yin and blood deficiencies
- ❧ *Gardenia Complex* – excess fire in all three *jiaos*
- ❧ *Gastrodia Complex* – hypertension with Liver yang rising and underlying Liver and Kidney yin deficiencies
- ❧ *Gentiana Complex* – hypertension and lower *jiao* disorders caused by damp–heat and fire in the Liver and Gallbladder channels
- ❧ *GI Care* – gastrointestinal disorders with Liver overacting on the Spleen and the Stomach
- ❧ *GI Harmony* – prevents and treats irritable bowel syndrome (IBS) by harmonizing the gastrointestinal tract
- ❧ *Herbal ABX* – all types of infection or inflammation with or without fever, inflammation, redness and swelling
- ❧ *Herbal DTX* – pathogenic accumulation of chemical compounds and environmental toxins from chronic exposure
- ❧ *Imperial Tonic* – weak constitution with qi, blood, yin and yang deficiencies
- ❧ *Liver DTX* – liver damage with elevated liver enzymes from toxic damp–heat in the Liver and Gallbladder
- ❧ *Menotrol* – amenorrhea, infertility, irregular, and delayed or scanty menstruation
- ❧ *Migratrol* – prevention and treatment of migraine headache
- ❧ *Neck & Shoulder (Chronic)* – chronic neck and shoulder pain
- ❧ *Nourish* – Various signs and symptoms of Liver and Kidney yin deficiencies
- ❧ *Osteo 8* – decreased bone density with soreness, weakness and pain
- ❧ *Polygonum 14* – gray hair, hair loss, and other hair disorders caused by deficiencies of Liver blood and Kidney *jing* (essence)
- ❧ *Resolve (AI)* – resolves hardness and nodules arising from swelling and inflammation
- ❧ *Resolve (Upper)* – benign breast disorders from stagnation of Liver qi, phlegm, blood and heat
- ❧ *Shine* – depression because of stagnation of blood, phlegm, food, and Liver qi with heat
- ❧ *Thyrodex* – hyperthyroidism from Liver fire and phlegm stagnation, with underlying qi and yin deficiencies
- ❧ *V–Statin* – vaginitis, pelvic inflammatory disease and urogenital infections

2. **GALLBLADDER (WOOD ELEMENT)**

- ❧ *Dissolve (GS)* – gallstones or cholecystitis from damp–heat in the Liver and Gallbladder
- ❧ *Gentiana Complex* – damp–heat and fire in the Liver and Gallbladder channels
- ❧ *Herbal ABX* – all types of infection or inflammation with or without fever, inflammation, redness and swelling
- ❧ *Liver DTX* – liver damage with elevated liver enzymes caused by toxic damp–heat in the Liver and Gallbladder
- ❧ *V–Statin* – vaginitis, pelvic inflammatory disease and urogenital infections

3. **HEART (FIRE ELEMENT)**

- ❧ *Balance (Heat)* – menopause and other women's disorders with *shen* (spirit) disturbance, yin deficiency and deficiency heat
- ❧ *Calm (ES)* – restlessness, anger, insomnia and severe emotional imbalance because of Liver fire with *shen* (spirit) disturbance

CHINESE DIAGNOSTIC INDEX

- ☯ *Calm (Jr)* – attention deficit disorder (ADD) or attention deficit hyperactivity disorder (ADHD)
- ☯ *Circulation* – cardiovascular disorders from phlegm and blood stagnation in the chest with Heart yang deficiency
- ☯ *Enhance Memory* – improves memory and mental functions
- ☯ *Schisandra ZZZ* – fatigue and *shen* (spirit) disturbance with Spleen and Heart deficiencies
- ☯ *Shine* – depression from stagnation of blood, phlegm, food, and Liver qi with heat
- ☯ *Thyrodex* – hyperthyroidism because of *shen* (spirit) disturbance, stagnation of Liver fire and phlegm with underlying qi and yin deficiencies

4. SMALL INTESTINE (FIRE ELEMENT)

- ☯ *Herbal ABX* – all types of infection or inflammation with or without fever, inflammation, redness and swelling
- ☯ *GI Care* – gastric or duodenal ulcers caused by Stomach fire
- ☯ *GI Care II* – diarrhea, foul–smelling stools with burning sensations of the anus, mucus, abdominal discomfort, pain, borborygmus, possible nausea, vomiting and feelings of incomplete defecation
- ☯ *GI Harmony* – prevents and treats irritable bowel syndrome (IBS) by harmonizing the gastrointestinal tract

5. SPLEEN (EARTH ELEMENT)

- ☯ *Adrenoplex* – fatigue, lack of interest, lack of drive and satisfaction, 'burned out,' with diminished mental and physical performance
- ☯ *Balance (Cold)* – women's disorders with deficiencies of the Liver and Spleen
- ☯ *C/R Support* – nausea and vomiting associated with Spleen and Stomach deficiencies caused by chemotherapy and radiation
- ☯ *Calm* – gastrointestinal disorders, stress, irritability and other emotional disturbances caused by Liver (wood element) overacting on the Spleen and the Stomach (earth elements)
- ☯ *GI Care* – stomach pain, gastritis or ulcers from heat in the middle *jiao* with Liver overacting on the Spleen and the Stomach
- ☯ *GI Care II* – diarrhea, foul–smelling stools with burning sensations of the anus, mucus, abdominal discomfort, pain, borborygmus, possible nausea, vomiting and feelings of incomplete defecation
- ☯ *GI Care (UC)* – prevents and treats ulcerative colitis (UC) characterized by diarrhea with mucus, pus and blood
- ☯ *GI Harmony* – prevents and treats irritable bowel syndrome (IBS) by harmonizing the gastrointestinal tract
- ☯ *GI Tonic* – strengthens Spleen and Stomach to stop diarrhea, indigestion, lethargy, and addresses general disorders of the gastrointestinal tract
- ☯ *Immune +* – weakened immune system with *wei* (defensive) *qi* deficiency
- ☯ *Imperial Tonic* – weak constitution with qi, blood, yin and yang deficiencies
- ☯ *Menotrol* – amenorrhea, infertility, irregular, and delayed or scanty menstruation
- ☯ *Schisandra ZZZ* – fatigue and *shen* (spirit) disturbance with Spleen and Heart deficiencies

6. STOMACH (EARTH ELEMENT)

- ☯ *Adrenoplex* – fatigue, lack of interest, lack of drive and satisfaction, 'burned out,' with diminished mental and physical performance
- ☯ *C/R Support* – nausea and vomiting associated with chemotherapy and radiation causing Spleen and Stomach deficiencies
- ☯ *Calm* – gastrointestinal disorders from stress from Liver (wood element) overacting on the Spleen and the Stomach (earth elements)

- *Equilibrium* – diabetes with yin deficiency of the Lung, Stomach and Kidneys
- *Gardenia Complex* – excess fire in all three *jiaos*
- *GI Care* – stomach pain, gastritis, and ulcers with Stomach fire and Stomach yin deficiencies
- *GI Care II* – diarrhea, foul–smelling stools with burning sensations of the anus, mucus, abdominal discomfort, pain, borborygmus, possible nausea, vomiting and feelings of incomplete defecation
- *Herbalite* – obesity with excessive hunger and appetite caused by Stomach heat
- *Herbal ABX* – all types of infection or inflammation with or without fever, inflammation, redness and swelling
- *GI Care (UC)* – prevents and treats ulcerative colitis (UC) characterized by diarrhea with mucus, pus and blood
- *GI Harmony* – prevents and treats irritable bowel syndrome (IBS) by harmonizing the gastrointestinal tract
- *GI Tonic* – strengthens Spleen and Stomach to stop diarrhea, indigestion, lethargy, and addresses general disorders of the gastrointestinal tract
- *Nourish (Fluids)* – yin and body fluid deficiency with dryness

7. LUNG (METAL ELEMENT)

- *Cordyceps 3* – lung, kidney, immune, reproductive, and chronic fatigue disorders remedied by tonifying the Lung and Kidney to strengthen the body and relieve underlying coldness and deficiency
- *Equilibrium* – diabetes with yin deficiency of the Lung, Stomach and Kidneys
- *Herbal ABX* – all types of infection or inflammation, with or without fever, inflammation, redness and swelling
- *Herbal DTX* – pathogenic accumulation of chemical compounds and environmental toxins following chronic exposure
- *Herbal ENT* – ear, nose, throat and lung infection
- *Immune +* – weakened immune system with *wei* (defensive) *qi* deficiency
- *Imperial Tonic* – weak constitution with qi, blood, yin and yang deficiencies
- *Lonicera Complex* – common cold, flu, sore throat from invasion of wind–heat
- *Poria XPT* – cough with yellow sputum arising from heat and phlegm in the Lungs
- *Magnolia Clear Sinus* – allergy, stuffy nose and other nasal disorders because of cold and fluid congestion in the Lungs
- *Nourish (Fluids)* – yin and body fluid deficiency with dryness
- *Pueraria Clear Sinus* – sinusitis, rhinitis, and other nasal disorders with yellow discharge caused by heat
- *Respitrol (CF)* – cough
- *Respitrol (Cold)* – common cold, flu, runny nose, and other respiratory disorders from Lung cold and phlegm
- *Respitrol (Deficient)* – asthma, dyspnea, cough and other respiratory disorders arising from deficiencies of the Lung and Kidney yang
- *Respitrol (Heat)* – cough, dyspnea, and other respiratory disorders caused by Lung heat
- *Silerex* – rash, itching, and other dermatological disorders from wind–heat or heat in the blood

8. LARGE INTESTINE (METAL ELEMENT)

- *Gentle Lax (Deficient)* – deficient type constipation with heat and dryness in the Large Intestine
- *Gentle Lax (Excess)* – excess type constipation with heat in the Large Intestine
- *GI Care II* – diarrhea, foul–smelling stools with burning sensations of the anus, mucus, abdominal discomfort, pain, borborygmus, possible nausea, vomiting and feelings of incomplete defecation
- *GI Care (HMR)* – hemorrhoids

- *GI Care (UC)* – prevents and treats ulcerative colitis (UC) characterized by diarrhea with mucus, pus and blood
- *GI Harmony* – prevents and treats irritable bowel syndrome (IBS) by harmonizing the gastrointestinal tract
- *Herbal ABX* – all types of infection or inflammation with or without fever, inflammation, redness and swelling
- *Herbalite* – obesity and constipation with excessive hunger and appetite caused by Stomach heat

9. KIDNEY (WATER ELEMENT)

- *Adrenoplex* – fatigue, lack of interest, lack of drive and satisfaction, 'burned out,' with diminished mental and physical performance
- *Back Support (Chronic)* – chronic back pain and weak knees from Kidney deficiency
- *Balance (Heat)* – menopause and other women's disorders with yin deficiency and deficiency heat
- *Blossom (Phase 1)* – female infertility: menstrual phase
- *Blossom (Phase 2)* – female infertility: follicular phase
- *Blossom (Phase 3)* – female infertility: ovulatory phase
- *Blossom (Phase 4)* – female infertility: luteal phase
- *Cordyceps 3* – lung, kidney, immune, reproductive, and chronic fatigue disorders remedied by tonifying the Lung and Kidney to strengthen the body and relieve underlying coldness and deficiency
- *Dissolve (KS)* – kidney or urinary stones with difficult urination
- *Equilibrium* – diabetes with yin deficiency of the Lung, Stomach and Kidneys
- *Flex (CD)* – bi zheng (painful obstruction syndrome) because of Kidney yin and yang deficiencies
- *Gardenia Complex* – excess fire in all three *jiaos*
- *Gastrodia Complex* – hypertension with Liver yang rising and Liver and Kidney yin deficiencies
- *Herbal DTX* – pathogenic accumulation of chemical compounds and environmental toxins from chronic exposure
- *Kidney DTX* – strengthens the kidney and improves its ability to excrete and eliminate toxins
- *Immune +* – weakened immune system with *wei* (defensive) *qi* deficiency
- *Imperial Tonic* – weak constitution with qi, blood, yin and yang deficiencies
- *Menotrol* – amenorrhea, infertility, irregular, and delayed or scanty menstruation
- *Neuro Plus* – Alzheimer's, Parkinson's, or stroke complications with deteriorating mental and physical functions (neurodegenerative disorders) caused by Kidney deficiency with phlegm and blood stagnation
- *Nourish* – various signs and symptoms of Liver and Kidney yin deficiencies
- *Osteo 8* – decreased bone density with soreness, weakness and pain
- *Polygonum 14* – gray hair, hair loss, and other hair disorders from deficiencies of Liver blood and Kidney *jing* (essence)
- *P–Statin* – benign prostatic hyperplasia (BPH) with dysuria and incontinence
- *Respitrol (Deficient)* – asthma, dyspnea, cough and other respiratory disorders arising from deficiencies of the Lung and Kidney yang
- *Saw Palmetto Complex* – prostatic enlargement because of damp–heat in the lower *jiao*
- *Venus* – increases the size and improves the shape of breasts
- *Vitality* – male sexual disorders from deficiencies of Kidney yang and Kidney *jing* (essence)
- *Vital Essence* – male infertility

CHINESE DIAGNOSTIC INDEX

10. URINARY BLADDER (WATER ELEMENT)

- ☯ *Dissolve (KS)* – kidney or urinary stones with difficult urination
- ☯ *Gentiana Complex* – lower *jiao* disorders of damp–heat and fire in the Liver and Gallbladder channels
- ☯ *Herbal ABX* – all types of infection or inflammation with or without fever, inflammation, redness and swelling
- ☯ *Herbal DRX* – edema and swelling
- ☯ *Neck & Shoulder (Acute)* – acute neck and shoulder pain along the Urinary Bladder channel
- ☯ *Neck & Shoulder (Chronic)* – chronic neck and shoulder pain
- ☯ *P–Statin* – benign prostatic hyperplasia (BPH) with dysuria and incontinence
- ☯ *Saw Palmetto Complex* – prostatic enlargement from damp–heat in the lower *jiao*

III.   *WEI QI YING XUE BIAN ZHENG* (DEFENSIVE, QI, NUTRITIVE, BLOOD DIFFERENTIATION)

1. *WEI (DEFENSE) LEVEL*

- ☯ *C/R Support* – weakened *wei* (defensive) *qi* and generalized deficiency in patients receiving chemotherapy and radiation
- ☯ *Corydalin* – headache because of wind invasion
- ☯ *Dermatrol (PS)* – addresses psoriasis
- ☯ *Herbal ABX* – all types of infection or inflammation with or without fever, inflammation, redness and swelling
- ☯ *Herbal Analgesic* – pain in various parts of the body caused by qi and blood stagnation
- ☯ *Herbal DTX* – pathogenic accumulation of chemical compounds and environmental toxins after chronic exposure
- ☯ *Herbal ENT* – ear, nose, throat and lung infection
- ☯ *Immune +* – weakened immune system with *wei* (defensive) *qi* deficiency
- ☯ *Lonicera Complex* – common cold, flu, sore throat caused by wind–heat
- ☯ *Magnolia Clear Sinus* – allergy, stuffy nose and other nasal disorders because of wind–cold
- ☯ *Migratrol* – prevention and treatment of migraine headache
- ☯ *Neck & Shoulder (Acute)* – acute neck and shoulder pain along the Urinary Bladder channel
- ☯ *Pueraria Clear Sinus* – sinusitis, rhinitis, and other nasal disorders with yellow discharge from wind–heat
- ☯ *Resolve (AI)* – resolves hardness and nodules caused by swelling and inflammation
- ☯ *Respitrol (CF)* – cough
- ☯ *Respitrol (Cold)* – common cold, flu, runny nose, and other respiratory disorders caused by wind–cold
- ☯ *Respitrol (Heat)* – cough, dyspnea, and other respiratory disorders caused by wind–heat
- ☯ *Silerex* – rash, itching, and other dermatological disorders arising from wind–heat

2. *QI (ENERGY) LEVEL*

- ☯ *Calm* – stress, irritability and other emotional imbalances from Liver qi stagnation with heat
- ☯ *Calm (Jr)* – attention deficit disorder (ADD) or attention deficit hyperactivity disorder (ADHD)
- ☯ *Dissolve (GS)* – gallstones or cholecystitis from damp–heat in the Liver and Gallbladder
- ☯ *Flex (Spur)* – resolves bone spurs to alleviate pain and inflammation
- ☯ *Gentiana Complex* – hypertension and lower *jiao* disorders caused by damp–heat and fire in the Liver and Gallbladder channels
- ☯ *Gentle Lax (Excess)* – excess type constipation with heat in the Large Intestine
- ☯ *GI Care* – stomach pain, gastritis, and ulcers with Stomach fire and Stomach yin deficiencies

☾ *GI Care II* – <u>diarrhea</u>, foul–smelling stools with burning sensations of the anus, mucus, abdominal discomfort, pain, borborygmus, possible nausea, vomiting and feelings of incomplete defecation

☾ *GI Care (UC)* – prevents and treats <u>ulcerative</u> <u>colitis</u> (<u>UC</u>) characterized by diarrhea with mucus, pus and blood

☾ *GI Harmony* – prevents and treats <u>irritable</u> <u>bowel</u> <u>syndrome</u> (<u>IBS</u>) by harmonizing the gastrointestinal tract

☾ *GI Tonic* – strengthens <u>Spleen</u> and <u>Stomach</u> to stop <u>diarrhea</u>, <u>indigestion</u>, <u>lethargy</u>, and addresses general disorders of the gastrointestinal tract

☾ *Herbal ABX* – all types of <u>infection</u> <u>or</u> <u>inflammation</u> with or without fever, inflammation, redness and swelling

☾ *Herbal Analgesic* – <u>pain</u> in various parts of the body caused by qi and <u>blood</u> <u>stagnation</u>

☾ *Herbal DTX* – pathogenic accumulation of <u>chemical</u> <u>compounds</u> and <u>environmental</u> <u>toxins</u> caused by chronic exposure

☾ *Herbal ENT* – ear, nose, throat and lung <u>infection</u>

☾ *Herbalite* – <u>obesity</u> <u>with</u> <u>excessive</u> <u>hunger</u> and <u>appetite</u> arising from Stomach heat

☾ *Kidney DTX* – strengthens the <u>kidney</u> and improves its ability to <u>excrete</u> and <u>eliminate</u> <u>toxins</u>

☾ *Liver DTX* – <u>liver</u> <u>damage</u> <u>with</u> <u>elevated</u> <u>liver</u> <u>enzymes</u> caused by Liver and Gallbladder toxic damp–heat

☾ *Migratrol* – prevention and treatment of <u>migraine</u> <u>headache</u>

☾ *P–Statin* – <u>benign</u> <u>prostatic</u> <u>hyperplasia</u> (<u>BPH</u>) with dysuria and incontinence

☾ *Resolve (AI)* – resolves <u>hardness</u> and <u>nodules</u> caused by <u>swelling</u> and <u>inflammation</u>

☾ *V–Statin* – <u>vaginitis</u>, <u>pelvic</u> <u>inflammatory</u> <u>disease</u> and <u>urogenital</u> <u>infections</u>

3. *YING* (NUTRITIVE) LEVEL

☾ *Balance (Heat)* – <u>menopause</u> and other <u>women's</u> <u>disorders</u> with yin deficiency and deficiency heat

☾ *Equilibrium* – <u>diabetes</u> with yin and body fluid deficiencies

☾ *Herbal DTX* – pathogenic accumulation of <u>chemical</u> <u>compounds</u> and <u>environmental</u> <u>toxins</u> arising from chronic exposure

☾ *Kidney DTX* – strengthens the <u>kidney</u> and improves its ability to <u>excrete</u> and <u>eliminate</u> <u>toxins</u>

☾ *LPS Support* – <u>systemic</u> <u>lupus</u> <u>erythematosus</u> (<u>SLE</u>)

☾ *Nourish* – various signs and symptoms of Liver and Kidney yin deficiencies

☾ *Resolve (Lower)* – <u>fibroids</u>, <u>endometriosis</u>, or <u>infertility</u> caused by blood and phlegm stagnation with cold in the lower *jiao*

☾ *Resolve (Upper)* – <u>benign</u> <u>breast</u> <u>disorders</u> arising from stagnation of Liver qi, phlegm, blood and heat

☾ *Silerex* – <u>rash</u>, <u>itching</u>, and other <u>dermatological</u> <u>disorders</u> manifesting heat in the *ying* (nutritive) level

4. *XUE* (BLOOD) LEVEL

☾ *Balance (Heat)* – <u>menopause</u> and other <u>women's</u> <u>disorders</u> with yin deficiency and deficiency heat

☾ *Herbal DTX* – accumulation of <u>chemical</u> <u>compounds</u> and <u>environmental</u> <u>toxins</u> caused by chronic exposure

☾ *Dermatrol (PS)* – addresses psoriasis

☾ *LPS Support* – <u>systemic</u> <u>lupus</u> <u>erythematosus</u> (<u>SLE</u>)

• Please refer to other diagnostic criteria for additional information

CHINESE DIAGNOSTIC INDEX

IV.   *LIU JING BIAN ZHENG* (SIX STAGES DIFFERENTIATION)

1. *TAIYANG*

- ❧ *Corydalin* – taiyang (parietal/occipital) headache
- ❧ *Dermatrol (PS)* – psoriasis
- ❧ *GI Care II* – diarrhea, foul–smelling stools with burning sensations of the anus, mucus, abdominal discomfort, pain, borborygmus, possible nausea, vomiting and feelings of incomplete defecation
- ❧ *Herbal ABX* – all types of infection or inflammation with or without fever, inflammation, redness and swelling
- ❧ *Herbal Analgesic* – pain in various parts of the body because of qi and blood stagnation
- ❧ *Herbal DTX* – pathogenic accumulation of chemical compounds and environmental toxins from chronic exposure
- ❧ *Herbal ENT* – ear, nose, throat and lung infection
- ❧ *Immune +* – weakened immune system with *wei* (defensive) *qi* deficiency
- ❧ *Lonicera Complex* – common cold, flu, sore throat because of wind–heat
- ❧ *Magnolia Clear Sinus* – allergy, stuffy nose, and other nasal disorders caused by wind–cold
- ❧ *Migratrol* – prevention and treatment of migraine headache
- ❧ *Neck & Shoulder (Acute)* – acute neck and shoulder pain along the *taiyang* Urinary Bladder channel
- ❧ *Neck & Shoulder (Chronic)* – chronic neck and shoulder pain along the *taiyang* Urinary Bladder channel
- ❧ *Pueraria Clear Sinus* – sinusitis, rhinitis, and other nasal disorders with yellow discharge because of wind–heat
- ❧ *Respitrol (CF)* – cough
- ❧ *Respitrol (Cold)* – common cold, flu, runny nose, and other respiratory disorders arising from wind–cold
- ❧ *Respitrol (Heat)* – cough, dyspnea, and other respiratory disorders of wind–heat
- ❧ *Silerex* – rash, itching, and other dermatological disorders arising from wind–heat

2. *YANGMING*

- ❧ *Corydalin* – yangming (frontal/orbital) headache
- ❧ *Equilibrium* – diabetes accompanied by Stomach fire and yin deficiency
- ❧ *Gentle Lax (Excess)* – excess type constipation with heat in the Large Intestine [*yangming fu* (hollow organ)]
- ❧ *GI Care* – stomach pain, gastritis, and ulcers with Stomach fire and Stomach yin deficiencies
- ❧ *Herbalite* – obesity with excessive hunger and appetite arising from Stomach heat
- ❧ *Herbal DTX* – pathogenic accumulation of chemical compounds and environmental toxins following chronic exposure
- ❧ *GI Harmony* – prevents and treats irritable bowel syndrome (IBS) by harmonizing the gastrointestinal tract
- ❧ *GI Tonic* – strengthens Spleen and Stomach to stop diarrhea, indigestion, lethargy, and addresses general disorders of the gastrointestinal tract
- ❧ *Herbal DTX* – pathogenic accumulation of chemical compounds and environmental toxins following chronic exposure
- ❧ *Resolve (AI)* – resolves hardness and nodules caused by swelling and inflammation

---

CHINESE DIAGNOSTIC INDEX

3. SHAOYANG

- ☙ **Calm** – <u>stress</u>, <u>irritability</u> and other <u>emotional</u> <u>imbalances</u> from Liver qi stagnation with heat
- ☙ **Calm (Jr)** – attention deficit disorder (<u>ADD</u>) or attention deficit hyperactivity disorder (<u>ADHD</u>)
- ☙ **Corydalin** – *shaoyang* (temporal) <u>headache</u>
- ☙ **Dissolve (GS)** – <u>gallstones</u> or <u>cholecystitis</u> caused by damp–heat in the Liver and Gallbladder
- ☙ **GI Harmony** – prevents and treats <u>irritable</u> <u>bowel</u> <u>syndrome</u> (<u>IBS</u>) by harmonizing the gastrointestinal tract
- ☙ **Herbal DTX** – pathogenic accumulation of <u>chemical</u> <u>compounds</u> and <u>environmental</u> <u>toxins</u> from chronic exposure
- ☙ **Herbalite** – <u>obesity</u> <u>with</u> <u>excessive</u> <u>hunger</u> and <u>appetite</u> arising from heat in the middle *jiao*
- ☙ **Kidney DTX** – strengthens the <u>kidney</u> and improves its ability to <u>excrete</u> and <u>eliminate</u> <u>toxins</u>
- ☙ **Liver DTX** – <u>liver</u> <u>damage</u> <u>with</u> <u>elevated</u> <u>liver</u> <u>enzymes</u> caused by toxic damp–heat in the Liver and Gallbladder
- ☙ **Resolve (AI)** – resolves <u>hardness</u> and <u>nodules</u> arising from <u>swelling</u> and <u>inflammation</u>

4. TAIYIN

- ☙ **GI Tonic** – strengthens <u>Spleen</u> and <u>Stomach</u> to stop <u>diarrhea</u>, <u>indigestion</u>, <u>lethargy</u>, and addresses general disorders of the gastrointestinal tract
- ☙ **Imperial Tonic** – *taiyin* syndrome with <u>Spleen</u> yang deficiency
- ☙ **Herbal DRX** – <u>edema</u> and <u>swelling</u>

5. SHAOYIN

- ☙ **Calm (Jr)** – attention deficit disorder (<u>ADD</u>) or attention deficit hyperactivity disorder (<u>ADHD</u>)
- ☙ **Circulation** – <u>cardiovascular</u> disorders of phlegm and blood stagnation in the chest, with Heart yang deficiency
- ☙ **Corydalin** – *shaoyin* (migraine) <u>headache</u>
- ☙ **Enhance Memory** – improves <u>memory</u> and <u>mental</u> <u>functions</u> deficiencies
- ☙ **Schisandra ZZZ** – <u>fatigue</u> and *shen* (<u>spirit</u>) <u>disturbance</u> characteristic of *shaoyin* syndrome with Heart and <u>Spleen</u>

6. JUEYIN

- ☙ **Corydalin** – *jueyin* (vertex) <u>headache</u>
- ☙ **Migratrol** – prevention and treatment of <u>migraine</u> <u>headache</u>

V. *SAN JIAO BIAN ZHENG* (TRIPLE BURNER DIFFERENTIATION)

1. UPPER *JIAO*

- ☙ **Calm (Jr)** – attention deficit disorder (<u>ADD</u>) or attention deficit hyperactivity disorder (<u>ADHD</u>)
- ☙ **Circulation** – <u>cardiovascular</u> disorders from phlegm and blood stagnation, with Heart yang deficiency
- ☙ **Cordyceps 3** – <u>lung</u>, <u>kidney</u>, <u>immune</u>, <u>reproductive</u>, and <u>chronic</u> <u>fatigue</u> disorders remedied by tonifying the <u>Lung</u> and <u>Kidney</u> to strengthen the body and relieve underlying coldness and deficiency
- ☙ **Dermatrol (PS)** – psoriasis
- ☙ **Enhance Memory** – improves <u>memory</u> and <u>mental</u> <u>functions</u>
- ☙ **Equilibrium** – <u>diabetes</u> characterized by <u>upper</u>, middle or lower

CHINESE DIAGNOSTIC INDEX

- ☙ *Herbal ABX* – all types of <u>infection</u> or <u>inflammation</u> with or without fever, inflammation, redness and swelling
- ☙ *Herbal ENT* – ear, nose, throat and lung <u>infection</u>
- ☙ *Lonicera Complex* – <u>common</u> <u>cold</u>, <u>flu</u>, <u>sore</u> <u>throat</u> because of wind–heat
- ☙ *Poria XPT* – <u>cough</u> with yellow sputum from heat and phlegm in the Lungs
- ☙ *Magnolia Clear Sinus* – <u>allergy</u>, <u>stuffy</u> <u>nose</u> and other <u>nasal</u> <u>disorders</u> because of wind–cold and fluid congestion in the Lungs
- ☙ *Migratrol* – prevention and treatment of <u>migraine</u> <u>headache</u>
- ☙ *Pueraria Clear Sinus* – <u>sinusitis</u>, <u>rhinitis</u>, and other <u>nasal</u> <u>disorders</u> with yellow discharge caused by heat
- ☙ *Resolve (AI)* – resolves <u>hardness</u> and <u>nodules</u> arising from <u>swelling</u> and <u>inflammation</u>
- ☙ *Resolve (Upper)* – <u>benign</u> <u>breast</u> <u>disorders</u> characteristic of stagnation of Liver qi, phlegm, blood and heat
- ☙ *Respitrol (CF)* – cough
- ☙ *Respitrol (Cold)* – <u>common</u> <u>cold</u>, <u>flu</u>, <u>runny</u> <u>nose</u>, and other <u>respiratory</u> <u>disorders</u> from Lung cold and phlegm
- ☙ *Respitrol (Deficient)* – <u>asthma</u>, <u>dyspnea</u>, <u>cough</u> and other <u>respiratory</u> <u>disorders</u> arising from deficiencies of the Lung and Kidney yang
- ☙ *Respitrol (Heat)* – <u>cough</u>, <u>dyspnea</u>, and other <u>respiratory</u> <u>disorders</u> caused by Lung heat
- ☙ *Symmetry* – <u>Bell's</u> <u>palsy</u>, <u>TMJ</u> (temporo-mandibular joint pain), <u>trigeminal</u> <u>neuralgia</u> due to wind
- ☙ *Venus* – increases the <u>size</u> and improves the <u>shape</u> of <u>breasts</u>

2. MIDDLE *JIAO*

- ☙ *C/R Support* – <u>nausea</u>, <u>vomiting</u> and <u>fatigue</u> from chemotherapy and radiation
- ☙ *Calm* – <u>gastrointestinal</u> <u>disorders</u>, stress, irritability and other emotional disturbances arising from Liver (wood element) overacting on the Spleen and the Stomach (earth elements)
- ☙ *Dermatrol (HZ)* – <u>shingles</u> caused by damp–heat
- ☙ *Dissolve (GS)* – <u>gallstones</u> or <u>cholecystitis</u> because of damp–heat in the Liver and Gallbladder
- ☙ *Equilibrium* – <u>diabetes</u> characteristic of Upper, <u>Middle</u> or Lower *xiao ke* (wasting and thirsting) syndrome
- ☙ *GI Care* – <u>stomach</u> <u>pain</u>, <u>gastritis</u>, and <u>ulcers</u> with Stomach fire and Stomach yin deficiencies
- ☙ *GI Care II* – <u>diarrhea</u>, foul–smelling stools with burning sensations of the anus, mucus, abdominal discomfort, pain, borborygmus, possible nausea, vomiting and feelings of incomplete defecation
- ☙ *GI Care (UC)* – prevents and treats <u>ulcerative</u> <u>colitis</u> (<u>UC</u>) characterized by diarrhea with mucus, pus and blood
- ☙ *GI Harmony* – prevents and treats <u>irritable</u> <u>bowel</u> <u>syndrome</u> (<u>IBS</u>) by harmonizing the gastrointestinal tract
- ☙ *GI Tonic* – strengthens <u>Spleen</u> and <u>Stomach</u> to stop <u>diarrhea</u>, <u>indigestion</u>, <u>lethargy</u>, and addresses general disorders of the gastrointestinal tract
- ☙ *Herbal ABX* – all types of <u>infection</u> or <u>inflammation</u> with or without fever, inflammation, redness and swelling
- ☙ *Herbalite* – <u>obesity</u> <u>with</u> <u>excessive</u> <u>hunger</u> and <u>appetite</u> arising from heat in the middle *jiao*
- ☙ *Liver DTX* – <u>liver</u> <u>damage</u> with <u>elevated</u> <u>liver</u> <u>enzymes</u> due to toxic damp–heat in the Liver and Gallbladder
- ☙ *Resolve (AI)* – resolves <u>hardness</u> and <u>nodules</u> caused by <u>swelling</u> and <u>inflammation</u>

3. LOWER *JIAO*

- ☙ *Adrenoplex* – fatigue, lack of interest, lack of drive and satisfaction, '<u>burned</u> <u>out</u>,' with diminished mental and physical performance

---

CHINESE DIAGNOSTIC INDEX

- ☯ *Cordyceps 3* – lung, kidney, immune, reproductive, and chronic fatigue disorders remedied by tonifying the Lung and Kidney to strengthen the body and relieve underlying coldness and deficiency
- ☯ *Dissolve (KS)* – kidney or urinary stones with difficult urination
- ☯ *Equilibrium* – diabetes characteristic of Upper, Middle or Lower *xiao ke* (wasting and thirsting) syndrome
- ☯ *Gentiana Complex* – lower *jiao* disorders of damp–heat and fire in the Liver and Gallbladder channels
- ☯ *Gentle Lax (Deficient)* – deficient type constipation with heat and dryness in the Large Intestine
- ☯ *Gentle Lax (Excess)* – excess type constipation with heat in the Large Intestine
- ☯ *GI Care II* – diarrhea, foul–smelling stools with burning sensations of the anus, mucus, abdominal discomfort, pain, borborygmus, possible nausea, vomiting and feelings of incomplete defecation
- ☯ *GI Care (HMR)* – hemorrhoids
- ☯ *Herbal ABX* – all types of infection or inflammation with or without fever, inflammation, redness and swelling
- ☯ *Herbal DTX* – pathogenic accumulation of chemical compounds and environmental toxins following chronic exposure
- ☯ *Kidney DTX* – strengthens the kidney and improves its ability to excrete and eliminate toxins
- ☯ *Menotrol* – amenorrhea, infertility, irregular, and delayed or scanty menstruation
- ☯ *Mense–Ease* – dysmenorrhea with cold and blood stagnation and yang deficiency
- ☯ *P–Statin* – benign prostatic hyperplasia (BPH) with dysuria and incontinence
- ☯ *Resolve (AI)* – resolves hardness and nodules caused by swelling and inflammation
- ☯ *Resolve (Lower)* – fibroids, endometriosis, or infertility because of blood and phlegm stagnation with cold in the lower *jiao*
- ☯ *Saw Palmetto Complex* – prostatic enlargement arising from damp–heat in the lower *jiao*
- ☯ *Thyro–forte* – hypothyroidism with fatigue, lack of energy, coldness of the body
- ☯ *V–Statin* – vaginitis, pelvic inflammatory disease and urogenital infections
- ☯ *Venus* – increases libido
- ☯ *Vitality* – male sexual disorders from deficiencies of Kidney yang and Kidney *jing* (essence)

VI. QI, BLOOD, BODY FLUIDS AND *JING* (ESSENCE)

1. QI DEFICIENCY

- ☯ *CA Support* – cancer support for weak patients who cannot tolerate chemotherapy or radiation
- ☯ *C/R Support* – weakness and poor appetite associated with qi deficiency caused by chemotherapy or radiation
- ☯ *Cordyceps 3* – lung, kidney, immune, reproductive, and chronic fatigue disorders remedied by tonifying the Lung and Kidney to strengthen the body and relieve underlying coldness and deficiency
- ☯ *Flex (MLT)* – degeneration of muscle, ligament, tendons and cartilage
- ☯ *GI Tonic* – strengthens Spleen and Stomach to stop diarrhea, indigestion, lethargy, and addresses general disorders of the gastrointestinal tract
- ☯ *Immune +* – weakened immune system with *wei* (defensive) *qi* deficiency
- ☯ *Imperial Tonic* – weak constitution with qi, blood, yin and yang deficiencies
- ☯ *Neuro Plus* – Alzheimer's, Parkinson's, or stroke complications with deteriorating mental and physical functions (neurodegenerative disorders) arising from Kidney deficiency with phlegm and blood stagnation
- ☯ *Osteo 8* – decreased bone density with soreness, weakness and pain
- ☯ *Schisandra ZZZ* – fatigue and *shen* (spirit) disturbance with qi, blood, Spleen and Heart deficiencies

CHINESE DIAGNOSTIC INDEX

- ☯ *Thyrodex* – <u>hyperthyroidism</u> because of Liver fire and phlegm stagnation with underlying qi and yin deficiencies
- ☯ *Vibrant* –<u>fatigue</u> and <u>lack of energy</u> characteristic of qi deficiency

2. REVERSED FLOW OF QI

- ☯ *C/R Support* – <u>nausea</u> and <u>vomiting</u> associated with chemotherapy or radiation
- ☯ *GI Care* – <u>acid reflux</u> and <u>belching</u> with Stomach fire and Stomach yin deficiencies
- ☯ *Poria XPT* – <u>cough</u> with yellow sputum from heat and phlegm in the Lungs
- ☯ *Respitrol (CF)* – cough
- ☯ *Respitrol (Cold)* – <u>flu</u>, <u>sneezing</u>, and other <u>respiratory disorders</u> arising from Lung cold and phlegm
- ☯ *Respitrol (Deficient)* – <u>asthma</u>, <u>dyspnea</u>, <u>cough</u> and other <u>respiratory disorders</u> from deficiencies of the Lung and Kidney yang
- ☯ *Respitrol (Heat)* – <u>cough</u>, <u>dyspnea</u>, and other <u>respiratory disorders</u> with Lung heat

3. QI STAGNATION

- ☯ *Back Support (Acute)* – <u>acute pain of the lower back</u>
- ☯ *Blossom (Phase 4)* – female infertility: luteal phase
- ☯ *Calm* – <u>stress</u>, <u>irritability</u> and other <u>emotional disturbances</u> characteristic of Liver (wood element) overacting on the Spleen and Stomach (earth elements)
- ☯ *Calm (ES)* – <u>restlessness</u>, <u>anger</u>, <u>insomnia</u> and <u>severe emotional imbalances</u> arising from Liver qi stagnation and fire with *shen* (spirit) disturbance
- ☯ *Circulation* –<u>cardiovascular</u> disorders of qi, phlegm and blood stagnation in the chest with Heart yang deficiency
- ☯ *Corydalin* – <u>headache</u> typical of qi and blood stagnation
- ☯ *Dissolve (GS)* – <u>gallstones</u> or <u>cholecystitis</u> arising from qi stagnation and damp–heat in the Liver and Gallbladder
- ☯ *Dissolve (KS)* – <u>kidney</u> or <u>urinary stones</u> with difficult urination
- ☯ *Flex (CD)* – *bi zheng* (<u>painful obstruction syndrome</u>) of cold and damp with qi and blood stagnation
- ☯ *Flex (NP)* – <u>peripheral neuropathy</u> with pain, numbness, tingling, swelling and muscle wasting, especially at the extremities
- ☯ *Flex (Heat)* – *bi zheng* (<u>painful obstruction syndrome</u>) typified by heat with qi and blood stagnation
- ☯ *GI Harmony*– <u>irritable bowel syndrome</u> from Liver qi stagnation
- ☯ *Flex (Spur)* – resolves <u>bone spurs</u> to alleviate pain and inflammation
- ☯ *Herbal Analgesic* – <u>pain</u> in various parts of the body affected by qi and <u>blood stagnation</u>
- ☯ *Mense–Ease* – <u>dysmenorrhea</u> with cold, qi and blood stagnation
- ☯ *Migratrol* – prevention and treatment of <u>migraine headache</u>
- ☯ *Neck & Shoulder (Acute)* – <u>acute neck</u> and <u>shoulder pain</u> with qi and blood stagnation
- ☯ *Neck & Shoulder (Chronic)* – <u>chronic neck</u> and <u>shoulder pain</u> from qi and blood stagnation
- ☯ *Neuro Plus* – <u>Alzheimer's</u>, <u>Parkinson's</u>, or <u>stroke complications</u> with deteriorating mental and physical functions (neurodegenerative disorders) because of Kidney deficiency with qi, phlegm and blood stagnation
- ☯ *Resolve (AI)* – resolves <u>hardness</u> and <u>nodules</u> arising from <u>swelling</u> and <u>inflammation</u>
- ☯ *Resolve (Lower)* – <u>fibroids</u>, <u>endometriosis</u>, or <u>infertility</u> created by qi, blood and phlegm stagnation with cold in the lower *jiao*
- ☯ *Resolve (Upper)* – <u>benign breast disorders</u> of stagnation of Liver qi, phlegm, blood and heat
- ☯ *Shine* – <u>depression</u> from stagnation of blood, phlegm, food, and Liver qi with heat

CHINESE DIAGNOSTIC INDEX

❧ *Thyrodex* – <u>hyperthyroidism</u> arising from qi stagnation, Liver fire and phlegm stagnation with underlying qi and yin deficiencies
❧ *Traumanex* – <u>injuries</u> with qi and blood stagnation

4.   QI AND BLOOD STAGNATION

❧ *Arm Support* – <u>shoulder</u>, <u>elbow</u> and <u>wrist</u> pain
❧ *Back Support (Acute)* – <u>acute</u> <u>lower</u> <u>back</u> <u>pain</u>
❧ *Back Support (Chronic)* – <u>chronic</u> <u>lower</u> <u>back</u> <u>pain</u> with Kidney deficiency, qi and blood stagnation
❧ *Back Support (HD)* – back pain due to a <u>herniated</u> <u>disk</u>
❧ *Back Support (Upper)* – <u>upper</u> <u>back</u> <u>pain</u>
❧ *Blossom (Phase 1)* – female infertility: menstrual phase
❧ *Circulation* –<u>cardiovascular</u> disorders of qi, phlegm and blood stagnation in the chest with Heart yang deficiency
❧ *Circulation (SJ)* – moves blood in all three *jiaos*
❧ *Corydalin* – <u>headache</u> typified by qi and blood stagnation
❧ *Flex (CD)* – *bi zheng* (<u>painful</u> <u>obstruction</u> <u>syndrome</u>) from cold and damp with qi and blood stagnation
❧ *Flex (Heat)* – *bi zheng* (<u>painful</u> <u>obstruction</u> <u>syndrome</u>) caused by heat with qi and blood stagnation
❧ *Flex (NP)* – <u>peripheral</u> <u>neuropathy</u> with pain, numbness, tingling, swelling and muscle wasting, especially at the extremities
❧ *Flex (SC)* – muscle <u>spasms</u> and <u>cramps</u> from qi and blood stagnation
❧ *Flex (Spur)* – resolves <u>bone</u> <u>spurs</u> to alleviate pain and inflammation
❧ *Herbal Analgesic* – <u>pain</u> in various parts of the body blocked by qi and <u>blood</u> <u>stagnation</u>
❧ *Knee & Ankle (Acute)* – <u>acute</u> <u>knee</u> <u>and</u> <u>ankle</u> <u>pain</u>
❧ *Knee & Ankle (Chronic)* – <u>chronic</u> <u>knee</u> <u>and</u> <u>ankle</u> <u>pain</u>
❧ *Menotrol* – <u>amenorrhea</u>, <u>infertility</u>, <u>irregular</u>, and <u>delayed</u> <u>or</u> <u>scanty</u> <u>menstruation</u>
❧ *Mense–Ease* – <u>dysmenorrhea</u> with cold, qi and blood stagnation
❧ *Migratrol* – prevention and treatment of <u>migraine</u> <u>headache</u>
❧ *Neck & Shoulder (Acute)* – <u>acute</u> <u>neck</u> and <u>shoulder</u> <u>pain</u> with qi and blood stagnation
❧ *Neck & Shoulder (Chronic)* – <u>chronic</u> <u>neck</u> and <u>shoulder</u> <u>pain</u> with qi and blood stagnation
❧ *Neuro Plus* – <u>Alzheimer's</u>, <u>Parkinson's</u>, or <u>stroke</u> <u>complications</u> with deteriorating mental and physical functions (neurodegenerative disorders) arising from Kidney deficiency with qi, phlegm and blood stagnation
❧ *Resolve (AI)* – resolves <u>hardness</u> and <u>nodules</u> formed by <u>swelling</u> and <u>inflammation</u>
❧ *Resolve (Lower)* – <u>fibroids</u>, <u>endometriosis</u>, or <u>infertility</u> because of qi, blood and phlegm stagnation with cold in the lower *jiao*
❧ *Resolve (Upper)* – <u>benign</u> <u>breast</u> <u>disorders</u> manifesting stagnation of Liver qi, phlegm, blood and heat
❧ *Shine* – <u>depression</u> from stagnation of blood, phlegm, food, and Liver qi with heat
❧ *Symmetry* – <u>Bell's</u> <u>palsy</u>, <u>TMJ</u> (temporo-mandibular joint pain), <u>trigeminal</u> <u>neuralgia</u> due to qi and blood stagnation
❧ *Traumanex* – <u>injuries</u> with qi and blood stagnation

5.   BLOOD DEFICIENCY

❧ *Balance (Cold)* – <u>women's</u> <u>disorders</u> with cold and blood deficiency
❧ *CA Support* – <u>cancer</u> <u>support</u> for weak patients who cannot tolerate chemotherapy or radiation

CHINESE DIAGNOSTIC INDEX

- ❂ **Calm** – <u>stress</u>, <u>irritability</u> and other <u>emotional</u> <u>imbalances</u> caused by Liver qi stagnation with blood deficiency
- ❂ **Dermatrol (PS)** – <u>psoriasis</u>
- ❂ **Flex (SC)** – <u>spasms</u> and <u>cramps</u> arising from Liver yin and blood deficiencies
- ❂ **Imperial Tonic** – <u>weak</u> <u>constitution</u> with qi, blood, yin and yang deficiencies
- ❂ **Menotrol** – <u>amenorrhea</u>, <u>infertility</u>, <u>irregular</u>, and <u>delayed</u> or <u>scanty</u> <u>menstruation</u>
- ❂ **Migratrol** – prevention and treatment of <u>migraine</u> <u>headache</u>
- ❂ **Osteo 8** – <u>decreased</u> <u>bone</u> <u>density</u> with soreness, weakness and pain
- ❂ **Polygonum 14** – <u>gray hair</u>, hair <u>loss</u>, and other <u>hair</u> <u>disorders</u> showing deficiencies of Liver blood and Kidney *jing* (essence)
- ❂ **Schisandra ZZZ** – <u>fatigue</u> and *shen* (spirit) <u>disturbance</u> with qi, blood, Spleen and Heart deficiencies
- ❂ **Venus** – increases the <u>size</u> and improves the <u>shape</u> of <u>breasts</u>

6. BLOOD STAGNATION

- ❂ **Back Support (Acute)** – <u>acute</u> pain <u>of</u> the <u>lower</u> <u>back</u>
- ❂ **Circulation** – <u>cardiovascular</u> disorders of phlegm and blood stagnation in the chest with Heart yang deficiency
- ❂ **Circulation (SJ)** – moves blood in all three *jiaos*
- ❂ **Corydalin** – <u>headache</u> typical of qi and blood stagnation
- ❂ **Flex (CD)** – <u>bi zheng</u> (<u>painful</u> <u>obstruction</u> <u>syndrome</u>) caused by cold and damp with qi and blood stagnation
- ❂ **Flex (Heat)** – <u>bi zheng</u> (<u>painful</u> <u>obstruction</u> <u>syndrome</u>) caused by heat with qi and blood stagnation
- ❂ **Flex (NP)** – <u>peripheral</u> <u>neuropathy</u> with pain, numbness, tingling, swelling and muscle wasting, especially at the extremities
- ❂ **Flex (Spur)** – resolves <u>bone</u> <u>spurs</u> to alleviate pain and inflammation
- ❂ **Herbal Analgesic** – <u>pain</u> in various parts of the body affected by qi and <u>blood</u> <u>stagnation</u>
- ❂ **Menotrol** – <u>amenorrhea</u>, <u>infertility</u>, <u>irregular</u>, and <u>delayed</u> or <u>scanty</u> <u>menstruation</u>
- ❂ **Mense–Ease** – <u>dysmenorrhea</u> with cold, qi and blood stagnation
- ❂ **Migratrol** – prevention and treatment of <u>migraine</u> <u>headache</u>
- ❂ **Neck & Shoulder (Acute)** – <u>acute</u> <u>neck</u> and <u>shoulder</u> <u>pain</u> with qi and blood stagnation
- ❂ **Neck & Shoulder (Chronic)** – <u>chronic</u> <u>neck</u> and <u>shoulder</u> <u>pain</u> from qi and blood stagnation
- ❂ **Neuro Plus** – <u>Alzheimer's</u>, <u>Parkinson's</u>, or <u>stroke</u> <u>complications</u> with deteriorating mental and physical functions (neurodegenerative disorders) because of Kidney deficiency with phlegm and blood stagnation
- ❂ **Notoginseng 9** – stops <u>bleeding</u>
- ❂ **Resolve (AI)** – resolves <u>hardness</u> and <u>nodules</u> caused by <u>swelling</u> and <u>inflammation</u>
- ❂ **Resolve (Lower)** – <u>fibroids</u>, <u>endometriosis</u>, or <u>infertility</u> because of blood and phlegm stagnation with cold in the lower *jiao*
- ❂ **Resolve (Upper)** – <u>benign</u> <u>breast</u> <u>disorders</u> from stagnation of Liver qi, phlegm, blood and heat
- ❂ **Shine** – <u>depression</u> caused by stagnation of blood, phlegm, food, and Liver qi with heat
- ❂ **Traumanex** – <u>injuries</u> with qi and blood stagnation

7. BLEEDING

- ❂ **Gentle Lax (Deficient)** – deficient types of <u>constipation</u> and hemorrhoids arising from heat in the Large Intestine
- ❂ **Gentle Lax (Excess)** – excess types of <u>constipation</u> and hemorrhoids from heat in the Large Intestine

CHINESE DIAGNOSTIC INDEX

- ❧ *GI Care* – <u>gastric</u> and <u>duodenal</u> <u>bleeding</u> because of Stomach fire and Stomach yin deficiencies
- ❧ *GI Care II* – <u>diarrhea</u>, foul–smelling stools with burning sensations of the anus, mucus, abdominal discomfort, pain, borborygmus, possible nausea, vomiting and feelings of incomplete defecation
- ❧ *GI Care (HMR)* – <u>hemorrhoids</u>
- ❧ *GI Care (UC)* – prevents and treats <u>ulcerative</u> <u>colitis</u> (<u>UC</u>) characterized by diarrhea with mucus, pus and blood
- ❧ *Notoginseng 9* – stops <u>bleeding</u>

8. BODY FLUIDS

- ❧ *Equilibrium* – <u>diabetes</u> with body fluid deficiencies
- ❧ *Flex (SC)* – <u>spasms</u> and <u>cramps</u> arising from body fluid deficiencies
- ❧ *Gentle Lax (Deficient)* – deficient type <u>constipation</u> with heat, body fluid deficiency and dryness in the Large Intestine
- ❧ *Gentle Lax (Excess)* – excess type <u>constipation</u> with heat in the Large Intestine
- ❧ *GI Care II* – <u>diarrhea</u>, foul–smelling stools with burning sensations of the anus, mucus, abdominal discomfort, pain, borborygmus, possible nausea, vomiting and feelings of incomplete defecation
- ❧ *Imperial Tonic* – <u>weak</u> <u>constitution</u> with qi, blood, yin and yang deficiencies
- ❧ *Nourish* – Various signs and symptoms of Liver and Kidney yin deficiencies
- ❧ *Nourish (Fluids)* – yin and <u>body</u> <u>fluid</u> <u>deficiency</u> with <u>dryness</u>

9. JING (ESSENCE)

- ❧ *Adrenoplex* – fatigue, lack of interest, lack of drive and satisfaction, '<u>burned</u> <u>out</u>,' with diminished mental and physical performance
- ❧ *Blossom (Phase 2)* – female infertility: follicular phase
- ❧ *Blossom (Phase 3)* – female infertility: ovulatory phase
- ❧ *CA Support* – <u>cancer</u> <u>support</u> for weak patients who cannot tolerate chemotherapy or radiation
- ❧ *Neuro Plus* – <u>Alzheimer's</u>, <u>Parkinson's</u>, or <u>stroke</u> <u>complications</u> with deteriorating mental and physical functions (neurodegenerative disorders) because of wind–stroke, Kidney deficiency with phlegm and blood stagnation
- ❧ *Osteo 8* – <u>decreased</u> <u>bone</u> <u>density</u> with soreness, weakness and pain
- ❧ *Thyro–forte* – <u>hypothyroidism</u> with fatigue, lack of energy, coldness of the body
- ❧ *Vitality* – <u>male</u> <u>sexual</u> <u>disorders</u> from deficiencies of Kidney yang and Kidney *jing* (essence)
- ❧ *Cordyceps 3* – <u>lung</u>, <u>kidney</u>, <u>immune</u>, <u>reproductive</u>, and <u>chronic</u> <u>fatigue</u> disorders remedied by tonifying the <u>Lung</u> and <u>Kidney</u> to strengthen the body and relieve underlying coldness and deficiency
- ❧ *Venus* – increases the <u>size</u> and improves the <u>shape</u> of <u>breasts</u>
- ❧ *Vital Essence* – <u>male</u> <u>infertility</u>

VII. LIU YIN (SIX EXOGENOUS FACTORS)

1. WIND

1.1 Exterior Wind

- ❧ *Corydalin* – <u>headache</u> because of wind
- ❧ *Flex (CD)* – <u>bi</u> <u>zheng</u> (<u>painful</u> <u>obstruction</u> <u>syndrome</u>) that worsens with exposure to wind, cold or damp
- ❧ *Flex (Heat)* – <u>bi</u> <u>zheng</u> (<u>painful</u> <u>obstruction</u> <u>syndrome</u>) from wind, heat and damp

CHINESE DIAGNOSTIC INDEX

- ❧ *Herbal ABX* – all types of infection or inflammation with or without fever, inflammation, redness and swelling
- ❧ *Herbal ENT* – ear, nose, throat and lung infection
- ❧ *Lonicera Complex* – common cold, flu, sore throat arising from wind–heat
- ❧ *Magnolia Clear Sinus* – allergy, stuffy nose and other nasal disorders because of wind–cold
- ❧ *Neck & Shoulder (Acute)* – acute neck and shoulder pain from wind–cold
- ❧ *Pueraria Clear Sinus* – sinusitis, rhinitis, and other nasal disorders with yellow discharge due to wind–heat
- ❧ *Respitrol (Cold)* – common cold, flu, runny nose, and other respiratory disorders from wind–cold
- ❧ *Respitrol (Heat)* – cough, dyspnea, and other respiratory disorders arising from Lung heat
- ❧ *Silerex* – rash, itching, and other dermatological disorders manifesting as wind
- ❧ *Dermatrol (PS)* – addresses psoriasis
- ❧ *Migratrol* – prevention and treatment of migraine headache
- ❧ *Symmetry* – Bell's palsy, TMJ (temporo-mandibular joint pain), trigeminal neuralgia due to wind

1.2 Internal Liver Wind

- ❧ *Calm (Jr)* – attention deficit disorder (ADD) or attention deficit hyperactivity disorder (ADHD)
- ❧ *Gastrodia Complex* – hypertension with Liver wind and underlying Liver and Kidney yin deficiencies
- ❧ *Gentiana Complex* – hypertension and lower *jiao* disorders of damp–heat, fire and wind in the Liver
- ❧ *Neuro Plus* – Alzheimer's, Parkinson's, or stroke complications with deteriorating mental and physical functions (neurodegenerative disorders) because of wind–stroke, Kidney deficiency with phlegm and blood stagnation

2. COLD

- ❧ *Adrenoplex* – fatigue, lack of interest, lack of drive and satisfaction, 'burned out,' with diminished mental and physical performance
- ❧ *Balance (Cold)* – women's disorders characterized by cold and deficiency
- ❧ *Corydalin* – headache caused by cold
- ❧ *Cordyceps 3* – lung, kidney, immune, reproductive, and chronic fatigue disorders remedied by tonifying the Lung and Kidney to strengthen the body and relieve underlying coldness and deficiency
- ❧ *Flex (CD)* – *bi zheng* (painful obstruction syndrome) typified by cold and damp
- ❧ *GI Tonic* – strengthens Spleen and Stomach to stop diarrhea, indigestion, lethargy, and addresses general disorders of the gastrointestinal tract
- ❧ *Herbal Analgesic* – pain in various parts of the body affected by qi and blood stagnation with cold
- ❧ *Magnolia Clear Sinus* – allergy, stuffy nose and other nasal disorders from cold and fluid congestion in the Lungs
- ❧ *Menotrol* – amenorrhea, infertility, irregular, and delayed or scanty menstruation
- ❧ *Mense–Ease* – dysmenorrhea with cold and blood stagnation
- ❧ *Neck & Shoulder (Acute)* – acute neck and shoulder pain
- ❧ *Neck & Shoulder (Chronic)* – chronic neck and shoulder pain
- ❧ *Neuro Plus* – Alzheimer's, Parkinson's, or stroke complications with deteriorating mental and physical functions (neurodegenerative disorders) from Kidney deficiency with phlegm and blood stagnation
- ❧ *Osteo 8* – decreased bone density with soreness, weakness and pain
- ❧ *Resolve (Lower)* – fibroids, endometriosis, or infertility because of blood and phlegm stagnation with cold in the lower *jiao*

CHINESE DIAGNOSTIC INDEX

- *Respitrol (Cold)* – <u>common</u> <u>cold</u>, <u>flu</u>, <u>runny</u> <u>nose</u>, and other respiratory disorders from Lung cold
- *Thyro–forte* – <u>hypothyroidism</u> with fatigue, lack of energy, coldness of the body
- *Venus* – increases the <u>size</u> and improves the <u>shape</u> of <u>breasts</u>

3. SUMMER–HEAT

- *Respitrol (Heat)* – heat in the Lungs
- *GI Care II* – <u>diarrhea</u>, foul–smelling stools with burning sensations of the anus, mucus, abdominal discomfort, pain, borborygmus, possible nausea, vomiting and feelings of incomplete defecation
- *Herbal ABX* – all types of <u>infection</u> or <u>inflammation</u> with or without fever, inflammation, redness and swelling
- *V–Statin* – <u>vaginitis</u>, <u>pelvic</u> <u>inflammatory</u> <u>disease</u> and <u>urogenital</u> <u>infections</u>

4. DAMP

- *Arm Support* – <u>shoulder</u>, <u>elbow</u> and <u>wrist</u> pain
- *Balance (Cold)* – <u>women's</u> <u>disorders</u> affected by cold, damp and water retention
- *Cholisma* – <u>high</u> <u>cholesterol</u> showing accumulation of damp and phlegm
- *Cholisma (ES)* – <u>high</u> <u>cholesterol</u> with <u>fatty</u> <u>liver</u> and <u>obesity</u>
- *Circulation* – <u>cardiovascular</u> <u>disorders</u> of phlegm and blood stagnation in the chest with Heart yang deficiency
- *Dermatrol (HZ)* – <u>shingles</u> caused by damp–heat
- *Dissolve (GS)* – <u>gallstones</u> or <u>cholecystitis</u> caused by damp–heat in the Liver and Gallbladder
- *Dissolve (KS)* – <u>kidney</u> or <u>urinary</u> <u>stones</u> with difficult urination
- *Equilibrium* – <u>diabetes</u> typified by yin deficiency and damp–heat
- *Flex (CD)* – *bi zheng* (<u>painful</u> <u>obstruction</u> <u>syndrome</u>) from cold and damp
- *Gentiana Complex* – <u>hypertension</u> and <u>lower</u> *jiao* <u>disorders</u> arising from damp–heat and fire in the Liver and Gallbladder channels
- *GI Care II* – <u>diarrhea</u>, foul–smelling stools with burning sensations of the anus, mucus, abdominal discomfort, pain, borborygmus, possible nausea, vomiting and feelings of incomplete defecation
- *GI Care (HMR)* – <u>hemorrhoids</u>
- *GI Care (UC)* – prevents and treats <u>ulcerative</u> <u>colitis</u> (<u>UC</u>) characterized by diarrhea with mucus, pus and blood
- *GI Harmony* – prevents and treats <u>irritable</u> <u>bowel</u> <u>syndrome</u> (<u>IBS</u>) by harmonizing the gastrointestinal tract
- *Herbal DRX* – <u>edema</u> and <u>swelling</u>
- *Herbalite* – <u>obesity</u> from damp and Stomach heat characterized by sensations of heaviness and excessive hunger and appetite
- *Liver DTX* – <u>liver</u> <u>damage</u> <u>with</u> <u>elevated</u> <u>liver</u> <u>enzymes</u> caused by toxic damp–heat in the Liver and Gallbladder
- *Kidney DTX* – chronic nephritis or nephritic syndrome
- *Poria XPT* – <u>cough</u> with yellow sputum from heat and phlegm in the Lungs
- *P–Statin* – <u>benign</u> <u>prostatic</u> <u>hyperplasia</u> (<u>BPH</u>) with dysuria and incontinence
- *Resolve (AI)* – resolves <u>hardness</u> and <u>nodules</u> caused by <u>swelling</u> and <u>inflammation</u>
- *Resolve (Lower)* – <u>fibrocystic</u> <u>disorders</u> <u>of</u> <u>the</u> <u>female</u> <u>reproductive</u> <u>organs</u> because of blood, damp, qi and blood stagnation
- *Resolve (Upper)* – <u>benign</u> <u>breast</u> <u>disorders</u> arising from stagnation of Liver qi, phlegm, blood and heat
- *Saw Palmetto Complex* – <u>prostatic</u> <u>enlargement</u> because of damp–heat in the lower *jiao*
- *Shine* – <u>depression</u> from stagnation of blood, damp, food, and Liver qi with heat
- *Silerex* – <u>rash</u>, <u>itching</u>, and other <u>dermatological</u> <u>disorders</u> of heat in the blood with damp

- *Thyrodex* – <u>hyperthyroidism</u> arising from Liver fire and phlegm stagnation with underlying qi and yin deficiencies
- *V–Statin* – <u>vaginitis</u>, <u>pelvic</u> <u>inflammatory</u> <u>disease</u> and <u>urogenital</u> <u>infections</u>

5. DRYNESS

- *Dermatrol (PS)* – <u>psoriasis</u>
- *Gentle Lax (Deficient)* – deficient type <u>constipation</u> with heat and dryness in the Large Intestine
- *Gentle Lax (Excess)* – excess type <u>constipation</u> with heat in the Large Intestine
- *Nourish* – various signs and symptoms of Liver and Kidney yin deficiencies
- *Nourish (Fluids)* – yin and <u>body</u> <u>fluid</u> <u>deficiency</u> with <u>dryness</u>
- *Polygonum 14* – <u>gray hair</u>, <u>hair</u> <u>loss</u>, and other <u>hair</u> <u>disorders</u> from deficiencies of Liver blood and Kidney *jing* (essence)
- *Respitrol (CF)* – <u>cough</u>
- *Respitrol (Deficient)* – <u>asthma</u>, <u>dyspnea</u>, <u>coughing</u> and other <u>respiratory</u> <u>disorders</u> with dryness in the Lung

6. HEAT

6.1 Deficiency Heat

- *Balance (Heat)* – <u>menopause</u> and other <u>women's</u> <u>disorders</u> with yin deficiency and deficiency heat
- *CA Support* – cancer support for weak patients who cannot tolerate chemotherapy or radiation
- *Calm (Jr)* – attention deficit disorder (<u>ADD</u>) or attention deficit hyperactivity disorder (<u>ADHD</u>)
- *Dissolve (KS)* – <u>kidney</u> or <u>urinary</u> <u>stones</u> with difficult urination
- *Equilibrium* – <u>diabetes</u> with yin deficiency and deficiency heat
- *Gentle Lax (Deficient)* – deficient type <u>constipation</u> with heat and dryness in the Large Intestine
- *Gastrodia Complex* – <u>hypertension</u> with Liver yang rising and underlying Liver and Kidney yin deficiencies
- *Herbal ABX* – all types of <u>infection</u> <u>or</u> <u>inflammation</u> with or without fever, inflammation, redness and swelling
- *Herbal DTX* – pathogenic accumulation of <u>chemical</u> <u>compounds</u> and <u>environmental</u> <u>toxins</u> from chronic exposure
- *Kidney DTX* – strengthens the <u>kidney</u> and improves its ability to <u>excrete</u> and <u>eliminate</u> <u>toxins</u>
- *LPS Support* – <u>systemic</u> <u>lupus</u> <u>erythematosus</u> (<u>SLE</u>)
- *Migratrol* – prevention and treatment of <u>migraine</u> <u>headache</u>
- *Nourish* – various signs and symptoms of Liver and Kidney yin deficiencies
- *Neck & Shoulder (Acute)* – <u>acute</u> <u>neck</u> and <u>shoulder</u> <u>pain</u>
- *Resolve (Lower)* – <u>endometriosis</u> with pain and cramps
- *V–Statin* – <u>vaginitis</u>, <u>pelvic</u> <u>inflammatory</u> <u>disease</u> and <u>urogenital</u> <u>infections</u>

6.2 Excess Heat

- *Calm* – <u>stress</u>, <u>irritability</u> and other <u>emotional</u> <u>imbalances</u> from Liver qi stagnation and heat
- *Calm (ES)* – <u>restlessness</u>, <u>anger</u>, <u>insomnia</u> and <u>severe</u> <u>emotional</u> <u>imbalance</u> showing Liver fire with *shen* (spirit) disturbance
- *Dermatrol (HZ)* – <u>shingles</u> caused by damp–heat
- *Dissolve (GS)* – <u>gallstones</u> or <u>cholecystitis</u> formed by damp–heat in the Liver and Gallbladder
- *Dissolve (KS)* – <u>kidney</u> or <u>urinary</u> <u>stones</u> with difficult urination
- *Flex (Heat)* – <u>bi</u> <u>zheng</u> (<u>painful</u> <u>obstruction</u> <u>syndrome</u>) with heat

- *Flex (Spur)* – resolves bone spurs to alleviate pain and inflammation
- *Gardenia Complex* – excess fire in all three *jiaos*
- *Gentiana Complex* – hypertension and lower *jiao* disorders of damp–heat and fire in the Liver and Gallbladder channels
- *Gentle Lax (Excess)* – excess type constipation with heat in the Large Intestine
- *GI Care* – stomach pain, gastritis, and ulcers with Stomach fire and Stomach yin deficiencies
- *GI Care II* – diarrhea, foul–smelling stools with burning sensations of the anus, mucus, abdominal discomfort, pain, borborygmus, possible nausea, vomiting and feelings of incomplete defecation
- *GI Care (HMR)* – hemorrhoids
- *GI Care (UC)* – prevents and treats ulcerative colitis (UC) characterized by diarrhea with mucus, pus and blood
- *GI Harmony* – prevents and treats irritable bowel syndrome (IBS) by harmonizing the gastrointestinal tract
- *Herbalite* – obesity with Stomach heat characterized by excessive hunger and appetite
- *Herbal ABX* – all types of infection or inflammation with or without fever, inflammation, redness and swelling
- *Herbal ENT* – ear, nose, throat and lung infection
- *Liver DTX* – liver damage with elevated liver enzymes from toxic damp–heat in the Liver and Gallbladder
- *Lonicera Complex* – common cold, flu, sore throat caused by wind–heat
- *Poria XPT* – cough with yellow sputum because of heat and phlegm in the Lungs
- *Resolve (AI)* – resolves hardness and nodules formed by swelling and inflammation
- *Resolve (Upper)* – benign breast disorders from stagnation of Liver qi, phlegm, blood and heat
- *Respitrol (Heat)* – cough, dyspnea, and other respiratory disorders of Lung heat
- *Saw Palmetto Complex* – prostatic enlargement because of damp–heat in the lower *jiao*
- *Shine* – depression from stagnation of blood, phlegm, food, and Liver qi with heat
- *Silerex* – rash, itching, and other dermatological disorders arising from heat in the blood
- *Pueraria Clear Sinus* – sinusitis, rhinitis, and other nasal disorders with yellow discharge caused by heat
- *P–Statin* – benign prostatic hyperplasia (BPH) with dysuria and incontinence
- *Thyrodex* – hyperthyroidism from Liver fire and phlegm stagnation with underlying qi and yin deficiencies
- *V–Statin* – vaginitis, pelvic inflammatory disease and urogenital infections

6.3 Toxic Heat

- *CA Support* – cancer support for weak patients who cannot tolerate chemotherapy or radiation
- *GI Care (HMR)* – hemorrhoids
- *Herbal ABX* – all types of infection or inflammation with or without fever, inflammation, redness and swelling
- *Herbal ENT* – ear, nose, throat and lung infection
- *LPS Support* – systemic lupus erythematosus (SLE)

VIII.   *QI QING* (SEVEN EMOTIONS)

1.   JOY

- *Schisandra ZZZ* – excess joy causing *shen* (spirit) disturbance with Spleen and Heart deficiencies

---

CHINESE DIAGNOSTIC INDEX

2. ANGER

- *Balance (Heat)* – menopause and other women's disorders with *shen* (spirit) disturbance, yin deficiency and deficiency heat
- *Calm* – stress, irritability and other emotional disturbances from Liver qi stagnation and heat
- *Calm ZZZ* – insomnia due to stress and deficiency
- *Calm (ES)* – restlessness, anger, insomnia and severe emotional imbalance arising from Liver fire with *shen* (spirit) disturbance
- *Corydalin* – tension headache because of stress
- *Gastrodia Complex* – hypertension with emotional disturbance and Liver yang rising
- *Gentiana Complex* – hypertension and lower *jiao* disorders from damp–heat and fire in the Liver and Gallbladder channels
- *GI Care* – gastrointestinal disorders with Liver overacting on the Spleen and the Stomach
- *GI Care (UC)* – prevents and treats ulcerative colitis (UC) characterized by diarrhea with mucus, pus and blood
- *GI Harmony* – prevents and treats irritable bowel syndrome (IBS) by harmonizing the gastrointestinal tract
- *Liver DTX* – liver damage with elevated liver enzymes from toxic damp–heat in the Liver and Gallbladder
- *Resolve (Upper)* – benign breast disorders because of stagnation of Liver qi, phlegm, blood and heat
- *Shine* – depression from stagnation of blood, phlegm, food, and Liver qi with heat
- *Thyrodex* – hyperthyroidism caused by Liver fire and phlegm stagnation with underlying qi and yin deficiencies

3. MELANCHOLY

- *Liver DTX* – liver damage with elevated liver enzymes from toxic damp–heat in the Liver and Gallbladder
- *Shine* – depression arising from stagnation of blood, phlegm, food, and Liver qi with heat

4. MEDITATION (OVER–THINKING)

- *Enhance Memory* – improves memory and mental functions
- *Schisandra ZZZ* – fatigue and *shen* (spirit) disturbance with Spleen and Heart deficiencies
- *Shine* – depression arising from stagnation of blood, phlegm, food, and Liver qi with heat

5. GRIEF

- *Shine* – depression because of stagnation of blood, phlegm, food, and Liver qi with heat

6. FEAR – Refer to other diagnostic criteria for additional information

7. FRIGHT – Refer to other diagnostic criteria for additional information

IX. OTHER FACTORS

1. FOOD (DIET)

- *Dissolve (GS)* – gallstones or cholecystitis formed by excessive consumption of fatty and greasy foods

---

CHINESE DIAGNOSTIC INDEX

- ☯ *Equilibrium* – <u>diabetes</u> with improper dietary intake
- ☯ *Gentle Lax (Excess)* – excess type <u>constipation</u> with heat and food stagnation
- ☯ *GI Care* – <u>gastrointestinal</u> <u>disorders</u> arising from improper diet
- ☯ *GI Care II* – <u>diarrhea</u>, foul–smelling stools with burning sensations of the anus, mucus, abdominal discomfort, pain, borborygmus, possible nausea, vomiting and feelings of incomplete defecation
- ☯ *GI Care (UC)* – prevents and treats <u>ulcerative</u> <u>colitis</u> (<u>UC</u>) characterized by diarrhea with mucus, pus and blood
- ☯ *GI Harmony* – prevents and treats <u>irritable</u> <u>bowel</u> <u>syndrome</u> (<u>IBS</u>) by harmonizing the gastrointestinal tract
- ☯ *GI Tonic* – strengthens <u>Spleen</u> and <u>Stomach</u> to stop <u>diarrhea</u>, <u>indigestion</u>, <u>lethargy</u>, and addresses general disorders of the gastrointestinal tract
- ☯ *Herbal ABX* – all types of <u>infection</u> or <u>inflammation</u> with or without fever, inflammation, redness and swelling
- ☯ *Herbal DTX* – pathogenic accumulation of <u>chemical</u> <u>compounds</u> and <u>environmental</u> <u>toxins</u> from chronic exposure
- ☯ *Herbalite* – <u>obesity</u> <u>with</u> <u>excessive</u> <u>hunger</u> and <u>appetite</u>
- ☯ *Liver DTX* – <u>liver</u> <u>damage</u> with <u>elevated</u> <u>liver</u> <u>enzymes</u> because of toxic damp–heat in the Liver and Gallbladder
- ☯ *Shine* – <u>depression</u> from stagnation of blood, phlegm, food, and Liver qi with heat

2. TRAUMATIC INJURIES

- ☯ *Arm Support* – <u>shoulder</u>, <u>elbow</u> and <u>wrist</u> pain
- ☯ *Back Support (Acute)* – <u>acute</u> <u>pain</u> of the <u>lower</u> <u>back</u> with qi and blood stagnation
- ☯ *Back Support (Chronic)* – <u>chronic</u> <u>lower</u> <u>back</u> <u>pain</u> with Kidney deficiency, qi and blood stagnation
- ☯ *Back Support (Upper)* – <u>Upper</u> <u>back</u> <u>pain</u>, <u>rib</u> injury, thoracic pain
- ☯ *Corydalin* – <u>headache</u> caused by injuries
- ☯ *Flex (CD)* – <u>bi zheng</u> (painful <u>obstruction</u> <u>syndrome</u>) because of cold and deficiency
- ☯ *Flex (MLT)* – <u>degeneration</u> of muscle, ligament, tendons and cartilage
- ☯ *Flex (NP)* – <u>peripheral</u> <u>neuropathy</u> with pain, numbness, tingling, swelling and muscle wasting especially at the extremities
- ☯ *Flex (Heat)* – <u>bi zheng</u> (painful <u>obstruction</u> <u>syndrome</u>) from heat
- ☯ *Flex (SC)* – muscle <u>spasms</u> and <u>cramps</u> arising from qi and blood stagnation
- ☯ *Flex (Spur)* – resolves <u>bone</u> <u>spurs</u> to alleviate pain and inflammation
- ☯ *Herbal Analgesic* – <u>pain</u> in various parts of the body affected by qi and <u>blood</u> <u>stagnation</u>
- ☯ *Knee & Ankle (Acute)* – Acute knee and ankle pain
- ☯ *Knee & Ankle (Chronic)* – Chronic knee and ankle pain
- ☯ *Neck & Shoulder (Acute)* – <u>acute</u> <u>neck</u> and <u>shoulder</u> <u>pain</u> with qi and blood stagnation
- ☯ *Neck & Shoulder (Chronic)* – <u>chronic</u> <u>neck</u> and <u>shoulder</u> <u>pain</u> caused by qi and blood stagnation
- ☯ *Migratrol* – prevention and treatment of <u>migraine</u> <u>headache</u>
- ☯ *Neuro Plus* – <u>Alzheimer's</u>, <u>Parkinson's</u>, or <u>stroke</u> <u>complications</u> with deteriorating mental and physical functions (neurodegenerative disorders after stroke) because of Kidney deficiency with phlegm and blood stagnation
- ☯ *Notoginseng 9* – stops <u>bleeding</u>
- ☯ *Osteo 8* – <u>decreased</u> <u>bone</u> <u>density</u> with soreness, weakness and pain
- ☯ *Traumanex* – <u>injuries</u> with qi and blood stagnation

CHINESE DIAGNOSTIC INDEX

3. PHLEGM

- *Cholisma* – high cholesterol because of accumulation of damp and phlegm
- *Cholisma (ES)* – high cholesterol with fatty liver and obesity
- *Circulation* – cardiovascular disorders of phlegm and blood stagnation in the chest with Heart yang deficiency
- *Poria XPT* – cough with yellow sputum from heat and phlegm in the Lungs
- *Neuro Plus* – Alzheimer's, Parkinson's, or stroke complications with deteriorating mental and physical functions (neurodegenerative disorders) because of Kidney deficiency with phlegm and blood stagnation
- *P–Statin* – benign prostatic hyperplasia (BPH) with dysuria and incontinence
- *Pueraria Clear Sinus* – sinusitis, rhinitis, and other nasal disorders with yellow discharge caused by heat and phlegm
- *Resolve (AI)* – resolves hardness and nodules formed by swelling and inflammation
- *Resolve (Lower)* – fibroids, endometriosis, or infertility from blood and phlegm stagnation with cold in the lower *jiao*
- *Resolve (Upper)* – benign breast disorders of stagnation of Liver qi, phlegm, blood and heat
- *Respitrol (CF)* – cough
- *Respitrol (Cold)* – common cold, flu, runny nose, and other respiratory disorders from Lung cold and phlegm
- *Respitrol (Deficient)* – asthma, dyspnea, cough and other chronic respiratory disorders with phlegm accumulation because of Lung and Kidney deficiencies
- *Respitrol (Heat)* – cough, dyspnea, and other respiratory disorders of Lung heat and phlegm
- *Shine* – depression from stagnation of blood, phlegm, food, and Liver qi with heat
- *Thyrodex* – hyperthyroidism because of Liver fire and phlegm stagnation with underlying qi and yin deficiencies

4. *BI ZHENG* (PAINFUL OBSTRUCTION SYNDROME)

- *Back Support (Acute)* – acute pain of the lower back
- *Back Support (Chronic)* – chronic lower back pain with Kidney deficiency, qi and blood stagnation
- *Back Support (Upper)* – upper back pain
- *Flex (CD)* – bi zheng (painful obstruction syndrome) because of cold and damp with qi and blood stagnation
- *Flex (GT)* – gout
- *Flex (Heat)* – bi zheng (painful obstruction syndrome) from heat with qi and blood stagnation
- *Flex (MLT)* – degeneration of muscle, ligament, tendons and cartilage
- *Flex (NP)* – peripheral neuropathy with pain, numbness, tingling, swelling and muscle wasting, especially at the extremities
- *Flex (Spur)* – Pain of bone spurs
- *Herbal Analgesic* – pain in various parts of the body affected by qi and blood stagnation
- *Knee and Ankle (Acute)* – acute knee and ankle pain
- *Knee and Ankle (Chronic)* – chronic knee and ankle pain
- *Neck & Shoulder (Acute)* – acute neck and shoulder pain with qi and blood stagnation
- *Neck & Shoulder (Chronic)* – chronic neck and shoulder pain from qi and blood stagnation
- *Neuro Plus* – Alzheimer's, Parkinson's, or stroke complications with deteriorating mental and physical functions (neurodegenerative disorders) arising from Kidney deficiency with phlegm and blood stagnation

CHINESE DIAGNOSTIC

5. *SHEN* (SPIRIT)

- ☺ *Calm* – <u>stress</u>, <u>irritability</u>, and other <u>emotional</u> <u>imbalances</u> arising from Liver qi stagnation with *shen* (spirit) disturbance
- ☺ *Calm (ES)* – <u>restlessness</u>, <u>anger</u>, <u>insomnia</u> and <u>severe</u> <u>emotional</u> <u>imbalance</u> because of Liver fire with *shen* (spirit) disturbance
- ☺ *Calm (Jr)* – attention deficit disorder (<u>ADD</u>) or attention deficit hyperactivity disorder (<u>ADHD</u>)
- ☺ *Calm ZZZ* – <u>insomnia</u> due to stress and deficiency
- ☺ *Enhance Memory* – improves <u>memory</u> and <u>mental</u> <u>functions</u>
- ☺ *GI Harmony* – <u>irritable</u> <u>bowel</u> <u>syndrome</u> from Liver qi stagnation
- ☺ *Neuro Plus* – <u>Alzheimer's</u>, <u>Parkinson's</u>, or <u>stroke</u> <u>complications</u> with deteriorating mental and physical functions (neurodegenerative disorders) arising from Kidney deficiency with phlegm and blood stagnation
- ☺ *Schisandra ZZZ* – <u>fatigue</u> and *shen* (spirit) disturbance with qi, blood, Spleen and Heart deficiencies
- ☺ *Shine* – <u>depression</u> from stagnation of blood, phlegm, food, and Liver qi with heat
- ☺ *Thyrodex* – <u>hyperthyroidism</u> because of *shen* (spirit) disturbance, Liver fire and phlegm stagnation with underlying qi and yin deficiencies

Section 4

Drug – Herb Index

中西藥索引

INTRODUCTION

It is estimated that 25% of all drugs originate from natural sources. From this information, we can draw two conclusions. One, herbal medicine possesses tremendous healing powers. Two, the use of herbal medicine should never be taken lightly. Even though herbs are classified by the U.S. Food and Drug Administration as "dietary supplements," they do possess strong medicinal properties. When used correctly, they can treat a wide variety of diseases and ailments; but if used incorrectly, they may contribute to unwanted side effects and adverse reactions.

The ultimate responsibility of a health care practitioner is to prevent illness and heal individuals who have become ill or injured. We are blessed today with a wide selection of treatment modalities, including herbs and drugs. It is our duty as health care practitioners to inform the patients of the treatment options available, as well as the advantages and disadvantages of each course of action.

In recent years the use of Chinese herbs has become a more and more popular option. To facilitate professional understanding of the choices between drugs and herbs, we have created this section entitled the *Drug-Herb Index*. Our goal in creating this section is to point out the similarities between drug and herbal treatments, so if a patient wishes to discontinue drug treatment, the practitioner has alternative treatment options available. *Knowing herbal alternatives to drugs gives the practitioner treatment options so they can decide with their patients on the best therapy possible.*

There are two sections in the Drug-Herb Index:

1. **Recognition and Prevention of Herb-Drug Interactions:**
   This section includes an excerpt on the fundamental concepts of herb-drug from *Chinese Medical Herbology and Pharmacology* published by Art of Medicine Press, Inc. It also includes a chart of drugs that have higher risks of interactions with herbs. It is important to note that the study of herb-drug interaction is still in its infancy, and the absence of information does not imply lack of interactions. Rather, the practitioners are strongly urged to check other sources for more detailed and updated information.

2. **Drug-Herb Index:**
   Drugs are listed alphabetically according to **Brand Names** or *Generic Names*. The *"Clinical Application"* column describes common uses of each drug. The *"Herb Alternative"* column lists the herbal formula having functions similar to the drug. Detailed information on the herbal formula(s) can be found in Section 5 Exemplar Formulas.

This section provides valuable information for doctors and patients who prefer to use herbs rather than drugs, or to use herbs as supplements to the regular prescription medication. The indexes compare the similarities between drugs and herbs. However, it is important to note that the indexes do not imply therapeutic equivalence, and the herbal alternatives as listed are not substitutes for their corresponding drugs. Informed professional judgment and careful evaluation must be exercised prior to recommending any herbal formulas to patients.

DRUG / HERB

RECOGNITION OF DRUGS WITH HIGHER RISK OF INTERACTION

The practice of medicine is now at a crossroad: countless patients are being treated simultaneously with both Western and Oriental medicine. It is quite common for a patient to seek herbal treatment while taking several prescription medications. According to Journal of American Medical Association (JAMA), an estimated 15 million adults in the United States (representing 18.4% of all prescription pharmaceutical users) took prescription drugs concurrently with herbal remedies and/or vitamins in 1997.[1]

As the general public grows increasingly open to the use of herbs and supplements, both patients and the health professionals who care for them are becoming more alert to the potential for occasional adverse herb-drug interactions. Safety has become a major topic of discussion. Even though herbal remedies are classified as dietary supplements, it must be noted that if used incorrectly, herbs, like any substance, may affect patients adversely. The safest route of access to herbal therapy is through a well-qualified herbalist.

Although Chinese herbal medicine has been prescribed safely by professionals in the West for many years now and a great deal of research has been amassed in China, there are still few formal studies published in English to document the safety and efficacy of combining herbs with prescription drugs. Some questions posed by Western healthcare professionals or patients are difficult to answer quickly with documented specifics. However, with some general insights into pharmacology, one can foresee possible interactions and take appropriate precautions to prevent incompatible combinations.

The concept of 'interaction' refers to the possibility that, when two (or more) substances are given concurrently, one substance may interact with another, or alter its bioavailability or clinical action. The net result may be an increase or a decrease in the effectiveness of one or both substances. It is important to note that interactions may yield positive effects (achieving better therapeutic effects at lower dosage) or negative results (creating unwanted side effects or adverse reactions). Most of the possible interactions may be classified in two major categories: pharmacokinetic and pharmacodynamic.[2,3]

PHARMACOKINETIC INTERACTIONS

'Pharmacokinetic interaction' refers to the fluctuation in bioavailability of herb/drug molecules in the body as a result of changes in absorption, distribution, metabolism and elimination.[4,5]

Absorption

Absorption is the term that describes the process of the physical passage of herbs or drugs from the outside to the inside of the body. The majority of all absorption occurs in the intestines, where herbs or drugs must pass through the intestinal wall to enter the bloodstream. Several mechanisms may interfere with the absorption of drugs through the intestines.[6,7]

The absorption of herbs may be adversely affected if herbs are administered with drugs that may promote binding in the gastrointestinal (G.I.) tract. Drugs such as cholestyramine (Questran), colestipol (Colestid) and sucralfate (Carafate) may bind to certain herbs, forming an insoluble complex that decreases absorption of both substances. Because of the large size of the insoluble complex, few or no molecules of either substance pass through the intestinal wall.[8,9,10]

Herb absorption may be adversely affected in the presence of drugs that change the pH of the stomach. Antacids, cimetidine (Tagamet), famotidine (Pepcid), nizatidine (Axid), ranitidine (Zantac) and omeprazole (Prilosec) may neutralize, decrease or inhibit the secretion of stomach acids.[11,12] With this subsequent decrease in stomach acidity,

RECOGNITION OF DRUGS WITH HIGHER RISK OF INTERACTION

herbs may not be broken down properly in the stomach, leading to poor absorption in the intestines. To minimize this interaction, herbs are best taken separately from these drugs by approximately two hours.

Drugs that affect gastrointestinal motility may also affect the absorption of herbs. G.I. motility is the rate at which the intestines contract to push food products from the stomach to the rectum. Slower G.I. motility means that the herbs stay in the intestines for a longer period of time, thereby increasing the potential absorption. Conversely, more rapid G.I. motility means that the herbs stay in the intestines for a shorter time, which may decrease absorption. Drugs such as haloperidol (Haldol) decrease G.I. motility and may increase herb absorption; while drugs such as metoclopramide (Reglan) increase G.I. motility and possibly decrease herb absorption.

Therefore, it may be necessary to decrease the dosage of herbs when the patient is taking a drug that decreases G.I. motility and increases overall absorption. Likewise, it is probably helpful to increase the dosage of herbs when the patient is taking a drug that increases G.I. motility and thus decreases overall absorption.

Distribution

After absorption, herbs or drugs must be delivered to the targeted area in order to exert their influence. 'Distribution' refers to the processes by which herbs or drugs (once absorbed) are carried and released to different parts of the body. Currently, it appears that the majority of herbs and drugs do not have any clinically-significant interactions affecting distribution and thus can safely be taken together. The exception seems to be if a drug has a narrow range-of-safety index, and is highly protein-bound, in which case interaction with other substances might occur during the distribution phase. Examples of drugs that have both a narrow range-of-safety index and a high protein-bound ratio include warfarin (Coumadin) and phenytoin (Dilantin). Unfortunately, it is very difficult to predict whether an individual herb will interact with either one of these drugs because there are no known tests or experiments documenting such interactions.[13,14]

Metabolism

Once metabolized by the liver, most herbs and drugs become inactive derivatives. The rate at which the liver metabolizes a substance determines the length of time it stays active in the body. If the liver were induced to speed up its metabolic rate, herbs and drugs would be deactivated at a more rapid pace, and the overall effectiveness of ingested substances would be lower. On the other hand, if the liver were made to slow its metabolism, herbs and drugs would be deactivated at a slower pace and the overall impact of the substances would be greater.

In general, drugs that induce greater liver metabolism do not exert an immediate effect. The metabolism rate of the liver changes slowly, over several weeks. Therefore, the effect of accelerated liver metabolism is not seen until weeks after the initiation of drug therapy. Some examples of pharmaceuticals that speed hepatic metabolism are: phenytoin (Dilantin), carbamazepine (Tegretol), phenobarbitals and rifampin (Rifadin).[15,16] Therefore, herbs given in the presence of one of these products may be deactivated more rapidly, and their overall effectiveness lowered. Under these circumstances, a higher dose of herbs may be required to achieve the desired effect.

In great contrast, drugs that inhibit liver metabolism have an immediate onset of action. The rate of liver metabolism may be greatly impaired within a few days. Pharmaceuticals that slow or inhibit liver metabolism include: cimetidine (Tagamet), erythromycin, ethanol, fluconazole (Diflucan), itraconazole (Sporanox) and ketoconazole (Nizoral), among others.[17,18] When a patient takes these drugs concurrently with herbs, there is a higher risk of herbal components accumulating in the body, as the ability of the liver to neutralize them is compromised. If the

DRUG / HERB

RECOGNITION OF DRUGS WITH HIGHER RISK OF INTERACTION

herbs are metabolized more slowly, their overall effectiveness may be prolonged. In this case, one may need to lower the dosage of herbs to avoid unwanted side effects.

Depending on the half-life in the body of drugs that influence liver metabolism, it may be necessary to increase or decrease the dosages of herbs for weeks or even months after discontinuation of the pharmaceutical substance, along with consistent monitoring.

Elimination

While the liver neutralizes incoming drugs and herbs, the kidneys are responsible for eliminating the substances and their metabolites from the body. If the kidneys are damaged, then the rate of elimination is slowed, leading to an accumulation of active substances in the body. Important examples of drugs that damage the kidneys include amphotericin B, methotrexate, tobramycin and gentamicin.[19,20] As a safety precaution, when prescribing herbs for a patient who is currently taking or has recently taken one of these drugs, it may be wise to lower the dose of herbs to avoid unnecessary and unwanted side effects.

SUMMARY OF PHARMACOKINETIC INTERACTIONS

The pharmacokinetic interactions listed above include both theoretical and actual interactions. Though such interactions are possible, the extent and severity of each interaction will vary depending on the specific circumstances, such as the dosages of all substances, the inherent sensitivity of each patient, individual body weight, and metabolic rate.

PHARMACODYNAMIC INTERACTIONS

The study of pharmacodynamics gives us insight into the dynamic behavior of drugs inside the human body. The phrase 'pharmacodynamic interactions' refers in our context to fluctuations in the bioavailability of ingested substances as a result of synergistic or antagonistic interactions between herb and drug molecules. Pharmacodynamic interactions are generally more difficult to predict and prevent than pharmacokinetic interactions. Most of the currently-known pharmacodynamic interactions have been documented through actual cases, not by laboratory experiments. The best way to prevent pharmacodynamic interactions is to follow the patient closely and monitor all clinical signs and symptoms, and particularly any abnormal reactions.

A *synergistic* interaction occurs when two drugs with similar properties show an additive or even exponential increase in clinical impact when given together. An *antagonistic* interaction occurs when two drugs with similar properties are administered simultaneously and show lessened or no clinical effectiveness.[21]

Synergistic or antagonistic interactions may occur with any concurrent use of medicinal substances, regardless of whether they are herbs, drugs, or both.

Herb-to-Herb Interactions

Oriental Medicine has tracked cases of herb-to-herb pharmacodynamic interactions for centuries. The additive effect is generally referred to as *xiang xu* (mutual accentuation) or *xiang shi* (mutual enhancement), such as takes place in the combination of *Shi Gao* (Gypsum Fibrosum) and *Zhi Mu* (Radix Anemarrhenae) to clear heat and purge fire. The antagonistic effect is generally referred to as *xiang wei* (mutual counteraction), *xiang sha* (mutual suppression) or

RECOGNITION OF DRUGS WITH HIGHER RISK OF INTERACTION

xiang wu (mutual antagonism), such as happens in the combination of *Lai Fu Zi* (Semen Raphani) and *Ren Shen* (Radix Ginseng), in which the therapeutic action of the latter herb is decreased by the addition of *Lai Fu Zi*.

Classic Chinese texts describe numerous other herb-to-herb interactions, such as the *Shi Ba Fan* (Eighteen Incompatibles) and *Shi Jiu Wei* (Nineteen Counteractions), discussed in greater detail in most textbooks of Chinese herbology. Ill-advised combinations of these herbs will likely lead to adverse side effects and/or toxic reactions.

Herb-to-Drug Interactions

Pharmacodynamic herb-to-drug interactions are best identified by analyzing the therapeutic profile of the herbs as well as that of the drugs. Concurrent use of herbs and drugs with similar therapeutic actions poses potential for herb-drug interactions. In these cases, the increased potency of treatment may interfere with optimal outcome, as the desired effect becomes less predictable and harder to obtain with precision. The highest risk of clinically-significant interactions occurs between herbs and drugs that have **sympathomimetic, anticoagulant, antiplatelet, diuretic** and **antidiabetic** effects.[22]

Herbs that exert **sympathomimetic** effects may interfere with antihypertensive and antiseizure drugs. The classic example of this type of herb is *Ma Huang* (Herba Ephedrae), containing ephedrine, pseudoephedrine, norephedrine and other ephedrine alkaloids. *Ma Huang* may interact with other drugs and disease conditions and should always be used with caution in patients vulnerable to hypertension, seizures, diabetes, thyroid conditions, and similar regulatory imbalances.[23]

Herbs with **anticoagulant** and **antiplatelet** effects include herbs that have blood-activating and blood-stasis-removing functions, such as *Dan Shen* (Radix Salviae Miltiorrhizae), *Dang Gui* (Radix Angelicae Sinensis), *Chuan Xiong* (Rhizoma Ligustici Chuanxiong), *Tao Ren* (Semen Persicae), *Hong Hua* (Flos Carthami) and *Shui Zhi* (Hirudo). These herbs may interfere with anticoagulant and antiplatelet drugs, including warfarin (Coumadin), enoxaparin (Lovenox), aspirin, dipyridamole (Persantine), and clopidogrel (Plavix). Without proper supervision, concurrent use of these herbs and drugs may lead to prolonged and excessive bleeding. Thus, individuals taking anticoagulant or antiplatelet drugs must be very cautious about concurrently using herbs, and would be wise to do so only under the supervision of well-trained healthcare professionals.[24]

Concomitant use of **diuretic** herbs and diuretic drugs may create additive or synergistic effects, making hypertension more difficult to control, or hypotensive episodes more likely.[25] The dosage of herbs and/or drugs must be adjusted to achieve optimal treatment outcome. Commonly-used diuretic herbs include *Fu Ling* (Poria), *Zhu Ling* (Polyporus), *Che Qian Zi* (Semen Plantaginis), and *Ze Xie* (Rhizoma Alismatis).

Antidiabetic herbs may interfere with antidiabetic drugs by accentuating the decrease of plasma glucose levels. The dosage of these herbs and drugs must be balanced carefully to effectively control blood glucose levels without causing hyper- or hypo-glycemia.[26] Herbs with definite antidiabetic effects include the following pairs of herbs: *Zhi Mu* (Radix Anemarrhenae) and *Shi Gao* (Gypsum Fibrosum); *Xuan Shen* (Radix Scrophulariae) and *Cang Zhu* (Rhizoma Atractylodis); and *Shan Yao* (Rhizoma Dioscoreae) and *Huang Qi* (Radix Astragali).

SUMMARY OF PHARMACODYNAMIC INTERACTIONS

Understanding synergistic and antagonistic interactions from both an Oriental medicine perspective and the realm of pharmaceutical medicines helps practitioners to anticipate, prevent, and/or monitor for unwanted interactions in patients who need or elect to rely on multiple therapeutic substances.

RECOGNITION OF DRUGS WITH HIGHER RISK OF INTERACTION

SUMMARY: CONCURRENT USE OF HERBAL MEDICINES AND PHARMACEUTICALS

Historically, herbs and drugs have been presumed to be very different treatment modalities, that have rarely, if ever, been used together. The line that separates use of herbs and drugs, however, has blurred in recent decades as the lay public gains increased accessibility to multiple treatment modalities. It is not uncommon for one patient to seek care from several health professionals for an ailment. As a result, a patient may easily be taking multiple drugs, herbs, supplements, and vitamins concurrently. It becomes difficult to predict whether the combination of all these substances will lead to unwanted side effects and/or interactions. It is imprudent to assume that there will be no interactions. On the other hand, it is just as unwise to abandon treatment simply for fear of possible interactions. The solution to this situation is in the understanding of pharmacokinetic and pharmacodynamic herb-drug interactions. By understanding these mechanisms, one can recognize potential interactions and take proper actions to prevent their occurrence.

[1] David M. Eisenberg, et al. *Trends in Alternative Medicine Use in the United States, 1990-1997.* JAMA. November 11, 1998

[2] Robert Berkow and Andrew J. Fletcher: *The Merck Manual of Diagnosis and Therapy 16th Edition.* Merck Research Laboratories, 1992

[3] Anthony S. Fauci, et al: *Harrison's Principles of Internal Medicine 14th Edition.* McGraw-Hill Health Professions Division, 1998

[4] Robert Berkow and Andrew J. Fletcher: *The Merck Manual of Diagnosis and Therapy 16th Edition.* Merck Research Laboratories, 1992

[5] Anthony S. Fauci, et al: *Harrison's Principles of Internal Medicine 14th Edition.* McGraw-Hill Health Professions Division, 1998

[6] Philip D. Hansten: *Understanding Drug-Drug Interactions. Science and Medicine* 16-25. January-February 1998

[7] Philip D. Hansten: *Chapter Three Drug Interactions. Applied Therapeutics.* Applied Therapeutics, Inc. 1993

[8] Philip D. Hansten: *Understanding Drug-Drug Interactions. Science and Medicine* 16-25. January-February 1998

[9] Philip D. Hansten: *Chapter Three Drug Interactions. Applied Therapeutics.* Applied Therapeutics, Inc. 1993

[10] Sophia Segal and Susan Kaminski: *Drug-Nutrient Interactions.* American Druggist 42-49. July 1996

[11] Philip D. Hansten: *Understanding Drug-Drug Interactions. Science and Medicine* 16-25. January-February 1998

[12] Philip D. Hansten: *Chapter Three Drug Interactions. Applied Therapeutics.* Applied Therapeutics, Inc. 1993

[13] Philip D. Hansten: *Understanding Drug-Drug Interactions. Science and Medicine* 16-25. January-February 1998

[14] Philip D. Hansten: *Chapter Three Drug Interactions. Applied Therapeutics.* Applied Therapeutics, Inc. 1993

[15] Philip D. Hansten: *Understanding Drug-Drug Interactions. Science and Medicine* 16-25. January-February 1998

[16] Philip D. Hansten: *Chapter Three Drug Interactions. Applied Therapeutics.* Applied Therapeutics, Inc. 1993

[17] Philip D. Hansten: *Understanding Drug-Drug Interactions. Science and Medicine* 16-25. January-February 1998

[18] Philip D. Hansten: *Chapter Three Drug Interactions. Applied Therapeutics.* Applied Therapeutics, Inc. 1993

[19] Philip D. Hansten: *Understanding Drug-Drug Interactions. Science and Medicine* 16-25. January-February 1998

[20] Philip D. Hansten: *Chapter Three Drug Interactions. Applied Therapeutics.* Applied Therapeutics, Inc. 1993

[21] Harold Kalant and Walter H.E. Roschlau: *Principles of Medical Pharmacology Sixth Edition.* Oxford University Press, 1998

[22] P.F.D'Arcy: Adverse Reactions and Interactions With Herbal Medicine. Part 2 – Drug Interactions. *Adverse Drug React. Toxicol.* Rev. 1993, 12(3) 147-162 Oxford University Press

[23] P.F.D'Arcy: Adverse Reactions and Interactions With Herbal Medicine. Part 2 – Drug Interactions. *Adverse Drug React. Toxicol.* Rev. 1993, 12(3) 147-162 Oxford University Press

[24] P.F.D'Arcy: Adverse Reactions and Interactions With Herbal Medicine. Part 2 – Drug Interactions. *Adverse Drug React. Toxicol.* Rev. 1993, 12(3) 147-162 Oxford University Press

[25] P.F.D'Arcy: Adverse Reactions and Interactions With Herbal Medicine. Part 2 – Drug Interactions. *Adverse Drug React. Toxicol.* Rev. 1993, 12(3) 147-162 Oxford University Press

[26] P.F.D'Arcy: Adverse Reactions and Interactions With Herbal Medicine. Part 2 – Drug Interactions. *Adverse Drug React. Toxicol.* Rev. 1993, 12(3) 147-162 Oxford University Press

RECOGNITION OF DRUGS WITH HIGHER RISK OF INTERACTION

BRAND NAME	GENERIC NAME	TYPE OF DRUGS	EFFECT OF INTERACTION	COMMENT
Amphotericin	Amphotericin	antifungal	may reduce elimination of herbs	decrease dose of herbs if necessary
Axid	Nizatidine	acid-reducer	may interfere with absorption of herbs	adjust herb doses accordingly
Carafate	Sucralfate	anti-ulcer	may interfere with absorption of herbs	separate taking herbs and drugs by two hours
Cholestid	Colestipol	antihyperlipidemic	may interfere with absorption of herbs	separate taking herbs and drugs by two hours
Coumadin	Warfarin	anticoagulant	this effect may change with herbs	monitor Coumadin effectiveness closely
Diflucan	Fluconazole	antifungal	may slow the metabolism of herbs	decrease dose of herbs if necessary
Dilantin	Phenytoin	anticonvulsant	may increase the metabolism of herbs	increase dose of herbs if necessary
E-Mycin	Erythromycin	antibiotic	may slow the metabolism of herbs	decrease dose of herbs if necessary
EES	Erythromycin	antibiotic	may slow the metabolism of herbs	decrease dose of herbs if necessary
Eryc	Erythromycin	antibiotic	may slow the metabolism of herbs	decrease dose of herbs if necessary
Ethanol	Alcohol	alcohol	may slow the metabolism of herbs	decrease dose of herbs if necessary
Haldol	Haloperidol	antipsychotic	may interfere with absorption of herbs	decrease dose of herbs if necessary
Maalax	Antacid	antacid	may interfere with absorption of herbs	separate taking herbs and drugs by two hours
Methotrexate	Methotrexate	antineoplastic	may reduce elimination of herbs	decrease dose of herbs if necessary
Mylanta	Antacid	antacid	may interfere with absorption of herbs	separate taking herbs and drugs by two hours
Nexium	Esomeprazole	acid-reducer	may interfere with absorption of herbs	adjust herb doses accordingly
Nizoral	Ketoconazole	antifungal	may slow the metabolism of herbs	decrease dose of herbs if necessary
Pepcid	Famotidine	acid-reducer	may interfere with absorption of herbs	adjust herb doses accordingly
Phenobarbital	Phenobarbital	anticonvulsant	may increase the metabolism of herbs	increase dose of herbs if necessary
Prevacid	Lansoprazole	acid-reducer	may interfere with absorption of herbs	adjust herb doses accordingly
Prilosec	Omeprazole	acid-reducer	may interfere with absorption of herbs	adjust herb doses accordingly
Propulsid	Cisapride	GI stimulant	may interfere with absorption of herbs	increase dose of herbs if necessary
Protonix	Pantoprazole	GI stimulant	may interfere with absorption of herbs	increase dose of herbs if necessary
Questran	Cholestyramine	antihyperlipidemic	may decrease absorption of herbs	separate taking herbs and drugs by two hours
Reglan	Metoclopramide	GI stimulant	may interfere with absorption of herbs	increase dose of herbs if necessary
Rifadin	Rifampin	antibiotic	may increase the metabolism of herbs	increase dose of herbs if necessary
Sporonox	Itraconazole	antifungal	may slow the metabolism of herbs	decrease dose of herbs if necessary
Tagamet	Cimetidine	acid-reducer	may interfere with absorption of herbs	adjust herb doses accordingly
Tagamet	Cimetidine	acid-reducer	may slow the metabolism of herbs	decrease dose of herbs if necessary
Tegretol	Carbamazepine	anticonvulsant	may increase the metabolism of herbs	increase dose of herbs if necessary
Tums	Antacid	antacid	may interfere with absorption of herbs	separate taking herbs and drugs by two hours
Zantac	Ranitidine	acid-reducer	may interfere with absorption of herbs	adjust herb doses accordingly

DRUG / HERB

DRUG – HERB INDEX

NAMES (BRAND / GENERIC)		CLINICAL APPLICATIONS	HERB ALTERNATIVES
Abreva	Docosanol	Cold sores	Lonicera Complex
Acamprosate	Campral	See Campral	
Accolate	Zafirlukast	Dyspnea and shortness of breath in cases of chronic asthma	Respitrol (Deficient)
		Management and prevention of chronic asthma	Cordyceps 3
Accupril	Quinapril	Cardiovascular disorders	Gastrodia Complex
Acetaminophen / Codeine	Tylenol / Codeine	See Tylenol with Codeine	
Aciphex	Rabeprazole	Various gastrointestinal disorders	GI Care
Actigall	Ursodiol	To dissolve and expel gallstones; cholecystitis	Dissolve (GS)
Actos	Pioglitazone	Elevated blood glucose levels in non-insulin dependent diabetics	Equilibrium
Acutrim	Phenylpropanolamine	Elevated body weight; slow basal metabolism; lack of energy	Herbalite
Acyclovir	Zovirax	See Zovirax	
Adefovir	Hepsera	See Hepsera	
Advil	Ibuprofen	Various types of headaches: migraine, tension, stress, vertex, occipital	Corydalin, Migratrol
		Musculoskeletal pain with redness, swelling and inflammation	Flex (Heat)
		Musculoskeletal pain that worsens during cold and rainy days	Flex (CD)
		Neuropathy	Flex (NP)
		Chronic injuries of soft tissues (muscles, ligaments and tendons)	Flex (MLT)
		Acute and chronic pain of the arm (shoulder, elbow and wrist)	Arm Support
		Acute or chronic pain of the leg (knee and ankle)	Knee & Ankle (Acute) or (Chronic)
		Acute or chronic upper and lower back pain	Back Support (Acute), (Chronic), or (Upper)
		Acute or chronic neck and shoulder pain	Neck & Shoulder (Acute) or (Chronic)
		Menstrual pain and cramps in dysmenorrhea	Mense-Ease
		Pain associated with amenorrhea	Menotrol
		Pain associated with endometriosis	Resolve (Lower)
		Severe pain of other herbal formulas	Use Herbal Analgesic with other formulas
Albuterol	Proventil / Ventolin	See Proventil / Ventolin	
Alefacept	Amevive	See Amevive	

DRUG – HERB INDEX

NAMES (BRAND / GENERIC)		CLINICAL APPLICATIONS	HERB ALTERNATIVES
Alendronate		*See Fosamax*	
Aleve	*Naproxen*	Various headaches: migraine, tension, stress, vertex, occipital	*Corydalin, Migratrol*
		Musculoskeletal pain with redness, swelling and inflammation	*Flex (Heat)*
		Musculoskeletal pain that worsens during cold and rainy days	*Flex (CD)*
		Neuropathy	*Flex (NP)*
		Chronic injuries of soft tissues (muscles, ligaments and tendons)	*Flex (MLT)*
		Acute and chronic pain of the arm (shoulder, elbow and wrist)	*Arm Support*
		Acute or chronic pain of the leg (knee and ankle)	*Knee & Ankle (Acute)* or *(Chronic)*
		Acute or chronic upper and lower back pain	*Back Support (Acute), (Chronic), or (Upper)*
		Acute or chronic neck and shoulder pain	*Neck & Shoulder (Acute)* or *(Chronic)*
		Menstrual pain and cramps in dysmenorrhea	*Mense-Ease*
		Pain associated with amenorrhea	*Menotrol*
		Pain associated with endometriosis	*Resolve (Lower)*
		Severe pain	*Herbal Analgesic*
Alfuzosin		*See Uroxatral*	
Allegra	*Fexofenadine*	Chronic and severe nasal congestion due to sinusitis or rhinitis	*Pueraria Clear Sinus*
		Nasal congestion due to allergies or common cold	*Magnolia Clear Sinus*
		Allergic or hypersensitive skin problems such as rash, itching, eczema, etc.	*Silerex*
Allopurinol	*Zyloprim*	Gout	*Flex (GT)*
Almotriptan	*Axert*	*See Axert*	
Alprazolam	*Xanax*	*See Xanax*	
Aluminum / Magnesium	*Maalax / Mylanta*	*See Maalax / Mylanta*	
Alupent	*Metaproterenol*	Heat-type asthma with fever, dry mouth, thirst, red face and red tongue	*Respitrol (Heat)*
		Cold-type asthma with chills, intolerance to cold, cyanotic complexion of the face and body	*Respitrol (Cold)*
		Chronic asthma with frequent attacks of wheezing and dyspnea	*Respitrol (Deficient), Cordyceps 3*
Amantadine	*Symmetrel*	*See Symmetrel*	
Ambien	*Zolpidem*	Insomnia and improve the overall quality of sleep	*Schisandra ZZZ*
		Insomnia due to stress and anxiety	*Calm ZZZ*

DRUG – HERB INDEX

NAMES (BRAND / GENERIC)		CLINICAL APPLICATIONS	HERB ALTERNATIVES
Amevive	Alefacept	Psoriasis	Dermatrol (PS)
Amitriptyline	Elavil	See Elavil	
Amlodipine	Norvasc	See Norvasc	
Amoxicillin	Amoxil	See Amoxil	
Amoxicillin / Clavulanic Acid	Augmentin	See Augmentin	
Amoxil	Amoxicillin	Generalized bacterial, viral and fungal infection	Herbal ABX
		Upper respiratory tract infection with fever, headache, sore throat	Lonicera Complex
		Respiratory tract infection with sinus congestion, watery nasal discharge, sneezing and chills	Respitrol (Cold)
		Lower respiratory tract infection with high fever, copious yellow sputum, cough and perspiration	Respitrol (Heat)
		Lower respiratory tract infection with chest congestion, cough, yellow phlegm and fever	Poria XPT
		Infection in the oral region, such as ulceration, sore throat, and herpes	Lonicera Complex
		Genito-urinary infections, such as herpes, urinary tract infection, or sexually-transmitted diseases	Gentiana Complex or V-Statin
		Ear, nose, throat and lung infections	Herbal ENT
		Cough and dyspnea	Respitrol (CF)
Ampicillin	Principen	See Principen	
Anaprox...	Naproxen...	Various headaches: migraine, tension, stress, vertex, occipital	Corydalin, Migratrol
		Musculoskeletal pain with redness, swelling and inflammation	Flex (Heat)
		Musculoskeletal pain that worsens during cold and rainy days	Flex (CD)
		Neuropathy	Flex (NP)
		Chronic injuries of soft tissues (muscles, ligaments and tendons)	Flex (MLT)
		Acute and chronic pain of the arm (shoulder, elbow and wrist)	Arm Support
		Acute or chronic pain of the leg (knee and ankle)	Knee & Ankle (Acute) or (Chronic)
		Acute or chronic upper and lower back pain	Back Support (Acute), (Chronic), or (Upper)
		Acute or chronic neck and shoulder pain	Neck & Shoulder (Acute) or (Chronic)
		Menstrual pain and cramps in dysmenorrhea	Mense-Ease
		Pain associated with amenorrhea	Menotrol

DRUG – HERB INDEX

NAMES (BRAND / GENERIC)		CLINICAL APPLICATIONS	HERB ALTERNATIVES
		Pain associated with endometriosis	Resolve (Lower)
		Severe pain	Herbal Analgesic
Ansaid	Flurbiprofen	Various headaches: migraine, tension, stress, vertex, occipital	Corydalin, Migratrol
		Musculoskeletal pain with redness, swelling and inflammation	Flex (Heat)
		Musculoskeletal pain that worsens during cold and rainy days	Flex (CD)
		Neuropathy	Flex (NP)
		Chronic injuries of soft tissues (muscles, ligaments and tendons)	Flex (MLT)
		Acute and chronic pain of the arm (shoulder, elbow and wrist)	Arm Support
		Acute or chronic pain of the leg (knee and ankle)	Knee & Ankle (Acute) or (Chronic)
		Acute or chronic upper and lower back pain	Back Support (Acute), (Chronic), or (Upper)
		Acute or chronic neck and shoulder pain	Neck & Shoulder (Acute) or (Chronic)
		Menstrual pain and cramps in dysmenorrhea	Mense-Ease
		Pain associated with amenorrhea	Menotrol
		Pain associated with endometriosis	Resolve (Lower)
		Severe pain	Herbal Analgesic
Antitussive Combination	Phenergan / Poly-Histine / Robitussin	See Phenergan / Poly-Histine / Robitussin	
Anusol-HC	Hydrocortisone	Hemorrhoids	GI Care (HMR)
Apidra	Insulin Glulisine	Diabetes	Equilibrium
Aprepitant	Emend	See Emend	
Aredia	Pamidronate	Osteoporosis	Osteo 8
Aricept	Donepezil	Both mental and physical functions in Alzheimer's disease	Neuro Plus, Enhance Memory
Armour Thyroid	Thyroid Desiccated	Hypothyroidism	Thyro-forte
Asacol	Mesalamine	Inflammatory bowel disease with diarrhea	GI Care II, GI Harmony
Aspirin...	Aspirin...	Various headaches: migraine, tension, stress, vertex, occipital	Corydalin, Migratrol
		Musculoskeletal pain with redness, swelling and inflammation	Flex (Heat)
		Musculoskeletal pain that worsens during cold and rainy days	Flex (CD)
		Neuropathy	Flex (NP)
		Chronic injuries of soft tissues (muscles, ligaments and tendons)	Flex (MLT)

DRUG / HERB

DRUG – HERB INDEX

NAMES (BRAND / GENERIC)		CLINICAL APPLICATIONS	HERB ALTERNATIVES
		Acute and chronic pain of the arm (shoulder, elbow and wrist)	*Arm Support*
		Acute or chronic pain of the leg (knee and ankle)	*Knee & Ankle (Acute)* or *(Chronic)*
		Acute or chronic upper and lower back pain	*Back Support (Acute), (Chronic),* or *(Upper)*
		Acute or chronic neck and shoulder pain	*Neck & Shoulder (Acute)* or *(Chronic)*
		Menstrual pain and cramps in dysmenorrhea	*Mense-Ease*
		Pain associated with amenorrhea	*Menotrol*
		Pain associated with endometriosis	*Resolve (Lower)*
		Severe pain	*Herbal Analgesic*
Atarax	*Hydroxyzine*	Allergic or hypersensitive skin problems such as rash, itching, eczema, etc.	*Silerex*
Atenolol		See **Tenormin**	
Ativan	*Lorazepam*	Moderate-to-severe emotional and psychological disorders	*Calm (ES)*
		Moderate levels of stress, anxiety, nervousness, tension, etc.	*Calm*
		Moderate levels of stress, anxiety, and insomnia	*Calm ZZZ*
Atomoxetine		See **Strattera**	
Augmentin	*Amoxicillin / Clavulanic Acid*	Infection	*Herbal ABX*
		Ear, nose, throat and lung infections	*Herbal ENT*
Avandia	*Rosiglitazone*	Elevated blood glucose levels in non-insulin dependent diabetics	*Equilibrium*
Axert	*Almotriptan*	Various headaches: migraine, tension, stress, vertex, occipital	*Corydalin*
		Migraine headache	*Migratrol*
Azithromycin		See **Zithromax**	
Bactrim…	*Sulfamethoxazole / Trimethoprim…*	Generalized bacterial, viral and fungal infection	*Herbal ABX*
		Upper respiratory tract infection with fever, headache, sore throat	*Lonicera Complex*
		Respiratory tract infection with sinus congestion, watery nasal discharge, sneezing and chills	*Respitrol (Cold)*
		Lower respiratory tract infection with high fever, copious yellow sputum, cough and perspiration	*Respitrol (Heat)*
		Lower respiratory tract infection with chest congestion, cough, yellow phlegm and fever	*Poria XPT*
		Infection in the oral region, such as ulceration, sore throat, and herpes	*Lonicera Complex*

Lotus Institute of Integrative Medicine

DRUG – HERB INDEX

NAMES (BRAND / GENERIC)		CLINICAL APPLICATIONS	HERB ALTERNATIVES
		Genito-urinary infections, such as herpes, urinary tract infection, or sexually-transmitted diseases	*Gentiana Complex* or *V-Statin*
Benadryl	Diphenhydramine	Ear, nose, throat and lung infections	*Herbal ENT*
		Cough and dyspnea	*Respitrol (CF)*
		Allergic or hypersensitive skin problems such as rash, itching, eczema, etc.	*Silerex*
		Chronic and severe nasal congestion due to sinusitis or rhinitis	*Pueraria Clear Sinus*
		Nasal congestion due to allergies or common cold	*Magnolia Clear Sinus*
Benicar	Olmesartan	Cardiovascular disorders	*Gastrodia Complex*
Benazepril	Lotensin	*See Lotensin*	
Biaxin	Clarithromycin	Generalized bacterial, viral and fungal infection	*Herbal ABX*
		Upper respiratory tract infection with fever, headache, sore throat	*Lonicera Complex*
		Respiratory tract infection with sinus congestion, watery nasal discharge, sneezing and chills	*Respitrol (Cold)*
		Lower respiratory tract infection with high fever, copious yellow sputum, cough and perspiration	*Respitrol (Heat)*
		Lower respiratory tract infection with chest congestion, cough, yellow phlegm and fever	*Poria XPT*
		Infection in the oral region, such as ulceration, sore throat, and herpes	*Lonicera Complex*
		Genito-urinary infections, such as herpes, urinary tract infection, or sexually-transmitted diseases	*Gentiana Complex* or *V-Statin*
		Ear, nose, throat and lung infections	*Herbal ENT*
		Cough and dyspnea	*Respitrol (CF)*
Bisacodyl	Dulcolax	*See Dulcolax*	
Brethine	Terbutaline	Heat-type asthma with fever, dry mouth, thirst, red face and red tongue	*Respitrol (Heat)*
		Cold-type asthma with chills, intolerance to cold, cyanotic complexion of the face and body	*Respitrol (Cold)*
		Chronic asthma with frequent attacks of wheezing and dyspnea	*Respitrol (Deficient), Cordyceps 3*
Bromfed	Pseudoephedrine / Brompheniramine	Lower respiratory tract infection with chest congestion, cough, yellow phlegm and fever	*Poria XPT*
		Chronic and severe nasal congestion due to sinusitis or rhinitis	*Pueraria Clear Sinus*
		Nasal congestion due to allergies or common cold	*Magnolia Clear Sinus*
		Cough and dyspnea	*Respitrol (CF)*
Bumex	Bumetanide	Edema and fluid retention	*Herbal DRX*
Bupropion	Wellbutrin	*See Wellbutrin*	

DRUG – HERB INDEX

NAMES (BRAND / GENERIC)		CLINICAL APPLICATIONS	HERB ALTERNATIVES
Buspar	*Buspirone*	Moderate-to-severe emotional and psychological disorders	*Calm (ES)*
		Moderate levels of stress, anxiety, nervousness, tension, etc.	*Calm*
		Moderate levels of stress, anxiety, and insomnia	*Calm ZZZ*
Buspirone	**Buspar**	*See BuSpar*	
Caffeine	Nodoz / Vivarin	*See NoDoz / Vivarin*	
Calan	*Verapamil*	Cardiovascular disorders	*Gastrodia Complex*
Calcium Carbonate	**Tums**	*See Tums*	
Calcium Sennosides	**Ex-Lax**	*See Ex-Lax*	
Campral	*Acamprosate*	Alcohol dependence	*Calm (ES)*
Capoten	*Captopril*	Cardiovascular disorders	*Gastrodia Complex*
Captopril	**Capoten**	*See Capoten*	
Carbamazepine	**Tegretol**	*See Tegretol*	
Carbidopa / Levodopa	**Sinemet**	*See Sinemet*	
Cardizem	*Diltiazem*	Cardiovascular disorders	*Gastrodia Complex*
Carisoprodol	**Soma**	*See Soma*	
Cartia XT	*Diltiazem*	Cardiovascular disorders	*Gastrodia Complex*
Catapres	*Clonidine*	Elevated blood pressure in patients with hyperactive adrenergic system	*Gentiana Complex*
Ceclor	*Cefaclor*	Generalized bacterial, viral and fungal infection	*Herbal ABX*
		Upper respiratory tract infection with fever, headache, sore throat	*Lonicera Complex*
		Respiratory tract infection with sinus congestion, watery nasal discharge, sneezing and chills	*Respitrol (Cold)*
		Lower respiratory tract infection with high fever, copious yellow sputum, cough and perspiration	*Respitrol (Heat)*
		Lower respiratory tract infection with chest congestion, cough, yellow phlegm and fever	*Poria XPT*
		Infection in the oral region, such as ulceration, sore throat, and herpes	*Lonicera Complex*
		Genito-urinary infections, such as herpes, urinary tract infection, or sexually-transmitted diseases	*Gentiana Complex* or *V-Statin*
		Ear, nose, throat and lung infections	*Herbal ENT*
		Cough and dyspnea	*Respitrol (CF)*
Cefaclor	**Ceclor**	*See Ceclor*	
Cefadroxil	**Duricef**	*See Duricef*	

Lotus Institute of Integrative Medicine

160

DRUG – HERB INDEX

NAMES (BRAND / GENERIC)		CLINICAL APPLICATIONS	HERB ALTERNATIVES
Cefixime	Suprax	See Suprax	
Cefprozil	Cefzil	See Cefzil	
Ceftin	Cefuroxime	Generalized bacterial, viral and fungal infection	Herbal ABX
		Upper respiratory tract infection with fever, headache, sore throat	Lonicera Complex
		Respiratory tract infection with sinus congestion, watery nasal discharge, sneezing and chills	Respitrol (Cold)
		Lower respiratory tract infection with high fever, copious yellow sputum, cough and perspiration	Respitrol (Heat)
		Lower respiratory tract infection with chest congestion, cough, yellow phlegm and fever	Poria XPT
		Infection in the oral region, such as ulceration, sore throat, and herpes	Lonicera Complex
		Genito-urinary infections, such as herpes, urinary tract infection, or sexually-transmitted diseases	Gentiana Complex or V-Statin
		Ear, nose, throat and lung infections	Herbal ENT
		Cough and dyspnea	Respitrol (CF)
Cefuroxime	Ceftin	See Ceftin	
Cefzil	Cefprozil	Generalized bacterial, viral and fungal infection	Herbal ABX
		Upper respiratory tract infection with fever, headache, sore throat	Lonicera Complex
		Respiratory tract infection with sinus congestion, watery nasal discharge, sneezing and chills	Respitrol (Cold)
		Lower respiratory tract infection with high fever, copious yellow sputum, cough and perspiration	Respitrol (Heat)
		Lower respiratory tract infection with chest congestion, cough, yellow phlegm and fever	Poria XPT
		Infection in the oral region, such as ulceration, sore throat, and herpes	Lonicera Complex
		Genito-urinary infections, such as herpes, urinary tract infection, or sexually-transmitted diseases	Gentiana Complex or V-Statin
		Ear, nose, throat and lung infections	Herbal ENT
		Cough and dyspnea	Respitrol (CF)
Celebrex…	Celecoxib…	Various headaches: migraine, tension, stress, vertex, occipital	Corydalin, Migratrol
		Musculoskeletal pain with redness, swelling and inflammation	Flex (Heat)
		Musculoskeletal pain that worsens during cold and rainy days	Flex (CD)
		Neuropathy	Flex (NP)
		Chronic injuries of soft tissues (muscles, ligaments and tendons)	Flex (MLT)
		Acute and chronic pain of the arm (shoulder, elbow and wrist)	Arm Support

DRUG / HERB

DRUG – HERB INDEX

NAMES (BRAND / GENERIC)		CLINICAL APPLICATIONS	HERB ALTERNATIVES
		Acute or chronic pain of the leg (knee and ankle)	*Knee & Ankle (Acute)* or *(Chronic)*
		Acute or chronic upper and lower back pain	*Back Support (Acute)*, *(Chronic)*, or *(Upper)*
		Acute or chronic neck and shoulder pain	*Neck & Shoulder (Acute)* or *(Chronic)*
		Menstrual pain and cramps in dysmenorrhea	*Mense-Ease*
		Pain associated with amenorrhea	*Menotrol*
		Pain associated with endometriosis	*Resolve (Lower)*
		Severe pain	*Herbal Analgesic*
Celecoxib	Celebrex	*See Celebrex*	
Celexa	*Citalopram*	Depression by inhibiting the re-uptake of serotonin	*Shine*
Cephalexin	Keflex	*See Keflex*	
Cetirizine	Zyrtec	*See Zyrtec*	
Chlorpromazine	Thorazine	*See Thorazine*	
Chlorzoxazone	Parafon Forte DSC	*See Parafon Forte DSC*	
Cialis	*Tadalafil*	To enhance male sexual and reproductive functions	*Vitality*
		Male sexual and reproductive dysfunctions with cold signs and symptoms	*Kidney Tonic (Yang)*
		Male infertility (not an indication of Viagra)	*Vital Essence*
Cimetidine	Tagamet	*See Tagamet*	
Cipro	Ciprofloxacin	Generalized bacterial, viral and fungal infection	*Herbal ABX*
		Upper respiratory tract infection with fever, headache, sore throat	*Lonicera Complex*
		Respiratory tract infection with sinus congestion, watery nasal discharge, sneezing and chills	*Respitrol (Cold)*
		Lower respiratory tract infection with high fever, copious yellow sputum, cough and perspiration	*Respitrol (Heat)*
		Lower respiratory tract infection with chest congestion, cough, yellow phlegm and fever	*Poria XPT*
		Infection in the oral region, such as ulceration, sore throat, and herpes	*Lonicera Complex*
		Genito-urinary infections, such as herpes, urinary tract infection, or sexually-transmitted diseases	*Gentiana Complex* or *V-Statin*
		Ear, nose, throat and lung infections	*Herbal ENT*
		Cough and dyspnea	*Respitrol (CF)*
Ciprofloxacin	Cipro	*See Cipro*	

DRUG – HERB INDEX

NAMES (BRAND / GENERIC)		CLINICAL APPLICATIONS	HERB ALTERNATIVES
Citalopram	Celexa	See Celexa	
Clarithromycin	Biaxin	See Biaxin	
Clarinex	Desloratadine	Chronic and severe nasal congestion due to sinusitis or rhinitis	Pueraria Clear Sinus
		Nasal congestion due to allergies or common cold	Magnolia Clear Sinus
Claritin	Loratadine	Chronic and severe nasal congestion due to sinusitis or rhinitis	Pueraria Clear Sinus
		Nasal congestion due to allergies or common cold	Magnolia Clear Sinus
Clinoril	Sulindac	Various headaches: migraine, tension, stress, vertex, occipital	Corydalin, Migratrol
		Musculoskeletal pain with redness, swelling and inflammation	Flex (Heat)
		Musculoskeletal pain that worsens during cold and rainy days	Flex (CD)
		Neuropathy	Flex (NP)
		Chronic injuries of soft tissues (muscles, ligaments and tendons)	Flex (MLT)
		Acute and chronic pain of the arm (shoulder, elbow and wrist)	Arm Support
		Acute or chronic pain of the leg (knee and ankle)	Knee & Ankle (Acute) or (Chronic)
		Acute or chronic upper and lower back pain	Back Support (Acute), (Chronic), or (Upper)
		Acute or chronic neck and shoulder pain	Neck & Shoulder (Acute) or (Chronic)
		Menstrual pain and cramps in dysmenorrhea	Mense-Ease
		Pain associated with amenorrhea	Menotrol
		Pain associated with endometriosis	Resolve (Lower)
		Severe pain	Herbal Analgesic
Clomid	Clomiphene	Amenorrhea or ovulatory failure	Menotrol
		Female infertility due to ovulatory failure	Blossom (Phase 1-4)
Clomiphene	Clomid	See Clomid	
Clonidine	Catapres	See Catapres	
Clotrimazole	Gyne-Lotrimin / Mycelex	See Gyne-Lotrimin / Mycelex	
Cognex	Tacrine	Both mental and physical functions in Alzheimer's disease	Neuro Plus, Enhance Memory
Colace	Docusate	Moderate-to-severe constipation	Gentle Lax (Excess) or (Deficient)
Colchicine	Colchicine	Gout	Flex (GT)
Cyclobenzaprine	Flexeril	See Flexeril	

Lotus Institute of Integrative Medicine

DRUG – HERB INDEX

NAMES (BRAND / GENERIC)		CLINICAL APPLICATIONS	HERB ALTERNATIVES
Dalmane	Flurazepam	Insomnia and the overall quality of sleep	Schisandra ZZZ
		Insomnia due to stress and anxiety	Calm ZZZ
Danazol	Danocrine	See Danocrine	
Danocrine	Danazol	To resolve fibrocystic benign breast disorder or cysts in the uterus and ovaries	Resolve (Upper) or (Lower)
		Endometriosis	Resolve (Lower)
Darvocet	Propoxyphene / Acetaminophen	Various headaches: migraine, tension, stress, vertex, occipital	Corydalin, Migratrol
		Musculoskeletal pain due to sports or traumatic injuries	Traumanex
		Arthritis, especially if condition worsens with cold and dampness	Flex (CD)
		Acute or chronic upper and lower back pain	Back Support (Acute) or (Upper)
		Acute or chronic neck and shoulder pain	Neck & Shoulder (Acute)
		Severe pain	Herbal Analgesic
		Acute and chronic pain of the arm (shoulder, elbow and wrist)	Arm Support
		Acute pain from herniated disk in the back	Back Support (HD)
		Acute pain of the leg (knee and ankle)	Knee & Ankle (Acute)
Darvon	Propoxyphene	Various headaches: migraine, tension, stress, vertex, occipital	Corydalin, Migratrol
		Musculoskeletal pain due to sports or traumatic injuries	Traumanex
		Arthritis, especially if condition worsens with cold and dampness	Flex (CD)
		Acute or chronic upper and lower back pain	Back Support (Acute) or (Upper)
		Acute or chronic neck and shoulder pain	Neck & Shoulder (Acute)
		Severe pain	Herbal Analgesic
		Acute and chronic pain of the arm (shoulder, elbow and wrist)	Arm Support
		Acute pain from herniated disk in the back	Back Support (HD)
		Acute pain of the leg (knee and ankle)	Knee & Ankle (Acute)
Daypro…	Oxaprozin…	Various headaches: migraine, tension, stress, vertex, occipital	Corydalin, Migratrol
		Musculoskeletal pain with redness, swelling and inflammation	Flex (Heat)
		Musculoskeletal pain that worsens during cold and rainy days	Flex (CD)
		Neuropathy	Flex (NP)
		Chronic injuries of soft tissues (muscles, ligaments and tendons)	Flex (MLT)
		Acute and chronic pain of the arm (shoulder, elbow and wrist)	Arm Support
		Acute or chronic pain of the leg (knee and ankle)	Knee & Ankle (Acute) or (Chronic)

DRUG – HERB INDEX

NAMES (BRAND / GENERIC)		CLINICAL APPLICATIONS	HERB ALTERNATIVES
		Acute or chronic upper and lower back pain	*Back Support (Acute), (Chronic), or (Upper)*
		Acute or chronic neck and shoulder pain	*Neck & Shoulder (Acute) or (Chronic)*
		Menstrual pain and cramps in dysmenorrhea	*Mense-Ease*
		Pain associated with endometriosis	*Resolve (Lower)*
		Severe pain	*Herbal Analgesic*
Demadex	*Torsemide*	Edema and fluid retention	*Herbal DRX*
Denavir	*Penciclovir*	Genital herpes	*Gentiana Complex*
		Treatment and / or prevention of oral herpes	*Lonicera Complex*
		Recurrent genital herpes	*Nourish*
		Shingles	*Dermatrol (HZ)*
Desloratadine	**Clarinex**	See Clarinex	
Dexedrine	*Dextroamphetamine*	To increase concentration and focus	*Calm (Jr)*
Dextroamphetamine	**Dexedrine**	See Dexedrine	
Diabeta	*Glyburide*	Elevated blood glucose levels in non-insulin dependent diabetics	*Equilibrium*
Diazepam	*Valium*	See Valium	
Dicolfenac	**Voltaren**	See Voltaren	
Didronel	*Etidronate*	Osteoporosis	*Osteo 8*
Diethylpropion	**Tenuate**	See Tenuate	
Diflunisal	**Dolobid**	See Dolobid	
Dilantin	*Phenytoin*	Nerve related pain, such as neuralgia and neuropathy	*Flex (NP)*
		Seizure and epilepsy	*Gastrodia Complex*
Diltiazem	**Cardizem**	See Cardizem	
Dimetapp	*Phenylpropanolamine / Brompheniramine*	Chronic and severe nasal congestion due to sinusitis or rhinitis	*Pueraria Clear Sinus*
		Nasal congestion due to allergies or common cold	*Magnolia Clear Sinus*
Diphenhydramine	**Benadryl / Sominex**	See Benadryl / Sominex	
Abreva	*Docosanol*	See Abreva	
Colace	*Docusate*	See Colace	
Dolobid…	*Diflunisal…*	Various headaches: migraine, tension, stress, vertex, occipital	*Corydalin, Migratrol*

DRUG / HERB

DRUG – HERB INDEX

NAMES (BRAND / GENERIC)	CLINICAL APPLICATIONS	HERB ALTERNATIVES
	Musculoskeletal pain with redness, swelling and inflammation	Flex (Heat)
	Musculoskeletal pain that worsens during cold and rainy days	Flex (CD)
	Neuropathy	Flex (NP)
	Chronic injuries of soft tissues (muscles, ligaments and tendons)	Flex (MLT)
	Acute and chronic pain of the arm (shoulder, elbow and wrist)	Arm Support
	Acute or chronic pain of the leg (knee and ankle)	Knee & Ankle (Acute) or (Chronic)
	Acute or chronic upper and lower back pain	Back Support (Acute), (Chronic), or (Upper)
	Acute or chronic neck and shoulder pain	Neck & Shoulder (Acute) or (Chronic)
	Menstrual pain and cramps in dysmenorrhea	Mense-Ease
	Pain associated with amenorrhea	Menotrol
	Pain associated with endometriosis	Resolve (Lower)
	Severe pain	Herbal Analgesic
Donepezil	See Aricept	
Doxylamine	See Unisom	
Dulcolax	Moderate-to-severe constipation	Gentle Lax (Excess) or (Deficient)
Duphalac	Moderate-to-severe constipation	Gentle Lax (Excess) or (Deficient)
Lactulose		
Duratuss	Lower respiratory tract infection with chest congestion, cough, yellow phlegm and fever	Poria XPT
Expectorant Combination	Cough and dyspnea	Respitrol (CF)
	Generalized bacterial, viral and fungal infection	Herbal ABX
Duricef	Upper respiratory tract infection with fever, headache, sore throat	Lonicera Complex
Cefadroxil	Respiratory tract infection with sinus congestion, watery nasal discharge, sneezing and chills	Respitrol (Cold)
	Lower respiratory tract infection with high fever, copious yellow sputum, cough and perspiration	Respitrol (Heat)
	Lower respiratory tract infection with chest congestion, cough, yellow phlegm and fever	Poria XPT
	Infection in the oral region, such as ulceration, sore throat, and herpes	Lonicera Complex
	Genito-urinary infections, such as herpes, urinary tract infection, or sexually-transmitted diseases	Gentiana Complex or V-Statin
	Ear, nose, throat and lung infections	Herbal ENT
	Cough and dyspnea	Respitrol (CF)

DRUG – HERB INDEX

NAMES (BRAND / GENERIC)		CLINICAL APPLICATIONS	HERB ALTERNATIVES
Dyazide	Triamterene / Hydrochlorothiazide	Edema and fluid retention	*Herbal DRX*
E-Mycin	Erythromycin	Respiratory tract infection with nose congestion, watery nasal discharge, sneezing, and chills	*Respitrol (Cold)*
		Lower respiratory tract infection with high fever, copious yellow sputum, cough and perspiration	*Respitrol (Heat)*
		Lower respiratory tract infection with chest congestion, cough, yellow phlegm and fever	*Poria XPT*
		Upper respiratory tract infection with fever, headache, sore throat	*Lonicera Complex*
		Infection	*Herbal ABX*
		Ear, nose, throat and lung infections	*Herbal ENT*
EES	Erythromycin	*See E-Mycin*	
Efalizumab	Raptiva	*See Raptiva*	
Effexor	Venlafaxine	Depression by inhibiting the re-uptake of serotonin	*Shine*
Elavil	Amitriptyline	Nerve related pain, such as neuralgia and neuropathy	*Flex (NP)*
Eldepryl	Selegiline	Both mental and physical functions in Parkinson's disease	*Neuro Plus*
		Cough and dyspnea	*Respitrol (CF)*
Elidel	Pimecrolimus	Allergic or hypersensitive skin problems such as rash, itching, eczema, etc.	*Silerex*
Eletriptan	Relpax	*See Relpax*	
Emend	Aprepitant	Chemotherapy-induced emesis	*C/R Support*
Enalapril	Vasotec	*See Vasotec*	
Entex	Phenylephrine / Phenylpropanolamine / Guaifenesin	Lower respiratory tract infection with chest congestion, cough, yellow phlegm and fever	*Poria XPT*
		Cough and dyspnea	*Respitrol (CF)*
Erythromycin	E-Mycin / EES / PCE	*See E-Mycin*	
Esomeprazole	Nexium	*See Nexium*	
Estrace	Estradiol	Menopausal symptoms such as hot flashes, irritability and mood swings	*Balance (Heat)*
		Osteoporosis	*Osteo 8*
Estradiol		*See Estrace*	
Estratab	Estrogens, Esterified	Menopausal symptoms such as hot flashes, irritability and mood swings	*Balance (Heat)*
		Osteoporosis	*Osteo 8*
Estrogens / Progestins	Prempro	*See Prempro*	

DRUG – HERB INDEX

NAMES (BRAND / GENERIC)		CLINICAL APPLICATIONS	HERB ALTERNATIVES
Estrogens, Conjugated	Premarin	See Premarin	
Estrogens, Esterified	Estratab	See Estratab	
Estropipate	Ogen	See Ogen	
Etidronate	Didronel	See Didronel	
Etodolac	Lodine	See Lodine	
Ex-Lax	Calcium Sennosides	Moderate-to-severe constipation	Gentle Lax (Excess) or (Deficient)
Exelon	Rivastigmine	Both mental and physical functions in Alzheimer's disease	Neuro Plus, Enhance Memory
Expectorant Combination	Duratuss / Zephrex	See Duratuss / Zephrex	
Ezetimibe	Zetia	See Zetia	
Famciclovir	Famvir	See Famvir	
Famotidine	Pepcid	See Pepcid	
Famvir	Famciclovir	Genital herpes	Gentiana Complex
		Genital herpes recurrences	Nourish
		Colds / flu with fever, headache, sore throat	Lonicera Complex
		Shingles	Dermatrol (HZ)
Fastin	Phentermine	Elevated body weight; slow basal metabolism; lack of energy	Herbalite
Feldene...	Piroxicam...	Various headaches: migraine, tension, stress, vertex, occipital	Corydalin, Migratrol
		Musculoskeletal pain with redness, swelling and inflammation	Flex (Heat)
		Musculoskeletal pain that worsens during cold and rainy days	Flex (CD)
		Neuropathy	Flex (NP)
		Chronic injuries of soft tissues (muscles, ligaments and tendons)	Flex (MLT)
		Acute and chronic pain of the arm (shoulder, elbow and wrist)	Arm Support
		Acute or chronic pain of the leg (knee and ankle)	Knee & Ankle (Acute) or (Chronic)
		Acute or chronic upper and lower back pain	Back Support (Acute), (Chronic), or (Upper)
		Acute or chronic neck and shoulder pain	Neck & Shoulder (Acute) or (Chronic)
		Menstrual pain and cramps in dysmenorrhea	Mense-Ease
		Pain associated with amenorrhea	Menotrol

DRUG – HERB INDEX

NAMES (BRAND / GENERIC)		CLINICAL APPLICATIONS	HERB ALTERNATIVES
		Pain associated with endometriosis	Resolve (Lower)
		Severe pain	Herbal Analgesic
Felodipine	Plendil	See Plendil	
Fexofenadine	Allegra	See Allegra	
Filgrastim	Neupogen	See Neupogen	
Finasteride	Proscar	See Proscar	
Flexeril	Cyclobenzaprine	Muscle stiffness and pain of the neck and shoulder	Neck & Shoulder (Acute)
		General relief of muscle spasm and cramps	Flex (SC)
Floxin	Ofloxacin	Generalized bacterial, viral and fungal infection	Herbal ABX
		Upper respiratory tract infection with fever, headache, sore throat	Lonicera Complex
		Respiratory tract infection with sinus congestion, watery nasal discharge, sneezing and chills	Respitrol (Cold)
		Lower respiratory tract infection with high fever, copious yellow sputum, cough and perspiration	Respitrol (Heat)
		Lower respiratory tract infection with chest congestion, cough, yellow phlegm and fever	Poria XPT
		Infection in the oral region, such as ulceration, sore throat, and herpes	Lonicera Complex
		Genito-urinary infections, such as herpes, urinary tract infection, or sexually-transmitted diseases	Gentiana Complex or V-Statin
		Ear, nose, throat and lung infections	Herbal ENT
		Cough and dyspnea	Respitrol (CF)
Fluoxetine	Prozac	See Prozac	
Flurazepam	Dalmane	See Dalmane	
Flurbiprofen	Ansaid	See Ansaid	
Fluvastatin	Lescol	See Lescol	
Fosamax	Alendronate	Osteoporosis	Osteo 8
Fosinopril	Monopril	See Monopril	
Frova	Frovatriptan	Various headaches: migraine, tension, stress, vertex, occipital	Corydalin
		Migraine headache	Migratrol
Frovatriptan	Frova	See Frova	
Gabapentin	Neurontin	See Neurontin	
Galantamine	Reminyl	See Reminyl	

DRUG / HERB

DRUG – HERB INDEX

NAMES (BRAND / *GENERIC*)		CLINICAL APPLICATIONS	HERB ALTERNATIVES
Gemfibrozil	Lopid	*See Lopid*	
Glipizide	Glucotrol	*See Glucotrol*	
Glucophage	*Metformin*	Elevated blood glucose levels in non-insulin dependent diabetics	*Equilibrium*
Glucotrol	*Glipizide*	Elevated blood glucose levels in non-insulin dependent diabetics	*Equilibrium*
Glyburide	Diabeta / Micronase	*See DiaBeta / Micronase*	
Guanfacine	Tenex	*See Tenex*	
Gyne-Lotrimin	*Clotrimazole*	Vaginitis, candidiasis, vaginal yeast infection	*V-Statin*
Haldol	*Haloperidol*	Moderate-to-severe emotional and psychological disorders	*Calm (ES)*
Haloperidol	Haldol	*See Haldol*	
Hamamelis	Tucks	*See Tucks*	
Hepsera	*Adefovir*	Hepatitis B	*Liver DTX*
Hydrochlorothiazide / Triamterene	Maxzide / Dyazide	*See Maxzide or Dyazide*	
Hydrocodone / Acetaminophen	Lorcet / Lortab / Vicodin	*See Lorcet / Lortab / Vicodin*	
Hydrocortisone	Anusol-HC	*See Anusol-HC*	
Hydroxyzine	Atarax	*See Atarax*	
Hytrin	*Terazosin*	Benign prostatic hypertrophy (BPH)	*Saw Palmetto Complex, P-Statin*
		Elevated blood pressure in patients with hyperactive adrenergic system	*Gentiana Complex*
Ibuprofen	Advil / Motrin	*See Advil / Motrin*	
Imitrex	*Sumatriptan*	Various headaches: migraine, tension, stress, vertex, occipital	*Corydalin, Migratrol*
		Migraine headache	*Gastrodia Complex*
Imodium	*Loperamide*	Acute diarrhea	*GI Care II*
		Chronic diarrhea	*GI Tonic*
Inderal	*Propranolol*	Elevated blood pressure in patients with hyperactive adrenergic system	*Gentiana Complex*
Indocin...	*Indomethacin...*	Various headaches: migraine, tension, stress, vertex, occipital	*Corydalin, Migratrol*
		Musculoskeletal pain with redness, swelling and inflammation	*Flex (Heat)*
		Musculoskeletal pain that worsens during cold and rainy days	*Flex (CD)*
		Neuropathy	*Flex (NP)*
		Chronic injuries of soft tissues (muscles, ligaments and tendons)	*Flex (MLT)*

Lotus Institute of Integrative Medicine

DRUG – HERB INDEX

NAMES (BRAND / GENERIC)	CLINICAL APPLICATIONS	HERB ALTERNATIVES
	Acute and chronic pain of the arm (shoulder, elbow and wrist)	*Arm Support*
	Acute or chronic pain of the leg (knee and ankle)	*Knee & Ankle (Acute)* or *(Chronic)*
	Acute or chronic upper and lower back pain	*Back Support (Acute)*, *(Chronic)*, or *(Upper)*
	Acute or chronic neck and shoulder pain	*Neck & Shoulder (Acute)* or *(Chronic)*
	Menstrual pain and cramps in dysmenorrhea	*Mense-Ease*
	Pain associated with amenorrhea	*Menotrol*
	Pain associated with endometriosis	*Resolve (Lower)*
	Severe pain	*Herbal Analgesic*
	Gout	*Flex (GT)*
Indomethacin	**Indocin**	*See Indocin*
Insulin Glulisine	**Apidra**	*See Apidra*
Ionamine	*Phentermine*	Elevated body weight; slow basal metabolism; lack of energy	*Herbalite*
Isometheptene / Apap / Dichloraphenazone	**Midrin**	*See Midrin*
Isoptin	*Verapamil*	Cardiovascular disorders	*Gastrodia Complex*
Keflex	*Cephalexin*	Generalized bacterial, viral and fungal infection	*Herbal ABX*
		Upper respiratory tract infection with fever, headache, sore throat	*Lonicera Complex*
		Respiratory tract infection with sinus congestion, watery nasal discharge, sneezing and chills	*Respirol (Cold)*
		Lower respiratory tract infection with high fever, copious yellow sputum, cough and perspiration	*Respirol (Heat)*
		Lower respiratory tract infection with chest congestion, cough, yellow phlegm and fever	*Poria XPT*
		Infection in the oral region, such as ulceration, sore throat, and herpes	*Lonicera Complex*
		Genito-urinary infections, such as herpes, urinary tract infection, or sexually-transmitted diseases	*Gentiana Complex* or *V-Statin*
		Ear, nose, throat and lung infections	*Herbal ENT*
		Cough and dyspnea	*Respirol (CF)*
Telithromycin...	**Ketek...**	Respiratory tract infection with nose congestion, watery nasal discharge, sneezing, and chills	*Respirol (Cold)*
		Lower respiratory tract infection with high fever, copious yellow sputum, cough and perspiration	*Respirol (Heat)*

DRUG / HERB

DRUG – HERB INDEX

NAMES (BRAND / *GENERIC*)		CLINICAL APPLICATIONS	HERB ALTERNATIVES
		Lower respiratory tract infection with chest congestion, cough, yellow phlegm and fever	*Poria XPT*
		Upper respiratory tract infection with fever, headache, sore throat	*Lonicera Complex*
		Infection	*Herbal ABX*
		Ear, nose, throat and lung infections	*Herbal ENT*
		Cough and dyspnea	*Respitrol (CF)*
Ketoprofen	**Orudis**	*See Orudis*	
Lactulose	**Duphalac**	*See Duphalac*	
Lansoprazole	**Prevacid**	*See Prevacid*	
Lasix	*Furosemide*	Edema and fluid retention	
Lescol	*Fluvastatin*	Elevated serum cholesterol and triglycerides levels	*Herbal DRX*
		Elevated serum cholesterol and triglycerides levels	*Cholisma*
		Elevated serum cholesterol and triglycerides levels with fatty liver and obesity	*Cholisma (ES)*
Leuprolide	**Lupron**	*See Lupron*	
Levaquin	*Levofloxacin*	Generalized bacterial, viral and fungal infection	*Herbal ABX*
		Upper respiratory tract infection with fever, headache, sore throat	*Lonicera Complex*
		Respiratory tract infection with sinus congestion, watery nasal discharge, sneezing and chills	*Respitrol (Cold)*
		Lower respiratory tract infection with high fever, copious yellow sputum, cough and perspiration	*Respitrol (Heat)*
		Lower respiratory tract infection with chest congestion, cough, yellow phlegm and fever	*Poria XPT*
		Infection in the oral region, such as ulceration, sore throat, and herpes	*Lonicera Complex*
		Genito-urinary infections, such as herpes, urinary tract infection, or sexually-transmitted diseases	*Gentiana Complex* or *V-Statin*
		Ear, nose, throat and lung infections	*Herbal ENT*
		Cough and dyspnea	*Respitrol (CF)*
Levitra	*Vardenafil*	To enhance male sexual and reproductive functions	*Vitality*
		Male sexual and reproductive dysfunctions with cold signs and symptoms	*Kidney Tonic (Yang)*
		Male infertility (not an indication of Viagra)	*Vital Essence*
Levofloxacin	**Levaquin**	*See Levaquin*	
Levothyroxine	**Synthroid / Levoxyl**	*See Synthroid or Levoxyl*	
Levoxyl	*Levothyroxine*	Hypothyroidism	
Liotrix	**Thyrolar**	*See Thyrolar*	*Thyro-forte*

Lotus Institute of Integrative Medicine

DRUG – HERB INDEX

NAMES (BRAND / GENERIC)		CLINICAL APPLICATIONS	HERB ALTERNATIVES
Lipitor	Atorvastatin	Elevated serum cholesterol and triglycerides levels	Cholisma
		Elevated serum cholesterol and triglycerides levels with fatty liver and obesity	Cholisma (ES)
Lisinopril	Prinivil / Zestril	See Prinivil or Zestril	
Lodine	Etodolac	Various headaches: migraine, tension, stress, vertex, occipital	Corydalin, Migratrol
		Musculoskeletal pain with redness, swelling and inflammation	Flex (Heat)
		Musculoskeletal pain that worsens during cold and rainy days	Flex (CD)
		Neuropathy	Flex (NP)
		Chronic injuries of soft tissues (muscles, ligaments and tendons)	Flex (MLT)
		Acute and chronic pain of the arm (shoulder, elbow and wrist)	Arm Support
		Acute or chronic pain of the leg (knee and ankle)	Knee & Ankle (Acute)
		Acute or chronic upper and lower back pain	Back Support (Acute) or (Upper)
		Acute or chronic neck and shoulder pain	Neck & Shoulder (Acute)
		Menstrual pain and cramps in dysmenorrhea	Mense-Ease
		Pain associated with amenorrhea	Menotrol
		Pain associated with endometriosis	Resolve (Lower)
		Severe pain	Herbal Analgesic
Loperamide	Imodium	See Imodium	
Lopid	Gemfibrozil	Elevated serum cholesterol and triglycerides levels	Cholisma
		Elevated serum cholesterol and triglycerides levels with fatty liver and obesity	Cholisma (ES)
Lopressor	Metoprolol	Elevated blood pressure in patients with hyperactive adrenergic system	Gentiana Complex
Lorabid…	Loracarbef…	Generalized bacterial, viral and fungal infection	Herbal ABX
		Upper respiratory tract infection with fever, headache, sore throat	Lonicera Complex
		Respiratory tract infection with sinus congestion, watery nasal discharge, sneezing and chills	Respitrol (Cold)
		Lower respiratory tract infection with high fever, copious yellow sputum, cough and perspiration	Respitrol (Heat)
		Lower respiratory tract infection with chest congestion, cough, yellow phlegm and fever	Poria XPT
		Infection in the oral region, such as ulceration, sore throat, and herpes	Lonicera Complex
		Genito-urinary infections, such as herpes, urinary tract infection, or sexually-transmitted diseases	Gentiana Complex or V-Statin
		Ear, nose, throat and lung infections	Herbal ENT

DRUG / HERB

DRUG – HERB INDEX

NAMES (BRAND / GENERIC)		CLINICAL APPLICATIONS	HERB ALTERNATIVES
Loracarbef		Cough and dyspnea	Respirol (CF)
Loratadine	Lorabid	See Lorabid	
Lorazepam	Claritin	See Claritin	
	Ativan	See Ativan	
Lorcet	Hydrocodone / Acetaminophen	Acute or chronic neck and shoulder pain	Neck & Shoulder (Acute)
		Musculoskeletal pain due to sports or traumatic injuries	Traumanex
		Arthritis, especially if condition worsens with cold and dampness	Flex (CD)
		Acute or chronic upper and lower back pain	Back Support (Acute) or (Upper)
		Acute or chronic neck and shoulder pain	Neck & Shoulder (Acute)
		Severe pain	Herbal Analgesic
		Acute and chronic pain of the arm (shoulder, elbow and wrist)	Arm Support
		Acute pain from herniated disk in the back	Back Support (HD)
		Acute pain of the leg (knee and ankle)	Knee & Ankle (Acute)
Lortab	Hydrocodone / Acetaminophen	Acute or chronic neck and shoulder pain	Neck & Shoulder (Acute)
		Musculoskeletal pain due to sports or traumatic injuries	Traumanex
		Arthritis, especially if condition worsens with cold and dampness	Flex (CD)
		Acute or chronic upper and lower back pain	Back Support (Acute) or (Upper)
		Acute or chronic neck and shoulder pain	Neck & Shoulder (Acute)
		Severe pain	Herbal Analgesic
		Acute and chronic pain of the arm (shoulder, elbow and wrist)	Arm Support
		Acute pain from herniated disk in the back	Back Support (HD)
		Acute pain of the leg (knee and ankle)	Knee & Ankle (Acute)
Lotensin	Benazepril	Cardiovascular disorders	Gastrodia Complex
Lovastatin	Mevacor	See Mevacor	
Lozol	Indapamide	Edema and fluid retention	Herbal DRX
Lupron	Leuprolide	To resolve cysts in the uterus and ovaries	Resolve (Lower)
Maalox	Aluminum / Magnesium	Various gastrointestinal disorders	GI Care
Magnesia	Milk of Magnesia	See Milk of Magnesia	
Maxzide	Triamterene / Hydrochlorothiazide	Edema and fluid retention	Herbal DRX

DRUG – HERB INDEX

NAMES (BRAND / GENERIC)		CLINICAL APPLICATIONS	HERB ALTERNATIVES
Memantine	Namenda	See Namenda	
Mephyton	Vitamin K	Bleeding disorders	Notoginseng 9
Mesalamine	Asacol	See Asacol	
Metaproterenol	Alupent	See Alupent	
Metaxalone	Skelaxin	See Skelaxin	
Metformin	Glucophage	See Glucophage	
Methimazole	Tapazole	See Tapazole	
Methocarbamol	Robaxin	See Robaxin	
Metoprolol	Lopressor / Toprol	See Lopressor / Toprol	
Mevacor	Lovastatin	Elevated serum cholesterol and triglycerides levels	Cholisma
		Elevated serum cholesterol and triglycerides levels with fatty liver and obesity	Cholisma (ES)
Miconazole	Monistat	See Monistat	
Micronase	Glyburide	Elevated blood glucose levels in non-insulin dependent diabetics	Equilibrium
Midrin	Isometheptene / Apap / Dichloraphenazone	Various headaches: migraine, tension, stress, vertex, occipital	Corydalin
		Migraine headache	Migratrol
Milk of Magnesia	Magnesia	Moderate-to-severe constipation	Gentle Lax (Excess) or (Deficient)
Minipress	Prazosin	Benign prostatic hypertrophy (BPH)	Saw Palmetto Complex, P-Statin
		Elevated blood pressure in patients with hyperactive adrenergic system	Gentiana Complex
Minoxidil	Rogaine	See Rogaine	
Monistat	Miconazole	Vaginitis, candidiasis, vaginal yeast infection	V-Statin
Monopril	Fosinopril	Cardiovascular disorders	Gastrodia Complex
Montelukast	Singulair	See Singulair	
Motrin…	Ibuprofen…	Various headaches: migraine, tension, stress, vertex, occipital	Corydalin, Migratrol
		Musculoskeletal pain with redness, swelling and inflammation	Flex (Heat)
		Musculoskeletal pain that worsens during cold and rainy days	Flex (CD)
		Neuropathy	Flex (NP)
		Chronic injuries of soft tissues (muscles, ligaments and tendons)	Flex (MLT)
		Acute and chronic pain of the arm (shoulder, elbow and wrist)	Arm Support
		Acute or chronic pain of the leg (knee and ankle)	Knee & Ankle (Acute) or (Chronic)

DRUG – HERB INDEX

NAMES (BRAND / GENERIC)		CLINICAL APPLICATIONS	HERB ALTERNATIVES
		Acute or chronic upper and lower back pain	Back Support (Acute), (Chronic), or (Upper)
		Acute or chronic neck and shoulder pain	Neck & Shoulder (Acute) or (Chronic)
		Menstrual pain and cramps in dysmenorrhea	Mense-Ease
		Pain associated with amenorrhea	Menotrol
		Pain associated with endometriosis	Resolve (Lower)
		Severe pain	Herbal Analgesic
Mycelex	Clotrimazole	Vaginitis, candidiasis, vaginal yeast infection	V-Statin
Mylanta	Aluminum / Magnesium	Various gastrointestinal disorders	GI Care
Nabumetone	Relafen	See Relafen	
Nafarelin	Synarel	See Synarel	
Namenda	Memantine	Both mental and physical functions in Alzheimer's disease	Neuro Plus, Enhance Memory
Naprosyn	Naproxen	Various headaches: migraine, tension, stress, vertex, occipital	Corydalin, Migratrol
		Musculoskeletal pain with redness, swelling and inflammation	Flex (Heat)
		Musculoskeletal pain that worsens during cold and rainy days	Flex (CD)
		Neuropathy	Flex (NP)
		Chronic injuries of soft tissues (muscles, ligaments and tendons)	Flex (MLT)
		Acute and chronic pain of the arm (shoulder, elbow and wrist)	Arm Support
		Acute or chronic pain of the leg (knee and ankle)	Knee & Ankle (Acute) or (Chronic)
		Acute or chronic upper and lower back pain	Back Support (Acute), (Chronic), or (Upper)
		Acute or chronic neck and shoulder pain	Neck & Shoulder (Acute) or (Chronic)
		Menstrual pain and cramps in dysmenorrhea	Mense-Ease
		Pain associated with amenorrhea	Menotrol
		Pain associated with endometriosis	Resolve (Lower)
		Severe pain	Herbal Analgesic
Naproxen	Naprosyn / Anaprox	See Naprosyn / Anaprox	
Starlix		See Starlix	
Neupogen…	Filgrastim…	To strengthen the overall constitution of the person	Imperial Tonic, Cordyceps 3

DRUG – HERB INDEX

NAMES (BRAND / GENERIC)		CLINICAL APPLICATIONS	HERB ALTERNATIVES
		To boost the immune system; prevents bacterial and viral infections	Cordyceps 3, Immune +
		To enhance the immune system during chemotherapy and radiation treatment	C/R Support
		To tonify the body for individuals who are too weak to receive chemotherapy and radiation treatment	CA Support
Neurontin	Gabapentin	Nerve related pain, such as neuralgia and neuropathy	Flex (NP)
		Seizure and epilepsy	Gastrodia Complex
Nexium	Esomeprazole	Various gastrointestinal disorders	GI Care
Niacin	Niacin	Elevated serum cholesterol and triglycerides levels	Cholisma
		Elevated serum cholesterol and triglycerides levels with fatty liver and obesity	Cholisma (ES)
Nifedipine	Procardia	See Procardia	
Nodoz	Caffeine	Lack of energy levels; decreased mental and physical performance	Vibrant
Nolvadex	Tamoxifen	To resolve fibrocystic benign breast disorder	Resolve (Upper)
Norflex	Orphenadrine	Muscle stiffness and pain of the neck and shoulder	Neck & Shoulder (Acute)
		General relief of muscle spasm and cramps	Flex (SC)
Norvasc	Amlodipine	Cardiovascular disorders	Gastrodia Complex
Floxin	Ofloxacin	See Floxin	
Ogen	Estropipate	Menopausal symptoms such as hot flashes, irritability and mood swings	Balance (Heat)
Olmesartan	Benicar	See Benicar	
Omeprazole	Prilosec	See Prilosec	
Orinase	Tolbutamide	Elevated blood glucose levels in non-insulin dependent diabetics	Equilibrium
Orlistat	Xenical	See Xenical	
Orphenadrine	Norflex	See Norflex	
Orudis…	Ketoprofen…	Various headaches: migraine, tension, stress, vertex, occipital	Corydalin, Migratrol
		Musculoskeletal pain with redness, swelling and inflammation	Flex (Heat)
		Musculoskeletal pain that worsens during cold and rainy days	Flex (CD)
		Neuropathy	Flex (NP)
		Chronic injuries of soft tissues (muscles, ligaments and tendons)	Flex (MLT)
		Acute and chronic pain of the arm (shoulder, elbow and wrist)	Arm Support
		Acute or chronic pain of the leg (knee and ankle)	Knee & Ankle (Acute) or (Chronic)

DRUG / HERB

DRUG – HERB INDEX

NAMES (BRAND / GENERIC)	CLINICAL APPLICATIONS	HERB ALTERNATIVES
	Acute or chronic upper and lower back pain	Back Support (Acute), (Chronic), or (Upper)
	Acute or chronic neck and shoulder pain	Neck & Shoulder (Acute) or (Chronic)
	Menstrual pain and cramps in dysmenorrhea	Mense-Ease
	Pain associated with amenorrhea	Menotrol
	Pain associated with endometriosis	Resolve (Lower)
	Severe pain	Herbal Analgesic
Oxaprozin	See Daypro	
Pamidronate	See Aredia	
Pantoprazole	See Protonix	
Parafon Forte DSC	Muscle stiffness and pain of the neck and shoulder	Neck & Shoulder (Acute)
Chlorzoxazone	General relief of muscle spasm and cramps	Flex (SC)
Paroxetine	See Paxil	
Paxil	Depression by inhibiting the re-uptake of serotonin	Shine
PCE	See E-Mycin	
Erythromycin		
Pen VK	Generalized bacterial, viral and fungal infection	Herbal ABX
Penicillin	Upper respiratory tract infection with fever, headache, sore throat	Lonicera Complex
	Respiratory tract infection with sinus congestion, watery nasal discharge, sneezing and chills	Respitrol (Cold)
	Lower respiratory tract infection with high fever, copious yellow sputum, cough and perspiration	Respitrol (Heat)
	Lower respiratory tract infection with chest congestion, cough, yellow phlegm and fever	Poria XPT
	Infection in the oral region, such as ulceration, sore throat, and herpes	Lonicera Complex
	Genito-urinary infections, such as herpes, urinary tract infection, or sexually-transmitted diseases	Gentiana Complex or V-Statin
	Ear, nose, throat and lung infections	Herbal ENT
	Cough and dyspnea	Respitrol (CF)
Penciclovir	See Denavir	
Pen VK	See Pen VK	
Penicillin		
Pepcid	Various gastrointestinal disorders	GI Care
Famotidine		

DRUG – HERB INDEX

NAMES (BRAND / GENERIC)		CLINICAL APPLICATIONS	HERB ALTERNATIVES
Phenergan	*Antitussive Combination*	Lower respiratory tract infection with chest congestion, cough, yellow phlegm and fever	*Poria XPT*
		Cough and dyspnea	*Respitrol (CF)*
Phentermine	**Fastin / Ionamine**	*See Fastin / Ionamine*	
Phenylephrine / Guaifenesin / Phenyl-propanolamine	**Entex**	*See Entex*	
Phenyl-propanolamine	**Acutrim**	*See Acutrim*	
Phenyl-propanolamine / Brompheniramine	**Dimetapp**	*See Dimetapp*	
Phenytoin	**Dilantin**	*See Dilantin*	
Pimecrolimus	**Elidel**	*See Elidel*	
Pioglitazone	**Actos**	*See Actos*	
Piroxicam	**Feldene**	*See Feldene*	
Plendil	*Felodipine*	Cardiovascular disorders	*Gastrodia Complex*
Poly-Histine	*Antitussive Combination*	Lower respiratory tract infection with chest congestion, cough, yellow phlegm and fever	*Poria XPT*
		Cough and dyspnea	*Respitrol (CF)*
Pravachol	*Pravastatin*	Elevated serum cholesterol and triglycerides levels	*Cholisma*
		Elevated serum cholesterol and triglycerides levels with fatty liver and obesity	*Cholisma (ES)*
Pravastatin	**Pravachol**	*See Pravachol*	
Prazosin	**Minipress**	*See Minipress*	
Prednisone		Arthritis	*Flex (Heat), Flex (CD), Flex (NP)*
		Skin rash and eczema	*Silerex*
		Sinusitis or rhinitis	*Magnolia Clear Sinus, Pueraria Clear Sinus*
		Acute asthma	*Respitrol (Heat), Respitrol (Cold)*
		Management and prevention of asthma	*Respitrol (Deficient), Cordyceps 3*
		Inflammatory bowel disorders in general	*GI Care II*
		Irritable bowel syndrome	*GI Harmony*
		Ulcerative colitis	*GI Care (UC)*

Lotus Institute of Integrative Medicine

DRUG – HERB INDEX

NAMES (BRAND / GENERIC)		CLINICAL APPLICATIONS	HERB ALTERNATIVES
Premarin	*Estrogens, Conjugated*	Menopausal symptoms such as hot flashes, irritability and mood swings	*Balance (Heat)*
		Osteoporosis	*Osteo 8*
Prempro	*Estrogens / Progestins*	Menopausal symptoms such as hot flashes, irritability and mood swings	*Balance (Heat)*
		Osteoporosis	*Osteo 8*
Prevacid	*Lansoprazole*	Various gastrointestinal disorders	*GI Care*
Prilosec	*Omeprazole*	Various gastrointestinal disorders	*GI Care*
Principen	*Ampicillin*	Generalized bacterial, viral and fungal infection	*Herbal ABX*
		Upper respiratory tract infection with fever, headache, sore throat	*Lonicera Complex*
		Respiratory tract infection with sinus congestion, watery nasal discharge, sneezing and chills	*Respirol (Cold)*
		Lower respiratory tract infection with high fever, copious yellow sputum, cough and perspiration	*Respirol (Heat)*
		Lower respiratory tract infection with chest congestion, cough, yellow phlegm and fever	*Poria XPT*
		Infection in the oral region, such as ulceration, sore throat, and herpes	*Lonicera Complex*
		Genito-urinary infections, such as herpes, urinary tract infection, or sexually-transmitted diseases	*Gentiana Complex* or *V-Statin*
		Ear, nose, throat and lung infections	*Herbal ENT*
		Cough and dyspnea	*Respirol (CF)*
Prinivil	*Lisinopril*	Cardiovascular disorders	*Gastrodia Complex*
Procardia	*Nifedipine*	Cardiovascular disorders	*Gastrodia Complex*
Propoxyphene	**Darvon**	See **Darvon**	
Propoxyphene / Acetaminophen	**Darvocet**	See **Darvocet**	
Propranolol	**Inderal**	See **Inderal**	
Propylthiouracil	**PTU**	See **PTU**	
Proscar	*Finasteride*	Benign prostatic hypertrophy (BPH)	*Saw Palmetto Complex, P-Statin*
Protonix	*Pantoprazole*	Various gastrointestinal disorders	*GI Care*
Proventil	*Albuterol*	Heat-type asthma with fever, dry mouth, thirst, red face and red tongue	*Respirol (Heat)*
		Cold-type asthma with chills, intolerance to cold, cyanotic complexion of the face and body	*Respirol (Cold)*
		Chronic asthma with frequent attacks of wheezing and dyspnea	*Respirol (Deficient), Cordyceps 3*
Prozac	*Fluoxetine*	Depression by inhibiting the re-uptake of serotonin	*Shine*
Pseudoephedrine	**Sudafed**	See **Sudafed**	

DRUG – HERB INDEX

NAMES (BRAND / GENERIC)		CLINICAL APPLICATIONS	HERB ALTERNATIVES
Pseudoephedrine / Brompheniramine	Bromfed	See Bromfed	
PTU	Propylthiouracil	Mild-to-moderate cases of hyperthyroidism	Thyrodex
Quinapril	Accupril	See Accupril	
Rabeprazole	Aciphex	See Aciphex	
Ranitidine	Zantac	See Zantac	
Raptiva	Efalizumab	Psoriasis	Dermatrol (PS)
Relafen	Nabumetone	Various headaches: migraine, tension, stress, vertex, occipital	Corydalin, Migratrol
		Musculoskeletal pain with redness, swelling and inflammation	Flex (Heat)
		Musculoskeletal pain that worsens during cold and rainy days	Flex (CD)
		Neuropathy	Flex (NP)
		Chronic injuries of soft tissues (muscles, ligaments and tendons)	Flex (MLT)
		Acute and chronic pain of the arm (shoulder, elbow and wrist)	Arm Support
		Acute or chronic pain of the leg (knee and ankle)	Knee & Ankle (Acute) or (Chronic)
		Acute or chronic upper and lower back pain	Back Support (Acute), (Chronic), or (Upper)
		Acute or chronic neck and shoulder pain	Neck & Shoulder (Acute) or (Chronic)
		Menstrual pain and cramps in dysmenorrhea	Mense-Ease
		Pain associated with amenorrhea	Menotrol
		Pain associated with endometriosis	Resolve (Lower)
		Severe pain	Herbal Analgesic
Relpax	Eletriptan	Various headaches: migraine, tension, stress, vertex, occipital	Corydalin
		Migraine headache	Migratrol
Reminyl	Galantamine	Both mental and physical functions in Alzheimer's disease	Neuro Plus, Enhance Memory
Restoril	Temazepam	Insomnia and improve the overall quality of sleep	Schisandra ZZZ
		Insomnia due to stress and anxiety	Calm ZZZ
Rifaximin	Xifaxan	See Xifaxan	
Ritalin	Methylphenidate	To promote concentration and focus	Calm (Jr)
Rivastigmine	Exelon	See Exelon	

DRUG / HERB

DRUG – HERB INDEX

NAMES (BRAND / GENERIC)		CLINICAL APPLICATIONS	HERB ALTERNATIVES
Robaxin	Methocarbamol	Muscle stiffness and pain of the neck and shoulder	Neck & Shoulder (Acute)
		General relief of muscle spasm and cramps	Flex (SC)
Robitussin	Antitussive Combination	Lower respiratory tract infection with chest congestion, cough, yellow phlegm and fever	Poria XPT
		Cough and dyspnea	Respitrol (CF)
Rogaine	Minoxidil	To promote growth of healthy and shiny new hair	Polygonum 14
Rosiglitazone	Avandia	See Avandia	
Selegiline	Eldepryl	See Eldepryl	
Senna	Senokot	See Senokot	
Senokot	Senna	Moderate-to-severe constipation	Gentle Lax (Excess) or (Deficient)
Sertraline	Zoloft	See Zoloft	
Sildenafil	Viagra	See Viagra	
Simvastatin	Zocor	See Zocor	
Sinemet	Carbidopa / Levodopa	Both mental and physical functions in Parkinson's disease	Neuro Plus
Singulair	Montelukast	Dyspnea and shortness of breath in cases of chronic asthma	Respitrol (Deficient)
		Management and prevention of chronic asthma	Cordyceps 3
Skelaxin	Metaxalone	Muscle stiffness and pain of the neck and shoulder	Neck & Shoulder (Acute)
		General relief of muscle spasm and cramps	Flex (SC)
Slo-Phylline	Theophylline	See Theo-Dur	
Soma	Carisoprodol	Muscle stiffness and pain of the neck and shoulder	Neck & Shoulder (Acute)
		General relief of muscle spasm and cramps	Flex (SC)
Sominex	Diphenhydramine	Insomnia and improve the overall quality of sleep	Schisandra ZZZ
		Insomnia due to stress and anxiety	Calm ZZZ
Starlix	Nateglinide	Elevated blood glucose levels in non-insulin dependent diabetics	Equilibrium
Strattera	Atomoxetine	ADHD	Calm (Jr)
Sudafed	Pseudoephedrine	Chronic and severe nasal congestion due to sinusitis or rhinitis	Pueraria Clear Sinus
		Nasal congestion due to allergies or common cold	Magnolia Clear Sinus
Sulfamethoxazole / Trimethoprim	Bactrim	See Bactrim	
Sulindac	Clinoril	See Clinoril	
Sumatriptan	Imitrex	See Imitrex	

Lotus Institute of Integrative Medicine

DRUG – HERB INDEX

NAMES (BRAND / GENERIC)		CLINICAL APPLICATIONS	HERB ALTERNATIVES
Suprax	Cefixime	Generalized bacterial, viral and fungal infection	Herbal ABX
		Upper respiratory tract infection with fever, headache, sore throat	Lonicera Complex
		Respiratory tract infection with sinus congestion, watery nasal discharge, sneezing and chills	Respitrol (Cold)
		Lower respiratory tract infection with high fever, copious yellow sputum, cough and perspiration	Respitrol (Heat)
		Lower respiratory tract infection with chest congestion, cough, yellow phlegm and fever	Poria XPT
		Infection in the oral region, such as ulceration, sore throat, and herpes	Lonicera Complex
		Genito-urinary infections, such as herpes, urinary tract infection, or sexually-transmitted diseases	Gentiana Complex or V-Statin
		Ear, nose, throat and lung infections	Herbal ENT
		Cough and dyspnea	Respitrol (CF)
Symmetrel	Amantadine	Colds / flu with fever, headache, sore throat	Lonicera Complex
Synarel	Nafarelin	Endometriosis	Resolve (Lower)
		Amenorrhea	Menotrol
Synthroid	Levothyroxine	Hypothyroidism	Thyro-forte
Tacrine	Cognex	See Cognex	
Tadalafil	Cialis	See Cialis	
Tagamet	Cimetidine	Various gastrointestinal disorders	GI Care
Tamoxifen	Nolvadex	See Nolvadex	
Tapazole	Methimazole	Mild-to-moderate cases of hyperthyroidism	Thyrodex
Tegaserod	Zelnorm	See Zelnorm	
Tegretol	Carbamazepine	Nerve related pain, such as neuralgia and neuropathy	Flex (NP)
		Seizure and epilepsy	Gastrodia Complex
Telithromycin	Ketek	See Ketek	
Temazepam	Restoril	See Restoril	
Tenex	Guanfacine	Elevated blood pressure in patients with a hyperactive adrenergic system	Gentiana Complex
Tenormin	Atenolol	Elevated blood pressure in patients with hyperactive adrenergic system	Gentiana Complex
Tenuate	Diethylpropion	Elevated body weight; slow basal metabolism; lack of energy	Herbalite
Terazosin	Hytrin	See Hytrin	

DRUG – HERB INDEX

NAMES (BRAND / GENERIC)		CLINICAL APPLICATIONS	HERB ALTERNATIVES
Terbutaline	Brethine	See Brethine	
Theo-24	Theophylline	See Theo-Dur	
Theo-Dur	Theophylline	Heat-type asthma with fever, dry mouth, thirst, red face and red tongue	Respirol (Heat)
		Cold-type asthma with chills, intolerance to cold, cyanotic complexion of the face and body	Respirol (Cold)
		Chronic asthma with frequent attacks of wheezing and dyspnea	Respirol (Deficient), Cordyceps 3
Theophylline	Slo-Phylline / Theo-24 / Theo-Dur	See Slo-Phylline / Theo-24 / Theo-Dur	
Thorazine	Chlorpromazine	Moderate-to-severe emotional and psychological disorders	Calm (ES)
Thyroid Desiccated	Armour Thyroid	See Armour Thyroid	
Thyrolar	Liotrix	Hypothyroidism	Thyro-forte
Tolbutamide	Orinase	See Orinase	
Tolectin	Tolmetin	Various headaches: migraine, tension, stress, vertex, occipital	Corydalin, Migratrol
		Musculoskeletal pain with redness, swelling and inflammation	Flex (Heat)
		Musculoskeletal pain that worsens during cold and rainy days	Flex (CD)
		Neuropathy	Flex (NP)
		Chronic injuries of soft tissues (muscles, ligaments and tendons)	Flex (MLT)
		Acute and chronic pain of the arm (shoulder, elbow and wrist)	Arm Support
		Acute or chronic pain of the leg (knee and ankle)	Knee & Ankle (Acute) or (Chronic)
		Acute or chronic upper and lower back pain	Back Support (Acute), (Chronic), or (Upper)
		Acute or chronic neck and shoulder pain	Neck & Shoulder (Acute) or (Chronic)
		Menstrual pain and cramps in dysmenorrhea	Mense-Ease
		Pain associated with amenorrhea	Menotrol
		Pain associated with endometriosis	Resolve (Lower)
		Severe pain	Herbal Analgesic
Tolmetin	Tolectin	See Tolectin	
Toprol	Metoprolol	Elevated blood pressure in patients with hyperactive adrenergic system	Gentiana Complex
Tramadol	Ultram	See Ultram	
Triamterene / Hydrochlorothiazide	Maxzide / Dyazide	See Maxzide or Dyazide	

DRUG – HERB INDEX

NAMES (BRAND / GENERIC)		CLINICAL APPLICATIONS	HERB ALTERNATIVES
Trimox	*Amoxicillin*	*See Amoxil*	
Tums	*Calcium Carbonate*	Various gastrointestinal disorders	*GI Care*
Tucks	*Hamamelis*	Hemorrhoids	*GI Care (HMR)*
Tylenol / Codeine	*Acetaminophen / Codeine*	Various headaches: migraine, tension, stress, vertex, occipital	*Corydalin, Migratrol*
		Musculoskeletal pain due to sports or traumatic injuries	*Traumanex*
		Arthritis, especially if condition worsens with cold and dampness	*Flex (CD)*
		Acute or chronic upper and lower back pain	*Back Support (Acute)* or *(Upper)*
		Acute or chronic neck and shoulder pain	*Neck & Shoulder (Acute)*
		Acute and chronic pain of the arm (shoulder, elbow and wrist)	*Arm Support*
		Acute pain from herniated disk in the back	*Back Support (HD)*
		Acute pain of the leg (knee and ankle)	*Knee & Ankle (Acute)*
Ultram	*Tramadol*	Various headaches: migraine, tension, stress, vertex, occipital	*Corydalin, Migratrol*
		Musculoskeletal pain with redness, swelling and inflammation	*Flex (Heat)*
		Chronic injuries of soft tissues (muscles, ligaments and tendons)	*Flex (MLT)*
		Acute and chronic pain of the arm (shoulder, elbow and wrist)	*Arm Support*
		Acute or chronic pain of the leg (knee and ankle)	*Knee & Ankle (Acute)* or *(Chronic)*
		Acute or chronic upper and lower back pain	*Back Support (Acute), (Chronic),* or *(Upper)*
		Acute or chronic neck and shoulder pain	*Neck & Shoulder (Acute)* or *(Chronic)*
		Severe pain	*Herbal Analgesic*
		Acute pain from herniated disk in the back	*Back Support (HD)*
Unisom	*Doxylamine*	Insomnia and the overall quality of sleep	*Schisandra ZZZ*
		Insomnia due to stress and anxiety	*Calm ZZZ*
Uroxatral	*Alfuzosin*	Benign prostatic hypertrophy (BPH)	*Saw Palmetto Complex, P-Statin*
Ursodiol	**Actigall**	*See Actigall*	
Valtrex	*Valacyclovir*	*See Valtrex*	
Valium	*Diazepam*	Moderate-to-severe emotional and psychological disorders	*Calm (ES)*
		Moderate levels of stress, anxiety, nervousness, tension, etc.	*Calm*
		Moderate levels of stress, anxiety, and insomnia	*Calm ZZZ*

Lotus Institute of Integrative Medicine

DRUG / HERB

DRUG – HERB INDEX

NAMES (BRAND / GENERIC)		CLINICAL APPLICATIONS	HERB ALTERNATIVES
Valtrex	Valacyclovir	Genital herpes	Gentiana Complex
		Treatment and / or prevention of oral herpes	Lonicera Complex
		Recurrent genital herpes	Nourish
		Shingles	Dermatrol (HZ)
Vardenafil		See Levitra	
Vasotec	Enalapril	Cardiovascular disorders	Gastrodia Complex
Venlafaxine		See Effexor	
Ventolin	Albuterol	Heat-type asthma with fever, dry mouth, thirst, red face and red tongue	Respirol (Heat)
		Cold-type asthma with chills, intolerance to cold, cyanotic complexion of the face and body	Respirol (Cold)
		Chronic asthma with frequent attacks of wheezing and dyspnea	Respirol (Deficient), Cordyceps 3
Verapamil	Calan / Isoptin	See Calan or Isoptin	
Viagra	Sildenafil	Male sexual and reproductive dysfunctions	Vitality
		Male sexual and reproductive dysfunctions with cold signs and symptoms	Kidney Tonic (Yang)
		Male infertility (not an indication of Viagra)	Vital Essence
Vicodin	Hydrocodone / Acetaminophen	Various headaches: migraine, tension, stress, vertex, occipital	Corydalin, Migratrol
		Musculoskeletal pain due to sports or traumatic injuries	Traumanex
		Arthritis, especially if condition worsens with cold and dampness	Flex (CD)
		Acute or chronic upper and lower back pain	Back Support (Acute) or (Upper)
		Acute or chronic neck and shoulder pain	Neck & Shoulder (Acute)
		Acute and chronic pain of the arm (shoulder, elbow and wrist)	Arm Support
		Acute pain from herniated disk in the back	Back Support (HD)
		Acute pain of the leg (knee and ankle)	Knee & Ankle (Acute)
Vistaril	Hydroxyzine	Allergic or hypersensitive skin problems such as rash, itching, eczema, etc.	Silerex
Vitamin K	Mephyton	See Mephyton	
Vivarin	Caffeine	Lack of energy levels; decreased mental and physical performance	Vibrant
Voltaren...	Dicolfenac...	Various headaches: migraine, tension, stress, vertex, occipital	Corydalin, Migratrol
		Musculoskeletal pain with redness, swelling and inflammation	Flex (Heat)
		Musculoskeletal pain that worsens during cold and rainy days	Flex (CD)
		Neuropathy	Flex (NP)
		Chronic injuries of soft tissues (muscles, ligaments and tendons)	Flex (MLT)

DRUG – HERB INDEX

NAMES (BRAND / *GENERIC*)	CLINICAL APPLICATIONS	HERB ALTERNATIVES
	Acute and chronic pain of the arm (shoulder, elbow and wrist)	*Arm Support*
	Acute or chronic pain of the leg (knee and ankle)	*Knee & Ankle (Acute)* or *(Chronic)*
	Acute or chronic upper and lower back pain	*Back Support (Acute)*, *(Chronic)*, or *(Upper)*
	Acute or chronic neck and shoulder pain	*Neck & Shoulder (Acute)* or *(Chronic)*
	Menstrual pain and cramps in dysmenorrhea	*Mense-Ease*
	Pain associated with amenorrhea	*Menotrol*
	Pain associated with endometriosis	*Resolve (Lower)*
	Severe pain	*Herbal Analgesic*
Wellbutrin *Bupropion*	Depression by inhibiting the re-uptake of serotonin	*Shine*
Xanax *Alprazolam*	Moderate-to-severe emotional and psychological disorders	*Calm (ES)*
	Moderate levels of stress, anxiety, nervousness, tension, etc.	*Calm*
	Moderate levels of stress, anxiety, and insomnia	*Calm ZZZ*
Xenical *Orlistat*	Obesity	*Herbalite*
Xifaxan *Rifaximin*	Traveler's diarrhea	*GI Care II, Herbal ABX*
Yocon *Yohimbine*	To enhance male sexual and reproductive functions	*Vitality*
	Male sexual and reproductive dysfunctions with cold signs and symptoms	*Kidney Tonic (Yang)*
	Male infertility (not an indication of Viagra)	*Vital Essence*
Yohimbine	*See Yocon*	
Zafirlukast	*See Accolate*	
Zantac *Ranitidine*	Various gastrointestinal disorders	*GI Care*
Zelnorm *Tegaserod*	Irritable bowel syndrome	*GI Harmony*
Zephrex *Expectorant Combination*	Lower respiratory tract infection with chest congestion, cough, yellow phlegm and fever	*Poria XPT*
	Cough and dyspnea	*Respitrol (CF)*
Zestril *Lisinopril*	Cardiovascular disorders	*Gastrodia Complex*
Zetia *Ezetimibe*	Hypercholesterolemia	*Cholisma, Cholisma (ES)*
Zileuton	*See Zyflo*	
Zyflo	Generalized bacterial, viral and fungal infection	*Herbal ABX*
Zithromax... *Azithromycin...*	Upper respiratory tract infection with fever, headache, sore throat	*Lonicera Complex*

DRUG / HERB

DRUG – HERB INDEX

NAMES (BRAND / GENERIC)		CLINICAL APPLICATIONS	HERB ALTERNATIVES
		Respiratory tract infection with sinus congestion, watery nasal discharge, sneezing and chills	*Respirol (Cold)*
		Lower respiratory tract infection with high fever, copious yellow sputum, cough and perspiration	*Respirol (Heat)*
		Lower respiratory tract infection with chest congestion, cough, yellow phlegm and fever	*Poria XPT*
		Infection in the oral region, such as ulceration, sore throat, and herpes	*Lonicera Complex*
		Genito-urinary infections, such as herpes, urinary tract infection, or sexually-transmitted diseases	*Gentiana Complex* or *V-Statin*
		Ear, nose, throat and lung infections	*Herbal ENT*
		Cough and dyspnea	*Respirol (CF)*
Zocor	*Simvastatin*	Elevated serum cholesterol and triglycerides levels	*Cholisma*
		Elevated serum cholesterol and triglycerides levels with fatty liver and obesity	*Cholisma (ES)*
Zoloft	*Sertraline*	Depression by inhibiting the re-uptake of serotonin	*Shine*
Zolpidem	*Ambien*	*See Ambien*	
		Genital herpes	*Gentiana Complex*
Zovirax	*Acyclovir*	Treatment and / or prevention of oral herpes	*Lonicera Complex*
		Recurrent genital herpes	*Nourish*
		Shingles	*Dermatrol (HZ)*
Zyflo	*Zileuton*	Dyspnea and shortness of breath in cases of chronic asthma	*Respirol (Deficient)*
		Management and prevention of chronic asthma	*Cordyceps 3*
Zyloprim	*Allopurinol*	Gout	*Flex (GT)*
Zyrtec	*Cetirizine*	Allergic or hypersensitive skin problems such as rash, itching, eczema, etc.	*Silerex*
		Chronic and severe nasal congestion due to sinusitis or rhinitis	*Pueraria Clear Sinus*
		Nasal congestion due to allergies or common cold	*Magnolia Clear Sinus*

Lotus Institute of Integrative Medicine

Section 5

Exemplar Formulas

方劑解釋

GUIDE TO FORMULA EXPLANATION

The information regarding herbal formulas on the following pages is intended for use by licensed health care practitioners only, as professional training and expertise are essential to correct interpretation of the material and optimal use of the herbs. All information is presented in an accurate and truthful manner. Therapeutic claims are supported by modern research and referenced accordingly throughout the entire text. The advantages and disadvantages of each herbal formula are disclosed in full so that the practitioners and their patients can make informed decisions.

Traditional Chinese Medicine (TCM) terminology. Because traditional Chinese medicine and western medicine have distinct cultural and philosophical influences, it is challenging to accurately convey some TCM terms and concepts by using English or allopathic clinical language. We have made sincere efforts to provide consistent standards for terms and concepts to bridge the gap, as follows:

- Terms that have become an accepted part of English language discourse and are well understood by the general public, such as qi, yin and yang, are not italicized nor capitalized.
- Terms unique to the profession, understood primarily by TCM practitioners, are given in pinyin, italicized and translated but not capitalized; such as *bi zheng* (painful obstruction syndrome), *xiao ke* (wasting and thirsting) syndrome, and *lin zheng* (dysuria syndrome).
- Nouns distinct to herbal medicine are italicized, capitalized and translated, such as *Ren Shen* (Radix Ginseng) and *Bu Zhong Yi Qi Tang* (Tonify the Middle and Augment the Qi Decoction).
- It is important to note that anatomical organ names in TCM imply functions distinct from their common understanding in western medicine. Therefore, organ names are capitalized when discussed within the context of traditional Chinese medicine but <u>not</u> when referring exclusively to anatomical function. For example, *Huang Qin* (Radix Scutellariae) is commonly used to clear **Lung** heat because the herb has shown antibiotic effectiveness to treat infection of the **lungs**.

CLINICAL APPLICATIONS

This section outlines the indications for use of the herbal formulas, including symptoms, diseases, and diagnoses according to Western and Oriental medicine.

WESTERN THERAPEUTIC ACTIONS

The functions of the herbal formulas are summarized according to allopathic criteria. Therapeutic functions and clinical effects stated are supported by modern research and clinical studies. Additional information and detailed explanation are discussed in the Modern Research section.

CHINESE THERAPEUTIC ACTIONS

This section summarizes the functions of the herbal formulas according to traditional Chinese medicine. Diagnoses, therapeutic functions and clinical effects are stated in Chinese medical terminology and are supported by historical references and modern textbooks.

DOSAGE

- The dosage of herbal extract for an average adult ranges from 4 to 8 capsules [2 to 4 grams] three to four times daily, taken with warm water on an empty stomach, one hour before or two hours after meals. However, it is important to keep in mind that the dosage must be adjusted to reflect the age and body weight of the patient, and the severity and nature of the illnesses.
- The average adult is roughly defined as an individual between 18 and 60 years of age, with a body weight of 120 to 180 pounds. However, since not everybody is an "average adult," dosing of herbs must be individualized based on age and body weight. Generally speaking, the dosage should be reduced if the patient is younger than

GUIDE TO FORMULA EXPLANATION

18 years of age or weighs less than 120 pounds. Conversely, the dosage should be increased if the patient weighs more than 180 pounds. For more information on dosing, please refer to *Strategic Dosing Guidelines* on page 13.

☙ The dosage should be adjusted according to the type and severity of the illness. For treating acute or severe illnesses, such as severe low back pain, the dosage may be doubled to enhance the therapeutic effect. Depending on the patient and the disease, some herbal formulas may be taken in dosages of up to 40 capsules [20 grams] per day. Similarly, the dosage frequency may be adjusted to reflect the nature of the illness. For example, a person with insomnia should take more herbs before bedtime and less during the day.

INGREDIENTS

The ingredients of the formulas are listed in alphabetic order by their *pinyin* and pharmaceutical names. The nomenclature of herbs and formulas are taken from the following primary sources:

☙ *Zhong Hua Ren Min Gong He Guo Yao Dian* (Chinese Herbal Pharmacopoeia by People's Republic of China), People's Republic of China, 2000. Our standard reference for nomenclature of pinyin and pharmaceutical names, this text offers the most precise, accurate and current information on the identification of Chinese herbs and other medicinal substances.

☙ *Xian Dai Zhong Yao Yao Li Xue* (Contemporary Pharmacology of Chinese Herbs) by Wang Ben-Yang, Tianjing Science and Technology Press, 1999.

☙ *Chinese Herbal Medicine Materia Medica*, by Dan Bensky and Andrew Gamble, Eastland Press, 1993.

☙ *Chinese Herbal Medicine Formulas & Strategies*, by Dan Bensky and Randall Barolet, Eastland Press, 1990.

☙ *A Practical Dictionary of Chinese Medicine* 2nd Edition, by Nigel Wiseman and Feng Ye, Paradigm Publications, 1998.

FORMULA EXPLANATION

This section explains the rationale for and the treatment strategy of the herbal formula. The therapeutic function of each ingredient is discussed in detail to provide a comprehensive understanding of each herbal formula. The explanations include both Chinese and Western medical terminology and are intended for readers with medical training.

SUPPLEMENTARY FORMULAS

☙ This section emphasizes the modification of herbal treatment. As two or more patients having the same disease may have different clinical manifestations, it is often necessary to choose an alternate formula, combine two formulas for synergistic effects, or add another formula to treat complications or progression of the disease.

NUTRITION

☙ This section describes the dietary changes recommended to facilitate short- and long-term recovery. Detailed information is available on what foods to consume and what foods to avoid.

The Tao of Nutrition by Ni and McNease

☙ This section highlights foods and nutrients that should be consumed and avoided. Recommendations include that are common foods, as well as those that are unique to the Chinese culture and traditional Chinese medicine.

☙ For more information, please refer to *The Tao of Nutrition* by Dr. Maoshing Ni and Cathy McNease.

GUIDE TO FORMULA EXPLANATION

LIFESTYLE INSTRUCTIONS

☯ This section highlights lifestyle changes recommended to enhance herbal treatment. Lifestyle instructions are recommended to enhance the effectiveness of herbal treatment and to prevent re-occurrence of illnesses.

CLINICAL NOTES

☯ This section includes quick and easy tips for practitioners to boost the effectiveness and overall success of the treatment.

☯ This section also provides valuable information on differential diagnosis, treatment and prognosis, based on the clinical experience of masters of traditional Chinese medicine.

Pulse Diagnosis by Dr. Jimmy Wei-Yen Chang:

☯ Dr. Chang is one of the best TCM practitioners in both Taiwan and the United States. Dr. Chang treated approximately 100 patients per day in Taiwan, and after practicing for over 20 years in Taiwan, he developed a keen understanding of pulse diagnosis and herbal therapeutics. In this section, Dr. Chang highlights the unique pulses associated with certain formulas and diseases.

☯ Note: Dr. Chang takes the pulse in slightly different positions. He places his index finger directly over the wrist crease, and his middle and ring fingers alongside to locate *cun*, *guan* and *chi* positions.

☯ For additional information and explanation, please attend his seminars or refer to *Pulsynergy* by Dr. Jimmy Wei-Yen Chang and Marcus Brinkman.

CAUTIONS

☯ This section discusses relevant cautions for use of the herbal formula, including (but not limited to) side effects, adverse reactions, contraindications and herb-drug interactions.

☯ In addition, this section addresses how to discern circumstances in which to treat or *not* to treat with a particular formula. It provides valuable information for prevention of wrong diagnosis and malpractice.

☯ Information is presented in an accurate and truthful manner so health care practitioners can evaluate risks versus benefits and the patients can make informed decisions.

☯ Use of herbs during pregnancy or while nursing is *not* recommended.

ACUPUNCTURE POINTS

Traditional Points:
☯ These are textbook recommendations for body and ear points.

Balance Method by Dr. Richard Tan:
☯ Balance Method by Dr. Richard Tan: Balance Method is a specialized system developed and presented by Dr. Tan. Additional information can be found by attending his seminars [hosted by Lotus Institute], visiting his website [www.drtanshow.com], or by reading his books [*Twelve and Twelve in Acupuncture, Twenty-Four More in Acupuncture, Dr. Tan's Strategy of Twelve Magical Points* and Acupuncture 1, 2, 3].

Auricular Acupuncture by Dr. Li-Chun Huang:
☯ Auricular Acupuncture by Dr. Li-Chun Huang: Auricular Acupuncture is a highly effective system of ear acupuncture contributed by Dr. Huang. Additional information can be found by attending her seminars [hosted by Lotus Institute] or reading her book *Auricular Treatment Formula and Prescriptions*.

FORMULAS

GUIDE TO FORMULA EXPLANATION

Note: This section lists and explains the suggested acupuncture treatments to be used with herbal therapy. The abbreviations of the meridians follow the system established by World Health Organization (WHO).

Lung (LU)
Large Intestine (LI)
Stomach (ST)
Spleen (SP)
Heart (HT)
Small Intestine (SI)
Bladder (BL)

Kidney (KI)
Pericardium (PC)
Triple Heater [*San Jiao*] (TH)
Gallbladder (GB)
Liver (LR)
Governor Vessel [*Du* channel] (GV)
Conception Vessel [*Ren* channel] (CV)

MODERN RESEARCH

This section summarizes clinical and laboratory studies on the effectiveness of the herbs. Therapeutic claims are explained in detail and referenced accordingly in this section.

- **References:** The references cited include human clinical trials that are randomized, double blind, placebo-controlled, with a large number of subjects and sound statistical design. Such studies provide meaningful results with conclusions that can be extrapolated to patients with similar conditions. In addition to human clinical trials, references cited include clinical observations, case studies, credible textbooks, *in-vivo* and *in-vitro* studies, and clinical and laboratory studies.
- **Scientific and Medical Terminology:** For the occasional allopathic term that readers might find puzzling, we recommend accessing any standard allopathic medical dictionary (see next entry for example). Since there is no need for translation or interpretation of these terms, we concluded that it was unnecessary to explain such terms in this text.
- **Medical Abbreviations and Symbols** are used in accordance with *Dorland's Illustrated Medical Dictionary*, 28th Edition, by Saunders.
- **Drug Names** are designated in this text by generic names only, or the combination of Proprietary (Generic) names. The Proprietary (Generic) names are referenced according to *Drug Facts and Comparisons*, updated monthly by Facts and Comparisons, a Wolters Kluwer Company.
- **Pharmacological Effects:** Most pharmacological studies focus on the anatomical and physiological influences of the herbs 1) on the body or 2) against pathogens. For example, many herbs are described as having antihypertensive effects, as the administration of the herbs leads directly to a decrease in blood pressure. Others are said to have antibacterial effects, as the introduction of the herb leads to the inhibition or death of bacteria. However, the exact mechanisms of action for many herbs are still not well understood at this time.

PHARMACEUTICAL DRUGS & CHINESE MEDICINE: A COMPARATIVE ANALYSIS

- Written by Dr. John Chen who has doctorate degrees in both western pharmacology and traditional Chinese medicine, this section compares and contrasts the advantages and disadvantages of drug and herbal medicines. Dr. Chen strongly believes in "medicine with no border," and concludes without bias the "bottom line" on the treatment options for any given conditions, whether it is drugs, herbs, or both. Learning the benefit and risk of both medicines empowers practitioners and patients to make more educated and informed decisions for optimal treatment.
- Dr. Chen is the author of Chinese Medical Herbology and Pharmacology, and the founder and president of Art of Medicine Press. For more information, please visit his website at www.aompress.com. He is also a regular speaker of Lotus Institute, as well as many colleges and professional associations.

FORMULAS

GUIDE TO FORMULA EXPLANATION

CASE STUDIES

This section includes actual case reports submitted by healthcare practitioners. It enables the readers to understand the response to, and efficacy of, the herbal formulas in clinical rather than research settings. As these are original reports, the formality of the presentation varies from one case study to another.

GENERAL DISCLAIMER

Great care has been taken to maintain the accuracy of the information contained in this *Clinical Manual*. The information as presented in this *Clinical Manual* is for educational purposes only. We cannot anticipate all conditions under which this may be used. In view of ongoing research, changes in governmental regulation, and the constant flow of information relating to Chinese and western medicine, the reader is urged to check with other sources for all up-to-date information. The staff and authors of Lotus Institute of Integrative Medicine recognize that practitioners accessing this information will have varying levels of training and expertise; therefore, we accept no responsibility for the results obtained by the application of the information within this *Clinical Manual*. Nor are we liable for the safety and suitability of the products, either alone or in combination with others, with single herbs or with the products of other manufacturers. Neither the Lotus Institute of Integrative Medicine nor the authors of this *Clinical Manual* can be held responsible for errors of fact or omission, nor for any consequences arising from the use or misuse of the information herein.

PROFESSIONAL USE ONLY

This *Clinical Manual of Oriental Medicine* is intended as an educational guide for licensed health care practitioners only, as professional training and expertise are essential to the safe recommendation of and effective guidance for use of herbs. All herbal products discussed within this *Clinical Manual* must be used only through licensed health care practitioners.

The information in this *Clinical Manual* is presented in an accurate, truthful and non-misleading manner. The information is supported by modern research whenever possible and referenced accordingly throughout the entire *Clinical Manual*. Nonetheless, the FDA requires the following statements:

These statements have not been evaluated by the Food and Drug Administration. These products are not intended to diagnose, treat, cure or prevent any disease.

FORMULAS

ADRENOPLEX ™

CLINICAL APPLICATIONS

- ☙ Adrenal insufficiency or low adrenal functions
- ☙ Premature aging
- ☙ Patients who are "burned out," with fatigue, no energy, lack of interest, lack of drive and satisfaction
- ☙ Diminished sexual and physical functions

WESTERN THERAPEUTIC ACTIONS

- ☙ Regulates and improves the functioning of the adrenal glands and the endocrine system
- ☙ Improves mental acuity and physical performance
- ☙ Restores normal sexual and reproductive function
- ☙ Enhances the immune system

CHINESE THERAPEUTIC ACTIONS

- ☙ Tonifies Kidney yin, yang, and *jing* (essence)
- ☙ Tonifies the qi and blood
- ☙ Strengthens the Spleen and Stomach

DOSAGE

Take 3 to 4 capsules three times daily on an empty stomach with warm water. The dosage may be increased to 6 to 8 capsules three times daily, if necessary. For maintenance, take 1 to 2 capsules daily.

INGREDIENTS

Ba Ji Tian (Radix Morindae Officinalis)
Da Zao (Fructus Jujubae)
Du Zhong (Cortex Eucommiae)
Fu Ling (Poria)
Fu Zi (Radix Aconiti Lateralis Praeparata)
Gou Qi Zi (Fructus Lycii)
Huai Niu Xi (Radix Achyranthis Bidentatae)
Mu Dan Pi (Cortex Moutan)
Ren Shen (Radix Ginseng)
Rou Gui (Cortex Cinnamomi)

Shan Yao (Rhizoma Dioscoreae)
Shan Zhu Yu (Fructus Corni)
Shi Chang Pu (Rhizoma Acori)
Shu Di Huang (Radix Rehmanniae Preparata)
Suo Yang (Herba Cynomorii)
Wu Wei Zi (Fructus Schisandrae Chinensis)
Xiao Hui Xiang (Fructus Foeniculi)
Yuan Zhi (Radix Polygalae)
Ze Xie (Rhizoma Alismatis)
Zhi Gan Cao (Radix Glycyrrhizae Preparata)

FORMULA EXPLANATION

Adrenoplex is designed to treat patients who are "burned out," with symptoms of premature aging, fatigue, no energy, lack of interest, drive, and satisfaction. Such conditions may be caused by excessive stress, anxiety, tension, overwork, and lack of rest. From the traditional Chinese medicine perspective, there is an excessive consumption of qi, blood, yin, yang, and Kidney *jing* (essence), accompanied by deficiency of Spleen, Stomach, Heart and Kidney. Deficiency of the Spleen and Stomach leads to an inadequate supply of qi, shown by symptoms of generalized weakness, fatigue, and anorexia. Deficiency of Heart qi and blood may contribute to forgetfulness, being easily frightened, low-grade fever, and night sweats. Deficiency of yin and yang lead to premature aging. Lastly, the lack of *jing* (essence) contributes further to Kidney deficiency, leading to decreased libido, spermatorrhea, and other sexual disorders.

FORMULAS

ADRENOPLEX ™

In this formula, a large portion of *Ren Shen* (Radix Ginseng) is used because it is the most effective and potent herb to tonify qi, strengthen the Lung and the Spleen, and improve mental functioning. It has excellent adaptogenic functions to help the body adjust to various stressful situations. Studies have shown that *Ren Shen* (Radix Ginseng) improves both mental and physical functions.

In addition to *Ren Shen* (Radix Ginseng), *Suo Yang* (Herba Cynomorii), *Ba Ji Tian* (Radix Morindae Officinalis), and *Xiao Hui Xiang* (Fructus Foeniculi) strengthen the Spleen and the Kidney. *Shu Di Huang* (Radix Rehmanniae Preparata) and *Gou Qi Zi* (Fructus Lycii) nourish the Kidney and benefit qi. *Du Zhong* (Cortex Eucommiae) and *Huai Niu Xi* (Radix Achyranthis Bidentatae) tonify the Kidney and strengthen the knees and the lower back. *Fu Ling* (Poria) and *Shan Yao* (Rhizoma Dioscoreae) strengthen the Spleen and dissolve dampness. *Shan Yao* (Rhizoma Dioscoreae) and *Wu Wei Zi* (Fructus Schisandrae Chinensis) tonify the Lung and prevent leakage of Lung qi. Furthermore, they reduce the loss of fluids from the Kidney, particularly via spermatorrhea. *Yuan Zhi* (Radix Polygalae) tonifies the Heart and calms the *shen* (spirit). *Shi Chang Pu* (Rhizoma Acori) opens the sensory orifices, improves mental functioning, and increases alertness. *Da Zao* (Fructus Jujubae) tonifies both qi and blood, and strengthens the Lung and Spleen systems.

Ze Xie (Rhizoma Alismatis) settles turbidity in the Kidney and controls the potential stagnation that may be associated with the use of *Shu Di Huang* (Radix Rehmanniae Preparata). *Mu Dan Pi* (Cortex Moutan) is used to sedate deficiency fire of the Liver; hence, it is used in conjunction with *Shan Zhu Yu* (Fructus Corni). *Fu Ling* (Poria), as the sedating herb used with *Shan Yao* (Rhizoma Dioscoreae), dispels damp through urination and tonifies the middle *jiao*.

Hot in nature, *Fu Zi* (Radix Aconiti Lateralis Praeparata) and *Rou Gui* (Cortex Cinnamomi) revitalize Kidney yang and warm the lower body. *Fu Zi* (Radix Aconiti Lateralis Praeparata) is excellent for treatment of various chronic cold type disorders associated with the endocrine, cardiovascular and musculoskeletal systems. *Rou Gui* (Cortex Cinnamomi) strengthens the Spleen and tonifies Kidney yang.

Zhi Gan Cao (Radix Glycyrrhizae Preparata) tonifies qi and harmonizes the action of the other herbs. Furthermore, the addition of a small amount of salt functions as a channel-guiding substance to enhance the Kidney-tonic properties of the formula.

SUPPLEMENTARY FORMULAS

- For an immediate boost of energy, use with *Vibrant*.
- For long-term restoration of vitality, use with *Imperial Tonic*.
- For patients with hypothyroidism, use with *Thyro-forte*.
- For sexual and reproductive disorders, use with *Vitality*.
- For compromised immune system, use with *Immune +*.
- For stomach and duodenal ulcers, use with *GI Care*.
- For stress and anxiety, use with *Calm*.
- For severe stress and anxiety, use with *Calm (ES)*.
- For stress, anxiety and insomnia, use with *Calm ZZZ*.
- For insomnia, use with *Schisandra ZZZ*.
- For obesity, use with *Herbalite*.
- For weakness and deficiency of the Lung, use with *Cordyceps 3*.
- For poor memory, use with *Enhance Memory*.
- For general Kidney yang deficiency, add *Kidney Tonic (Yang)*.
- For general Kidney yin deficiency, add *Kidney Tonic (Yin)*.
- For male infertility, add *Vital Essence*.

ADRENOPLEX ™

NUTRITION

☯ Increase the consumption of fresh fruits, vegetables, grains, seeds and nuts.

☯ Eat more fish and fish oils, onions, garlic, olives, olive oil, herbs, spices, yogurt, fiber, and tofu or other soy products.

☯ Sea vegetables, such as kelp and dulse, replenish the body with minerals like magnesium, potassium, calcium, iodine and iron.

☯ Ensure adequate intake of vitamin B complex to process and utilize energy.

☯ Decrease intake of red meat, alcohol, fats, and highly processed foods.

☯ Avoid the use of stimulants, such as coffee, caffeine, and high-sugar products.

☯ Food allergies or chemical hypersensitivity can drain energy and cause fatigue. Additional tests are necessary to rule out allergy and/or hypersensitivity.

LIFESTYLE INSTRUCTIONS

☯ Get regular exercise and adequate rest.

☯ For relaxation and better sleep, take a warm bath for about 20 minutes before bedtime. Sea salts or epsom salts can also be added.

☯ Engage in activities such as *Tai Chi Chuan*, walking, or meditation that allow calming of the mind without creating stagnation or excessive fatigue.

☯ Avoid exposure to heavy metals such as lead, cadmium, aluminum, copper, and arsenic, all of which can suppress the immune system and cause fatigue. Those who have already been exposed should take **Herbal DTX** to eliminate these toxins.

CAUTIONS

☯ This formula is contraindicated during pregnancy and nursing.

☯ This formula is not recommended in cases with exterior or excess conditions. It should not be used in cases of infections and inflammations.

☯ Patients who wear a pacemaker, or individuals who take anti-arrhythmic drugs or cardiac glycosides such as Lanoxin (Digoxin), should not take this formula. *Fu Zi* (Radix Aconiti Lateralis Praeparata) may interact with these drugs by affecting the rhythm and potentiating the contractile strength of the heart.

ACUPUNCTURE POINTS

Traditional Points:

☯ Apply moxa to *Mingmen* (GV 4), *Shenshu* (BL 23), and *Guanyuan* (CV 4).

☯ Needle *Shenshu* (BL 23), *Sanyinjiao* (SP 6), *Zusanli* (ST 36), *Qihai* (CV 6), *Mingmen* (GV 4), and *Shenque* (CV 8).

Balance Method by Dr. Richard Tan:

☯ Left side: *Hegu* (LI 4), *Fuliu* (KI 7), *Ligou* (LR 5), and Kidney point on the ear.

☯ Right side: *Zusanli* (ST 36), *Yanglingquan* (GB 34), and *Tongli* (HT 5).

☯ Left and right side can be alternated from treatment to treatment.

☯ For additional information on the Balance Method, please refer to *Dr. Tan's Strategy of Twelve Magical Points* by Dr. Richard Tan.

ADRENOPLEX ™

Auricular Acupuncture by Dr. Li-Chun Huang:

❧ Addison's Disease: Adrenal Gland, Endocrine, Pituitary, Exciting Point, Thalamus, *San Jiao*, Kidney, and Liver.

❧ For additional information on the location and explanation of these points, please refer to *Auricular Treatment Formula and Prescriptions* by Dr. Li-Chun Huang.

MODERN RESEARCH

Adrenoplex is designed to treat patients who are "burned out," with fatigue and lethargy accompanied by premature aging and a decline in mental acuity and physical performance. It contains herbs that stimulate the mind, improve physical strength, restore sexual prowess, and enhance the immune system.

According to *Dorland's Medical Dictionary*, the endocrine system has a significant impact on various glands of the body, including, but not limited to, the hypothalamus, pituitary, thyroid, parathyroid, the adrenal glands, gonads, pancreas, and paraganglia.[1] Normal functioning of the endocrine system is essential for good health. Imbalance of the endocrine system will lead to disease. Decline of the endocrine system also leads to premature aging and decreased mental and physical performance. To properly address such conditions, this formula uses many herbs to regulate and enhance the endocrine system. For example, *Shu Di Huang* (Radix Rehmanniae Preparata) has been shown to increase plasma levels of adrenal cortical hormone.[2] *Ba Ji Tian* (Radix Morindae Officinalis) has a stimulating effect on the pituitary gland and the adrenal cortex, and its administration has been associated with an increase in plasma levels of corticosteroids.[3] Administration of glycyrrhizin and glycyrrhetinic, two active ingredients in *Zhi Gan Cao* (Radix Glycyrrhizae Preparata), clearly enhances the overall duration and influence of cortisone as demonstrated by various laboratory studies.[4] One clinical trial showed that patients with declining pituitary gland function were successfully treated by continuous use of *Ren Shen* (Radix Ginseng) and *Zhi Gan Cao* (Radix Glycyrrhizae Preparata) for two to three months.[5] Since the long-term use of *Zhi Gan Cao* (Radix Glycyrrhizae Preparata) is sometimes associated with cellular accumulation of water, *Ze Xie* (Rhizoma Alismatis) is added for its diuretic action to alleviate this potential side effect.[6] Other herbs that affect and improve the endocrine system include *Shan Zhu Yu* (Fructus Corni), *Du Zhong* (Cortex Eucommiae), and *Ba Ji Tian* (Radix Morindae Officinalis).[7,8]

In addition to regulating the endocrine system, it is also important to restore optimal mental and physical functioning. *Shi Chang Pu* (Rhizoma Acori) and *Ren Shen* (Radix Ginseng) improve mental acuity. In laboratory studies, administration of *Shi Chang Pu* (Rhizoma Acori) is associated with improvement of memory.[9] In clinical studies, use of *Ren Shen* (Radix Ginseng) is associated with marked effectiveness in improving memory and learning ability.[10] In one study on mental retardation, 30 children with low IQ's took a formula comprised of *Ren Shen* (Radix Ginseng) and three other herbs and showed mild to moderate improvement in classroom performance.[11] Furthermore, *Da Zao* (Fructus Jujubae) and *Ba Ji Tian* (Radix Morindae Officinalis) improve physical performance. In comparison with placebo substances, both of these herbs showed significant capacity to increase body weight, muscle strength, and physical endurance.[12,13]

Furthermore, many herbs in this formula function to improve sexual and reproductive functions. Use of *Gou Qi Zi* (Fructus Lycii) is highly effective to improve low sperm count and poor motility.[14] *Wu Wei Zi* (Fructus Schisandrae Chinensis) has a stimulating effect on reproductive organs, increasing the weight of the testicles in males and inducing ovulation in females.[15] Lastly, in one clinical study, patients with impotence were treated with *Ren Shen* (Radix Ginseng) with marked success. Out of 27 patients, 15 regained normal function, 9 had moderate improvement, and 3 showed no effect. In another study, 24 patients with low sperm count, treated with a preparation of *Ren Shen* (Radix Ginseng), demonstrated an increase in sperm count in 70% of the patients, and an increase in sperm motility in 67% of the patients.[16]

FORMULAS

ADRENOPLEX ™

Since patients who are weak and deficient often have a suppressed immune system, herbs are included in this formula to strengthen the body and enhance the immune system. This herbal formula has dual effects on the immune system. Not only does it increase the white blood cell count, but it also increases the activity of the macrophages. According to studies, use of a *Rou Gui* (Cortex Cinnamomi) preparation for five days increased white blood cell count by 150 to 200%, and use of *Ren Shen* (Radix Ginseng) increased the total count of IgM.[17,18] Additionally, *Gou Qi Zi* (Fructus Lycii) and *Du Zhong* (Cortex Eucommiae) increase non-specific immunity, as they promote phagocytic activity by the macrophages, and increase the total number of T cells.[19,20,21]

In summary, *Adrenoplex* contains herbs that have excellent effects of regulating the adrenal glands and balance the endocrine system. It is a key formula to treat patients experiencing premature aging, declining mental and physical functioning, or who are simply "burned out" with fatigue, no energy, lack of interest, lack of drive and satisfaction.

PHARMACEUTICAL DRUGS & CHINESE MEDICINE: A COMPARATIVE ANALYSIS

Adrenal insufficiency or low adrenal functions are general terms used to describe individuals who have premature aging or are "burned out," with fatigue, no energy, lack of interest, lack of drive and satisfaction. These conditions affect overall health, and often lead to diminished mental and physical functions.

Western Medical Approach: Adrenal insufficiency technically and specifically refers to conditions such as Addison's disease. Such serious conditions are often treated with various types of intravenous or oral adrenocortical hormones. Though effective, they often have a great number of side effects, including immune suppression, increased frequency and decreased resistance to infections, decreased or blurred vision, filling or rounding out of the face, frequent urination, increased thirst, abdominal or stomach pain, acne, bloody or black [tarry] stools, headache, irregular heartbeat, menstrual problems, muscle cramps or pain, muscle weakness, nausea, pain throughout the body, sensitivity of eyes to light, stunting of growth (in children), swelling of feet or lower legs, tearing of eyes, thin and shiny skin, difficulty sleeping, unusual bruising, unusual increase in hair growth, unusual tiredness or weakness, rapid weight gain, and non-healing wounds. Therefore, unless the patients are diagnosed with the biomedical condition of adrenal cortical hypofunction, potent drugs such as adrenocortical hormones are not used.

Traditional Chinese Medicine Approach: Adrenal insufficiency is used to describe the general signs and symptoms of qi, blood, yin, yang, and Kidney *jing* (essence) depletion accompanied by Spleen, Stomach, Heart and Kidney deficiencies. As described above, *Adrenoplex* has excellent functions to regulate the endocrine system, stimulate the adrenal glands, and improve mental and physical functions. Though herbs do not treat specific and serious conditions such as Addison's disease, they do offer excellent preventative and treatment effects for individuals who are "burned out," with fatigue, no energy, lack of interest, lack of drive and satisfaction. Most importantly, herbal therapy has significantly better safety profile in comparison with drug treatments.

CASE STUDY

L.D., a 31-year-old female, presented with fatigue, dizziness, low body temperature, coldness and muscle weakness. Her blood pressure was 100/60 mmHg and her heart rate was 65 beats per minute. Her western diagnosis was hypotension and hypoglycemia. Laboratory result showed she had decreased thyroid activity and adrenal medullary insufficiency. The diagnosis was yang deficiency. She was prescribed *Thyro-forte* and *Adrenoplex* at 2.5 and 1.5 grams per day, respectively. She did not receive any acupuncture. After two months, she felt much more energized and the dizziness was gone. She no longer felt cold.

W.F., Bloomfield, New Jersey

ADRENOPLEX ™

[1] *Dorland's Illustrated Medical Dictionary, 28th Edition*. W.B.Saunders Company, 1994.
[2] *Zhong Yao Xue* (Chinese Herbology), 1998; 156:158
[3] *Guo Wai Yi Xue Zhong Yi Zhong Yao Fen Ce* (Monograph of Chinese Herbology from Foreign Medicine), 1990; 12(6):48
[4] *Zhong Yao Zhi* (Chinese Herbology Journal), 1993; 358
[5] *Zhong Hua Yi Xue Za Zhi* (Chinese Journal of Medicine), 1975; 10:718
[6] *Sheng Yao Xue Za Zhi* (Journal of Raw Herbology), 1982; 36(2):150
[7] *Zhong Yao Yao Li Yu Lin Chuang* (Pharmacology and Clinical Applications of Chinese Herbs), 1989; 5(1):36
[8] *Zhong Yi Xue* (Chinese Herbal Medicine), 1982; 13(6):24
[9] *Zhong Yi Xue* (Chinese Herbal Medicine), 1992; 23(8):417
[10] *Zhong Yao Ci Hai* (Encyclopedia of Chinese Herbs), 1994
[11] *Zhong Cheng Yao Yan Jiu* (Research of Chinese Patent Medicine), 1982; 6:22
[12] *Guo Wai Yi Xue Zhong Yi Zhong Yao Fen Ce* (Monograph of Chinese Herbology from Foreign Medicine), 1985; 7(4):48
[13] *Zhong Xi Yi Jie He Za Zhi* (Journal of Integrated Chinese and Western Medicine), 1991; 11(7):415
[14] *Xin Zhong Yi* (New Chinese Medicine), 1988; 2:20
[15] *Shang Hai Zhong Yi Yao Za Zhi* (Shanghai Journal of Chinese Medicine and Herbology), 1989; 2:43
[16] *Ji Lin Yi Xue* (Jilin Medicine), 1983; 5:54
[17] *Zhong Yao Yao Li Yu Ying Yong* (Pharmacology and Applications of Chinese Herbs), 1983;443
[18] *Zhong Yao Xue* (Chinese Herbology), 1998; 729:736
[19] *Zhong Yi Xue* (Chinese Herbal Medicine), 1983;19(7):25
[20] *Zhong Yi Xue* (Chinese Herbal Medicine), 1983;14(8):27
[21] *Zhong Xi Yi Jie He Za Zhi* (Journal of Integrated Chinese and Western Medicine), 1988; 8(12):736

FORMULAS

ARM SUPPORT ™

CLINICAL APPLICATIONS

- **Shoulder**: periarthritis of the shoulder, frozen shoulder, capsulitis, rotator cuff tear, rotator cuff tendonitis, bursitis, inflammation and pain of the shoulder, subluxation or dislocation, AC (acromioclavicular) separation
- **Elbow**: lateral epicondylitis (tennis elbow), medial epicondylitis (golfer's elbow), olecranon bursitis, tendonitis
- **Wrist**: carpal tunnel syndrome, tendonitis, sprain and strain
- General musculoskeletal injuries: tendonitis, bursitis, arthritis of the arm
- Numbness, decreased range of motion and atrophy of the arm

WESTERN THERAPEUTIC ACTIONS

- Analgesic effect to relieve pain
- Anti-inflammatory effect to reduce swelling and inflammation

CHINESE THERAPEUTIC ACTIONS

- Dispels cold and damp
- Activates qi and blood circulation
- Opens peripheral channels and collaterals
- Relieves pain

DOSAGE

Take 3 to 4 capsules, three times daily as needed to relieve pain. The dosage may be increased up to 6 to 8 capsules every four to six hours if necessary, especially in the early stages of injury when there is severe and excruciating pain. When the pain subsides, the dosage should be reduced to 3 or 4 capsules, three times daily. For maximum effectiveness, take the herbs on an empty stomach with two tall glasses of warm water. In chronic cases or for consolidation of treatment efficacy, the dosage can be reduced to 2 capsules twice daily on an empty stomach.

INGREDIENTS

Bai Shao (Radix Paeoniae Alba)
Dan Shen (Radix Salviae Miltiorrhizae)
E Zhu (Rhizoma Curcumae)
Ge Gen (Radix Puerariae)
Gui Zhi (Ramulus Cinnamomi)
Ji Xue Teng (Caulis Spatholobi)
Jiang Huang (Rhizoma Curcumae Longae)

Luo Shi Teng (Caulis Trachelospermi)
Sang Shen Zi (Fructus Mori)
Sang Zhi (Ramulus Mori)
Shan Zha (Fructus Crataegi)
Wu Jia Pi (Cortex Acanthopanacis)
Xi Xian Cao (Herba Siegesbeckiae)
Yan Hu Suo (Rhizoma Corydalis)

FORMULA EXPLANATION

Arm Support is designed specifically to treat disorders of the arms, including shoulders, elbows, and wrists. Disorders of the arms are usually characterized by swelling, inflammation, pain, decreased range of motion with movement difficulty, and in severe cases, atrophy of the muscles and soft tissues. To successfully treat this condition, herbs are used to activate qi and blood circulation, dispel qi and blood stagnation, open channels and collaterals, and relieve pain.

In this formula, *Dan Shen* (Radix Salviae Miltiorrhizae), *E Zhu* (Rhizoma Curcumae), and *Yan Hu Suo* (Rhizoma Corydalis) activate qi and blood circulation, and dispel qi and blood stagnation. *Shan Zha* (Fructus Crataegi) enters the *xue* (blood) level, moves blood and reduces inflammation and swelling. *Sang Shen Zi* (Fructus Mori), *Ji Xue Teng* (Caulis Spatholobi) and *Wu Jia Pi* (Cortex Acanthopanacis) tonify yin and blood, and strengthen soft tissues (muscles, tendons, and ligaments). *Gui Zhi* (Ramulus Cinnamomi), *Sang Zhi* (Ramulus Mori), *Xi Xian Cao* (Herba Siegesbeckiae), *Jiang Huang* (Rhizoma Curcumae Longae) and *Luo Shi Teng* (Caulis Trachelospermi) open the channels and collaterals and relieve pain. *Bai Shao* (Radix Paeoniae Alba) relaxes muscles and *Ge Gen* (Radix Puerariae) relieves pain in the upper *jiao*. Lastly, *Gui Zhi* (Ramulus Cinnamomi) and *Sang Zhi* (Ramulus Mori) act as channel-guiding herbs, leading the effect of the formula to the upper body and the extremities to directly treat the affected area.

In summary, *Arm Support* is an excellent formula to treat all types of musculoskeletal disorders affecting the arms, including shoulders, elbows, and wrists.

SUPPLEMENTARY FORMULAS

- With acute pain or numbness of neck and shoulders, combine with *Neck & Shoulder (Acute)*.
- With radiating or tingling pain of the arm caused by cervical spondylosis, combine with *Neck & Shoulder (Acute)*.
- With chronic pain of neck and shoulders, combine with *Neck & Shoulder (Chronic)*.
- For acute disorders of the arm with severe pain, combine with *Herbal Analgesic*.
- For chronic disorders of the arm with atrophy and tearing of soft tissues (muscles, ligaments, tendons), combine with *Flex (MLT)*.
- For headache, combine with *Corydalin*.
- For arthritis or *bi zheng* (painful obstruction syndrome) due to heat, add *Flex (Heat)*.
- For arthritis or *bi zheng* (painful obstruction syndrome) due to cold, add *Flex (CD)*.
- For tightness and spasms of the muscles, tendons and ligaments, add *Flex (SC)*.
- For bone spurs and calcific tendonitis, add *Flex (Spur)*.
- For nerve pain, add *Flex (NP)*.
- For bone fractures or bruises, add *Traumanex*.
- For osteoarthritis, add *Osteo 8*.

NUTRITION

- Eat plenty of whole grains, seafood, dark green vegetables, and nuts. These foods are rich in vitamin B complex and magnesium, which are essential for nerve health and relaxation of tense muscles, respectively.
- Adequate intake of minerals, such as calcium and potassium, are essential for pain management. A deficiency of these minerals will lead to spasms, cramps, and tense muscles.

LIFESTYLE INSTRUCTIONS

- Patients should avoid exposing affected areas to cold or drafts. Wear adequate clothing to cover the arms and shoulders to avoid exposure to cold.
- Patients with disorders of the elbows or wrists should be encouraged to gently exercise the affected area as much as possible.
- Frozen shoulder is one condition in which the patient should be advised to exercise the joint frequently. Because the shoulder has the greatest range of motion of any joint in the body, stretching and strengthening exercises are essential in keeping the shoulders healthy. Prolonged immobilization causes adhesions, which makes treatment very difficult and painful. Patients should be advised to move their shoulder(s) in all directions (external and internal rotation, abduction and extension) to improve pain free range of motion. Heat packs are often helpful in this condition.
- Hot baths with Epsom salts help to relax tense muscles and draw toxins from tissues. Rest and relax in the bath for about 30 minutes.

FORMULAS

ARM SUPPORT ™

ARM SUPPORT

❧ Patients should note their sleeping position, as poor sleeping position may lead to shoulder and neck pain in the morning.

CLINICAL NOTES

❧ This formula is most effective when used an adjunct formula to acupuncture treatment. Optimal results will show when acupuncture, electro-stimulation and herbs are included in the treatment regimen.

❧ Avoid repetitive movements that may contribute to further injuries, such as in cases of inflammation of the joint, tennis elbow or carpal tunnel syndrome.

❧ Cold packs may be used for acute injuries to reduce swelling and inflammation. In general, only during the first 24 to 48 hours of the injury where there is prominent inflammation should ice be used. On the other hand, hot packs should be used for chronic injuries to promote blood circulation and enhance healing in the affected area.

❧ *Tui-Na* and acupuncture can add tremendous relief for the patient immediately. Herbs can then be administered to consolidate the effect.

❧ This formula is designed for pain in the arm starting from the shoulder down to the wrist. ***Neck & Shoulder (Acute)*** and ***Neck & Shoulder (Chronic)*** are formulated for pain in the cervical and shoulder area.

CAUTIONS

❧ This formula has strong qi and blood activating herbs and is contraindicated during pregnancy and nursing.

❧ *Dan Shen* (Radix Salviae Miltiorrhizae) may enhance the overall effectiveness of Coumadin (Warfarin), an anticoagulant drug. Patients who take anticoagulant or antiplatelet medications should ***not*** take this herbal formula without supervision by a licensed health care practitioner.

❧ Shoulder pain that originates from a heart condition is known as referred pain. The left shoulder is mostly affected and there will be other accompanying symptoms of chest pain, palpitation or shortness of breath. Referred pain due to liver or gallbladder problems may also reflect in the shoulder, but especially the right shoulder. These potential differential diagnoses should be investigated and ruled out during initial evaluations. This formula is ***not*** designed for referred pain caused by acute internal organ problems.

ACUPUNCTURE POINTS

Traditional Points:
❧ Shoulder pain: *Jianyu* (LI 15), *Jianliao* (TH 14), *Jianzhen* (SI 9) and any other *ah shi* points.
❧ Elbow pain: *Quchi* (LI 11), *Xiaohai* (SI 8), *Tianjing* (TH 10), *Shousanli* (LI 10), *Hegu* (LI 4) and any other *ah shi* points.
❧ Wrist pain: *Yangchi* (TH 4), *Yangxi* (LI 5), *Yanggu* (SI 5) and any other *ah shi* points.

Balance Method by Dr. Richard Tan:
❧ Shoulder pain:
- Needle *ah shi* points on the opposite wrist. *Yangxi* (LI 5), *Yangchi* (TH 4), *Wangu* (SI 4) to *Yanggu* (SI 5), *Jingqu* (LU 8) to *Taiyuan* (LU 9), *Shenmen* (HT 7), and *Daling* (PC 7).
- Needle all *ah shi* points on the opposite ankle. *Zhongfeng* (LR 4), *Shangqiu* (SP 5), *Taixi* (KI 3), *Kunlun* (BL 60), *Qiuxu* (GB 40), and *Jiexi* (ST 41).
❧ Elbow pain:
- Needle *ah shi* points on the opposite knee. *Yinlingquan* (SP 9) to *Xuehai* (SP 10), *Ququan* (LR 8), *Yingu* (KI 10), *Weiyang* (BL 39) to *Weizhong* (BL 40), *Xiyangguan* (GB 33) to *Yanglingquan* (GB 34), and *Dubi* (ST 35) to *Zusanli* (ST 36).
❧ Wrist pain:
- Needle the opposite side of the pain. *Shangqiu* (SP 5), *Zhongfeng* (LR 4), *Rangu* (KI 2) and *Taixi* (KI 3), *Yangxi* (LI 5), *Yanggu* (SI 5), and *Yangchi* (TH 4).

- ▪ Needle the same side of the pain. *Kunlun* (BL 60), *Qiuxu* (GB 40), and *Jiexi* (ST 41).
- ☯ For additional information on the Balance Method, please refer to Acupuncture 1, 2, 3 by Dr. Richard Tan.

Auricular Acupuncture by Dr. Li-Chun Huang:
- ☯ Tennis elbow (external humeral epicondylitis)
  - ▪ Main point: Tennis Elbow
  - ▪ Supplementary points: Elbow; bleed Helix 2
- ☯ Carpal tunnel
  - ▪ Main point: Wrist (front and back of ear)
  - ▪ Supplementary point: Lesser Occipital Nerve
- ☯ For additional information on the location and explanation of these points, please refer to *Auricular Treatment Formula and Prescriptions* by Dr. Li-Chun Huang.

MODERN RESEARCH

Arm Support is designed specifically to treat disorders of the arms, including shoulders, elbows, and wrists. Clinical manifestations of such disorders include swelling, inflammation and pain, decreased range of motion with movement difficulties, and in severe cases, atrophy of the muscles and soft tissues. Clinical applications of this formula include periarthritis of the shoulder, frozen shoulder, tennis elbow, carpal tunnel syndrome, and general conditions such as tendonitis, bursitis, and arthritis.

One of the most important herbs in this formula is *Yan Hu Suo* (Rhizoma Corydalis), generally considered the herb with the most potent analgesic and anti-inflammatory effect in the traditional Chinese pharmacopoeia. It is used to ensure the overall efficacy to relieve pain and reduce inflammation.[1] The potency of *Yan Hu Suo* (Rhizoma Corydalis) has been compared to that of morphine. Though the herb has a slower onset and weaker analgesic effect, it is associated with far less side effects, including absence of addiction and a much slower development of tolerance.[2] Furthermore, the analgesic effect of *Yan Hu Suo* (Rhizoma Corydalis) can be enhanced significantly when combined with electro-acupuncture.[3]

In addition to *Yan Hu Suo* (Rhizoma Corydalis), this formula contains many other herbs with analgesic and anti-inflammatory effects, such as *Xi Xian Cao* (Herba Siegesbeckiae),[4] *Wu Jia Pi* (Cortex Acanthopanacis),[5] *Gui Zhi* (Ramulus Cinnamomi),[6] and *Jiang Huang* (Rhizoma Curcumae Longae).[7] Furthermore, some of these herbs have a long duration of action that last up to five hours.[8] Others have adaptogenic effects that enhance physical endurance and performance.[9]

In terms of clinical applications, these herbs have shown marked effects to treat a wide variety of disorders. According to one clinical study, use of herbs such as *Sang Zhi* (Ramulus Mori), *Ji Xue Teng* (Caulis Spatholobi), *Gui Zhi* (Ramulus Cinnamomi) and others was associated with marked success to treat 15 patients with tendonitis of the elbow.[10] According to another study, herbs such as *Gui Zhi* (Ramulus Cinnamomi) were used with good success in a study of 30 patients with arthritis.[11] Lastly, one study reported that use of *Xi Xian Cao* (Herba Siegesbeckiae) and others resulted in positive effect to treat generalized *bi zheng* (painful obstruction syndrome) characterized by wind-damp.[12]

Overall, *Arm Support* is considered as one of the best formulas to treat various musculoskeletal disorders of the arms. Clinical applications of this formula include, but are not limited to, periarthritis of the shoulder, frozen shoulder, tennis elbow, carpal tunnel syndrome, and general conditions such as tendonitis, bursitis, and arthritis.

PHARMACEUTICAL DRUGS & CHINESE MEDICINE: A COMPARATIVE ANALYSIS

Western Medical Approach: Pain is a basic bodily sensation induced by a noxious stimulus that causes physical discomfort (as pricking, throbbing, or aching). Pain may be of acute or chronic state, and may be of nociceptive, neuropathic, or psychogenic type. NSAID's are generally prescribed for musculoskeletal disorders of the arm, including shoulders, elbows, and wrists. NSAID's [such as Motrin (Ibuprofen) and Voltaren (Diclofenac)] treat pain of mild to moderate intensity, and are most effective to reduce inflammation and swelling. Though effective, these drugs cause serious side effects such as gastric ulcer, duodenal ulcer, gastrointestinal bleeding, tinnitus, blurred vision, dizziness and headache. Furthermore, the newer NSAID's, also known as Cox-2 inhibitors [such as Celebrex (Celecoxib)], are associated with significantly higher risk of cardiovascular events, including heart attack and stroke. Therefore, practitioners and patients must evaluate the potential benefit versus risk before prescribing and taking these drugs. In short, it is important to remember that while drugs offer reliable and potent symptomatic pain relief, they should be used only if and when needed. Frequent use and abuse leads to unnecessary side effects and complications.

Traditional Chinese Medicine Approach: Treatment of pain is a sophisticated balance of art and science. Proper treatment of pain requires a careful evaluation of the type of disharmony (excess or deficiency, cold or heat, exterior or interior), characteristics (qi and/or blood stagnations), and locations (upper body, lower body, extremities, or internal organs). Furthermore, optimal treatment requires integrative use of herbs, acupuncture and *Tui-Na* therapies. All these therapies work together to tonify underlying deficiencies, strengthen the body, and facilitate recovery from chronic pain. TCM pain management targets both the symptom and the cause of pain, and as such, often achieves immediate and long-term success. Furthermore, TCM pain management is often associated with few or no side effects.

Summation: For treatment of mild to severe pain due to various causes, TCM pain management offers similar treatment effects with significantly fewer side effects.

---

[1] *Biol Pharm Bull*, 1994:Feb; 17(2):262-5
[2] *Zhong Yao Yao Li Yu Ying Yong* (Pharmacology and Applications of Chinese Herbs), 1983; 447
[3] *Chen Tzu Yen Chiu* (Acupuncture Research), 1994; 19(1):55-8
[4] *Zhong Yao Yao Li Yu Ying Yong* (Pharmacology and Applications of Chinese Herbs), 1983; 1221
[5] *Zhong Guo Yao Li Xue Tong Bao* (Journal of Chinese Herbal Pharmacology), 1986; 2(2):21
[6] *Zhong Yao Xue* (Chinese Herbology), 1998; 65:67
[7] *Zhong Cao Yao* (Chinese Herbal Medicine), 1991; 22(3):141
[8] *Zhong Cheng Yao Yan Jiu* (Research of Chinese Patent Medicine), 1984; 10:22
[9] *Zhong Cao Yao* (Chinese Herbal Medicine), 1987; 18(3):28
[10] *Hei Long Jiang Zhong Yi Yao* (Heilongjiang Chinese Medicine and Herbology), 1991; (1):27
[11] *Shi Zhen Guo Yao Yan Jiu* (Research of Shizhen Herbs), 1991; 5(4):36
[12] *Shang Hai Zhong Yi Yao Za Zhi* (Shanghai Journal of Chinese Medicine and Herbology), 1982; 9:33

FORMULAS

BACK SUPPORT (Acute) ™

CLINICAL APPLICATIONS

- Acute low back pain
- Back pain from sports or traumatic injuries, sprains and strains, subluxation
- Back pain due to strenuous exercise or repetitive movements (e.g., grocery checkers/packers, warehouse and assembly-line workers, and others in similarly demanding occupations)
- Back pain with inflammation, swelling or redness
- Chronic back pain with acute exacerbation or re-injury

WESTERN THERAPEUTIC ACTIONS

- Anti-inflammatory action to reduce pain and inflammation
- Analgesic influence to relieve pain
- Antispasmodic effects to relax muscles and tendons

CHINESE THERAPEUTIC ACTIONS

- Relieves pain
- Opens channels
- Disperses qi and blood stagnation

DOSAGE

Take 3 to 4 capsules, three times daily as needed to relieve pain. The dosage may be increased up to 6 to 8 capsules every four to six hours if necessary, especially in the early stages of injury when there is severe and excruciating pain. When the pain subsides, the dosage can then be decreased to 3 or 4 capsules three times daily. For maximum effectiveness, take the herbs on an empty stomach with two tall glasses of warm water.

INGREDIENTS

Bai Shao (Radix Paeoniae Alba)
Chuan Niu Xi (Radix Cyathulae)
Du Zhong (Cortex Eucommiae)
Ge Gen (Radix Puerariae)
Gui Zhi (Ramulus Cinnamomi)
Huang Jin Gui (Caulis Vanieriae)
Ji Xue Teng (Caulis Spatholobi)

Liu Zhi Huang (Herba Solidaginis)
Mo Gu Xiao (Caulis Hyptis Capitatae)
Mu Gua (Fructus Chaenomelis)
Wei Ling Xian (Radix Clematidis)
Yan Hu Suo (Rhizoma Corydalis)
Zhi Gan Cao (Radix Glycyrrhizae Preparata)

FORMULA EXPLANATION

Back Support (Acute) is formulated specifically to relieve acute low back pain, caused by sports or traumatic injuries, strenuous exercise, repetitive movements, or accidents. *Back Support (Acute)* contains herbs that regulate qi and blood circulation, remove qi and blood stagnation, and relieve pain.

Yan Hu Suo (Rhizoma Corydalis) activates qi and blood circulation, and is one of the strongest analgesic herbs to relieve pain. *Mo Gu Xiao* (Caulis Hyptis Capitatae), *Liu Zhi Huang* (Herba Solidaginis) and *Huang Jin Gui* (Caulis Vanieriae) have anti-inflammatory and analgesic properties and are often used to treat the acute pain associated with traumatic injuries or sprains and strains. *Gui Zhi* (Ramulus Cinnamomi) warms the channels, facilitates the flow of qi and relieves painful obstruction. *Ge Gen* (Radix Puerariae) alleviates muscle tightness. *Bai Shao* (Radix Paeoniae

FORMULAS

BACK SUPPORT (Acute) ™

Alba) has analgesic, antispasmodic and anti-inflammatory actions. Furthermore, the combination of *Bai Shao* (Radix Paeoniae Alba) and *Zhi Gan Cao* (Radix Glycyrrhizae Preparata) nourish and relax the tendons and the muscles of the back. *Mu Gua* (Fructus Chaenomelis), *Wei Ling Xian* (Radix Clematidis) and *Ji Xue Teng* (Caulis Spatholobi) increase qi and blood circulation to relax the muscles and the tendons. *Chuan Niu Xi* (Radix Cyathulae) invigorates the blood. *Du Zhong* (Cortex Eucommiae) acts as a channel-guiding herb to focus the actions of the formula on the lumbar region.

SUPPLEMENTARY FORMULAS

- For simultaneous upper and lower back pain, use with *Back Support (Upper)*.
- For acute back pain due to herniated disk, use with *Back Support (HD)*.
- To enhance the analgesic action, use with *Herbal Analgesic*.
- For traumatic injuries with bruises and bone fractures, use with *Traumanex*.
- For pain due to bone spurs, add *Flex (Spur)*.
- For back pain associated with osteoporosis, use with *Osteo 8*.
- For back pain with severe cramps, take with *Flex (SC)*.
- For arthritic pain that worsens during cold and rainy weather, use with *Flex (CD)*.
- For arthritis with redness, swelling and inflammation, use with *Flex (Heat)*.
- For back pain due to menstrual discomfort, use *Mense-Ease*.
- For back pain aggravated by obesity, *Herbalite* may be used for weight loss.
- For back pain caused by kidney stones, use *Dissolve (KS)*.
- For back pain or soreness resulting from chronic nephritis, use *Kidney DTX*.
- For chronic, stubborn back pain with blood stagnation, add *Circulation (SJ)*.

NUTRITION

- Eat a diet with a wide variety of raw vegetables and fruits, and whole grain cereals to ensure a complete supply of nutrients for the bones, nerves, and muscles.
- Adequate intake of calcium is essential for the repair and rebuilding of bones, tendons, cartilage, and connective tissues.
- Fresh pineapples are recommended as they contain bromelain, an enzyme that is excellent in reducing inflammation. If the consumption of fresh pineapples causes stomach upset, eat it after meals.
- To relieve cramps and spasms, eat plenty of fruits and vegetables, especially those high in potassium, such as bananas and oranges. Also drink an adequate amount of warm water.
- Adequate intake of minerals, such as calcium and potassium, is essential for pain management. Deficiency of these minerals will lead to spasms, cramps, and tense muscles.
- Avoid red meat and seafood in the diet as they contain high levels of uric acid, which puts added strain on the kidneys.
- Avoid cold beverages, ice cream, caffeine, sugar, tomatoes, milk, and dairy products.
- The following is a folk remedy to treat acute back pain from sprain and strain. Crack open 2 crabs (ocean) with a wooden stick (do not use a knife or any metal instruments) and put them into a clay pot with enough vodka or whiskey to cover both crabs. Place the clay pot into another larger pot with water, and steam it for one hour. Serve the crab meat along with the liquor soup.

LIFESTYLE INSTRUCTIONS

- Patients are advised to use their knees (instead of bending from the waist or back) when lifting heavy objects.
- Stretching and strengthening exercises for the back muscles are essential for long-term recovery. Strengthening the abdominal muscles is also beneficial to reduce strain on the lower back.

BACK SUPPORT (Acute) ™

  ☙ Mild exercise such as swimming, yoga, or *Tai Chi Chuan* <u>on a regular basis</u> is recommended.

  ☙ For those who are overweight, weight loss is strongly recommended to decrease pressure on the joints and relieve pain.

  ☙ Proper balance of work and rest is very important. While sitting, make sure the back is straight and the elbows and knees are bent at a 90° angle. Take a break at least once every hour to alleviate pressure on the vertebrae and disks.

  ☙ Hot baths with Epsom salts help to relax tense muscles and draw toxins from tissues. Rest and relax in the bath for about 30 minutes, but avoid becoming over-tired from the heat and soaking.

  ☙ Finally, adequate rest is essential to recovery. It is wise to review the sleeping postures to ensure that the back is being appropriately supported and relaxed.

CLINICAL NOTES

  ☙ Take *Back Support (Acute)* with 2 tall glasses of warm water, as back pain can be related to dehydration.

  ☙ There are several causes for back pain. This formula is designed to treat back pain due to musculoskeletal injuries. For back pain resulting from other causes, please refer to the Supplementary Formula section for appropriate formulas.

  ☙ Many patients may seek treatment for a chronic back condition that has recently been exacerbated. In such cases, *Back Support (Acute)* should be prescribed for one or two weeks to relieve the acute pain. After the pain subsides, switch to *Back Support (Chronic)* to consolidate the effect.

  ☙ Clinical Tip: For musculoskeletal injuries to the back, *Back Support (Acute)* can be given to the patient prior to each acupuncture treatment. The muscle-relaxant influence from the herbs will take effect within about half an hour. By relaxing the muscles and invigorating qi and blood circulation with the herbs, there will be less stagnation in the channels, and the acupuncture and *Tui Na* treatments will be more effective.

CAUTIONS

  ☙ Because of the blood-invigorating nature of this formula, *Back Support (Acute)* is not recommended during pregnancy and nursing.

  ☙ *Back Support (Acute)* is not designed for long-term use. If the pain lasts for a long period of time and becomes chronic in nature, *Back Support (Chronic)* should be used.

  ☙ If the patient presents with fever and a one-sided back pain, consider a possible kidney infection and do not use this herbal formula. Patients with acute nephritis should be referred to their medical doctor immediately.

  ☙ Patients who have pain radiating to the extremities accompanied by a sudden loss of bladder or bowel control may have a pinched nerve or spinal injury, and must be referred out to emergency care. This condition, known as Cauda Equina syndrome, can lead to permanent disability and must be evaluated and treated immediately.

ACUPUNCTURE POINTS

Traditional Points:

  ☙ *Yaotongxue, Huantiao* (GB 30), *Yaoyan* (Extra 9), *Shenshu* (BL 23), and *Weizhong* (BL 40).

Balance Method by Dr. Richard Tan:

  ☙ Needle the following points on the side opposite the pain: *Hegu* (LI 4), *Houxi* (SI 3), *Wangu* (SI 4), *Lingku, Dabai, Zhongbai, Dazhong* (KI 4) or *ah shi* points nearby, and *Dazhong* (KI 4), and *Fuliu* (KI 7) or *ah shi* points nearby.

  ☙ Needle the following points on the same side as the pain: *Chize* (LU 5), *Shugu* (BL 65), and *Kongzui* (LU 6) or *ah shi* points nearby.

BACK SUPPORT (Acute) ™

- Note: *Lingku, Dabai* and *Zhongbai* are Master Tong's points on both hands. *Lingku* is located in the depression just distal to the junction of the first and second metacarpal bones, approximately 0.5 *cun* proximal to *Hegu* (LI 4), on the *yangming* line. *Dabai* is located at about 0.5 *cun* proximal to *Sanjian* (LI 3), on the *yangming* line. *Zhongbai* is located at about 0.5 *cun* proximal to *Zhongzhu* (TH 3), on the *shaoyang* line.

- For additional information on the Balance Method, please refer to *Twelve and Twelve in Acupuncture, Twenty-Four More in Acupuncture*, and *Acupuncture 1, 2, 3* by Dr. Richard Tan.

Ear Points:

- Sciatic pain: Lower Back, Hip, Sciatic, and Pituitary Gland. Embed needles or use ear seeds in both ears, and instruct the patient to massage the points three to four times daily for two to three minutes each time.

- Tailbone injury: Coccyx, Adrenal Gland, and Pituitary Gland.

Auricular Acupuncture by Dr. Li-Chun Huang:

- Low back pain
  - Main point: Lumbar Vertebral of the groove of spinal posterior
  - Supplementary point: Lumbar Vertebral of the antihelix middle line on the upper 4/5 positive area (front and back of ear)
- Sciatic nerve pain
  - Main point: Triangle Area Sciatic Nerve of the posterior.
  - Supplementary points: Corresponding Points (to the area of pain), Sacrolumbar, Buttock, Hip Joint, Popliteal Fossa, Calf, Ankle, Heel, and Toe.
- Sacroiliac joint pain: Sacroiliac Joint (front and back of ear).
- Lumbar muscle pain (strain): Select the outside of Antihelix of upper 1/5 and 2/5 area. Positive point or area (front and back of ear).
- Low back pain due to Kidney qi deficiency: Corresponding points (to the area of pain in the Lumbar and Lumbar Muscle Area), Kidney, Liver, Spleen, Endocrine, Coronary Vascular Subcortex, Large Auricular Nerve, and Lumbar Area.

MODERN RESEARCH

Back Support (Acute) is formulated with herbs that have strong analgesic, anti-inflammatory and muscle-relaxant functions, as confirmed by independent research.

Yan Hu Suo (Rhizoma Corydalis), containing corydaline, exerts strong anti-inflammatory activities and is effective in both the acute and chronic phases of inflammation.[1] *Yan Hu Suo* (Rhizoma Corydalis) also possesses strong analgesic activities that act directly on the central nervous system.[2] Because of this action, *Yan Hu Suo* (Rhizoma Corydalis) works synergistically with acupuncture to relieve pain. One study demonstrated that when combined with *Yan Hu Suo* (Rhizoma Corydalis), the analgesic potency of electro-acupuncture increased significantly when compared with the control group that received electro-acupuncture only.[3]

Bai Shao (Radix Paeoniae Alba) and *Zhi Gan Cao* (Radix Glycyrrhizae Preparata) are two of the most effective herbs to relieve pain, reduce inflammation, and alleviate spasms and cramps. Pharmacologically, these two herbs have shown marked analgesic effect, anti-inflammatory effect, and muscle-relaxant effects.[4,5] Clinically, these two herbs have been used to treat a wide variety of musculoskeletal disorders. According to one study, use of these herbs via intramuscular injection was associated with 84.67% rate of effectiveness (105 out of 124 subjects) to treat the general complaint of pain.[6] More specifically, these two herbs have also been found to effectively treat pain in the lower back and legs among 33 elderly patients,[7] as well as severe pain of the back and legs in 27 patients.[8] Furthermore, the combination of these two herbs was effective in relieving nerve pain (neuralgia) in 30 out of 42 patients.[9] According to another study, the use of these two herbs was also effective for muscle spasms and cramps in

BACK SUPPORT (Acute) ™

various areas of the body, including muscle spasms and twitching in the facial region in 11 patients,[10] intestinal spasms in 254 patients,[11] and intestinal cramps and spasms in 85 patients.[12]

Lastly, this formula uses several herbs for their adjunct effect to relieve pain and alleviate spasms and cramps. *Gui Zhi* (Ramulus Cinnamomi) has an analgesic effect to relieve pain. According to one study, it has been used successfully to treat arthritis among 30 patients.[13] According to another study, use of this herb is effective to treat numbness among 30 patients.[14] Lastly, *Ge Gen* (Radix Puerariae) has also been shown to have muscle-relaxant effect to relieve muscle spasms and cramps.[15]

In conclusion, this is an excellent formula for acute and severe pain in the lower back region, as it contains herbs with excellent analgesic effect to relieve pain, anti-inflammatory effect to reduce swelling and inflammation, and muscle-relaxant effect to alleviate spasms and cramps.

PHARMACEUTICAL DRUGS & CHINESE MEDICINE: A COMPARATIVE ANALYSIS

Western Medical Approach: Pain is a basic bodily sensation induced by a noxious stimulus that causes physical discomfort (as pricking, throbbing, or aching). Pain may be of acute or chronic states. For acute back pain, two classes of drugs commonly used for treatment include non-steroidal anti-inflammatory agents (NSAID) and opioid analgesics. NSAID's [such as Motrin (Ibuprofen) and Voltaren (Diclofenac)] are generally used for mild to moderate pain, and are most effective to reduce inflammation and swelling. Though effective, they may cause such serious side effects as gastric ulcer, duodenal ulcer, gastrointestinal bleeding, tinnitus, blurred vision, dizziness and headache. Furthermore, the newer NSAID's, also known as Cox-2 inhibitors [such as Celebrex (Celecoxib)], are associated with significantly higher risk of cardiovascular events, including heart attack and stroke. Opioid analgesics [such as Vicodin (APAP/Hydrocodone) and morphine] are usually used for severe to excruciating pain. While they may be the most potent agents for pain, they also have the most serious risks and side effects, including but not limited to dizziness, lightheadedness, drowsiness, upset stomach, vomiting, constipation, stomach pain, rash, difficult urination, and respiratory depression resulting in difficult breathing. Furthermore, long-term use of these drugs leads to tolerance and addiction. In brief, it is important to remember that while drugs offer reliable and potent symptomatic pain relief, they should be used only if and when needed. Frequent use and abuse leads to unnecessary side effects and complications.

Traditional Chinese Medicine Approach: Treatment of pain is a sophisticated balance of art and science. Proper treatment of pain requires a careful evaluation of the type of disharmony (excess or deficiency, cold or heat, exterior or interior), characteristics (qi and/or blood stagnations), and locations (upper body, lower body, extremities, or internal organs). Furthermore, optimal treatment requires integrative use of herbs, acupuncture and *Tui-Na* therapies. All these therapies work together to tonify the underlying deficiencies, strengthen the body, and facilitate recovery from chronic pain. TCM pain management targets both the symptom and the cause of pain, and as such, often achieves immediate and long-term success. Furthermore, TCM pain management is often associated with few or no side effects.

Summation: For treatment of mild to severe pain due to various causes, TCM pain management offers similar treatment effects with significantly fewer side effects.

CASE STUDIES

A 50-year-old female acupuncturist sustained an injury to her sacrum and coccyx. She fell from a chair hammock 3-4 feet above ground onto cement. A sensation similar to a lightening bolt was felt in the sacral area as well as a feeling of electricity from her sacrum to her knees. She was in acute pain and thought she was paralyzed. As an acupuncturist, she diagnosed herself as qi and blood stagnation resulting from trauma. She was immediately treated by a chiropractor. She also took 6 capsules of **Back Support (Acute)** three times a day. After just 2 doses, the patient

FORMULAS

BACK SUPPORT (Acute) ™

experienced tremendous relief. Although the patient still complained of slight lingering pain that persisted for a while, she stated that *Back Support (Acute)* made a remarkable difference in her recovery process. Within one month, the patient improved almost 95%.

M.T.B., Alpine, California

An injury caused by a fall resulted in acute low back pain to a 29-year-old male blackjack dealer. Sequelae included local swelling, redness and limited lumbar range of motion. Skin and muscle bruising was quite noticeable. The TCM diagnosis of qi and blood stagnation was confirmed through tongue analysis that showed a pale, purple tongue body, a wiry pulse, as well as pain upon palpation. Administration of *Back Support (Acute)* reduced the pain immediately the same day. Low back pain was completely resolved within a week, with full lumbar range of motion recovery within only four days.

T.G., Albuquerque, NM

D.D., a 41-year-old nurse, presented with a work-related injury. She had severe back pain that was the result of a fall from lifting a patient. She said she heard a popping sound in her back when she fell. MRI confirmed her diagnosis of lumbar herniated disc. By the time she came for treatment, she was 9 weeks post-injury and had scheduled for steroid epidurals. She refused injections and came to our clinic for 'safe and non-invasive care.' Her blood pressure was 140/80 mmHg and the heart rate was 80 beats per minute. The TCM diagnoses include qi and blood stagnation and soft tissue damage. *Back Support (Acute)*, *Flex (SC)* and *Traumanex* were prescribed at 3 capsules each three times a day. After the herbs, the patient was able to reduce Vicodin (APAP/Hydrocodone) use from 2 to 0.5 tablets per day, and none at all on some days. She had increased blood pressure from stress over the injury, which was up to 170/110 mmHg. After the herbs and massage, the blood pressure came down to normal and is staying down. She had received no additional physical therapy. She did remarkably well in a short period of time.

M.H., West Palm Beach, Florida

J.M., a 36-year-old female massage therapist, presented with pain from a recent automobile accident (second accident in 6 months). She exhibited neck, back, arm, and leg pain. Airbags bent her right thumb. Her blood pressure was 120/70 mmHg and her heart rate was 72 beats per minute. X-rays showed herniation and soft tissue damage. She also complained of muscle spasms, hot sensation on trigger points, inability to move the right thumb and the range of motion for the neck and trunk were both decreased. *Traumanex*, *Neck & Shoulder (Acute)* and *Back Support (Acute)* were all prescribed at 2 capsules each three times daily. J.M. responded quickly to these formulas and acupuncture treatments. Pain levels were reduced by half in a short period of time.

M.H., West Palm Beach, Florida

A 36-year-old female college professor reported back pain for a period of one week. The cause of injury involved her reaching for an item and a sudden severe back pain followed. Tenderness upon palpation was noted at T12 to L2 region along with paraspinal hypertonicity. Although no X-rays were taken, she initially got chiropractic treatment for a slipped disc, which included ultrasound and chiropractic manipulative adjustments. Though her back pain was still present, it was not as severe. Her pulse was wiry, slippery and slightly weak. The TCM diagnoses for her condition include Liver qi stagnation, local qi and blood stagnation, and qi deficiency. After taking a prescription of *Back Support (Acute)* for a couple of days, the patient noticed slight improvement. By the fourth and fifth day on the formula, her mobility had markedly improved along with a decrease in pain.

N.M., Torrance, CA

A 47-year-old female office manager complained of neck pain and low back pain that were aggravated by prolonged sitting. She has a past history of two whiplash injuries that can also have attributed to causing her neck pain. Upon

FORMULAS

BACK SUPPORT (Acute) ™

examination, the practitioner found extreme spasms of the erector muscles, bilateral weakness of her sternocleidomastoid muscles and a lack of muscle tone in her lower back. With these symptoms, the patient was diagnosed with right-sided sciatica, arthralgia of the spine and stress-induced muscle spasms. The TCM diagnosis was concluded to be Liver qi stagnation. The treatment included acupuncture, moxa, and infrared heat. *Back Support (Acute)* and *Neck & Shoulder (Acute)* were prescribed for this patient. The results were as follows:

> 3/29/01: stress: 8; pain: 9-10 (on a scale of 1 to 10; 10 rating = worse condition)
> 5/05/01: 50% improvement
> 5/19/01: 70% improvement
> 8/16/01: No more pain. However, slight intermittent flaring of her condition was noted.

The practitioner and the patient both concluded that the *Back Support (Acute)* and *Neck & Shoulder (Acute)* have really helped.

T.W., Santa Monica, California

G.A., a 51-year-old female patient, presented with bilateral lower back pain ranging from 7 to 9 out of 10 on a pain scale. She described the pain as stabbing and spasmodic. She could barely walk or sit, and even lying down was uncomfortable. In fact, the patient stated she couldn't find relief in any position. She'd had intermittent back pain and spasms for much of her adult life, with the first serious episode occurring in her late twenties. The patient had recently missed several days of work and could concentrate on nothing but the pain. Objective findings included X-rays that revealed arthritis at L4 possibly as the result of trauma. The patient reported that she had injured her back when she was in first grade – a classmate had pulled a chair out from under her as she prepared to sit down. Tongue body color was unremarkable with scalloped edges. The tongue coating was thick and white with hairline cracks. Pulse was deep and small on both sides. Her lower back pain was too painful to palpate.

The TCM diagnosis was severe qi and blood stagnation in the lower back with mild Kidney qi and yang deficiencies. *Back Support (Chronic)* was prescribed at 4 capsules three to four times a day. The practitioner wanted to prescribe *Back Support (Acute)*, but had only *Back Support (Chronic)* in the pharmacy. Rather than wait a few days for the herbs to arrive, *Back Support (Chronic)* was given first to begin the herbal therapy. *Back Support (Chronic)* reduced the patient's pain level dramatically within 24 hours. This case exemplifies the principle of therapeutic diagnosis – the patient's excellent response to this formula demonstrated the degree to which underlying Kidney deficiency played a role in the pathology. However, she wasn't conscientious about taking the herbs and when the pain was gone and the bottle was empty, she didn't resume taking the herbs and the deficiency persisted.

The same patient returned some months later with another flare-up of stabbing and spasmodic bilateral lower back pain. Again, she could hardly walk nor could she find a position that relieved her pain at all. This time she reported that the pain was probably the result of her new job as an esthetician – she was now spending her workdays sitting on a stool bending over customers, giving them facials. Tongue appeared pale and scalloped, and peeled on the edges with thin white coating and hairline cracks. Pulses were still deep on both sides. The blood pressure was 118/72 mmHg and the heart rate was 62 beats per minute. The TCM diagnosis was severe qi and blood stagnation of the lumbar region, which probably resulted from working under ergonomically unsound conditions. She also suffered from mild Kidney qi and yang deficiencies. This time, *Back Support (Acute)* was prescribed at 4 capsules three to four times a day. Though the patient responded well to *Back Support (Chronic)* during her previous lumbar pain flare-up, the practitioner chose to give the patient *Back Support (Acute)* instead this time. Though the formula reduced her pain, it took longer to do so and the pain, though milder, lingered. This case was submitted by the practitioner as an example of the importance of treating the underlying deficiency in chronic cases.

H.H., San Francisco, California

BACK SUPPORT (Acute) ™

[1] Kubo, M. et al. Anti-inflammatory activities of methanolic extract and alkaloidal components from corydalis tuber. *Biol Pharm Bull*. 17(2):262-5 February 1994

[2] Zhu, XZ. Development of natural products as drugs acting on central nervous system. *Memorias do Instituto Oswaldo Cruz*. 1991;86 Suppl 2:173-5.

[3] Hu, J. et al. Effect of some drugs on electroacupuncture analgesia and cytosolic free Ca2+ concentration of mice brain. *Chen Tzu Yen Chiu* 1994;19(1):55-8

[4] *Zhong Yao Xue* (Chinese Herbology), 1998; 759:765

[5] *Zhong Cao Yao* (Chinese Herbal Medicine), 1991; 22(10):452

[6] *Shang Hai Zhong Yi Yao Za Zhi* (Shanghai Journal of Chinese Medicine and Herbology), 1983; 4:14

[7] *Yun Nan Zhong Yi* (Yunnan Journal of Traditional Chinese Medicine), 1990; 4:15

[8] *Zhe Jiang Zhong Yi Za Zhi* (Zhejiang Journal of Chinese Medicine), 1980; 2:60

[9] *Zhong Yi Za Zhi* (Journal of Chinese Medicine), 1983; 11:9

[10] *Hu Nan Zhong Yi* (Hunan Journal of Traditional Chinese Medicine), 1989; 2:7

[11] *Zhong Hua Nei Ke Za Zhi* (Chinese Journal of Internal Medicine), 1960; 4:354

[12] *Zhong Yi Za Zhi* (Journal of Chinese Medicine), 1985; 6:50

[13] *Zhong Yao Xue* (Chinese Herbology), 1998; 65:67

[14] *Hu Nan Zhong Yi Za Zhi* (Hunan Journal of Chinese Medicine), 1987; 8(2):4

[15] *Zhong Yao Xue* (Chinese Herbology), 1998; 101:103

BACK SUPPORT (Chronic) ™

CLINICAL APPLICATIONS

- ☯ Chronic low back pain
- ☯ Weakness and soreness of the lower back and knees
- ☯ Slow and incomplete recovery from back injuries
- ☯ Sciatica, osteoarthritis, lumbago, lower back pain resulting from osteoporosis

WESTERN THERAPEUTIC ACTIONS

- ☯ Antirheumatic effect to treat disorders associated with joints, muscles, bursae, tendons and fibrous tissue
- ☯ Antispasmodic effect to stop muscle spasm and cramping
- ☯ Anti-inflammatory function to reduce pain, swelling and redness

CHINESE THERAPEUTIC ACTIONS

- ☯ Disperses painful obstruction
- ☯ Relieves pain
- ☯ Invigorates qi and blood circulation
- ☯ Tonifies Liver and Kidney deficiencies

DOSAGE

Take 3 to 4 capsules three times daily. Depending on the nature and severity of the illness, the dosage may be increased up to 8 to 10 capsules three times daily for three or four days to tonify and relieve pain. For maximum effectiveness, take the herbs on an empty stomach with warm water.

INGREDIENTS

Bai Shao (Radix Paeoniae Alba)
Chuan Niu Xi (Radix Cyathulae)
Du Huo (Radix Angelicae Pubescentis)
Du Zhong (Cortex Eucommiae)
Ji Xue Teng (Caulis Spatholobi)
Mu Gua (Fructus Chaenomelis)

Qian Nian Jian (Rhizoma Homalomenae)
Sang Ji Sheng (Herba Taxilli)
Sheng Di Huang (Radix Rehmanniae)
Wei Ling Xian (Radix Clematidis)
Zhi Gan Cao (Radix Glycyrrhizae Preparata)

FORMULA EXPLANATION

Back Support (Chronic) is formulated to treat general disorders of the lower back, including pain and inflammation, weakness and soreness, lumbago, sciatica, and osteoarthritis. *Back Support (Chronic)* contains herbs that activate qi and blood circulation, remove qi and blood stagnation, relieve pain, and nourish the muscles and tendons.

Du Huo (Radix Angelicae Pubescentis) has antirheumatic, anti-inflammatory, and analgesic functions. It expels wind, dampness and cold from the lower back and removes painful obstructions. *Du Zhong* (Cortex Eucommiae), *Sang Ji Sheng* (Herba Taxilli), *Qian Nian Jian* (Rhizoma Homalomenae) and *Sheng Di Huang* (Radix Rehmanniae) replenish the vital functions of the Liver and the Kidney, which are responsible for strengthening the bones, sinews and muscles of the lower back and knees. *Bai Shao* (Radix Paeoniae Alba) has analgesic, antispasmodic and anti-inflammatory effects. Together with the harmonizing effect of *Zhi Gan Cao* (Radix Glycyrrhizae Preparata), they nourish and relax the tendons and muscles in the back. *Mu Gua* (Fructus Chaenomelis), *Wei Ling Xian* (Radix Clematidis), and *Ji Xue Teng* (Caulis Spatholobi) increase qi and blood circulation in order to relax the muscles and

FORMULAS

tendons in the back. *Chuan Niu Xi* (Radix Cyathulae) invigorates the blood and acts as a channel-guiding herb to focus the action of the formula on the lumbar region.

SUPPLEMENTARY FORMULAS

❧ For chronic pain affecting upper and lower back, add *Back Support (Upper)*.

❧ For chronic low back pain due to herniated disk, use with *Back Support (HD)*.

❧ For chronic low back pain with weakness and soreness of the knees, add *Knee & Ankle (Chronic)*.

❧ For chronic low back pain with weakened soft tissues (muscles, tendons and ligaments), add *Flex (MLT)*.

❧ To enhance the analgesic effect, add *Herbal Analgesic*.

❧ For osteoporosis or weakness of the bones, add *Osteo 8*.

❧ For soreness and weakness of the lower back and knees and/or low sex drive because of Kidney yang deficiency, add *Kidney Tonic (Yang)*.

❧ For soreness and weakness of the lower back and knees due to yin deficiency, add *Kidney Tonic (Yin)*.

❧ For bone fractures and internal bruises, add *Traumanex*.

❧ For arthritis that worsens during cold or rainy seasons, add *Flex (CD)*.

❧ For arthritis with redness, inflammation, swelling, and burning pain, add *Flex (Heat)*.

❧ For muscle spasms and cramps, add *Flex (SC)*.

❧ For pain related to bone spurs, add *Flex (Spur)*.

❧ For back pain due to kidney stones, use *Dissolve (KS)*.

❧ For back pain or soreness because of nephritis, use *Kidney DTX*.

❧ For dull back pain with menstruation, add *Mense-Ease*.

❧ For back pain resulting from obesity, use *Herbalite* may help with weight loss.

NUTRITION

❧ Eat a diet with a wide variety of raw vegetables and fruits, and whole grain cereals to ensure a complete supply of nutrients for the bones, nerves, and muscles.

❧ Adequate intake of calcium is essential for the repair and rebuilding of bones, tendons, cartilage, and connective tissues.

❧ Fresh pineapples are recommended as they contain bromelain, an enzyme that is excellent in reducing inflammation.

❧ To relieve cramps and spasms, eat plenty of fruits and vegetables, especially those high in potassium such as bananas and oranges. Also drink an adequate amount of water, as back pain may be due in part to dehydration.

❧ Adequate intake of minerals, such as calcium and potassium, are essential for pain management. Deficiency of these minerals will lead to spasms, cramps, and tense muscles.

❧ Avoid red meat and seafood in the diet as they contain high levels of uric acid, which adds strain on the kidneys.

❧ Avoid cold beverages, ice cream, caffeine, sugar, tomatoes, milk, dairy products and red meat.

LIFESTYLE INSTRUCTIONS

❧ Patients are advised to use their knees (instead of bending their back) when lifting heavy objects.

❧ Exercises for stretching and strengthening the back muscles are essential for long-term recovery. Strengthening the stomach muscles is also beneficial as it reduces the strain on the lower back.

❧ Mild exercise such as swimming, yoga, or *Tai Chi Chuan* is recommended.

❧ Weight loss is suggested, to decrease the pressure on the joints and relieve pain.

FORMULAS

BACK SUPPORT (Chronic) ™

- Proper balance of work and rest is very important. While sitting, make sure the back is straight and the elbows and knees are bent at a 90° angle. Take a break at least once every hour to alleviate the pressure on the vertebrae and disks.
- Mild back pain can be relieved with application of heat to stimulate the blood circulation. Massage, hot packs, saunas and whirlpools are recommended.
- Hot baths with Epsom salts help to relax tense muscles and draw toxins from the tissues. Rest and relax in the bath for about 30 minutes.
- Finally, adequate rest is essential to recovery.

CLINICAL NOTES

- Patients who have chronic back pain from repetitive movement from their job should take this formula at a maintenance dose of two capsules a day to strengthen the muscles and the tendons in the back to prevent injury.
- *Back Support (Acute)* is for acute cases with inflammation and pain. It is the best formula for recent injury or acute exacerbation with excruciating pain.
- *Back Support (Chronic)* is usually used for chronic pain or dull pain. In addition to having herbs that relieve pain, *Back Support (Chronic)* also has herbs to nourish and strengthen the underlying structures and tissues so the back becomes less fragile.

CAUTIONS

- Because of the blood-invigorating nature of this formula, *Back Support (Chronic)* is not recommended during pregnancy and nursing.
- *Back Support (Chronic)* is a warm formula, and use of this warm formula may be associated with a slight increase in blood pressure. Therefore, blood pressure should be monitored while taking this formula.
- Patients who have pain radiating to the extremities accompanied by a sudden loss of bladder or bowel control may have a pinched nerve or spinal injury, and must be treated accordingly.
- If the patient presents with fever and one-sided back pain, consider a possible kidney infection and do not use this herbal formula. Patients with acute nephritis should be referred to their medical doctor immediately.

ACUPUNCTURE POINTS

Traditional Points:
- *Huatuojiaji* points (Extra 15) in the back from L3 to L5 for lower back pain. *Huatuojiaji* points (Extra 15) from T1 to T12 for upper back pain.
- *Hegu* (LI 4), *Yaotongxue* (Extra 29), *Huantiao* (GB 30), *Yaoyen* (Extra 21), *Shenshu* (BL 23), and *Weizhong* (BL 40)

Balance Method by Dr. Richard Tan:
- Needle the following points on the side opposite of the pain: *Hegu* (LI 4), *Houxi* (SI 3), *Wangu* (SI 4), *Rangu* (KI 2), *Dazhong* (KI 4) or *ah shi* points nearby, and *Fuliu* (KI 7) or *ah shi* points nearby.
- Needle the following points on the same side as the pain: *Chize* (LU 5), *Kongzui* (LU 6) and *Shugu* (BL 65) or *ah shi* points nearby.
- To read more about Dr. Tan's theories behind acupuncture, see his book *Dr. Tan's Strategy of Twelve Magic Points*.
- For additional information on the Balance Method, please refer to *Dr. Tan's Strategy of Twelve Magical Points* by Dr. Richard Tan.

FORMULAS

BACK SUPPORT (Chronic) ™

Ear Points:
- Back, Lumbago, Small Intestine, Adrenal Gland, and Pituitary Gland. Embed ear needles or use ear seeds. Ten treatments equal one course.

Auricular Acupuncture by Dr. Li-Chun Huang:
- Low Back Pain
  - Main point: Lumbar Vertebral of the groove of spinal posterior
  - Supplementary point: Lumbar Vertebral of the antihelix middle line on the upper 4/5 positive area (front and back of ear)
- Sciatic nerve pain
  - Main point: Triangle Area Sciatic Nerve of the posterior
  - Supplementary points: Corresponding Points (to the area of pain), Sacrolumbar, Buttock, Hip Joint, Popliteal Fossa, Calf, Ankle, Heel, and Toe.
- Sacroiliac joint pain: Sacroiliac Joint (front and back of ear).
- Lumbar muscle pain (strain): Select the outside of Antihelix of upper 1/5 and 2/5 area. Positive point or area (front and back of ear).
- Low back pain due to Kidney qi deficiency: Corresponding points (to the area of pain in the Lumbar and Lumbar Muscle Area), Kidney, Liver, Spleen, Endocrine, Coronary Vascular Subcortex, Large Auricular Nerve, and Lumbar Area.

MODERN RESEARCH

Back Support (Chronic) is formulated based on *Du Huo Ji Sheng Tang* (Angelica Pubescens and Taxillus Decoction), the historical herbal formula used to treat chronic low back pain, sciatica, rheumatoid arthritis and osteoarthritis.[1] *Back Support (Chronic)* contains herbs with antirheumatic, antispasmodic and anti-inflammatory functions confirmed by modern research.

Du Huo (Radix Angelicae Pubescentis) and *Sang Ji Sheng* (Herba Taxilli) have antirheumatic and anti-inflammatory functions and are commonly used together to treat upper and lower back pain.[1]

Bai Shao (Radix Paeoniae Alba) and *Zhi Gan Cao* (Radix Glycyrrhizae Preparata) are two of the most effective herbs to relieve pain, reduce inflammation, and alleviate spasms and cramps. Pharmacologically, these two herbs have shown marked analgesic effects, anti-inflammatory effects, and muscle-relaxant effects.[2,3] *Bai Shao* (Radix Paeoniae Alba), containing paeoniflorin and daisein, has a strong antispasmodic effect to alleviate muscle spasms and cramps. *Bai Shao* (Radix Paeoniae Alba) and *Zhi Gan Cao* (Radix Glycyrrhizae Preparata) have historically been combined to relieve muscle spasms and cramps. They may be used for muscle spasms and leg cramps associated with external or sports injuries. Recently, the antispasmodic and anti-inflammatory effects of *Bai Shao* (Radix Paeoniae Alba) and *Zhi Gan Cao* (Radix Glycyrrhizae Preparata) have been confirmed by several clinical trials.[1,4]

For treatment of musculoskeletal disorders, the combination of *Bai Shao* (Radix Paeoniae Alba) and *Zhi Gan Cao* (Radix Glycyrrhizae Preparata) relieved trigeminal pain in 30 out of 42 patients;[5] it relieved muscle spasm and twitching in the facial region in 11 out of 11 patients;[6] and in 33 elderly patients with pain in the lower back and legs, 12 patients reported significant improvement, 16 reported moderate improvement, 4 reported slight improvement and 1 reported no effect.[7]

For treatment of smooth muscle disorders, the combination of *Bai Shao* (Radix Paeoniae Alba) and *Zhi Gan Cao* (Radix Glycyrrhizae Preparata) relieved abdominal pain and cramps caused by intestinal parasites in 11 out of 11 patients;[8] and in 185 patients with epigastric and abdominal pain, 139 patients reported significant improvement, 41 reported moderate improvement, and 5 reported no effect.[9] Lastly, *Bai Shao* (Radix Paeoniae Alba) has tranquilizing and analgesic effects to relieve pain.

PHARMACEUTICAL DRUGS & CHINESE MEDICINE: A COMPARATIVE ANALYSIS

Western Medical Approach: Pain is a basic bodily sensation induced by a noxious stimulus that causes physical discomfort (as pricking, throbbing, or aching). Pain may be of acute or chronic state, and may be of nociceptive, neuropathic, or psychogenic type. For acute pain, use of non-steroidal anti-inflammatory agents (NSAID) and opioid analgesics offer immediate and reliable effects to relieve pain. Though these drugs have serious side effects, short-term use can be justified because the benefits often outweigh the risks. For chronic pain, on the other hand, use of NSAID's and opioid analgesics are usually not the desired treatment options, as they symptomatically relieve pain, but do not change the underlying course of illness. Unfortunately, the convenience of these drugs contributes to the vicious cycle of pain, followed by continuous and repetitive use of drugs to symptomatically relieve pain. When the effect of the drugs dissipates, patients are often left with nothing but more pain and more complications from side effects. Therefore, it is important to understand that while these drugs may be beneficial for acute pain, they do not adequately address most cases of chronic pain. Additional treatment modalities must be incorporated to ensure effective and complete recovery from chronic pain conditions. [Note: Common side effects of NSAID's include gastric ulcer, duodenal ulcer, gastrointestinal bleeding, tinnitus, blurred vision, dizziness and headache. Serious side effects of newer NSAID's, also known as Cox-2 inhibitors [such as Celebrex (Celecoxib)], include significantly higher risk of cardiovascular events, including heart attack and stroke. Side effects of opioid analgesics [such as Vicodin (APAP/Hydrocodone) and morphine] include dizziness, lightheadedness, drowsiness, upset stomach, vomiting, constipation, stomach pain, rash, difficult urination, and respiratory depression resulting in difficult breathing. Furthermore, long-term use of these drugs leads to tolerance and addiction.]

Traditional Chinese Medicine Approach: Treatment of chronic pain is a sophisticated balance of art and science. Proper treatment of pain requires a careful evaluation of the type of disharmony (excess or deficiency, cold or heat, exterior or interior), characteristics (qi and/or blood stagnations), and locations (upper body, lower body, extremities, or internal organs). Furthermore, optimal treatment requires integrative use of herbs, acupuncture and *Tui-Na* therapies. All these therapies work together to tonify the underlying deficiencies, strengthen the body, and facilitate recovery from chronic pain. All these therapies work together to tonify the underlying deficiencies, strengthen the body, and facilitate recovery from chronic pain. TCM pain management targets both the symptom and the cause of pain, and as such, often achieves immediate and long-term success. Furthermore, TCM pain management is often associated with few or no side effects.

Summation: For treatment of mild to severe pain due to various causes, TCM pain management offers similar treatment effects with significantly fewer side effects. Though TCM therapies may not be as potent as the drugs for acute pain management, they are often superior [better effects with fewer side effects] for chronic pain management.

CASE STUDIES

A 58-year-old female presented with back pain she'd had for 15 years, that was worse upon waking and better with activity. Most recently, she had hip pain for 5 months that felt deep in the acetabulum region. Tendon pain located antero-medially near the groin was also noted. No structural abnormalities were found upon further investigation. The practitioner diagnosed the condition as qi and blood stagnation in the Urinary Bladder and Gallbladder channels. After taking **Back Support (Chronic)**, her back pain decreased and since then, she experienced less muscle stiffness, especially in the morning. Her previous radiating hip pain is now less severe and infrequent. She has also noticed that walking, which was painful for her in the past, has become almost pain-free. In addition to **Back Support (Chronic)**, she also took Wobenzyme and has improved her diet.

J.M., Baltimore, Maryland

FORMULAS

BACK SUPPORT (Chronic) ™

A 56-year-old female presented with severe back pain, joint pain, morning stiffness, and difficulty walking, which were all attributed to degenerative joint disease. Standing and bending aggravated her pain. She found relief with rest. Severe irritation and discomfort were evoked during lumbar range of motion. The practitioner diagnosed the condition as cold-damp stagnation in the Urinary Bladder channel with underlying Kidney deficiency. The patient was treated with *Back Support (Chronic)* along with acupuncture. Soon after, the patient reported that she was able to walk without difficulty and stand without pain for longer periods of time (30 to 60 minutes). Eventually she was able to return to a painless level of activity and function.

M.I., San Pedro, California

A 45-year-old male presented with pain in the low back and buttocks. On a pain scale from 0-10 (with 10 being the most painful), the patient rated his pain as a 7. There was decreased range of motion in the lumbar spine, and radicular pain on the right side. He was diagnosed with a herniated disc in the lumbar spine. After taking *Back Support (Chronic)*, the patient stated that the severity of the pain decreased on a daily basis from 7 to 4.

G.P., Lawndale, California

A female patient suffering from lower back (L4 area) pain radiating down the left hip was unable to lie on her back. On examination, her left leg was shorter than the right. The patient reported that the pain was caused by a twisted pelvis from a tailbone injury years before: her tailbone projected outwards, and her knees were swollen and painful. She also suffered from gout. X-ray showed bone spurs in the lower spine. After taking *Back Support (Chronic)*, she was able to lie on her back for almost an hour without pain, sit for a long period of time with less pain, and sleep restfully. She also experienced more flexibility in the lower spine while doing yoga.

S.M., Midline, Michigan

G.A., a 51-year-old female patient, presented with bilateral lower back pain ranging from 7 to 9 out of 10 on a pain scale. She described the pain as stabbing and spasmodic. She could barely walk or sit, and even lying down was uncomfortable. In fact, the patient stated she couldn't find relief in any position. She'd had intermittent back pain and spasms for much of her adult life, with the first serious episode occurring in her late twenties. The patient had recently missed several days of work and could concentrate on nothing but the pain. Objective findings included X-rays that revealed arthritis at L4 possibly as the result of trauma. The patient reported that she had injured her back when she was in first grade – a classmate had pulled a chair out from under her as she prepared to sit down. Tongue body color was unremarkable with scalloped edges. The tongue coating was thick and white with hairline cracks. Pulse was deep and small on both sides. Her lower back pain was too painful to palpate.

The TCM diagnosis was severe qi and blood stagnation in the lower back with mild Kidney qi and yang deficiencies. *Back Support (Chronic)* was prescribed at 4 capsules three to four times a day. The practitioner wanted to prescribe *Back Support (Acute)*, but had only *Back Support (Chronic)* in the pharmacy. Rather than wait a few days for the herbs to arrive, *Back Support (Chronic)* was given first to begin the herbal therapy. *Back Support (Chronic)* reduced the patient's pain level dramatically within 24 hours. This case exemplifies the principle of therapeutic diagnosis – the patient's excellent response to this formula demonstrated the degree to which underlying Kidney deficiency played a role in the pathology. However, she wasn't conscientious about taking the herbs and when the pain was gone and the bottle was empty, she didn't resume taking the herbs and the deficiency persisted.

The same patient returned some months later with another flare-up of stabbing and spasmodic bilateral lower back pain. Again, she could hardly walk nor could she find a position that relieved her pain at all. This time she reported that the pain was probably the result of her new job as an esthetician – she was now spending her workdays sitting on a stool bending over customers, giving them facials. Tongue appeared pale and scalloped, and peeled on the edges with thin white coating and hairline cracks. Pulses were still deep on both sides. The blood pressure was 118/72 mmHg and the heart rate was 62 beats per minute. The TCM diagnosis was severe qi and blood stagnation of the lumbar region, which probably resulted from working under ergonomically unsound conditions. She also suffered from mild Kidney qi and yang deficiencies. This time, *Back Support (Acute)* was prescribed at 4 capsules three to four times a day. Though the patient responded well to *Back Support (Chronic)* during her previous lumbar pain flare-up, the practitioner chose to give the patient *Back Support (Acute)* instead this time. Though the formula reduced her pain, it took longer to do so and the pain, though milder, lingered. This case was submitted by the practitioner as an example of the importance of treating the underlying deficiency in chronic cases.

H.H., San Francisco, California

[1] Bensky, D. et al. *Chinese Herbal Medicine Formulas & Strategies*. Eastland Press. 1990
[2] *Zhong Yao Xue* (Chinese Herbology), 1998; 759:765
[3] *Zhong Cao Yao* (Chinese Herbal Medicine), 1991; 22(10):452
[4] Tan, H. et al. Chemical components of decoction of radix paeoniae and radix glycyrrhizae. *China Journal of Chinese Materia Medica*. 20(9):550-1,576, September 1995
[5] Huang, DD. *Zhong Yi Za Zhi* (Journal of Chinese Medicine). 1983; 11:9
[6] Luo, DP. *Hu Nan Zhong Yi* (Hunan Journal of Traditional Chinese Medicine). 1989; 2:7
[7] Chen, Hong. *Yun Nan Zhong Yi* (Yunnan Journal of Traditional Chinese Medicine). 1990; 4:15
[8] Zhang, RB. Jiang Su Zhong Yi (Jiangsu Journal of Traditional Chinese Medicine). 1966; 5:38-39
[9] You, JH. *Guang Xi Zhong Yi Yao* (Guangxi Chinese Medicine and Herbology). 1987; 5:5-6

FORMULAS

BACK SUPPORT (HD) ™

(Herniated Disk)

CLINICAL APPLICATIONS

- Herniated disk, lumbar radiculopathy, prolapsed or bulging disk, or slipped disk with possible severe back pain which may worsen with coughing, straining or laughing, tingling or numbness in the legs or feet, muscle spasm or weakness
- Pain originating from the spinal cord and radiating down the legs

WESTERN THERAPEUTIC ACTIONS

- Analgesic effect to relieve pain
- Anti-inflammatory effect to reduce swelling and inflammation

CHINESE THERAPEUTIC ACTIONS

- Activates blood circulation and eliminates blood stasis
- Reduces swelling and inflammation
- Strengthens soft tissues and relieves pain

DOSAGE

Take 3 to 4 capsules, three times daily, as needed to relieve pain. The dosage may be increased up to 6 to 8 capsules every four to six hours if necessary, especially in the early stages of injury when there is severe and excruciating pain. When the pain subsides, reduce the dosage to 3 or 4 capsules, three times daily. For maximum effectiveness, take the herbs on an empty stomach, with two tall glasses of warm water.

INGREDIENTS

Bai Shao (Radix Paeoniae Alba)
Che Qian Zi (Semen Plantaginis)
Chuan Niu Xi (Radix Cyathulae)
Chuan Xiong (Rhizoma Ligustici Chuanxiong)
Dan Shen (Radix Salviae Miltiorrhizae)
Dang Gui (Radicis Angelicae Sinensis)
Du Zhong (Cortex Eucommiae)
E Zhu (Rhizoma Curcumae)

Gan Cao (Radix Glycyrrhizae)
Gui Zhi (Ramulus Cinnamomi)
San Leng (Rhizoma Sparganii)
Shen Jin Cao (Herba Lycopodii)
Yan Hu Suo (Rhizoma Corydalis)
Yi Yi Ren (Semen Coicis)
Ze Xie (Rhizoma Alismatis)

FORMULA EXPLANATION

Back Support (HD) is designed to treat herniated disk, also commonly known as prolapsed or slipped disk. The herbs activate blood circulation and eliminate blood stasis, reduce swelling and inflammation, strengthen soft tissue and relieve pain. It is most effective for acute injuries that are mild to moderate in severity.

Dang Gui (Radicis Angelicae Sinensis), *Chuan Xiong* (Rhizoma Ligustici Chuanxiong) and *Dan Shen* (Radix Salviae Miltiorrhizae) tonify blood and activate blood circulation. *Yan Hu Suo* (Rhizoma Corydalis), *San Leng* (Rhizoma Sparganii) and *E Zhu* (Rhizoma Curcumae) are among the strongest pain-relieving herbs that also eliminate blood stasis. *Bai Shao* (Radix Paeoniae Alba) and *Gan Cao* (Radix Glycyrrhizae) nourish yin to relieve muscle spasms and cramps. They also nourish Liver yin and benefit soft tissues. *Ze Xie* (Rhizoma Alismatis), *Che Qian Zi* (Semen Plantaginis) and *Yi Yi Ren* (Semen Coicis) drain water accumulation to reduce swelling and inflammation associated with herniated disk. *Shen Jin Cao* (Herba Lycopodii) and *Gui Zhi* (Ramulus Cinnamomi) open the channels and collaterals to unblock obstructions, especially of the extremities to treat radiating pain and/or numbness. *Du Zhong* (Cortex Eucommiae) and *Chuan Niu Xi* (Radix Cyathulae) are channel-guiding herbs that

BACK SUPPORT (HD)™

(Herniated Disk)

direct to the back and strengthen soft tissues, such as muscles, tendons, and ligaments. They also tonify the Kidney, dominate the marrow and directly benefit the bones and disks.

Back Support (HD) is an excellent formula to treat herniated disk, prolapsed disk, or slipped disk. It is most effective for acute injuries that are mild to moderate in severity.

SUPPLEMENTARY FORMULAS

- For acute neck, shoulder and upper back pain, add *Neck & Shoulder (Acute)*.
- For severe back pain, add *Back Support (Acute)* and *Herbal Analgesic*.
- For neuropathy, add *Flex (NP)*.
- For bone spurs, add *Flex (Spur)*.
- For external or traumatic injuries, use with *Traumanex*.
- For degeneration of disks, add *Osteo 8*.
- To enhance and support soft tissues and cartilages, add *Flex (MLT)*.

NUTRITION

- Eat whole grain cereals and a wide variety of raw vegetables and fruits to ensure a complete supply of nutrients for the bones, nerves, and muscles.
- Fresh pineapples are recommended as they contain bromelain, an enzyme that is excellent in reducing inflammation. If the consumption of fresh pineapples causes stomach upset, eat it after meals.
- To relieve cramps and spasms, eat plenty of fruits and vegetables, especially those high in potassium, such as bananas and oranges. Also, drink an adequate amount of warm water.
- Adequate intake of minerals, such as calcium and potassium, is essential for pain management. Deficiency of these minerals leads to spasms, cramps, and tense muscles.
- Avoid cold beverages, ice cream, caffeine, sugar, tomatoes, milk, and dairy products.

LIFESTYLE INSTRUCTIONS

- Stretching and strengthening exercises for the back muscles are essential for long-term recovery.
- Mild exercise such as swimming, yoga, or *Tai Chi Chuan* on a regular basis is recommended.
- Avoid engaging in activities that may lead to re-injury, such as improper lifting with turning or twisting, or excessive strain on the back. Advise the patient that lifting should involve the use of the knees, not the back. Avoid all strenuous physical activity.
- For those who are overweight, weight loss is strongly recommended to decrease pressure on the joints and relieve pain.
- Finally, adequate rest is essential to recovery. It is wise to review sleeping postures to ensure that the back is appropriately supported and relaxed in sleep.

CLINICAL NOTES

- Herniated disk can be caused by a prolapsed or slipped disk pressing on the nerves. As a result, there may be shooting pain that starts from the vertebrae and travels outwards to the extremities. While the use of herbs and acupuncture are helpful to relieve pain and reduce inflammation, physical treatment (such as *Tui-Na* or chiropractic adjustments) may be necessary to correct the underlying problem. In overt cases of radiculopathy, manipulation to the spinal area is contraindicated.
- To maximize the therapeutic effect, this formula should be given to patients before acupuncture treatments. The muscle-relaxant influence from the herbs takes effect within about half an hour. By relaxing the muscles and

BACK SUPPORT (HD) ™

(Herniated Disk)

invigorating qi and blood circulation, there is less stagnation in the channels, and the acupuncture and *Tui-Na* treatments can be more effective.

- Cold packs may be used for acute injuries during the first 24 to 48 hours to reduce swelling and inflammation. Afterwards, hot packs should be used afterwards to promote blood circulation and enhance healing in the affected area.
- L4-L5 and L5-S1 are the most common area of injury for herniated disk.
- This formula is an adjunct to acupuncture treatment. Optimal results are obtained when acupuncture, electro-stimulation and herbs are included in the treatment regimen.
- The following is a folk remedy to treat acute back pain from sprain and strain: Crack open 2 ocean crabs with a wooden stick (do not use a knife or any metal instruments) and put them into a clay pot with enough vodka or whiskey to cover both crabs. Place the clay pot into another bigger pot with water and steam it for one hour. Serve the crab meat along with the liquor soup.

CAUTIONS

- Because of the blood-invigorating nature of this formula, it is contraindicated during pregnancy and nursing.
- Patients who have pain radiating to the extremities accompanied by a sudden loss of bladder or bowel control may have a pinched nerve or spinal injury and must be referred out to emergency care if they have not already been evaluated by a specialist. This condition, known as Cauda Equina syndrome, can lead to permanent disability and must be evaluated and treated immediately.
- *Dan Shen* (Radix Salviae Miltiorrhizae) and *Dang Gui* (Radicis Angelicae Sinensis) may enhance the overall effectiveness of Coumadin (Warfarin), an anticoagulant drug. Patients who take anticoagulant or antiplatelet medications should ***not*** take this herbal formula without supervision by a licensed health care practitioner.

ACUPUNCTURE POINTS

Traditional Points:
- *Ah shi* points on the back, *Yinmen* (BL 37), and *Chengshan* (BL 57). Strongly stimulate and remove the needles.
- *Shenshu* (BL 23), *Yaoyangguan* (GV 3), *Weizhong* (BL 40), *Huantiao* (GB 30), and *Chengfu* (BL 36).

Balance Method by Dr. Richard Tan:
- *Lingku, Dabai* and *Zhongbai*. Needle all three points bilaterally 1.0 to 1.5 *cun*. Leave the needles in for 15 minutes and have the patient move the affected area in the back to help with circulation of qi and blood.
- All *ah shi* points from *Houding* (GV 19) to *Xuanji* (CV 21). Needle obliquely towards the back.
- Needle the following points on the side opposite of the pain: *Hegu* (LI 4), *Houxi* (SI 3), *Wangu* (SI 4), *Dazhong* (KI 4) or *ah shi* points nearby, and *Fuliu* (KI 7) or *ah shi* points nearby.
- Needle the following points on the same side as the pain: *Chize* (LU 5), *Shugu* (BL 65), and *Kongzui* (LU 6) or *ah shi* point nearby.
- Note: *Lingku, Dabai* and *Zhongbai* are Master Tong's points on both hands. *Lingku* is located in the depression just distal to the junction of the first and second metacarpal bones, approximately 0.5 *cun* proximal to *Hegu* (LI 4), on the *yangming* line. *Dabai* is located at about 0.5 *cun* proximal to *Sanjian* (LI 3), on the *yangming* line. *Zhongbai* is located at about 0.5 *cun* proximal to *Zhongzhu* (TH 3), on the *shaoyang* line.
- For additional information on the Balance Method, please refer to *Twelve and Twelve in Acupuncture* and *Twenty-Four More in Acupuncture* by Dr. Richard Tan.

Ear Points:
- Lower back (search for most sensitive and painful point), *Shenmen*, and Adrenals.

BACK SUPPORT (HD) ™

(Herniated Disk)

MODERN RESEARCH

Back Support (HD) was developed specifically to treat herniated, prolapsed, or slipped disk. It contains herbs with marked analgesic effects to relieve pain, and anti-inflammatory effects to reduce swelling and inflammation. Furthermore, many of these herbs have effect to treat other related conditions, such as sciatica, arthritis, and neuralgia.

One of the most important herbs in this formula is *Yan Hu Suo* (Rhizoma Corydalis), generally considered the herb with most potent analgesic and anti-inflammatory effect in the traditional Chinese pharmacopoeia. It is used to ensure the overall efficacy to relieve pain and reduce inflammation.[1] The effectiveness of *Yan Hu Suo* (Rhizoma Corydalis) is similar to that of morphine. Though the herb has a slower onset and weaker analgesic effect, it is associated with far fewer side effects, including absence of addiction and much slower development of tolerance.[2] In addition, the analgesic effect of *Yan Hu Suo* (Rhizoma Corydalis) can be enhanced significantly when combined with electroacupuncture.[3]

Dang Gui (Radicis Angelicae Sinensis) has marked analgesic and anti-inflammatory effect, with potency similar to or stronger than that of acetylsalicylic acid.[4,5] *Du Zhong* (Cortex Eucommiae) also has marked anti-inflammatory action. Its mechanisms are attributed to a stimulating effect on the endocrine system and the consequent secretion of endogenous steroids from the adrenal cortex.[6] Another herb in this formula that has analgesic and anti-inflammatory effects is *Du Huo* (Radix Angelicae Pubescentis).[7]

With regards to clinical applications, many herbs in this formula have been used with great success to specifically treat nerve pain. For example, *Du Zhong* (Cortex Eucommiae) has been used in various formulas with good results to treat sciatica.[8] *Chuan Xiong* (Rhizoma Ligustici Chuanxiong), *Dang Gui* (Radicis Angelicae Sinensis), *Dan Shen* (Radix Salviae Miltiorrhizae) and others have been used with a greater than 90% rate of effectiveness to treat trigeminal nerve pain.[9] *Chuan Xiong* (Rhizoma Ligustici Chuanxiong) may be used to treat nerve pain from bone spurs.[10] *Gui Zhi* (Ramulus Cinnamomi) is commonly used in many herbal formulas to treat arthritis.[11] *Bai Shao* (Radix Paeoniae Alba) and *Gan Cao* (Radix Glycyrrhizae) are effective in treating neuralgia.[12] *Bai Shao* (Radix Paeoniae Alba) and *Zhi Gan Cao* (Radix Glycyrrhizae Preparata) have also demonstrated effectiveness to treat pain in the entire body, especially lower back and legs.[13]

In conclusion, ***Back Support (HD)*** is developed specifically to treat herniated disk, prolapsed disk, or slipped disk. It contains herbs with marked analgesic effect to relieve pain, and anti-inflammatory effect to reduce swelling and inflammation.

PHARMACEUTICAL DRUGS & CHINESE MEDICINE: A COMPARATIVE ANALYSIS

Western Medical Approach: Pain is a basic bodily sensation induced by a noxious stimulus that causes physical discomfort (as pricking, throbbing, or aching). Pain may be of nociceptive, neuropathic, or psychogenic types. For neuropathic pain due to herniated disks, drugs [aspirin, non-steroidal anti-inflammatory agents (NSAID) and opioid analgesics] offer few benefits. Use of drugs do not change the underlying condition [herniated disk], they only mask the symptom [pain]. Most patients are simply told to relax at home, stay confined to bed, and take drugs as needed for pain. If the pain persists, more and more drugs are needed, thereby creating more side effects and complications. If the pain becomes worse, invasive treatment such as surgery is often suggested. In other words, western medicine offers few or no options. [Note: Common side effects of aspirin and NSAID's include gastric ulcer, duodenal ulcer, gastrointestinal bleeding, tinnitus, blurred vision, dizziness and headache. Serious side effects of newer NSAID's, also known as Cox-2 inhibitors [such as Celebrex (Celecoxib)], include significantly higher risk of cardiovascular events, including heart attack and stroke. Side effects of opioid analgesics [such as Vicodin (APAP/Hydrocodone) and morphine] include dizziness, lightheadedness, drowsiness, upset stomach, vomiting, constipation, stomach pain, rash, difficult urination, and respiratory depression resulting in difficult breathing. Furthermore, long-term use of these drugs leads to tolerance and addiction.]

BACK SUPPORT (HD) ™

(Herniated Disk)

Traditional Chinese Medicine Approach: Treatment of pain is a sophisticated balance of art and science. Proper treatment of pain requires a careful evaluation of the type of disharmony (excess or deficiency, cold or heat, exterior or interior), characteristics (qi and/or blood stagnations), and locations (upper body, lower body, extremities, or internal organs). Furthermore, optimal treatment requires integrative use of herbs, acupuncture and *Tui-Na* therapies. All these therapies work together to tonify the underlying deficiencies, strengthen the body, and facilitate recovery from chronic pain. Herbs and acupuncture are effective to treat the symptom (pain), and *Tui-Na* is effective to correct the underlying cause (herniation). By addressing both symptom and cause, TCM therapies often achieves immediate and long-term success. Furthermore, TCM therapies are often associated with few or no side effects. However, it is important to also recognize the limitation of TCM therapies. Integrative use of herbs, acupuncture and *Tui-Na* are excellent for initial stages of herniated disks of mild to moderate severity. When applied properly, they are often very successful to treat pain, correct the underlying problem, and restore normal physical functions. However, certain conditions may still require surgical treatment, such as in severe cases of herniated disks (such as ruptured disk) or chronic conditions where all other options have failed.

Summation: Optimal treatment of herniated disks is to understand all available options (from western and traditional Chinese medicine), and utilize the most effective modality for each specific condition.

[1] *Biol Pharm Bull*, 1994; Feb; 17(2):262-5
[2] *Zhong Yao Yao Li Yu Ying Yong* (Pharmacology and Applications of Chinese Herbs), 1983; 447
[3] *Chen Tzu Yen Chiu* (Acupuncture Research), 1994; 19(1):55-8
[4] *Xin Yi Yao Xue Za Zhi* (New Journal of Medicine and Herbology), 1975; (6):34
[5] *Yao Xue Za Zhi* (Journal of Medicinals), 1971; (91):1098
[6] *Zhong Cao Yao* (Chinese Herbal Medicine), 1983; 14(8):27
[7] *Zhong Yao Yao Li Yu Ying Yong* (Pharmacology and Applications of Chinese Herbs), 1983; 796
[8] *Zhong Yao Xue* (Chinese Herbology), 1998; 797:799
[9] *He Bei Zhong Yi Za Zhi* (Hebei Journal of Chinese Medicine), 1982; 4:34
[10] *Xin Yi Xue* (New Medicine), 1975; 6(1):50
[11] *Shi Zhen Guo Yao Yan Jiu* (Research of Shizhen Herbs), 1991; 5(4):36
[12] *Zhong Yi Za Zhi* (Journal of Chinese Medicine), 1983; 11:9
[13] *Yun Nan Zhong Yi* (Yunnan Journal of Traditional Chinese Medicine), 1990; 4:15

FORMULAS

BACK SUPPORT (Upper) ™

CLINICAL APPLICATIONS

- ❧ Acute injury or trauma to the chest, ribs, or thoracic area with pain, inflammation, swelling, or bruises
- ❧ Upper back stiffness and pain, scapular pain and/or pain between the scapulae
- ❧ Subluxation of the thoracic vertebrae
- ❧ Rib fracture

WESTERN THERAPEUTIC ACTIONS

- ❧ Analgesic effect to relieve pain
- ❧ Anti-inflammatory effect to reduce swelling and inflammation

CHINESE THERAPEUTIC ACTIONS

- ❧ Activates qi and blood circulation
- ❧ Dispels qi and blood stagnation
- ❧ Opens channels and collaterals
- ❧ Relieves pain

DOSAGE

Take 3 or 4 capsules, three times daily, or as needed to relieve pain. The dosage may be increased: up to 6 to 8 capsules every four to six hours if necessary, especially in the early stages of injury when there is severe and excruciating pain. When the pain subsides, drop the dosage to 3 or 4 capsules, three times daily. For maximum effectiveness, take the herbs on an empty stomach with two tall glasses of warm water. In chronic cases, or for consolidation of treatment effect, the dosage can be reduced to 2 capsules per day on an empty stomach.

INGREDIENTS

Chai Hu (Radix Bupleuri)
Chuan Xiong (Rhizoma Ligustici Chuanxiong)
Dan Shen (Radix Salviae Miltiorrhizae)
Dang Gui Wei (Extremitas Radicis Angelicae Sinensis)
Fu Ling (Poria)
Hong Hua (Flos Carthami)
Jiang Xiang (Lignum Dalbergiae Odoriferae)

Mu Xiang (Radix Aucklandiae)
Si Gua Luo (Retinervus Luffae Fructus)
Xiang Fu (Rhizoma Cyperi)
Yan Hu Suo (Rhizoma Corydalis)
Yu Jin (Radix Curcumae)
Zhi Ke (Fructus Aurantii)

FORMULA EXPLANATION

Back Support (Upper) is designed to treat acute injury and trauma to the chest, ribs, scapula, upper back and/or thoracic area. These types of injuries result from car accidents, sports injuries, external trauma, work injuries such as lifting heavy objects, or simply discomfort of the upper back from sitting or standing in one position for too long. Signs and symptoms include pain, stiffness, inflammation, swelling, and bruising. To successfully treat these conditions, herbs must activate qi and blood circulation, dispel qi and blood stagnation, open channels and collaterals, and relieve pain.

Back Support (Upper) dispels qi and blood stagnation and relieves pain in the upper *jiao*, which manifests in shortness of breath or oppression in the chest, and the chronic sensation of wanting to take a deep breath and sigh. *Dang Gui Wei* (Extremitas Radicis Angelicae Sinensis), *Dan Shen* (Radix Salviae Miltiorrhizae), *Chuan Xiong* (Rhizoma Ligustici Chuanxiong), *Hong Hua* (Flos Carthami) and *Yan Hu Suo* (Rhizoma Corydalis) activate blood

BACK SUPPORT (Upper) ™

circulation, dispel blood stasis and relieve pain. *Yu Jin* (Radix Curcumae), *Zhi Ke* (Fructus Aurantii), *Chai Hu* (Radix Bupleuri), *Xiang Fu* (Rhizoma Cyperi), and *Mu Xiang* (Radix Aucklandiae) activate Liver qi circulation and relieve qi stagnation in the chest area. Proper qi flow and blood circulation are extremely important, as stagnation and stasis directly contribute to discomfort, stiffness and pain. *Si Gua Luo* (Retinervus Luffae Fructus) and *Jiang Xiang* (Lignum Dalbergiae Odoriferae) open the channels and collaterals to relieve pain. *Bai Fu Ling* (Poria Alba) strengthens the middle *jiao*, and protects the Stomach from the potent qi and blood moving herbs. It also dispels dampness and prevents accumulation of phlegm in the Lungs. Lastly, *Chai Hu* (Radix Bupleuri) also works as a channel-guiding herb, and directs the effect of the formula to the chest, ribs, and thoracic area, domains of the Liver.

Back Support (Upper) is an excellent formula to treat acute injury and trauma to the chest, ribs, upper back or thoracic area. It helps to restore the body's ability to move fully, freely and without pain.

SUPPLEMENTARY FORMULAS

- For severe pain, combine with *Herbal Analgesic*.
- For pain that also affects the neck and shoulder areas, combine with *Neck & Shoulder (Acute)*.
- For pain that also affects the lower back, combine with *Back Support (Acute)*.
- In pain of acute injuries or trauma, combine with *Traumanex*.
- For chronic injuries affecting the soft tissues (muscles, tendons and ligaments), combine with *Flex (MLT)*.
- For bone spurs, add *Flex (Spur)*.
- For arthritis or *bi zheng* (painful obstruction syndrome) caused by heat, add *Flex (Heat)*.
- For arthritis or *bi zheng* (painful obstruction syndrome) caused by cold, add *Flex (CD)*.
- For osteoarthritis, osteoporosis or degeneration, add *Osteo 8*.
- For arm pain, add *Arm Support*.

NUTRITION

- Eat a wide variety of raw vegetables and fruits, and whole grain cereals to ensure a complete supply of nutrients for the bones, nerves, and muscles.
- Adequate intake of calcium is essential for the repair and rebuilding of bones, tendons, cartilage, and connective tissues.
- Fresh pineapples are recommended as they contain bromelain, an enzyme that is excellent in reducing inflammation. Serve after meals if the consumption of fresh pineapples causes stomach upset.
- To relieve cramps and spasms, eat plenty of fruits and vegetables, especially those high in potassium, such as bananas and oranges. Also, drink an adequate amount of warm water.
- Adequate intake of minerals, such as calcium and potassium, is essential for pain management. Deficiency of these minerals leads to spasms, cramps, and tense muscles.
- Avoid cold beverages, ice cream, caffeine, sugar, tomatoes, milk, and dairy products.

LIFESTYLE INSTRUCTIONS

- Use the knees (instead of bending from their waist or back) when lifting heavy objects.
- Stretching and strengthening exercises are essential for long-term recovery.
- Mild exercise such as swimming, yoga, or *Tai Chi Chuan* on a regular basis is recommended.
- Proper balance of work and rest is very important. While sitting, make sure the back is straight and the elbows and knees are bent at a 90° angle. Take a break at least once every hour to alleviate pressure on the vertebrae.
- Hot baths with Epsom salts help to relax tense muscles and draw toxins from the tissues. Rest and relax in the bath for about 30 minutes, but avoid becoming over-tired from the heat and soaking.
- Do not work in front of the computer for an extended period without rest. Stretch every 30 to 40 minutes and walk around to relax the muscles and re-balance muscle tone.

FORMULAS

BACK SUPPORT (Upper) ™

- Cycling with an improper position may contribute or aggravate mid- or upper back pain, and should be limited or stopped while undergoing treatment.
- Finally, adequate rest is essential to recovery. It is wise to review the patient's sleeping postures to ensure that the back is being appropriately supported and relaxed in sleep.

CLINICAL NOTES

- There may be several causes for pain in the chest, ribs, and thoracic region. This formula is designed to treat pain due to musculoskeletal injuries.
- Clinical tip: Give this formula to the patient before acupuncture and *Tui-Na* treatments. The muscle-relaxant influence of the herbs takes effect within about half an hour. By relaxing the muscles and invigorating qi and blood circulation, there is less stagnation in the channels, and the acupuncture and *Tui-Na* treatments are thus more effective.

CAUTIONS

- Because of its blood-invigorating nature of this formula, it is not recommended during pregnancy and nursing.
- Patients who have pain radiating to the extremities accompanied by a sudden loss of bladder or bowel control may have a pinched nerve or a spinal injury, and must be dealt with accordingly and referred out to emergency care if they have not already been evaluated by a specialist. Regardless, it may be necessary to seek urgent care or evaluation at the emergency room in severe cases of slipped disk, also known as Cauda Equina Syndrome, where symptoms include bilateral leg pain, loss of perianal sensation and bladder paralysis.
- *Dan Shen* (Radix Salviae Miltiorrhizae) and *Dang Gui Wei* (Extremitas Radicis Angelicae Sinensis) may enhance the overall effectiveness of Coumadin (Warfarin), an anticoagulant drug. Patients who take anticoagulant or antiplatelet medications should **not** take this herbal formula without supervision by a licensed health care practitioner.

ACUPUNCTURE POINTS

Traditional Points:
- Needle *ah shi* points around the upper back.

Balance Method by Dr. Richard Tan:
- *Chung Tze*: This point is located on the palmar surface of the hand, about 1 *cun* medial to the midpoint of the web-margin between the thumb and index finger, on a line drawn from this intersection to *Daling* (PC 7). Finding the *Ah shi* point is best. This point is especially effective for pain between the scapulae. Needle on both hands.
- *Chung-Hsien*: Along the same line as described in the location for *Chung Tze*, about 1 *cun* proximal or medial to *Chung Tze*. Needle on both sides.
- Needle *Chize* (LU 5), *Kongzui* (LU 6) and *Zhubin* (KI 9) on the same or opposite side of the pain. Needle *Jiaoxin* (KI 8) on the opposite side of the pain. If the pain is bilateral, needle both sides.
- For additional information on the Balance Method, please refer to *Twelve and Twelve in Acupuncture* and *Twenty-Four More in Acupuncture* by Dr. Richard Tan.

MODERN RESEARCH

Back Support (Upper) is designed to treat acute injury and trauma to the chest, ribs, and thoracic and upper back area. It contains herbs with remarkable analgesic effects to relieve pain, and anti-inflammatory effects to reduce swelling and inflammation.

FORMULAS

BACK SUPPORT (Upper) ™

One of the most important herbs in this formula is *Yan Hu Suo* (Rhizoma Corydalis), generally considered to have the most potent analgesic and anti-inflammatory effect among commonly-available herbs. It is used to ensure overall efficacy to relieve pain and reduce inflammation.[1] The effectiveness of *Yan Hu Suo* (Rhizoma Corydalis) has been compared to that of morphine. Though the herb has a slower onset and weaker analgesic effect, it is associated with far fewer side effects, the absence of addiction and much slower development of tolerance.[2] Furthermore, the analgesic effect of *Yan Hu Suo* (Rhizoma Corydalis) can be enhanced significantly when combined with electro-acupuncture.[3]

In addition to *Yan Hu Suo* (Rhizoma Corydalis), this formula uses many herbs with marked analgesic and anti-inflammatory effects to relieve pain and reduce swelling and inflammation. For example, *Dang Gui Wei* (Extremitas Radicis Angelicae Sinensis) has potency similar to or stronger than that of acetylsalicylic acid.[4,5] In addition, *Chai Hu* (Radix Bupleuri), *Xiang Fu* (Rhizoma Cyperi) and *Jiang Xiang* (Lignum Dalbergiae Odoriferae) all enhance the overall effect to relieve pain and reduce inflammation.[6,7,8,9]

Back Support (Upper) is designed with herbs with remarkable analgesic effects to relieve pain and anti-inflammatory effect to reduce swelling and inflammation, and is an excellent formula to treat acute injury and trauma to the chest, ribs, upper back or thoracic area.

PHARMACEUTICAL DRUGS & CHINESE MEDICINE: A COMPARATIVE ANALYSIS

Western Medical Approach: Pain is a basic bodily sensation induced by a noxious stimulus that causes physical discomfort (as pricking, throbbing, or aching). Pain may be of acute or chronic state, and may be of nociceptive, neuropathic, or psychogenic type. NSAID's are generally prescribed for musculoskeletal disorders of the arm, including shoulders, elbows, and wrists. NSAID's [such as Motrin (Ibuprofen) and Voltaren (Diclofenac)] treat pain of mild to moderate intensity, and are most effective to reduce inflammation and swelling. Though effective, these drugs cause serious side effects such as gastric ulcer, duodenal ulcer, gastrointestinal bleeding, tinnitus, blurred vision, dizziness and headache. Furthermore, the newer NSAID's, also known as Cox-2 inhibitors [such as Celebrex (Celecoxib)], are associated with significantly higher risk of cardiovascular events, including heart attack and stroke. Therefore, practitioners and patients must evaluate the potential benefit versus risk before prescribing and taking these drugs. In short, it is important to remember that while drugs offer reliable and potent symptomatic pain relief, they should be used only if and when needed. Frequent use and abuse leads to unnecessary side effects and complications.

Traditional Chinese Medicine Approach: Treatment of pain is a sophisticated balance of art and science. Proper treatment of pain requires a careful evaluation of the type of disharmony (excess or deficiency, cold or heat, exterior or interior), characteristics (qi and/or blood stagnations), and locations (upper body, lower body, extremities, or internal organs). Furthermore, optimal treatment requires integrative use of herbs, acupuncture and *Tui-Na* therapies. All these therapies work together to tonify the underlying deficiencies, strengthen the body, and facilitate recovery from chronic pain. TCM pain management targets both the symptom and the cause of pain, and as such, often achieves immediate and long-term success. Furthermore, TCM pain management is often associated with few or no side effects.

Summation: For treatment of mild to severe pain due to various causes, TCM pain management offers similar treatment effects with significantly fewer side effects.

[1] *Biol Pharm Bull*, 1994; Feb; 17(2):262-5
[2] *Zhong Yao Yao Li Yu Ying Yong* (Pharmacology and Applications of Chinese Herbs), 1983; 447
[3] *Chen Tzu Yen Chiu* (Acupuncture Research), 1994; 19(1):55-8
[4] *Xin Yi Yao Xue Za Zhi* (New Journal of Medicine and Herbology), 1975; (6):34
[5] *Yao Xue Za Zhi* (Journal of Medicinals), 1971; (91):1098
[6] *Shen Yang Yi Xue Yuan Xue Bao* (Journal of Shenyang University of Medicine), 1984; 1(3):214

BACK SUPPORT (Upper) ™

[7] *Zhong Yao Yao Li Yu Ying Yong* (Pharmacology and Applications of Chinese Herbs), 1983; 888
[8] *Gui Yang Yi Xue Yuan Xue Bao* (Journal of Guiyang Medical University), 1959; 113
[9] *Zhong Yao Xue* (Chinese Herbology), 1998; 576:577

BALANCE (Cold) ™

CLINICAL APPLICATIONS

- Menstrual disorders with overall cold manifestations, such as cold extremities, dull menstrual pain alleviated by warmth, and/or generalized weakness, pale face, anemia or edema
- Maintenance therapy to balance female hormones and promote overall wellness
- General menstrual disorders, such as amenorrhea, dysmenorrhea or irregular menstruation
- Female infertility, or habitual or threatened miscarriage because of deficiency

WESTERN THERAPEUTIC ACTIONS

- Hematopoietic effect to treat anemia, dizziness, generalized weakness [5,6]
- Diuretic effect to treat edema, water accumulation and bloating sensation [5]
- Balances female hormones to ease common symptoms associated with PMS [1,2,3,4]
- Analgesic and anti-inflammatory effects to relieve pain and cramps associated with PMS [4]

CHINESE THERAPEUTIC ACTIONS

- Nourishes the Liver blood
- Strengthens the Spleen
- Dispels dampness
- Spreads the Liver qi

DOSAGE

Take 3 to 4 capsules three times daily. Dosage may be increased, up to 6 to 8 capsules every four hours as needed, in cases of severe deficiency and/or water retention.

INGREDIENTS

Bai Shao (Radix Paeoniae Alba)
Bai Zhu (Rhizoma Atractylodis Macrocephalae)
Chuan Xiong (Rhizoma Ligustici Chuanxiong)

Dang Gui (Radicis Angelicae Sinensis)
Fu Ling (Poria)
Ze Xie (Rhizoma Alismatis)

FORMULA EXPLANATION

According to traditional Chinese medicine, blood is generally considered the root of female physiology. Deficiency of blood is characterized by anemia, dizziness, and generalized weakness; stagnation of blood is characterized by pain and cramps; and poor circulation of blood may lead to water accumulation and edema. Therefore, it is necessary to focus on nourishing blood and regulating blood circulation in the *chong* (thoroughfare) channel when treating female disorders.

Dang Gui (Radicis Angelicae Sinensis) and *Chuan Xiong* (Rhizoma Ligustici Chuanxiong) are used here to nourish the blood and invigorate its circulation. *Dang Gui* (Radicis Angelicae Sinensis) tonifies the blood to treat blood deficiency. *Chuan Xiong* (Rhizoma Ligustici Chuanxiong) regulates blood circulation to relieve pain. *Bai Shao* (Radix Paeoniae Alba) has analgesic effects to relieve pain and inflammation. It also has antispasmodic effects to alleviate spasms and cramps in the lower abdominal region.

FORMULAS

BALANCE (Cold) ™

Fu Ling (Poria) and *Bai Zhu* (Rhizoma Atractylodis Macrocephalae) strengthen the Spleen and facilitate water metabolism. *Ze Xie* (Rhizoma Alismatis) is a diuretic, which eliminates dampness and treats edema. When used together, these three herbs remove water accumulation and treat edema.

SUPPLEMENTARY FORMULAS

- ❧ For female infertility, use **Blossom (Phase 1-4)** instead.
- ❧ For dysmenorrhea, use **Mense-Ease** instead.
- ❧ For edema, add **Herbal DRX**.
- ❧ For irritability arising from menopause, use with **Calm (ES)** or **Calm ZZZ**.
- ❧ For hot flashes and/or sweating because of menopause, use with **Balance (Heat)**.
- ❧ For insomnia and anemia, add **Schisandra ZZZ**.
- ❧ For dull, lusterless hair or hair loss, add **Polygonum 14**.
- ❧ To tonify the overall constitution, add **Imperial Tonic**.
- ❧ For poor appetite, loose stool, add **GI Tonic**.
- ❧ For infertility due Kidney yang deficiency and blood stagnation, add **Menotrol**.
- ❧ For dysmenorrhea with headache, use with **Migratrol** or **Corydalin**.
- ❧ For low libido, add **Vitality**.

NUTRITION

- ❧ Adequate intake of calcium is important to prevent menstrual cramps. Calcium level in the body is decreased about 10 days before a period.
- ❧ Increase the intake of vegetable oil and fish. They are rich resources of prostaglandin, which relieves cramping and pain associated with painful menstruation.
- ❧ Soy products are also beneficial as they help to regulate hormone imbalance.
- ❧ Increase the intake of foods that are warm in nature, such as onions, garlic, mutton, chili or chives.
- ❧ Avoid cold or raw foods as they impair the Spleen function and create more dampness and stagnation.

LIFESTYLE INSTRUCTIONS

- ❧ Avoid vigorous exercise, cigarette smoking and second-hand smoke.
- ❧ Exercise, rest and relaxation will relieve tension and prevent menstrual cramps.
- ❧ A hot water shower directed at the abdomen, or heat packs, are helpful to relieve pain.

CAUTION

- ❧ Patients who are on anticoagulant or antiplatelet therapies, such as Coumadin (Warfarin), should use this formula with caution, as there may be a slightly higher risk of bleeding and bruising.

ACUPUNCTURE POINTS

Traditional Points:
- ❧ *Zusanli* (ST 36), *Sanyinjiao* (SP 6). Apply moxa to *Guanyuan* (CV 4) and *Qihai* (CV 6).
- ❧ *Shigou* (TH 6), *Guanyuan* (CV 4), *Xuehai* (SP 10), *Geshu* (BL 17), *Tianshu* (ST 25), *Zusanli* (ST 36), *Sanyinjiao* (SP 6), *Zhongwan* (CV 12), and *Shongji* (CV 3).

BALANCE (Cold) ™

Balance Method by Dr. Richard Tan:

- ☙ Left side: *Zusanli* (ST 36) and *Lieque* (LU 7).
- ☙ Right side: *Hegu* (LI 4), *Yinlingquan* (SP 9), *Lougu* (SP 7) or *ah shi* points nearby, and *Sanyinjiao* (SP 6).
- ☙ Left and right side can be alternated from treatment to treatment.
- ☙ For additional information on the Balance Method, please refer to *Dr. Tan's Strategy of Twelve Magical Points* by Dr. Richard Tan.

Auricular Acupuncture by Dr. Li-Chun Huang:

- ☙ Menstrual disorder (menoxenia): Uterus, Kidney, Liver, Pituitary, Ovary, and Endocrine.
- ☙ Amenorrhea and hypomenorrhea: Uterus, Ovary, Gonadotropin, Exciting Point, Pituitary Point, Endocrine, Kidney, Liver, and Sympathetic.
- ☙ Dysmenorrhea: Uterus, Pelvic, Liver, Sympathetic, Kidney, Ovary, Endocrine, Pituitary, and Lower *Jiao*.
- ☙ For additional information on the location and explanation of these points, please refer to *Auricular Treatment Formula and Prescriptions* by Dr. Li-Chun Huang.

MODERN RESEARCH

Balance (Cold) is based on a classic Chinese formula designed specifically to address female imbalances. The clinical applications of this formula include primary dysmenorrhea, pelvic inflammatory disease, chronic nephritis, beriberi, and habitual or threatened miscarriage.[9] *Balance (Cold)* is formulated with herbs with blood tonic, diuretic, analgesic, anti-inflammatory, and hormone-regulating functions.

Dang Gui (Radicis Angelicae Sinensis) has demonstrated a wide variety of clinical functions. It has been reported in many textbooks and numerous clinical studies that *Dang Gui* (Radicis Angelicae Sinensis) treats a variety of women's disorders, such as menstrual cramps and anemia with dizziness and palpitation.[1,2,3,4,5] Furthermore, it regulates female hormones to relieve amenorrhea, dysmenorrhea and menorrhalgia.[6,7,8,9] The reported functions of *Dang Gui* (Radicis Angelicae Sinensis) include activation of blood circulation, regulation of menstruation, spasmolytic, anti-inflammatory and analgesic actions. [1,2,3,4]

Bai Shao (Radix Paeoniae Alba), containing daisein, has a strong antispasmodic effect to alleviate abdominal muscle spasms and cramps.[10] *Fu Ling* (Poria) and *Ze Xie* (Rhizoma Alismatis) have diuretic functions to eliminate water accumulation and treat edema and bloating. [11]

PHARMACEUTICAL DRUGS & CHINESE MEDICINE: A COMPARATIVE ANALYSIS

Western Medical Approach: Menstrual disorders, including premenstrual syndrome (PMS), dysmenorrhea, and amenorrhea are conditions that affect all women on occasional basis. As common as these conditions are, there are few drug treatments available. Over-the-counter (OTC) drugs, such as Midol, may be used to reduce swelling and relieve edema. Non-steroidal anti-inflammatory agents (NSAID) are effective to relieve pain and reduce inflammation, but cause serious side effects such as gastric ulcer, duodenal ulcer, gastrointestinal bleeding, tinnitus, blurred vision, dizziness and headache. Lastly, hormone drugs, such as birth control pills or patches, are prescribed to regulate menstrual cycles. Though they are more effective, they often cause serious side effects, such as weight gain, hyperkalemia, clotting disorders, retinal thrombosis, cancer, liver damage, hypertriglyceridemia, hypertension, bleeding, and fertility impairment. In short, drug treatment options are very limited between those that treat only symptoms and do not work well, and those that work well but may have significant side effects.

Traditional Chinese Medicine Approach: Herbal therapy is extremely effective to regulate menstruation and treat various menstrual disorders. These herbs have analgesic effect to relieve pain, anti-inflammatory effect to reduce swelling and inflammation, and antispasmodic effect to relieve cramping. Furthermore, many herbs have been shown to have marked effect to regulate hormones to promote normal menstruation. However, this effect requires

BALANCE (Cold) ™

continuous use of herbs for at least one to two cycles. In short, herbal therapy is extremely beneficial for treatment of menstrual disorder as it treats both the symptoms and the cause of PMS, dysmenorrhea, irregular menstruation, amenorrhea, and others..

Summation: Drug offers limited options for treatment of PMS, dysmenorrhea, and amenorrhea. NSAIDs relieve pain, but should be used as needed for only a short period of time. Birth controls are effective, but these drugs carry significant short- and long-term side effects. Herbs, on the other hand, are extremely effective for both immediate and prolonged benefits. Furthermore, they are very safe and are associated with few or no side effects. Individuals with such menstrual disorders should definitely explore these non-drug treatment options.

---

[1] *Pharmacopoeia of the People's Republic of China*. English version edited from the Pharmacopoeia of PRC 1990 edition. Guangzhou: Guangdong Science and Technology Press. 1990

[2] Tang, W. and Eisenbrand, G. Chinese Drugs of Plant Origin: Chemistry, Pharmacology, and Use in Traditional and Modern Medicine. Berlin: Springer-Verlag. 1992

[3] Hsu, HY. et al. *Oriental Material Medica: A Concise Guide*. Long Beach: Oriental Healing Arts Press. 1986

[4] Huang, KC. *The Pharmacology of Chinese Herbs*. Boca Raton: CRC Press. 1993

[5] Murray, MT. *The Healing Power of Herbs*. Rocklin, CA: Prima Publishing. 1991

[6] Shi, MY. et al. *China J Chinese Materia Medica*. 1995; 20(3):173-175

[7] Olin et al. The Lawrence Review of Natural Products by Facts and Comparisons. Dong Quai. March 1997

[8] Li, HY. et al. *China J. Chinese Materia Medica*. 1991; 16(9):560-562

[9] Bensky, D. et al. Chinese Herbal Medicine Formulas & Strategies. Eastland Press. 1990

[10] Bensky, D. et al. *Chinese Herbal Medicine Materia Medica*. Eastland Press. 1993

[11] Yeung, HC. *Handbook of Chinese Herbal Formulas*. Institute of Chinese Medicine. 1996

FORMULAS

BALANCE (Heat) ™

CLINICAL APPLICATIONS

- Symptoms associated with menopause
- Hot flashes or night sweats
- Mood swings, emotional instability and irritability
- Related symptoms such as restless sleep, crying spells and disorientation

WESTERN THERAPEUTIC ACTIONS

- Endocrine effect to balance female hormones and ease common symptoms associated with menopause [1,2,4,5,6]
- Antiperspirant function to stop sweating [3,7,8]
- Mild sedative action to settle the emotions and stabilize moods [1,2]
- Mild sedative action to treat insomnia and restless sleep [1,2,3]

CHINESE THERAPEUTIC ACTIONS

- Nourishes yin
- Clears deficiency heat
- Calms the *shen* (spirit)
- Stops perspiration

DOSAGE

Take 3 to 4 capsules three times daily on an empty stomach with warm water. Take the last dose half an hour before bedtime if hot flashes, insomnia, restless sleep or night sweating are especially worse at night. For severe conditions gradually increase the dosage to 8 to 10 capsules three times daily until symptoms are controlled. After relief of symptoms, dosage can then be reduced to 3 to 4 capsules daily.

INGREDIENTS

Bai Shao (Radix Paeoniae Alba)
Bie Jia (Carapax Trionycis)
Chai Hu (Radix Bupleuri)
Da Zao (Fructus Jujubae)
Di Gu Pi (Cortex Lycii)
Fu Xiao Mai (Semen Tritici Aestivi Levis)
Gan Cao (Radix Glycyrrhizae)

Hu Huang Lian (Rhizoma Picrorhizae)
Mu Dan Pi (Cortex Moutan)
Qing Hao (Herba Artemisiae Annuae)
Sheng Di Huang (Radix Rehmanniae)
Xiao Mai (Fructus Tritici)
Ye Jiao Teng (Caulis Polygoni Multiflori)
Zhi Mu (Radix Anemarrhenae)

FORMULA EXPLANATION

The chief cause of imbalance in women during menopause is Kidney yin deficiency with deficiency heat. The treatment protocol to address the hot flashes, mood swings and night sweats is to clear the deficiency heat and nourish the yin. The patient may also have irritability and emotional instability because of Liver qi stagnation.

Xiao Mai (Fructus Tritici) nourishes the *shen* (spirit) of the Heart and treats excessive worrying or anxiety. *Chai Hu* (Radix Bupleuri) works with *Xiao Mai* (Fructus Tritici) to regulate nervousness, irritability, and mood swings by spreading the stagnant Liver qi. *Qing Hao* (Herba Artemisiae Annuae), *Zhi Mu* (Radix Anemarrhenae) and *Mu Dan Pi* (Cortex Moutan) reduce hot flashes and heat sensations by clearing deficiency heat. *Bie Jia* (Carapax Trionycis) and *Sheng Di Huang* (Radix Rehmanniae) nourish the Kidney *jing* (essence) and replenish vitality that is lost

FORMULAS

BALANCE (Heat) ™

through normal aging. *Fu Xiao Mai* (Semen Tritici Aestivi Levis) stops abnormal perspiration. *Ye Jiao Teng* (Caulis Polygoni Multiflori) nourishes the Heart blood, pacifies nerves and treats insomnia and nervousness. *Bai Shao* (Radix Paeoniae Alba), *Gan Cao* (Radix Glycyrrhizae) and *Da Zao* (Fructus Jujubae), the three herbs that make up the formula *Gan Mai Da Zao Tang* (Licorice, Wheat, and Jujube Decoction), nourish the blood of the Heart and moisten internal organ dryness. Finally, *Di Gu Pi* (Cortex Lycii) and *Hu Huang Lian* (Rhizoma Picrorhizae) drain yin-deficient fire to control flare-ups of hot flashes.

In summary, ***Balance (Heat)*** is an excellent formula to address all imbalance associated with menopause.

SUPPLEMENTARY FORMULAS

- To address the cause of menopause by tonifying the Kidney yin and reduce deficiency heat, add ***Nourish***.
- To only tonify Kidney yin and *jing* (essence), add ***Kidney Tonic (Yin)***.
- For prevention and treatment of osteoporosis, add ***Osteo 8***.
- For emotional instability, irritability, and mood swings, combine with ***Calm***.
- For severe *shen* (spirit) disturbance with insomnia, combine with ***Calm (ES)***.
- For menopause with stress, insomnia and fatigue, add ***Calm ZZZ***.
- For depression, add ***Shine***.
- For fibrocystic disorders of the female reproductive organs, use ***Resolve (Lower)***.
- For benign breast tumors, mastitis and nodules, use ***Resolve (Upper)***.
- For hair loss, combine with ***Polygonum 14***.
- For constipation, use ***Gentle Lax (Deficient)***.
- For lack of libido, add ***Vitality***.
- For poor memory and forgetfulness, use with ***Enhance Memory***.
- For hypertension, add ***Gastrodia Complex***.
- For vaginitis, add ***V-Statin***.
- For thirst and dryness, add ***Nourish (Fluids)***.

NUTRITION

- Encourage a diet with a high content of raw foods, fruits and vegetables to stabilize blood sugar. Wild yam is very helpful to nourish yin and reduce menopause symptoms.
- Discourage dairy products and red meats, as they promote hot flashes.
- Avoid alcohol, sugar, spicy foods, and caffeine as they trigger hot flashes and aggravate mood swings.
- Increase the intake of soy products such as tofu, soymilk and soy nuts. Soy products regulate the estrogen levels and are beneficial for menopause.
- Take *Gou Qi Zi* (Fructus Lycii) on a daily basis (mix with cereal or trail mix) to nourish Kidney yin.
- *Gan Mai Da Zao Tang* (Licorice, Wheat, and Jujube Decoction) can be used as tea on a daily basis.

The Tao of Nutrition by Ni and McNease
- Menopause
  - Recommendations: black beans, sesame seeds, soybeans, walnuts, lycium berries, mulberries, yams, licorice, lotus seeds, and chrysanthemum flowers.
  - Avoid stress, tension, and all stimulants.
- For more information, please refer to *The Tao of Nutrition* by Dr. Maoshing Ni and Cathy McNease.

FORMULAS

BALANCE (Heat) ™

LIFESTYLE INSTRUCTIONS

- Avoid stress, tension and anxiety as much as possible.
- Avoid cigarette smoking or exposure to second-hand smoke, as they may dry yin and body fluids.
- Natural progesterone cream can be applied every 15 minutes to help relieve hot flashes.
- Vaginal dryness can be alleviated with sitz-baths, application of natural progesterone cream, aloe-vera gel or KY jelly.

CLINICAL NOTES

- *Balance (Heat)* and *Nourish* are two of the most commonly used formulas for menopause.
  - *Balance (Heat)* is stronger to clear deficiency heat, and relieve symptoms such as hot flashes and emotional disturbance.
  - *Nourish* is more effective to tonify the underlying Kidney yin deficiency, and alleviate conditions such as thirst, dryness, and atrophy of genitourinary tissues.
- *Balance (Heat)* and *Nourish* are both safe formulas that can be used throughout the entire menopause period.

ACUPUNCTURE POINTS

Traditional Points:
- *Taixi* (KI 3) and *Taichong* (LR 3).
- *Shenmen* (HT 7), *Sanyinjiao* (SP 6), *Xinshu* (BL 15), *Ganshu* (BL 18), *Pishu* (BL 20), *Feishu* (BL 13), *Shenshu* (BL 23), *Taixi* (KI 3), and *Yinlingquan* (SP 9).

Balance Method by Dr. Richard Tan:
- Left side: *Zusanli* (ST 36) and *Lieque* (LU 7).
- Right side: *Hegu* (LI 4), *Yinlingquan* (SP 9), *Lougu* (SP 7) or *ah shi* points nearby, and *Sanyinjiao* (SP 6).
- Left and right side can be alternated from treatment to treatment.
- For additional information on the Balance Method, please refer to *Dr. Tan's Strategy of Twelve Magical Points* by Dr. Richard Tan.

Ear Points:
- Uterus, Ovary, Endocrine, Sympathetic, and Subcortex.
  - Add *Shenmen* and Heart for emotional disorders.
  - Add Heart and Small Intestine for palpitations and irregular heartbeat.
  - Add Sympathetic, Cheeks and Lung for flushed cheeks, excess perspiration.

Auricular Acupuncture by Li-Chun Huang:
- Menopause
  - Main points: Uterus, Endocrine, Ovary, Gonadotropin, Pituitary, Sympathetic, Anxious
  - Supplementary points: Kidney, Liver, Heart
- For additional information on the location and explanation of these points, please refer to *Auricular Treatment Formula and Prescriptions* by Dr. Li-Chun Huang.

MODERN RESEARCH

Balance (Heat) is formulated based on a classical Chinese formula. It is designed specifically for female imbalances and disorders such as menopausal syndrome with hot flashes, irritability, insomnia, and mood swings.[1,2]

BALANCE (Heat) ™

Zhi Mu (Radix Anemarrhenae) and *Mu Dan Pi* (Cortex Moutan) are used to regulate body temperature. *Sheng Di Huang* (Radix Rehmanniae) and *Gan Cao* (Radix Glycyrrhizae) regulate endocrine functions. *Ye Jiao Teng* (Caulis Polygoni Multiflori) treats insomnia. *Fu Xiao Mai* (Semen Tritici Aestivi Levis) and *Xiao Mai* (Fructus Tritici) stop perspiration.[3] Furthermore, *Gan Cao* (Radix Glycyrrhizae) has been used to treat adrenocorticoid insufficiency.[4,5,6]

It was demonstrated in one study of 21 patients that *Qing Hao* (Herba Artemisiae Annuae) reduced fever in 100% of the patients after having taken the herbs continuously for 7 days.[7] Another study showed *Qing Hao* (Herba Artemisiae Annuae) to effectively reduce body temperature in 126 patients with high fever with a success rate of approximately 68%.[8]

PHARMACEUTICAL DRUGS & CHINESE MEDICINE: A COMPARATIVE ANALYSIS

As life expectancy continues to increase, women are expected to spend more and more of their life in post-menopause years. Therefore, it is becoming increasingly important to ensure a smooth transition during the menopause years.

Western Medical Approach: Hormone replacement therapy (HRT) was long considered the standard treatment for menopause and related conditions. However, there is no longer a consensus as to when and how to use these drugs. While these drugs may alleviate hot flashes, they significantly increase the risk of breast cancer, ovarian cancer, uterine cancer, and have a number of significant side effects. For most physicians and patients, the risks are simply far greater than the potential benefits. The bottom line is – synthetic hormones can never replace endogenous hormones. Therefore, no matter how or when they are prescribed, the potential for adverse reactions is always present.

Traditional Chinese Medicine Approach: TCM offers a gentle yet effective way to address menopause and related conditions. Chinese herbs have demonstrated via numerous *in vivo* and *in vitro* study to have marked effect to alleviate hot flashes, vasomotor instability, loss of bone mass, and other conditions associated with menopause. Most importantly, they are much gentler and safer on the body.

Summation: Menopause is simply a transition in the journey of life. It is a not a disease, and therefore, should not be treated with synthetic drugs that pose significantly higher risks of cancer and other side effects. Herbs should be considered the primary option, and not the secondary alternative, as they are safe and natural, and more than sufficient to address almost all cases of menopause.

CASE STUDIES

M.K., a 50-year-old female, presented with a hot and flushed face, and very mild sweat one week before her menstrual cycle. Due to the sweating, she was unable to wear nylon or silk clothes. Blood pressure was 120/80 mmHg and her heart rate was 82 beats per minute. The pulse was thready and weak in the Kidney yin positions. The TCM diagnosis was Kidney yin deficiency with deficiency heat. *Balance (Heat)* was prescribed at 8 capsules twice daily. Symptoms resolved quickly after taking the herbs. She was then instructed to reduce the dosage to 4 capsules twice daily. Dietary changes were also made. Patient felt extremely grateful to the practitioner for prescribing the formula.

M.H., West Palm Beach, Florida

A 62-year-old saleslady initially presented with neck pain resulting from a car accident. She also had symptoms of night sweats and dry skin. The patient complained of feeling frustrated and had been gaining weight. Besides having smoked 1½ packs of cigarettes a day her whole life, the patient had been diagnosed with hypothyroid and was on 100 mcg of levothyroxin (Synthroid) per day. Her tongue was dusky red with a thick coat. Her pulse was choppy

FORMULAS

BALANCE (Heat) ™

and rapid. The TCM diagnosis included Liver qi stagnation, Kidney yin and yang deficiency, and qi and blood stagnation. After 2 weeks of taking *Balance (Heat)*, the patient commented, "I feel much better overall and I definitely sleep better and am less irritable."

F.A., Calabasas, California

C.B. was a 56-year-old female who suffered from weight gain, right-side sciatic pain, insomnia, hot flashes and night sweats. She exhibited rapid, thin and thready pulse with peeled and cracked tongue. The practitioner diagnosed her with Kidney yin and blood deficiency with deficiency heat and blood stagnation. *Neuro Plus* and *Balance (Heat)* were prescribed. The patient reported the sciatic pain went away completely. Night sweats and hot flashes were reduced, and therefore, insomnia was no longer an issue.

S.C., Santa Monica, California

A 44-year-old female nurse presented with irritability and approximately 60 hot flashes per day. Her tongue body was red with no coating and the pulse was slippery and rapid. The practitioner diagnosed this as Kidney and Liver yin deficiency. Because of the severity of her condition, she was given a higher dose of a modified *Balance (Heat)* formula. The formula contained *Balance (Heat)* along with 15 grams of *Gui Ban* (Plastrum Testudinis) and 9 grams of *Qing Hao* (Herba Artemisiae Annuae). The prescribed dosage was 6 capsules at 3 times a day. After taking *Balance (Heat)*, the frequency of hot flashes reduced dramatically, from 60 per day to 2 to 3 per week!

K.S., Encinitas, California

A 49-year-old female social worker presented with stress, anxiety, dizziness and irregular menses. The patient reported occasional irritability, hot flashes, night sweats and painful menses. Dry eyes and muscle cramps were also present. The patient was diagnosed with Kidney and Liver yin deficiency with Liver qi stagnation. With *Balance (Heat)* and *Calm (ES)*, the patient experienced a reduction of hot flashes and had less irritability, stress, anxiety and dizziness. She also stated that she slept much better and that her menses were not as painful. The practitioner concluded that the combination of *Balance (Heat)* and *Calm (ES)* was quite effective in treating the patient's condition.

D.W., Raton, New Mexico

M.M., a 41-year-old female, presented with "adrenaline-rush" sensations, characterized by heat flushes to her face, associated with mood swings and anxiety. Her tongue was red and purple, and her face was red. The Western diagnosis was stress-related anxiety attack; the TCM diagnosis was Liver stagnation and yin deficiency. After beginning herbal therapy with *Calm,* two capsules three times daily, and *Balance (Heat),* two capsules, three times daily, the patient stated that her affect and personality became calmer. Furthermore, she reported "feeling good," with increased energy levels and sound sleep.

C.L., Chino Hills, California

J.D., a 48-year-old post-menopausal female, complained of severe hot flashes. She stated that even during cooler temperatures at night, she needed to cool down by constantly using a hand-held battery-operated fan directed at her face. However, she did not complain of insomnia, mood swings, or palpitations. She confessed that, as a nurse, she was leery of trying herbal treatment. However, she had already tried hormone replacement therapy and OTC supplements with no success, and finally decided to try herbs. *Balance (Heat)* was prescribed, at three capsules, three times daily. During a follow-up visit two weeks later, the patient stated that the hot flashes were completely resolved.

C.L., Chino Hills, California

BALANCE (Heat) ™

A 51-year-old female nuclear medicine technician presented with hot flashes, night sweats and insomnia. The practitioner diagnosed her with Kidney yin and Heart yin deficiency with deficiency heat signs. Before the patient's treatment, she had irregular periods for 1½ year. During treatment, no periods occurred for 6 months. The practitioner had tried *Liu Wei Di Huang Wan* (Rehmannia Six Formula) with minimal results. Next, she tried *Zhi Bai Di Huang Wan* (Anemarrhena Phellodendron and Rehmannia Formula) and the hot flashes were reduced from 10-12 episodes to 4 episodes per day. The practitioner then switched to *Balance (Heat)* at 6 capsules twice a day. Within 1 week the hot flashes and night sweats were gone. *Tian Wan Bu Xin Dan* (Ginseng and Zizyphus Formula) was also supplemented, which in turn helped her to sleep better. *Balance (Heat)* proved to be very effective for clearing heat.

R.M., San Rafael, California

A 50-year-old female interior designer presented with peri-menopausal symptoms of hot flashes, night sweats, insomnia, and emotional fragility. The patient still had residual hot flashes despite correct dosing with hormone replacement therapy. With this clinical picture, the practitioner diagnosed this case as yin deficiency with deficiency heat. *Balance (Heat)* was prescribed at 3 capsules in the afternoon and 3 capsules before bedtime. Abatement of all residual heat symptoms occurred within one day. The practitioner found that *Balance (Heat)* was an excellent augment to the hormone replacement therapy.

C.W., San Diego, California

---

[1] Bensky, D. et al. *Chinese Herbal Medicine Formulas & Strategies*. Eastland Press. 1990
[2] Yeung, HC. *Handbook of Chinese Herbal Formulas*. Institute of Chinese Medicine. 1996
[3] Bensky, D. et al. *Chinese Herbal Medicine Materia Medica*. Eastland Press. 1993
[4] Bradley, P. (ed). British Herbal Compendium Vol. 1. Dorset, England: British Herbal Medicine Association. 1992
[5] Newall, CA. L.A. Anderson and J.D. Phillipson. *Herbal Medicines: A Guide for Health-care Professionals*. London: The Pharmaceutical Press. 1996
[6] Snow, JM. Monograph – Glycyrrhiza glabra L. (Leguminaceae). *The Protocol Journal of Botanical Medicine* Vol. 1, No.3. 1996
[7] Li, Kao Guo. et al. Effectiveness of artemisia (qing hao) in reducing fever. *Chinese Herbology*. 6:16. 1985
[8] Zhu, CH. Effectiveness of artemisia (qing hao) as injectables in reducing fever. *Hubei Journal of Traditional Chinese Medicine*. 2:17. 1983

FORMULAS

BLOSSOM ™

INTRODUCTION

Infertility is defined as failure to become pregnant after one or more years of regular sexual activity conducted during the time of ovulation. Infertility afflicts over 6 million American couples, of which approximately 40% is attributed to male and 60% to female partners.

For females, there are many reasons that contribute to infertility, including but not limited to ovulatory failure or defect, blocked fallopian tubes, endometriosis, uterine fibroids, polyps, pelvic adhesions, pelvic inflammatory diseases, chlamydia, hormonal imbalance, age (especially over 34 years of age), and psychological issues. Often, more than one cause contributes to infertility.

According to traditional Chinese medicine, treatment of female infertility must focus on regulation of the menses. Essential keys in becoming pregnant include a healthy menstrual cycle along with strong Kidney qi, an abundance of blood in the *chong* (thoroughfare) channel, and an unblocked *ren* (conception) channel.

The four principles of treatment for infertility are as follow:

- Phase 1 - Menstrual Phase (the week of menstruation): In this phase, it is important to regulate the menses and ensure proper shedding of the uterine lining. Qi and blood moving herbs are utilized to achieve this effect to clear and prevent any stagnation in the lower *jiao*.
- Phase 2 - Follicular Phase (the week following the last day of menstruation): During this phase, the key strategy is to tonify the Kidney yin, *jing* (essence) and blood, which are depleted during the period. This stage is essential in fortifying the body to ensure healthy conception.
- Phase 3 - Ovulatory Phase (week of ovulation): The primary treatment plan during the ovulatory phase is to help the eggs mature and to promote ovulation. Kidney yang tonic herbs have the effect to enhance the surge of luteinizing hormone (LH), which then stimulates ovulation. Herbs should be taken 3 days before and 3 days after ovulation.
- Phase 4 - Luteal Phase (the week before the onset of the menstruation): The focus during this phase is to regulate Liver qi and treat any possible premenstrual syndrome (PMS) and ensure proper flow of qi and blood in the Liver, *chong* (thoroughfare) and *ren* (conception) channels. When patients are more relaxed and at ease throughout the month, conception will more likely happen.

Herbal formulas designed for each phase:

Phase	Phase 1 - Menstrual Phase	Phase 2 - Follicular Phase	Phase 3 - Ovulatory Phase	Phase 4 - Luteal Phase
Primary formula (4-6 caps TID)	*Blossom (Phase 1)*	*Blossom (Phase 2)*	*Blossom (Phase 3)*	*Blossom (Phase 4)*
Supplementary formula (2-4 caps TID)	Supplementary Formula (throughout the entire month)			

Note: Specific information regarding each of the four primary formulas is listed in the following sections.

When treating infertility, ***Blossom (Phase 1-4)*** should be used as the primary formulas. A primary formula should be selected based on the corresponding phase of menstruation. When the phase changes, the primary formula should be changed as well. In addition, a supplementary formula may be necessary to treat the underlying imbalance if there is any. For example, if the patient suffers from infertility caused by fibroids, ***Resolve (Lower)***, a supplementary formula should be added throughout the month while taking ***Blossom (Phase 1-4)*** during the appropriate phases. The patient should be on 4 to 6 capsules of the primary formula and 2 to 4 capsules of the supplementary formula three times daily throughout the month. Only by treating the root cause of infertility in addition to regulating the hormones and menses can the patient achieve the best clinical result and become pregnant. Use of primary and supplementary formulas together will treat both the cause and symptoms, and enhance the overall efficacy. If there is unexplained infertility or there is no other significant underlying cause to the infertility, simply following the four formulas for each phase will be sufficient.

One course of treatment is three months. Efficacy can be seen ranging from one to three courses [3 to 9 months] of treatments. The couple should not try to conceive the first two months of herbal treatment. They should be patient, and be psychologically prepared to not expect results prematurely. Because there is only one window of chance of becoming pregnant each month, patients are advised to wait and give the herbs enough time to regulate the hormones, nourish the *jing* (essence) and bring the body to balance. Patients should be advised not feel so anxious, nervous, depressed or worried as these are contributors to qi stagnation and may lessen the chances of becoming pregnant. Advise patients that proper pre-conception care by taking herbs will enable the body to be at its optimal health, and is extremely important to ensure a healthy conception and course of pregnancy.

Use of these four fertility formulas will strengthen the underlying condition, regulate menstruation, balance hormones and significantly improve the probability of a successful pregnancy. These four formulas can be used for patients who suffer from habitual miscarriage, support patients who opt for IVF treatment or simply experience infertility for unknown reasons.

Note: Additional information, such as Supplementary Formulas, Nutrition, Lifestyle Instructions, and Clinical Notes, are listed after the text of *Blossom (Phase 1-4)*.

BLOSSOM (Phase 1) ™

CLINICAL APPLICATIONS

☙ Female infertility - **menstrual phase formula**

WESTERN THERAPEUTIC ACTIONS

☙ Regulates menstruation and treats related complications
☙ Relieves pain, reduces inflammation, and eliminates water accumulation

CHINESE THERAPEUTIC ACTIONS

☙ Invigorates blood and relieves pain
☙ Regulates the *chong* (thoroughfare) and *ren* (conception) channels
☙ Regulates menstruation

DOSAGE

Take 4 to 6 capsules three times daily on an empty stomach. Discontinue use when the patient becomes pregnant.

INGREDIENTS

Bai Shao (Radix Paeoniae Alba)
Chi Shao (Radix Paeoniae Rubrae)
Chong Wei Zi (Semen Leonuri)
Chuan Xiong (Rhizoma Ligustici Chuanxiong)

Dang Gui (Radicis Angelicae Sinensis)
Fu Ling (Poria)
Xiang Fu (Rhizoma Cyperi)
Ze Lan (Herba Lycopi)

FORMULA EXPLANATION

Blossom (Phase 1) is to be used during Phase 1 - menstrual phase, the week of menstruation. This formula contains herbs that are mild yet effective to regulate the menstrual flow and promote healthy shedding of endometrial tissue. *Dang Gui* (Radicis Angelicae Sinensis) tonifies and moves blood. *Chong Wei Zi* (Semen Leonuri) promotes blood circulation, regulates menstruation. When combined with *Dang Gui* (Radicis Angelicae Sinensis), they treat various types of gynecological disorders ranging from irregular menstruation, dysmenorrhea, and amenorrhea to postpartum abdominal pain. *Ze Lan* (Herba Lycopi) moves blood to dispel clots. It also works with *Fu Ling* (Poria) to reduce water retention and edema associated with menstruation. *Chi Shao* (Radix Paeoniae Rubrae) and *Chuan Xiong* (Rhizoma Ligustici Chuanxiong) also treat a wide variety of gynecological disorders by relieving pain. *Xiang Fu* (Rhizoma Cyperi) enters the Liver and regulates qi to relieve bloating and emotional imbalances during the menstrual period. *Bai Shao* (Radix Paeoniae Alba) nourishes blood, softens the Liver and has an antispasmodic effect to relax the uterus and relieve pain.

In summary, this formula moves qi and blood to regulate the menses and ensure proper shedding of the uterine lining during the menstrual phase.

NUTRITION

☙ During this stage, it is especially important to not eat foods that are cold (sushi, uncooked vegetables, salad, tomatoes, watermelon, cucumbers, wintermelon, strawberries, tofu, crabs, bananas, pear, soy milk, kiwi, ice cream, cold beverages) or sour (all citrus) in nature. They create stagnation and cause pain.

LIFESTYLE INSTRUCTION

- During menstruation, avoid sports that may expose the body to the cold environment, such as skiing or cold-water sports.
- Wear clothing that promotes warmth in cold weather, and covers the abdomen and low back.

CAUTIONS

- This formula should be discontinued when the patient becomes pregnant.
- This formula may cause more bleeding in some patients. In cases where there is excessive bleeding, reduce the dosage to half or discontinue its use temporarily.
- *Dang Gui* (Radicis Angelicae Sinensis) may enhance the overall effectiveness of Coumadin (Warfarin), an anticoagulant drug. Patients who take anticoagulant or antiplatelet medications should ***not*** take this herbal formula without supervision by a licensed health care practitioner.

ACUPUNCTURE POINTS

Traditional Points:
- *Guanyuan* (CV 4), *Qihai* (CV 6), *Sanyinjiao* (SP 6), *Zusanli* (ST 36), *Shenshu* (BL 23), *Taixi* (KI 3), *Taichong* (LR 3), *Neiguan* (PC 6)

Balance Method by Dr. Richard Tan:
- Left side: *Hegu* (LI 4), *Lingku*, *Yinlingquan* (SP 9), *Lougu* (SP 7), and *Sanyinjiao* (SP 6).
- Right side: *Neiguan* (PC 6), *Lieque* (LU 7), *Tongli* (HT 5), *Zusanli* (ST 36), and *Fenglong* (ST 40).
- Alternate sides from treatment to treatment.
- Note: *Lingku* is one of Master Tong's points. *Lingku* is located in the depression just distal to the junction of the first and second metacarpal bones, approximately 0.5 *cun* proximal to *Hegu* (LI 4), on the *yangming* line.
- For additional information on the Balance Method, please refer to *Twelve and Twelve in Acupuncture* and *Twenty-Four More in Acupuncture* by Dr. Richard Tan.

MODERN RESEARCH

Blossom (Phase 1) is the first of four formulas to treat infertility. It is formulated with herbs that have marked influence to regulate the menstruation. According to several studies, administration of *Dang Gui* (Radicis Angelicae Sinensis) is associated with both stimulating and inhibiting effects on the uterus, thereby exhibiting an overall regulatory effect on menstruation.[1] Furthermore, use of *Dang Gui* (Radicis Angelicae Sinensis) in essential oil form was effective in relieving menstrual pain with a 76.79% rate of effectiveness among 112 patients.[2] The mechanism of this action is attributed in part to the analgesic and anti-inflammatory effect of the herb, which has been cited to be similar or stronger than acetylsalicylic acid.[3]

In addition to *Dang Gui* (Radicis Angelicae Sinensis), many other herbs are used in this formula to treat menstruation-related symptoms. For example, *Xiang Fu* (Rhizoma Cyperi) has an inhibitory effect on the uterus to relax the muscles and relieve pain.[4] *Bai Shao* (Radix Paeoniae Alba) and *Chi Shao* (Radix Paeoniae Rubrae) have an antispasmodic effects to alleviate spasms and cramps.[5,6] *Xiang Fu* (Rhizoma Cyperi) and *Bai Shao* (Radix Paeoniae Alba) have analgesic effects to effectively relieve pain.[7,8] *Chi Shao* (Radix Paeoniae Rubrae) and *Chuan Xiong* (Rhizoma Ligustici Chuanxiong) have antiplatelet effects to reduce clotting and pain.[9,10] *Chuan Xiong* (Rhizoma Ligustici Chuanxiong) and *Xiang Fu* (Rhizoma Cyperi) have sedative effects to relieve stress, anxiety and general discomfort.[11,12] Lastly, *Fu Ling* (Poria) has diuretic effects, and is helpful to reduce water accumulation and treat edema.[13,14] In summary, ***Blossom (Phase 1)*** is an excellent formula for Phase 1 - menstrual phase. It contains herbs to regulate menstruation and treat related complications.

FORMULAS

[1] *Zhong Yao Xue* (Chinese Herbology), 1998; 815:823

[2] *Lan Zhou Yi Xue Yuan Xue Bao* (Journal of Lanzhou University of Medicine), 1988; 1:36

[3] *Yao Xue Za Zhi* (Journal of Medicinals), 1971; (91):1098

[4] *Zhong Hua Yi Xue Za Zhi* (Chinese Journal of Medicine), 1935; 12:1351

[5] *Zhong Cheng Yao Yan Jiu* (Research of Chinese Patent Medicine), 1980; 1:32

[6] *Zhong Yi Za Zhi* (Journal of Chinese Medicine), 1985; 6:50

[7] *Gui Yang Yi Xue Yuan Xue Bao* (Journal of Guiyang Medical University), 1959;113

[8] *Shang Hai Zhong Yi Yao Za Zhi* (Shanghai Journal of Chinese Medicine and Herbology), 1983; 4:14

[9] *Zhong Xi Yi Jie He Za Zhi* (Journal of Integrated Chinese and Western Medicine), 1984; 4(12):745

[10] *Hua Xi Yi Xue Za Zhi* (Huaxi Medical Journal), 1993; 8(3):170

[11] *Zhong Yao Yao Li Yu Ying Yong* (Pharmacology and Applications of Chinese Herbs), 1983;123

[12] *Zhong Guo Yao Ke Da Xue Xue Bao* (Journal of University of Chinese Herbology), 1989; 20(1):48

[13] *Chang Yong Zhong Yao Cheng Fen Yu Yao Li Shou Ce* (A Handbook of the Composition and Pharmacology of Common Chinese Drugs), 1994; 1383:1391

[14] *Shang Hai Zhong Yi Yao Za Zhi* (Shanghai Journal of Chinese Medicine and Herbology), 1986; 8:25

BLOSSOM (Phase 2) ™

CLINICAL APPLICATIONS

❂ Female infertility - **follicular phase formula**

WESTERN THERAPEUTIC ACTIONS

❂ Regulatory effect to promote normal menstruation
❂ Hematopoietic effect to promote the production of white and red blood cells
❂ Adaptogenic effect to address emotional and physical stress associated with menstruation

CHINESE THERAPEUTIC ACTIONS

❂ Nourishes blood
❂ Tonifies Kidney yin
❂ Replenishes Kidney *jing* (essence)

DOSAGE

Take 4 to 6 capsules three times daily on an empty stomach. Discontinue use when the patient becomes pregnant.

INGREDIENTS

Bai Zhu (Rhizoma Atractylodis Macrocephalae)
Chong Wei Zi (Semen Leonuri)
Chuan Xiong (Rhizoma Ligustici Chuanxiong)
Dang Gui (Radicis Angelicae Sinensis)
E Jiao (Colla Corii Asini)
Fu Ling (Poria)
Gou Qi Zi (Fructus Lycii)
Huai Niu Xi (Radix Achyranthis Bidentatae)
Lu Jiao Shuang (Cornu Cervi Degelatinatium)

Mu Dan Pi (Cortex Moutan)
Nu Zhen Zi (Fructus Ligustri Lucidi)
Shan Yao (Rhizoma Dioscoreae)
Shan Zhu Yu (Fructus Corni)
Shu Di Huang (Radix Rehmanniae Preparata)
Tu Si Zi (Semen Cuscutae)
Wu Wei Zi (Fructus Schisandrae Chinensis)
Ze Xie (Rhizoma Alismatis)

FORMULA EXPLANATION

Blossom (Phase 2) is designed to be used during Phase 2 - follicular phase, the week after finishing menstruation. This formula is formulated with herbs that tonify blood, nourish yin, and replenish *jing* (essence). Mild qi- and blood-moving herbs are also used to prevent stagnation as a result of the rich tonics.

In this formula, *Dang Gui* (Radicis Angelicae Sinensis), *Shu Di Huang* (Radix Rehmanniae Preparata) and *E Jiao* (Colla Corii Asini) are among the most effective blood-tonifying herbs to replenish what was lost through menstruation. *Bai Zhu* (Rhizoma Atractylodis Macrocephalae), *Fu Ling* (Poria) and *Shan Yao* (Rhizoma Dioscoreae) are used to strengthen the Spleen. A healthy Spleen is essential in the production of blood and extraction of post-natal qi from food. *Shan Zhu Yu* (Fructus Corni), *Nu Zhen Zi* (Fructus Ligustri Lucidi) and *Gou Qi Zi* (Fructus Lycii) nourish the Kidney yin and *jing* (essence). *Tu Si Zi* (Semen Cuscutae) and *Lu Jiao Shuang* (Cornu Cervi Degelatinatium) are two mild yang-tonic herbs to support the Kidney yang. Without yang tonics, yin tonics cannot achieve their maximum effect. *Wu Wei Zi* (Fructus Schisandrae Chinensis) is an astringent herb added to consolidate, bind and prevent the leakage of *jing* (essence). *Ze Xie* (Rhizoma Alismatis) is used to offset the stagnating nature of *Shu Di Huang* (Radix Rehmanniae Preparata). *Chuan Xiong* (Rhizoma Ligustici Chuanxiong), *Mu Dan Pi* (Cortex Moutan) and *Chong Wei Zi* (Semen Leonuri) are mild blood-moving herbs used to ensure that the tonics do not become stagnant. Finally, *Huai Niu Xi* (Radix Achyranthis Bidentatae) guides the effect of the herbs to the lower *jiao*, namely the Kidney.

In summary, this formula successfully tonifies the body to ensure healthy conception by using herbs that supplement the Kidney yin, *jing* (essence) and blood.

CAUTIONS

❧ This formula should be discontinued when the patient becomes pregnant.

❧ *Dang Gui* (Radicis Angelicae Sinensis) may enhance the overall effectiveness of Coumadin (Warfarin), an anticoagulant drug. Patients who take anticoagulant or antiplatelet medications should **not** take this herbal formula without supervision by a licensed health care practitioner.

ACUPUNCTURE POINTS

Traditional Points:

❧ *Guanyuan* (CV 4), *Qihai* (CV 6), *Sanyinjiao* (SP 6), *Zusanli* (ST 36), *Shenshu* (BL 23), *Taixi* (KI 3), *Taichong* (LR 3), and *Neiguan* (PC 6).

Balance Method by Dr. Richard Tan:

❧ Left side: *Hegu* (LI 4), *Lingku*, *Yinlingquan* (SP 9), *Lougu* (SP 7), and *Sanyinjiao* (SP 6).

❧ Right side: *Neiguan* (PC 6), *Lieque* (LU 7), *Tongli* (HT 5), *Zusanli* (ST 36), and *Fenglong* (ST 40).

❧ Alternate sides from treatment to treatment.

❧ Note: *Lingku* is one of Master Tong's points. *Lingku* is located in the depression just distal to the junction of the first and second metacarpal bones, approximately 0.5 *cun* proximal to *Hegu* (LI 4), on the *yangming* line.

❧ For additional information on the Balance Method, please refer to *Twelve and Twelve in Acupuncture* and *Twenty-Four More in Acupuncture* by Dr. Richard Tan.

MODERN RESEARCH

Blossom (Phase 2) is formulated with herbs that have marked influence to facilitate and restore normal health and well being after menstruation. This formula contains herbs with regulatory effects to promote normal menstruation, hematological effects to promote the production of white and red blood cells, and adaptogenic effects to address mental and physical stresses associated with menstruation.

According to several studies, administration of *Dang Gui* (Radicis Angelicae Sinensis) is associated with both stimulating and inhibiting effects on the uterus, thereby exhibiting an overall regulatory effect on menstruation.[1] Because of this regulatory effect, *Dang Gui* (Radicis Angelicae Sinensis) is beneficial and can be used before, during and after menstruation.

Since most women have pronounced weakness and deficiencies after their menstruation during the follicular phase, many herbs in this formula promote the production of the various types of blood cells. According to one study, *Gou Qi Zi* (Fructus Lycii) has a marked hematopoietic effect to increase the production of red blood cells and white blood cells.[2] According to another study, administration of *E Jiao* (Colla Corii Asini) is associated with marked hematopoietic effect to increase the production of red blood cells and white blood cells,[3] and its use has been shown to effectively treat leukopenia and anemia.[4] Furthermore, *Bai Zhu* (Rhizoma Atractylodis Macrocephalae) has an immunostimulant effect by increasing the activity of macrophages and the reticuloendothelial system, and it also increases the number of white blood cells, lymphocytes, and IgG.[5,6] *Wu Wei Zi* (Fructus Schisandrae Chinensis) has an immunostimulant effect to heighten non-specific immunity.[7] Lastly, *Gou Qi Zi* (Fructus Lycii) has an immunostimulant effect to increase non-specific immunity and the phagocytic activity of macrophages and the total number of T cells.[8]

As stated above, this formula contains herbs with an adaptogenic effect to help the body cope with mental and physical stress during and after menstruation. Examples of herbs with such effects include *Bai Zhu* (Rhizoma Atractylodis Macrocephalae) and *Tu Si Zi* (Semen Cuscutae).[9,10] In addition, *Shan Yao* (Rhizoma Dioscoreae) has a stimulating effect on the gastrointestinal tract to promote normal digestion and absorption of nutrients.[11] *Chuan Xiong* (Rhizoma Ligustici Chuanxiong) and *Mu Dan Pi* (Cortex Moutan) stimulate blood circulation and promote delivery of oxygen and essential nutrients to various parts of the body.[12,13] *Wu Wei Zi* (Fructus Schisandrae Chinensis) stimulates the central nervous system and increases mental alertness, improves work efficiency, and quickens reflexes.[14] *Fu Ling* (Poria) and *Ze Xie* (Rhizoma Alismatis) have diuretic effects, drain water, and treat edema frequently associated with menstruation.[15,16]

In conclusion, ***Blossom (Phase 2)*** is an excellent formula to facilitate and restore normal health and well being after menstruation. This formula contains herbs with regulatory effects to promote normal menstruation, hematopoietic effects to promote the production of white and red blood cells, and adaptogenic effects to address mental and physical stresses associated with menstruation.

---

[1] *Zhong Yao Xue* (Chinese Herbology), 1998; 815:823
[2] *Zhong Yao Xue* (Chinese Herbology), 1998; 860:862
[3] *Zhong Cheng Yao Yan Jiu* (Research of Chinese Patent Medicine), 1981; (5):31
[4] *Shan Dong Yi Yao Gong Ye* (Shandong Pharmaceutical Industry), 1986; 3:21
[5] *Jun Shi Yi Xue Jian Xun* (Military Medicine Notes), 1977; 2:5
[6] *Xin Yi Yao Xue Za Zhi* (New Journal of Medicine and Herbology), 1979; 6:60
[7] *Zhong Yao Xue* (Chinese Herbology), 1998; 878:881
[8] *Zhong Cao Yao* (Chinese Herbal Medicine), 19(7):25
[9] *Xin Yi Yao Xue Za Zhi* (New Journal of Medicine and Herbology), 1974; 8:13
[10] *Chang Yong Zhong Yao Cheng Fen Yu Yao Li Shou Ce* (A Handbook of the Composition and Pharmacology of Common Chinese Drugs), 1994; 1563:1564
[11] *Zhi Wu Zi Yuan Yu Huan Jing* (Source and Environment of Plants), 1992; 1(2):10
[12] *Zhong Yao Xue* (Chinese Herbology), 1989; 535:539
[13] *Guo Wai Yi Xue Zhong Yi Zhong Yao Fen Ce* (Monograph of Chinese Herbology from Foreign Medicine), 1983; (3):5,1984;(5):54
[14] *Zhong Yao Xue* (Chinese Herbology), 1998; 878:881
[15] *Sheng Yao Xue Za Zhi* (Journal of Raw Herbology), 1982; 36(2):150
[16] *Chang Yong Zhong Yao Cheng Fen Yu Yao Li Shou Ce* (A Handbook of the Composition and Pharmacology of Common Chinese Drugs), 1994; 1383:1391

FORMULAS

CLINICAL APPLICATIONS

❧ Female infertility - **ovulatory phase formula**

WESTERN THERAPEUTIC ACTIONS

❧ Regulatory effect to promote normal menstruation
❧ Regulatory effect on the endocrine system to promote production and secretion of hormones

CHINESE THERAPEUTIC ACTIONS

❧ Tonifies Kidney yang
❧ Replenishes Kidney *jing* (essence)
❧ Mildly moves blood in the lower *jiao*

DOSAGE

Take 4 to 6 capsules three times daily on an empty stomach. Patient should be on the herbs 3 days before and after ovulation. Discontinue use when the patient becomes pregnant.

INGREDIENTS

Ba Ji Tian (Radix Morindae Officinalis)
Bai Shao (Radix Paeoniae Alba)
Dang Gui (Radicis Angelicae Sinensis)
Gou Qi Zi (Fructus Lycii)
Lu Jiao Shuang (Cornu Cervi Degelatinatium)
Shan Zhu Yu (Fructus Corni)
Shu Di Huang (Radix Rehmanniae Preparata)

Suo Yang (Herba Cynomorii)
Tu Si Zi (Semen Cuscutae)
Xiao Hui Xiang (Fructus Foeniculi)
Xu Duan (Radix Dipsaci)
Yi Mu Cao (Herba Leonuri)
Yin Yang Huo (Herba Epimedii)

FORMULA EXPLANATION

Blossom (Phase 3) is developed specifically for Phase 3 - ovulatory phase, during the week of ovulation. The ovulatory stage is when Kidney yin is turning into yang and ovulation occurs with a peak in temperature. The primary treatment strategy is to help the eggs mature and promote ovulation. Kidney yang tonic herbs have the effect to enhance the surge of luteinizing hormone (LH), which then stimulates ovulation. To facilitate ovulation, mild blood-moving herbs are also added.

Suo Yang (Herba Cynomorii) is traditionally used for infertility, low libido, lack of Kidney *jing* (essence) and other Kidney yang deficiency conditions. It is used here with *Yin Yang Huo* (Herba Epimedii), *Lu Jiao Shuang* (Cornu Cervi Degelatinatium), *Xu Duan* (Radix Dipsaci) and *Ba Ji Tian* (Radix Morindae Officinalis) to boost the yang and promote ovulation. *Tu Si Zi* (Semen Cuscutae) tonifies both Kidney yin and yang and is an essential herb for treating infertility. *Xiao Hui Xiang* (Fructus Foeniculi) warms the Kidney and the womb in preparation for pregnancy. *Shu Di Huang* (Radix Rehmanniae Preparata), *Gou Qi Zi* (Fructus Lycii), *Bai Shao* (Radix Paeoniae Alba) and *Shan Zhu Yu* (Fructus Corni) support Kidney yin for two purposes: First, to enhance the effects of the yang tonics, as both Kidney yin and yang should always be tonified together for maximum effect; second, to prevent the yang tonics from creating deficiency Kidney fire. Yang tonics as described above promote the release of the egg. *Dang Gui* (Radicis Angelicae Sinensis) tonifies blood and *Yi Mu Cao* (Herba Leonuri) moves the blood, which increases blood supply to the ovaries to induce the contraction of the muscles pulling the ovaries closer to the fallopian tubes, thus facilitating the movement of the egg into the fallopian tube.

NUTRITION

- During the ovulatory phase, patients are advised to eat more lamb, which increases warmth of the body.

CAUTIONS

- This formula should be discontinued when the patient becomes pregnant.
- *Dang Gui* (Radicis Angelicae Sinensis) may enhance the overall effectiveness of Coumadin (Warfarin), an anticoagulant drug. Patients who take anticoagulant or antiplatelet medications should ***not*** take this herbal formula without supervision by a licensed health care practitioner.

ACUPUNCTURE POINTS

Traditional Points:
- *Guanyuan* (CV 4), *Qihai* (CV 6), *Sanyinjiao* (SP 6), *Zusanli* (ST 36), *Shenshu* (BL 23), *Taixi* (KI 3), *Taichong* (LR 3), and *Neiguan* (PC 6).

Balance Method by Dr. Richard Tan:
- Left side: *Hegu* (LI 4), *Lingku*, *Yinlingquan* (SP 9), *Lougu* (SP 7), and *Sanyinjiao* (SP 6).
- Right side: *Neiguan* (PC 6), *Lieque* (LU 7), *Tongli* (HT 5), *Zusanli* (ST 36), and *Fenglong* (ST 40).
- Alternate sides from treatment to treatment.
- Note: *Lingku* is one of Master Tong's points. *Lingku* is located in the depression just distal to the junction of the first and second metacarpal bones, approximately 0.5 *cun* proximal to *Hegu* (LI 4), on the *yangming* line.
- For additional information on the Balance Method, please refer to *Twelve and Twelve in Acupuncture* and *Twenty-Four More in Acupuncture* by Dr. Richard Tan.

MODERN RESEARCH

Blossom (Phase 3) is developed for Phase 3 - Ovulatory Phase, during the week of ovulation. To ensure proper maturation of eggs and subsequent ovulation, this formula uses herbs with a regulatory effect on the endocrine system to promote normal menstruation and the production and secretion of hormones.

According to several studies, administration of *Dang Gui* (Radicis Angelicae Sinensis) is associated with both stimulating and inhibiting effects on the uterus, thereby exhibiting an overall regulatory effect on menstruation.[1] Because of this regulatory effect, *Dang Gui* (Radicis Angelicae Sinensis) is beneficial and can be used before, during and after menstruation.

To regulate ovulation, *Blossom (Phase 3)* uses many herbs with marked endocrinological effects, to promote the production and secretion of various hormones. For example, use of *Shu Di Huang* (Radix Rehmanniae Preparata) is associated with marked stimulating effect on the endocrine system, with the mechanism of action attributed to inhibiting negative feedback signals to the pituitary gland.[2] According to another study, administration of *Ba Ji Tian* (Radix Morindae Officinalis) also has a stimulant effect on the endocrine system and increases the production and release of hormones.[3] Most importantly, use of *Yin Yang Huo* (Herba Epimedii) has a stimulant effect on the endocrine system by increasing the production and secretion of endogenous hormones such as corticosterone, cortisol, and testosterone.[4] Lastly, this formula uses many herbs to facilitate and enhance the overall effect of therapy. *Gou Qi Zi* (Fructus Lycii) and *Yi Mu Cao* (Herba Leonuri) both have stimulating effects on the reproductive organs, namely the uterus, to prepare for conception.[5,6]

In summary, this is an excellent formula specifically designed for women in Phase 3 – ovulatory phase of the menstrual cycle. It contains herbs that regulate menstruation, promote the production and secretion of hormones, and prepare the uterus for conception.

FORMULAS

[1] *Zhong Yao Xue* (Chinese Herbology), 1998; 815:823
[2] *Zhong Yao Xue* (Chinese Herbology), 1998; 156:158
[3] *Guo Wai Yi Xue Zhong Yi Zhong Yao Fen Ce* (Monograph of Chinese Herbology from Foreign Medicine), 1990; 12(6):48
[4] *Zhong Xi Yi Jie He Za Zhi* (Journal of Integrated Chinese and Western Medicine), 1989; 9(12):737-8,710
[5] *Zhong Yao Xue* (Chinese Herbology), 1998; 860:862
[6] *Zhong Yao Yan Jiu* (Research of Chinese Herbology), 1979; 581

FORMULAS

CLINICAL APPLICATIONS

⚚   Female infertility - **luteal phase formula**

WESTERN THERAPEUTIC ACTIONS

⚚   Regulates menstruation to relieve premenstrual syndrome (PMS)
⚚   Regulates menstruation to prepare for proper shedding of the uterine lining
⚚   Analgesic effect to relieve pain
⚚   Anti-inflammatory effect to relieve inflammation
⚚   Muscle-relaxant effect to relieve spasms and cramps.

CHINESE THERAPEUTIC ACTIONS

⚚   Moves Liver qi
⚚   Invigorates blood

DOSAGE

Take 4 to 6 capsules three times daily on an empty stomach. Discontinue use when the patient becomes pregnant.

INGREDIENTS

Bai Shao (Radix Paeoniae Alba)   *Gan Cao* (Radix Glycyrrhizae)
Bai Zhu (Rhizoma Atractylodis Macrocephalae)   *He Huan Pi* (Cortex Albiziae)
Chai Hu (Radix Bupleuri)   *Ju He* (Semen Citri Rubrum)
Chuan Niu Xi (Radix Cyathulae)   *Lu Lu Tong* (Fructus Liquidambaris)
Chuan Xiong (Rhizoma Ligustici Chuanxiong)   *Xiang Fu* (Rhizoma Cyperi)
Dang Gui (Radicis Angelicae Sinensis)   *Yi Mu Cao* (Herba Leonuri)
Fu Ling (Poria)   *Yu Jin* (Radix Curcumae)

FORMULA EXPLANATION

Blossom (Phase 4) is formulated specifically for Phase 4 - luteal phase, the week before the period. Regulating Liver qi is the most important treatment strategy during this stage. Liver qi stagnation is characterized by irregular menstruation, abdominal bloating, irritability, emotional instability, short temper and breast distension. This formula is designed to relieve premenstrual syndrome (PMS), release tension and stagnation, and prepare the uterus for proper shedding the following week.

In this formula, *Chai Hu* (Radix Bupleuri) and *Xiang Fu* (Rhizoma Cyperi) smooth the Liver qi and disperse qi stagnation. *He Huan Pi* (Cortex Albiziae) relieves Liver qi stagnation and reduces anxiety and irritability associated with PMS. *Dang Gui* (Radicis Angelicae Sinensis) tonifies blood and relieves pain. *Bai Shao* (Radix Paeoniae Alba) nourishes the blood to soften the Liver to relieve distention and pain. *Bai Zhu* (Rhizoma Atractylodis Macrocephalae) and *Fu Ling* (Poria) tonify the Spleen and dispel dampness to facilitate the transportation and transformation of nutrients. *Gan Cao* (Radix Glycyrrhizae) supplements qi and helps *Bai Shao* (Radix Paeoniae Alba) soften the Liver to relieve pain.

Yu Jin (Radix Curcumae), *Chuan Xiong* (Rhizoma Ligustici Chuanxiong), *Lu Lu Tong* (Fructus Liquidambaris) and *Yi Mu Cao* (Herba Leonuri) move blood and break blood stasis in the lower *jiao* to ensure proper shedding of the endometrial lining during the period. *Chuan Niu Xi* (Radix Cyathulae) and *Ju He* (Semen Citri Rubrum) are channel-guiding herbs that help direct the effect of the herbs to the lower *jiao*.

FORMULAS

BLOSSOM (Phase 4) ™

CAUTIONS

❧ This formula should be discontinued when the patient becomes pregnant.

❧ *Dang Gui* (Radicis Angelicae Sinensis) may enhance the overall effectiveness of Coumadin (Warfarin), an anticoagulant drug. Patients who take anticoagulant or antiplatelet medications should ***not*** take this herbal formula without supervision by a licensed health care practitioner.

ACUPUNCTURE POINTS

Traditional Points:

❧ *Guanyuan* (CV 4), *Qihai* (CV 6), *Sanyinjiao* (SP 6), *Zusanli* (ST 36), *Shenshu* (BL 23), *Taixi* (KI 3), *Taichong* (LR 3), and *Neiguan* (PC 6).

Balance Method by Dr. Richard Tan:

❧ Left side: *Hegu* (LI 4), *Lingku*, *Yinlingquan* (SP 9), *Lougu* (SP 7), and *Sanyinjiao* (SP 6).

❧ Right side: *Neiguan* (PC 6), *Lieque* (LU 7), *Tongli* (HT 5), *Zusanli* (ST 36), *Fenglong* (ST 40)

❧ Alternate sides from treatment to treatment.

❧ Note: *Lingku* is one of Master Tong's points. *Lingku* is located in the depression just distal to the junction of the first and second metacarpal bones, approximately 0.5 *cun* proximal to *Hegu* (LI 4), on the *yangming* line.

❧ For additional information on the Balance Method, please refer to *Twelve and Twelve in Acupuncture* and *Twenty-Four More in Acupuncture* by Dr. Richard Tan.

MODERN RESEARCH

Blossom (Phase 4) is formulated specifically for Phase 4 – luteal phase, the week before the period. This formula uses herbs to regulate menstruation to relieve premenstrual syndrome (PMS) and prepare for proper shedding. Furthermore, it incorporates additional herbs with an analgesic effects to relieve pain, anti-inflammatory effects to relieve inflammation, and spasmolytic effects to relieve spasms and cramps.

According to several studies, administration of *Dang Gui* (Radicis Angelicae Sinensis) is associated with both stimulating and inhibiting effects on the uterus, thereby exhibiting an overall regulatory effect on menstruation.[1] Furthermore, use of *Dang Gui* (Radicis Angelicae Sinensis) in essential oils form was effective in relieving menstrual pain with a 76.79% rate of effectiveness among 112 patients.[2] The mechanism of this action is attributed in part to the analgesic and anti-inflammatory effects of the herb, which has been cited to be similar to or stronger than acetylsalicylic acid.[3]

This formula contains many herbs to address premenstrual syndrome (PMS) with analgesic effects to relieve pain, anti-inflammatory effects to relieve inflammation, and muscle-relaxant effects to relieve spasms and cramps. Herbs with analgesic effect to relieve pain include *Xiang Fu* (Rhizoma Cyperi),[4] *Gan Cao* (Radix Glycyrrhizae),[5] *Chai Hu* (Radix Bupleuri),[6] and *Bai Shao* (Radix Paeoniae Alba).[7] Herbs with anti-inflammatory effects to reduce swelling and inflammation include *Gan Cao* (Radix Glycyrrhizae),[8] *Chai Hu* (Radix Bupleuri),[9] and *Bai Shao* (Radix Paeoniae Alba).[10] Lastly, herbs with muscle-relaxant effects to relieve spasms and cramps include *Bai Shao* (Radix Paeoniae Alba) and *Gan Cao* (Radix Glycyrrhizae).[11,12] In addition, *Fu Ling* (Poria) is added for its mild sedative effect to relieve the general pain and discomfort associated with PMS.[13] Lastly, *Yi Mu Cao* (Herba Leonuri) has been used specifically to treat irregular menstruation and hypermenorrhea.[14]

Furthermore, this formula uses many herbs to treat menstruation-related complications. For example, *Fu Ling* (Poria) and *Bai Zhu* (Rhizoma Atractylodis Macrocephalae) have diuretic effects, and are used to drain water accumulation and treat edema.[15,16,17] *Chuan Xiong* (Rhizoma Ligustici Chuanxiong), *Yi Mu Cao* (Herba Leonuri) and

Bai Zhu (Rhizoma Atractylodis Macrocephalae) have antiplatelet effects, and are used to prevent clotting and pain before and during menstruation.[18,19,20]

Lastly, *Yi Mu Cao* (Herba Leonuri) has a stimulating effect, while *Xiang Fu* (Rhizoma Cyperi) has an inhibiting effect, on the uterus. The regulatory effects of these two herbs ensure proper and smooth transition throughout changes in the menstrual cycle.[21,22]

In summary, this is a great formula to conclude the four phases of menstruation and promote fertility. It regulates menstruation to relieve premenstrual syndrome and prepare for proper shedding. Furthermore, it incorporates additional herbs with analgesic effect to relieve pain, anti-inflammatory effect to relieve inflammation, and muscle-relaxant effect to relieve spasms and cramps.

[1] *Zhong Yao Xue* (Chinese Herbology), 1998; 815:823
[2] *Lan Zhou Yi Xue Yuan Xue Bao* (Journal of Lanzhou University of Medicine), 1988; 1:36
[3] *Yao Xue Za Zhi* (Journal of Medicinals), 1971; (91):1098
[4] *Gui Yang Yi Xue Yuan Xue Bao* (Journal of Guiyang Medical University), 1959; 113
[5] *Zhong Yao Xue* (Chinese Herbology), 1998; 759:765
[6] *Shen Yang Yi Xue Yuan Xue Bao* (Journal of Shenyang University of Medicine), 1984; 1(3):214
[7] *Shang Hai Zhong Yi Yao Za Zhi* (Shanghai Journal of Chinese Medicine and Herbology), 1983; 4:14
[8] *Zhong Cao Yao* (Chinese Herbal Medicine), 1991; 22(10):452
[9] *Zhong Yao Yao Li Yu Ying Yong* (Pharmacology and Applications of Chinese Herbs), 1983; 888
[10] *Zhong Yao Zhi* (Chinese Herbology Journal), 1993; 183
[11] *Zhong Yi Za Zhi* (Journal of Chinese Medicine), 1985; 6:50
[12] *Hu Nan Zhong Yi* (Hunan Journal of Traditional Chinese Medicine), 1989; 2:7
[13] *Zhong Yao Da Ci Dian* (Dictionary of Chinese Herbs), 1977; 1596
[14] *Zhong Hua Fu Chan Ke Za Zhi* (*Chinese Journal of OB/GYN*), 1958; 1:1
[15] *Chang Yong Zhong Yao Cheng Fen Yu Yao Li Shou Ce* (A Handbook of the Composition and Pharmacology of Common Chinese Drugs), 1994; 1383:1391
[16] *Shang Hai Zhong Yi Yao Za Zhi* (Shanghai Journal of Chinese Medicine and Herbology), 1986; 8:25
[17] *Zhong Hua Yi Xue Za Zhi* (Chinese Journal of Medicine), 1961; 47(1):7
[18] *Hua Xi Yi Xue Za Zhi* (Huaxi Medical Journal), 1993; 8(3):170
[19] *Zhong Xi Yi Jie He Za Zhi* (Journal of Integrated Chinese and Western Medicine), 1986; 6(1):39
Chang Yong Zhong Yao Cheng Fen Yu Yao Li Shou Ce (A Handbook of the Composition and Pharmacology of Common Chinese Drugs), 1994; 739:742[20]
[21] *Zhong Yao Yan Jiu* (Research of Chinese Herbology), 1979; 581
[22] *Zhong Hua Yi Xue Za Zhi* (Chinese Journal of Medicine), 1935; 12:1351

FORMULAS

SUPPLEMENTARY FORMULAS

Supplementary formulas are crucial to successful treatment of infertility. In addition to taking the primary formulas, *Blossom (Phase 1-4)* for the four corresponding phases, one or two [maximum] supplementary formula(s) should be added for optimal effect. The following are some recommendations. The patient should take 4 to 6 capsules of the primary formula and 2 to 4 capsules of the supplementary formula three times daily throughout the month.

- ❧ With Kidney yang deficiency manifesting as cold body and extremities, low libido, polyuria, hair loss, pale and cold appearance, and other cold symptoms, add *Kidney Tonic (Yang)*.
- ❧ With Kidney yin deficiency or women over 40 manifesting heat sensations, dryness, scanty menstruation, flushed cheeks, thin appearance, night sweats or dry mouth, add *Kidney Tonic (Yin)*.
- ❧ With dampness accumulation where the patient shows overweight tendency or phlegm accumulation with thick tongue coating, heaviness sensation, add *Herbal DRX*.
- ❧ With uterine fibroids, polycystic ovaries, endometriosis, fallopian tube blockage, tuberculosis of the fallopian tube, post-surgical adhesions or other stagnations, add *Resolve (Lower)*.
- ❧ With generalized tiredness and fatigue due to qi and blood deficiencies, add *Imperial Tonic*.
- ❧ With high levels of stress and Liver qi stagnation, add *Calm*.
- ❧ With chronic pelvic inflammatory disease, add *Herbal ABX* and *Resolve (Lower)*.
- ❧ With post-abortion, post-surgical, or chronic infection/inflammation causing infertility, add *Herbal ABX*.
- ❧ For Liver qi stagnation causing infertility in patients who have had abortions or miscarriages, add *Calm*.
- ❧ For infertility with coldness and blood stagnation, add *Menotrol*.
- ❧ With anemia or blood deficiency, add *Schizandra ZZZ*.
- ❧ For painful menstruation, add *Mense-Ease*.
- ❧ For male infertility, use *Vital Essence* instead.

NUTRITION

- ❧ According to Dr. Richard Tan's mirror concept, a diet high in small eggs such as fish eggs may be beneficial to women who suffer from infertility due to ovulatory or ovarian dysfunctions.
- ❧ Foods that are cold (sushi, uncooked vegetables, salad, tomatoes, watermelon, cucumbers, wintermelon, strawberries, tofu, crabs, bananas, pear, soybean milk, kiwi, ice cream, cold beverages) or sour (all citrus) in nature should be avoided one week before and during menstruation. Cold and sour foods create stagnation and cause pain.
- ❧ Eat more nuts and seeds in their diet.
- ❧ Avoid overly spicy and pungent food as they may cause excessive bleeding.
- ❧ Decrease processed food and increase organic food.
- ❧ Avoid alcohol, coffee and cigarette smoking.

LIFESTYLE INSTRUCTIONS

- ❧ Avoid sports that may expose the body to cold environments, such as skiing and all water sports.
- ❧ It is important to understand that the body is like a garden. No seed can properly sprout and grow without fertilized soil, water and sunshine. Taking these herbs to regulate the menses and fortify the body with these nutrients and *jing* (essence) are steps one must take to ensure a healthy pregnancy. Because there is only one window of opportunity to become pregnant each month, it is important to be patient and to give herbs enough time to regulate and bring the body back to balance. Do not feel so anxious, nervous, depressed or worried. Engage in yoga, meditation, *Tai Chi Chuan* or other activities that help them relax and focus on something else other than constantly thinking about trying to become pregnant.
- ❧ A positive attitude and low stress level can contribute greatly to a successful pregnancy. If taking a vacation will help, they should be advised to do so.

CLINICAL NOTES

❧ There are many causes of infertility according to western medicine, all with corresponding TCM diagnosis. For example, an inability to ovulate often indicates Kidney yang deficiency while tubal obstruction means qi and blood or phlegm stagnation. A specific diagnosis is necessary in selecting the right herbal formula for the patient.

❧ One course of treatment is three months. Efficacy range from one to three courses. The couple should not try excessively to become pregnant during the first month of herbal treatment. They should be psychologically prepared to not expect results too soon, and therefore relax the Liver qi. In such cases, the chances of becoming pregnant would be greater. Advise patients that proper pre-conception care enables the body to be at its optimal health and is extremely important to ensure healthy conception and course of pregnancy.

❧ In cases where the period is irregular and there is no clear distinction of the phases, treat the underlying cause first by using a supplementary formula. When a pattern establishes, use *Blossom (Phase 1-4)* accordingly.

❧ Women who were on oral contraceptives previously may not become pregnant as quickly as those who did not take any because the body needs a period of time to re-adjust and begin to secrete hormones regularly without the interference of contraceptives. Herbs will help speed up this process.

❧ Pelvic inflammatory disease (PID), usage of intrauterine devices (IUDs), ruptured appendix, lower abdominal surgery, and ectopic pregnancy can all be causative factors to tubal dysfunction. A hysterosalpingogram is taken as a definitive test for tubal dysfunction. *See* Supplementary Formulas section for the most appropriate formula to use.

1. PID includes endometritis, salpingitis, mucopurulent cervicitis, oophoritis and upper female genital tract infection. Transmitted sexually through gonococcal, chlamydial, or bacterial infection, acute PID may present with no symptoms and in many instances be barely discernible. Consequently, pathogenic factors infiltrate and cause damage within the endocervix, as well as weaken tubal integrity.

2. IUD complications include bleeding and pain as well as potential for a perforated uterus. The most common side effects of IUDs include cramping and irregular vaginal bleeding. Complications ensue if other extenuating pathogens are introduced into the endometrial cavity. The possibility of rupturing a tubo-ovarian abscess may also occur during insertion.

3. Pre- and post-surgical impediments also impair tubal patency. A thorough medical history should be taken, including past surgical procedures, especially of the lower abdominal region, for complete diagnostic assessment.

❧ Taking the formulas throughout the four phases also enhance the success rate of *in vitro* fertilization (IVF). *Blossom (Phase 1-4)* formulas have the following effects:

1. Tonify the Kidney to help the ovaries produce better-quality eggs.
2. Increase blood flow to the lower *jiao*/uterus and prepare the uterine lining for implantation.
3. Regulate Liver qi for relaxation.
4. Help consolidate the pregnancy, to decrease the chances of miscarriage.

❧ If it is unexplained infertility or there is no other significant underlying cause to the infertility, simply following the four formulas for each phase will be sufficient.

❧ Note: For male sexual and reproductive disorders, please refer to *Vitality* and *Vital Essence*.

CAUTIONS

❧ *Blossom (Phase 1-4)* should be discontinued when the patient becomes pregnant.

❧ Women who take these fertility formulas may experience more bleeding during their period, which is a normal response of the herbs.

❧ It is important to remember that these formulas are designed to treat infertility. They do not offer any protection against sexually transmitted diseases.

❧ Herbs are ineffective for infertility caused by immune dysfunction.

FORMULAS

SUMMARY

Infertility is a common disorder that may be due to a wide variety of causes. Before treatment, both partners should be examined, evaluated, and treated if necessary. Each course of treatment is three months, and efficacy can usually be seen within one to three courses. Continuous and persistent use of these four fertility formulas will regulate menstruation, balance hormones, and strengthen the underlying condition. Not only will they significantly improve the possibility of successful fertilization, they will also increase the probability of a smooth pregnancy with minimal complications.

PHARMACEUTICAL DRUGS & CHINESE MEDICINE: A COMPARATIVE ANALYSIS

Western Medical Approach: Female infertility is a complicated disorder that has numerous causes. In western medicine, those with physiological disorders, such as irregular or absence of ovulation, are usually treated with Clomid (Clomiphene). Though it induces ovulation, it causes side effects such as hot flashes, abdominal swelling, breast tenderness, nausea, vision disturbance, and headaches. Furthermore, those with physical disorders, such as problems with the fallopian tubes or cervix, are treated with physical intervention, such as surgery, intrauterine insemination, and *in vitro* fertilization. Though these methods are effective, they are more invasive, more expensive, and have more risks.

Traditional Chinese Medicine Approach: Female infertility is very complicated, and requires multiple treatment plans to ensure optimal success. Therefore, four formulas are used to address all possible causes of infertility. Together, they regulate menstruation, promote ovulation, nourish the body, and ensure optimal conditions for fertilization. This comprehensive method has been used with tremendous success throughout the history of traditional Chinese medicine.

Summation: Western and traditional Chinese medicine are both effective for female infertility. In general, herbal therapy is an excellent option for mild to severe cases of infertility, as it is very effective and has few or no side effects. However, if the women do not respond to herbal therapy, physical intervention may be considered as the last alternative.

FORMULAS

CA SUPPORT ™

CLINICAL APPLICATIONS

❂ Cancer patients who suffer extreme weakness and deficiency and cannot receive surgery or chemotherapy and radiation treatments
❂ Late stage, terminally-ill cancer patients with pain and suffering

WESTERN THERAPEUTIC ACTIONS

❂ Immunostimulant effect to increase white blood cells
❂ Hematopoietic effect to increase red blood cells
❂ Antineoplastic effect to suppress cancer cells

CHINESE THERAPEUTIC ACTIONS

❂ Clears heat
❂ Eliminates toxins
❂ Tonifies the underlying deficiencies (qi, blood, yin and yang)

DOSAGE

Take 3 to 4 capsules three times daily. It should be taken on an empty stomach with warm water for maximum effectiveness.

INGREDIENTS

Bai Hua She She Cao (Herba Oldenlandia)
Bai Zhu (Rhizoma Atractylodis Macrocephalae)
Ban Zhi Lian (Herba Scutellariae Barbatae)
Dong Chong Xia Cao (Cordyceps)
E Zhu (Rhizoma Curcumae)
Fu Ling (Poria)

Huang Jing (Rhizoma Polygonati)
Huang Qi (Radix Astragali)
Ji Xue Teng (Caulis Spatholobi)
Xi Yang Shen (Radix Panacis Quinquefolii)
Yi Yi Ren (Semen Coicis)
Zao Xiu (Rhizoma Paridis)

FORMULA EXPLANATION

CA Support is developed specifically for individuals who have extreme weakness and deficiency after prolonged battles with cancer and its treatments (chemotherapy and radiation). This condition is characterized by both extreme excess (cancer is often considered as accumulation of phlegm, heat and toxins) and extreme deficiency (qi, blood, yin and yang deficiencies caused by chemotherapy and radiation). Therefore, optimal treatment requires use of herbs to gently clear heat, eliminate toxins, and greatly tonify the underlying deficiencies.

In this formula, *Huang Qi* (Radix Astragali) and *Xi Yang Shen* (Radix Panacis Quinquefolii) are both used to greatly tonify qi. Both tonics are light, have very strong immune-enhancing effects. Though potent, they do not create the general stagnating side-effects associated with tonics. *Bai Zhu* (Rhizoma Atractylodis Macrocephalae), *Fu Ling* (Poria), and *Yi Yi Ren* (Semen Coicis) strengthen the middle *jiao*, and further enhance the qi-tonifying effect of *Huang Qi* (Radix Astragali) and *Xi Yang Shen* (Radix Panacis Quinquefolii). By strengthening the middle *jiao*, the digestive system can function properly and appetite will increase. *Ji Xue Teng* (Caulis Spatholobi) tonifies blood, *Huang Jing* (Rhizoma Polygonati) nourishes yin, and *Dong Chong Xia Cao* (Cordyceps) strengthens yang. Together, these herbs tonify and treat the underlying qi, blood, yin and yang deficiencies. Small amounts of *E Zhu* (Rhizoma Curcumae), *Zao Xiu* (Rhizoma Paridis), *Ban Zhi Lian* (Herba Scutellariae Barbatae) and *Bai Hua She She Cao* (Herba Oldenlandia) clear heat, relieve pain and eliminate toxins, and have shown promising anticancer effects according to various *in vitro* and *in vivo* studies.[1,2]

FORMULAS

CA SUPPORT ™

In summary, *CA Support* is developed specifically to address the difficult and challenging cases of cancer in which the patients are too weak to continue with chemotherapy and/or radiation treatments. Use of this formula will strengthen the underlying constitution, improve quality of life, and decrease pain and suffering.

SUPPLEMENTARY FORMULAS

- To enhance the immune system and increase white blood cell count, take with *Cordyceps 3* or *Immune +*.
- To increase red blood cell count, add *Dang Gui Bu Xue Tang* (Tangkuei Decoction to Tonify the Blood) or *Schisandra ZZZ*.
- For hair loss from chemotherapy or radiation, take with *Polygonum 14*.
- For loose stool because of Spleen deficiency, add *GI Tonic*.
- For pain due to cancer, add *Herbal Analgesic*.
- With headache, add *Corydalin*.
- With migraine, add *Migratrol*.

NUTRITION

- A diet based on organic fresh fruits and vegetables is highly recommended. For patients who have breast cancer, the following foods are especially beneficial: all mushrooms, whole grains, broccoli, brussels sprouts, cabbage, cauliflower, yellow/orange vegetables (carrots, pumpkins, squash, sweet potatoes), fresh garlic, onions, fresh berries, apples, cherries, grapes, and plums.
- Avoid meat, processed food, junk food, alcohol, greasy food, caffeine, dairy products (except for unsweetened low-fat yogurt), tap water, iron-supplements and vegetables and fruits with pesticides.
- Foods with antioxidant effects, such as vitamin A, C and E are beneficial as they neutralize the free radicals and minimize damage to cells. Beneficial foods include citrus fruits, carrots, green leaf vegetables, and green tea.
- Ginger can always be used to relieve nausea. Boil ten slices of ginger for 5 minutes and mix with brown sugar. Slices of fresh ginger can also be chewed or sucked on for a stronger and immediate effect.

LIFESTYLE INSTRUCTIONS

- Avoid radiation from microwaves and limit prolonged exposure to appliances with high electromagnetic output, such as television, computer monitors, electric stoves, cellular phones, and other popular electronic components.
- Relax, exercise regularly (*Tai Chi Chuan, Qi Gong* or yoga), and have a positive outlook on life.
- Avoid consumption of alcohol and exposure to tobacco in any form.
- Avoid stress and anxiety whenever possible. They suppress the immune system, slow down the metabolic process, and foster development of cancer.
- Avoid wearing tight bras that can cut off lymphatic flow, obstruct elimination of toxins and increase risk of tumor growth.

CLINICAL NOTE

- Chinese or Korean *Ren Shen* (Radix Ginseng) should not be used in individuals who suffer from extreme weakness and deficiency from chemotherapy and radiation treatments. These individuals often have severe yin deficiency, and use of a warm herb [such as *Ren Shen* (Radix Ginseng)] may create more side effects such as dry nose and mouth, nosebleeds and ulcerations in the mouth. Therefore, instead of *Ren Shen* (Radix Ginseng), *Xi Yang Shen* (Radix Panacis Quinquefolii) will be much more beneficial.

CA SUPPORT ™

CAUTIONS

☾ This formula is *not* designed to treat cancer, nor is it designed to replace chemotherapy and/or radiation. The focus of this formula is to support patients with cancer who are too weak to continue with chemotherapy and radiation treatments. This formula contains herbs that tonify the underlying deficiencies to improve quality of life and reduce pain and suffering.

☾ This formula is contraindicated in patients with severe infection or inflammation with excess heat.

ACUPUNCTURE POINTS

Traditional Points:
☾ *Zusanli* (ST 36).
☾ Patients in many cases are too weak to receive acupuncture. It is recommended to just perform gentle massage or acupressure.

Balance Method by Dr. Richard Tan:
☾ Use the twelve magical points. See *Dr. Tan's Twelve Magical Points* for details.

MODERN RESEARCH

CA Support is developed specifically for individuals who have extreme weakness and deficiency after prolonged battles with cancer and its treatments (chemotherapy and radiation). At this moment, though the patient still has cancer, their constitution is too fragile to continue with chemotherapy and radiation. Optimal treatment requires use of herbs to suppress the growth of cancer cells while stimulating the production of healthy cells. To achieve this goal, this formula uses herbs with immunostimulant effect to increase white blood cells, hematopoietic effect to increase red blood cells, and antineoplastic effect to suppress cancer cells.

Huang Qi (Radix Astragali), one of the most commonly used herbs, has been shown via many clinical studies to effectively increase white blood cells, multinuclear leukocytes, and IgM.[3,4] Furthermore, use of *Huang Qi* (Radix Astragali) has been shown to restore normal immune system function in 115 patients with leukopenia,[5] and it also reverses immune suppression induced by cyclophosphamide, a chemotherapy drug.[6] Lastly, use of *Huang Qi* (Radix Astragali) is also associated with marked hematopoietic effect, as it stimulates the bone marrow and increases the production and maturity of blood cells.[7] In addition to *Huang Qi* (Radix Astragali), there are many other herbs in this formula with immunostimulant effect. *Ji Xue Teng* (Caulis Spatholobi) has been shown to increase both neutrophils and eosinophils as quickly as three days after the herbal therapy.[8] *Dong Chong Xia Cao* (Cordyceps) has a direct effect to enhance the phagocytic activities of macrophages.[9] *Bai Zhu* (Rhizoma Atractylodis Macrocephalae) increases the number of white blood cells, lymphocytes, and IgG, as well as enhancing the activity of the macrophages and the reticuloendothelial system.[10,11]

In addition to strengthening the body, *CA Support* also incorporates many herbs with antineoplastic effect to fight cancer. *E Zhu* (Rhizoma Curcumae) has a marked antineoplastic effect, and has been used with satisfactory results for treatment of stomach, lung, liver, and esophageal cancers.[12,13] *Bai Zhu* (Rhizoma Atractylodis Macrocephalae) has marked inhibitory action against esophageal cancer according to several *in vitro* studies.[14] *Yi Yi Ren* (Semen Coicis) and *Fu Ling* (Poria) have mild antineoplastic activity, and are generally more effective when combined with other therapies.[15,16] *Ban Zhi Lian* (Herba Scutellariae Barbatae) and *Bai Hua She She Cao* (Herba Oldenlandia) have potent antineoplastic effects, and have shown promising effect to treat various types of cancer according to both *in vitro* and *in vivo* studies.[17,18]

Overall, *CA Support* is developed specifically to address the difficult and challenging cases of cancer in which the patient is too weak to continue with chemotherapy and radiation treatments. Use of this formula will strengthen the underlying constitution and suppress the growth of cancer cells. In conclusion, this is an excellent formula to decrease pain and suffering, and improve quality of life for patients with cancer.

PHARMACEUTICAL DRUGS & CHINESE MEDICINE: A COMPARATIVE ANALYSIS

Despite all the advances in medicine, treatment of cancer is still in its relative infancy in both western and traditional Chinese medicine.

Western Medical Approach: Optimal treatment methods may include chemotherapy, radiation and/or surgery. Though they may be effective, they are extremely harsh and create a tremendous number of side effects, including severe nausea, vomiting, hair loss, and most importantly, bone marrow suppression with decreased count of red and white blood cells. Serious cases of bone marrow suppression often necessitate the termination of chemotherapy and radiation treatments, a scenario where the patient now suffers from both cancer and its treatments at the same time.

Traditional Chinese Medicine Approach: For patients with cancer who are too weak to receive chemotherapy, radiation, and/or surgery, use of herbal therapies is extremely beneficial to alleviate the side effects of drugs, strengthen the body, and improve overall quality of life.

Summation: Optimal therapy in cases of cancer is not to choose between western *or* traditional Chinese medicine, but to use western *and* traditional Chinese medicines together. These two modalities of medicine complement each others, and provide the brightest outlook and prognosis for successful treatment of cancer.

---

[1] Wong BY, Lau BH, Jia TY, Wan CP. Oldenlandia diffusa and Scutellaria barbata augment macrophage oxidative burst and inhibit tumor growth. *Cancer Biother Radiopharm* 1996 Feb; 11(1):51-6

[2] Wong BY, Lau BH, Jia TY, Wan CP. Oldenlandia diffusa and Scutellaria barbata augment macrophage oxidative burst and inhibit tumor growth. *Cancer Biother Radiopharm* 1996 Feb; 11(1):51-6

[3] *Shan Xi Yi Yao Za Zhi* (Shanxi Journal of Medicine and Herbology), 1974; 5-6:57

[4] *Biol Pharm Bull*, 1977; 20(11)-1178-82

[5] *Zhong Guo Zhong Xi Yi Jie He Za Zhi* (Chinese Journal of Integrative Chinese and Western Medicine), 1995 Aug.; 15(8):462-4

[6] *Journal of Clinical and Laboratory Immunology*, Mar. 1988; 25(3):125-9

[7] *Nan Jing Zhong Yi Xue Yuan Xue Bao* (Journal of Nanjing University of Traditional Chinese Medicine), 1989; 1:43

[8] *Shang Hai Zhong Yi Yao Za Zhi* (Shanghai Journal of Chinese Medicine and Herbology), 1965; 9:16

[9] *Shang Hai Yi Yao Za Zhi* (Shanghai Journal of Medicine and Herbology), 1988; 1:48

[10] *Xin Yi Yao Xue Za Zhi* (New Journal of Medicine and Herbology), 1979; 6:60

[11] *Jun Shi Yi Xue Jian Xun* (Military Medicine Notes), 1977; 2:5

[12] *Xin Yi Yao Xue Za Zhi* (New Journal of Medicine and Herbology), 1976; 12:28

[13] *Shan Dong Zhong Yi Xue Yuan Xue Bao* (Journal of Shandong University School of Chinese Medicine), 1980; 1:30

[14] *Zhong Liu Yu Zhi Tong Xun* (Journal of Prevention and Treatment of Cancer), 1976; 2:40

[15] *Zhong Cao Yao Xue* (Study of Chinese Herbal Medicine), 1976; 15

[16] *Zhong Xi Yi Jie He Za Zhi* (Journal of Integrated Chinese and Western Medicine), 1985; 2:115

[17] Wong BY, Lau BH, Jia TY, Wan CP. Oldenlandia diffusa and Scutellaria barbata augment macrophage oxidative burst and inhibit tumor growth. *Cancer Biother Radiopharm* 1996 Feb; 11(1):51-6

[18] Wong BY, Lau BH, Jia TY, Wan CP. Oldenlandia diffusa and Scutellaria barbata augment macrophage oxidative burst and inhibit tumor growth. *Cancer Biother Radiopharm* 1996 Feb; 11(1):51-6

C/R SUPPORT ™

(Chemotherapy/Radiation)

CLINICAL APPLICATIONS

☯ Side effects commonly associated with chemotherapy or radiation
☯ Myasthenia gravis
☯ Chronic fatigue syndrome
☯ Prolapse of organs such as the stomach, rectum, uterus and bladder
☯ Anorexia and wasting syndrome

WESTERN THERAPEUTIC ACTIONS

☯ Enhances the immune system by increasing the white blood cell count [1,2,3,8,9,10,11,14,15,16]
☯ Supports the an immune system during chemotherapy and radiation treatments [1,2,3,5,6]
☯ Inhibits the growth of cancer cells [5,12,13]
☯ Inhibits the growth of harmful bacteria [7]
☯ Boosts energy and vitality [1,2,3]

CHINESE THERAPEUTIC ACTIONS

☯ Tonifies the Spleen and the Stomach
☯ Tonifies yin and moistens dryness
☯ Tonifies the *wei* (defensive) *qi*
☯ Harmonizes the middle *jiao*

DOSAGE

Take 3 to 4 capsules three times daily as a maintenance dose. Dosage may be increased to 5 to 6 capsules three times daily for cancer patients receiving chemotherapy or radiation treatments. *C/R Support* should be taken on an empty stomach with warm water for maximum effectiveness. Honey can also be added to enhance the taste of the herbs, tonify qi and harmonize the middle *jiao*.

INGREDIENTS

Bai Zhu (Rhizoma Atractylodis Macrocephalae)
Chen Pi (Pericarpium Citri Reticulatae)
Dang Gui (Radicis Angelicae Sinensis)
Dong Chong Xia Cao (Cordyceps)
Gou Qi Zi (Fructus Lycii)
Huang Qi (Radix Astragali)
Ling Zhi (Ganoderma)

Mai Men Dong (Radix Ophiopogonis)
Ren Shen (Radix Ginseng)
Sheng Di Huang (Radix Rehmanniae)
Shi Di (Calyx Kaki)
Zhi Gan Cao (Radix Glycyrrhizae Preparata)
Zhu Ru (Caulis Bambusae in Taenia)

FORMULA EXPLANATION

C/R Support is an herbal formula specifically designed to support patients with cancer as they undergo chemotherapy and radiation treatments. Though effective against cancer cells, chemotherapy and radiation destroy normal tissue and healthy cells and cause a wide array of side effects and adverse reactions, including but not limited to nausea, vomiting, hair loss, weakness and fatigue. For cancer patients receiving chemotherapy and radiation, *C/R Support* complements the overall treatment by enhancing the immune system, reducing the side effects of the drug treatment, inhibiting the growth of cancer cells, and boosting the energy and vitality of the patient.

FORMULAS

C/R SUPPORT ™

(Chemotherapy/Radiation)

Huang Qi (Radix Astragali) is the chief herb in this formula. It replenishes the vital qi, consolidates the *wei* (defensive) *qi*, and protects against external pathogenic factors. It has anticancer effects to increase the content of cAMP and inhibit the growth of tumor cells. *Ling Zhi* (Ganoderma) tonifies blood and vital energy, increases the white blood cell count, and inhibits the growth of various viruses and bacterium. *Dong Chong Xia Cao* (Cordyceps) is essential in rebuilding the patient's constitution and is used for chronically debilitated patients. *Shi Di* (Calyx Kaki), *Zhi Gan Cao* (Radix Glycyrrhizae Preparata) and *Zhu Ru* (Caulis Bambusae in Taenia) tonify the Spleen and Stomach of the middle *jiao* to prevent nausea, vomiting and stomach discomfort. *Chen Pi* (Pericarpium Citri Reticulatae) strengthens the Spleen and dispels phlegm. *Sheng Di Huang* (Radix Rehmanniae), *Gou Qi Zi* (Fructus Lycii), and *Mai Men Dong* (Radix Ophiopogonis) treat thirst and dryness by replenishing body fluids. *Dang Gui* (Radicis Angelicae Sinensis) augments the yin and blood and relieves thirst and dryness. *Ren Shen* (Radix Ginseng) and *Bai Zhu* (Rhizoma Atractylodis Macrocephalae) tonify the Spleen qi to increase both energy and appetite during radiation treatments.

C/R Support can also be used to treat prolapse of internal organs, such as the stomach, rectum, bladder, or uterus. *Huang Qi* (Radix Astragali), *Ling Zhi* (Ganoderma), *Ren Shen* (Radix Ginseng), and *Bai Zhu* (Rhizoma Atractylodis Macrocephalae) tonify qi, ascend yang, and raise the prolapse of internal organs. Similarly, qi and yang tonic herbs in this formula help to relieve chronic fatigue syndrome, anorexia, wasting syndrome, and myasthenia gravis.

SUPPLEMENTARY FORMULAS

- For patients with cancer who have extreme weakness and deficiency and cannot tolerate chemotherapy or radiation treatment, use *CA Support*.
- Take with *Immune +* to enhance the immune system during or after chemotherapy or radiation treatment.
- For cancer of the lung and reproductive systems, *Cordyceps 3* can be added to strengthen the constitution of these two organs.
- Individuals who experience hair loss during chemotherapy or radiation treatment should take *Polygonum 14* to nourish qi and blood and prevent hair damage.
- For maintenance at the conclusion of chemotherapy or radiation treatment, take both *Immune +, Cordyceps 3* and *Imperial Tonic* on a long-term basis.
- For poor appetite and loose stools from Spleen deficiency caused by chemotherapy or radiation, add *GI Tonic*.
- For Kidney yin deficiency, add *Kidney Tonic (Yin)*.
- For Kidney yang deficiency, add *Kidney Tonic (Yang)*.
- For constipation, add *Gentle Lax (Deficient)*.
- For pain due to cancer, add *Herbal Analgesic*.
- For stress and anxiety, use *Calm*.
- For stress, anxiety and insomnia, use *Calm ZZZ*.
- For a quick boost of energy and vitality, use *Vibrant*.

NUTRITION

- A diet based on organic fresh fruits and vegetables is highly recommended. For patients who have breast cancer, the following foods are especially beneficial: all mushrooms, whole grains, broccoli, brussels sprouts, cabbage, cauliflower, yellow/orange vegetables (carrots, pumpkins, squash, sweet potatoes), fresh garlic, onions, fresh berries, apples, cherries, grapes, and plums.
- Avoid meat, processed foods, junk foods, alcohol, greasy foods, caffeine, dairy products (except for unsweetened low-fat yogurt), tap water, iron-supplements and vegetables and fruits grown with pesticides.
- Foods with antioxidant effects, such as vitamin A, C and E are beneficial as they neutralize the free radicals and minimize damages to cells. Beneficial foods include citrus fruits, carrots, green leafy vegetables, and green tea.

C/R SUPPORT ™

(Chemotherapy/Radiation)

☯ Ginger can always be used to relieve nausea. It can be taken as a tea with some brown sugar or honey. Slices of fresh ginger can also be chewed or sucked on for a stronger and more immediate effect.

The Tao of Nutrition by Ni and McNease
☯ Recommendations: Blend shitake or ganoderma mushrooms and white fungus, boil and drink the soup three times a day.
☯ Recommendations: Boil together mung beans, pearl barley, azuki beans, and figs. This makes a delicious dessert that will aid appetite and sustain energy level.
☯ Avoid meat, chicken, coffee, cinnamon, anise, pepper, dairy products, spicy foods (except garlic), high fat foods, cooked oils, chemical additives, moldy foods, smoking, constipation, stress, and all irritations.
☯ For more information, please refer to *The Tao of Nutrition* by Dr. Maoshing Ni and Cathy McNease.

LIFESTYLE INSTRUCTIONS

☯ Avoid radiation from microwaves and limit prolonged exposure to appliances with high electromagnetic output, such as television, computer monitors, electric stoves, cellular phones, and other popular electronic components.
☯ Relax, exercise regularly (*Tai Chi Chuan, Qi Gong* or yoga), and have a positive outlook on life.
☯ Avoid the consumption of alcohol and exposure to tobacco or nicotine in any form.
☯ Avoid stress and anxiety whenever possible. They suppress the immune system, slow down the metabolic process, and foster development of cancer.
☯ Avoid wearing tight bras, which can cut off lymphatic flow, obstruct elimination of toxins and increase risk of tumor growth.

CLINICAL NOTES

☯ *C/R Support* has a wide range of clinical applications. Its use is not limited to cancer patients receiving chemotherapy and radiation.
☯ *C/R Support* contains herbs with immune-enhancing, anticancer activities, and energy-boosting properties. It will benefit cancer patients, whether or not they are receiving chemotherapy and radiation treatments.

CAUTIONS

☯ *C/R Support* is *not* designed to treat cancer or replace chemotherapy and radiation (C/R). Its main focus is to complement chemotherapy and radiation treatments by strengthening the overall constitution of the patient and minimize the side effects.
☯ Patients who are on anticoagulant or antiplatelet therapies, such as Coumadin (Warfarin), should use this formula with caution as there may be a slightly higher risk of bleeding and bruising.

ACUPUNCTURE POINTS

Traditional Points:
☯ *Zusanli* (ST 36), *Fuliu* (KI 7), and *Neiguan* (PC 6).
☯ *Pishu* (BL 20), *Weishu* (BL 21), *Neiguan* (PC 6), *Zusanli* (ST 36), *Hegu* (LI 4), and *Shanzhong* (CV 17).

Balance Method by Dr. Richard Tan:
☯ Left side: *Zusanli* (ST 36) and *Neiguan* (PC 6).
☯ Right side: *Yinlingquan* (SP 9), *Waiguan* (TH 5), and *Hegu* (LI 4).
☯ Left and right side can be alternated from treatment to treatment.

FORMULAS

C/R SUPPORT ™

(Chemotherapy/Radiation)

- For additional information on the Balance Method, please refer to *Dr. Tan's Strategy of Twelve Magical Points* by Dr. Richard Tan.

Ear Points:
- Pain due to cancer:
  - Main points: Subcortex, Heart and correlating diseased organ.
  - Adjunct points: Sympathetic, Liver, *Shenmen*.
- Select four to six points each time. Alternate the ear treatments every two days.

MODERN RESEARCH

C/R Support is formulated specifically for cancer patients who are receiving chemotherapy or radiation. *C/R Support* contains herbs that have been found to have antitumor, immune-enhancing, antibiotic, and antinauseant effects.

Huang Qi (Radix Astragali) is one of the most frequently used Chinese herbs and has historically been used for its function to tonify the *wei* (defensive) *qi*. In Western medicine, modern research has proven repeatedly that *Huang Qi* (Radix Astragali) increases both specific and non-specific immunity.[1,2,3] In a clinical study of 115 leucopenic patients, it was found that the use of *Huang Qi* (Radix Astragali) is associated with an "obvious rise of the white blood cell (WBC) count" with a dose-dependent relationship.[4] In addition, *Huang Qi* (Radix Astragali) works well with current drug therapy in enhancing the overall effectiveness of the treatment. *Huang Qi* (Radix Astragali) potentiates the antitumor effect of chemotherapy drugs,[5] while reversing drug-induced immune suppression.[6] Finally, *Huang Qi* (Radix Astragali) also demonstrates anticancer activity as it increases the content of cAMP and inhibits the growth of tumor cells.[7]

Ling Zhi (Ganoderma) has a wide range of therapeutic effects in the treatment of cancer. Various clinical studies have demonstrated the effects of *Ling Zhi* (Ganoderma) to enhance the immune system.[8,9,10,11] The specific effects of *Ling Zhi* (Ganoderma) include an increase in monocytes, macrophages and T lymphocytes as well as an increased production of cytokine, interleukin, tumor-necrosis-factor and interferon.[8] In addition, *Ling Zhi* (Ganoderma) has a broad spectrum of antibacterial activity, and inhibits the growth of *pneumococci*, *streptococci* (type A), *staphylococci*, *E. coli*, B. *dysenteriae*, *pseudomonas*, and others.[7]

Dong Chong Xia Cao (Cordyceps) is another herb that has demonstrated antitumor and immunomodulatory functions. *Dong Chong Xia Cao* (Cordyceps) was found to significantly inhibit the proliferation of cancer cells;[12] and in some instances, the growth inhibition rate of the cancer cells reached up to 78 to 83%.[13] In addition to the antitumor activities, *Dong Chong Xia Cao* (Cordyceps) also enhances the overall immunity by increasing the number of lymphocytes and natural killer cells, and the production of interleukin, interferon and tumor-necrosis-factor.[14,15,16,17,18]

PHARMACEUTICAL DRUGS & CHINESE MEDICINE: A COMPARATIVE ANALYSIS

Despite all the advances in medicine, treatment of cancer is still in its relative infancy in both western and traditional Chinese medicine.

Western Medical Approach: Optimal treatment methods may include chemotherapy, radiation and/or surgery. Though they may be effective, they are extremely harsh and create a huge number of side effects, including severe nausea, vomiting, hair loss, and most importantly, bone marrow suppression with decreased count of red and white blood cells. Serious cases of bone marrow suppression often necessitate the termination of chemotherapy and radiation treatments, a scenario where the patient now suffers from both cancer and its treatments at the same time.

C/R SUPPORT ™

(Chemotherapy/Radiation)

Traditional Chinese Medicine Approach: Use of herbs is extremely effective to complement chemotherapy and radiation. Not only do they alleviate many side effects of chemotherapy and radiation, they strengthen the overall constitution of the body so they can tolerate and finish the entire course of therapies.

Summation: Optimal therapy in cases of cancer is not to choose between western *or* traditional Chinese medicine, but to integrate western *and* traditional Chinese medicines together. These two modalities of medicine complement each others, and provide the brightest outlook and prognosis for successful treatment of cancer.

CASE STUDIES

In July 1999, a 66-year-old retired business woman was brought in for acupuncture and herbal treatment, seriously ill from severe chronic anorexia triggered by intolerance to chemotherapeutic treatment following radiation and surgery for cancer of the vocal cords. Approximately 5'4" tall, the woman was curled up in fetal position, weighing 85 lbs., cold, lethargic, nauseous and exceedingly anxious. She had had one previous occurrence of the cancer 2 years before, and felt she was in danger of dying, if not from the cancer, then from the treatment. She began taking small doses of *C/R Support* granules stirred into warm water, as she could not swallow anything but liquids. She continued with *C/R Support* for several weeks, later augmented with *Bu Zhong Yi Qi Tang* (Tonify the Middle and Augment the Qi Decoction), but found it difficult to incorporate a second herbal formula, so relied on *C/R Support* for approximately eight months. No further chemotherapeutic or radiation treatment was attempted, at the direction of her M.D. oncologist and at the patient's wishes. Within three weeks of beginning treatment, the woman was able to resume eating small meals of well-cooked foods, and within 2 months, she was gaining weight noticeably and regaining color in her face. Her voice was a strained whisper initially, gradually regaining some volume and tone. Because the underlying pathogens in her case were Lung heat, Heart fire, and dryness with persistent phlegm, her herbal formula was gradually changed to half *C/R Support*, and half additional ingredients to address the heat, dryness and phlegm. At approximately 24 months into treatment, *C/R Support* was discontinued, although the patient continues to take herbs specific to her imbalance and seek acupuncture weekly. Because of emotional issues related to her throat, compliance with her herbal regime is difficult for the patient: she seldom takes the full dosage or recommended frequency, however, she states she tries to become more and more consistent. She has regained normal weight and vitality, returning to an active 'retired' home and social life. As of January 2002, she continues to receive 'cancer free' reports from her oncologist and surgeon, and is seeing gradual improvement in her voice, thirst levels and phlegm.

L.C., Santa Monica, California

A 69-year-old male presented in July 1999 with advanced multiple myeloma, brittle bones, chronic intense pain in his back and hips, digestive difficulties, deficient constipation and hair loss. He is an entertainment professional and concerned about being able to preserve his career in the face of medical expenses and the emotional satisfaction of continuing to work. His blood cancer count was high and remained somewhat high through February 2001, when it was 2,100. He began taking *C/R Support* at the normal dosage in July 1999, combined over time with a normal dosage of either *Nourish*, *Shou Wu Pian* (Polygonum Pills), or *You Gui Wan* (Restore the Right [Kidney] Pill), depending on the symptoms presented at his weekly visits for acupuncture and herbal consultation. He continued on *C/R Support* through the middle of 2001, transitioning at that point to individualized formulas specific to his underlying digestive weakness, osteoporosis and pain. Although the osteoporotic aspects of his illness continue to make him vulnerable to skeletal injury and pain, he has maintained 80% of the hairline he had upon presenting for treatment, and has been able to continue working in his profession. His blood cancer counts in December 2001 were below 300. He states he continues to feel he is improving.

L.C., Santa Monica, California

C/R SUPPORT ™
(Chemotherapy/Radiation)

K.E., a 45-year-old female, presented with ovarian cancer and *C/R Support* was prescribed at 2 grams three times a day. She was instructed to take 4 grams three times daily if her white blood cell count was low. She also received acupuncture treatment in addition to the herbs. Patient reported that she felt okay during the chemotherapy and stayed relatively healthy and kept the white blood cell count healthy.

W.F., Bloomfield, New Jersey

[1] Chu, DT. et al. Immunotherapy with Chinese medicinal herbs. I. immune restoration of local xenogenetic graft-versus-host reaction in cancer patients by fractionated astragalus membranaceus in vitro. *Journal Of Clinical & Laboratory Immunology.* Mar. 1988; 25(3):119-23

[2] Sun, Y. et al. Immune restoration and/or augmentation of local graft versus host reaction by traditional Chinese medicinal herbs. *Cancer.* July 1983; 52(1):70-3

[3] Sun, Y. et al. Preliminary observations on the effects of the Chinese medicinal herbs astragalus membranaceus and ganoderma lucidum on lymphocyte blastogenic responses. *Journal Of Biological Response Modifiers.* 1983; 2(3):227-37

[4] Weng, XS. *Chung Juo Chung Hsia I Chieh Ho Tsa Chih.* August 1995

[5] Chu, DT. et al. Fractionated extract of astragalus membranaceus, a Chinese medicinal herb, potentiates LAK cell cytotoxicity generated by a low dose of recombinant interleukin-2. *Journal Of Clinical & Laboratory Immunology.* Aug. 1988; 26(4):183-7

[6] Chu, DT. et al. Immunotherapy with Chinese medicinal herbs. II. Reversal of cyclophosphamide-induced immune suppression by administration of fractionated astragalus membranaceus in vivo. *Journal Of Clinical & Laboratory Immunology.* Mar. 1988; 25(3):125-9

[7] Yeung, HC. *Handbook Of Chinese Herbs.* Institute Of Chinese Medicine. 1996

[8] Wang, SY. et al. The anti-tumor effect of ganoderma lucidum is mediated by cytokines released from activated macrophages and t-lymphocytes. *International Journal Of Cancer.* Mar 17. 1997; 70(6):699-705

[9] Van Der Hem, LG. et al. Ling Zhi-8: Studies of a new immunomodulating agent. *Transplantation.* Sep 15. 1995; 60(5):438-43

[10] Haak-Frendscho, M. et al. Ling Zhi-8: A novel t-cell mitogen induces cytokine production and up-regulation of ICAM-1 expression. *Cellular Immunology.* Aug. 1993; 150(1):101-13

[11] Tanaka, S. et al. Complete amino acid sequence of a novel immuno-modulatory protein, ling zhi-9. an immuno-modulator from a fungus, ganoderma lucidum, having similar effect to immunoglobulin variable regions.

[12] Kuo, YC. et al. Growth inhibitors against tumor cells in cordyceps sinensis other than cordycepin and polysaccharides. *Cancer Investigation.* 1994; 12(6):611-5

[13] Chen, YJ. et al. Effect of cordyceps sinensis on the proliferation and differentiation of human leukemic U937 Cells. *Life Sciences.* 1997; 60(25):2349-59

[14] Kuo,YC. et al. Cordyceps sinensis as an immuno-modulatory agent. *American Journal Of Chinese Medicine.* 24(2):111-25, 1996

[15] Guan, YJ. et al. Effect of cordyceps sinensis on T-lymphocyte subsets in chronic renal failure. *Chung-Kuo Chung His I Chieh Ho Tsa Chih.* Jun. 1992; 12(6):338-9,323

[16] Liu, C. et al. Effects of cordyceps sinensis (CS) on in vitro natural killer cells. *Chung-Kuo Chung His I Chieh Ho Tsa Chih.* May. 1992; 12(5):267-9,259

[17] Xu, RH. et al. Effects of cordyceps sinensis on natural killer activity and colony formation of B16 melanoma. *Chinese Medical Journal.* Feb. 1992; 105(2):97-101

[18] Liu, P. et al. Influence of cordyceps sinensis (berk.) sacc. and rat serum containing same medicine on IL-1, IFN and TNF produced by rat Kupffer's cells. *Chung Kuo Chung Yao Tsa Chih*, June 1996; 21(6):367-9, 384

FORMULAS

CALM ™

CLINICAL APPLICATIONS

❧ Stress, anxiety, nervousness, restlessness
❧ General symptoms associated with stress, such as poor appetite, headache, tension, insomnia, etc.
❧ Premenstrual syndrome (PMS) with breast distention, irritability and/or mood swings

WESTERN THERAPEUTIC ACTIONS

❧ Mild sedative effect to relieve nervousness and irritability [2,3]
❧ Anxiolytic function to relieve stress and anxiety [2,3]
❧ Analgesic action to relieve pain, headache and muscle tension associated with stress [2]

CHINESE THERAPEUTIC ACTIONS

❧ Spreads the Liver qi
❧ Nourishes Liver blood
❧ Clears heat
❧ Harmonizes middle *jiao*

DOSAGE

Take 3 to 4 capsules three times daily on an empty stomach with warm water. Dosage may be increased to 6 to 8 capsules three times daily if necessary to alleviate symptoms for a few days. Once stabilized, reduce dosage back down to 3 to 4 capsules three times daily.

INGREDIENTS

Bai Shao (Radix Paeoniae Alba)
Bai Zhu (Rhizoma Atractylodis Macrocephalae)
Bo He (Herba Menthae)
Chai Hu (Radix Bupleuri)
Dang Gui (Radicis Angelicae Sinensis)

Fu Ling (Poria)
Mu Dan Pi (Cortex Moutan)
Sheng Jiang (Rhizoma Zingiberis Recens)
Zhi Gan Cao (Radix Glycyrrhizae Preparata)
Zhi Zi (Fructus Gardeniae)

FORMULA EXPLANATION

According to the Five-Elements Theory, the Liver is the most sensitive of all organs to emotional distress. Stress and pressure can easily lead to Liver qi stagnation, which can overact on the Spleen and the Stomach. The treatment protocol is to spread the Liver qi, harmonize the middle *jiao*, and nourish the blood.

Chai Hu (Radix Bupleuri) enters the Liver and disperses stagnant qi. *Bai Shao* (Radix Paeoniae Alba) and *Dang Gui* (Radicis Angelicae Sinensis) nourish the blood and soften the Liver. *Bai Zhu* (Rhizoma Atractylodis Macrocephalae) and *Fu Ling* (Poria) strengthen the Spleen and the Stomach to prevent the overacting of the Liver (Wood element) on the Spleen and the Stomach (Earth element). The fragrant and acrid properties of *Bo He* (Herba Menthae) and *Sheng Jiang* (Rhizoma Zingiberis Recens) help disperse Liver qi stagnation. The combination of *Zhi Gan Cao* (Radix Glycyrrhizae Preparata) and *Bai Shao* (Radix Paeoniae Alba) produces an analgesic effect to treat hypochondriac distention. *Zhi Zi* (Fructus Gardeniae) and *Mu Dan Pi* (Cortex Moutan) clear heat and reduce irritability, anger and other heat signs.

FORMULAS

CALM ™

SUPPLEMENTARY FORMULAS

- For stomach pain, heartburn, gastric and duodenal ulcers, add *GI Care*.
- For severe emotional disturbance with anger and neurosis or insomnia, use *Calm (ES)*.
- For stress, anxiety and insomnia in patients with deficiency, use *Calm ZZZ*.
- For excess worrying with insomnia, combine with *Schisandra ZZZ*.
- For hypertension, combine with *Gastrodia Complex* or *Gentiana Complex*.
- For women experiencing hot flashes and night sweating during menopause, add *Balance (Heat)*.
- For infertility due to stress, use *Blossom (Phase 1-4)*.
- In cases of prolonged Liver qi stagnation causing benign breast lumps, breast tumor and/or mastitis, use *Resolve (Upper)*.
- For dysmenorrhea, add *Mense-Ease*.
- If the patient has hyperthyroidism, add *Thyrodex*.
- For migraine, add *Migratrol* or *Corydalin*.
- For ADD/ADHD, add *Calm (Jr)*.
- For irritable bowel syndrome (IBS) due to stress, add *GI Harmony*.
- For ulcerative colitis due to stress, add *GI Care (UC)*.
- For excess heat, add *Gardenia Complex*.
- With blood stagnation, add *Circulation (SJ)*.

NUTRITION

- A diet high in calcium, magnesium, phosphorus, potassium, and vitamins B and E is recommended. These nutrients are easily depleted by stress.
- Encourage the consumption of fruits and vegetables such as apricots, wintermelon, asparagus, avocados, bananas and broccoli in addition to brown rice, dried fruit, figs, salmon, garlic, green leafy vegetables, soy products, and yogurt.
- Avoid caffeine (coffee, tea, cola, chocolate), tobacco, alcohol and sugar whenever possible.[1]

The Tao of Nutrition by Ni and McNease
- Premenstrual syndrome (PMS)
  - Recommendations: At least one week prior to the usual onset time of PMS symptoms, consume some of the following: ginger, green onions, fennel, orange peel, spinach, walnuts, hawthorn berries, cinnamon, and black pepper, and Chinese date.
  - Avoid cold foods, raw foods, excessive consumption of fruits, vinegar, all shellfish, coffee, stimulants, sugar, dairy products, and smoking.
- For more information, please refer to *The Tao of Nutrition* by Dr. Maoshing Ni and Cathy McNease.

LIFESTYLE INSTRUCTIONS

- Regular exercise, adequate rest, and normal sleep patterns are beneficial for stress reduction.
- Practice meditation exercises at least twice daily.
- Get away from the daily routine to do something different and enjoyable to relieve stress whenever possible.
- Noise can be disturbing to mental health and cause stress. Noise greater than 65-decibels can cause psychological disturbance, greater than 90-decibels can cause emotional and vegetative consequences, and greater than 120-decibels can cause nervous system and hearing damages.
- Shift outlook on life and look at changes in a positive way and as challenges, rather than threats.

CALM ™

CLINICAL NOTES

❧ *Calm* is one of the most effective and popular herbal formulas for stress. It relieves Liver qi stagnation, which manifests in a wide range of clinical signs and symptoms, including but not limited to stress, anxiety, nervousness, restlessness, PMS, insomnia, fidgeting, and irritability.

❧ *Calm* has a quick onset of action. Most patients experience relief within a few hours, though it may take a few days to reach maximum effect.

CAUTIONS

❧ *Calm* is a qi-regulating formula, and prolonged use (4 to 6 months) may cause qi deficiency in some patients. Such patients with stressful lifestyles or jobs who cannot be without *Calm* should be advised to take a qi tonic formula, such as *Immune +* or *Cordyceps 3* at 1 to 2 capsules daily, to help maintain optimal qi levels in the body.

❧ Patients who are on anticoagulant or antiplatelet therapies, such as Coumadin (Warfarin), should use this formula with caution, as there may be a slightly higher risk of bleeding and bruising.

ACUPUNCTURE POINTS

Traditional Points:
❧ *Hegu* (LI 4), *Taichong* (LR 3) and *Yintang*.
❧ *Taichong* (LR 3), *Xingjian* (LR 2), *Qimen* (LR 14), *Zhangmen* (LR 13), *Feishu* (BL 13), *Shangwan* (CV 13), and *Shanzhong* (CV 17).

Balance Method by Dr. Richard Tan:
❧ Left side: *Zulinqi* (GB 41), *Yanglingquan* (GB 34), *Shaohai* (HT 3), and *Shenmen* (HT 7).
❧ Right side: *Taichong* (LR 3), *Ququan* (LR 8), *Zhongzhu* (TH 3), and *Tianjing* (TH 10).
❧ Left and right side can be alternated from treatment to treatment.
❧ For additional information on the Balance Method, please refer to *Dr. Tan's Strategy of Twelve Magical Points* by Dr. Richard Tan.

Ear Points:
❧ *Shenmen*.

MODERN RESEARCH

Calm is formulated based on *Xiao Yao San* (Rambling Powder), a classic Chinese formula for Liver qi stagnation. It has a wide range of therapeutic actions, but is most commonly used for treating stress and nerve-related disorders with such symptoms as irritability, bad temper, lower abdominal rigidity, difficult and painful urination, increased menstrual flow or uterine bleeding.[2] Other uses of *Calm* include the treatment of chronic hepatitis, menopausal syndrome, chronic gastritis and peptic ulcers.[2,3]

Calm contains herbs that have good effects in treating PMS. In a study of 52 patients with PMS who began to take herbs three to five days prior to menstruation, it was reported that 14 patients experienced no signs and symptoms of PMS, 32 experienced significant improvement, and 6 experienced no effect.[4] Furthermore, ingredients of *Calm* were reported to have effects in treating menopause as well. In a study with 102 patients with menopause, 92 reported significant improvement, 8 reported some improvement, and 2 discontinued the herbal treatment.[5]

FORMULAS

CALM ™

Dang Gui (Radicis Angelicae Sinensis) has demonstrated a wide variety of clinical functions. It has been reported in many textbooks and numerous clinical studies that *Dang Gui* (Radicis Angelicae Sinensis) treats a variety of women's disorders, such as anemia with dizziness and palpitation, and menstrual cramps. [6,7,8,9,10] Furthermore, it regulates female hormones to relieve amenorrhea, dysmenorrhea and menorrhalgia.[11,12,13,14] The reported functions of *Dang Gui* (Radicis Angelicae Sinensis) include activation of blood circulation, regulation of menstruation, spasmolytic, anti-inflammatory and analgesic.[6,7,8,9,10]

In addition, *Bai Shao* (Radix Paeoniae Alba), containing paeoniflorin and daisein, has a strong antispasmodic effect to alleviate muscle spasms and cramping and to reduce stress and anxiety.[2,15]

PHARMACEUTICAL DRUGS & CHINESE MEDICINE: A COMPARATIVE ANALYSIS

Stress and anxiety are two of the most common emotional disorders. Clinical signs and symptoms include recurrent and intrusive thoughts, insomnia, disturbed sleep, illusions, hallucinations, difficulty concentrating, hypervigilance, restlessness, anger, and irritability.

Western Medical Approach: Pharmaceutical drug treatment for stress and anxiety focus primarily on use of sedative and hypnotic drugs, such as Valium (Diazepam) and Ativan (Lorazepam). Though these drugs are very potent and have immediate effect to sedate patients, they do not address the underlying conditions. Furthermore, long-term use of these medications are associated with many side effects, including drowsiness, dizziness, tiredness, blurred vision, changes in sex drive or ability, shuffling walk, persistent, fine tremor or inability to sit still, difficulty breathing or swallowing, severe skin rash, yellowing of the skin or eyes, irregular heartbeat, and addiction. Therefore, these drugs should only be used when necessary, and only for a short period of time.

Traditional Chinese Medicine Approach: Use of herbs is extremely effective to treat stress and anxiety. Herbs regulate mood and emotions, and alleviate stress and anxiety by enhancing the body's own ability to deal with these external factors. Unlike drugs that have immediate effect to treat stress and anxiety by "sedating the mind and decreasing its responsiveness," herbs do not have an immediate effect, and require two or more weeks of continuous use to gradually treat these conditions. In contrast, one of the main advantages of herbs is they are safe and natural, and do not have negative side effects like drugs.

Summation: Stress and anxiety are two very common disorders. While drugs and herbs are both effective, they have contrasting differences of benefits and risks. While drugs are more effective for shot-term treatment, herbs are more successful for long-term management. Furthermore, counseling (behavior and psychotherapy) is extremely important toward the understanding of, and complete recovery from, these conditions.

CASE STUDIES

A 35-year-old male manager presented with stress, anxiety and anger. His pulse was rapid and face was red. The practitioner diagnosed the condition as Liver qi stagnation and Liver yang rising. When the patient began the initial treatment one year ago, he and his wife noticed a significant improvement. Through the course of the one-year treatment, the patient noticed a regression of his improvement when not taking his dose of *Calm* and felt as though he had "less control of his life." The patient was recommended to continue taking *Calm* at 4 capsules two times a day. Consequently, his condition showed signs of improvement.

K.S., San Diego, California

A new job and concurrent relationship problems had created quite a stressful situation for a 27-year-old female restaurant cook, who was diagnosed with Liver qi stagnation. Her tongue was purple and her pulse was wiry. Constantly thinking about her problems made her unable to relax. Placed on a two week regimen of *Calm* has improved her condition tremendously. Although the patient reported that her stress has not changed, she felt more relaxed after taking **Calm**.

T.G., Albuquerque, New Mexico

A 40-year-old housewife presented with migraines, stress, and a lack of sleep. She woke up frequently and had many stress-related headaches for years. The practitioner diagnosed the condition as Liver qi stagnation with heat rising. The practitioner felt the treatment should revolve around calming the *shen* (spirit). After two weeks of taking **Calm**, the headaches were less severe and less frequent, however sleeping was still poor. At four weeks, her headaches were very mild and under control. She no longer needed to take any western medications. The patient appeared more calm and reported sleeping better and feeling less stressful. She was recommended to continue taking **Calm** for two to three more months. As an adjunct to the treatment, the practitioner also suggested taking **Corydalin** for her headaches, as well as reducing her caffeine intake.

D.S., Flagstaff, Arizona

A 38-year-old female administrator presented with insomnia and TMJ. The practitioner diagnosed her as having Liver fire rising, Kidney and Heart not communicating, and depression. When the patient initially came to the office, she had not slept that same night. She was nervous and had jawbone pain, which was caused by sleeping with a clenched jaw. The acupuncture treatment calmed the patient. To reinforce her acupuncture treatment, **Calm** was also given at a dose of 3 capsules, three times a day. On the second treatment, the patient was much calmer and more relaxed. The same acupuncture treatment was given, with the advice to continue taking **Calm**. As a result, the practitioner concluded that **Calm** was effective for her depression, anxiety and other symptoms of Liver fire.

A.D., La Crescenta, California

S.C., a 42-year-old female, presented with stress due to domestic situations. Clinical manifestations included constipation, bloating, neck tension, insomnia, anorexia, fatigue, tearfulness and sadness. Her tongue was pale and scalloped, with a mid-line crack; her pulse was soft and soggy. The Western diagnosis was depressive disorder; the TCM diagnosis was Liver qi stagnation. After taking **Calm** at three capsules, three times daily, the patient reported feeling much better. Her voice became more animated, there was more character in her face, and more shine to her eyes. Furthermore, the patient stated that her neck tension, insomnia, constipation and sadness were gone.

C.L., Chino Hills, California

M.M., a 41-year-old female, presented with "adrenaline-rush" sensations, characterized by heat flushes to her face, associated with mood swings and anxiety. Her tongue was red and purple, and her face was red. The Western diagnosis was stress-related anxiety attack; the TCM diagnosis was Liver stagnation and yin deficiency. After beginning herbal therapy with **Calm**, two capsules three times daily, and **Balance (Heat)**, two capsules, three times daily, the patient stated that her affect and personality became calmer. Furthermore, she reported "feeling good," with increased energy levels and sound sleep.

C.L., Chino Hills, California

L.A., a 37-year-old female patient, presented with insomnia, with difficulty falling and staying asleep. Other symptoms included neck and shoulder stiffness, TMJ pain, heavy menstrual flow, and cramping with blood clots. She complained of marital problems and held the stress and sadness inside. She was also seeing a psychotherapist. The blood pressure was 123/86 mmHg and her heart rate was 88 beats per minute. The tongue appeared to be salmon pink in color, moist with numerous fissures from the center to the tip. The tongue was swollen and the tip was red. The pulse was slippery and thin. The TCM diagnosis was Spleen qi and Heart blood deficiencies with Liver qi stagnation. **Calm** was prescribed. **Calm** alone eased her tension, but did not help much with her energy. Her sleep improved slightly. The TMJ resolved after eight acupuncture treatments. After two months, **Schisandra ZZZ** was

FORMULAS

added. The patient then slept through the night much more soundly. However, she still complained about the neck and shoulder pain.

J.C.O., Whittier, California

A female presented with stress, irritability, premenstrual syndrome (PMS), loose stool, crying for no reason, muscle tension, and nervous trembling in the hands. She stated that she felt overwhelmed in life and worried incessantly. Her blood pressure was 115/75 mmHg and her heart rate was 87 beats per minute. Her tongue was pink with a red tip and a thin white coating. Pulse was wiry on the left side and slippery on the right side. The TCM diagnosis was Spleen qi deficiency with Liver qi stagnation. *Calm* was prescribed. The patient responded immediately, stating her "nerves" calmed down, stomach settled, and began to feel more "emotionally stable." She took only 3 capsules three times a day the week before her period.

J.C., Whittier, California

D.S., a 45-year-old female, presented with insomnia, mood swings, cramps and fatigue. The tongue was slightly purplish and pale with teeth marks. The coating was thin and white. The pulse was deep and wiry. She was diagnosed with Spleen qi deficiency and blood deficiency. *Nourish*, *Calm*, and *Schisandra ZZZ* were prescribed. The patient reported her sleep pattern improved, her moods balanced, and her energy level increased. She was very happy with the herbs.

B.F., Newport Beach, California

A 36-year-old female patient presented with a long history of anxiety, irritability, insomnia, mood swings, and dream-disturbed sleep. Her pulse was slow, full and wiry; tongue red on the tip and sides. The TCM diagnosis was Liver qi stagnation. After taking three capsules of *Calm* three times daily, the patient reported subtle changes in moods, including that she was not as irritable, and was able to focus on work and maintain higher productivity. She was also able to sleep better, without disturbing dreams.

C.L., Chino Hills, California

J.W., a 44-year-old patient, presented with infertility and a history of miscarriage. She experienced high stress which she "bottled up" inside. Her hands and feet were cold. She also had back pain, low energy, severe menstrual cramps and premenstrual syndrome (PMS). Her tongue was pale and purplish, swollen with teeth marks. The tip was red. Pulses were wiry on both sides and slippery on the right. Her blood pressure was 125/86 mmHg and heart rate was 83 beats per minute. Lab report showed she had low FSH levels. The diagnosis was Spleen and Kidney yang deficiencies with Liver qi and blood stagnation. *Menotrol* was prescribed. After one month on *Menotrol*, the patient reported her menstrual cramping "miraculously disappeared" and her estrogen levels increased dramatically. She was afraid the herbs would interfere with her *in vitro* fertilization (IVF) procedure so she stopped taking them for six weeks. After the IVF was not successful and her tongue color became very purple in the center, the practitioner suggested she take the formula *Calm*. She was open to it. Within a week, her stress level decreased and her energy level increased. Her tongue color changed from purple to pink and slightly dusky. She is presently continuing to take *Calm* and is actively trying to conceive naturally.

J.C.O., Whittier, California

E.P., a 32-year-old female, presented with a 2½-year history of vertigo, associated with insomnia, palpitations, anxiety and nausea. She also suffered from irritable bowel syndrome with alternating diarrhea and constipation. She had an unsteady gait and was unable to drive. For the Western diagnosis of anxiety disorder, the TCM diagnosis was Liver fire. Initially, *Calm* and *Gentiana Complex* were prescribed at two capsules each, three times daily, but then the dosage was increased to three capsules of each, three times daily. After three weeks, the signs and symptoms of irritable bowel syndrome were resolved, and *Gentiana Complex* was discontinued. On the sixth treatment, the patient reported all symptoms improved. However, work-related stress anxiety remained. On the 15th visit, *Calm* was changed to *Schisandra ZZZ* to help with her insomnia. After taking this formula for nine days, the patient

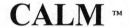

CALM ™

reported much improvement in her sleeping patterns, from 5 to 6 hours of interrupted sleep to 6 to 7 hours of uninterrupted sleep. The patient was treated with acupuncture five times throughout the course of herbal treatment.

C.L., Chino Hills, California

[1] Balch, JF. et al. *Prescription for Nutritional Healing*. Avery Publishing Group. 1997
[2] Bensky, D. et al. *Chinese Herbal Medicine Formulas & Strategies*. Eastland Press. 1990
[3] Yeung, HC. *Handbook of Chinese Herbal Formulas*. Institute of Chinese Medicine. 1995
[4] Gong, LL. et al. *Guiyang Traditional Chinese Medical Journal*. 1985; 3:42.
[5] Huang, ZL. et al. *Modern Applications of Traditional Chinese Medicine*. 1990; 1:17
[6] *Pharmacopoeia of the People's Republic of China*. English version edited from the Pharmacopoeia of PRC 1990 edition. Guangzhou: Guangdong Science and Technology Press. 1990
[7] Tang, W. and Eisenbrand, G. *Chinese Drugs of Plant Origin: Chemistry, Pharmacology, and Use in Traditional and Modern Medicine*. Berlin: Springer-Verlag. 1992
[8] Hsu, HY. et al. *Oriental Material Medica: A Concise Guide*. Long Beach: Oriental Healing Arts Press. 1986.
[9] Huang, KC. *The Pharmacology of Chinese Herbs*. Boca Raton: CRC Press. 1993
[10] Murray, MT. *The Healing Power of Herbs*. Rocklin, CA: Prima Publishing. 1991
[11] Shi, MY. et al. *China J Chinese Materia Medica*. 1995; 20(3):173-175
[12] Olin et al. *The Lawrence Review of Natural Products by Facts and Comparisons*. Dong Quai. March 1997
[13] Li, HY. et al. *China J. Chinese Materia Medica*. 1991; 16(9):560-562
[14] Bensky, D. et al. *Chinese Herbal Medicine Formulas & Strategies*. Eastland Press. 1990
[15] Bensky, D. et al. *Chinese Herbal Medicine Materia Medica*. Eastland Press. 1993

FORMULAS

CALM (ES) ™

CLINICAL APPLICATIONS

- Stress with poor appetite, headache, tension, insomnia, and similar stress responses
- Extreme or severe emotional and psychological disorders such as hysteria, neurosis, schizophrenia, and others
- Withdrawal signs and symptoms associated with alcohol, drug and smoking addiction
- Insomnia with disturbed sleep and night awakenings

WESTERN THERAPEUTIC ACTIONS

- Sedative effect to relieve nervousness and irritability
- Anxiolytic function to relieve stress and anxiety
- Tranquilizing effect to alleviate severe emotional and psychological disorders
- Calming effect to ease withdrawal signs and symptoms associated with alcohol, drug and smoking addiction
- Antispasmodic effect to relieve muscle tension and cramping

CHINESE THERAPEUTIC ACTIONS

- Spreads Liver qi, purges excess Liver fire
- Calms the *shen* (spirit) and tranquilizes the Heart

DOSAGE

For stress- and anxiety-related disorders, take 3 to 4 capsules three times daily. For severe emotional and psychological disorders, or patients with withdrawal signs and symptoms because of drug or alcohol addiction, the dosage may be increased to 6 to 8 capsules every four to six hours or as needed. Dosage can then be dropped down to 3 to 4 capsules three times daily when symptoms are stabilized.

INGREDIENTS

Bai Zhu (Rhizoma Atractylodis Macrocephalae)
Chai Hu (Radix Bupleuri)
Chuan Xiong (Rhizoma Ligustici Chuanxiong)
Da Huang (Radix et Rhizoma Rhei)
Da Zao (Fructus Jujubae)
Dang Gui (Radicis Angelicae Sinensis)
Fu Ling (Poria)
Gan Cao (Radix Glycyrrhizae)
Gou Teng (Ramulus Uncariae cum Uncis)

Gui Zhi (Ramulus Cinnamomi)
Huang Qin (Radix Scutellariae)
Long Gu (Os Draconis)
Mu Li (Concha Ostreae)
Sheng Jiang (Rhizoma Zingiberis Recens)
Suan Zao Ren (Semen Zizyphi Spinosae)
Xi Yang Shen (Radix Panacis Quinquefolii)
Xie Cao (Radix et Rhizoma Valerianae)
Zhu Ru (Caulis Bambusae in Taenia)

FORMULA EXPLANATION

Calm (ES) is one of the strongest herbal formulas to treat emotional and psychological disorders. In addition to regulating Liver qi and purging Liver fire, it also calms the *shen* (spirit) and tranquilizes the Heart. Clinically, it is commonly used for patients with severe emotional distress or mild psychological disorders. Furthermore, it can also be used to treat withdrawal signs and symptoms commonly associated with substance addiction.

Long Gu (Os Draconis) and *Mu Li* (Concha Ostreae) are mineral medicinal substances commonly used to anchor the floating *shen* (spirit). They have tranquilizing and sedative effects, which can subdue the hyperactivity of Liver fire. *Gou Teng* (Ramulus Uncariae cum Uncis) treats headache associated with a sudden rise of blood pressure. *Huang*

CALM (ES) ™

Qin (Radix Scutellariae) and *Da Huang* (Radix et Rhizoma Rhei) clear heat and relieve irritability. *Chai Hu* (Radix Bupleuri) disperses stagnant Liver qi and *Dang Gui* (Radicis Angelicae Sinensis) nourishes Liver blood. *Xi Yang Shen* (Radix Panacis Quinquefolii), *Bai Zhu* (Rhizoma Atractylodis Macrocephalae), *Fu Ling* (Poria), *Sheng Jiang* (Rhizoma Zingiberis Recens), and *Da Zao* (Fructus Jujubae) strengthen and harmonize the middle *jiao* and prevent the Liver from overacting on the Spleen. *Gui Zhi* (Ramulus Cinnamomi) and *Chuan Xiong* (Rhizoma Ligustici Chuanxiong) promote qi and blood circulation. *Suan Zao Ren* (Semen Zizyphi Spinosae) and *Xie Cao* (Radix et Rhizoma Valerianae) calm the Heart and nourish the *shen* (spirit). *Gan Cao* (Radix Glycyrrhizae) harmonizes all the herbs in the formula and protects the stomach against harshness of the mineral medicinal substances in this formula.

SUPPLEMENTARY FORMULAS

- For moderate amounts of stress and anxiety or PMS, use **Calm**.
- For stress and anxiety with insomnia in deficiency patients, use **Calm ZZZ**.
- For insomnia arising from blood deficiency, add **Schisandra ZZZ**.
- For menopausal signs, add **Balance (Heat)**.
- For hypertension, add **Gentiana Complex** or **Gastrodia Complex**.
- For headache, add **Corydalin** or **Migratrol**.
- For crying spells or depression, add **Shine**.
- For constipation, combine with **Gentle Lax (Excess)**.
- If the patient has hyperthyroidism, add **Thyrodex**.
- For ADD/ADHD, add **Calm (Jr)**.
- For heartburn or gastric ulcers, add **GI Care**.
- For stress-related irritable bowel syndrome (IBS), add **GI Harmony**.
- For stress-related ulcerative colitis, add **GI Care (UC)**.
- For chronic, stubborn insomnia with blood stagnation, add **Circulation (SJ)**.
- For excess fire in the body, add **Gardenia Complex**.
- For thirst and dryness, add **Nourish (Fluids)**.

NUTRITION

- A diet high in calcium, magnesium, phosphorus, potassium, and vitamins B and E is recommended. These vitamins and minerals are easily depleted by stress.
- Encourage the consumption of fruits and vegetables such as apricots, asparagus, avocados, bananas and broccoli. Brown rice, dried fruit, figs, salmon, garlic, green leafy vegetables, soy products, and yogurt are also recommended.
- Avoid caffeine (coffee, tea, cola, chocolate), tobacco, alcohol and sugar whenever possible.[1]

LIFESTYLE INSTRUCTIONS

- If insomnia is related to work or stress, advised the patients not to work in the bedroom and remove anything that may be a reminder of the office or work. A warm bath or light snack before bedtime may also be helpful.
- Regular exercise, adequate rest, and normal sleep patterns are beneficial for stress reduction.
- Practice meditation exercises at least twice daily.
- Get away from daily routines to do something enjoyable to relieve stress whenever possible.
- Noise can be disturbing to mental health and cause stress. Noise greater than 65-decibels can cause psychological disturbance, greater than 90-decibels can cause emotional and vegetative consequences, and greater than 120-decibels can cause nervous system and hearing damages.

FORMULAS

CALM (ES) ™

CAUTIONS

❧ Patients with a weak digestive system may experience mild gastrointestinal disturbances. In such cases, reduce the dosage or take the herbs with *GI Care* for nausea, and *Gentle Lax (Deficient)* for constipation.

❧ Patients who are on anticoagulant or antiplatelet therapies, such as Coumadin (Warfarin), should use this formula with caution as there may be a slightly higher risk of bleeding and bruising.

❧ This formula is contraindicated during pregnancy and nursing.

CLINICAL NOTE

❧ In addition to using *Calm (ES)*, efforts should be made to identify the underlying cause of illness. Both the symptoms and the cause should be treated concurrently to ensure optimal results.

ACUPUNCTURE POINTS

Traditional Points:

❧ *Yintang* (Extra 1) and *Xingjian* (LR 2).

❧ *Shenmen* (HT 7), *Taichong* (LR 3), *Ganshu* (BL 18), *Baihui* (GV 20), *Xinshu* (BL 15), and *Pishu* (BL 20).

Balance Method by Dr. Richard Tan:

❧ Left side: *Zulinqi* (GB 41), *Yanglingquan* (GB 34), *Shaohai* (HT 3), and *Shenmen* (HT 7).

❧ Right side: *Taichong* (LR 3). *Ququan* (LR 8), *Zhongzhu* (TH 3), and *Tianjing* (TH 10).

❧ *Yintang* (Extra 1) and ear *Shenmen*.

❧ Left and right side can be alternated from treatment to treatment.

❧ For additional information on the Balance Method, please refer to *Dr. Tan's Strategy of Twelve Magical Points* by Dr. Richard Tan.

Ear Points:

❧ Insomnia: Heart, Kidney, and Parietal Lobe. Place magnetic ear balls or embedded ear needles on one or both sides of the ear every evening and remove in the morning. Five days of consecutive therapy equals one treatment course.

❧ Controlling cigarette smoking urges: Mouth, Bronchi, Lung, Pituitary Gland, *Shenmen*, and Subcortex. Switch ears every five days. Instruct the patient to massage the points for 1 to 2 minutes when smoking urges occur.

❧ Psychiatric disorders: *Shenmen*, Heart, Subcortex, Brain Stem. Strongly stimulate the points every other day. Fifteen treatments equal one course. Ear seeds can also be used. Alternate ears every week.

❧ Select six points from the following and needle both ears: Stomach, Adrenal Gland, *Shenmen*, Kidney, Subcortex to Endocrine, Brain Stem, and Heart.

Auricular Acupuncture by Dr. Li-Chun Huang:

❧ Psychosis: Forehead, Nervous Subcortex, Heart, Liver, Shenmen, Occiput, and Anxious. Bleed Ear Apex.
  ▪ For manic type, add Brain Stem
  ▪ For depressive type, add Be Happy

❧ Hysteria: Heart, Liver, *Shenmen*, Brain Stem, Anxious Point, Forehead, and Nervous Subcortex. Bleed Ear Apex.
  ▪ For hysterical paralysis, add Knee Joint, Hip Joint, and Lumbosacral.
  ▪ For hysterical aphasia, add Mouth, Glottis, and *San Jiao*.
  ▪ For hysterical blindness, add Vision 2, Eyes, and Occiput.

❧ Addiction
  ▪ Smoking addiction: Sympathetic, *Shenmen*, Mouth, and Lower Lung.

CALM (ES) ™

- Alcohol addiction: Sympathetic, *Shenmen*, Drunk Point, Liver, Nervous Subcortex, and Anxious Point.
- Drug addiction: Sympathetic, *Shenmen*, Kidney, Liver, Lower Lung, Anxious Point, Nervous Subcortex
- For additional information on the location and explanation of these points, please refer to *Auricular Treatment Formula and Prescriptions* by Dr. Li-Chun Huang.

MODERN RESEARCH

Calm (ES) is formulated based on careful research and includes herbs that have sedative, hypnotic and muscle-relaxant effects. Common applications of *Calm (ES)* include the treatment of stress, anxiety, insomnia, emotional and psychiatric disorders, and addiction.

Xie Cao (Radix et Rhizoma Valerianae) also has a wide range of functions, including but not limited to antispasmodic and sedative/hypnotic properties.[2, 3] In a double-blind crossover study of 128 people, it was found that those who took *Xie Cao* (Radix et Rhizoma Valerianae) had a significant improvement in sleep quality with less awakenings during the night, and less somnolence the next morning.[4] The clinical effects of *Xie Cao* (Radix et Rhizoma Valerianae) are thought to be similar to those of short-acting benzodiazepines.[5]

Calm (ES) is formulated based on a traditional herbal formula that is commonly used to treat stress, anxiety and sleep disorders. Furthermore, clinical trials have proven this formula to be effective in treating such disorders as neurosis, schizophrenia, hysteria, epilepsy, and withdrawal signs and symptoms associated with drug, alcohol and smoking cessation.[6,7,8]

PHARMACEUTICAL DRUGS & CHINESE MEDICINE: A COMPARATIVE ANALYSIS

Stress and anxiety are two of the most common emotional disorders. Clinical signs and symptoms include recurrent and intrusive thoughts, insomnia, disturbed sleep, illusions, hallucinations, difficulty concentrating, hypervigilance, restlessness, anger, and irritability.

Western Medical Approach: Pharmaceutical drug treatment for stress and anxiety focus primarily on use of sedative and hypnotic drugs, such as Valium (Diazepam) and Ativan (Lorazepam). Though these drugs are very potent and have immediate effect to sedate patients, they do not address the underlying conditions. Furthermore, long-term use of these medications are associated with many side effects, including drowsiness, dizziness, tiredness, blurred vision, changes in sex drive or ability, shuffling walk, persistent, fine tremor or inability to sit still, difficulty breathing or swallowing, severe skin rash, yellowing of the skin or eyes, irregular heartbeat, and addiction. Therefore, these drugs should only be used when necessary, and only for a short period of time.

Traditional Chinese Medicine Approach: Use of herbs is extremely effective to treat stress and anxiety. Herbs regulate mood and emotions, and alleviate stress and anxiety by enhancing the body's own ability to deal with these external factors. Unlike drugs that have immediate effect to treat stress and anxiety by "sedating the mind and decreasing its responsiveness," herbs do not have an immediate effect, and require two or more weeks of continuous use to gradually treat these conditions. In contrast, one of the main advantages of herbs is they are safe and natural, and do not have negative side effects like drugs.

Summation: Stress and anxiety are two very common disorders. While drugs and herbs are both effective, they have contrasting differences of benefits and risks. While drugs are more effective for shot-term treatment, herbs are more successful for long-term management. Furthermore, counseling (behavior and psychotherapy) is extremely important toward the understanding of, and complete recovery from, these conditions.

CALM (ES) ™

CASE STUDIES

L.L., a 56-year-old female, presented with frustration, anger and sadness over losing her home in the hurricanes. She was unable to move through these emotions. She was also diagnosed with hypertension, high cholesterol, and post-traumatic stress syndrome recently, and refused to take medications. Her blood pressure was 138/78 mmHg and her heart rate was 82 beats per minute. She also suffered from headaches in the temporal region and the vertex. Other symptoms included twitching of the eyes, agitation, red eyes, and a scalloped tongue with thick yellow tongue coating. TCM diagnoses were damp-heat in the Liver and Gallbladder, Kidney yin deficiency, and excess fire and wind rising. She was prescribed the following formulas: *Calm (ES)* at 1 to 3 capsules, as needed, *Cholisma* at 4 capsules twice daily, and *Gentiana Complex* at 5 capsules twice daily. The patient gained control of her emotions immediately after taking *Calm (ES)*. Blood pressure gradually reduced over time to 120/72 mmHg. The practitioner commented that the combination of these formulas are phenomenal.

M.H., West Palm Beach, Florida

A 49-year-old female social worker presented with stress, anxiety, dizziness and irregular menses. The patient reported occasional irritability, hot flashes, night sweats and dysmenorrhea. Dry eyes and muscle cramps were also present. The patient was diagnosed with Kidney and Liver yin deficiency with Liver qi stagnation. With *Balance (Heat)* and *Calm (ES)*, the patient experienced a reduction of hot flashes and had less irritability, stress, anxiety and dizziness. She also stated that she slept better and her menses were not as painful. The practitioner concluded that *Balance (Heat)* and *Calm (ES)* were an excellent combination for the condition.

D.M., Raton, New Mexico

A 44-year-old female police officer presented with chronic headaches located in the occipital/temporal regions. She stated that stress aggravated the problem. There was acute tenderness at the *Fengchi* (GB 20) area as well as in the cervical spine. She also experienced pain on her zygoma. The practitioner diagnosed the condition as qi and blood stagnation in Gallbladder, Urinary Bladder, and Small Intestine channels in addition to myofascial syndrome, which was stress-induced because of the nature of her job. She was treated with *Corydalin*, *Neck & Shoulder (Acute)* and *Calm (ES)*, which were all so effective that they subsequently replaced her medication, Imitrex (Sumatriptan). The practitioner concluded that a critical aspect in the treatment was to assist the patient in coping with stress, which in turn made the herbal treatment more effective.

S.C., La Crescenta., CA

An 18-year-old female presents with vivid visual hallucinations at night, mainly when going alone from her car to the house. The Western diagnosis was paranoia with visual hallucination; the TCM diagnosis was Liver qi stagnation with *shen* (spirit) disturbance. The practitioner prescribed three capsules of *Calm (ES)*, three times daily for two weeks, and taught the patient to engage in positive visual imagery and mental clarification. After the integrative therapies, the patient reported that her hallucinations and fears had resolved.

C.L., Chino Hills, California

A 40-year-old male presented with severe insomnia, restlessness and hyperactivity. Tongue body appeared red while his pulse felt rapid and wiry. Western assessment of his condition was schizophrenia. TCM diagnosis was Heart fire and Liver fire. Within a week of taking *Calm (ES)*, his sleep time increased from 2 to 3 hours a night to 7 to 8 hours a night. His restlessness and hyperactivity also subsided.

T.G., Albuquerque, New Mexico

FORMULAS

CALM (ES) ™

M.C., a 53-year-old female, presented with anxiety. She was very anxious and fearful of flying. Otherwise healthy, she had to take her son up north to begin college and had to fly, and came to my office for treatment. Her blood pressure was 120/78 mmHg and her heart rate was 76 beats per minute. TCM diagnosis was Liver fire. *Calm (ES)* was prescribed at 4 to 6 capsules before the flight. She reported later that she took 4 capsules 1 hour before her flight, and that her anxiety was under control. She was able to fly out more often to see her son as she felt she could handle the flights when she takes *Calm (ES)*.

M.H., West Palm Beach, Florida

A 53-year-old male miner presented with insomnia, depression, stress, anxiety and fatigue. He had difficulty falling asleep, which was aggravated by relentless worrying. Other symptoms included palpitations and occasional dizziness. A choppy pulse and a pale tongue were present, along with a pale complexion. The practitioner diagnosed the condition as Heart and Spleen blood deficiency. After the initial treatment, his sleep improved from 2 to 3 hours per night to 5 to 6 hours per night. The patient was no longer fatigued and felt much calmer. Because of his occupation and the nature of his condition, he was unable to take the western medication since drowsiness was one side effect. The combination of *Schisandra ZZZ* and *Calm (ES)* made it possible to manage his condition with no known side effects. The practitioner recommended continuous application of the herbal combination of *Schisandra ZZZ* and *Calm (ES)* for his medical condition.

D.M., Raton, New Mexico

A 78-year-old female with a past history of stroke presented with memory loss, insomnia, and nightmares. She was easily frightened and frequently woke up in the middle of the night because of her dreams. Her western medical diagnosis was dementia. TCM diagnosis included qi and blood stagnation, Liver and Kidney yin deficiency, and Heart fire. She was given *Calm (ES)* and *Neuro Plus*. After taking the herbs for approximately one month, the patient was able to recall the practitioner's name for the very first time! In addition, her sleep, mood, complexion, and energy level improved greatly. The patient was much calmer and less irritable. Despite the fact that she still did not know the name of her town or the correct month, there were many improvements in all other areas. The practitioner concluded that the combination of *Calm (ES)* and *Neuro Plus* has enhanced the patient's quality of life.

P.R., Encinitas, California

An 85-year-old retired female presented with excruciating pain in the neck and shoulder that causes difficulty sleeping. Objective findings included limited range of motion of the neck. The tongue had a dirty yellow coat and a red tip. The western diagnosis included psoriatic arthritis, arthritis, fibromyalgia, hiatal hernia, hypertension, depression, chronic constipation, leaky gut syndrome, sciatica and insomnia. The patient was instructed to take *Neck & Shoulder (Acute)* and *Corydalin*, 3 capsules of each three times daily in between meals. *Calm (ES)* was given at night to help sleep. The patient responded that the formulas were effective in reducing the acute pain in the neck and shoulder region. After the acute phase two weeks later, the patient was switched to *Gan Mai Da Zao Tang* (Licorice, Wheat, and Jujube Decoction) and *Shao Yao Gan Cao Tang* (Peony and Licorice Decoction), a combination recommended by Dr. Richard Tan that consistently helped patients with fibromyalgia.

J.B., Camarillo, California

B.B., a 51-year-old female, presented with daily, moderate headaches. She suffered from breast tenderness and a headache that worsened before each period. She also had insomnia and would waken and stay awake for an hour, several times a night. She suffered from irritability that may have arisen from her recent quitting of tobacco smoking. Her tongue was purplish red; her pulse was rapid and wiry. The TCM diagnosis was Liver fire and Liver qi stagnation. *Jia Wei Xiao Yao San* (Augmented Rambling Powder) and *Calm (ES)* were prescribed at 2 grams each, daily. After taking the herbs, the patient reported the breast soreness was gone. Her headache began to diminish, especially after she was past nicotine detox. Irritability was also greatly reduced. The patient continued

CALM (ES) ™

taking the herbs for a year, and noticed that if she stopped taking the herbs, the irritability would return but not the headache or sore breasts. She continues with the formulas at 1 gram per day each, and is very impressed with the results.

C.D., Phoenix, Oregon

[1] Balch, JF. et al. *Prescription for Nutritional Healing*. Avery Publishing Group. 1997

[2] Hazelhoff, B. et al. Antispasmodic effects of valeriana compounds: an in-vivo and in-vitro study on the guinea pig ileum. *Arch Int Pharmacodyn*. 1982; 257:274

[3] Hendriks, H. et al. Central nervous depressant activity of valerenic acid in the mouse. *Planta Med*. (Feb):28. 1985

[4] Leathwood, PD. et al. Aqueous extract of valerian root (valeriana officinalis l.) Improves sleep quality in man. *Pharmacal Biochem Behav*. 1982; 17:65

[5] Von Eickstedt, KW. *Arzneimittelforschung*. 1969; 19:995.

[6] Bensky, D. et al. *Chinese Herbal Medicine Materia Medica*. Eastland Press. 1993

[7] Bensky, D. et al. *Chinese Herbal Medicine Formulas and Strategies*. Eastland Press. 1990

[8] Feng, E. Radix bupleuri added to the os draconis and concha ostreae decoction in the treatment of neuropsychopathies -- a report of 4 cases. *J Tradit Chin Med*. Dec 1994 ; 14(4):243-6

CALM (Jr) ™

CLINICAL APPLICATIONS

- ADD (Attention Deficit Disorder)
- ADHD (Attention Deficit Hyperactivity Disorder)
- Autism
- Hyperactivity, impulsiveness, difficulty in focusing, inattentiveness, restlessness
- Childhood convulsions, epilepsy, seizures and twitching of muscles

WESTERN THERAPEUTIC ACTIONS

- Improves memory and learning abilities [1,2]
- Eliminates toxic substances or allergens which increase the risk of ADD/ADHD [3,4]
- Balances the central nervous system to relieve hyperactivity [5,6,7,8]
- Harmonizes the cardiovascular system [9,10,11,12]
- Regulates the endocrine system [13]

CHINESE THERAPEUTIC ACTIONS

- Extinguishes Liver wind
- Nourishes Liver yin
- Tranquilizes the *shen* (spirit)

DOSAGE

For adults, take 3 to 4 capsules three times daily. For children, please refer to the Strategic Dosing Guidelines section to determine the proper dose based on age. For maximum effect, take the herbs on an empty stomach. The herbs should be taken for 3 months continuously prior to an evaluation on the progress of the individual.

INGREDIENTS

Bai Shao (Radix Paeoniae Alba)
Bie Jia (Carapax Trionycis)
Chuan Xiong (Rhizoma Ligustici Chuanxiong)
Gou Teng (Ramulus Uncariae cum Uncis)
Gui Ban (Plastrum Testudinis)
Jue Ming Zi (Semen Cassiae)
Mai Men Dong (Radix Ophiopogonis)

Mu Li (Concha Ostreae)
Sheng Di Huang (Radix Rehmanniae)
Shi Chang Pu (Rhizoma Acori)
Tai Zi Shen (Radix Pseudostellariae)
Yu Jin (Radix Curcumae)
Yuan Zhi (Radix Polygalae)
Zhi Gan Cao (Radix Glycyrrhizae Preparata)

BACKGROUND

Introduction: ADD/ADHD is a developmental condition in which the affected person is unable to concentrate and is easily distracted, with or without accompanying hyperactivity. Adults or children must have had an onset of symptoms before the age of 7 that caused significant social or academic impairment. More recently, increasing attention has been focused on adult forms of ADHD, which have probably been under-diagnosed.

Pathophysiology: The pathology of ADHD is not clear. Findings indicating that psychostimulants (which facilitate dopamine release) and noradrenergic tricyclics treat this condition have led to speculation that certain areas of the brain related to attention are deficient in neural transmission. The neurotransmitters dopamine and norepinephrine have been associated with ADD/ADHD.

FORMULAS

CALM (Jr) ™

Frequency: The incidence is 3 to 7% in school-age children, and 2 to 7% in adults.

Mortality/Morbidity: There is no clear correlation with mortality in ADD/ADHD. However, studies suggest that childhood ADD/ADHD is a risk factor for subsequent conduct and substance abuse problems, which can carry significant mortality and morbidity. ADD/ADHD may lead to difficulties with academic or employment performance and social difficulties that can profoundly affect normal development. However, exact morbidity has not been established.

Gender Distribution: In children, ADD/ADHD is 3 to 5 times more common in boys than girls. Some studies report incidences as high as 5:1. In adults, the gender ratio is closer to even.

Age: ADD/ADHD is a developmental disorder diagnosis that requires an onset of symptoms before age 7. After childhood, symptoms may persist into adolescence and adulthood, or they may ameliorate or disappear. The percentages in each group are not well established, but at least an estimated 15-20% of children with ADD/ADHD will maintain the full diagnosis in adulthood. Up to 65% of these children will have ADD/ADHD or some residual symptoms of ADD/ADHD as adults.

Treatment: Stimulants such as Ritalin (Methylphenidate) and Dexedrin (Dextroamphetamine), are generally prescribed for treatment of ADD/ADHD. Though they may be effective, there are certain risks involved. Common short-term side effects include significant insomnia, appetite suppression and weight loss, headaches, mood fluctuations (depression, irritability), and these substances can exacerbate tics in children. Long-term risks include possible growth retardation, especially with prolonged use. Furthermore, stimulants such as Ritalin (Methylphenidate) and Dexedrin (Dextroamphetamine) have significant abuse potential and must be used and regulated carefully.

FORMULA EXPLANATION

According to traditional Chinese medicine, ADD/ADHD is diagnosed as Liver wind rising with *shen* (spirit) disturbance arising from Liver yin deficiency. To treat these disorders, both sedative and tonic herbs must be used together to restore normal balance in the body.

To extinguish Liver wind and calm down Liver yang rising (manifesting in muscle twitching or restlessness), *Mu Li* (Concha Ostreae), *Jue Ming Zi* (Semen Cassiae) and *Gou Teng* (Ramulus Uncariae cum Uncis) are used. These three herbs neutralize the mood, addressing the emotional aspects of ADD/ADHD such as irritability, hyperactivity and short temper. *Bie Jia* (Carapax Trionycis) and *Gui Ban* (Plastrum Testudinis) are used to tonify Liver yin and further assist the first three herbs in extinguishing Liver wind. To address yin deficiency, *Bai Shao* (Radix Paeoniae Alba), *Sheng Di Huang* (Radix Rehmanniae) and *Mai Men Dong* (Radix Ophiopogonis) are used. *Bai Shao* (Radix Paeoniae Alba) also softens the Liver to relieve spasms, cramps and stiffness that may be associated with convulsion or seizure. *Mai Men Dong* (Radix Ophiopogonis) also sedates Heart fire to relieve *shen* (spirit) disturbance. *Shi Chang Pu* (Rhizoma Acori) and *Yuan Zhi* (Radix Polygalae) are two aromatic herbs used to disperse phlegm obstructing the orifices and help restore cognitive and sensory functions. They are often used for forgetfulness and inability to concentrate. *Yu Jin* (Radix Curcumae) clears Heart heat, opens orifices and promotes consciousness. *Tai Zi Shen* (Radix Pseudostellariae) is neutral and tonifies both qi and yin. *Chuan Xiong* (Rhizoma Ligustici Chuanxiong) promotes blood circulation and relieves stagnation and pain in the channels that may be caused by the long-term stiffening or twitching of the muscles. *Zhi Gan Cao* (Radix Glycyrrhizae Preparata) nourishes the Heart and harmonizes the entire formula.

CALM (Jr) ™

In short, *Calm (Jr)* is an effective and sophisticated formula with many herbs that address different aspects of ADD/ADHD. Herbs are used to tonify qi to treat the underlying deficiency, calm the *shen* (spirit) to improve focus and concentration, and sedate Liver wind and fire, to reduce hyperactivity.

SUPPLEMENTARY FORMULAS

- With excess heat in the body, add *Gardenia Complex*.
- With anger and/or insomnia, add *Calm (ES)*.
- For stress, add *Calm*.
- For stress and insomnia with underlying deficiency and weakness, add *Calm ZZZ*.
- For depression, add *Shine*.
- With muscle stiffness, cramps and spasms, add *Flex (SC)*.
- With headache, add *Corydalin*.
- With constipation, add *Gentle Lax (Excess)*.
- With fatigue, blood deficiency and excessive worrying or restless sleep, add *Schisandra ZZZ*.
- For Liver and Kidney yin deficiency, add *Nourish*.
- For individuals with constant exposure to toxic substances, add *Herbal DTX*.
- For poor memory or forgetfulness caused by Kidney deficiency, use *Enhance Memory*.
- With blood stagnation, add *Circulation (SJ)*.

NUTRITION

- Avoid exposure to toxic substances, food additives or coloring, or allergens, which increase the risk of developing ADD/ADHD.
- Make sure the diet has an adequate amount of calcium and magnesium, which have a calming effect.
- Cold-water fish, such as tuna, salmon, and herring, are great sources of docosahexaenoic acid (DHA). This essential fatty acid is vital for proper development of the brain.
- Increase consumption of complex carbohydrates, such as fresh vegetables, fresh fruits, beans, and whole grains. Decrease consumption of simple carbohydrates, such as glucose, fructose, sugars, and processed grains.
- Eliminate from the diet: sugar, candy, junk food, foods with artificial color and flavor, and fried foods. Also avoid antacids, cough drops, throat lozenges, and carbonated beverages.
- Limit exposure to television, video games, and loud music. Encourage reading and outdoor activities.

LIFESTYLE INSTRUCTIONS

- Psychosocial support is extremely important for complete and long-term treatment of ADD/ADHD. Such approaches include contingency management (e.g., reward and timeout systems), parent training (educating the parent on child management skills), clinical behavior therapy (coordinated contingency management by both parents and teachers), and cognitive-behavioral treatment (e.g., self-monitoring, verbal self-instruction, problem-solving strategies, self-reinforcement).

CLINICAL NOTES

- It has been proposed that the environment is one of the major factors contributing to the cause of ADD/ADHD. In utero exposures to toxic substances, food additives or colorings, or allergens may increase the risk of the disorder. Environmental factors, such as diet, education and media influences (such as television), may also influence behavior in children.

FORMULAS

CALM (Jr) ™

- Proper treatment of ADD/ADHD is important to ensure proper academic performance, vocational success, and social-emotional development. Lack of or delayed treatment may contribute to incomplete development of such skills.
- There is great controversy on whether children with ADD/ADHD should receive drug treatment because of the possible risks and side effects. Herbs are a safe alternative as they restore the natural balance in the body without being addictive.
- It is important to educate and/or treat the parents who are over-anxious about the academic achievements of their children. If necessary, *Calm* or *Calm (ES)* can be used to calm the *shen* (spirit) of the parents.
- This formula should be used as needed during school. However, use of this formula is not necessary during vacations, such as summer and winter vacations.

CAUTIONS

- This formula is contraindicated in individuals with yang deficiency or coldness.
- This formula should be discontinued once the condition is stabilized, or when the desired effects are achieved.
- This formula is contraindicated during pregnancy and nursing.

ACUPUNCTURE POINTS

Traditional Points:
- *Baihui* (GV 20) and *Si Shen Cong*.
- *Neiguan* (PC 6), *Taichong* (LR 3), *Dazhui* (GV 14), *Quchi* (LI 11), *Baihui* (GV 20), *Mingmen* (GV 4), and *Daling* (PC 7).

Balance Method by Dr. Richard Tan:
- Left side: *Taichong* (LR 3), *Ligou* (LR 5), *Ququan* (LR 8), *Houxi* (SI 3), and Ear *Shenmen*.
- Right side: *Qiuxu* (GB 40), *Yanglingquan* (GB 34), and *Shenmen* (HT 7).
- Left and right side can be alternated from treatment to treatment.
- For additional information on the Balance Method, please refer to *Dr. Tan's Strategy of Twelve Magical Points* by Dr. Richard Tan.

Auricular Acupuncture by Dr. Li-Chun Huang:
- Epilepsy: Epilepsy Point, Brain, Brain Stem, Nervous Subcortex, Occiput, *Shenmen*, Kidney, and Liver.

MODERN RESEARCH

Calm (Jr) is an herbal formula developed by Dr. Feng Bu-Zhen, a master of traditional Chinese medicine in Shanxi, China. *Calm (Jr)* contains herbs that nourish yin, regenerate pulse, calm wind, and sedate fire. From a western perspective, such herbs improve memory and reduce hyperactivity.

In general, Chinese herbs have been used with excellent success for treatment of ADD/ADHD. Most of the herbs that show promising effects include ones that calm the *shen* (spirit), control Liver wind, and sedate Liver fire. Pharmacologically, utilization of the herbs has shown to improve memory and treat mental retardation. In one laboratory study, administration of *Shi Chang Pu* (Rhizoma Acori) is associated with a dose-dependent effect in improving memory. [1] Furthermore, in one clinical trial, 30 children with low IQ were treated, resulting in mild to moderate improvement in classroom performance using an herbal formula containing such herbs as *Shi Chang Pu* (Rhizoma Acori) and *Yuan Zhi* (Radix Polygalae). The treatment protocol was to administer the formula twice daily for two weeks per course of treatment, for a total of three months of treatment. [2]

CALM (Jr) ™

Since exposure to toxic substances, food additives or colorings has been proposed by the Merck Manual as one of the main causes of ADD/ADHD, the importance of eliminating environmental toxins cannot be over-emphasized. In *Calm (Jr)*, herbs are added to specifically protect the liver and improve the detoxification of environmental toxins. *Zhi Gan Cao* (Radix Glycyrrhizae Preparata) has been used successfully for thousands of years for detoxification. More recently, it has been documented that *Zhi Gan Cao* (Radix Glycyrrhizae Preparata) has a marked detoxifying effect to treat a variety of poisonings, including but not limited to drug poisoning (chloral hydrate, urethane, cocaine, picrotoxin, caffeine, pilocarpine, nicotine, barbiturates, mercury and lead), food poisoning (tetrodotoxin, snake, and mushrooms), and others (enterotoxin, herbicides, pesticides). [3] Furthermore, *Zhi Gan Cao* (Radix Glycyrrhizae Preparata) and *Yu Jin* (Radix Curcumae) have also been shown to have hepatoprotective effects against chemical- or tetrachloride-induced liver damage and liver cancer. [4]

Since ADD/ADHD is characterized by an imbalance of neurotransmitters leading to a disharmony of the entire body, herbs that harmonize and balance the entire body have been used for treatment with good success. *Mai Men Dong* (Radix Ophiopogonis), *Bai Shao* (Radix Paeoniae Alba), *Shi Chang Pu* (Rhizoma Acori) and *Chuan Xiong* (Rhizoma Ligustici Chuanxiong) balance the central nervous system and calm hyperactivity. They have been used to effectively reverse drug-induced excitation.[5,6,7,8] *Mai Men Dong* (Radix Ophiopogonis), *Bai Shao* (Radix Paeoniae Alba) and *Chuan Xiong* (Rhizoma Ligustici Chuanxiong) harmonize the cardiovascular system and minimize the fluctuation of heart rate and blood pressure. [9,10,11,12] *Sheng Di Huang* (Radix Rehmanniae) regulates the endocrine system to ensure normal production and release of endogenous hormones.[13]

In summary, *Calm (Jr)* treats ADD/ADHD by improving memory and learning ability, relieving hyperactivity, and balancing the entire body. The effects of the formula have been documented with clinical trials, and the functions of the individual herbs have been shown by numerous clinical studies.

PHARMACEUTICAL DRUGS & CHINESE MEDICINE: A COMPARATIVE ANALYSIS

ADD/ADHD is a developmental condition in which the affected person is unable to concentrate and is easily distracted, with or without accompanying hyperactivity.

Western Medical Approach: Stimulants such as Ritalin (Methylphenidate) and Dexedrin (Dextroamphetamine) are generally prescribed for treatment of ADD/ADHD. Though they may be effective, there are certain risks involved. Common short-term side effects include significant insomnia, appetite suppression and weight loss, headaches, mood fluctuations (depression, irritability), and exacerbation of tics in children. Long-term risks include possible growth retardation, especially with prolonged use. Furthermore, stimulants such as Ritalin (Methylphenidate) and Dexedrin (Dextroamphetamine) have significant abuse potentials and must be used and regulated carefully.

Traditional Chinese Medicine Approach: From traditional Chinese medicine perspectives, ADD and ADHD are characterized by Liver wind rising with *shen* (spirit) disturbance arising from Liver yin deficiency. Therefore, herbs calm the mind and nourish the underlying deficiencies. Many herbs in this formula have been shown via *in vitro* and *in vivo* studies to be effective to enhance concentration and memory. Furthermore, these herbs are safe and natural, and do not have the harsh side effects of drugs.

Summation: it is important to realize that though drugs may be effective, they have serious short- and long-term side effects. Furthermore, these drugs have significant abuse potentials, and their use must be monitored carefully. On the other hand, use of herbs is not only effective to improve focus and attention, they also improve memory and learning ability. Furthermore, herbs are much safer than drugs, both for short- and long-term uses. Lastly, practitioners and parents must both recognize that optimal treatment of ADD and ADHD requires more than just taking drugs or herbs, it also requires dietary, environmental and behavior changes. Combination of all these modalities ensures long-term success.

FORMULAS

CALM (Jr) ™

CASE STUDIES

J.S., a 9-year-old male, presented with inability to complete tasks, inability to focus on school work, irritability and restlessness. He was easily angered and also had insomnia. He was skinny and had a pale complexion and dark circles under his eyes. Western diagnosis was ADHD. The TCM diagnosis was Liver wind rising, Liver yin deficiency, *shen* (spirit) disturbance. *Calm (Jr)* was prescribed, and he showed great improvement in his ability to stay on tasks, with less irritability and fewer outbursts of anger. Sleep also improved. This patient continued to eat a diet high in simple carbohydrates and fats. His parents have not reached a point where they are willing to consider dietary changes. However, with *Calm (Jr)* and acupuncture, the child is improving.

J.S., Milwaukee, OR

Calm (Jr) is commonly used in China to reduce hyperactivity, improve memory and increase attention span. According to one clinical trial published in *Shanxi Medicine and Herbology* in 1990, children with ADD/ADHD were treated daily for 1 month with herbs in *Calm (Jr)*. At the end of the clinical trial, it was reported that out of 68 children, 61 showed no presentation of ADD/ADHD, 3 showed some improvement, and 4 had no response. No side effects were reported.

B.F., Shanxi, China

S.A., a 5-year-old female, was diagnosed with her first seizure attack on May 2, 2002 and spent two days in the hospital. She was put on Tegretol (Carbamazepine). Shortly after beginning the medication, the child started to have stomachaches and was not her usual self. The mother thought the seizure might have been caused by immunization shots the child had received earlier. The TCM diagnosis was Liver wind. While taking *Calm (Jr)*, the child was able to decrease the dosage of Tegretol (Carbamazepine). The mother noticed the seizures diminishing in frequency and intensity. The child was able to endure the seizures in a more relaxed manner. The patient also received cranio-sacral therapy.

M.C., Sarasota, Florida

[1] *Zhong Cao Yao* (Chinese Herbal Medicine), 1992; 23(8):417
[2] *Zhong Cheng Yao Yan Jiu* (Research of Chinese Patent Medicine), 1982; 6:22
[3] *Zhong Yao Tong Bao* (Journal of Chinese Herbology), 1986; 11(10):55
[4] *Zhong Guo Mian Yi Xue Za Zhi* (Chinese Journal of Immunology), 1989; 5(2):121
[5] *Guang Zhou Zhong Yi Xue Yuan Xue Bao* (Journal of Guangzhou University of Chinese Medicine), 1986; (23):29
[6] *Zhong Yao Tong Bao* (Journal of Chinese Herbology), 1985; 10(6):43
[7] *Zhong Yao Yao Li Yu Ying Yong* (Pharmacology and Applications of Chinese Herbs), 1983; 477
[8] *Zhong Yao Yao Li Yu Ying Yong* (Pharmacology and Applications of Chinese Herbs), 1983; 123
[9] *Zhong Yao Yao Li Yu Ying Yong* (Pharmacology and Applications of Chinese Herbs); 1983; 35
[10] *Hua Xi Yao Xue Za Zhi* (Huaxi Herbal Journal), 1991; 6(1):13
[11] *Zhong Guo Yao Li Xue Tong Bao* (Journal of Chinese Herbal Pharmacology), 1986; 2(5):26
[12] *Zhong Yao Yao Li Yu Ying Yong* (Pharmacology and Applications of Chinese Herbs), 1989; (2):40
[13] *Zhong Yao Xue* (Chinese Herbology), 1998; 156:158

CALM ZZZ ™

CLINICAL APPLICATIONS

- ☙ Patients with underlying deficiency who suffer from chronic and constant stress, irritability, anxiety and emotional instability
- ☙ Insomnia with difficulty falling or staying asleep in patients who are stressed or have things on their minds
- ☙ Type "A" personality with excessive competitive drive, impatience, sense of urgency without the body strength and constitution to cope with their stress

WESTERN THERAPEUTIC ACTIONS

- ☙ Anxiolytic effect to relieve stress and anxiety
- ☙ Sedative and hypnotic effect to treat insomnia
- ☙ Muscle-relaxant effect to alleviate tension and stiffness

CHINESE THERAPEUTIC ACTIONS

- ☙ Calms the *shen* (spirit)
- ☙ Regulates Liver qi
- ☙ Sedates Liver fire
- ☙ Tonifies the deficiencies

DOSAGE

Take 3 to 4 capsules three times daily for stress, anxiety, emotional instability and similar mental disorders. For insomnia, another dose may be taken 30 minutes before bedtime. This formula is safe for long-term use.

INGREDIENTS

Bai Shao (Radix Paeoniae Alba)
Chai Hu (Radix Bupleuri)
Da Zao (Fructus Jujubae)
Deng Xin Cao (Medulla Junci)
Fu Shen (Poria Paradicis)
Gan Cao (Radix Glycyrrhizae)
Gou Teng (Ramulus Uncariae cum Uncis)

He Huan Hua (Flos Albiziae)
Suan Zao Ren (Semen Zizyphi Spinosae)
Xiang Fu (Rhizoma Cyperi)
Xiao Mai (Fructus Tritici)
Ye Jiao Teng (Caulis Polygoni Multiflori)
Zhi Mu (Radix Anemarrhenae)

FORMULA EXPLANATION

Calm ZZZ is designed to treat individuals who are under constant stress but also have a deficient constitution. This is one of the best formulas to treat *shen* (spirit) disturbance both during the day and at night. *Shen* (spirit) disturbance during the day can manifest as stress, anxiety and emotional instability. *Shen* (spirit) disturbance at night manifests as insomnia with difficulty falling asleep and/or staying asleep. Many of these patients will also have underlying deficiencies, as a result of Liver excess consuming yin and body fluids on a long-term basis. Therefore, optimal treatment requires use of herbs to calm the *shen* (spirit), regulate Liver qi, sedate Liver fire, and tonify the deficiencies.

In this formula, *Chai Hu* (Radix Bupleuri) and *Xiang Fu* (Rhizoma Cyperi) are used to regulate qi circulation and relieve Liver qi stagnation. *Gou Teng* (Ramulus Uncariae cum Uncis) calms Liver yang, *Deng Xin Cao* (Medulla Junci) sedates Heart fire, and *Zhi Mu* (Radix Anemarrhenae) clears deficiency fire. These three herbs treat the excess aspects of *shen* (spirit) disturbance and relieve irritability.

CALM ZZZ ™

In addition, *Bai Shao* (Radix Paeoniae Alba), *Fu Shen* (Poria Paradicis), *Suan Zao Ren* (Semen Zizyphi Spinosae), *He Huan Hua* (Flos Albiziae), and *Ye Jiao Teng* (Caulis Polygoni Multiflori) calm the *shen* (spirit) and relieve stress and anxiety by nourishing the Heart. *Xiao Mai* (Fructus Tritici), *Gan Cao* (Radix Glycyrrhizae) and *Da Zao* (Fructus Jujubae) calm the *shen* (spirit) and control emotional instability and prevent the drastic shifting of moods. Together, these eight herbs address the deficiency aspects of *shen* (spirit) disturbance.

In short, *Calm ZZZ* uses an integrative approach to treat both the excess and deficient aspects of *shen* (spirit) disturbance. Clinical applications include stress, anxiety, emotional or mental disorders, and insomnia.

SUPPLEMENTARY FORMULAS

- For mild to moderate cases of stress and anxiety, combine with *Calm*.
- For moderate to severe cases of stress and anxiety, combine with *Calm (ES)*.
- For severe cases of insomnia, combine with *Schisandra ZZZ*.
- For headache, add *Corydalin* or *Migratrol*.
- For heartburn or gastric ulcers, add *GI Care*.
- For depression, add *Shine*.
- For constipation, combine with *Gentle Lax (Deficient)*.
- For irritable bowel syndrome (IBS) due to stress, add *GI Harmony*.
- For ulcerative colitis due to stress, add *GI Care (UC)*.
- For menopausal symptoms, combine with *Balance (Heat)*.
- For forgetfulness, add *Enhance Memory*.
- For hypertension, combine with *Gastrodia Complex* or *Gentiana Complex*.
- To tonify the overall body constitution, combine with *Imperial Tonic*.

NUTRITION

- A diet high in calcium, magnesium, phosphorus, potassium, and vitamins B and E is recommended. These vitamins and minerals are easily depleted by stress.
- Encourage the consumption of fruits and vegetables such as apricots, wintermelon, asparagus, avocados, bananas and broccoli in addition to brown rice, dried fruit, figs, salmon, garlic, green leafy vegetables, soy products, and yogurt.
- Avoid caffeine (coffee, tea, cola, chocolate), tobacco, alcohol and sugar whenever possible.
- Advise the patient to avoid foods that contain tyramine near bedtime. Tyramine increases the release of the brain stimulant norepinephrine. Food with high content of tyramine include bacon, cheese, chocolate, eggplant, ham, potatoes, sugar, sausage, spinach, and tomatoes.
- A glass of warm milk with honey before bedtime is helpful for mild insomnia.

LIFESTYLE INSTRUCTIONS

- Regular exercise, adequate rest, and normal sleep patterns are beneficial for stress reduction.
- Practice meditation exercises at least twice daily.
- Get away from the daily routine to do something different and enjoyable to relieve stress whenever possible.
- Noise can be disturbing to mental health and cause stress.
- If insomnia is due to overwork, do not to work in the bedroom, and remove anything that may be a reminder of the office or work. A warm bath or light snack before bedtime may also be helpful.
- Advise the patients not worry and to do their best to prepare for upcoming events they know may be stressful. Try to ask for help from friends, family and colleagues when stress in life becomes intolerable.
- Shift outlook on life and look at changes in a positive way and as challenges, rather than threats.

CALM ZZZ ™

CLINICAL NOTES

☾ *Calm ZZZ* is an excellent formula to treat insomnia associated with stress and anxiety. However, it will generally take a few days before this formula nourishes the underlying deficiency and restores the normal sleeping patterns accordingly.

CAUTIONS

☾ This herbal formula may cause drowsiness in individuals who are sensitive to herbs. Patients are advised not to drive or operate heavy machinery while taking this herbal formula. Similarly, alcohol is not recommended as it may intensify the effect.

☾ *Calm ZZZ* is *not* to be used as "sleeping pills." Do *not* ingest a large amount of this formula, as this will only increase the risk of potential side effects.

ACUPUNCTURE POINTS

Traditional Points:
☾ *Shenmen* (HT 7), *Sanyinjiao* (SP 6), *Ganshu* (BL 18), *Danshu* (BL 19), *Wangu* (GB 12), *Anmian*, *Yintang*, and ear *Shenmen*.

Balance Method by Dr. Richard Tan:
☾ Left side: *Zulinqi* (GB 41), *Yanglingquan* (GB 34), *Shaohai* (HT 3), and *Shenmen* (HT 7).
☾ Right side: *Taichong* (LR 3), *Ququan* (LR 8), *Zhongzhu* (TH 3), and *Tianjing* (TH 10).
☾ Left and right side can be alternated from treatment to treatment.
☾ For additional information on the Balance Method, please refer to *Dr. Tan's Strategy of Twelve Magical Points* by Dr. Richard Tan.

Ear Points:
☾ *Shenmen*

MODERN RESEARCH

Calm ZZZ is an excellent formula to treat both the emotional and physical aspects of mental and psychological disorders. Pharmacological effects of this formula include anxiolytic effect to relieve stress and anxiety, sedative and hypnotic effects to treat insomnia, and muscle-relaxant effects to relieve tension and stiffness. Clinical applications include stress, anxiety, neurasthenia, hysteria, and insomnia.

Many herbs in this formula have marked sedative and hypnotic effects, which is one of the many proposed mechanisms of action for treating stress, anxiety and insomnia. For example, *Chai Hu* (Radix Bupleuri) and its saikosaponin both have sedative effect to prolong sleeping time.[1] *Suan Zao Ren* (Semen Zizyphi Spinosae) has marked sedative and hypnotic effects,[2] and has been shown to effectively treat insomnia.[3,4] Other herbs with similar sedative and hypnotic effects include *Bai Shao* (Radix Paeoniae Alba),[5] *Xiang Fu* (Rhizoma Cyperi),[6] and *Gou Teng* (Ramulus Uncariae cum Uncis).[7]

Bai Shao (Radix Paeoniae Alba) and *Gan Cao* (Radix Glycyrrhizae) are two herbs that have excellent muscle-relaxant effects.[8,9] They help to relieve muscle tension and stiffness, which often occur as a result of prolonged stress, anxiety and insomnia.

Gan Cao (Radix Glycyrrhizae), *Xiao Mai* (Fructus Tritici) and *Da Zao* (Fructus Jujubae) are the three principle herbs in this formula. Together, these three herbs have been shown to have excellent anxiolytic effect to treat

FORMULAS

disorders such as neurasthenia, hysteria, and insomnia. For neurasthenia, use of *Gan Cao* (Radix Glycyrrhizae), *Xiao Mai* (Fructus Tritici), *Da Zao* (Fructus Jujubae) and others was shown to effectively treat 92 out of 100 patients.[10] For hysteria, concurrent use of acupuncture and these herbs effectively stabilized the condition and resolved clinical signs and symptoms in all 60 patients, with no recurrence in follow-up visits 6 months after the conclusion of treatments.[11] For insomnia, use of *Gan Cao* (Radix Glycyrrhizae), *Xiao Mai* (Fructus Tritici), *Da Zao* (Fructus Jujubae) and others was associated with a 74.2% overall rate of effectiveness in 110 patients.[12]

In conclusion, **Calm ZZZ** is an excellent formula that treats both the emotional and physical aspects of mental and psychological disorders. Treatment of the emotional aspects of mental disorder includes use of herbs with anxiolytic effect to relieve stress and anxiety, and sedative and hypnotic effects to treat insomnia. Furthermore, treatment of the physical aspects of mental disorder includes use of herbs with muscle-relaxant effects to relieve tension and stiffness.

PHARMACEUTICAL DRUGS & CHINESE MEDICINE: A COMPARATIVE ANALYSIS

Stress, anxiety and insomnia are three conditions that often contribute to and aggravate each others. Clinical signs and symptoms include intrusive thoughts, illusions, hallucinations, difficulty concentrating, hypervigilance, restlessness, anger, irritability, and inability to fall and/or stay asleep.

Western Medical Approach: Pharmaceutical drug treatment for stress, anxiety and insomnia focus primarily on use of benzodiazepines such as Valium (Diazepam), Ativan (Lorazepam), Halcion (triazolam), Restoril (temazepam), and Dalmane (flurazepam). Though these drugs are very potent and have immediate effect to sedate patients, they do not address the underlying conditions. Furthermore, long-term use of these medications are associated with many side effects, including drowsiness, dizziness, tiredness, blurred vision, changes in sex drive or ability, shuffling walk, persistent, fine tremor or inability to sit still, difficulty breathing or swallowing, severe skin rash, yellowing of the skin or eyes, irregular heartbeat, and addiction. Therefore, these drugs should only be used when necessary, and only for a short period of time.

Traditional Chinese Medicine Approach: Use of herbs is extremely effective to treat stress, anxiety and insomnia. Herbs regulate mood and emotions, and alleviate stress and anxiety by enhancing the body's own ability to deal with these external factors. Furthermore, many herbs calm the *shen* (spirit), and help to restore normal sleeping patterns. Unlike benzodiazepine drugs that have immediate and potent sedative effects, herbs are moderate in potency, and may require 1 to 2 weeks to relieve stress, anxiety and insomnia. In contrast, one of the main advantages of herbs is they are safe and natural, and do not have negative side effects like drugs.

Summation: Stress, anxiety and insomnia are very common disorders. While drugs and herbs are both effective, they have contrasting differences of benefits and risks. While drugs are more effective for shot-term treatment, herbs are more successful for long-term management. Furthermore, counseling (behavior and psychotherapy) is extremely important toward the understanding of, and complete recovery from, these conditions.

[1] *Zhong Yao Yao Li Yu Ying Yong* (Pharmacology and Applications of Chinese Herbs), 1983; 888
[2] *Chang Yong Zhong Yao Xian Dai Yan Jiu Yu Lin Chuan* (Recent Study & Clinical Application of Common Traditional Chinese Medicine), 1995; 489:491
[3] *Xin Zhong Yi* (New Chinese Medicine), 1982; (11):35
[4] *Shang Hai Zhong Yi Yao Za Zhi* (Shanghai Journal of Chinese Medicine and Herbology), 1984; (10):30
[5] *Zhong Yao Tong Bao* (Journal of Chinese Herbology), 1985; 10(6):43
[6] *Zhong Guo Yao Ke Da Xue Xue Bao* (Journal of University of Chinese Herbology), 1989; 20(1):48
[7] *Zhong Yao Yao Li Yu Ying Yong* (Pharmacology and Applications of Chinese Herbs), 1983; 786
[8] *Guo Wai Yi Xue* (Foreign Medicine), 1984; 6(1):58
[9] *He Nan Zhong Yi* (Henan Chinese Medicine), 1986; (6):15
[10] *Jiang Su Yi Yao* (Jiangsu Journal of Medicine and Herbology), 1976; 1:47
[11] *Shan Dong Zhong Yi Za Zhi* (Shandong Journal of Chinese Medicine), 1994; 5:237
[12] *Zhe Jiang Zhong Yi Za Zhi* (Zhejiang Journal of Chinese Medicine), 1982; 9:412

CHOLISMA ™

CLINICAL APPLICATIONS

☯ High cholesterol level
☯ High triglycerides level
☯ Hypertension with arteriosclerosis and atherosclerosis

WESTERN THERAPEUTIC ACTIONS

☯ Antihyperlipidemic effect to reduce plasma levels of cholesterol and triglycerides[1,2,3,4,7,8]
☯ Reduces absorption of fatty food and enhances breakdown of fatty tissues[6,13]
☯ Lowers serum glucose level and reduces synthesis of cholesterol and triglycerides[4,6,14]
☯ Diuretic effect to reduce blood pressure[2,3]

CHINESE THERAPEUTIC ACTIONS

☯ Dissolves dampness and eliminates phlegm
☯ Invigorates the circulation of blood

DOSAGE

Take 3 to 4 capsules three times daily on an empty stomach. For maximum effectiveness, take the last dose one hour prior to bedtime, as synthesis of cholesterol is most active at night. Maintenance dose is 1 to 2 capsules a day.

INGREDIENTS

Cang Zhu (Rhizoma Atractylodis)
Dan Shen (Radix Salviae Miltiorrhizae)
Ge Gen (Radix Puerariae)
He Shou Wu (Radix Polygoni Multiflori)
He Ye (Folium Nelumbinis)
Hu Zhang (Rhizoma Polygoni Cuspidati)
Jiao Gu Lan (Rhizoma seu Herba Gynostemmatis)

Ju Hua (Flos Chrysanthemi)
Jue Ming Zi (Semen Cassiae)
Shan Zha (Fructus Crataegi)
Yi Yi Ren (Semen Coicis)
Ze Xie (Rhizoma Alismatis)
Zi Mu Xu (Herba Medicago Sativa)

FORMULA EXPLANATION

According to traditional Chinese medicine, cholesterol is considered as an excess deposit of dampness and phlegm in the blood vessels. To effectively reduce plasma levels of cholesterol and triglycerides, treatment must focus on dissolving damp, eliminating phlegm, and invigorating blood circulation.

To dissolve dampness, diuretic and digestive herbs are used. *Shan Zha* (Fructus Crataegi) is the primary digestive herb used to break down animal fat. It has been found to be effective in lowering serum cholesterol and blood pressure. *Ze Xie* (Rhizoma Alismatis) and *Yi Yi Ren* (Semen Coicis) are two diuretic herbs that have actions similar to choline and lecithin to lower blood sugar and cholesterol. *Jue Ming Zi* (Semen Cassiae) and *He Ye* (Folium Nelumbinis), *Ju Hua* (Flos Chrysanthemi) and *Jiao Gu Lan* (Rhizoma seu Herba Gynostemmatis) clear damp-heat, lower serum cholesterol and blood pressure. *He Shou Wu* (Radix Polygoni Multiflori) is a unique herb that tonifies Kidney *jing* (essence) and reduces cholesterol and triglycerides at the same time. With its aromatic property, *Cang Zhu* (Rhizoma Atractylodis) dries up dampness and eliminates phlegm. *Dan Shen* (Radix Salviae Miltiorrhizae) invigorates blood circulation, improves microcirculation, inhibits coagulation of blood, and lowers blood cholesterol. *Hu Zhang* (Rhizoma Polygoni Cuspidati) detoxifies the Liver and lowers the cholesterol. *Ge Gen* (Radix

---

CHOLISMA ™

Puerariae) dilates blood vessels to lower blood pressure. *Zi Mu Xu* (Herba Medicago Sativa) may reduce cholesterol absorption from food and atherosclerotic formation.

SUPPLEMENTARY FORMULAS

- For obese patients with an excess appetite, add *Herbalite*.
- For fatty liver and obesity, use *Cholisma (ES)*.
- For diabetes mellitus and high blood glucose, add *Equilibrium*.
- For hypertension with dizziness or vertigo, combine with *Gastrodia Complex*.
- For hypertension with anger or flushed face, combine with *Gentiana Complex*.
- For edema, add *Herbal DRX*.
- For excess heat in the body, add *Gardenia Complex*.
- For excessive blood stagnation in the body, add *Circulation (SJ)*.
- For coronary heart disorders, add *Circulation*.

NUTRITION

- Increase the daily intake of cholesterol-lowering foods such as apples, bananas, carrots, cold-water fish, dried beans, garlic, grapefruit, olive oil, and fibers such as bran and oats.
- Increase the intake of niacin, which can lower total cholesterol levels by up to 18%, increase HDL cholesterol by up to 32%, and lower triglycerides by up to 26%. Do not overdose on niacin to avoid flushing and stomach pain.
- Other supplements that are beneficial are vitamin B5, vitamin C, vitamin E, chromium picolinate, lecithin, and coenzyme Q10.
- Decrease the intake of food that will raise cholesterol levels, including but not limited to beer, wine, cheese, tobacco products, aged and cured meats, sugar, and greasy or fried foods.
- Increase the intake of vinegar, as it will help to soften the blood vessels and prevent atherosclerosis.

LIFESTYLE INSTRUCTIONS

- Exercise is the best way to decrease the buildup of cholesterol in the arteries. It also helps to reduce weight.
- Drink tea on a daily basis, especially after meals, to facilitate the elimination of fatty foods from the diet. Beneficial teas include black, *oolong* or green tea.
- Avoid the use of alcohol and exposure to tobacco. They increase cholesterol buildup and hardening of the arteries.

CLINICAL NOTES

- Hyperlipidemia is a disorder of lipoprotein metabolism and not a cardiovascular malfunction. It may lead to various cardiovascular disorders such as arteriosclerosis, coronary artery disease, hypertension, angina pectoris, etc. Optimal treatment must address both the cause and the symptoms. *See* Supplementary Formulas for more details.
- The baseline cholesterol level should be established prior to the initiation of herbal therapy; and the first follow-up test should be done one month after the initiation of herbal therapy. Subsequent follow-ups can be done every 2 to 3 months to determine overall effectiveness. Cholesterol testing kits are available over-the-counter in most pharmacies. Results may vary from patient to patient. Lifestyle and dietary changes are also crucial for satisfactory results.
- *Cholisma* is specifically formulated to reduce blood cholesterol and triglyceride levels. Patients must take this herbal formula on a long-term basis for maximum results.

CHOLISMA ™

Pulse Diagnosis by Dr. Jimmy Wei-Yen Chang:
- Deep and forceful on all positions.
- Note: Dr. Chang takes the pulse in slightly different positions. He places his index finger directly over the wrist crease, and his middle and ring fingers alongside to locate *cun*, *guan* and *chi* positions. For additional information and explanation, please refer to *Pulsynergy* by Dr. Jimmy Wei-Yen Chang and Marcus Brinkman.

CAUTIONS

- *Dan Shen* (Radix Salviae Miltiorrhizae) may enhance the overall effectiveness of Coumadin (Warfarin), an anticoagulant drug. Patients who take anticoagulant or antiplatelet medications should ***not*** take this herbal formula without supervision by a licensed health care practitioner.
- *Jue Ming Zi* (Semen Cassiae), *He Shou Wu* (Radix Polygoni Multiflori) and *Ju Hua* (Flos Chrysanthemi) may cause loose stool or diarrhea for those with sensitive gastro-intestinal tracts. Should this occur, reduce the dosage to 2 to 3 capsules three times daily.
- Hypertension should also be suspected if the patient has high cholesterol. Treat both hypertension and hyperlipidemia simultaneously for maximum results.

ACUPUNCTURE POINTS

Traditional Points:
- Bleed *Weizhong* (BL 40) or wherever there is dilated visible vein in the area of the transverse crease of the popliteal fossa.
- *Taichong* (LR 3), *Xingjian* (LR 2), *Zusanli* (ST 36), *Quchi* (LI 11), and *Fenglong* (ST 40)

Balance Method by Dr. Richard Tan:
- Left side: *Yinlingquan* (SP 9), *Xuehai* (SP 10), and *Waiguan* (TH 5).
- Right side: *Zusanli* (ST 36), *Fenglong* (ST 40), *Daling* (PC 7), and *Laogong* (PC 8).
- Alternate sides from treatment to treatment.
- For additional information on the Balance Method, please refer to *Dr. Tan's Strategy of Twelve Magical Points* by Dr. Richard Tan.

MODERN RESEARCH

Cholisma is formulated with both Chinese and Western herbs which have been proven to reduce cholesterol and/or triglyceride levels. All the herbs work synergistically to reduce blood cholesterol and triglycerides levels by reducing the absorption of fatty food, enhancing the breakdown of fatty tissue and decreasing the synthesis of cholesterol.

Ze Xie (Rhizoma Alismatis) is historically used as a diuretic herb. It was noted recently that in addition to resolving dampness and promoting diuresis, *Ze Xie* (Rhizoma Alismatis) has an excellent function to lower serum lipids and cholesterol levels, as demonstrated through various clinical trials.[1,2,3]

Shan Zha (Fructus Crataegi) offers cardio-protective functions by increasing coronary circulation and lowering blood triglycerides, cholesterol and blood sugar levels.[4,5] *Shan Zha* (Fructus Crataegi) has been shown to exert these effects through various mechanisms of action: enhancement in LDL-receptor activity and increasing hepatic breakdown of cholesterol while decreasing its synthesis.[6] In a study of 130 patients on the treatment of hyperlipidemia, an herbal formulation with *Shan Zha* (Fructus Crataegi) and other herbs lowered serum cholesterol and triglycerides in 87% and 80.8% of the patients, respectively.[7]

FORMULAS

CHOLISMA ™

Jiao Gu Lan (Rhizoma seu Herba Gynostemmatis) is another herb well known for its effect on the cardiovascular system. It was given to 30 patients in a study, and 86.7% showed a reduction in serum lipid levels.[8] Another study reported the combination of *Jiao Gu Lan* (Rhizoma seu Herba Gynostemmatis) and *Shan Zha* (Fructus Crataegi) to reduced both cholesterol and triglycerides levels.[9]

Zi Mu Xu (Herba Medicago Sativa), a western herb also known as alfalfa, may reduce cholesterol absorption and atherosclerotic formation.[10,11,12] It significantly reduces cholesterol absorption through direct binding in the gastrointestinal tract.[13] *Zi Mu Xu* (Herba Medicago Sativa) also reduces the cholesterol level by reducing the accumulation and synthesis of cholesterol in the liver.[14]

PHARMACEUTICAL DRUGS & CHINESE MEDICINE: A COMPARATIVE ANALYSIS

Hyperlipidemia is the accumulation of abnormally high levels of fats (cholesterols, triglycerides, or both) in the blood. If untreated, hyperlipidemia can significantly increase the risk of coronary artery disease (CAD). One of the most common misconceptions about hyperlipidemia is that this condition is "genetically predetermined," and therefore, can only be treated with pharmaceutical drugs. This is incorrect because diet and lifestyle changes are the most effective prevention and treatment modalities. However, most practitioners and patients are "commercially preconditioned" into believing drugs are the best and only treatment. As such, drugs for hyperlipidemia are now the most commonly prescribed drugs in the United States.

Western Medical Approach: There are several categories of drugs that may be used to treat hyperlipidemia. The most commonly used category is HMG-CoA reductase inhibitors, with examples such as Lipitor (Atorvastatin), Zocor (Simvastatin), and Pravachol (Pravastatin). Also known as "statin" drugs, these drugs reduce plasma cholesterol and triglyceride levels by reducing their synthesis in the liver. In most cases, these drugs are effective and are well tolerated. However, these drugs have been shown to cause serious and potentially life-threatening side effects in a small number of patients, such as rhabdomyolysis with kidney failure (0.5%), liver impairment (2.3%), and increased risk of liver cancer.[15] Furthermore, discontinuation of these drugs is frequently associated with a rebound increase of cholesterol and triglyceride levels. Given the potential risks versus benefits, it is important to take drugs only when necessary, and once on drug therapy, be monitored closely by the medical doctor so the drug can be discontinued immediately if these serious side effects begin to develop.

Traditional Chinese Medicine Approach: Hyperlipidemia is diagnosed as the accumulation of damp and phlegm in the blood vessels. This condition may be treated effectively with herbs, with gradual and consistent reduction of plasma cholesterol levels by an average of 10 to 15 mg/dL per month. However, the therapeutic effects of herbs may require 2 to 3 months before they become more noticeable. The herbs in this formula are very well tolerated by patients, and are associated with no known side effects.

Summation: hyperlipidemia is a serious condition that requires treatment. The best and most effective treatment is diet and lifestyle changes, as outlined earlier in this monograph. Herbal therapy may be added to facilitate and enhance the overall results. Lastly, and only if necessary, drug therapy may be used but only with careful screening and supervision.

CASE STUDIES

E.S., a 48-year-old male, presented with hypercholesterolemia and hypertension. His pulse was deep and slippery; his tongue was normal. The patient refused acupuncture treatment, requesting only herbal treatment. *Cholisma* was prescribed at two grams, three times daily on November 4, 2004, along with recommendations for improved diet and exercise habits. After two months of herbal therapy, lab reports showed significant reduction of total cholesterol, LDL and triglyceride levels, and an increase of healthy HDL. There was also a reduction of blood pressure. The patient continues to take herbs. Lab reports before and after commencement of herbal treatments are as follows:

CHOLISMA ™

Lab Tests	10-21-2004	11-04-2004	01-13-2005
Cholesterol	221	Herbal Treatment	206
HDL	66		69
LDL	141		123
Triglycerides	73		68
Blood Pressure	140/100		118/80

C.L., Chino Hills, California

R.L., a 79-year-old female, presented with post-stroke symptoms of paralysis on the right side (leg, arm and face). Her blood pressure was 140/80 mmHg and the heart rate was 90 beats per minute. She also had high cholesterol. She was diagnosed with wind-stroke with blood stagnation. *Neuro Plus* and *Cholisma* were prescribed at 4.5 grams and 1.5 grams each day, respectively. This patient also received acupuncture. After 10 weeks of treatment, the patient regained movement of her leg and partial movement of her arm and almost full movement of her face and mouth. *Neuro Plus* also helped the patient regain strength. These were very quick results. In addition, the cholesterol level dropped from 250 to 180 mg/dL.

W.F., Bloomfield, New Jersey

A 46-year-old female speech therapist presented with weight gain, pain in the left arm and a slow metabolism. Her cholesterol reading was noted at 280 mg/dL. The TCM diagnosis included damp and phlegm stagnation as well as blood stagnation as indicated by a red tongue body with a thick tongue coating and a "rolling" pulse. Within three months of taking *Cholisma*, her cholesterol reading decreased to 220 mg/dL. Within six months of exclusively taking *Cholisma*, her cholesterol reading fell to 198 mg/dL.

T.G., Albuquerque, New Mexico

A 22-year-old female presented with high triglycerides and high ALT. The patient appeared thin and pale. Her limbs were always cold and she was easily agitated. Her blood pressure was 115/70 mmHg and the heart rate was 72 beats per minute. The TCM diagnosis was yang deficiency with heat in the Liver. She was prescribed *Liver DTX* at 3 capsules three times a day with *Cholisma* at 2 capsules twice a day. She also received acupuncture. After six weeks, her liver enzymes and triglycerides levels returned to normal.

W.F., Bloomfield, New Jersey

A 31-year-old female who went to her medical doctor for a postpartum check-up had a blood cholesterol level of 375 mg/dL. Since she was nursing, her doctor refused to prescribe any drugs. She decided to begin herbal treatment with marked changes to the diet and lifestyle. She was instructed to take *Cholisma*, 2 grams three times daily. In addition, she exercised for 30 minutes three times per week. Furthermore, she avoided red meat and carbohydrate as much as possible, and increased the intake of fresh fruits and vegetables. Two months after the initial check-up, her cholesterol was reduced from 375 to 266 mg/dL. The patient continued to take *Cholisma*.

J.C., Diamond Bar, California

C.B., a 72-year-old female, presented with gallstones, pain under the right ribcage, poor digestion, and pain in the right shoulder. Her blood pressure was 180/95 mmHg and the heart rate was 85 beats per minute. Ultrasound was performed which confirmed the stone. The western diagnosis was gallstones and high cholesterol. The TCM diagnosis was damp-heat accumulation with Liver qi stagnation. She was prescribed *Dissolve (GS)* at 4.5 grams daily and *Cholisma* at 1.5 grams daily. The patient also received acupuncture. After eight weeks, the patient

CHOLISMA ™

reported the pain in the right shoulder has improved fully. Digestion was much better with no more bloating or constipation.

W.F., Bloomfield, New Jersey

A 50-year-old unemployed male presented with a family history of heart disease and diabetes. He was also described as overweight and extremely irritated. With increased levels of triglycerides, cholesterol and VLDL, the practitioner diagnosed the patient with hyperlipidemia. The TCM diagnosis was Liver and Kidney yin deficiency. The patient took *Cholisma* continuously for one year, but refused to do another laboratory test in order to note any significant changes. Without any changes to his diet and physical activities, he was still able to lose weight. The practitioner recommended *Cholisma* to his other patients with similar conditions. He also noted that *Cholisma* worked slower in comparison with drugs such as Lipitor (Atorvastatin) and Zocor (Simvastatin).

F.A., Calabasas, California

J.L., a 86-year-old male, presented with hypertension, insomnia, anxiety and high cholesterol. His blood pressure was 180/90 mmHg and the heart rate was 60 beats per minute. The blood pressure was higher in the morning (180-190/90-95 mmHg) than in the evening (170-180/85-90 mmHg). The TCM diagnosis was damp-heat accumulation. *Gastrodia Complex* at 4.5 grams a day and *Cholisma* at 1.5 grams a day were prescribed. This patient also received acupuncture. After six weeks of treatment, both morning and evening blood pressure were down to an average of 147/80 mmHg.

W.F., Bloomfield, New Jersey

L.L., a 56-year-old female, presented with frustration, anger and sadness over losing her home in the hurricanes. She was unable to move through these emotions. She was also diagnosed with hypertension, high cholesterol, and post-traumatic stress syndrome recently, and refused to take medications. Her blood pressure was 138/78 mmHg and her heart rate was 82 beats per minute. She also suffered from headaches in the temporal region and the vertex. Other symptoms included twitching of the eyes, agitation, red eyes, and a scalloped tongue with thick yellow tongue coating. TCM diagnoses were damp-heat in the Liver and Gallbladder, Kidney yin deficiency, and excess fire and wind rising. She was prescribed the following formulas: *Calm (ES)* at 1 to 3 capsules, as needed, *Cholisma* at 4 capsules twice daily, and *Gentiana Complex* at 5 capsules twice daily. The patient gained control of her emotions immediately after taking *Calm (ES)*. Blood pressure gradually reduced over time to 120/72 mmHg. The practitioner commented that the combination of these formulas are phenomenal.

M.H., West Palm Beach, Florida

P.Z., a 61-year-old male, presented with high triglycerides. His tongue was red with yellow tongue coating. His pulse was wiry and slippery. The patient was overweight. *Cholisma* was prescribed at 4 capsules three times daily. His triglycerides dropped from 250 to 136 mg/dL after herbal and acupuncture treatments.

W.F., Bloomfield, New Jersey

M.C., a 49-year-old highly-stressed executive, presented with elevated SGPT, LDL and cholesterol levels. He stated he frequently checked his blood pressure and it ranged from 135-148/85-91 mmHg. He was never diagnosed with hypertension but had an upcoming insurance physical and wanted to lower his blood pressure naturally [without using drugs]. He also complained of low-grade temporal headaches, a pressured feeling in the head, neck and shoulder tension. His blood pressure at the time of examination was 148/94 mmHg and his heart rate was 72 beats per minute. He worried excessively, in part because his son was diagnosed with a brain tumor ten years ago. He also suffered from insomnia, and fist clenching that lasted throughout the day. He said that his stress caused numbness and tension of his left shoulder and rhomboid area. TCM diagnoses include Liver qi stagnation and Spleen qi

FORMULAS

CHOLISMA ™

deficiency. *Cholisma* at 4 capsules three times daily and *Liver DTX* at 5 capsules at night were prescribed. He reported after taking the herbs, he passed his insurance exam. Blood pressure has stayed down at 120/72 mmHg. His stress was manageable and there were no more headaches. His energy level was also excellent. His cholesterol levels also dropped from 216 to 186 mg/dL. The practitioner reported that the patient is now a believer of herbs.

M.H., West Palm Beach, Florida

[1] He, XY. Effects of alisma plantago l. on hyperlipidemia, atherosclerosis and fatty liver. *Chinese Journal of Modern Developments in Traditional Medicine*. Oct. 1981; 1(2):114-7

[2] Bensky, D. et al. *Chinese Herbal Medicine Materia Medica*. Eastland Press. 1993

[3] Yeung, HC. *Handbook of Chinese Herbs*. Institute of Chinese Medicine. 1996

[4] Harmon NW. Hawthorns. *Canad Pharm J*. 108,724. Nov 1988

[5] He, G. Effects of the prevention and treatment of atherosclerosis of a mixture of hawthorn and motherwort. *Chung His I Choe Ho Tsa Chih*. 1990; 10:361

[6] Rajendran, S. et al. Effect of tincture of crataegus on the LDL-receptor activity of hepatic plasma membrane of rats fed on atherogenic diet. *Atherosclerosis*. June 1997; 123(1-2):235-41

[7] Guan, Y. et al. Yishou Jiangshi (de-blood-lipid) tablets in the treatment of hyperlipidemia. *Journal of Traditional Chinese Medicine*. Sep. 1995; 15(3):178-9

[8] Yu, R. et al. Clinical and experimental study on effects of Yinchen Wuling powder in preventing and treating hyperlipoproteinemia. *Chung Kuo Chung Hsi I Chieh Ho Tsa Chih*. Aug. 1996; 16(8):470-3

[9] la Cour, B. et al. Traditional Chinese medicine in treatment of hyperlipidemia. *Journal of Ethnopharmacology*. May 1996; 46(2):125-9

[10] Malinow, MR. et al. Effect of alfalfa saponins on intestinal cholesterol absorption in rats. *Am J Clin Nutr*. 1977; 30:2061

[11] Malinow, MR. et al. Cholesterol and bile acid balance in macaca fascicularis; effects of alfalfa saponins. *J Clin Invest*. 1981; 67:156

[12] Wilcox, MR. et al. Serum and liver cholesterol, total lipids and lipid phosphorus levels of rats under various dietary regimes. *Am J Clin Nutr*. 1961; 9:236

[13] Story, JA. et al. Adsorption of bile acids by components of alfalfa and wheat bran in vitro. *J Food Sci*. 1982; 47:1276

[14] Story, JA. et al. Interactions of alfalfa plant and sprout saponins with cholesterol in vitro and in cholesterol-fed rats. *Am J Clin Nutr*. 1984; 39:917

[15] Drug Facts and Comparisons, Updated Monthly. A Wolters Kluwer Company. Page 538. June 2001.

FORMULAS

CHOLISMA (ES) ™

CLINICAL APPLICATIONS

- ❧ High cholesterol and triglycerides levels
- ❧ Fatty liver
- ❧ Obesity
- ❧ Prevention and treatment for the conditions above

WESTERN THERAPEUTIC ACTIONS

- ❧ Antihyperlipidemic effect to reduce plasma levels of cholesterol and triglycerides
- ❧ Prevents and treats fatty liver
- ❧ Reduces body weight to treat obesity

CHINESE THERAPEUTIC ACTIONS

- ❧ Dissolves damp
- ❧ Eliminates phlegm
- ❧ Invigorates blood circulation
- ❧ Clears heat

DOSAGE

Take 3 to 4 capsules three times daily on an empty stomach. For maximum effectiveness, take the last dose one hour before bedtime, as synthesis of cholesterol is most active at night. As a preventative formula, take 2 capsules twice daily on an empty stomach.

INGREDIENTS

Da Huang (Radix et Rhizoma Rhei)
Dan Shen (Radix Salviae Miltiorrhizae)
Ge Gen (Radix Puerariae)
Hai Zao (Sargassum)
Huang Qin (Radix Scutellariae)

Jue Ming Zi (Semen Cassiae)
Shan Zha (Fructus Crataegi)
Yin Chen Hao (Herba Artemisiae Scopariae)
Yu Jin (Radix Curcumae)
Ze Xie (Rhizoma Alismatis)

FORMULA EXPLANATION

According to traditional Chinese medicine, cholesterol and triglycerides are considered as excess accumulations of dampness and phlegm in the blood vessels (hyperlipidemia), liver (fatty liver), and body (obesity). To effectively reduce plasma levels of cholesterol and triglycerides, treat fatty liver, and reduce body weight, treatment must focus on dissolving damp, eliminating phlegm, invigorating blood circulation, and clearing heat.

In this formula, Ze Xie (Rhizoma Alismatis) resolves dampness and Hai Zao (Sargassum) eliminates phlegm. Dan Shen (Radix Salviae Miltiorrhizae), Yu Jin (Radix Curcumae), and Shan Zha (Fructus Crataegi) activate blood circulation and eliminate blood stasis; keeping the flow of blood smooth will prevent plaque build-up on the vessel walls and ensure a healthy cardiovascular system. In addition, the liver has a remarkable power to regenerate itself, and it does so even faster when blood movers are used to ensure the proper supply of nutrients and elimination of waste. Long-term stagnation of damp, phlegm and blood will create heat. Therefore, several herbs are used to clear heat, such as Jue Ming Zi (Semen Cassiae), Da Huang (Radix et Rhizoma Rhei), Yin Chen Hao (Herba Artemisiae Scopariae), Ge Gen (Radix Puerariae) and Huang Qin (Radix Scutellariae). Yin Chen Hao (Herba Artemisiae Scopariae) and Da Huang (Radix et Rhizoma Rhei) ensure the healthy function of the liver and gallbladder by

CHOLISMA (ES) ™

promoting the secretion of bile, digestion of fat and the dispelling of damp-heat accumulation in the Liver and Gallbladder.

In summary, *Cholisma (ES)* is an excellent formula to treat individuals with an overall condition characterized by elevated cholesterol and triglyceride levels, accompanied by a fatty liver and obesity.

SUPPLEMENTARY FORMULAS

- For high cholesterol and triglyceride levels without fatty liver, obesity or risk of cardiovascular disorder, use *Cholisma* instead.
- For obese patients with an excess appetite, add *Herbalite*.
- For patients with diabetes mellitus and high blood glucose, add *Equilibrium*.
- For deficient-type hypertension with dizziness or vertigo, combine with *Gastrodia Complex*.
- For excess-type hypertension with anger or flushed face, combine with *Gentiana Complex*.
- For coronary heart disorders, add *Circulation*.
- For excess heat everywhere in the body, add *Gardenia Complex*.
- For hepatitis or other liver dysfunction, add *Liver DTX*.

NUTRITION

- Increase the daily intake of cholesterol-lowering foods such as apples, bananas, carrots, cold-water fish, dried beans, garlic, grapefruit, olive oil, and fibers such as bran and oat.
- Advise the patients to consume large quantities of fresh fruits and vegetables.
- Decrease the intake of food that will raise cholesterol levels, including but not limited to beer, wine, cheese, aged and cured meats, sugar, and greasy or fried foods. Avoid eating red meat, fatty foods, processed or fried foods, soda, pastries, pies, doughnuts, candy, etc.
- Stop drinking alcohol and smoking cigarettes.
- Eat small, frequent meals throughout the day instead of a few large ones. Eat slowly and chew thoroughly.
- Drink tea on a daily basis, especially after meals, to decrease the absorption of fatty foods from the diet. Beneficial teas include *pu-er*, black, *oolong* or green tea.
- Increase the intake of niacin, which can lower total cholesterol levels by up to 18%, increase HDL cholesterol by up to 32%, and lower triglycerides by up to 26%. Do not overdose on niacin to avoid stomach pain and flushing.
- Other supplements that are beneficial are vitamin B5, vitamin C, vitamin E, chromium picolinate, lecithin, and coenzyme Q10.
- Avoid greasy, fatty and oily foods. Seafood should also be reduced if cholesterol/triglycerides levels are high.

LIFESTYLE INSTRUCTIONS

- Avoid the consumption of alcohol and exposure to tobacco. They increase cholesterol buildup and hardening of arteries.
- The importance of a regular exercise routine cannot be over-emphasized. Exercise will improve energy levels, normalize metabolic functions, reduce fat, and burn calories.
- Change dietary and exercise habits, to avoid rebound weight gain.
- Do not to lose weight drastically. Rapid weight loss may be hazardous and is more likely to lead to rebound weight gain.

FORMULAS

CHOLISMA (ES) ™

CLINICAL NOTES

☙ Hyperlipidemia is a disorder of lipoprotein metabolism and not a cardiovascular malfunction. It may lead to various cardiovascular disorders such as arteriosclerosis, coronary artery disease, hypertension, angina pectoris, etc. Optimal treatment must address both the cause and the symptoms. See Supplementary Formulas for more details.

☙ The baseline cholesterol levels should be established before the initiation of herbal therapy; the first follow-up test should be done one month after the initiation of herbal therapy. Subsequent follow-ups can be done every two to three months to determine overall effectiveness. Cholesterol testing kits are available over-the-counter in most pharmacies. Results may vary from patient to patient. Lifestyle and dietary changes are also crucial for satisfactory result.

☙ *Cholisma (ES)* is specifically formulated to reduce blood cholesterol and triglyceride levels in individuals with fatty liver and/or obesity. Patients must take this herbal formula on a long-term basis for maximum results.

CAUTIONS

☙ *Dan Shen* (Radix Salviae Miltiorrhizae) may enhance the overall effectiveness of Coumadin (Warfarin), an anticoagulant drug. Patients who take anticoagulant or antiplatelet medications should *not* take this herbal formula without supervision by a licensed health care practitioner.

☙ *Jue Ming Zi* (Semen Cassiae) and *Da Huang* (Radix et Rhizoma Rhei) may cause loose stool or diarrhea for those with sensitive gastrointestinal tracts. Should this occur, reduce the dosage to 2 to 3 capsules three times daily.

☙ *Cholisma (ES)* is contraindicated during pregnancy.

ACUPUNCTURE POINTS

Traditional Points:
☙ High cholesterol and triglycerides levels
  ▪ Bleed *Weizhong* (BL 40) or wherever there is dilated visible vein in the transverse crease of the popliteal fossa.
  ▪ *Taichong* (LR 3), *Xingjian* (LR 2), *Zusanli* (ST 36), *Quchi* (LI 11), and *Fenglong* (ST 40)

Balance Method by Dr. Richard Tan:
☙ High cholesterol and triglycerides levels
  ▪ Left side: *Yinlingquan* (SP 9), *Xuehai* (SP 10), and *Waiguan* (TH 5).
  ▪ Right side: *Zusanli* (ST 36), *Fenglong* (ST 40), *Daling* (PC 7), and *Laogong* (PC 8).
  ▪ Alternate sides from treatment to treatment.
  ▪ For additional information on the Balance Method, please refer to *Dr. Tan's Strategy of Twelve Magical Points* by Dr. Richard Tan.
☙ Fatty liver
  ▪ Right side, needle the *ah shi* points around *Quze* (PC 3) to *Ximen* (PC 4), and *Yanglingquan* (GB 34).
  ▪ Left side, *Tianjing* (TH 10), *Shanglian* (LI 9) and *Shousanli* (LI 10), *Xiguan* (LR 7), and *Yinlingquan* (SP 9).
  ▪ Alternate sides from treatment to treatment.
  ▪ For additional information on the Balance Method, please refer to *Dr. Tan's Strategy of Twelve Magical Points* by Dr. Richard Tan.

CHOLISMA (ES) ™

Auricular Acupuncture by Dr. Li-Chun Huang:

☯ Weight loss

- Pituitary, Endocrine, Forehead, Exciting Point, Hunger Point, Thalamus, Sanjiao, Kidney, Large Intestine, Lung, and areas that have fat deposit such as the Abdomen or Buttock.
- For additional information on the location and explanation of these points, please refer to Auricular Treatment Formula and Prescriptions by Dr. Li-Chun Huang.

MODERN RESEARCH

Cholisma (ES) incorporates many herbs with excellent antihyperlipidemic effect to reduce plasma levels of cholesterol and triglycerides. Furthermore, many herbs have been shown in various clinical studies to effectively treat related conditions, such as fatty liver, obesity, arteriosclerosis and coronary artery disease.

Ze Xie (Rhizoma Alismatis) has a remarkable antihyperlipidemic effect, and has been shown in various clinical studies to effectively treat hyperlipidemia, hypercholesterolemia, arteriosclerosis and fatty liver.[1,2] *Jue Ming Zi* (Semen Cassiae) is very beneficial in treating hyperlipidemia, as the use of this herb has been shown to lower LDL and increase the HDL level.[3,4] According to one clinical study, use of *Jue Ming Zi* (Semen Cassiae) effectively reduced cholesterol levels to normal within 6 weeks in 98 of 100 patients.[5] According to another clinical study, use of *Jue Ming Zi* (Semen Cassiae) in 48 patients was associated with reduction in blood cholesterol in 95.8% of the patients, reduction in triglycerides in 86.7%, and reduction of beta-lipoprotein in 89.5%.[6]

Yu Jin (Radix Curcumae), *Da Huang* (Radix et Rhizoma Rhei) and *Yin Chen Hao* (Herba Artemisiae Scopariae) are all effective in lowering plasma and liver content of cholesterol and triglycerides.[7,8,9] Clinical applications of these herbs include hyperlipidemia, hypercholesterolemia, and coronary artery disease.[10,11,12]

Lastly, *Ge Gen* (Radix Puerariae) and *Shan Zha* (Fructus Crataegi) have both shown marked effectiveness for reduction of plasma cholesterol levels, with mechanisms of action attributed to enhancement of LDL-receptor activity, increased hepatic breakdown and decreased synthesis of cholesterol.[13,14] Furthermore, these two herbs also have a vasodilating effect on the coronary artery, and are definitely beneficial in severe cases of elevated cholesterol and triglyceride levels accompanied by such illnesses as atherosclerosis or coronary artery disease.[15,16]

In conclusion, *Cholisma (ES)* is one of the best formulas to treat complicated conditions of elevated cholesterol and triglyceride levels, fatty liver, and obesity. The formula is most effective if combined with lifestyle and dietary changes as described above.

PHARMACEUTICAL DRUGS & CHINESE MEDICINE: A COMPARATIVE ANALYSIS

Hyperlipidemia, obesity and fatty liver are three conditions that are often closed linked to each others. Hyperlipidemia is the accumulation of abnormally high levels of fats (cholesterols, triglycerides, or both) in the blood, fatty liver is the excess accumulation of fat in the liver cells, and obesity is the abnormal increase in body weight. If untreated, these conditions increase risk of diabetes, coronary artery disease, and cardiovascular and cerebrovascular disorders.

Western Medical Approach: Hyperlipidemia is usually treated with HMG-CoA reductase inhibitors, a category of drugs that includes Lipitor (Atorvastatin), Zocor (Simvastatin), and Pravachol (Pravastatin). Also known as "statin" drugs, these drugs reduce plasma cholesterol and triglyceride levels by reducing their synthesis in the liver. In most cases, these drugs are effective and are well tolerated. However, these drugs have been shown to cause serious and potentially life-threatening side effects in a small number of patients, such as rhabdomyolysis with kidney failure (0.5%), liver impairment (2.3%), and increased risk of liver cancer.[17] Furthermore, discontinuation of these drugs is frequently associated with a rebound increase of cholesterol and triglyceride levels. Given the potential risks versus

FORMULAS

CHOLISMA (ES) ™

benefits, it is important to take drugs only when necessary, and once on drug therapy, be monitored closely by the medical doctor so the drug can be discontinued immediately if these serious side effects begin to develop.

Obesity, a common health problem that is quickly becoming an epidemic, has few treatment options available. There are only two drugs approved by the Food and Drug Administration for long-term weight loss, and they both have serious side effects. Xenical (Orlistat) reduces body weight by blocking absorption of fat in the digestive tract. Because it interferes with the normal absorption process, this drug is known to cause many gastrointestinal side effects, such as fecal incontinence, fecal urgency, flatulence with discharge, increased defecation, oily evacuation, oily rectal leakage, steatorrhea, and projectile diarrhea. Meridia (Sibutramine) is a stimulant agent that causes weight loss by increasing metabolism and suppressing appetite. Similar to many other stimulant weight-loss drugs, use of Meridia (Sibutramine) may cause anorexia, anxiety, constipation, dizziness, headache, insomnia, irritability, nervousness, rhinitis, xerostomia, hypertension, congestive heart failure, arrhythmias, seizure and stroke.

Fatty liver is a potentially serious condition that, if untreated, may lead to liver cirrhosis. Unfortunately, there is no drug treatment for fatty liver in western medicine.

Traditional Chinese Medicine Approach: Hyperlipidemia, obesity and fatty liver are all characterized by the presence of damp and phlegm affecting various parts of the body. Use of herbs has been shown to be extremely effective to slowly and steadily improve all three of these conditions.

Summation: For treatment of hyperlipidemia and obesity, drugs are more potent but have significantly more side effects, in comparison with herbs. However, the higher potency of the drugs is not necessary advantages, because these conditions are chronic in nature, and require persistent and long-term treatment, not aggressive and short-term treatment. Therefore, long-term evaluation will often show comparable efficacy of both treatments. For fatty liver, herbal treatment is superior, especially as there are no treatment options available in western medicine. Lastly, it is extremely important to remember there is no magic bullet. Without commitment to changing diet and lifestyles, use of either drugs or herbs will have limited effectiveness. The practitioners and patients must work together to achieve significant and sustainable clinical results.

[1] He, XY. Effects of alisma plantago l. on hyperlipidemia, arteriosclerosis and fatty liver. *Chinese Journal of Modern Developments in Traditional Medicine*. 1(2):114-7, Oct. 1981

[2] *Zhong Hua Yi Xue Za Zhi* (Chinese Journal of Medicine), 1976; 11:693

[3] *Zhong Yao Zhi* (Chinese Herbology Journal), 1984; 352

[4] *Zhong Cao Yao* (Chinese Herbal Medicine), 1991; 22(2):72

[5] *Xin Yi Yao Xue Za Zhi* (New Journal of Medicine and Herbology), 1974; 3:30

[6] *Zhong Guo Yi Yuan Yao Xue Za Zhi* (Chinese Hospital Journal of Herbology), 1987; 9:395

[7] *Xin Yi Yao Xue Za Zhi* (New Journal of Medicine and Herbology), 1978; (9):540

[8] *Shang Hai Zhong Yi Yao Za Zhi* (Shanghai Journal of Chinese Medicine and Herbology), 1986; 12:40

[9] *Zhong Yao Yao Li Yu Ying Yong* (Pharmacology and Applications of Chinese Herbs), 1990; 15(6):52

[10] *Shang Hai Zhong Yi Yao Za Zhi* (Shanghai Journal of Chinese Medicine and Herbology), 1988; 8:2

[11] *Zhong Yi Za Zhi* (Journal of Chinese Medicine), 1980; 1:39

[12] *Shang Hai Zhong Yi Yao Za Zhi* (Shanghai Journal of Chinese Medicine and Herbology), 1986; 12:40

[13] *Zhong Yi Yao Xue Bao* (Report of Chinese Medicine and Herbology), 1989; 2:45

[14] Rajendran, S. et al. Effect of tincture of crataegus on the LDL-receptor activity of the hepatic plasma membrane of rats fed on atherogenic diet. *Atherosclerosis*. June 1997; 123(1-2):235-41

[15] *Guang Xi Zhong Yi Yao* (Guangxi Chinese Medicine and Herbology), 1990; 13(3):45

[16] *Zhong Hua Xin Xue Guan Bing Za Zhi* (Chinese Journal of Cardiology), 1985; 3:175

[17] Drug Facts and Comparisons, Updated Monthly. A Wolters Kluwer Company. Page 538. June 2001.

FORMULAS

CIRCULATION ™

CLINICAL APPLICATIONS

- Cardiovascular disorders, such as coronary heart disease, angina pectoris, arteriosclerosis, and radiating chest pain
- Circulatory disorders, such as poor cerebral and body circulation, numbness of the limbs, peripheral neuropathy and similar problems

WESTERN THERAPEUTIC ACTIONS

- Cardiotonic function to increase contractile strength and cardiac output [1,2,3]
- Anticoagulant function to reduce the risk of blood clots [5]
- Increases central and peripheral blood circulation [1,2,5]
- Improves blood circulation and treats ischemia of the brain, liver and kidney [6,7,8,9,10,11]

CHINESE THERAPEUTIC ACTIONS

- Invigorates blood circulation in the upper *jiao* and dispels blood stasis
- Unblocks meridians and relieves pain
- Warms Heart yang and dispels damp and phlegm

DOSAGE

Take 2 to 4 capsules three times daily on an empty stomach with warm water. This formula is to be taken on a daily basis for maintenance and/or prevention of cardiovascular disorders. Do **not** use this formula to treat acute myocardial infarction.

INGREDIENTS

Bai Shao (Radix Paeoniae Alba)
Chuan Xiong (Rhizoma Ligustici Chuanxiong)
Dan Shen (Radix Salviae Miltiorrhizae)
Dang Gui (Radicis Angelicae Sinensis)
Ge Gen (Radix Puerariae)
Gui Zhi (Ramulus Cinnamomi)
Hong Hua (Flos Carthami)

Hou Po (Cortex Magnoliae Officinalis)
Jiang Xiang (Lignum Dalbergiae Odoriferae)
Mao Dong Qing (Radix Ilicis Pubescentis)
Ren Shen (Radix Ginseng)
Sha Ren (Fructus Amomi)
Xie Bai (Bulbus Allii Macrostemonis)
Zhi Shi (Fructus Aurantii Immaturus)

FORMULA EXPLANATION

Cardiovascular disorders, such as coronary heart disease angina pectoris, are characterized by Heart yang deficiency with blood stagnation and damp and phlegm accumulation. To effectively treat cardiovascular disorders, treatment must focus on warming Heart yang, dissolving damp, eliminating phlegm, and invigorating blood circulation.

Ren Shen (Radix Ginseng) replenishes the vital qi and mimics the effect of cardiac glycosides, making the heart beat stronger and more rhythmically. *Xie Bai* (Bulbus Allii Macrostemonis) disperses painful obstructions due to turbid-phlegm congealing in the chest. *Xie Bai* (Bulbus Allii Macrostemonis) and *Gui Zhi* (Ramulus Cinnamomi) warm and facilitate the flow of yang qi in the chest to improve the function of the heart. *Dan Shen* (Radix Salviae Miltiorrhizae) improves microcirculation, strengthens myocardial contraction and adjusts the heart rate. *Mao Dong Qing* (Radix Ilicis Pubescentis) dilates the blood vessels, lowers blood pressure and reduces the oxygen consumption of cardiac muscles. *Ge Gen* (Radix Puerariae) dilates blood vessels to lower blood pressure. *Hong Hua*

CIRCULATION ™

(Flos Carthami), *Dang Gui* (Radicis Angelicae Sinensis), *Jiang Xiang* (Lignum Dalbergiae Odoriferae) and *Chuan Xiong* (Rhizoma Ligustici Chuanxiong) invigorate general blood circulation and dispel blood stasis. *Bai Shao* (Radix Paeoniae Alba) nourishes the blood and relieves pain. *Gui Zhi* (Ramulus Cinnamomi) promotes the peripheral blood circulation and unblocks stagnation in the channels and collaterals. *Sha Ren* (Fructus Amomi) regulates qi and dissolves dampness. *Zhi Shi* (Fructus Aurantii Immaturus) and *Hou Po* (Cortex Magnoliae Officinalis) regulate qi, expand the chest, and relieve congestion.

SUPPLEMENTARY FORMULAS

❧ For cardiovascular or circulatory disorders affecting the entire body, add *Circulation (SJ)*.

❧ For hypertension with dizziness or vertigo, combine with *Gastrodia Complex*.

❧ For hypertension with anger or flushed face, combine with *Gentiana Complex*.

❧ For edema and water accumulation, add *Herbal DRX*.

❧ For high cholesterol and triglycerides, add *Cholisma*.

❧ For high cholesterol and triglycerides with fatty liver and obesity, add *Cholisma (ES)*.

❧ For insomnia characterized by restlessness and disturbed *shen* (spirit) in excess conditions, add *Calm (ES)*

❧ For insomnia with excessive stress and underlying deficiency, add *Calm ZZZ*.

❧ For insomnia arising from deficiency, anemia or excessive worrying, add *Schisandra ZZZ*.

❧ For cigarette addiction, *Calm (ES)* may be used to ease the withdrawal signs and symptoms of addiction.

❧ For obesity, *Herbalite* may be used to suppress appetite and facilitate weight loss.

❧ For severe blood stagnation, add *Circulation (SJ)*.

❧ For excess heat accumulation, add *Gardenia Complex*.

NUTRITION

❧ Individuals with arteriosclerosis should eat foods high in fiber (fruits and vegetables) and low in fat and cholesterol. Avoid sweets, chips, fried and greasy foods, junk food, ice cream, and alcohol. Stay away from smoking and exposure to second-hand smoke. Shark cartilage is not recommended as it may inhibit the formation of new blood vessels. Regular exercise with close monitoring of weight is recommended.

❧ Increase intake of garlic and onions, as they can reduce serum cholesterol levels. Raw nuts (except peanuts), olive oil, pink salmon, trout, tuna, Atlantic herring, and mackerel are also rich in essential fatty acids that are good for patients with cardiovascular disorders.

❧ Eliminate sodium, MSG, baking soda, canned vegetables, diet soft drinks, junk food, preservatives, meat tenderizers, saccharin, and softened water from the diet.

❧ Patients on anticoagulants drugs, such as Coumadin (Warfarin), should not fluctuate the daily consumption of vitamin K, which is found in alfalfa, cauliflower, liver, and in all dark green vegetables including broccoli and spinach.

❧ Increase the intake of niacin, which can lower total cholesterol levels by up to 18%, increase HDL cholesterol by up to 32%, and lower triglycerides by up to 26%.

❧ Other supplements that are beneficial are vitamin B5, vitamin C, vitamin E, chromium picolinate, lecithin, and coenzyme Q10.

The Tao of Nutrition by Ni and McNease

❧ Coronary heart disease

- Recommendations: American ginseng, brown rice, black fungus, sea cucumber, vinegar, shitake mushrooms, celery, seaweed, lotus root, cassia seeds, jelly fish, chrysanthemums, hawthorn berries, water chestnuts, mung beans, pearl barley, peach kernels, ginger, soy sprouts, mung sprouts, other sprouts, wheat bran, persimmons, bananas, watermelon, sunflower seeds, and lotus seeds.

FORMULAS

CIRCULATION ™

- ▪ Avoid fatty foods, stimulating foods, spicy foods, coffee, smoking, alcohol, simple carbohydrates (sugar and white flour), slat, stress, tension, worrying, emotional stimulation, and lack of sleep.
- ☙ For more information, please refer to *The Tao of Nutrition* by Dr. Maoshing Ni and Cathy McNease.

LIFESTYLE INSTRUCTIONS

- ☙ Exercise helps blood circulation and is the key to keeping the blood vessels elastic, flexible and unclogged.
- ☙ Avoid the use of alcohol and exposure to tobacco. They increase cholesterol buildup and hardening of arteries.
- ☙ Healthy diet and lifestyle changes can reverse arteriosclerosis and its complications. However, they must be applied daily and continuously for a long time, without interruptions.

CLINICAL NOTES

- ☙ Maintenance of the herbal treatment is necessary for approximately six months in order to stabilize the condition. One should always address the secondary causes and/or complications of coronary artery disease.
- ☙ Patients with high risk of cardiovascular disorders may benefit from preventative treatments by taking low doses of *Circulation*. Risk factors of cardiovascular disorders include family history, obesity, sedentary lifestyle, cigarette smoking, etc.

Pulse Diagnosis by Dr. Jimmy Wei-Yen Chang:
- ☙ "Pulse within a pulse" on the left *cun* position. Feeling of fibrous, wire-like material inside the blood vessel that is extremely thin and forceful.
- ☙ Note: Dr. Chang takes the pulse in slightly different positions. He places his index finger directly over the wrist crease, and his middle and ring fingers alongside to locate *cun*, *guan* and *chi* positions. For additional information and explanation, please refer to *Pulsynergy* by Dr. Jimmy Wei-Yen Chang and Marcus Brinkman.

CAUTIONS

- ☙ Acute myocardial infarction is a medical emergency. Call 911 to sent patients to emergency room as soon as possible. Monitor their condition until emergency medical personnel arrive.
- ☙ Do *not* use this formula to treat myocardial infarction. *Circulation* is to be used for prevention of coronary artery disease; *not* for treatment of heart attacks.
- ☙ *Circulation* may enhance the overall effectiveness of Coumadin (Warfarin), an anticoagulant drug. Patients who take anticoagulants or blood-thinning medications should *not* take this herbal formula without the supervision of a licensed health care practitioner.
- ☙ *Circulation* is contraindicated during pregnancy and nursing.

ACUPUNCTURE POINTS

Traditional Points:
- ☙ *Liangqiu* (ST 34), *Renzhong* (GV 26), *Xinshu* (BL 15), *Tongli* (HT 5), *Qihai* (CV 6), and *Fenglong* (ST 40).
  - ▪ Acute: Needle *Ximen* (PC 4). Bleed *Quze* (PC 3) or the vein nearby.
  - ▪ Chronic: *Shanzhong* (CV 17) and *Neiguan* (PC 6).

Balance Method by Dr. Richard Tan:
- ☙ Left side: *Neiguan* (PC 6), and *Guanmen* (ST 22) or *ah shi* points nearby.
- ☙ Right side: *Sanjian* (LI 3), *Sanyinjiao* (SP 6), and *Ligou* (LR 5) or *ah shi* points nearby.
- ☙ Needle Heart point on the ear.

CIRCULATION ™

CIRCULATION

- ☙ For additional information on the Balance Method, please refer to *Dr. Tan's Strategy of Twelve Magical Points* by Dr. Richard Tan.

Ear Points:
- ☙ Main points: Heart, Small Intestine, Sympathetic, Carotid Artery, Prostate Gland, Anterior Pituitary, and Subcortex.
- ☙ Adjunct points: Brain Stem, Lung, Liver, Chest, and Occipital point.
- ☙ Needle every other day three to five points for an hour. Twelve treatments equal one course.

Auricular Acupuncture by Dr. Li-Chun Huang:
- ☙ Coronary Heart Disease: Heart, Liver, Chest, Small Intestine, Sympathetic, and Coronary Vascular Subcortex.
- ☙ For additional information on the location and explanation of these points, please refer to *Auricular Treatment Formula and Prescriptions* by Dr. Li-Chun Huang.

MODERN RESEARCH

Circulation is formulated with herbs that have been shown to improve both central and peripheral blood circulation. Though most of the herbs in this formula have such functions, *Dang Gui* (Radicis Angelicae Sinensis) and *Dan Shen* (Radix Salviae Miltiorrhizae) are the two herbs that have been studied most extensively.

Dang Gui (Radicis Angelicae Sinensis) historically has been used to tonify and invigorate blood circulation. Extracts of the herb have demonstrated a quinidine-like effect.[1] In one study, *Dang Gui* (Radicis Angelicae Sinensis) showed a clear protective effect on patients with myocardial dysfunction and injury induced by ischemia/reperfusion.[2] In another study of cirrhotic patients with portal hypertension, *Dang Gui* (Radicis Angelicae Sinensis) effectively decreased portal pressure without influencing the system's hemodynamics.[3] Finally, *Dang Gui* (Radicis Angelicae Sinensis) may improve overall blood circulation by decreasing the whole blood specific viscosity, or improving the hemorrheological changes in "blood stagnation."[4]

Dan Shen (Radix Salviae Miltiorrhizae) is a dynamic herb which has been shown to have a wide range of cardiovascular functions: it increases blood flow of the coronary artery, strengthens myocardial contraction, improves micro-circulation to peripheral parts of the body, and inhibits blood coagulation.[1,5] *Dan Shen* (Radix Salviae Miltiorrhizae) is commonly used to treat patients at risk of angina pectoris. In a study of 323 patients taking *Dan Shen* (Radix Salviae Miltiorrhizae) for 1-9 months, marked clinical improvement was noted in 20.3% and improvement in 62% of the patients.[1] In addition, *Dan Shen* (Radix Salviae Miltiorrhizae) improves circulation to various parts of the body overall, and is effective in treating cerebral ischemia,[6,7,8,9] hepatic ischemia,[10] and renal ischemia.[11] Lastly, *Dan Shen* (Radix Salviae Miltiorrhizae) decreases the risk of blood clots as it inhibits coagulation of blood and activates fibrinolysis.[5]

PHARMACEUTICAL DRUGS & CHINESE MEDICINE: A COMPARATIVE ANALYSIS

Western Medical Approach: Cardiovascular and circulatory disorders are complex illnesses that affect various parts of the body. In western medicine, these disorders are treated with medications such as antiplatelets [aspirin and Ticlid (Ticlopidine)] and anticoagulants [heparin and Coumadin (Warfarin)]. In emergencies, nitroglycerin and thrombolytic drugs may be used to dilate blood vessels and dissolve blood clots, respectively. Though these drugs have serious side effects, their use can be justified because they offer major benefits, especially in urgent situations.

Traditional Chinese Medicine Approach: Use of herbs is also beneficial to treat cardiovascular and circulatory disorders. In fact, many drugs used for treatment of cardiovascular and circulatory disorders are originally derived

FORMULAS

from natural sources. Similarly, these herbs have similar pharmacological effects to those of the drugs, such as antiplatelet, anticoagulant, thrombolytic, and vasodilating effects. Furthermore, herbs are much safer than drugs, as they have a regulatory effect on blood hemodynamics, thereby achieving desired effects with minimal side effects.

Summation: Both drugs and herbs are effective for prevention and treatment of mild to moderate cases of cardiovascular and circulatory disorders. Drug therapies are more potent, more precise, but do have more side effects. However, drugs are simply the most effective and most reliable therapy in emergency cases such as in acute heart attack. On the other hand, herbs are effective for both prevention and treatment of cardiovascular and circulatory disorders. However, they should not be used in emergencies, as they are not as potent and consistently reliable as the drugs.

CASE STUDY

A 58-year-old male presented with symptoms of chest oppression and a dry unproductive cough. Swelling was noted on the hands as well as around the eyes. Pain was felt at *Dabao* (SP 21) especially during movement. Other signs and symptoms included bright red blood in the stool, epistaxis, abdominal bloating, and tremors upon slight exertion. The tongue appeared swollen, pale, scalloped and wet with a thin coat and red tip. The pulse was superficial and forceful. The TCM diagnosis was phlegm retention in the Heart with an underlying deficiency of Spleen qi and Heart blood. The treatment protocol included the combination of three herbal formulas: *Circulation* at 1 capsule twice daily, *Gui Pi Tang* (Ginseng and Longan Combination) at 2 capsules twice daily, and a special formula at 1 capsule once daily. In addition, Cactus Comp [a homeopathic product] was used as needed, and magnet 10,000 gans was applied at site of discomfort nightly. The practitioner recommended this protocol for long-term treatment.

Note: The special formula included ingredients such as *Dan Shen* (Radix Salviae Miltiorrhizae), *Chuan Xiong* (Rhizoma Ligustici Chuanxiong), *Sheng Di Huang* (Radix Rehmanniae), *Bai Shao* (Radix Paeoniae Alba), *Fu Ling* (Poria), *Tao Ren* (Semen Persicae), *Huai Niu Xi* (Radix Achyranthis Bidentatae), *Hong Hua* (Flos Carthami), *Jie Geng* (Radix Platycodonis), *Chai Hu* (Radix Bupleuri), *Gan Cao* (Radix Glycyrrhizae), *Ge Gen* (Radix Puerariae), and *Yuan Zhi* (Radix Polygalae).

I.B., Miami, Florida

F.L., a 53-year-old female patient, presented with recent history of TIA (transient ischemic attack). Objective findings included right-sided pulling and numbness of the face with difficulty smiling and closing the right eye, as well as drooping of facial muscles on the right side when smiling, and partial facial flaccidity. Treatment using three capsules of *Circulation,* three times daily, was successful: no recurring episodes were noted during subsequent follow-up visits. This patient also had constipation with hard, difficult to move stools, abdominal pain, and cramps with bloating. All these gastrointestinal symptoms were resolved with **Gentle Lax (Deficient)** taken at four capsules, three times daily.

C.L., Chino Hills, California

[1] Bensky, D. et al. *Chinese Herbal Medicine Materia Medica.* Eastland Press. 1993
[2] Chen SG, et al. Protective effects of angelica sinensis injection on myocardial ischemia/reperfusion injury in rabbits. *Chung Kuo Chung His I Chieh Ho Tsa Chih.* Aug 1995; 15(8):485-8.
[3] Huang, Z. et al. Effects of radix angelicae sinensis on systemic and portal hemodynamics in cirrhotics with portal hypertension.
[4] Xue, JX. et al. Effects of the combination of astragalus membranaceus (Fisch.) Bge. (AM), angelica sinensis (Oliv.) Diels (TAS), cyperus rotundus L. (CR), ligusticum chuanxiong Hort (LC) and paeonia veitchii lynch (PV) on the hemorrheological changes in "blood stagnating" rats. *Chung Kuo Chung Yao Tsa Chih.* Feb 1994; 19(2):108-10, 128
[5] Yeung, HC. *Handbook Of Chinese Herbs.* Institute Of Chinese Medicine. 1996
[6] Wu, W. et al. The effect of radix salviae miltiorrhizae on the changes of ultrastructure in rat brain after cerebral ischemia. *J Tradit Chin Med,* Sep 1992; 12(3):183-6

CIRCULATION ™

[7] Kuang, PG. et al. The effect of radix salviae miltiorrhizae on vasoactive intestinal peptide in cerebral ischemia: an animal experiment. *J Tradit Chin Med*, Sep 1989; 9(3):203-6

[8] Kuang, P. et al. Salviae miltiorrhizae treatment results in decreased lipid peroxidation in reperfusion injury. Department Of Neurology' Chinese PLA General Hospital' Postgraduate Military Medical School' Beijing' China. *J Tradit Chin Med*, Jun 1996; 16(2):138-42

[9] Kuang, P. et al. Protective effect of radix salviae miltiorrhizae composita on cerebral ischemia. Department Of Neurology' Chinese PLA General Hospital Postgraduate Military Medical School' Beijing. *J Tradit Chin Med*, Jun 1995; 15(2):135-40

[10] Lu, Q. et al. An experimental and clinical study on radix salviae miltiorrhizae in the treatment of hepatocellular Ca2+ overload during hepatic ischemia/reperfusion injury. Wuhan General Hospital' Guangzhou Command Of People's Liberation Army. *Chung Hua Wai Ko Tsa Chih*, Feb 1996; 34(2):98-101

[11] Yokozawa, T. et al. Isolation of a renal function-facilitating constituent from the oriental drug, salviae miltiorrhizae radix. Nippon Jinzo Gakkai Shi, Oct 1989; 31(10):1091-8

FORMULAS

CIRCULATION (SJ) ™

CLINICAL APPLICATIONS

☙ Severe blood stasis and stagnant blood circulation in upper, middle and lower *jiaos* (*San Jiao*):
  - Severe blood stagnation in the <u>upper body</u>: headache, angina pectoris, rheumatic heart disease, thrombosis, embolism, cardiac ischemia, bradyarrhythmia, stroke, concussion, post-concussion syndrome, cerebral atherosclerosis, hyperlipidemia, and physical injury to the chest
  - Severe blood stagnation in the <u>middle body</u>: pleural adhesion, acute and chronic hepatitis, liver cirrhosis, hepatic hemangioma, cholecystitis, jaundice, and splenomegaly
  - Severe blood stagnation in the <u>lower body</u>: female infertility, male infertility, amenorrhea, dysmenorrhea, irregular menstruation, uterine bleeding, ectopic pregnancy, hysteromyoma, endometriosis, oophoritic cyst, ovarian cyst, pelvic inflammatory disease, hyperplastic tuberculosis of intestine, ulcerative colitis, and urinary stones
☙ Severe, chronic conditions that do not respond to standard herbal treatment [use *Circulation (SJ)* as an adjunct formula to boost the overall therapeutic effect]
☙ Chronic traumatic injury that wasn't treated properly back in the acute phase and now re-exacerbates off and on
☙ Cardiovascular, circulatory or clotting disorders
☙ Chronic musculoskeletal injuries, joint injuries (knee, ankle, wrist, elbow, shoulder, back, etc.)

WESTERN THERAPEUTIC ACTIONS

☙ Analgesic effect to relieve pain [1,2,3]
☙ Anti-inflammatory effects to reduce inflammation and swelling [4]
☙ Antiplatelet and anticoagulant effects to improve blood circulation and decrease blood viscosity [5,6,7]
☙ Cardiovascular effect to improve blood circulation to the heart and the blood vessels [8,9]

CHINESE THERAPEUTIC ACTIONS

☙ Invigorates blood and qi circulation in the upper, middle and lower *jiaos*
☙ Dispels blood stasis and qi stagnation
☙ Unblocks meridians and relieves pain

DOSAGE

Take 3 to 4 capsules three times daily. For severe cases, dosage may be increased to 7 to 8 capsules three times daily to relieve pain. This formula should be taken for no more than 1 month continuously. As an adjunct to another formula to invigorate blood, the recommended dose is 1 to 2 capsules in addition to the regular dose of the base formula.

INGREDIENTS

Bai Shao (Radix Paeoniae Alba)
Chai Hu (Radix Bupleuri)
Chi Shao (Radix Paeoniae Rubrae)
Chuan Niu Xi (Radix Cyathulae)
Chuan Xiong (Rhizoma Ligustici Chuanxiong)
Dang Gui (Radicis Angelicae Sinensis)
Gan Cao (Radix Glycyrrhizae)
Hong Hua (Flos Carthami)
Jie Geng (Radix Platycodonis)
Mo Yao (Myrrha)

Mu Dan Pi (Cortex Moutan)
Pu Huang (Pollen Typhae)
Rou Gui (Cortex Cinnamomi)
Sheng Di Huang (Radix Rehmanniae)
Shui Zhi (Hirudo)
Tao Ren (Semen Persicae)
Wu Yao (Radix Linderae)
Xiang Fu (Rhizoma Cyperi)
Yan Hu Suo (Rhizoma Corydalis)
Zhi Ke (Fructus Aurantii)

FORMULAS

CIRCULATION (SJ) ™

BACKGROUND INFORMATION

Circulation (SJ) is designed by Dr. Jimmy Wei-Yen Chang to treat a wide variety of disorders characterized by severe or chronic blood and qi stagnation. He calls this condition "dead blood syndrome" where there is chronic blood stasis in the body with no outlet. With this stagnation, the homeostasis of the body is disturbed and multiple symptoms may appear.

Circulation (SJ) has three main functions:

1. First, it treats chronic persistent pain that is the result of previous traumatic injuries, which were not treated properly. Chronic qi and blood stagnation lead to pain which worsens with exacerbation or when the body is not in optimal health. This formula contains strong blood-moving herbs, which effectively drive away chronic blood stasis.

2. Second, it treats multiple chronic disorders or complex patterns with no clear diagnosis. These cases have multiple symptoms and each is very severe. However, there may be conflicting signs and symptoms, which prevent clear diagnosis of the exact cause. Such cases are best treated with blood-moving herbs. By clearing away chronic "dead blood" that may be complicating the condition, the true illness will surface, which then makes it possible to diagnose and prescribe an appropriate formula.

3. Finally, it treats complex conditions where the diagnosis is clear but after using the correct herbs following differentiation principles, the condition still does not improve. For example, a patient may suffer from insomnia and appropriate *shen* (spirit) calming herbs are given but the patient shows no result after several treatments. Alternatively, a patient suffers from high fever and *Bai Hu Tang* (White Tiger Decoction) is given but the high fever persists. In such cases where the diagnostic signs clearly match the herbal prescription but the patient shows no result, then one might consider that there is underlying "dead blood" disrupting the balance of the body. "Dead blood" might be blocking the blood flow and preventing it from nourishing the Heart *shen* (spirit) in the first case. It might also be the "dead blood" that is creating so much stagnation that the fever persists because there is a lack of proper circulation. In any case, removing the root cause is the only long-term solution to the problem.

FORMULA EXPLANATION

Circulation (SJ) is an herbal formula specifically formulated with herbs that invigorate blood circulation, dispel blood stasis, unblock meridians, and relieve pain. It promotes normal blood circulation in the upper, middle, and lower *jiaos*. Its formulation follows the principles of three classic formulas: *Xue Fu Zhu Yu Tang* (Drive Out Stasis in the Mansion of Blood Decoction) to treat blood stagnation in the upper *jiao*, *Ge Xia Zhu Yu Tang* (Drive Out Blood Stasis Below the Diaphragm Decoction) to treat blood stagnation in the middle *jiao*, and *Shao Fu Zhu Yu Tang* (Drive Out Blood Stasis in the Lower Abdomen Decoction) to treat blood stagnation in the lower *jiao*.

Tao Ren (Semen Persicae) and *Hong Hua* (Flos Carthami) are used to activate the blood circulation. These two herbs have excellent synergistic effect and are often used together. *Shui Zhi* (Hirudo) is one of the strongest blood stasis removing herbs, and is added to enhance the overall effect to break down blood stagnation. *Dang Gui* (Radicis Angelicae Sinensis), *Chuan Xiong* (Rhizoma Ligustici Chuanxiong) and *Sheng Di Huang* (Radix Rehmanniae) nourish blood, activate blood circulation and eliminate blood stasis. *Mu Dan Pi* (Cortex Moutan) and *Chi Shao* (Radix Paeoniae Rubrae) clear heat, cool blood, and dispel blood stagnation. Since blood stagnation and qi stagnation often occur simultaneously, *Zhi Ke* (Fructus Aurantii), *Wu Yao* (Radix Linderae) and *Xiang Fu* (Rhizoma Cyperi) are used to activate and regulate qi circulation. To effectively treat qi and blood stagnation in all three *jiaos*, *Jie Geng* (Radix Platycodonis), *Chai Hu* (Radix Bupleuri), and *Chuan Niu Xi* (Radix Cyathulae) are used to guide the formula to the upper, middle and lower *jiaos*, respectively. In addition, because pain is often associated with qi and blood stagnation, *Yan Hu Suo* (Rhizoma Corydalis), *Mo Yao* (Myrrha), *Pu Huang* (Pollen Typhae) and *Rou Gui* (Cortex Cinnamomi) are used to unblock the channels and collaterals to relieve pain. Furthermore, the combination of *Bai Shao* (Radix Paeoniae Alba) and *Gan Cao* (Radix Glycyrrhizae) also has great effect to relieve spasms and cramps. Lastly, *Gan Cao* (Radix Glycyrrhizae) tonifies qi and harmonizes all the herbs in this formula.

In summary, *Circulation (SJ)* is an excellent formula to treat various types of disorders characterized by blood stagnation anywhere in the upper, middle, and lower *jiaos* of the body.

SUPPLEMENTARY FORMULAS

Circulation (SJ) can be used individually, or in combination with any other formulas that treat disorders of the *zang fu* organs or diseases of the body.

Cardiovascular Disorders:
- Angina, atherosclerosis: add *Circulation*.
- High cholesterol: add *Cholisma*.
- Hypertension with dizziness or vertigo, combine with *Gastrodia Complex*.
- Hypertension with anger or flushed face, combine with *Gentiana Complex*.

Gynecological Disorders:
- Dysmenorrhea: add *Mense-Ease*.
- Fibrocystic disorder in the breast: add *Resolve (Upper)*.
- Endometriosis or fibroids or cysts in the uterus or other mass: add *Resolve (Lower)*.

Musculoskeletal Disorders:
- Neck, shoulder and upper back pain: add *Neck & Shoulder (Acute)* or *Neck & Shoulder (Chronic)*.
- Back pain: add *Back Support (Acute)* or *Back Support (Chronic)*.
- Headache: add *Corydalin*.
- Neuropathy: add *Flex (NP)*.
- *Bi zheng* (painful obstruction syndrome) due to cold: add *Flex (CD)*.
- *Bi zheng* (painful obstruction syndrome) due to heat: add *Flex (Heat)*.
- Muscle stiffness, cramps and spasms: add *Flex (SC)*.
- For excruciating pain: add *Herbal Analgesic*.
- Bone spurs: add *Flex (Spur)*.
- Knee pain: add *Knee & Ankle (Acute)* or *Knee & Ankle (Chronic)*.
- Thoracic or upper back pain: add *Back Support (Upper)*.
- Gout: add *Flex (GT)*.
- Trauma, post-surgical recovery: add *Traumanex*.

Others:
- Post-stroke care: add *Neuro +*.
- For nodules or swelling: add *Resolve (AI)*.
- High fever: add *Gardenia Complex*.
- Insomnia: add *Calm (ES)*, *Calm ZZZ*, or *Schisandra ZZZ*.
- Depression: add *Shine*.
- Psoriasis or chronic skin condition: add *Dermatrol (PS)*.
- For edema or swelling, add *Herbal DRX*.
- Varicose veins: add *Shan Zha* (Fructus Crataegi)

CIRCULATION (SJ) ™

NUTRITION

- L-carnitine is helpful to strengthen the heart muscle and to promote circulation.
- Coenzyme Q10 improves tissue oxygenation.
- A multienzyme complex supplement helps enhance use of oxygen in body tissue.
- Multivitamins are very beneficial for various aspects of proper circulation, such as formation of red blood cells, restoration of normal blood viscosity, and prevention of blood clots.
- Minerals, such as calcium, magnesium and potassium, are essential for normal heartbeat.
- Refrain from drinking cold beverages and foods, such as ice water, watermelon, cucumbers, sushi and citrus.

LIFESTYLE INSTRUCTIONS

- Exercise helps blood circulation and is the key to keeping the blood vessels elastic, flexible and unclogged.
- Avoid the use of alcohol and exposure to tobacco. They increase cholesterol buildup and hardening of arteries.
- Healthy diet and lifestyle changes can reverse arteriosclerosis and its complications. However, they must be practiced daily and continuously for a long time without interruptions.

CLINICAL NOTES

- The sedentary lifestyle of modern society is characterized by sitting for long hours and lack of exercise. Most people spend many hours of the day sitting in their cars, office, and home. With lack of movement, blood circulation is impaired and gradually leads to a large number of illnesses. Therefore, this formula is not only an excellent formula to improve blood circulation and treat clot related disorders, it is also a wonderful formula for prevention of chronic illness. In addition, this formula can be combined with many other formulas to improve blood circulation and deliver the herbs to the affected areas that may be hard to reach.
- *Circulation (SJ)* has a wide range of therapeutic actions and may be used to treat many different diseases. One common presentation among all these diseases is blood stagnation characterized by either a light or dark purplish tongue. There are also cases where the tongue may appear normal but the sublingual vein are distended and dark in appearance. Patients face may appear dark and lusterless. Lips may be dark or purplish. Axillae, transverse cubital crease and the popliteal fossa may all appear slightly darker than the rest of the skin.
- Patients with intermittent claudication, chronic pain in the calf when walking, should check for cardiovascular disorders.
- *Circulation (SJ)* works similarly like the reset button on the computer. When too many programs are open and in function, the computer may freeze. The body works the same way in that it breaks down when there are too many aggravating factors or symptoms. The formula works like the reset button on the computer to clear away stagnation so the body has a chance to start new again. In breaking down the blood clot, it then should become clear what condition needs to be addressed instead of being confused with multiple symptoms that may not point to any clear diagnosis.

Pulse Diagnosis by Dr. Jimmy Wei-Yen Chang:

- Deep and forceful on all positions.
- Note: Dr. Chang takes the pulse in slightly different positions. He places his index finger directly over the wrist crease, and his middle and ring fingers alongside to locate *cun*, *guan* and *chi* positions. For additional information and explanation, please refer to *Pulsynergy* by Dr. Jimmy Wei-Yen Chang and Marcus Brinkman.

CAUTIONS

- This formula may enhance the overall effectiveness of Coumadin (Warfarin), an anticoagulant drug. Patients who take anticoagulants or blood-thinning medications should *not* take this herbal formula without the supervision of a licensed health care practitioner.

FORMULAS

CIRCULATION (SJ) ™

- Patients on anticoagulant drugs, such as Coumadin (Warfarin), should not fluctuate their daily consumption of vitamin K, which is found in alfalfa, cauliflower, liver, and in all dark green vegetables including broccoli and spinach.
- This formula is contraindicated during pregnancy and nursing. It should be used with caution during menstruation as it may cause excessive bleeding. In such cases, discontinue use immediately and resume after menstruation is over.
- This formula is contraindicated in patients with bleeding disorders, such as hypermenorrhea, uterine bleeding, and hemophilia.
- This formula should be discontinued 1 to 2 weeks before surgery.
- Avoid drinking cold beverages or eating cold or raw foods, since they constricting in nature and may cause more blood stagnation.
- Use with caution or add *GI Tonic* if the patient has a weak digestive system or Spleen qi deficiency with diarrhea.
- During the course of treatment with this formula, some patients with chronic "dead blood" might notice pain in places of past injuries. Advise the patient of this possible experience before giving the formula that it is a positive sign as it is clearing away the residual stagnation and bringing in fresh blood supply to the chronically injured place. In some cases where patients cannot tolerate the pain, reduce the dosage of the formula by 20%. After experiencing the initial pain, the patient will later experience a total clearing sensation. This is especially prevalent in those suffering from chronic headaches due to previous head injuries. Failure to advise the patient on the potential experience of pain may result in misunderstanding by the patient, who may think the herbal treatment is causing them more pain in an adverse way.
- This formula should be taken for no more than 1 month continuously.
- Due to its potent effect, this formula is contraindicated in weak and elderly patients.

ACUPUNCTURE POINTS

Traditional Points:
- For varicose veins, bleeding technique should be performed once a week on the distended vein while taking *Circulation (SJ)* and *Shan Zha* (Fructus Crataegi).

Balance Method by Dr. Richard Tan:
- Left side: *Shaoshang* (LU 11), *Zhongchong* (PC 9), *Shaochong* (HT 9), *Zusanli* (ST 36), *Yanglingquan* (GB 34), and *Weizhong* (BL 40).
- Right side: *Hegu* (LI 4), *Houxi* (SI 3), *Zhongzhu* (TH 3), *Sanyinjiao* (SP 6), *Zhongfeng* (LR 4), and *Taixi* (KI 3).
- Alternate sides from treatment to treatment.
- For additional information on the Balance Method, please refer to *Dr. Tan's Strategy of Twelve Magical Points* by Dr. Richard Tan.

Auricular Acupuncture by Dr. Li-Chun Huang:
- Thromboangiitis obliterans: Corresponding point (to the area affected), Sympathetic, Coronary Vascular Subcortex, Lesser Occipital Nerve, Large Auricular Nerve, Hot Point, and Heart.
  - Supplementary points: Lung, Liver, Spleen, Endocrine
- Thrombophlebitis: Corresponding point (to the area affected), Sympathetic, Endocrine, Sanjiao, Heart, Lung, Liver, Kidney, Spleen, Hot, and Coronary Vascular Subcortex. Bleed Ear Apex.
- For additional information on the location and explanation of these points, please refer to *Auricular Treatment Formula and Prescriptions* by Dr. Li-Chun Huang.

FORMULAS

CIRCULATION (SJ) ™

MODERN RESEARCH

Circulation (SJ) is designed to treat various types of illnesses characterized by cardiovascular and circulatory disorders. Pharmacologically, many herbs in this formula have marked antiplatelet, anticoagulant and thrombolytic effects, and are excellent for treating clotting disorders. Clinically, the herbs in the formula have been shown to treat cardiovascular, circulatory and clotting disorders as well as many other illnesses.

This formula incorporates many herbs with antiplatelet and anticoagulant effects to inhibit thrombus formation and treat clotting disorders. Herbs with antiplatelet effects include *Dang Gui* (Radicis Angelicae Sinensis),[10] *Hong Hua* (Flos Carthami),[11] and *Chi Shao* (Radix Paeoniae Rubrae).[12] Herbs with anticoagulant effects include *Shui Zhi* (Hirudo) and *Tao Ren* (Semen Persicae).[13,14] There are many herbs in this formula that also have marked influence on the cardiovascular system. For example, *Dang Gui* (Radicis Angelicae Sinensis) has a negative chronotropic and positive inotropic effect.[15] Furthermore, it has been shown to improve overall blood circulation by decreasing the whole blood specific viscosity, or improving the hemorrheological changes in "blood stagnation. "[16] Use of *Zhi Ke* (Fructus Aurantii) showed a marked ability to increase blood pressure and lower the oxygen requirement of cardiac muscle.[17] *Jie Geng* (Radix Platycodonis) has been shown to dilate blood vessels and increase blood perfusion to peripheral parts of the body.[18] Lastly, *Chuan Xiong* (Rhizoma Ligustici Chuanxiong) dilates blood vessels to lower blood pressure, increases blood perfusion to coronary arteries, and decreases oxygen consumption by the cardiac muscle.[19]

Clinically, this formula may be used individually, or as an adjunct to other formulas to treat a wide variety of cardiovascular, circulatory, clotting, and related disorders. *Dang Gui* (Radicis Angelicae Sinensis) has been used in formulas with good success to treat 40 patients with cerebral vascular accident.[20] *Hong Hua* (Flos Carthami) has been used in formulas with a 94.7% rate of effectiveness in treating 137 patients with cerebral thrombosis,[21] and a 80.8% rate of effectiveness in relieving chest pain in 100 patients with coronary artery disease.[22] *Chi Shao* (Radix Paeoniae Rubrae) has been used with 92.01% rate of effectiveness for prevention of thrombus formation in 263 patients.[23] *Chuan Xiong* (Rhizoma Ligustici Chuanxiong), when given via injection, was associated with relief of pain in 92.5% of patients with angina,[24] 94.5% rate of effectiveness among 400 patients with cerebral thrombosis,[25] and 90% rate of effectiveness for 50 patients with acute cerebral embolisms.[26] Lastly, coronary artery disorder may be effectively treated with formulas that contain *Yan Hu Suo* (Rhizoma Corydalis) or *Pu Huang* (Pollen Typhae).[27,28]

Circulation (SJ) is formulated following the principles of three classic formulas: *Xue Fu Zhu Yu Tang* (Drive Out Stasis in the Mansion of Blood Decoction), *Ge Xia Zhu Yu Tang* (Drive Out Blood Stasis Below the Diaphragm Decoction), and *Shao Fu Zhu Yu Tang* (Drive Out Blood Stasis in the Lower Abdomen Decoction). Because of this formulation strategy, *Circulation (SJ)* can also be explained from the perspective of how it is used to treat disorders of upper, middle, and lower *jiaos*.

Circulation (SJ) uses *Xue Fu Zhu Yu Tang* (Drive Out Stasis in the Mansion of Blood Decoction) to treat blood stagnation in the upper *jiao*, a condition characterized by circulatory disorders in the upper parts of the body. Clinically, *Xue Fu Zhu Yu Tang* (Drive Out Stasis in the Mansion of Blood Decoction) has been shown to have a 89.3% rate of effectiveness in treating cardiac ischemia in 84 patients,[29] 92.8% rate of effectiveness in treating bradyarrhythmia in 28 patients,[30] 90% rate of effectiveness in treating vascular headache in 50 patients,[31] 93.33% rate of effectiveness in treating headache in 15 patients,[32] 92.3% rate of effectiveness in treating concussion in 12 patients,[33] 87% rate of effectiveness in treating cerebral atherosclerosis in 63 patients,[34] and 95% rate of effectiveness to treat hyperlipidemia with elevated cholesterol and triglyceride levels in 20 patients.[35]

Circulation (SJ) uses *Ge Xia Zhu Yu Tang* (Drive Out Blood Stasis Below the Diaphragm Decoction) to treat blood stagnation in the middle *jiao*. Clinical researches have been shown that *Ge Xia Zhu Yu Tang* (Drive Out Blood Stasis Below the Diaphragm Decoction) has an 86% rate of effectiveness to treat hepatic hemangioma in 32 patients,[36] a marked effect to treat chronic active hepatitis in 25 patients,[37] good success to treat pleural adhesion in 60 patients,[38]

FORMULAS

a 90.6% rate of effectiveness to treat chronic pelvic inflammatory disease in 64 patients,[39] a 90% rate of effectiveness to treat prostatic hypertrophy in 22 patients,[40] a 96% rate of effectiveness to treat chronic colitis in 75 patients,[41] and a 90% rate of effectiveness to treat gastric or duodenal ulcer in 30 patients.[42]

Circulation (SJ) uses *Shao Fu Zhu Yu Tang* (Drive Out Blood Stasis in the Lower Abdomen Decoction) to treat blood stagnation in the lower *jiao*, a condition characterized by circulatory disorders in the lower parts of the body. According to numerous clinical research studies, *Shao Fu Zhu Yu Tang* (Drive Out Blood Stasis in the Lower Abdomen Decoction) has marked effect to treat both male and female infertility.[43,44,45] Furthermore, it may also be used to treat various other disorders, such as a 97.5% rate of effectiveness in 40 women with endometriosis,[46] 92% rate of effectiveness in 50 women with oophoritic cyst,[47] 97% rate of effectiveness in 100 patients with dysmenorrhea,[48] 94% rate of effectiveness in 14 patients with hysteromyoma,[49] 92% rate of effectiveness in 42 women with pelvic inflammatory disease,[50] and marked effect in 32 women with uterine bleeding associated with functional disorder.

In summary, though *Circulation (SJ)* is not designed to treat any one specific indication, it does have a wide range of therapeutic application to address numerous disorders characterized by blood and qi stagnation. Pharmacologically, many herbs in this formula have marked antiplatelet and anticoagulant effects. Clinically, the herbs in the formula have been shown to treat cardiovascular, circulatory, clotting disorders, and many other illnesses.

PHARMACEUTICAL DRUGS & CHINESE MEDICINE: A COMPARATIVE ANALYSIS

Western Medical Approach: Cardiovascular and circulatory disorders are complex illnesses that affect various parts of the body. In western medicine, these disorders are treated with medications such as antiplatelets [aspirin and Ticlid (Ticlopidine)] and anticoagulants [heparin and Coumadin (Warfarin)]. In emergencies, nitroglycerin and thrombolytic drugs may be used to dilate blood vessels and dissolve blood clots, respectively. Though these drugs have serious side effects, their use can be justified because they offer tremendous benefits, especially in urgent situations.

Traditional Chinese Medicine Approach: Use of herbs is also beneficial to treat cardiovascular and circulatory disorders. In fact, many drugs used for treatment of cardiovascular and circulatory disorders are originally derived from natural sources. Similarly, these herbs have similar pharmacological effects to those of the drugs, such as antiplatelet, anticoagulant, thrombolytic, and vasodilating effects. Furthermore, herbs are much safer than drugs, as they have a regulatory effect on blood hemodynamics, thereby achieving desired effects with minimal side effects.

Summation: Both drugs and herbs are effective for prevention and treatment of mild to moderate cases of cardiovascular and circulatory disorders. Drug therapies are more potent, more precise, but do have more side effects. However, drugs are simply the most effective and most reliable therapy in emergency cases such as in acute heart attack. On the other hand, herbs are effective for both prevention and treatment of cardiovascular and circulatory disorders. However, they should not be used in emergencies, as they are not as potent or consistently reliable as the drugs.

CASE STUDY

After recently attending Dr. Chang's seminar in Austin, Tx, I decided to try *Circulation SJ* with a client I had been working with since March. He is a 25 year old who has been diagnosed with Reflex Sympathetic Dystrophy (RSD) of the right ankle. This is the result of a fall from a cliff 5 years ago in which he sustained extensive crushing injury to the bones of the ankle and fibula. He had 3 surgeries to attempt to repair the damage that were unsuccessful to the extent that amputation just below the knee was strongly encouraged by his Physicians. Most of the time he cannot stand anything touching his rt. leg so he is in shorts and barefoot and in a wheelchair. I started working with him

FORMULAS

with acupuncture only using Dr. Tan's 12 Magic Points since he was reluctant to try herbs since he was using painkillers even though they were not very effective. We had made some progress, he had been able to reduce his Meds and sometimes he could put on a sock and loose shoe. Then 2 weeks ago I put him on Circulation SJ. The first week some diminishment of pain occurred but the 2nd week was the miracle! He came to his appointment with a shoe and sock on and was walking with a slight limp. His face and eyes were clearer then I had ever seen, he was laughing and calm. Later that day the Massage Therapist who had originally referred him to me called to tell me for the first time in the 2 years she had been working with him she was able to touch his leg without him screaming in pain. She said his entire body was different the tension and rigidity that was always there in the past was gone. Her statement to me was "it was like massaging a normal person". She stated that she had been contemplating discontinuing working with him because she "felt like all she was doing was grinding bone on bone and causing him pain".. My client and I thank you and Dr. Chang for your continuing efforts in the field of Asian Medicine. Please do not let him stop teaching. I plan to take Dr. Chang's Pulse seminar in 2006 since the one this week was already full and I am already committed during the time it is offered in Hawaii. I intend to attend anything Lotus offers with Dr. Chang in the future. I think we should refer to you, John and Jimmy as the Holy Trinity of Asian Medicine! Thanks Again,

As an update, this week when I saw this young man, he had continued improvement. While we were talking before his treatment he was sitting there with his legs crossed as only men can do, stroking and playing with his damaged ankle and toes. When I commented on this, he said that it was just so amazing to him to be able to be touched without it causing pain for the first time in years.

A.G., Austin, Texas

[1] Kubo, M. et al. Anti-inflammatory activities of methanolic extract and alkaloidal components from corydalis tuber. *Biol Pharm Bull.*; 17(2):262-5 February 1994

[2] Zhu, XZ. Development of natural products as drugs acting on central nervous system. *Memorias do Instituto Oswaldo Cruz*. 1991;86 Suppl 2:173-5

[3] Hu, J. et al. Effect of some drugs on electroacupuncture analgesia and cytosolic free Ca2+ concentration of mice brain. *Chen Tzu Yen Chiu*; 1994; 19(1):55-8

[4] *Zhong Yao Yao Li Yu Lin* Chuang (Pharmacology and Clinical Applications of Chinese Herbs), 1987; 37

[5] *Zhong Yao Yao Li Yu Lin Chuang* (Pharmacology and Clinical Applications of Chinese Herbs), 1993; 9(1):8

[6] *Zhong Hua Nei Ke Xue Za Zhi* (Journal of Chinese Internal Medicine), 1977; 2(2):79

[7] *Zhong Guo Yi Yao Xue Bao* (Chinese Journal of Medicine and Herbology), 1990; 5(4):33

[8] *Zhong Yao Yao Li Yu Lin Chuang* (Pharmacology and Clinical Applications of Chinese Herbs), 1993; 9(1):8

[9] *Zhong Guo Yi Yao Xue Bao* (Chinese Journal of Medicine and Herbology), 1990; 5(4):33

[10] *Zhong Guo Yao Li Xue Tong Bao* (Journal of Chinese Herbal Pharmacology), 1981; 2(1):35

[11] *Zhong Cheng Yao Yan Jiu* (Research of Chinese Patent Medicine), 1983; 12:31

[12] *Zhong Yao Xue* (Chinese Herbology), 1998; 831:836

[13] *Pharmazie*, 1988; 43:737

[14] *Shang Hai Zhong Yi Yao Za Zhi* (Shanghai Journal of Chinese Medicine and Herbology), 1985; 7:45

[15] *Jiang Su Zhong Yi* (Jiangsu Chinese Medicine), 1965; (3):22

[16] Xue, JX. et al. Effects of the combination of astragalus membranaceus (Fisch.) Bge. (AM), angelica sinensis (Oliv.) Diels (TAS), cyperus rotundus L. (CR), ligusticum chuanxiong Hort (LC) and paeonia veitchii lynch (PV) on the hemorrheological changes in "blood stagnating" rats. *Chung Kuo Chung Yao Tsa Chih*; Feb 1994; 19(2):108-10, 128

[17] *Zhi Wu Yao You Xiao Cheng Fen Shou Ce* (Manual of Plant Medicinals and Their Active Constituents), 1986; 725

[18] *Zhong Yao Yao Li Yu Ying Yong* (Pharmacology and Applications of Chinese Herbs), 1983; 866

[19] *Zhong Yao Xue* (Chinese Herbology), 1989; 535:539

[20] *Shen Jing Jing Shen Ji Bing Za Zhi* (Journal of Psychiatric Disorders), 1981; 4:222

[21] *Shan Xi Yi Yao Za Zhi* (Shanxi Journal of Medicine and Herbology), 1983; 5:297

[22] *Xin Zhang Xue Guan Ji Bing* (Cardiovascular Diseases), 1976; 4(4):265

[23] *Zhong Xi Yi Jie He Za Zhi* (Journal of Integrated Chinese and Western Medicine), 1986; 9:561

[24] *Xin Yi Yao Xue Za Zhi* (New Journal of Medicine and Herbology), 1977; 1:15

[25] *Zhong Xi Yi Jie He Za Zhi* (Journal of Integrated Chinese and Western Medicine), 1986; 6(4):234

[26] *Zhong Yi Yan Jiu Yuan* (Research Hospital of Chinese Medicine), 1976; 4(4):261

[27] *Zhong Yao Tong Bao* (Journal of Chinese Herbology), 1980; 4:192

[28] *Hu Nan Yi Yao Za Zhi* (Hunan Journal of Medicine and Herbology), 1982; 9:(3):6

FORMULAS

[29] *Zhe Jiang Zhong Yi Za Zhi* (Zhejiang Journal of Chinese Medicine), 1997; 10:445

[30] *Zhe Jiang Zhong Yi Xue Yuan Xue Bao* (Journal of Zhejiang University of Chinese Medicine), 1992; 16(3):19

[31] *Zhong Guo Zhong Xi Yi Jie He Za Zhi* (Chinese Journal of Integrative Chinese and Western Medicine), 1995; 15(7):438

[32] *Guang Xi Zhong Yi Yao* (Guangxi Chinese Medicine and Herbology), 1996; 5:22

[33] *Shan Xi Zhong Yi* (Shanxi Chinese Medicine), 1993; 14(5):222

[34] *Hu Nan Zhong Yi Za Zhi* (Hunan Journal of Chinese Medicine), 1993; 9(1):41

[35] *Zhong Xi Yi Jie He Za Zhi* (Journal of Integrated Chinese and Western Medicine), 1988; 8(10):601

[36] *Jiang Su Zhong Yi* (Jiangsu Chinese Medicine), 1997; 8:21

[37] *Xin Yi Yao Xue Za Zhi* (New Journal of Medicine and Herbology), 1978; 9:44

[38] *Bei Jing Zhong Yi* (Beijing Chinese Medicine), 1987; 4:24

[39] *Jiang Xi Zhong Yi Yao* (Jiangxi Chinese Medicine and Herbology), 1988; 2:28

[40] *Si Chuan Zhong Yi* (Sichuan Chinese Medicine), 1998; 1:36

[41] *Shan Xi Zhong Yi* (Shanxi Chinese Medicine), 1991; 7(5):16

[42] *Xin Zhong Yi* (New Chinese Medicine), 1976; 4:35

[43] *Hu Nan Yi Yao Za Zhi* (Hunan Journal of Medicine and Herbology), 1983; 3:52

[44] *He Nan Zhong Yi* (Henan Chinese Medicine), 1985; 3:29

[45] Yang CC. Chen JC. Chen GW. Chen YS. Chung JG. Effects of Shao-Fu-Zhu-Yu-Tang on motility of human sperm. American Journal of Chinese Medicine. 2003; 31(4):573-9

[46] *Zhong Xi Yi Jie He Za Zhi* (Journal of Integrated Chinese and Western Medicine), 1988; 10:639

[47] *Xin Zhong Yi* (New Chinese Medicine), 1995; 8:40

[48] *Zhe Jiang Zhong Yi Za Zhi* (Zhejiang Journal of Chinese Medicine), 1964; 11:17

[49] *Bei Jing Zhong Yi* (Beijing Chinese Medicine), 1987; 5:34

[50] *Hu Bei Zhong Yi Za Zhi* (Hubei Journal of Chinese Medicine), 1993; 15(3):23

FORMULAS

CORDYCEPS 3 ™

CLINICAL APPLICATIONS

- Chronic immune deficiency
- Chronic fatigue syndrome
- Sexual/reproductive dysfunction
- Respiratory dysfunction
- Chronic trachitis
- Allergic rhinitis
- Kidney impairment
- Tinnitus
- Arrhythmia
- Hyperlipidemia

WESTERN THERAPEUTIC ACTIONS

- Enhances energy and increases the basal metabolism [1,2,3,4]
- Increases sperm count and sperm motility [5,6,7,8]
- Improves kidney and ear function [9,10,11,12,13,14]
- Prevents and treats respiratory disorders [15,16,17,18,19,20,21]
- Prevents and treats elevated cholesterol levels [22,23,24,25]
- Prevents and treats cardiovascular disorders, such as arrhythmia and high blood pressure [26,27,28,29]
- Stimulates the immune system to fight against cancer [30,31,32,33,34,35,36]

CHINESE THERAPEUTIC ACTIONS

- Tonifies Kidney yang and augments Kidney *jing* (essence)
- Tonifies Lung, stops bleeding and dissolves phlegm
- Tonifies qi

DOSAGE

Take 3 to 4 capsules three times daily on an empty stomach with warm water. *Cordyceps 3* is safe for long-term use.

INGREDIENTS

Dong Chong Xia Cao (Cordyceps)   *Ren Shen* (Radix Ginseng)
Huang Qi (Radix Astragali)

FORMULA EXPLANATION

Dong Chong Xia Cao (Cordyceps), *Huang Qi* (Radix Astragali) and *Ren Shen* (Radix Ginseng) are three of the most precious herbs in Chinese herbal medicine. The combination of these three herbs has a wide spectrum of beneficial effects, including but not limited to increasing energy, strengthening the overall constitution of the body, and improving overall well being. Clinically, these herbs are commonly used to treat chronic fatigue syndrome, sexual and reproductive disorders, kidney impairment, chronic respiratory disorders, arrhythmia, hyperlipidemia and immune deficiency.

Dong Chong Xia Cao (Cordyceps) has a remarkable effect to tonify both the Lung and the Kidney, to treat chronic deficiency of both organs. *Dong Chong Xia Cao* (Cordyceps) tonifies the Kidney to treat impotence, spermatorrhea,

CORDYCEPS 3 ™

frequent urination, nocturnal emission, premature ejaculation, tinnitus, forgetfulness, and early signs of aging. Furthermore, it tonifies the Lung to treat chronic respiratory disorders, such as chronic cough and frequent respiratory infections. *Huang Qi* (Radix Astragali) tonifies the qi to improve energy levels, strengthens the Lung to prevent and treat infections, and enhances the immune system to fight against cancer. It is one of the most potent and effective herbs for patients with generalized weakness and deficiencies. *Ren Shen* (Radix Ginseng) is one of the oldest and most recognized herbs in Chinese herbal medicine. It has a tremendous effect to tonify qi to improve energy, strengthen the Spleen to improve digestion, tonify the Lung to prevent infection, and calm the *shen* (spirit) to improve mental function.

In conclusion, *Cordyceps 3* is formulated with three of the best tonic herbs in the Chinese herbal pharmacopoeia. The tonic effect is gentle and potent, allowing the herbs to be taken safely for a long time. *Cordyceps 3* has a wide range of therapeutic effects and can be used on a long-tem basis. Lastly, it is also an anti-aging tonic to ensure optimal health.

SUPPLEMENTARY FORMULAS

- To tonify the yin, yang, qi and blood of the body, add *Imperial Tonic*.
- For patients with cancer undergoing chemotherapy or radiation, add *C/R Support*.
- For patients with cancer who are unable to receive chemotherapy or radiation due to generalized weakness or deficiency, add *CA Support*.
- For Kidney yin deficiency, add *Kidney Tonic (Yin)*.
- For Kidney yang deficiency, add *Kidney Tonic (Yang)*.
- For dry, brittle, or gray hair, add *Polygonum 14*.
- To enhance the immune system or alleviate spontaneous sweating in recovery from chronic illness, add *Immune +*.
- For chronic cough or asthma arising from Kidney and Lung yin deficiencies, add *Respitrol (Deficient)*.
- For cough with unknown etiology, add *Respitrol (CF)*.
- For kidney disorders, add *Kidney (DTX)*.
- For tinnitus, add *Nourish*.
- For high cholesterol levels, add *Cholisma*.
- For coronary artery disease, add *Circulation*.
- For patients who are "burned out" with adrenal insufficiency, add *Adrenoplex*.
- For impotence and reproductive disorders in men, add *Vitality*.
- For lack of libido in women, add *Vitality*.
- For thirst or dryness, add *Nourish (Fluids)*.
- For anemia, add *Schisandra ZZZ*.
- For male infertility, add *Vital Essence*.
- For female infertility, add *Blossom (Phase 1-4)*.

LIFESTYLE INSTRUCTION

- Since there is such a wide range of therapeutic benefits associated with this formula, please refer to other related formulas for detailed descriptions of nutrition and lifestyle instructions pertinent to the specific imbalance under treatment.

CLINICAL NOTES

- *Cordyceps 3* is most effective when used on a long-term basis for prevention of various cardiovascular, reproductive and respiratory disorders. Furthermore, it is one of the best herbal formulas to stimulate the

CORDYCEPS 3 ™

immune system to fight against cancer. It should be taken continuously for at least 4 to 6 months for maximum effectiveness.

❧ *Cordyceps 3* is excellent for treating many disorders, such as cardiovascular, reproductive and respiratory diseases. However, though it is useful if taken individually, results can be enhanced by combining it with other appropriate formulas as listed in Supplementary Formulas.

CAUTIONS

❧ This formula should be used with caution with the following conditions: in the presence of an exterior pathogen, excess internal heat, or dampness; and with infectious or inflammatory diseases.

❧ Some patients may notice headache and irritability after taking *Cordyceps 3* because of its warm and tonic properties. If that is the case, reduce the dosage to 1 to 2 capsules three times daily.

ACUPUNCTURE POINTS

Traditional Points:
❧ *Shenshu* (BL 23) and *Feishu* (BL 13).

Ear Points:
❧ Nose, Spleen, and Bone Marrow.

MODERN RESEARCH

Cordyceps 3 has a wide spectrum of therapeutic effects and clinical applications. Historically, the herbs in this formula have been used to treat disorders of the Kidney, Lung and Heart. More recently, it has been used to support cancer patients with good results.

Increased energy, elevated metabolism, and improved general well-being are three of the most immediate and recognizable benefits of *Cordyceps 3*. *Huang Qi* (Radix Astragali) is an excellent tonic that raises the energy level by increasing the basal metabolic rate and cAMP.[1] *Ren Shen* (Radix Ginseng) awakens the central nervous system which improves both mental and physical performances.[2,3] It was demonstrated in one laboratory study that the administration of *Ren Shen* (Radix Ginseng) is associated with marked effect in improving memory and learning abilities.[4]

Cordyceps 3 has a marked influence on regulation of the reproductive system. Pharmacologically, it has been shown that the use of *Dong Chong Xia Cao* (Cordyceps) is associated with an increase in sperm count and sperm motility in mice.[5] In one clinical study, 197 patients with sexual disorders were treated with *Dong Chong Xia Cao* (Cordyceps) three times daily for 40 days, with an effective rate of 64.15%.[6] In addition, the use of *Ren Shen* (Radix Ginseng) is associated with stimulation of the pituitary gland to increase the secretion of gonadotropin. According to laboratory studies, it increases the production of sperm in males, and it lengthens the estrus period in females.[7] Furthermore, *Ren Shen* (Radix Ginseng) is also effective in the treatment of sexual dysfunction. According to one clinical study, 24 patients with low sperm count were treated with a preparation of *Ren Shen* (Radix Ginseng). An increase in sperm count was noted in 70% of patients, and an increase in sperm motility in 67% of the patients.[8]

Use of *Dong Chong Xia Cao* (Cordyceps) is also associated with marked improvement of Kidney and ear functions. In one report, 117 patients with compromised kidney function were treated with *Dong Chong Xia Cao* (Cordyceps) three times daily with good results.[9] In another study, 23 patients with tinnitus were treated with *Dong Chong Xia Cao* (Cordyceps) three times daily for four weeks with significant improvement.[10] Besides *Dong Chong Xia Cao* (Cordyceps), *Huang Qi* (Radix Astragali) is generally regarded as one of the most effective herbs for treatment of kidney-related disorders such as proteinuria, nephritis, and glomerulonephritis. According to clinical studies, use of *Huang Qi* (Radix Astragali) is associated with beneficial actions against nephropathy and glomerulonephritis.[11] In one clinical trial, 20 patients with nephritis were treated with *Huang Qi* (Radix Astragali) decoction for 15 to 90 days with improvements noted in 16 patients.[12] In another study, 56 patients with chronic glomerulonephritis were treated with intramuscular injections of *Huang Qi* (Radix Astragali) for one month with marked reduction of protein in the urine (effective rate of 61.7%) and an improvement of kidney functions.[13] The pharmacological efficacy of *Huang Qi* (Radix Astragali) in treating kidney disorders was attributed to decreased amount of protein in the urine, increased volume of urine, and decreased excretion of chloride and ammonia.[14]

Dong Chong Xia Cao (Cordyceps) is useful in treating various respiratory disorders. Pharmacologically, *Dong Chong Xia Cao* (Cordyceps) has demonstrated bronchodilating and antibiotic effects.[15,16] In one clinical trial, 656 patients with chronic respiratory tract disorders were treated with *Dong Chong Xia Cao* (Cordyceps) three times daily for 40 days with good success.[17] In another study, 43 patients with allergic rhinitis were treated with 6 grams of *Dong Chong Xia Cao* (Cordyceps) three times daily for four weeks with 93% effective rate.[18] Furthermore, the use of *Huang Qi* (Radix Astragali) was found through numerous clinical trials to be effective in prevention of respiratory tract disorders. In one study, the use of *Huang Qi* (Radix Astragali) was associated with a decreased risk of infection as well as shortened duration of infection.[19] In another study, daily use of *Huang Qi* (Radix Astragali) showed 94% effectiveness in prevention of respiratory tract infections in 100 children.[20] Lastly, in a clinical trial of 41 patients with asthma, injection of *Huang Qi* (Radix Astragali) daily for three months showed significant improvement in 85.4% of patients.[21]

Dong Chong Xia Cao (Cordyceps) is also effective in the treatment of hyperlipidemia.[22] In one clinical study, 273 patients with hyperlipidemia were treated with 1 gram of *Dong Chong Xia Cao* (Cordyceps) three times daily, showing a marked decrease of LDL and TG and increase of HDL.[23] Another study of 204 patients reported that *Dong Chong Xia Cao* (Cordyceps) is effective in lowering LDL.[24] Similarly, *Ren Shen* (Radix Ginseng) is effective in treating atherosclerosis and hypercholesterolemia. In one study, use of a *Ren Shen* (Radix Ginseng) preparation twice daily was beneficial in patients with hypertension, atherosclerosis, and chest pain. Furthermore, *Ren Shen* (Radix Ginseng) has also been found to have a moderate effect in lowering blood cholesterol levels, with a significant influence to lower triglycerides.[25]

Dong Chong Xia Cao (Cordyceps) is also effective in the prevention and treatment of a variety of cardiovascular disorders, such as arrhythmia and high blood pressure. In one study, 57 patients with arrhythmia were treated with *Dong Chong Xia Cao* (Cordyceps) three times daily for 2 weeks with an effective rate of 64.9%.[26] In another study, the administration of *Dong Chong Xia Cao* (Cordyceps) is associated with decreased heart rate and blood pressure lasting over one hour. In addition to *Dong Chong Xia Cao* (Cordyceps), the use of *Ren Shen* (Radix Ginseng) is effective for treating various cardiovascular disorders. According to numerous clinical trials, the use of *Ren Shen* (Radix Ginseng) is beneficial in cases of coronary artery disease, cardiac ischemia and cardiogenic shock.[27,28,29]

Most importantly, *Dong Chong Xia Cao* (Cordyceps) is one of the few herbs that have demonstrated exceptional stimulant effect on the immune system to fight cancer. *Dong Chong Xia Cao* (Cordyceps) enhances the immune system by stimulating and increasing the phagocytic activities of macrophages against foreign substances.[30] This effect is further potentiated with the addition of *Huang Qi* (Radix Astragali) and *Ren Shen* (Radix Ginseng). *Huang Qi* (Radix Astragali) is extremely effective in enhancing the immune system and reversing immune deficiency.[31,32,33] In patients with leukopenia, administration of *Huang Qi* (Radix Astragali) was associated with an obvious rise of white blood cell count in 115 patients.[34] *Ren Shen* (Radix Ginseng) also has an immune-enhancing effect of increasing the function of the reticuloendothelial system and the total IgM count.[35] In one clinical study, 52 cancer patients who have leukopenia caused by chemotherapy were able to continue and complete the entire course of chemotherapy treatment with the intake of *Ren Shen* (Radix Ginseng) to prevent bone marrow suppression.[36]

CORDYCEPS 3 ™

In summary, *Cordyceps 3* is a diversified formula that can be used for treatment and prevention of numerous conditions. It is also one of the best general tonic formulas to take on a long-term basis to ensure health and well being.

PHARMACEUTICAL DRUGS & CHINESE MEDICINE: A COMPARATIVE ANALYSIS

One striking difference between western and traditional Chinese medicine is that western medicine focuses and excels in crisis management, while traditional Chinese medicine emphasizes and shines in holistic and preventative treatments. Therefore, in emergencies, such as gun shot wounds or surgery, western medicine is generally the treatment of choice. However, for treatment of chronic idiopathic illness of unknown origins, where all lab tests are normal and a clear diagnosis cannot be made, traditional Chinese medicine is distinctly superior.

Cordyceps 3 is an herbal tonic that has a broad spectrum of therapeutic effects. It may be used as maintainance and preventive treatment for various conditions, including but not limited to chronic immune deficiency, chronic fatigue syndrome, and sexual and/or reproductive dysfunctions. For many of these conditions, traditional Chinese medicine is superior to western medicine, as there are limited drug options available.

[1] *Zhong Yao Yao Li Yu Lin Chuang* (Pharmacology and Clinical Applications of Chinese Herbs), 1985:193
[2] *Zhong Yao Yao Li Yu Ying Yong* (Pharmacology and Applications of Chinese Herbs), 1983; 16
[3] *Zhong Hua Yi Xue Za Zhi* (Chinese Journal of Medicine), 1985; 42(12):13
[4] *Zhong Yao Ci Hai* (Encyclopedia of Chinese Herbs), 1994
[5] *Zhong Yao Xue* (Chinese Herbology), 1998; 785:788
[6] *Jiang Su Zhong Yi Yao* (Jiangsu Medicine and Herbology), 1985; 5:46
[7] *Zhong Cheng Yao* (Study of Chinese Patent Medicine), 1989; 11(9):30
[8] *Ji Lin Yi Xue* (Jilin Medicine), 1983; 5:54
[9] *Shang Hai Zhong Yi Yao Za Zhi* (Shanghai Journal of Chinese Medicine and Herbology), 1986; 8:29
[10] *Fu Jian Yi Yao Za Zhi* (Fujian Journal of Medicine and Herbology), 1985; 6:42
[11] *Jiang Su Yi Xue* (Jiangsu Medical Journal), 1989; 15(1):12
[12] *Hei Long Jiang Zhong Yi Yao* (Heilongjiang Chinese Medicine and Herbology), 1982; 1:39
[13] *Zhong Xi Yi Jie He Za Zhi* (Journal of Integrated Chinese and Western Medicine), 1987; 7:403
[14] *Jiang Su Yi Xue* (Jiangsu Medical Journal), 1989; 15(1):12
[15] *Fu Jian Yi Yao Za Zhi* (Fujian Journal of Medicine and Herbology), 1983; 5:311
[16] *Ren Min Wei Sheng Chu Ban She* (Journal of People's Public Health), 1983; 358
[17] *Zhong Cao Yao* (Chinese Herbal Medicine), 1987; 10:8
[18] *Zhong Xi Yi Jie He Za Zhi* (Journal of Integrated Chinese and Western Medicine), 1987; 1:43
[19] *Zhong Yi Za Zhi* (Journal of Chinese Medicine), 1980; 1:71
[20] *Jiang Su Zhong Yi* (Jiangsu Chinese Medicine), 1988; 9:32
[21] *Zhong Hua Er Ke Za Zhi* (Chinese Journal of Pediatrics), 1978; 2:87
[22] *Zhong Yao Xue* (Chinese Herbology), 1998; 785:788
[23] *Zhong Xi Yi Jie He Za Zhi* (Journal of Integrated Chinese and Western Medicine), 1985; 11:652
[24] *Qing Hai Yi Yao Za Zhi* (Qinghai Journal of Medicine and Herbology), 1986; 3:22
[25] *Ji Lin Yi Xue* (Jilin Medicine), 1983; 5:54
[26] *Zhe Jiang Zhong Yi Xue Yuan Xue Bao* (Journal of Zhejiang University of Chinese Medicine), 1985; 6:28
[27] *CA*, 1992;116:34223d
[28] *Zhong Cao Yao Tong Xun* (Journal of Chinese Herbal Medicine), 1972; 4:21
[29] *An Hui Yi Xue* (Anhui Medicine), 1988; 3:51
[30] *Shang Hai Zhong Yi Za Zhi* (Shanghai Journal of Chinese Medicine), 1988; 1:48
[31] *Biol Pharm Bull*, 1977; 20(11)-1178-82
[32] *Yun Nan Zhong Yi Za Zhi* (Yunan Journal of Chinese Medicine), 1980; 2:28
[33] *Journal of Clinical and Laboratory Immunology*, 1988 Mar.; 25(3):125-9
[34] *Zhong Guo Zhong Xi Yi Jie He Za Zhi* (Chinese Journal of Integrative Chinese and Western Medicine), 1995 Aug.; 15(8):462-4
[35] *Zhong Yao Xue* (Chinese Herbology), 1998; 729:736
[36] *Te Chan Ke Xue Shi Yan* (Research of Special Scientific Projects), 1984; 4:24

FORMULAS

CORYDALIN ™

CLINICAL APPLICATIONS

- Headache
- Various kinds of headaches (according to western medicine): sinus, orbital, tension or migraine headaches
- Various types of headaches (according to traditional Chinese medicine): vertex, occipital, wind-cold, wind-heat and blood stagnation headaches

WESTERN THERAPEUTIC ACTIONS

- Analgesic effect to relieve pain [1,2,4,5,6,7]
- Anti-inflammatory effect to reduce swelling and pain [1]
- Antispasmodic function to relieve muscle spasm [5,9]
- Improves peripheral and micro-circulation to relieve headache and prevent cerebral ischemia [9,10]

CHINESE THERAPEUTIC ACTIONS

- Relieves pain
- Invigorates qi and blood circulation
- Removes qi and blood stagnation

DOSAGE

Take 3 to 4 capsules three times daily on an empty stomach. The dosage may be increased up to 6 to 8 capsules every four to six hours as needed for severe pain.

INGREDIENTS

Bai Zhi (Radix Angelicae Dahuricae)
Chuan Xiong (Rhizoma Ligustici Chuanxiong)
Dan Shen (Radix Salviae Miltiorrhizae)
Ge Gen (Radix Puerariae)
Yan Hu Suo (Rhizoma Corydalis)

FORMULA EXPLANATION

Corydalin is an empirical formula designed to relieve a variety of headaches. *Corydalin* contains herbs, which activate qi and blood circulation, remove qi and blood stagnation, and relieve pain.

Yan Hu Suo (Rhizoma Corydalis) is the principle herb in this formula and is used to activate qi and blood circulation, remove blood stasis, and relieve pain. It is one of the strongest analgesic herbs and its effectiveness has been compared with morphine and codeine.[9] *Bai Zhi* (Radix Angelicae Dahuricae) is used as a channel-guiding herb, which leads the effectiveness of the formula to the head. In addition, *Bai Zhi* (Radix Angelicae Dahuricae) has a strong effect to dispel wind and other exterior pathogenic factors. *Chuan Xiong* (Rhizoma Ligustici Chuanxiong) and *Dan Shen* (Radix Salviae Miltiorrhizae) activate blood circulation in the peripheral parts of the body and remove stasis. *Ge Gen* (Radix Puerariae) relieves pain in the upper body and dispels wind-cold or wind-heat from the exterior parts of the body.

FORMULAS

CORYDALIN ™

SUPPLEMENTARY FORMULAS

- ❧ For migraine headaches, add *Migratrol*.
- ❧ For headache caused by recent traumatic or musculoskeletal injury, add *Traumanex*.
- ❧ For severe, long-term headache from previous traumatic injury or blood stagnation, add *Circulation (SJ)*.
- ❧ For headache with excess heat, add *Gardenia Complex*.
- ❧ For headache due to stress and tension, add *Calm*, *Calm (ES)* or *Calm ZZZ*.
- ❧ For headache due to Liver fire, add *Gentiana Complex*.
- ❧ For migraine headache with Liver wind rising, combine with *Gastrodia Complex*.
- ❧ For headache due to wind-heat, add *Lonicera Complex*.
- ❧ For headache due to sinus congestion, add *Pueraria Clear Sinus* or *Magnolia Clear Sinus*.
- ❧ For headache with neck and shoulder stiffness, add *Neck & Shoulder (Acute)*.
- ❧ For headache with upper back pain, add *Back Support (Upper)*.
- ❧ For headache due to environmental or toxic poisoning, add *Herbal DTX*.

NUTRITION

- ❧ Avoid intake of ice drinks or cold food, as they constrict vessels, channels and collaterals.
- ❧ Drink plenty of water throughout the day to avoid dehydration.
- ❧ Diet is important to control and prevent headaches that are food related.
- ❧ Encourage the patient to consume an adequate amount of fruits, vegetables, grains and raw nuts and seeds.
- ❧ Caffeine withdrawal is one of the most common causes of headache. In such cases, gradually decrease and stop the consumption of caffeine-containing foods, such as coffee, tea, cola, etc.
- ❧ Avoid foods containing tyramine, which can cause headaches, such as alcohol, chocolate, banana, citrus fruits, avocado, cabbage, and potato. Also, avoid the consumption of cakes, coffee, dairy products (except yogurt), processed or packaged foods, tobacco, or any junk foods.
- ❧ Monosodium glutamate (MSG) should be avoided in individuals who are sensitive to it. MSG is generally found in canned soups, TV dinners, some meats, and restaurant foods.

The Tao of Nutrition by Ni and McNease
- ❧ Headache
  - ▪ Recommendations: chrysanthemum flowers, mint, green onions, oyster shells, pearl barley, carrots, prunes, buckwheat, peach kernels, and green tea.
  - ▪ Avoid spicy food, lack of sleep, alcohol, smoking, excess stimulation, eye strain, and stress.
- ❧ For more information, please refer to *The Tao of Nutrition* by Dr. Maoshing Ni and Cathy McNease.

LIFESTYLE INSTRUCTIONS

- ❧ Avoid allergens as much as possible if the headache is triggered by allergy. Installation of an air purifier will minimize the presence of allergens in the air and reduce the risk of allergy and headache.
- ❧ Avoid direct exposure to air conditioning, a fan or wind to the head or neck region.
- ❧ Avoid stressful situations and environments whenever possible. Ease the tension with massage, warm baths, and an exercise program.
- ❧ Tension headaches can be relieved by gentle massage of the neck and shoulders to relax the muscles. A hot Epsom salts bath is also helpful.
- ❧ Headache due to poor circulation will respond to vigorous scalp massage.
- ❧ Regular exercise, adequate rest, and normal sleeping habits are essential for optimal health.

CORYDALIN ™

CAUTIONS

- Patients with persistent pain not relieved by *Corydalin* should seek further examination to rule out structural or functional abnormalities.
- Should other prominent signs of diminishing eye-sight and vomiting occur in addition to the headache, refer the patient to a medical doctor immediately for a CT scan or MRI to rule out intra-cranial pressure due to tumor, aneurysms, or cerebral stenosis.
- Patients who are on anticoagulant or antiplatelet therapies, such as Coumadin (Warfarin), should use this formula with caution, as there may be a slightly higher risk of bleeding and bruising.
- This formula is contraindicated during pregnancy and nursing.
- *Corydalin* is designed for short-term management of acute pain, not for long-term treatment of chronic pain. Therefore, once the acute pain has subsided, *Corydalin* should be discontinued and another maintainance formula should be initiated.

CLINICAL NOTES

- *Corydalin* contains herbs that exert analgesic function directly on the central nervous system. *Corydalin* works synergistically with acupuncture to provide pain relief for various aches and pain.
- *Corydalin* is best for acute headaches with severe pain, and is most effective for symptomatic relief. *Migratrol* is most effective when taken on a long-term basis to control and prevent the recurrence of headaches.
- In addition to treating the acute symptom of pain, efforts should be made to identify the underlying cause of pain. For optimal results, another formula should be prescribed to target the cause while using *Corydalin* to address the symptoms.

ACUPUNCTURE POINTS

Traditional Points:
- *Hegu* (LI 4). Needle 1 to 1.5 *cun* deep. Massage the affected area on the head.
- *Renzhong* (GV 26), *Lieque* (LU 7), *Taichong* (LR 3), *Xingjian* (LR 2), *Geshu* (BL 17), *Baihui* (GV 20), *Taiyang* (Extra 2), and *Yintang* (Extra 1).

Balance Method by Dr. Richard Tan:
- Left Side: *Zhongchong* (PC 9), *Shaochong* (HT 9), *Shaoshang* (LU 11), *Zusanli* (ST 36), *Weizhong* (BL 40), and *Yanglingquan* (GB 34).
- Right Side: *Hegu* (LI 4), *Houxi* (SI 3), *Zhongzhu* (TH 3), *Taixi* (KI 3), *Zhongfeng* (LR 4), and *Sanyinjiao* (SP 6).
- Left and right side can be alternated from treatment to treatment.
- For additional information on the Balance Method, please refer to *Dr. Tan's Strategy of Twelve Magical Points* by Dr. Richard Tan.

Ear Points:
- *Taiyang*, Adrenal Gland, Hypothalamus, and Temporal Lobe.
- Use metal ear balls. Switch ears every three days. Five sessions equals one treatment course.

Auricular Acupuncture by Dr. Li-Chun Huang:
- Frontal headache: External Sympathetic, Forehead, and Nervous Subcortex.
  - For headache due to sinus or rhinitis, add Internal Nose.
  - For headache due to ametropia: add Vision II.
- Temporal headache: Temple, Sympathetic, External Sympathetic, Nervous Subcortex, and Coronary Vascular Subcortex. Bleed Ear Apex.

CORYDALIN ™

- ❦ Occipital headache: Occiput, Lesser Occipital Nerve, and Nervous Subcortex. Bleed Ear Apex.
  - ▪ For occiput headache due to cervical vertebral C3 and C4 degeneration, add Cervical Vertebral C3,4 (frontal and back of ear)
- ❦ Vertex headache: Vertex, External Sympathetic, and Nervous Subcortex. Bleed Ear Apex.
- ❦ For additional information on the location and explanation of these points, please refer to *Auricular Treatment Formula and Prescriptions* by Dr. Li-Chun Huang.

MODERN RESEARCH

Corydalin is an empirical formula designed to relieve various kinds of headaches, such as vertex, occipital, migraine, blood-stagnation, and wind-cold headaches. *Corydalin* contains herbs with strong effects to relieve pain, improve blood circulation, and prevent damage to the brain cells.

Yan Hu Suo (Rhizoma Corydalis), containing corydaline, exerts strong anti-inflammatory activity and is effective in both the acute and chronic phases of inflammation.[1] *Yan Hu Suo* (Rhizoma Corydalis) also possesses strong analgesic properties that act directly on the central nervous system.[2] Due to this action, *Yan Hu Suo* (Rhizoma Corydalis) works synergistically with acupuncture to relieve pain. It was demonstrated in a research study that when combined with *Yan Hu Suo* (Rhizoma Corydalis), the analgesic effect of electro-acupuncture increased significantly when compared to a control group that received electro-acupuncture only.[3] Furthermore, *Yan Hu Suo* (Rhizoma Corydalis) has been used as a local anesthetic for surgery. In a study with 105 patients who received *Yan Hu Suo* (Rhizoma Corydalis) as an anesthetic prior to surgery, 98 patients (93.4%) showed satisfactory results while 6 patients (5.7%) experienced mild pain.[4]

Bai Zhi (Radix Angelicae Dahuricae) has analgesic properties and is effective for treating various headaches. *Bai Zhi* (Radix Angelicae Dahuricae) is used to treat vertex headache, sinus headache, orbital headache, and headache due to wind-heat or wind-cold.[5] In a study of 73 patients with occipital headache, after receiving two doses of *Bai Zhi* (Radix Angelicae Dahuricae), 69 patients experienced complete relief, 3 patients experienced partial relief, and 1 patient noted no relief.[6] In another study involving 62 patients with chronic headache, 54 patients reported satisfactory results after approximately two weeks of herbal treatment.[7]

Chuan Xiong (Rhizoma Ligustici Chuanxiong) improves blood circulation and is commonly used with *Bai Zhi* (Radix Angelicae Dahuricae) for treating headache.[5] In one study with 50 patients, *Chuan Xiong* (Rhizoma Ligustici Chuanxiong) was used in conjunction with other herbs and was found to be especially effective in treating headache due to blood stagnation and wind-cold. Out of 20 patients with headache due to blood stagnation, 16 patients reported complete or dramatic improvement; and out of 12 patients with headache due to wind-cold; 10 reported complete or dramatic improvement.[8]

Dan Shen (Radix Salviae Miltiorrhizae) is used primarily to improve peripheral blood circulation.[9] *Dan Shen* (Radix Salviae Miltiorrhizae) improves microcirculation and is commonly used to increase blood perfusion to the brain.[10] Two studies showed *Dan Shen* (Radix Salviae Miltiorrhizae) to offer protection against cerebral ischemia by increasing cerebral perfusion and reducing ultra-structural abnormalities.[11,12] Other studies demonstrated that by increasing cerebral perfusion, *Dan Shen* (Radix Salviae Miltiorrhizae) reduces neurological deficits and repairs cellular damage.[13,14]

Lastly, *Ge Gen* (Radix Puerariae) is used to improve blood circulation and relieve muscle spasm, and is reported to be up to 83% effective in treating migraine headache.[5,9] In one study with 53 patients with migraines, 44 patients (83%) reported significant reduction in pain after taking *Ge Gen* (Radix Puerariae) three times daily for 2 to 22 days.[15]

CORYDALIN ™

PHARMACEUTICAL DRUGS & CHINESE MEDICINE: A COMPARATIVE ANALYSIS

Western Medical Approach: Pain is a basic bodily sensation induced by a noxious stimulus that causes physical discomfort (as pricking, throbbing, or aching). Pain may be of acute or chronic state, and may be of nociceptive, neuropathic, or psychogenic type. Two classes of drugs commonly used to treat pain include non-steroidal anti-inflammatory agents (NSAID) and opioid analgesics. NSAID's [such as Motrin (Ibuprofen) and Voltaren (Diclofenac)] are generally used for mild to moderate pain, and are most effective to reduce inflammation and swelling. Though effective, they may cause such serious side effects as gastric ulcer, duodenal ulcer, gastrointestinal bleeding, tinnitus, blurred vision, dizziness and headache. Furthermore, the newer NSAID's, also known as Cox-2 inhibitors [such as Celebrex (Celecoxib)], are associated with significantly higher risk of cardiovascular events, including heart attack and stroke. Opioid analgesics [such as Vicodin (APAP/Hydrocodone) and morphine] are usually used for severe to excruciating pain. While they may be the most potent agents for pain, they also have the most serious risks and side effects, including but not limited to dizziness, lightheadedness, drowsiness, upset stomach, vomiting, constipation, stomach pain, rash, difficult urination, and respiratory depression resulting in difficult breathing. Furthermore, long-term use of these drugs leads to tolerance and addiction. In brief, it is important to remember that while drugs offer reliable and potent symptomatic pain relief, they should be used only if and when needed. Frequent use and abuse leads to unnecessary side effects and complications.

Traditional Chinese Medicine Approach: Treatment of pain is a sophisticated balance of art and science. Proper treatment of pain requires a careful evaluation of the type of disharmony (excess or deficiency, cold or heat, exterior or interior), characteristics (qi and/or blood stagnations), and locations (upper body, lower body, extremities, or internal organs). Furthermore, optimal treatment requires integrative use of herbs, acupuncture and *Tui-Na* therapies. All these therapies work together to tonify the underlying deficiencies, strengthen the body, and facilitate recovery from chronic pain. TCM pain management targets both the symptom and the cause of pain, and as such, often achieves immediate and long-term success. Furthermore, TCM pain management is often associated with few or no side effects.

Summation: For treatment of mild to severe pain due to various causes, TCM pain management offers similar treatment effects with significantly fewer side effects. However, as in any therapeutic approach, it is important to recognize the limitations of TCM pain management. In some cases, such as excruciating cancer pain in terminally ill patients, drugs are simply superior to herbs. Under these circumstances, potent and consistently reliable pain relief is the main objective, and this can be accomplished more effectively by use of drugs such as intravenous injection of morphine. Herbs should be used to support the underlying constitution of the body, and to alleviate the side effects of the drugs.

CASE STUDIES

A 43-year-old female nurse presented with severe menstrual cramping and pain, along with nausea and vomiting. She was unable to work because of her illness. Tenderness and pain were felt in the abdominal region with *Zhongfeng* (LR 4) and *Ligou* (LR 5) being the most tender upon palpation. The practitioner diagnosed the condition as qi and blood stagnation in the abdomen and Liver qi stagnation. In addition to the stagnation were damp accumulation with multiple uterine fibroids (7.3 cm in size) and an ovarian cyst. She was instructed to take *Corydalin,* 6 to 8 capsules, 2 to 4 times a day, which helped to control the pain and, in turn, reduced the need for her missing more work. With the help of the herbs, not only did the severity and intensity of her menstrual cramping subsided, but the occurrence lasted only for a few hours instead of 1 to 2 days. Eventually the patient did not experience any more vomiting associated with pain. The practitioner concluded that *Corydalin* worked as a superb analgesic herbal formula during the treatment.

T.W., Santa Monica, CA

FORMULAS

CORYDALIN ™

A 31-year-old male administrative assistant with migraines since the age of 6 had been treated with Imitrex (Sumatriptan) with limited success. The migraines were diagnosed as qi and blood stagnation with Liver qi stagnation stirring up wind. The doctor prescribed *Corydalin*, upon which the patient experienced almost immediate and positive results! The patient subsequently stopped using Imitrex (Sumatriptan) completely which, in turn, reduced occurrences of rebound headaches.

J.K., Woodland Hills, California

A 47-year-old female acupuncturist presented with one-sided severely debilitating migraines, which occurred particularly during the weekends. The TCM diagnosis was Kidney yin deficiency leading to Liver yang rising. A dose of *Corydalin* relieved the pain especially when the drug Imitrex (Sumatriptan) was unsuccessful. Within two weeks of taking *Corydalin*, she was free from headaches. She supplemented her treatment with *Gastrodia Complex* in addition to acupuncture treatments. She has experienced no migraine episodes for more than six months, and continues using the herbal combination of *Corydalin* and *Gastrodia Complex*.

D.W., Hashbrouck Heights, New Jersey

A 44-year-old female police officer presented with chronic headaches located in the occipital/temporal regions. She stated that stress aggravated the problem. There was acute tenderness at the *Fengchi* (GB 20) area as well as in the cervical spine. She also experienced pain on her zygoma. The practitioner diagnosed the condition as qi and blood stagnation in Gallbladder, Urinary Bladder, and Small Intestine channels in addition to myofascial syndrome, which was stress-induced because of the nature of her job. She was treated with *Corydalin*, *Neck & Shoulder (Acute)* and *Calm (ES)*, which were all so effective that they subsequently replaced her medication, Imitrex (Sumatriptan). The practitioner concluded that a critical aspect in the treatment was to assist patient in coping with their stress, which in turn made the herbal treatment more effective.

S.C., La Crescenta., CA

A 64-year-old female retired editor presented with severe sinus headaches and acute/chronic sinusitis. There was severe sinus pain on palpation above and below her eyebrows. Her tongue had a reddish tip, and the coat was thin with a whitish yellow color. Pulse diagnosis was slightly elevated at the Lung position. The practitioner diagnosed the condition as damp-heat in the upper *jiao*. Administration of the recommended doses of *Corydalin* produced excellent results. The patient also reported that the most immediate relief from her sinus headaches occurred upon taking the *Corydalin* formula exclusively. The practitioner also noted similar positive outcomes from other patients.

R.K., San Diego, California

A 50-year-old female public information specialist who was emotionally labile presented with pain in the shoulder, neck, thoracic, lumbar and foot. Her lumbar discs at L4 and L5 were herniated. In addition to migraines and bouts of constipation, she also complained of anxiety, depression and insomnia, all of which may be attributed to some side effects of taking multiple pharmaceuticals. The practitioner diagnosed her condition as qi and blood stagnation as well as Liver depression. *Corydalin* and *Schisandra ZZZ* were given. *Corydalin* significantly reduced her pain. She was able to lessen the use of oxycontin and Duragesic (Fentanyl) patches significantly. In fact, the dosages of oxycontin and Duragesic (Fentanyl) patches were reduced by as much as 75%. Furthermore, the practitioner observed that *Corydalin* was also effective to maintain other patients who suffered from occasional pain. The majority of patients (about 90%) who took *Corydalin* responded favorably, especially since most were experiencing digestive side effects with ibuprofen.

F.G., Sykesville, Maryland

CORYDALIN ™

An 85-year-old retired female presented with excruciating pain in the neck and shoulder that causes difficulty sleeping. Objective findings included limited range of motion of the neck. The tongue had a dirty yellow coat and a red tip. The western diagnosis included psoriatic arthritis, arthritis, fibromyalgia, hiatal hernia, hypertension, depression, chronic constipation, leaky gut syndrome, sciatica and insomnia. The patient was instructed to take *Neck & Shoulder (Acute)* and *Corydalin*, 3 capsules of each three times daily in between meals. *Calm (ES)* was given at night to help sleep. The patient responded that the formulas were effective in reducing the acute pain in the neck and shoulder region. After the acute phase two weeks later, the patient was switched to *Gan Mai Da Zao Tang* (Licorice, Wheat, and Jujube Decoction) and *Shao Yao Gan Cao Tang* (Peony and Licorice Decoction), a combination recommended by Dr. Richard Tan that consistently helped patients with fibromyalgia.

J.B., Camarillo, California

A 40-year-old housewife presented with migraines, stress and a lack of sleep. She woke up frequently and has had many stress-related headaches for years. The practitioner diagnosed the condition as Liver qi stagnation with heat rising. The practitioner felt the treatment should revolve around calming the *shen* (spirit). After 2 weeks of taking *Calm*, the headaches were less severe and less frequent, however sleeping was still poor. At 4 weeks, her headaches were very mild and under control. She no longer needed to take any western medications. The patient appeared more calm and reported sleeping better and feeling less stressful. She was recommended to continue taking *Calm* for 2 to 3 more months. As an adjunct to the treatment, the practitioner also suggested taking *Corydalin* for her headaches as well as reducing her caffeine intake.

D.S., Flagstaff, Arizona

At a seminar in Providence, Rhode Island, a question was raised as whether *Yan Hu Suo* (Rhizoma Corydalis) would cause a person treated with this herb to test positive in a drug screen (as do a number of analgesic substances). A very small study was conducted in a laboratory at the Rhode Island Clinical Research Center: two people taking 6 capsules of *Corydalin* were screened for drugs 3 hours later. Both were completely negative in the seven drug panels. A solution of 5% *Yan Hu Suo* (Rhizoma Corydalis) powdered extract (freed from excessive carbohydrate) was also tested in the drug-screening test, again with negative results. It was concluded by the researchers that a person being treated for pain with the usual dosage of *Corydalin* would not risk testing positive for opiates, benzodiazepines, barbiturates, etc. [Note: *Yan Hu Suo* (Rhizoma Corydalis) is the main ingredient that is present in both *Corydalin* and *Herbal Analgesic*.]

D.W., Hadley, MA

L.N., a 42-year-old female, had a history of headache and migraine triggered by stress and/or environmental factors. She presented with sinus headache for two days following a migraine headache. Clinical manifestations included orbital pain with photophobia, and neck and shoulder pain. The TCM diagnosis was qi and blood stagnation. Acupuncture treatment was combined with *Corydalin* at three capsules, three times daily, or as needed for headache. The practitioner commented that all symptoms were resolved after treatments.

C.L., Chino Hills, California

[1] Kubo, M. et al. Anti-inflammatory activities of methanolic extract and alkaloidal components from corydalis tuber. *Biol Pharm Bull.*; February 1994; 17(2):262-5

[2] Zhu, XZ. Development of natural products as drugs acting on central nervous system. *Memorias do Instituto Oswaldo Cruz*. 1991; 86 2:173-5

[3] Hu, J. et al. Effect of some drugs on electroacupuncture analgesia and cytosolic free Ca2+ concentration of mice brain. *Chen Tzu Yen Chiu*; 1994; 19(1):55-8

[4] Use of corydalis (yan hu suo) injectables for surgical anesthesia. Tangshang Medical Hospital Second Branch. *Hebei Xin Yi Yao) Medical Journal of Hebei)*; 1973; 4:34

CORYDALIN ™

[5] Bensky, D. et al. *Chinese Herbal Medicine Materia Medica*. Eastland Press 1993.

[6] Effectiveness of angelica (bai zhi) in treating occipital headache: a report of 73 cases. Airforce Hospital in Hengyang, China. (Xin Zhong Yi) *Modern Medical Journal*; 1976; 3:128

[7] Effectiveness of angelica (bai zhi) in treating chronic headache: a report of 62 cases. National Defense Hospital. (Xin Yi Xue Yao Za Zi) *Journal of Modern* Medicine, 1976;8:35.

[8] Wang, LS. Treatment of headache using xiong zhi shi gao tang: 50 cases. *Shanxi Journal of Traditional Chinese Medicine*.;10:447. 1985

[9] Yeung, HC. *Handbook of Chinese Herbs*. Institute of Chinese Medicine. 1983.

[10] Nagai, M. et al. Vasodilator effects of des(alpha-carboxy-3'4-dihydroxyphenethyl)lithospermic acid (8-epiblechnic acid)' a derivative of lithospermic acids in Salviae miltiorrhizae radix. *Biol Pharm Bull*, Feb. 1996; 19(2):228-32

[11] Wu, W. et al. the effect of radix salviae miltiorrhizae on the changes of ultrastructure in rat brain after cerebral ischemia. *J. Tradit Chin Med*, Sept. 1992; 12(3):183-6

[12] Kuang, PG. et al. The effect of radix salviae miltiorrhizae on vasoactive intestinal peptide in cerebral ischemia: an animal experiment. *J Tradit Chin Med*, Sept. 1989; 9(3):203-6,

[13] Kuang, P. et al. Effect of radix salviae miltiorrhizae on nitric oxide in cerebral ischemia-reperfusion injury. *J Tradit Chin Med*, Sept. 1996; 16(3):224-7,

[14] Protective effect of radix saliva miltiorrhizae on nitric oxide in cerebral ischemia-reperfusion injury. *J Tradit Chin Med*, Jun. 1995; 15(2):135-40,

[15] Gao, XX. et al. Effectiveness of pueraria root (ge gen) in treating migraine headache: a case report of 53 patients. (Zhong Hua Nei Ke Za Zi) *Journal of TCM Internal Medicine*. 1977; 6:326.

DERMATROL (HZ) ™

(Herpes Zoster)

CLINICAL APPLICATIONS

- Shingles (herpes zoster)
- Shingles with skin lesions and nerve pain

WESTERN THERAPEUTIC ACTIONS

- Antiviral effect to shorten the duration and suppress the severity of shingles
- Analgesic effect to relieve pain
- Anti-inflammatory effect to reduce inflammation

CHINESE THERAPEUTIC ACTIONS

- Drains damp-heat
- Purges fire
- Eliminates toxins
- Tonifies the underlying deficiencies

DOSAGE

Take 4 capsules three times daily during the entire course of infection. The herbal therapy should begin immediately upon the notice of the first warning signs. If necessary, the dosage may be doubled on day one of herbal therapy to achieve faster onset of action. However, this formula should be discontinued when the course of infection is terminated.

INGREDIENTS

Chi Shao (Radix Paeoniae Rubrae)
Dao Di Wu Gong (Rhizoma Heliminthostachytis)
Gan Cao (Radix Glycyrrhizae)
Huang Bai (Cortex Phellodendri)
Huang Lian (Rhizoma Coptidis)
Huang Qin (Radix Scutellariae)
Jin Qian Cao (Herba Lysimachiae)
Jin Yin Hua (Flos Lonicerae)
Jing Jie (Herba Schizonepetae)

Lian Qiao (Fructus Forsythiae)
Long Dan Cao (Radix Gentianae)
Mu Dan Pi (Cortex Moutan)
Niu Bang Zi (Fructus Arctii)
Pu Gong Ying (Herba Taraxaci)
Sheng Di Huang (Radix Rehmanniae)
Zao Xiu (Rhizoma Paridis)
Zhi Zi (Fructus Gardeniae)
Zi Hua Di Ding (Herba Violae)

FORMULA EXPLANATION

Dermatrol (HZ) is an herbal formula specifically formulated to treat shingles. In traditional Chinese medicine, the history of treating shingles is well-documented, with the first recorded treatment in *Huang Di Nei Jing* (Yellow Emperor's Inner Classic) in the second century A.D. Shingles is generally diagnosed as the presence of damp-heat, fire and toxins, accompanied by underlying deficiencies. Therefore, *Dermatrol (HZ)* incorporates herbs specifically to drain damp-heat, purge fire, eliminate toxins, and tonify the underlying deficiencies.

In this formula, *Dao Di Wu Gong* (Rhizoma Heliminthostachytis) is used as the principle herb as it has a unique effect to clear heat and eliminate toxins. The use of this herb has been documented to effectively treat shingles, both in internal and topical formulations. *Long Dan Cao* (Radix Gentianae) and *Jin Qian Cao* (Herba Lysimachiae) clear damp-heat from the Liver and Gallbladder channels. Together, they drain out damp-heat through urination. *Huang Lian* (Rhizoma Coptidis), *Huang Qin* (Radix Scutellariae), *Huang Bai* (Cortex Phellodendri) and *Zhi Zi* (Fructus Gardeniae) clear damp-heat from upper, middle and lower *jiaos*, and enable this formula to treat shingles affecting

DERMATROL (HZ) ™

different parts of the body. *Jin Yin Hua* (Flos Lonicerae), *Lian Qiao* (Fructus Forsythiae) and *Jing Jie* (Herba Schizonepetae) clear heat and toxins from the exterior to treat lesions and sores. *Niu Bang Zi* (Fructus Arctii), *Pu Gong Ying* (Herba Taraxaci), *Zi Hua Di Ding* (Herba Violae) and *Zao Xiu* (Rhizoma Paridis) clear heat and eliminate toxins from the interior to treat lesions and sores. *Chi Shao* (Radix Paeoniae Rubrae) activates blood circulation and relieves pain. Adequate blood circulation will ensure proper healing of the lesions. *Sheng Di Huang* (Radix Rehmanniae) and *Mu Dan Pi* (Cortex Moutan) nourish yin and clear deficiency heat. They also prevent all the bitter and cold herbs from consuming the yin and fluids of the body. Lastly, *Gan Cao* (Radix Glycyrrhizae) harmonizes all the herbs in this formula.

In short, ***Dermatrol (HZ)*** is an herbal formula that utilizes thousands of years of clinical experiences to treat shingles. It shortens the duration and reduces the severity of illness by using herbs to drain damp-heat, purge fire, eliminate toxins and tonify the underlying deficiencies.

SUPPLEMENTARY FORMULAS

- To enhance the overall effect to treat genital herpes, combine with ***Gentiana Complex***.
- To enhance the overall effect to treat oral herpes, combine with ***Lonicera Complex***.
- For post-herpetic pain, combine with ***Flex (NP)***.
- To strengthen the immune system and minimize the recurrences of shingles, use ***Immune +*** and ***Nourish*** on a regular basis at low doses.
- For chronic pain without blisters but dark appearance at the place of the lesions, add ***Circulation (SJ)***.
- For fever, add ***Gardenia Complex***.

NUTRITION

- There are many nutrients that are essential for preventing, fighting, and healing of shingles. Some examples include garlic, L-lysine, calcium, magnesium, and vitamins A, B, C, and E.
- The following foods are also beneficial: brewer's yeast, brown rice, garlic, raw fruits and vegetables, whole grains, and foods rich in vitamins.
- Avoid foods that are spicy, fried or greasy. Refrain from foods that are high in L-carnitine, such as peanuts, chocolate, and corn. Shellfish and seafood are also contraindicated.
- Avoid alcohol and tobacco products.

LIFESTYLE INSTRUCTIONS

- Shingles attack may be triggered by many factors, including but not limited to emotional or physical stress, spinal cord injuries, and conditions that cause immunodeficiency. All these conditions and situations should be avoided, if at all possible.
- Individuals with shingles should avoid direct skin contact with others, as the fluid from shingles blisters is contagious, and exposure to it can cause chickenpox (but not shingles).
- It is important to take good general care of skin sores, such as not scratching blisters and keeping the skin clean and dry.
- Be careful at the gym, as the virus may be transmitted through physical contact, such as via exercise mats.

CLINICAL NOTES

- ***Dermatrol (HZ)*** is a potent herbal formula that treats shingles. It should be used immediately with the first warning signs of herpes outbreak, and continue until the remission. However, it should not be taken indefinitely as this formula is relatively strong, and may weaken the overall constitution if taken for a long period of time.

DERMATROL (HZ) ™

(Herpes Zoster)

Discontinue use after symptoms have cleared. However, if there is still pain, herbs can be continued for a few more days. Acupuncture is a more effective method for treating just the pain after herpetic lesions have cleared.

☙ Herbal therapy is most effective if it is started immediately, upon experiencing the first warning signs. The dosage may be doubled on the first day to speed up the initial onset of action. The herbal therapy should be continued until the course of infection is terminated. Possible warning signs and symptoms may include: headache, flu-like symptoms (usually without a fever), and sensitivity to light, followed by itching, tingling, or even severe pain in the area of the rash.

☙ Herpes lesions can also be treated topically, in conjunction with taking herbs orally. There are two topical treatments that are quite effective:

  ▪ The first topical treatment uses an herbal paste made from mixing the extract granules of 2 parts *Da Huang* (Radix et Rhizoma Rhei), 2 parts *Huang Bai* (Cortex Phellodendri), 1 part *Wu Bei Zi* (Galla Chinensis), and 1 part *Mang Xiao* (Natrii Sulfas) with 30% petroleum jelly. The herbal paste is to be applied topically and covered with gauze. The herbal paste should be changed on a daily basis.

  ▪ The second topical treatment uses *Hai Jin Sha* (Herba Lygodii) as an herbal wash. Mix 1 tablespoon of the extract granule of *Hai Jin Sha* (Herba Lygodii) with 1 cup of water and apply topically as a wash after shower.

☙ It is important to see an ophthalmologist if the shingles lesions appear near the eyes. If untreated, herpes zoster infection of the eye may lead to blindness.

CAUTIONS

☙ This formula is bitter and cold, and may cause nausea and vomiting in individuals who have a sensitive stomach. Therefore, it may be taken with food to minimize such adverse reactions.

☙ This formula should be stopped once symptoms are cleared. It is not recommended for long-term use.

ACUPUNCTURE POINTS

Traditional Points:

☙ *Hegu* (LI 4), *Zhigou* (TH 6), and *Yanglingquan* (GB 34). Insert needles 0.5 *cun* deep all along the sides of the shingles (use between 4 and 16 needles).

☙ Tap plum-blossom needles all along the sides of the shingles. Be careful ***not*** to tap directly on the lesions. Tap until there is slight bleeding from the skin.

  ▪ Shingles with more itching (wind): *Quchi* (LI 11), *Fengchi* (GB 20), *Hegu* (LI 4), *Waiguan* (TH 5), *Yanglingquan* (GB 34), and *Xuehai* (SP 10).

  ▪ Shingles with more burning sensations (toxic-heat): *ah shi* points, *Huatuojiaji*, *Quchi* (LI 11), *Waiguan* (TH 5), and *Yanglingquan* (GB 34).

  ▪ Shingles with more pain (qi and blood stagnation): *Zhangmen* (LR 13), *Yifeng* (TH 17), *Zhigou* (TH 6), and *Yanglingquan* (GB 34).

  ▪ Shingles with wet lesions (dampness and Spleen deficiency): *Zusanli* (ST 36), *Qimen* (LR 14), *Yuanye* (GB 22), *Fenglong* (ST 40), *Zhigou* (TH 6), and *ah shi* points.

Balance Method by Dr. Richard Tan:

☙ Shingles on the rib cage: Needle bilaterally *ah shi* points from *Chize* (LU 5) to *Kongzui* (LU 6), *Tongli* (HT 5) to *Shaohai* (HT 3), and from *Waiguan* (TH 5) to *Sidu* (TH 9), and *Yanggu* (SI 5) to *Xiaohai* (SI 8).

☙ For additional information on the Balance Method, please refer to *Twelve and Twelve in Acupuncture, Twenty-Four More in Acupuncture*, and *Dr. Tan's Strategy of Twelve Magical Points* by Dr. Richard Tan.

Ear Points:

☙ Herpes zoster: Lung (three needles), Subcortex, Endocrine, and affected area. Strong stimulation should be applied for two hours every other day. Ten to fifteen treatments equal one course of treatment.

FORMULAS

DERMATROL (HZ) ™

(Herpes Zoster)

☯ Herpes zoster: Lung, Sympathetic, Adrenal Gland, and *ah shi* points on the affected area. Leave in the needles for one hour.

Auricular Acupuncture by Dr. Li-Chun Huang:

☯ Herpes zoster: Corresponding point (to the area affected), Allergic Area, Endocrine, Adrenal Gland, *Shenmen*, Occiput, Liver, Gallbladder, Spleen, and Lung. Bleed Ear Apex.
  ▪ For herpes zoster due to insomnia, add Neurasthenia Area and Neurasthenia Point.
☯ For additional information on the location and explanation of these points, please refer to *Auricular Treatment Formula and Prescriptions* by Dr. Li-Chun Huang.

MODERN RESEARCH

Shingles, also known as chicken pox, herpes zoster, zona zoster, is caused by re-activation of the herpes virus. Shingles is an acute viral inflammation of the sensory ganglia of spinal and cranial nerves associated with a vesicular eruption and neuralgic pain. ***Dermatrol (HZ)*** is formulated with many herbs that address the overall condition of herpes infection, including use of herbs to treat the virus, reduce the inflammation, relieve pain, promote normal urination, and facilitate the healing of lesions and sores.

Since herpes is a viral infection, ***Dermatrol (HZ)*** is formulated with many herbs that have marked antiviral effect, such as *Long Dan Cao* (Radix Gentianae), *Huang Lian* (Rhizoma Coptidis), *Huang Qin* (Radix Scutellariae), *Huang Bai* (Cortex Phellodendri), and *Chi Shao* (Radix Paeoniae Rubrae). These herbs have been shown to effectively suppress the replication of virus, and reduce the duration of viral infections. [1,2,3,4,5]

To reduce inflammation and relieve pain, ***Dermatrol (HZ)*** incorporates many herbs with excellent anti-inflammatory and analgesic effects. *Mu Dan Pi* (Cortex Moutan), *Lian Qiao* (Fructus Forsythiae), *Jin Yin Hua* (Flos Lonicerae) and *Sheng Di Huang* (Radix Rehmanniae) have good effects to reduce swelling and inflammation. [6,7,8,9] *Zhi Zi* (Fructus Gardeniae) has a marked analgesic effect to relieve pain, and may be used either internally or externally. [10,11]

Furthermore, since herpes infection may affect the genital area and cause dysuria, this formula also contains many herbs with diuretic effect to relieve painful and difficult urination. The herbs with diuretic effects include *Long Dan Cao* (Radix Gentianae), [12] *Jin Qian Cao* (Herba Lysimachiae), [13] and *Pu Gong Ying* (Herba Taraxaci). [14]

Lastly, ***Dermatrol (HZ)*** uses many herbs to facilitate the healing of herpetic lesions and sores and to shorten the duration of illness, such as *Dao Di Wu Gong* (Rhizoma Heliminthostachytis), *Zi Hua Di Ding* (Herba Violae), and *Zao Xiu* (Rhizoma Paridis). *Jing Jie* (Herba Schizonepetae) is also added for its function to relieve itching and general skin discomfort. [15]

In summary, ***Dermatrol (HZ)*** is an herbal formula that treats both the cause and the symptoms of shingles. It contains herbs with antiviral effect to treat the herpes infection. Furthermore, it contains herbs with anti-inflammatory, analgesic, and diuretic effects to treat the symptoms of shingles.

PHARMACEUTICAL DRUGS & CHINESE MEDICINE: A COMPARATIVE ANALYSIS

Western Medical Approach: Shingles, also known as chicken pox or herpes zoster, is a viral infection with an acute inflammation of the sensory ganglia of spinal and cranial nerves associated with a vesicular eruption and neuralgic pain. There is no specific treatment in western medicine. However, certain drugs may be used to treat the symptoms. Wet compresses are soothing when applied topically. Aspirin and Elavil (Amitriptyline) are sometimes used to relieve pain. Antiviral drugs, such as Zovirax (Acyclovir), are recommended only in individuals with

DERMATROL (HZ) ™

(Herpes Zoster)

weakened immune systems, such as geriatric and pediatric patients. In short, most of these drugs relieve symptoms, but do not change the course of infection or reduce its severity.

Traditional Chinese Medicine Approach: Herbs are very effective to treat the cause and the symptoms of shingles. As described above, many herbs have been shown via *in vitro* and *in vivo* studies to effectively treat viral infections by reducing its severity and duration. Furthermore, many herbs have excellent analgesic effect to relieve pain and anti-inflammatory effect to reduce inflammation. Though there is no cure, herbs do offer excellent short- and long-term relief. Finally, after the shingles are resolved, patients should follow the guidelines established in Nutrition and Lifestyles Instructions sections to strengthen the body and reduce recurrences.

CASE STUDY

A 65-year-old male farmer complained of shingles lesions that started one week ago at the left chest area, which then spread throughout the ribs and the back. The pain was described as burning, stabbing, and extremely painful. The patient had yellow urine, normal bowel movement, and a wiry-forceful pulse. This condition was diagnosed as damp-heat and Liver fire. The patient was treated with *Dermatrol (HZ)* orally. The patient was also instructed to use *Hai Jin Sha* (Herba Lygodii) as an herbal wash topically to the affected area once daily. After 4 days of internal and external treatments, the shingles lesions decreased in size, and the pain was reduced significantly. After 7 days, the patient reported complete recovery.

Anonymous

[1] *Zhong Yao Yao Li Yu Ying Yong* (Pharmacology and Applications of Chinese Herbs), 1983; 295
[2] *Zhong Xi Yi Jie He Za Zhi* (Journal of Integrated Chinese and Western Medicine), 1989; 9(8):494
[3] *Zhong Yao Xue* (Chinese Herbology), 1988; 137:140
[4] *Zhong Yao Xue* (Chinese Herbology), 1998; 144:146
[5] *Zhong Yao Xue* (Chinese Herbology), 1998; 162:164
[6] *Sheng Yao Xue Za Zhi* (Journal of Raw Herbology), 1979; 33(3):178
[7] *Ke Yan Tong Xun* (Journal of Science and Research), 1982; (3):35
[8] *Shan Xi Yi Kan* (Shanxi Journal of Medicine), 1960;(10):22
[9] *Zhong Yao Yao Li Yu Ying Yong* (Pharmacology and Applications of Chinese Herbs), 1983: 400
[10] *Zhong Yao Zhi* (Chinese Herbology Journal), 1984; 578
[11] *Zhong Yi Za Zhi* (Journal of Chinese Medicine), 1964; 12:450
[12] *Zhong Yao Yao Li Yu Ying Yong* (Pharmacology and Applications of Chinese Herbs), 1983; 295
[13] *Guang Xi Zhong Yi Yao* (Guangxi Chinese Medicine and Herbology), 1990; 13(6):40
[14] *Zhong Yi Za Zhi* (Journal of Chinese Medicine), 1964; 12:450
[15] *Zhong Yi Za Zhi* (Journal of Chinese Medicine), 1964; 12:18

FORMULAS

DERMATROL (PS) ™

(Psoriasis)

CLINICAL APPLICATIONS

- ❧ Psoriasis
- ❧ Dermatological disorders with lesions, blisters or severe itching of the skin
- ❧ Acne with pus and redness

WESTERN THERAPEUTIC ACTIONS

- ❧ Suppresses proliferation of the psoriatic cells [2,3,4,5,6,7,8]
- ❧ Reduces tissue inflammation [9,10,11,12]
- ❧ General action to relieve dermatological disorders such as rash, itching and eczema [13,14,15,16]

CHINESE THERAPEUTIC ACTIONS

- ❧ Clears heat and detoxifies
- ❧ Invigorates blood circulation and nourishes blood

DOSAGE

Take 3 to 4 capsules three times daily on an empty stomach with warm water. In acute conditions, dosage may be increased to 8 to 10 capsules three times daily for one week, or until symptoms subside. After relief of symptoms, dosage then can be reduced to 3 or 4 capsules daily.

INGREDIENTS

Bai Hua She She Cao (Herba Oldenlandia)
Bai Xian Pi (Cortex Dictamni)
Ban Lan Gen (Radix Isatidis)
Chan Tui (Periostracum Cicadae)
Chi Shao (Radix Paeoniae Rubrae)
Da Qing Ye (Folium Isatidis)
Gan Cao (Radix Glycyrrhizae)

He Shou Wu (Radix Polygoni Multiflori)
Jin Yin Hua (Flos Lonicerae)
Ku Shen Gen (Radix Sophorae Flavescentis)
Lu Feng Fang (Nidus Vespae)
Mu Dan Pi (Cortex Moutan)
Quan Xie (Scorpio)
Wu Shao She (Zaocys)

FORMULA EXPLANATION

Psoriasis and severe skin itching in traditional Chinese medicine are amongst the most difficult disorders to treat since there may be various pathogenic factors involved. In addition, most conditions are chronic and may be complicated by the presence of both excess and deficient factors simultaneously, such as wind, toxic heat, dampness, and blood deficiency. To successfully treat such stubborn and complicated conditions, ***Dermatrol (PS)*** contains many strong and potent herbs to treat both the cause and the symptoms concurrently.

Dermatrol (PS) contains many animal and insect medicinal substances that have potent actions to eliminate the heat and toxins that contribute directly to psoriasis or other dermatological conditions. *Wu Shao She* (Zaocys) has excellent dispersing functions that enter the internal organs and travel to the skin to relieve itching. It disperses wind, which is the predominant cause for itching. To further assist the principle herb in relieving itching and dispersing wind, *Ku Shen Gen* (Radix Sophorae Flavescentis), *Bai Xian Pi* (Cortex Dictamni) and *Chan Tui* (Periostracum Cicadae) are used. *Da Qing Ye* (Folium Isatidis), *Ban Lan Gen* (Radix Isatidis) and *Bai Hua She She Cao* (Herba Oldenlandia) are used to clear heat and detoxify. *Jin Yin Hua* (Flos Lonicerae) is commonly used to treat toxic heat in the exterior characterized by all dermatological sores, lesions, ulcerations, warts and furuncles. To

DERMATROL (PS) ™

cool the blood and prevent further spreading of lesions, *Mu Dan Pi* (Cortex Moutan) and *Chi Shao* (Radix Paeoniae Rubrae) are used. *Quan Xie* (Scorpio) and *Lu Feng Fang* (Nidus Vespae) are used together to relieve toxicity, dispel wind and relieve pain. The use of these two substances is effective because in traditional Chinese medicine, it is sometimes necessary to "use toxin to attack toxin." These two herbs are used to treat a wide range of dermatological disorders ranging from toxic sores, mastitis, mumps, swellings and scrofula. *He Shou Wu* (Radix Polygoni Multiflori) tonifies blood and prevent flaring of wind associated with blood deficiency. Finally, *Gan Cao* (Radix Glycyrrhizae) is used to harmonize the formula, reduce the toxicity of *Quan Xie* (Scorpio) and also to protect the stomach from the cold properties of the heat-clearing herbs.

SUPPLEMENTARY FORMULAS

- For itching due to wind-heat, add *Silerex*.
- For acne with redness, pain and pus, add *Herbal ENT*.
- For excess heat manifesting in redness, add *Gardenia Complex*.
- For chronic skin condition with blood stagnation, add *Circulation (SJ)* or *Flex (NP)*.
- For blood or yin deficiency with dry skin, flaking, and dry throat, add *Schisandra ZZZ* and *Gardenia Complex*.
- For toxic heat with redness and pain, or skin infection, add *Herbal ABX*.
- For yin deficiency with heat and dryness, add *Nourish*.
- For ulcerations and wet lesions on the skin due to damp-heat, add *Gentiana Complex*.
- For dry stools or constipation, add *Gentle Lax (Excess)* or *Gentle Lax (Deficient)*.
- For conditions that worsen during winter or with coldness, add *Balance (Cold)*.
- For shingles, use *Dermatrol (HZ)* instead.
- For lupus, use *LPS Support* instead.

NUTRITION

- Successful treatment of psoriasis or any dermatological disorders with herbs is highly dependent on the patient's cooperation in maintaining a proper diet. During the treatment period, alcohol, spicy food, seafood and anything that may be stimulating, or that may cause allergies should be avoided completely.
- Fish oil, flax seed oil, and primrose oil help to reduce inflammation, and are beneficial for treatment of psoriasis.
- Make sure the diet contains adequate amount of fruits, vegetables, whole grains, and dietary fiber.
- Avoid citrus fruits, fried foods, processed foods, and saturated fats.

The Tao of Nutrition by Ni and McNease
- Psoriasis
  - Recommendations: Chinese prunes, guava skins, pearl barley, vinegar, garlic, walnuts, cucumber, beet tops, dandelions, squash, and mung beans.
  - Recommendations: Take 15 peeled and sliced water chestnuts and 1 vinegar (preferably aged rice vinegar), slowly simmer in a non-metal pot for 20 minutes until water chestnuts absorb most of the vinegar. Then mash into a paste and seal in a jar. Spread evenly on a gauze pad and apply to affected area, changing daily if not too serious, three times daily if serious condition. Mild cases should show improvement within 5 days, but serious conditions may take up to 2 weeks.
  - Avoid spicy food, stimulating food, alcohol, caffeine, smoking, and excessive sun exposure.
- Acne
  - Recommendations: Apply plain, low fat, no chemical yogurt to the affected area. Leave on for 20 minutes then wash off.
  - Recommendations: Roast buckwheat, grind to powder and mix with rice vinegar into a paste, then apply to area.

FORMULAS

DERMATROL (PS) ™

(Psoriasis)

- Recommendations: For oozing acne condition, cover area with pearl barley powder over night, wash off with water.
- Avoid: fried foods, fatty or oily foods, spicy foods, coffee, alcohol, sugar, smoking, stress, constipation, make-up, washing with chemicals, chocolate, ice cream, soft drinks, and emotional stress.
- For more information, please refer to *The Tao of Nutrition* by Dr. Maoshing Ni and Cathy McNease.

LIFESTYLE INSTRUCTIONS

- Prevention of respiratory infections is also important. Adequate rest is essential.
- Do not scratch the affected area, which increase risk of infection and scarring.

CLINICAL NOTES

- Because psoriasis is a difficult and stubborn disease, the treatment period is set at three months at a time, between intervals for evaluation and modification of the herbal formula(s).
- After the condition has stabilized, it is recommended that the patient take 2 capsules per day of *Dermatrol (PS)*. Furthermore, those with qi deficiency or blood deficiency should take *Immune +* or *Schisandra ZZZ*, respectively.

CAUTIONS

- Patients with weak Spleen and Stomach should take this formula with food to avoid stomach upset.
- Patients with yang deficiency or coldness should use this formula with caution. A yang-tonic formula such as *Kidney Tonic (Yang)* is recommended to be taken with *Dermatrol (PS)* for maximum effect.
- This formula is contraindicated during pregnancy and nursing.

ACUPUNCTURE POINTS

Traditional Points:
- *Quchi* (LI 11), *Xuehai* (SP 10), *Zusanli* (ST 36), *Neiguan* (PC 6), *Shenmen* (HT 7), *Sanyinjiao* (SP 6), and *Feiyang* (BL 58).

Balance Method by Dr. Richard Tan:
- Left side: *Dadun* (LR 1), *Zhongfeng* (LR 4), *Shangyang* (LI 1), and *Hegu* (LI 4).
- Right side: *Zuqiaoyin* (GB 44), *Qiuxu* (GB 40), *Shaoshang* (LU 11), and *Jingqu* (LU 8).
- Left and right side can be alternated from treatment to treatment.
- For additional information on the Balance Method, please refer to *Dr. Tan's Strategy of Twelve Magical Points* by Dr. Richard Tan.

Ear Points:
- Main points: Lung, Endocrine, *Shenmen*, and Occipital point.
- Adjunct points: Adrenal Gland, Liver, Spleen, Brain Stem, and Heart.
- Select four to five points each time, and needle for 30 to 60 minutes every other day. Ear seeds can also be used. Alternate ears every three to seven days.

Auricular Acupuncture by Dr. Li-Chun Huang:
- Psoriasis: Corresponding points (to the areas affected), Gallbladder, Liver, Spleen, Lung, Large Intestine, and Endocrine. Bleed Ear Apex.

DERMATROL (PS) ™

(Psoriasis)

❧ For additional information on the location and explanation of these points, please refer to *Auricular Treatment Formula and Prescriptions* by Dr. Li-Chun Huang.

MODERN RESEARCH

Psoriasis is defined as a chronic and recurrent disease characterized by dry, well-circumscribed, silvery, scaling papules and plaques of varying sizes.[1] Areas commonly affected by psoriasis include the scalp, sacral area, extensor surface of the extremities, buttocks, and penis. The exact cause of psoriasis is unknown, but the lesions are characterized by increased epidermal cell proliferation and inflammation. Therefore, optimal treatment must focus on suppressing cell proliferation and reducing tissue inflammation.

Dermatrol (PS) contains many herbs with marked characteristics to treat psoriasis by suppressing the proliferation of cells. The inhibitory effect of these herbs slows or stops the abnormally high rate of proliferation of cells, as in cases of psoriasis. Herbs with this inhibitory effect include *Quan Xie* (Scorpio),[2] *Ku Shen Gen* (Radix Sophorae Flavescentis),[3,4,5,6] *Da Qing Ye* (Folium Isatidis),[7] and *Bai Hua She She Cao* (Herba Oldenlandia).[8]

Dermatrol (PS) also employs many herbs with marked traits for treatment of psoriasis by suppressing the inflammation of tissue. The anti-inflammatory effect of the herbs helps to reduce swelling and facilitate recovery. Herbs with this anti-inflammatory activity include *Wu Shao She* (Zaocys),[9] *Jin Yin Hua* (Flos Lonicerae),[10] *Mu Dan Pi* (Cortex Moutan),[11] and *Gan Cao* (Radix Glycyrrhizae).[12] These herbs have excellent anti-inflammatory influences with differing mechanisms of action. Some reduce inflammation by inhibiting prostaglandin synthesis and decreasing the permeability of the blood vessels.[13] Others reduce swelling by stimulating the release of glucocorticoids and delaying their breakdown.[12]

In addition to herbs that suppress cell proliferation and tissue inflammation, *Dermatrol (PS)* contains many herbs that have excellent effects to treat general dermatological disorders, such as *Chan Tui* (Periostracum Cicadae), *Ku Shen Gen* (Radix Sophorae Flavescentis), and *Bai Xian Pi* (Cortex Dictamni). *Chan Tui* (Periostracum Cicadae) is excellent for generalized itching and discomfort of the skin, due to its antihistamine-like effect. According to one study, the use of *Chan Tui* (Periostracum Cicadae) was successful in treating 27 out of 30 patients with chronic urticaria.[14] In another study, use of *Ku Shen Gen* (Radix Sophorae Flavescentis) was found to have a 79% effective rate in treating 148 patients with dermatological disorders, such as rash, itching and eczema.[15] Lastly, topical application of *Bai Xian Pi* (Cortex Dictamni) was found to be 100% effective in treating 33 cases of suppurative dermatological disorders.[16]

In summary, *Dermatrol (PS)* is a well-balanced formula that addresses all aspects of psoriasis and other dermatological disorders with severe itching. *Dermatrol (PS)* contains herbs that suppress the proliferation of cells, reduce the inflammation of tissue, and relieve itching and discomfort. It is one of the most effective formulas for the treatment of the challenging and stubborn disorder of psoriasis.

PHARMACEUTICAL DRUGS & CHINESE MEDICINE: A COMPARATIVE ANALYSIS

Western Medical Approach: Successful treatment of psoriasis is one of the most challenging conditions for both western and traditional Chinese medicine. There is no cure in western medicine, and only a few effective treatments to control symptoms. Drug options include lubricants, keratolytics and corticosteroids. Lubricating cream is usually combined with coal tar, followed by exposure to ultraviolet (UV) light. Though this method may be effective, excessive exposure to UV light may cause sunburn and induce exacerbations. Keratolytics such as anthralin may be beneficial, but it is irritating and should not be used in intertriginous areas. Lastly, topical corticosteroids help to reduce itching and inflammation. However, they cause local side effects such as atrophy and telangiectases. Furthermore, continuous use of topical corticosteroids for just 1 to 2 weeks results in loss of steroid effectiveness.

FORMULAS

DERMATROL (PS) ™

(Psoriasis)

Traditional Chinese Medicine Approach: Herbs are effective to treat both the causes and the symptoms of psoriasis. However, despite both short- and long-term improvements, herbs do not cure psoriasis. Therefore, it is necessary to periodically re-initiate herbal therapy to control psoriasis and prevent flare-ups. With persistent prevention and aggressive treatments, it will be possible to control psoriasis by reducing the frequency and severity of recurrences.

CASE STUDY

A 33-year-old female presented with eczema on localized areas of the hands, wrists and face. The affected skin was itchy and dry, and appeared thicker and paler than surrounding areas. The woman had tried steroid creams and prescription drugs for four years without satisfactory results. The western diagnosis was eczema and atopic dermatitis; the TCM diagnosis was blood deficiency leading to blood dryness and wind. After taking *Dermatrol (PS)*, the patient reported complete resolution of eczema on the face and arms. The skin on the wrists and hands may remain discolored. Overall, *Dermatrol (PS)* helped tremendously. [Note: This formula should be used with caution in some yin deficient patients as it might cause hot flashes.]

M.M., Randolph, New Jersey

L.W., a 22-year-old male, presented with septic facial acne. Very depressed, he did not want to be seen in public. The TCM diagnosis was damp-heat with Liver qi stagnation. After one week of taking *Dermatrol PS* and *Shine*, the acne was 80% resolved and the depression improving. After washing his face with a mild soap, the patient applied a topical skin wash (Yin Care) diluted with tea tree oil. The acne was gone in 28 days. The patient now socializes happily with family and friends.

H.C., Stephens City, Virginia

A 26-year-old farmer with a history of alcohol consumption reported a rash and itchiness of the body without any obvious cause. He was initially diagnosed with a skin rash, and treated with topical steroids without success. As the condition continued to deteriorate, with formation of white skin flakes, the diagnosis was changed to psoriasis. After 3 months of unsuccessful treatment with drugs, the patient then sought herbal treatment. The patient subsequently presented with severe itching, thirst, irritability, constipation, dysuria, and the presence of psoriatic flakes throughout his head and body. Open lesions resulted as a consequence of constant scratching. The tongue was red with a yellow, greasy coat, while the pulse was thready and rapid. The TCM diagnosis was accumulation of heat and toxins. After two weeks of herbal treatment with *Dermatrol (PS)*, the patient reported marked improvement with reduction of itching and skin irritation, healing of skin lesions, and less psoriatic flakes. The patient was advised to continue with the herbs for another week until the psoriasis resolved completely.

C. S., Jilin, China.

A 31-year-old female presented with a family history of chronic psoriasis, and outbreaks mainly on her elbows, knees and sacrum. She also suffered from vaginal itching and burning sensations. The TCM diagnosis was toxic damp-heat in the Liver. *V-Statin* and *Dermatrol (PS)* were prescribed. A topical wash, Yin Care, was prescribed for external application for the psoriasis and vaginally for local itching. The patient had acupuncture treatments and was on the herbal formulas for two years. The patient was advised to stop smoking, eat less spicy food, and refrain from alcohol intake, but was unable to change her lifestyle. Nonetheless, her condition continued to improve, and she noticed that if she did not take the herbs, the symptoms would return.

M.C., Sarasota, Florida

---

[1] Beers, M. and Berkow, R. *The Merck Manual of Diagnosis and Therapy 17th Edition.* 1999.
[2] *Jiang Su Yi Yao* (Jiangsu Journal of Medicine and Herbology), 1990; 16(9):513

DERMATROL (PS) ™

(Psoriasis)

[3] *Yao Xue Za Zhi* (Journal of Medicinals), 1961; 81:1635

[4] *Bei Jing Yi Ke Da Xue Xue Bao* (Journal of Beijing University of Medicine), 1986; 18(2):127

[5] *Zhong Hua Xue Yi Xue Za Zhi* (Chinese Journal on Study of Hematology), 1991; 12(2):89

[6] *Zhong Guo Zhong Yao Za Zhi* (People's Republic of China Journal of Chinese Herbology), 1990; 15(10):49

[7] *Zhi Wu Yao You Xiao Cheng Fen Shou Ce* (Manual of Plant Medicinals and Their Active Constituents), 1986: 608,1084

[8] *Zhong Yao Xue* (Chinese Herbology), 1998; 204:205

[9] *Zhe Jiang Yao Xue* (Zhejiang Journal of Chinese Herbology), 1986; 3(4):4

[10] *Shan Xi Yi Kan* (Shanxi Journal of Medicine), 1960; (10):22

[11] *Sheng Yao Xue Za Zhi* (Journal of Raw Herbology), 1979; 33(3):178

[12] *Zhong Yao Zhi* (Chinese Herbology Journal), 1993; 358

[13] *Zhong Guo Yao Ke Da Xue Xue Bao* (Journal of University of Chinese Herbology), 1990; 21(4):222

[14] *Pi Fu Bing Fang Zhi Yan Jiu Tong Xun* (Research Journal on Prevention and Treatment of Dermatological Disorders), 1972; 3:215

[15] *Zhong Cao Yao Tong Xun* (Journal of Chinese Herbal Medicine), 1976; 1:35

[16] *Chi Jiao Yi Sheng Za Zhi* (Journal of Barefoot Doctors), 1975; 6:21

FORMULAS

DISSOLVE (GS) ™

(Gallstones)

CLINICAL APPLICATIONS

- ☯ Cholecystitis – inflammation of the gallbladder and bile duct
- ☯ Cholelithiasis – gallstones
- ☯ Signs and symptoms of cholecystitis and cholelithiasis include fullness and pain in the right hypochondriac region, low-grade fever, constipation and leukorrhea. Acute onset is characterized by jaundice, severe colicky pain in the upper right quadrant that may radiate to the right shoulder and back, nausea, vomiting, aversion to oily and greasy foods, lack of appetite, anxiety and related symptoms. Diagnostic signs and symptoms include a positive response to Murphy's sign and tenderness at the inferior right scapula.

WESTERN THERAPEUTIC ACTIONS

- ☯ Reduces inflammation of the gallbladder [1,2,3,6]
- ☯ Dissolves gallstones [1,2,3,4,5]
- ☯ Facilitates the passage of gallstones [1]

CHINESE THERAPEUTIC ACTIONS

- ☯ Dissolves smaller gallstones
- ☯ Facilitates the passage of larger gallstones
- ☯ Spreads Liver qi
- ☯ Clears damp-heat

DOSAGE

Take 4 capsules three times daily on an empty stomach with warm water. **Dissolve (GS)** must be taken continuously for at least three months. In cases of multiple or large stones, the treatment should be continued until the stones are dissolved or passed out. **Dissolve (GS)** can also be taken after surgery to prevent formation of new stones. In such cases, take 2 capsules a day for three months and 1 capsule a day for another six months.

INGREDIENTS

Da Huang (Radix et Rhizoma Rhei)
Hai Jin Sha (Herba Lygodii)
Jin Qian Cao (Herba Lysimachiae)
Li Zhi He (Semen Litchi)

Long Dan Cao (Radix Gentianae)
Wei Ling Xian (Radix Clematidis)
Yin Chen Hao (Herba Artemisiae Scopariae)
Zhi Ke (Fructus Aurantii)

FORMULA EXPLANATION

The fundamental etiology of cholecystitis and cholelithiasis is damp-heat. Cholecystitis is characterized by damp-heat in the Gallbladder and cholelithiasis is characterized by damp-heat drying up fluids in the Gallbladder.

Long Dan Cao (Radix Gentianae) enters the Liver and the Gallbladder to clear damp-heat. *Yin Chen Hao* (Herba Artemisiae Scopariae), an empirical herb for treating hepatic and gallbladder disorders, has a cholagogic function that increases the secretion of bile and the excretion of bile salt and bilirubin. It also lowers serum cholesterol and beta-lipoprotein. *Jin Qian Cao* (Herba Lysimachiae) dissolves gallstones and increases the secretion of bile by the liver cells. *Wei Ling Xian* (Radix Clematidis) unblocks the channels and helps to dissolve stones. *Li Zhi He* (Semen Litchi) relieves abdominal and epigastric pain due to Liver qi constraint. *Zhi Ke* (Fructus Aurantii) unblocks qi obstruction and facilitates the passage of gallstones. *Hai Jin Sha* (Herba Lygodii) transforms hardness and dissolves

DISSOLVE (GS) ™

(Gallstones)

stones. *Da Huang* (Radix et Rhizoma Rhei) lowers cholesterol and eliminates damp-heat accumulation by its purgative action.

SUPPLEMENTARY FORMULAS

- ☙ For hepatitis, jaundice, or high liver enzyme levels, combine with *Liver DTX*.
- ☙ For constipation, combine with *Gentle Lax (Excess)*.
- ☙ With blood stagnation, add *Circulation (SJ)*.
- ☙ With excess heat, add *Gardenia Complex*.
- ☙ With prominent signs and symptoms of Liver fire or damp-heat in the Liver and Gallbladder, combine with *Gentiana Complex*.
- ☙ To reduce blood cholesterol and triglyceride levels, use *Cholisma*.
- ☙ To reduce cholesterol and triglyceride levels in individuals with fatty liver and obesity, use *Cholisma (ES)*.
- ☙ For peptic ulcers or gastritis, combine with *GI Care*.
- ☙ For severe pain, use with *Herbal Analgesic*.
- ☙ For bloating and distention, add *GI Harmony*.
- ☙ For angina or chest pain, combine with *Circulation*.

NUTRITION

- ☙ For patients with cholecystitis, advise against eating solid foods for a few days. They should drink distilled water and fresh juices. Liquid foods can be introduced slowly after three or four days.
- ☙ For patients with gallstones, advise taking three tablespoons of olive oil with lemon juice before going to bed and upon awakening. Gallstones are sometimes passed and eliminated with this method.
- ☙ Increase the consumption of apple-sauce, yogurt, fresh apples and beets.
- ☙ Avoid eating red meat, shrimps, lobsters, oysters, fatty or greasy foods, fried foods, spicy foods, margarine, soft drinks, commercial oils and processed foods.
- ☙ Food allergies can cause inflammation and obstruction of the bile duct. Avoid foods that commonly cause gallbladder disorders, such as eggs, pork, onion, fowl, milk, coffee, and citrus fruits.

LIFESTYLE INSTRUCTIONS

- ☙ Individuals with gallbladder colic should fast, keep warm and rest in bed.
- ☙ Detoxification of liver and colon are helpful for long-term management.
- ☙ Sitz bath is helpful to decongest and detoxify the intestines.

CLINICAL NOTES

- ☙ Cholecystitis and cholelithiasis commonly occur simultaneously. They are most commonly seen in women over 30 to 40 years of age, and in individuals who are obese. Often times they are un-diagnosed or mis-diagnosed as gastritis, peptic ulcers, viral hepatitis, angina or acute pancreatitis. X-ray results are not always accurate. Ultrasound of the gallbladder is more reliable and has approximately 90 to 95% accuracy. Conditions most suitable for Chinese herbal treatment include chronic cholecystitis, the presence of gallstones in the liver, gallstones composed primarily of calcium, small gallstones, and the presence of gallstones after removal of the gallbladder. Elderly or weak patients not suitable for surgical treatment can also benefit from Chinese herbal treatment.
- ☙ Individuals with high risk of developing cholecystitis or gallstones will benefit from prophylactic treatment by taking *Dissolve (GS)* on a preventative basis. Risk factors of cholecystitis or gallstones include the 4 F's: female, fair, fertile, and fat.

FORMULAS

DISSOLVE (GS) ™

(Gallstones)

Pulse Diagnosis by Dr. Jimmy Wei-Yen Chang:
- "Pen-tip" like feeling on the deep level of the left *guan* position.
- Note: Dr. Chang takes the pulse in slightly different positions. He places his index finger directly over the wrist crease, and his middle and ring fingers alongside to locate *cun*, *guan* and *chi* positions. For additional information and explanation, please refer to *Pulsynergy* by Dr. Jimmy Wei-Yen Chang and Marcus Brinkman.

CAUTIONS

- This formula is contraindicated during pregnancy and nursing.
- *Dissolve (GS)* is not suitable for the following conditions:
  - Acute onset with severe colic
  - Large stones with obstruction of the bile duct (surgery is the treatment of choice)
  - Sudden deterioration in the overall health of the patient
  - Sudden deterioration in cholecystitis/cholelithiasis
  - Poor results from previous treatments and initial signs of liver damage

ACUPUNCTURE POINTS

Traditional Points:
- *Zulinqi* (GB 41) and *Zhigou* (TH 6).
- *Dannangxue*, *Zusanli* (ST 36), *Zhangmen* (LR 13), *Qimen* (LR 14), *Ganshu* (BL 18), *Danshu* (BL 19), and *Zhongwan* (CV 12).

Balance Method by Dr. Richard Tan:
- Left side: *Hegu* (LI 4) or *ah shi* points nearby, *Sanyangluo* (TH 8) or *ah shi* points nearby, and *Zhongdu* (LR 6) or *ah shi* points nearby.
- Right Side: *Yanglingquan* (GB 34) or *ah shi* points nearby, *Yangjiao* (GB 35) or *ah shi* points nearby, and *Quze* (PC 3) or *ah shi* points nearby.
- For additional information on the Balance Method, please refer to *Dr. Tan's Strategy of Twelve Magical Points* by Dr. Richard Tan.

Ear Points:
- Pancreas, Gallbladder, Duodenum, Liver. Use ear seeds.
- Liver, Gallbladder, Abdomen. Strongly stimulate the points or use electric stimulation.
- Set 1: *Shenmen*, Abdomen, Endocrine, and Gallbladder. Set 2: Liver, Adrenal Gland, Upper Abdomen, and Shoulder. Alternate sets between ears every seven days and instruct the patient to massage the points several times a day.
- On the right ear, needle *Shenmen* towards the Abdomen, Sympathetic, and Gallbladder, needle .2 mm below the Gallbladder towards the Duodenum. On the left ear, needle Gallbladder towards the Duodenum.

Auricular Acupuncture by Dr. Li-Chun Huang:
- Cholelithiasis (gallstones): Sympathetic, Sanjiao, Digestive Subcortex, Gallbladder, Gallbladder Node of the posterior, Bile Duct, and Duodenum.
  - Supplementary points: Ear Center and Endocrine.
- Cholecystitis and Cholangitis: Bile Duct, Liver, Duodenum, Stomach, Spleen, Hepatitis, *San Jiao*, Endocrine, and Digestive Subcortex.
- For additional information on the location and explanation of these points, please refer to *Auricular Treatment Formula and Prescriptions* by Dr. Li-Chun Huang.

DISSOLVE (GS) ™

(Gallstones)

MODERN RESEARCH

Dissolve (GS) is an herbal formula developed by Professor Xiao-Ping Zhang of Anhui Hospital of Traditional Chinese Medicine. *Dissolve (GS)* is an empirical formula designed to treat cholecystitis and cholelithiasis. It has been used for over 30 years in China and has helped several thousand patients with cholecystitis and cholelithiasis. It is imperative, however, that patients comply with instructions and continue to take the herbal formula for at least three months for optimal results.

Long Dan Cao (Radix Gentianae), the principle herb in the formula *Long Dan Xie Gan Tang* (Gentiana Longdancao Decoction to Drain the Liver), is an herb commonly used to treat various hepatic and gallbladder disorders including but not limited to hepatitis, and acute and chronic cholecystitis.[1] *Yin Chen Hao* (Herba Artemisiae Scopariae) and *Da Huang* (Radix et Rhizoma Rhei) are used in conjunction with *Long Dan Cao* (Radix Gentianae) for their synergistic effects to treat jaundice, cholecystitis and cholelithiasis.[2] In addition, the combination of *Yin Chen Hao* (Herba Artemisiae Scopariae) and *Da Huang* (Radix et Rhizoma Rhei) also treat hepatitis. It was demonstrated in a study of 32 cases of icteric hepatitis that after seven days of treatment, the patients showed dramatic improvement, with reduction of fever, disappearance of jaundice, and normalization of liver enzymes.[1] It was found in another study that *Yin Chen Hao* (Herba Artemisiae Scopariae) and *Da Huang* (Radix et Rhizoma Rhei) have excellent effects in the treatment of neonatal jaundice.[3]

Jin Qian Cao (Herba Lysimachiae), *Wei Ling Xian* (Radix Clematidis), *Li Zhi He* (Semen Litchi), and *Zhi Ke* (Fructus Aurantii) regulate qi circulation and dissolve gallstones.[4] In addition, it has been reported that *Jin Qian Cao* (Herba Lysimachiae) had dramatic effects in the treatment of cholelithiasis through case reports of 4 patients.[5] Furthermore, in a study involving 52 patients with cholecystitis, *Jin Qian Cao* (Herba Lysimachiae) was given for two to three months and over 76% of patients showed significant improvement.[6]

PHARMACEUTICAL DRUGS & CHINESE MEDICINE: A COMPARATIVE ANALYSIS

Western Medical Approach: Cholelithiasis and cholecystitis are two conditions that often occur together. In western medicine, if these two conditions are asymptomatic, treatment may not be necessary, as risks often outweigh the benefits. If symptomatic, bile acids [such as Ursodiol (Ursodeoxycholic acid)] are usually given to dissolve stones. However, these drugs must be given for a long period of time, and have only limited success rate of about 30%. Furthermore, these drugs may cause side effects such as bladder pain, bloody or cloudy urine, burning or painful urination, dizziness, fast heartbeat, indigestion, lower back or side pain, severe nausea, shortness of breath, skin rash, stomach pain, vomiting, weakness, wheezing, and others. Lastly, if drugs fail, invasive treatments such as surgery and sonic shock wave are the last alternatives.

Traditional Chinese Medicine Approach: Cholelithiasis and cholecystitis are two conditions that are successfully treated with herbs. The mechanisms of action of herbs are to dissolve and expel stones from the gallbladder and bile duct. Herbal therapies are effective to treat and to prevent stones. Depending on the number and size of the stones, the duration of treatment ranges from days to months. Nonetheless, use of herbs should be limited to individuals with mild to moderate cases of cholelithiasis and cholecystitis. If there is acute manifestations, or if herbal therapy is ineffective after 3 months, then patients should be referred to western medicine for surgery and sonic shock wave treatments.

CASE STUDIES

S.T., a 54-year-old female, presented with complaints of waking at 3 A.M., feeling cold easily, craving sweets, overweight, and hot flashes in the morning. Her blood pressure was 125/80 mmHg and her heart rate was 75 beats per minute. Her lab report revealed gallstones and elevated liver enzymes. The TCM diagnosis was cold and damp in the Spleen with Spleen deficiency, and damp-heat in the Liver. *Dissolve (GS)* was prescribed at 12 grams a day

FORMULAS

DISSOLVE (GS) ™

for a week. The patient reported she passed two gallstones, which were recovered, through the stool. The practitioner concluded that patients with gallstones should take *Dissolve (GS)* prior to considering surgery because it is less invasive and less expensive.

S.C., Colonie, New York

A 51-year-old female housekeeper presented with pain in the upper right quadrant of the abdomen within the gallbladder region. The practitioner diagnosed the condition as damp-heat in the Gallbladder. After taking *Dissolve (GS)* for a period of 9 months, there was a complete cessation of upper right quadrant pain.

D.K., Forestville, California

C.B., a 72-year-old female, presented with gallstones, pain under the right ribcage, poor digestion, and pain in the right shoulder. Her blood pressure was 180/95 mmHg and the heart rate was 85 beats per minute. Ultrasound was performed to confirm the stone. The western diagnosis was gallstones and high cholesterol. The TCM diagnosis was damp-heat accumulation with Liver qi stagnation. She was prescribed *Dissolve (GS)* at 4.5 grams daily and *Cholisma* at 1.5 grams daily. The patient also received acupuncture. After eight weeks, the patient reported the pain in the right shoulder had improved fully. Digestion was much better with no more bloating or constipation.

W.F., Bloomfield, New Jersey

[1] Bensky, D. et al. *Chinese Herbal Medicine Materia Medica*, Eastland Press, 1993.
[2] Yeung, HC. *Handbook of Chinese Herbs*, Institute of Chinese Medicine, 1996.
[3] Traditional Chinese medicine and treatment of neonatal jaundice. Department of Neonatology 1, Kandang Kerbau Hospital, Singapore. *Singapore Med J*; Dec 1996; 37(6):645-651
[4] Zhang, XP. Treatment of Endocrine Disorders with Herbs. Presentation given by Professor Zhang at the Seminar hosted by California Association of Acupuncture and Oriental Medicine. July 1998
[5] Observation on the effectiveness of Jinqiancao in treating Cholelithiasis, *Journal of Traditional Chinese Medicine*, 1958; 11:749.
[6] Li, J. et al. Effectiveness of Jinqiancao in treating Cholecystitis: a case report with 52 patients. *Beijing, People's Republic of China*. 1985; 1:26.

DISSOLVE (KS) ™

(Kidney Stones)

CLINICAL APPLICATIONS

☯ Kidney and/or bladder stones

☯ Painful urination, with difficulty initiating or maintaining a good urinary stream; sudden stopping or blockage of urination with passage of a stone(s); lower abdominal pain

☯ Renal colic, characterized by excruciating, one-sided, intermittent pain in the flank area that spreads across the abdomen and to the genital area and inner thigh

WESTERN THERAPEUTIC ACTIONS

☯ Dissolves and facilitates the passage of stones [1,2,3,4]

☯ Promotes normal urination [5,6,7]

☯ Relieves pain [8,9]

CHINESE THERAPEUTIC ACTIONS

☯ Dissolves stones

☯ Treats dysuria due to *shi lin* (stone dysuria)

☯ Promotes normal urination

☯ Relieves spasms and pain

DOSAGE

Take 3 to 4 capsules three times daily on an empty stomach, with two glasses of warm water. Dosage may be increased up to 6 to 8 capsules three times daily, when necessary. Patients should continue to take these herbs until the stones are dissolved or passed out in the urine. The passage/absence of stones can be confirmed via X-ray or other imaging techniques. For maintenance purposes, herbs can be taken at 1 to 2 capsules a day for six months to prevent the formation of new stones.

INGREDIENTS

Chuan Lian Zi (Fructus Toosendan)   *Wei Ling Xian* (Radix Clematidis)
Fu Ling (Poria)   *Yan Hu Suo* (Rhizoma Corydalis)
Hai Jin Sha (Herba Lygodii)   *Ze Xie* (Rhizoma Alismatis)
Jin Qian Cao (Herba Lysimachiae)   *Zhi Ke* (Fructus Aurantii)
Shi Wei (Folium Pyrrosiae)   *Zhu Ling* (Polyporus)

FORMULA EXPLANATION

Dissolve (KS) is an effective formula to dissolve and facilitate the passage of kidney and bladder stones, relieve pain and promote normal urination.

According to traditional Chinese medicine, kidney and urinary stones are known as *"shi lin,"* which literally means dysuria due to stones. *Jin Qian Cao* (Herba Lysimachiae), *Hai Jin Sha* (Herba Lygodii), and *Shi Wei* (Folium Pyrrosiae), are three principle herbs used in this formula to dissolve and pass the stones. *Jin Qian Cao* (Herba Lysimachiae) dissolves stones and helps to clear damp-heat in the lower *jiao* to relieve burning dysuria. *Hai Jin Sha* (Herba Lygodii) dissolves and dispels stones. *Hai Jin Sha* (Herba Lygodii) also reduces swelling caused by obstruction. *Shi Wei* (Folium Pyrrosiae) softens and dissolves stones.

FORMULAS

DISSOLVE (KS) ™

(Kidney Stones)

Ze Xie (Rhizoma Alismatis), *Zhu Ling* (Polyporus) and *Fu Ling* (Poria) are diuretic herbs used here to facilitate the passage and elimination of stones. Together, they promote urination, flush out the stones, and reduce edema and/or water retention in the body caused by kidney stone obstruction.

Zhi Ke (Fructus Aurantii) relieves the distention and pressure caused by kidney stones by activating qi circulation. It also breaks up stagnant qi to resolve accumulations in the abdomen. *Wei Ling Xian* (Radix Clematidis) is one of the strongest herbs to enter and open all the channels and collaterals in the body. With its penetrating characteristics, it breaks up stagnation to relieve pain caused by obstruction(s).

To relieve pain, *Yan Hu Suo* (Rhizoma Corydalis) and *Chuan Lian Zi* (Fructus Toosendan) are added to the formula. *Yan Hu Suo* (Rhizoma Corydalis) is one of the strongest analgesic herbs for pain relief, while *Chuan Lian Zi* (Fructus Toosendan) has antispasmodic effects to relieve spasms of the smooth muscle of the ureter.

SUPPLEMENTARY FORMULAS

- For struvite stones, use with ***Herbal ABX***.
- For kidney or bladder stones with infection and inflammation, use with ***Herbal ABX***.
- For burning dysuria, dark yellow urine, urinary tract infection, use with ***V-Statin***.
- For kidney or bladder stones with edema, use with ***Herbal DRX***.
- For excess heat or fever, add ***Gardenia Complex***.
- For hypertension, use ***Gastrodia Complex*** or ***Gentiana Complex***
- For flank or back pain and spasms, use with ***Flex (SC)***.
- To relieve pain, use with ***Herbal Analgesic***.
- For bleeding, add ***Notoginseng 9***.
- For chronic nephritis, chronic nephrotic syndrome or proteinuria, use ***Kidney DTX*** instead.
- For benign prostatic hypertrophy, use ***P-Statin*** instead.

NUTRITION

- Patients with calcium stones should refrain from eating foods containing high amounts of oxalates, such as rhubarb, spinach (especially in combination with calcium-rich foods), nuts, cocoa, tea and pepper. These foods contribute to calcium stone formation in the body.
- Patients with uric acid stones should refrain from foods that increase the level of uric acid in the urine, such as meat, poultry, pork, liver, beef, sardines, meat broth, clams, crabs, peas, various beans, cauliflower, coffee and tea.
- Patients who are prone to forming kidney stones should drink 8 to 10 glasses of water a day. Chronic dehydration increases the risk of stone formation.
- Minimize the intake of salt to avoid water retention. A diet high in salt will also increase the loss of calcium from the urine, and increase the risk of stone formation.
- Potassium citrate makes the urine more alkaline, and helps to flush out uric acid. Fruits and vegetables should be increased, while protein, eggs and milk should be reduced in the diet.
- Vitamin A is essential to prevent formation and deposit of stones in the kidneys. Increase the consumption of foods high in vitamin A, such as carrots, yams, apricots, peaches, and mango.

The Tao of Nutrition by Ni and McNease

- Recommendations: corn-silk, water chestnuts, seaweed, beet tops, watermelon, celery, watercress, winter melon, pearl barley, walnuts, watermelon rind, winter melon rind, green tea powder, and distilled water.
- Avoid spicy foods, fried foods, oily foods, coffee, hard water, spinach, citrus, tomatoes, spinach combined with tofu or dairy products.

DISSOLVE (KS) ™

(Kidney Stones)

❧ For more information, please refer to *The Tao of Nutrition* by Dr. Maoshing Ni and Cathy McNease.

LIFESTYLE INSTRUCTIONS

❧ Patients should drink plenty of water throughout the day to help flush out the stones.

❧ Patients should urinate whenever necessary (or more frequently than usual, if they do not feel strong urges to urinate), and not hold their urine.

❧ Sitz-baths may be helpful if there is shooting pain in kidney and bladder area with fever and chills. However, if the condition is not alleviated, the patient should seek medical help immediately.

CLINICAL NOTES

❧ Patients with kidney stones may be asymptomatic. They may or may not experience pain, bleeding, obstruction of urine flow or any sign of infection. Patients who are asymptomatic but have stones may take this formula to dissolve kidney stones.

❧ Kidney stones without pain usually indicates that the stone is still in the kidney. When pain is experienced in the flank area, radiating across the abdomen down to the genitals, it is an indication that the stone is passing or is obstructed in its passage from the kidney to the ureter.

❧ If the stones are too big to pass through the ureter and urethra, sonic waves is one treatment option to break the stones into smaller fragments, in combination with taking the herbal formula to facilitate elimination. The patient should drink plenty of fluids regularly, to help flush stone fragments out of the kidney and urinary tract.

❧ If the stones are too big to pass through the ureter and urethra, surgery may be the best treatment option, as herbal treatment often requires a prolonged period of time to show effectiveness.

❧ If the stones are small enough to pass through the urinary ducts, the patient may begin taking this formula. Some patients may feel slight pain or discomfort during this process, as the herbs work to dispel the stones. Continue taking the herbs until the stones pass out of the body.

❧ The presence of kidney stones may be detected by pulse diagnosis. Upon pressure, one can feel a tiny rock- or bean-like protrusion on the *chi* position of the right hand. If there is also inflammation, the pulse will be forceful.

❧ Pain associated with kidney stones may occur after rigorous exercise that promotes movement of the stone.

❧ Back pain due to kidney stone(s) should be differentiated from sprain, strain or trauma. Colicky pain due to kidney stones is usually one-sided, and radiates across the abdomen down to the genitals. Patients with sprain and strain will report that the pain is due to trauma or over-exertion. Reports from current X-rays or other imaging can also provide a clue to the cause of the pain.

❧ Recurrences of kidney stone(s) may be prevented by taking *Dissolve (KS)* 2 to 3 capsules, once a day.

Pulse Diagnosis by Dr. Jimmy Wei-Yen Chang:

❧ "Pen-tip" like feeling on the deep level of the left or right *chi* positions. Detection of the specific side indicates the respective location of the stone (right or left side).

❧ Note: Dr. Chang takes the pulse in slightly different positions. He places his index finger directly over the wrist crease, and his middle and ring fingers alongside to locate *cun*, *guan* and *chi* positions. For additional information and explanation, please refer to *Pulsynergy* by Dr. Jimmy Wei-Yen Chang and Marcus Brinkman.

CAUTIONS

❧ This formula is not suitable for stones that are too big to be passed. The size can be determined by X-ray or ultrasound, or by the severity of pain.

❧ Patients with kidney infection or acute pain from the kidney stone should seek medical help immediately.

❧ This formula is contraindicated during pregnancy and nursing.

FORMULAS

DISSOLVE (KS) ™

(Kidney Stones)

ACUPUNCTURE POINTS

Traditional Points:
- Needle and strongly stimulate *Quanliao* (SI 18) and *Yangchi* (TH 4).
- *Shenshu* (BL 23), *Yaoyan* (Extra 9), *Renzhong* (GV 26), *Guanyuan* (CV 4), *Zusanli* (ST 36), *Zhongji* (CV 3), and *Sanyinjiao* (SP 6).

Balance Method by Dr. Richard Tan:
- Left side: *Chengshan* (BL 57), *Jinggu* (BL 64), *Chize* (LU 5) or *ah shi* points nearby, and *Kongzui* (LU 6) or *ah shi* points nearby.
- Right side: *Sanyinjiao* (SP 6), *Rangu* (KI 2), *Dazhong* (KI 4), *Fuliu* (KI 7), *Zhubin* (KI 9), *Hegu* (LI 4), and Kidney point on the ear.
- Sides can be alternated between treatments.
- For additional information on the Balance Method, please refer to *Dr. Tan's Strategy of Twelve Magical Points* by Dr. Richard Tan.

Ear Points:
- Kidney, Abdomen, Sympathetic, and Subcortex. Stimulate these points strongly for 20 to 40 minutes.
- Kidney, Ureter, and Urethra. Needle bilaterally.

Auricular Acupuncture by Dr. Li-Chun Huang:
- Urinary System Stone: Sympathetic, Lower *Jiao*, *San Jiao*, Nervous Subcortex, *Shenmen*, and Corresponding point (to the area of pain).
  - For kidney stone, add Kidney and External Abdomen
  - For ureter stone, detect positive point Ureter, add Lower Sanjiao
  - For bladder stone, add Bladder
- For additional information on the location and explanation of these points, please refer to *Auricular Treatment Formula and Prescriptions* by Dr. Li-Chun Huang.

MODERN RESEARCH

Dissolve (KS) is formulated specifically for the treatment of stones present in the kidney and urinary bladder. It contains herbs that have shown great effectives in dissolving stones, facilitating the passage of stones, promoting normal urination, relieving pain, and treating infection.

Jin Qian Cao (Herba Lysimachiae), *Hai Jin Sha* (Herba Lygodii) and *Shi Wei* (Folium Pyrrosiae) are three herbs with marked capacity to dissolve stones and facilitate the passage of stones. These three herbs are extremely effective for treatment of kidney and urinary stones, because they break apart existing stones and facilitate the elimination of substances that cause the formation of stones, such as calcium, sodium, and other minerals.[1,2,3] Several clinical studies concluded that these herbs demonstrate high effectiveness in treating kidney and urinary stones. In one study, 7 patients with urinary stones showed complete dissolution of the stones within ten days of herbal treatment. The presence of the stones before and the absence of the stones after treatment were confirmed by X-ray.[4] In another study, it was found that *Jin Qian Cao* (Herba Lysimachiae) is effective for treatment of both kidney and urinary stones.[1]

Restoration of normal urination is also important: many patients with a history of stones or current kidney or urinary stones may have difficult and painful urination. *Jin Qian Cao* (Herba Lysimachiae), *Ze Xie* (Rhizoma Alismatis), *Zhu Ling* (Polyporus) and *Fu Ling* (Poria) are four herbs that have excellent diuretic functions. They facilitate the passage of urine, reduce accumulation of water, and minimize difficulty with urination. Furthermore, they also

(Kidney Stones)

increase the elimination of many minerals and salt so these substances do not adhere to the stones and further increase stone size.[5,6,7]

While many patients with kidney and urinary stones may be asymptomatic, some experience pain ranging from mild back pain to severe renal colic. *Chuan Lian Zi* (Fructus Toosendan) and *Yan Hu Suo* (Rhizoma Corydalis) are added to this formula for their excellent pain-relieving properties. *Chuan Lian Zi* (Fructus Toosendan) is used to relieve the mild back pain while *Yan Hu Suo* (Rhizoma Corydalis) is used to alleviate the severe renal colic. *Yan Hu Suo* (Rhizoma Corydalis) is one of the most effective and most potent herbs for treating pain. In fact, with the appropriate dose adjustment, the analgesic effect of *Yan Hu Suo* (Rhizoma Corydalis) has been described to be comparable to morphine, with fewer side effects, no evidence of dependency, and 100% slower development of tolerance.[8] Furthermore, the analgesic effect of acupuncture is potentiated when combined with *Yan Hu Suo* (Rhizoma Corydalis).[9] With the addition of these two herbs, one can successfully address the pain commonly associated with kidney and urinary stones.

Some herbs in this formula also have antibiotic activities to treat infections of the urinary tract. Herbs with antibiotic influence include *Jin Qian Cao* (Herba Lysimachiae), *Zhu Ling* (Polyporus), and *Fu Ling* (Poria).[10,11,12]

PHARMACEUTICAL DRUGS & CHINESE MEDICINE: A COMPARATIVE ANALYSIS

Western Medical Approach: Urinary stones (kidney and bladder stones) are two conditions that often occur together. In western medicine, if these two conditions are asymptomatic, treatment may not be necessary, as risks often outweigh the benefits. If symptomatic, alkalinization of the urine may be effective for uric acid stones, but not for other types of stones. In most cases, urinary stones (kidney and bladder stones) can only be treated with invasive treatments such as surgery or ultrasound disruption therapy.

Traditional Chinese Medicine Approach: Kidney and bladder stones are two conditions that are successfully treated with herbs. The mechanisms of action of herbs are to dissolve and expel stones from the kidney and urinary bladder. Herbal therapies are effective to treat and to prevent stones. Depending on the number and size of the stones, the duration of treatment ranges from days to months. Nonetheless, use of herbs should be limited to individuals with mild to moderate cases of kidney and bladder stones. If there is acute manifestations, or if herbal therapy is ineffective after 3 months, then patients should be referred to western medicine for surgery or ultrasound disruption therapy.

CASE STUDIES

A 21-year-old female art gallery manager complained of kidney pain, which was severe at times. Other symptoms included lumbar pain and heat. The diagnosis for her case was renal lithiasis. After taking *Dissolve (KS)* for 6 months, there was a complete cessation of the heat sensation and pain.

D.K., estville, California

A 42-year-old male computer specialist presented with pain indicative of kidney stones. The patient's medical doctor suggested immediate surgery. The patient was placed on a treatment plan with *Dissolve (KS)* for 10 days. He was checked by his medical doctor two weeks later and discovered that the stones were completely gone. The practitioner also commented that many of her colleagues have used *Dissolve (KS)* on their patients with similar results.

C.B., Santa Barbara, California

FORMULAS

DISSOLVE (KS) ™

(Kidney Stones)

A 38-year-old female had 20 years of history of kidney stones. Her kidney stones condition had a familiar cycle that started with low back pain, retention of urine, and ended with passing of a stone 5 to 6 months later. She was in her first two weeks of the cycle when she came for treatment. Her condition included low back pain, edema in her lower legs, swollen eyes, retention of urine, and night sweats. Her western medical diagnosis was kidney stones with pyelonephritis. Her TCM diagnosis was Kidney yang deficiency. After taking *Dissolve (KS)* for 3 days, her condition began to improve. Edema in the lower legs disappeared with only slight swelling in the eyes. Night sweats and tearing in the eyes resolved. Her low back pain diminished. Furthermore, her lab analysis tested negative for any presence of kidney stones.

M.J., Brooklyn, New York

A female came to the practitioner's office for treatment of kidney stones. A chronic low back pain condition had plagued the patient for five years, shuffling in and out of the E.R. and being treated with painkillers. The practitioner prescribed *Dissolve (KS)* formula along with two other homeopathic compositions. Within 36 hours, she was able to pass a kidney stone. Another patient with the same condition was given the same treatment protocol. Again, a kidney stone was passed within the same time-frame.

I.B., Miami, Florida

A 73-year-old female veterinarian presented with severe low back and abdominal pain due to renal calculi [kidney stone]. There was redness and swelling over the right kidney on her back. Tenderness over the right kidney region was also noted upon palpation. The pain referred along the belt channel, which traveled around the lower abdomen. The patient's pulse was wiry, particularly on the right side with the kidney pulse weak but tight. The practitioner diagnosed the condition as Kidney deficiency resulting in damp-heat in the lower *jiao* along with qi obstruction. After the patient took *Dissolve (KS)* for 4 weeks, she began experiencing a cessation of pain and an increased urine flow. Subsequent X-ray findings showed a decrease in size of stones in her right kidney, the site that originally contained much larger and a higher number of renal calculi. There was no apparent change in the stones in her left kidney. Upon discontinuing treatment of *Dissolve (KS)*, the severe pain returned and urination again became scanty. The patient re-started her treatment with *Dissolve (KS)*, which immediately stopped the pain and an easy urine flow resumed. The patient's condition continued to fluctuate before it finally returned to some form of normalcy three months later.

V.W., Princeville, Hawaii

A 25-year-old male computer technician presented with left-sided low back pain radiating to the left testicle. There was also frequent painful urination with dribbling. The symptoms had been present for 6 days. Kidney stones tested positive by way of Computerized Electrodermal Screening (EAV). The practitioner diagnosed the condition as damp-heat in the lower *jiao*. After three days of taking *Dissolve (KS)* at 3 capsules three times daily with meals, the low back pain and dysuria were completely relieved. Frequency of urination and dribbling were also resolved. Application of *Dissolve (KS)* appeared to have accelerated the patient's recovery.

D.H., Fort Myers, Florida

A female patient presented with severe right-sided lumbar pain that she described as 'cutting' in nature. She also had frequent, painful and yellow urination. The Western diagnosis was kidney stones; the TCM diagnosis was *lin zheng* (dysuria syndrome), with damp-heat in the Urinary Bladder. After two bottles of *Dissolve (KS)* and *Ba Zheng San* (Eight-Herb Powder for Rectification), the pain subsided and urine was clear. The patient felt some stones may have passed in her urine.

M.C., Sarasota, Florida

DISSOLVE (KS) ™

(Kidney Stones)

1 *Guang Xi Zhong Yi Yao* (Guangxi Chinese Medicine and Herbology), 1990; 13(6):40
2 *Xin Zhong Yi* (New Chinese Medicine), 1985; (6):51
3 *Zhong Yao Cai* (Study of Chinese Herbal Material), 1990; 13(11):30
4 *Zhe Jiang Zhong Yi Za Zhi* (Zhejiang Journal of Chinese Medicine), 1983; (11):493
5 *Sheng Yao Xue Za Zhi* (Journal of Raw Herbology), 1982; 36(2):150
6 *Yao Xue Xue Bao* (Journal of Herbology), 1964; 11(12):815
7 *Chang Yong Zhong Yao Cheng Fen Yu Yao Li Shou Ce* (A Handbook of the Composition and Pharmacology of Common Chinese Drugs), 1994; 1383:1391
8 *Zhong Yao Yao Li Yu Ying Yong* (Pharmacology and Applications of Chinese Herbs), 1983; 447
9 *Chen Tzu Yen Chiu* (Acupuncture Research), 1994;19(1):55-8
10 *Zhong Yao Yao Li Yu Ying Yong* (Pharmacology and Applications of Chinese Herbs), 1983; 696
11 *Zhong Yao Xue* (Chinese Herbology), 1998; 334:336
12 *Zhong Yao Cai* (Study of Chinese Herbal Material), 1985; (2):36

FORMULAS

ENHANCE MEMORY ™

CLINICAL APPLICATIONS

☯ Forgetfulness, poor memory, difficulty concentrating or focusing
☯ Delayed mental development in children
☯ Deteriorating cognition in elderly patients
☯ Adjunct formula for individuals who wish to improve their memory, cognitive function, and mental alertness
☯ Support formula for periods of mental stress, such as long work hours, impending deadlines, and exams

WESTERN THERAPEUTIC ACTIONS

☯ Improves memory and learning ability [4,5,6]
☯ Treats dementia by improving cognitive performance and social behaviors [7]
☯ Prevents and treats drug-induced memory impairment [8]
☯ Improves micro-circulation of blood to deliver oxygen and essential nutrients to the brain tissue [1,2]
☯ Improves cognition in cases of mental retardation [3]

CHINESE THERAPEUTIC ACTIONS

☯ Nourishes the Heart
☯ Tonifies the Kidney *jing* (essence)
☯ Invigorates blood circulation to the head

DOSAGE

For adults, take 3 to 4 capsules three times daily with warm water for treatment. For maintenance, take 2 capsules twice daily. For children, take 2 capsules twice daily. This formula is most effective when taken on a continuous basis for three to six months.

INGREDIENTS

Bai Zi Ren (Semen Platycladi)
Dan Shen (Radix Salviae Miltiorrhizae)
Dang Gui (Radicis Angelicae Sinensis)
Fu Ling (Poria)
Jie Geng (Radix Platycodonis)
Mai Men Dong (Radix Ophiopogonis)
Ren Shen (Radix Ginseng)
Sheng Di Huang (Radix Rehmanniae)

Shi Chang Pu (Rhizoma Acori)
Suan Zao Ren (Semen Zizyphi Spinosae)
Tian Men Dong (Radix Asparagi)
Wu Wei Zi (Fructus Schisandrae Chinensis)
Xuan Shen (Radix Scrophulariae)
Yin Guo Ye (Folium Ginkgo)
Yuan Zhi (Radix Polygalae)

FORMULA EXPLANATION

According to traditional Chinese medicine, the Kidney produces marrow and the brain is the sea of marrow. Strong Kidney *jing* (essence) is vital to the nourishment of the brain, memory, concentration and alertness. Kidney is also essential in helping the Heart house the *shen* (spirit) and maintain clear mental activity, consciousness, memory and thinking.

Forgetfulness and inability to concentrate or focus are usually the result of deficiency and lack of nourishment due to overwork, lack of rest, or aging. *Enhance Memory* contains herbs that tonify the Kidney and Heart, invigorate blood circulation to the head, and open orifices to improve alertness. *Sheng Di Huang* (Radix Rehmanniae), *Xuan*

ENHANCE MEMORY ™

Shen (Radix Scrophulariae), *Mai Men Dong* (Radix Ophiopogonis) and *Tian Men Dong* (Radix Asparagi) nourish Kidney yin and *jing* (essence). *Ren Shen* (Radix Ginseng) and *Fu Ling* (Poria) tonify Heart qi. *Dan Shen* (Radix Salviae Miltiorrhizae) and *Dang Gui* (Radicis Angelicae Sinensis) invigorate the blood, and *Yin Guo Ye* (Folium Ginkgo) acts as a channel-guiding herb to the brain. Furthermore, the flavonoids in *Yin Guo Ye* (Folium Ginkgo) provide antioxidant protection to the brain and its related vascular structure. These blood-moving herbs keep adequate amounts of oxygenated blood to the brain cells to ensure healthy brain functions. *Yuan Zhi* (Radix Polygalae) and *Shi Chang Pu* (Rhizoma Acori) improve mental alertness because they have aromatic dispelling functions to clear phlegm obstructing the orifices. *Bai Zi Ren* (Semen Platycladi), *Suan Zao Ren* (Semen Zizyphi Spinosae) and *Wu Wei Zi* (Fructus Schisandrae Chinensis) tranquilize the *shen* (spirit) and prevent the leakage of Heart qi. *Jie Geng* (Radix Platycodonis) acts as a channel-guiding herb to bring other herbs to the Heart.

In conclusion, *Enhance Memory* is a well-balanced formula to improve memory and increase cognition. *Enhance Memory* contains herbs that nourish the Heart, tonify the Kidney *jing* (essence), and invigorate blood circulation to the head.

SUPPLEMENTARY FORMULAS

- With Alzheimer's disease, add *Neuro Plus*.
- With Kidney yang deficiency, add *Kidney Tonic (Yang)*.
- With Kidney yin deficiency, add *Kidney Tonic (Yin)*.
- With patients who are "burned-out", add *Adrenoplex*.
- With stress or Liver qi stagnation, add *Calm*.
- With stress and insomnia in patients with deficiency, add *Calm ZZZ*.
- With ADD/ADHD and poor memory, add *Calm (Jr)*.
- With blood stagnation, add *Circulation (SJ)*.

NUTRITION

- Smoking and alcoholic beverages are not recommended.
- Make sure the diet contains an adequate amount of lecithin, which is essential for transmission of nerve impulses that control memory. Good sources of lecithin include flax seed oil, walnut oil, sesame oil, egg yolk, soybean, and raw wheat germ.
- The B vitamins are also important for energy and proper brain function.

LIFESTYLE INSTRUCTIONS

- Patients are recommended to have a good balance between exercise, rest, and relaxation.
- Encourage patients to continuously stay mentally active. Go back to school, take a part time job, solve crossword puzzles, play chess, etc.
- Avoid a stressful and hectic lifestyle. A poor memory is often related to an excessive amount of stress on a daily basis.

CLINICAL NOTES

- It is important to note that the maximum benefit of *Enhance Memory* is derived from continuous use, not from one excessive dose. In other words, use the normal dose continuously for 3 to 6 months for optimal effect. Increasing the dose will not necessarily accelerate the desired effect.
- This formula is safe for long-term use.

FORMULAS

ENHANCE MEMORY ™

CAUTIONS

- This formula is contraindicated in cases of excess heat or existing exterior pathogenic conditions.
- This formula is contraindicated during pregnancy and nursing.
- Patients who are on anticoagulant or antiplatelet therapies, such as Coumadin (Warfarin), should use this formula with caution, as there may be a slightly higher risk of bleeding and bruising.

ACUPUNCTURE POINTS

Traditional Points:
- *Si Shen Cong* and Scalp Points.
- *Taichong* (LR 3), *Xingjian* (LR 2), *Yinlingquan* (SP 9), *Yanglingquan* (GB 34), *Renzhong* (GV 26), and *Baihui* (GV 20).

Balance Method by Dr. Richard Tan:
- Left side: *Shenmen* (HT 7), *Lingdao* (HT 4), *Qiuxu* (GB 40), and *Yanglingquan* (GB 34).
- Right side: *Taichong* (LR 3), *Zhongdu* (LR 6), *Zhongzhu* (TH 3), *Zhizheng* (SI 7), and Ear *Shenmen*.
- Alternate sides in needle placement from treatment to treatment.
- For additional information on the Balance Method, please refer to *Dr. Tan's Strategy of Twelve Magical Points* by Dr. Richard Tan.

MODERN RESEARCH

Enhance Memory is carefully crafted with herbs that have shown marked ability to treat compromised mental functions. Herbs in *Enhance Memory* have been shown to improve blood circulation to deliver oxygen and essential nutrients to the brain. Furthermore, herbs in *Enhance Memory* have shown to be effective for treatment of mental retardation in children, to enhance memory in adults, and to delay dementia in the elderly. Lastly, many herbs in *Enhance Memory* have been found to be effective in treating drug-induced memory impairments.

Dang Gui (Radicis Angelicae Sinensis) and *Dan Shen* (Radix Salviae Miltiorrhizae) are two herbs in *Enhance Memory* that have shown pronounced ability to improve blood circulation. *Dang Gui* (Radicis Angelicae Sinensis) improves overall blood circulation by decreasing blood viscosity, or improving the hemorrheological changes in "blood stagnation."[1] Administration of *Dan Shen* (Radix Salviae Miltiorrhizae) in various laboratory animals is associated with marked vasodilation of the coronary arteries, a negative chronotropic and inotropic effect, and a reduction of blood pressure.[2] Both herbs act to improve microcirculation, thus delivering oxygen and essential nutrients to the brain to ensure the health and optimal performance of brain cells.

In clinical trials of children with mental retardation, 30 children with low IQ were treated with mild to moderate improvement in classroom performance using an herbal formula containing *Ren Shen* (Radix Ginseng) along with other herbs. The children were given 10 to 15 grams of the formula twice daily for 2 weeks per course of the treatment, for a total of three months.[3]

Enhance Memory contains many herbs that have been shown to improve memory. According to one laboratory study, the administration of *Shi Chang Pu* (Rhizoma Acori) has a dose-dependent effect on improving cognition and memory.[4] In another study, a preparation of *Wu Wei Zi* (Fructus Schisandrae Chinensis) has a stimulating effect on the central nervous system to increase mental alertness, improve work efficiency, and quicken reflexes.[5] Furthermore, administration of *Ren Shen* (Radix Ginseng) for 3 days has demonstrated marked impact in improving memory and learning ability.[6]

ENHANCE MEMORY ™

For prevention and treatment of dementia, *Yin Guo Ye* (Folium Ginkgo) is generally considered the herb of choice. In a placebo-controlled, double-blind, randomized clinical trial with 309 patients over 52 weeks, *Yin Guo Ye* (Folium Ginkgo) was concluded to be "safe" and capable of "improving the cognitive performance and the social functioning of demented patients for 6 months to 1 year."[7]

Lastly, the use of herbs in *Enhance Memory* has also been found to be effective in preventing and treating drug-induced memory impairment. In an *in vitro* study, a traditional Chinese medicinal preparation [composed of *Ren Shen* (Radix Ginseng), *Yuan Zhi* (Radix Polygalae), *Shi Chang Pu* (Rhizoma Acori), and *Fu Ling* (Poria)] reduced the ethanol-induced impairment of memory registration. It also ameliorated the scopolamine-induced memory registration deficit. These results suggest that the herbal preparation ameliorates the impairment effect of ethanol on learning and the memory processes.[8]

In summary, *Enhance Memory* is an excellent formula to improve cognition and treat memory-related disorders such as mental retardation, dementia, and memory impairment.

PHARMACEUTICAL DRUGS & CHINESE MEDICINE: A COMPARATIVE ANALYSIS

One striking difference between western and traditional Chinese medicine is that western medicine focuses and excels in crisis management, while traditional Chinese medicine emphasizes and shines in holistic and preventative treatments. Therefore, in emergencies, such as gun shot wounds or surgery, western medicine is generally the treatment of choice. However, for treatment of chronic idiopathic illness of unknown origins, where all lab tests are normal and a clear diagnosis cannot be made, traditional Chinese medicine is distinctly superior.

In cases of gradual deterioration of mental acuity (with forgetfulness and poor memory), there are no diagnostic signs or symptoms, no laboratory abnormalities, and no functional or anatomical disorders. Under these circumstances, western medicine struggles to identify a specific diagnosis and offers no drug treatments. On the other hand, traditional Chinese medicine is beneficial as it excels in maintainance and preventative therapies. Herbs can be used to improve blood circulation to the brain, nourish underlying deficiencies, and improve cognitive functions. In comparison with western medicine, traditional Chinese medicine offers safe and effective treatment options. Therefore, herbal therapy should definitely be employed to prevent deterioration of this condition, and to restore optimal health.

---

[1] Xue, JX. et al. Effects of the combination of astragalus membranaceus (Fisch.) Bge. (AM), angelica sinensis (Oliv.) Diels (TAS), cyperus rotundus L. (CR), ligusticum chuanxiong Hort (LC) and paeonia veitchii lynch (PV) on the hemorrheological changes in "blood stagnating" rats. *Chung Kuo Chung Yao Tsa Chih*; 19(2): Feb 1994; 108-10, 128.

[2] *Shang Hai Di Yi Xue Yuan Xue Bao (Journal of First Shanghai Medical College)*, 1980; 7(5):347

[3] *Zhong Cheng Yao Yan Jiu (Research of Chinese Patent Medicine)*, 1982; 6:22

[4] *Zhong Yi Xue (Chinese Herbal Medicine)*, 1992; 23(8):417

[5] *Zhong Yao Xue (Chinese Herbology)*, 1998; 878:881

[6] *Zhong Yao Ci Hai (Encyclopedia of Chinese Herbs)*, 1994

[7] Le Bars, P. et al. A placebo-controlled, double-blind, randomized trial of an extract of ginkgo biloba for dementia. *Journal of American Medical Association;* October 22, 1997; 278:1327-1332.

[8] *Biological and Pharmaceutical Bulletin*. 1994 Nov.; 17(11):1472-6,

FORMULAS

EQUILIBRIUM ™

CLINICAL APPLICATIONS

- Diabetes mellitus
- High blood glucose levels and/or high urine ketone levels
- Polyuria, polydypsia and/or polyphagia

WESTERN THERAPEUTIC ACTIONS

- Lowers blood glucose levels [1,2]
- Lowers blood cholesterol levels [3,4]
- Improves blood circulation to the coronary arteries and peripheral parts of the body [3,4]

CHINESE THERAPEUTIC ACTIONS

- Nourishes Lung, Stomach and Kidney yin
- Clears deficiency fire
- Dries damp

DOSAGE

Take 3 to 4 capsules three times daily on an empty stomach, either one hour before or two hours after meals. To effectively control blood glucose level, it is important to keep in mind that dosing must be adjusted to reflect the condition of the patient, as the severity of diabetes is different in every case.

INGREDIENTS

Bai Zhu (Rhizoma Atractylodis Macrocephalae)
Cang Zhu (Rhizoma Atractylodis)
Dan Shen (Radix Salviae Miltiorrhizae)
Hong Hua (Flos Carthami)
Huang Qi (Radix Astragali)
Lian Xu (Stamen Nelumbinis)
Lian Zi Xin (Plumula Nelumbinis)

Shan Yao (Rhizoma Dioscoreae)
Shi Gao (Gypsum Fibrosum)
Xi Yang Shen (Radix Panacis Quinquefolii)
Xuan Shen (Radix Scrophulariae)
Zhi Mu (Radix Anemarrhenae)

FORMULA EXPLANATION

According to traditional Chinese medicine, diabetes mellitus is classified as upper, middle or lower *xiao ke* (wasting and thirsting) syndromes. Upper *xiao ke* (wasting and thirsting) syndrome is characterized by Lung heat drying up the moisture, leading to polydypsia; middle *xiao ke* (wasting and thirsting) syndrome is characterized by Stomach heat damaging fluid, leading to polyphagia; and lower *xiao ke* (wasting and thirsting) syndrome is characterized by Kidney deficiency, leading to polyuria. Furthermore, patients with high blood glucose commonly show signs of damp accumulation and Spleen deficiency. Overall, the clinical presentation of patients with diabetes can be summarized as yin deficiency with damp and heat.

Xi Yang Shen (Radix Panacis Quinquefolii) greatly replenishes the vital essence of the body and promotes the secretion of body fluids to treat polydypsia. *Shi Gao* (Gypsum Fibrosum) and *Zhi Mu* (Radix Anemarrhenae) are a pair commonly used to treat heat in the middle *jiao*. They sedate Stomach fire and suppress appetite to relieve polyphagia. *Xuan Shen* (Radix Scrophulariae) enters the Lung, the Stomach and the Kidney to replenish the vital essence and clear heat simultaneously. *Huang Qi* (Radix Astragali) and *Shan Yao* (Rhizoma Dioscoreae) strengthen

FORMULAS

the Spleen and enhance its function of transportation and transformation. *Bai Zhu* (Rhizoma Atractylodis Macrocephalae) and *Cang Zhu* (Rhizoma Atractylodis) strengthen the Spleen and dry up dampness. *Dan Shen* (Radix Salviae Miltiorrhizae) and *Hong Hua* (Flos Carthami) activate blood circulation and enhance the overall effectiveness of the herbs. Activation of blood circulation also reduces the risk of atherosclerosis by preventing buildup of cholesterol on the inner walls of blood vessels. Proper blood circulation also helps to prevent diabetic neuropathy. Lastly, *Lian Zi Xin* (Plumula Nelumbinis) and *Lian Xu* (Stamen Nelumbinis) tonify the Kidney and control frequent urination.

SUPPLEMENTARY FORMULAS

- For high cholesterol and triglycerides, add **Cholisma**.
- For high cholesterol and triglycerides with fatty liver and obesity, add **Cholisma (ES)**.
- For hypertension, add **Gastrodia Complex**.
- For chronic buildup of cholesterol leading to coronary artery disease, add **Circulation**.
- With thirst and dry mouth, add **Nourish (Fluids)**.
- For blurred vision or vision impairment, combine with **Nourish**.
- For impotence, combine with **Circulation (SJ)**.
- For infection, add **Herbal ABX**.
- For recurrent yeast infection, add **V-Statin**.
- For urinary tract infection, add **Gentiana Complex**.
- For infection of ear, nose and throat, add **Herbal ENT**.
- For diabetes with compromised kidney functions, add **Kidney DTX**.

NUTRITION

- Avoid the consumption of simple sugars, which have an adverse effect on glucose tolerance.
- Eat a low-fat, high-fiber diet including plenty of raw fruits and vegetables.
- Avoid supplements containing the amino acid cysteine, which interferes with absorption of insulin by the cells.
- Avoid excessive amounts of vitamin B1 (thiamine) and C, which may inactivate insulin.
- Avoid the consumption of alcohol and use of tobacco in any form as they increase nerve damage.

The Tao of Nutrition by Ni and McNease

- Recommendations: pumpkin, wheat, mung beans, winter melon, celery, pears, spinach, yams, peas, sweet rice, soybeans, tofu, mulberries, squash, daikon radish, cabbage, peach, and organic pig or chicken pancreas.
- Avoid sweets, sugar, honey, molasses, smoking, alcohol, caffeine, spicy foods, and most raw fruits.
- For more information, please refer to *The Tao of Nutrition* by Dr. Maoshing Ni and Cathy McNease.

LIFESTYLE INSTRUCTIONS

- Make lifestyle adjustments – include regular daily exercise, and eliminate sugar and carbohydrates from the diet.
- Regular exercise, a sensible, healthy diet and weight control are essential for long-term management of diabetes.
- Hot baths may be beneficial to regulate pancreatic functions.

EQUILIBRIUM ™

CLINICAL NOTES

- For patients with type II diabetes, *Equilibrium* in combination with diet and exercise provide excellent clinical results. Most patients will experience satisfactory clinical results within 3 to 4 weeks of herbal treatment. Clinical effects include a significant reduction in blood glucose levels and less fluctuations throughout the day.

- In western medicine, diabetes is defined simply as an increase in blood glucose levels. Diagnosis, however, can be difficult because diabetes has many complications, including impairment of vision, impotence, chronic infections, neuropathy, poor healing of wounds, and risk of coma, among others.

- In traditional Chinese medicine, diabetes is commonly referred as *xiao ke* (wasting and thirsting) syndrome. However, it is important to keep in mind that even though these two conditions share many similarities, they are not equivalent. Both diabetes and *xiao ke* (wasting and thirsting) syndrome are characterized by the presence of three P's: polyuria, polydypsia and polyphagia. Diabetes is defined as an increase in blood glucose level, with or without the presence of the three P's. In addition, diabetes may have many complications that are not present in *xiao ke* (wasting and thirsting) syndrome, such as visual disturbance, impotence, amenorrhea, and frequent or chronic infections. Conversely, *xiao ke* (wasting and thirsting) syndrome is diagnosed based on the presence of three P's. Polyuria, polydypsia and polyphagia may be caused by factors other than diabetes, such as fever, dehydration, or kidney diseases. Understanding the similarities and differences between the two is essential to achieving optimal treatment of the patient.

CAUTIONS

- This formula is contraindicated during pregnancy and nursing.

- Patients should not stop using their drug treatment abruptly as there is a risk of hyperglycemia or diabetic ketoacidosis. Herbal and drug treatments should overlap for one to two weeks before patients begin tapering off their drug treatment, in order to ensure adequate control of blood glucose levels.

- *Equilibrium* may reduce the dosage and frequency of insulin injection needed; however, *Equilibrium* can never replace insulin, especially in type I diabetes mellitus patients. Patients with type I diabetes mellitus should always be treated by insulin, or the combination of insulin and herbs, and should continue to test their blood glucose regularly.

- Patients who are on anticoagulant or antiplatelet therapies, such as Coumadin (Warfarin), should use this formula with caution as there may be a slightly higher risk of bleeding and bruising.

ACUPUNCTURE POINTS

Traditional Points:
- *Quchi* (LI 11), *Sanyinjiao* (SP 6), and *Yanglingquan* (GB 34).
- *Shenshu* (BL 23) and *Taixi* (KI 3).
- *Pishu* (BL 20), *Shenshu* (BL 23), *Qihai* (CV 6), *Sanyinjiao* (SP 6), *Yanglingquan* (GB 34), and *Shenque* (CV 8).

Balance Method by Dr. Richard Tan:
- Left side: *Sanyinjiao* (SP 6) *Yinlingquan* (SP 9) or *ah shi* points nearby, *Fuliu* (KI 7), *Hegu* (LI 4), and *Waiguan* (TH 5).
- Right side: *Zusanli* (ST 36), *Weizhong* (BL 40), and *Zulinqi* (GB 41).
- Left and right side can be alternated from treatment to treatment.
- For additional information on the Balance Method, please refer to *Dr. Tan's Strategy of Twelve Magical Points* by Dr. Richard Tan.

FORMULAS

EQUILIBRIUM ™

Ear Points:
- ꙮ Main points: Pancreas and Endocrine.
- ꙮ Adjunct points: Kidney, Sanjiao, *Shenmen*, Heart, and Liver.
- ꙮ Select three to four points for three to seven days.

Auricular Acupuncture by Dr. Li-Chun Huang:
- ꙮ Diabetes mellitus: Diabetes Point, Pancreas, Ear Center, Pituitary, Thalamus, *San Jiao*, and Endocrine.
  - ▪ For excessive thirst, add Thirst Point and Mouth.
  - ▪ For hunger, add Hunger Point.
  - ▪ For polyuria, add Bladder and Urethra.
  - ▪ For cutaneous pruritus, add Allergic Area.
  - ▪ For numbness in the extremities, add Lesser Occipital Nerve, and Large Auricular Nerve.
  - ▪ For blurry vision, add Vision II. Bleed Ear Apex.
- ꙮ For additional information on the location and explanation of these points, please refer to *Auricular Treatment Formula and Prescriptions* by Dr. Li-Chun Huang.

MODERN RESEARCH

Equilibrium is an herbal formula developed by Professor Xiao-Ping Zhang of Anhui Hospital of Traditional Chinese Medicine. It is an empirical formula designed to treat patients with diabetes mellitus. It has been used for over 30 years in China and has helped several thousand patients with diabetes by lowering their blood glucose level and reducing the long-term risks and complications associated with diabetes.

Diabetes mellitus is defined simply as a rise in blood glucose levels. The clinical manifestation, however, is much more complicated than its definition. Patients with chronic diabetes mellitus are frequently plagued by various complications, such as visual disturbances, prolonged delay in healing of wounds, frequent recurrence of infections, impotence, and others. Treatment of diabetes mellitus, therefore, must focus on treating both the cause and the symptoms simultaneously.

Xi Yang Shen (Radix Panacis Quinquefolii) is most commonly used for its strong effect to tonify qi. In terms of western physiology, tonification of qi enhances the ability of cells to utilize glucose as energy and prevent excessive synthesis of fat. Clinically, *Xi Yang Shen* (Radix Panacis Quinquefolii) has demonstrated effectiveness to lower blood glucose and cholesterol levels.[1]

In addition to *Xi Yang Shen* (Radix Panacis Quinquefolii), Anhui Hospital of Traditional Chinese Medicine frequently uses two pairs of herbs with excellent hypoglycemic effects: *Shi Gao* (Gypsum Fibrosum) and *Zhi Mu* (Radix Anemarrhenae) lower blood glucose levels and control polyphagia; and *Xuan Shen* (Radix Scrophulariae) and *Cang Zhu* (Rhizoma Atractylodis) lower blood glucose levels and reduce buildup of cholesterol within blood vessels. The combination of these herbs has excellent hypoglycemic effects and reduces the risk of long-term atherosclerosis.[2]

Dan Shen (Radix Salviae Miltiorrhizae) and *Hong Hua* (Flos Carthami) are used in this formula to improve the blood circulation and minimize long-term complications of diabetes. Studies have demonstrated that *Dan Shen* (Radix Salviae Miltiorrhizae) improves micro-circulation to the peripheral parts of the body, increases blood flow to the coronary artery, and lowers blood cholesterol and blood glucose levels. [3,4]

PHARMACEUTICAL DRUGS & CHINESE MEDICINE: A COMPARATIVE ANALYSIS

Western Medical Approach: Diabetes mellitus is one of the most common disorders in developed countries. The disease is well understood, and there are numerous treatment options. For type I diabetes (juvenile onset), insulin is

FORMULAS

the drug of choice. For type II (adult onset), drug treatment usually begins with oral medications, followed by insulin if necessary. Oral medications, such as Glucotrol (Glipizide) and Diabeta (Glyburide), are beneficial to control blood glucose levels, but may cause side effects such as seizures, loss of consciousness, skin rash, itching or redness, exaggerated sunburn, yellowing of the skin or eyes, light-colored stools, dark urine, unusual bleeding or bruising, fever, and sore throat. Furthermore, long-term use of these medications may lead to weight gain and insulin resistance, thereby decreasing overall effectiveness. Insulin is an effective and reliable drug to control blood glucose. However, once insulin injection therapy begins, endogenous production of insulin slowly decreases and the body becomes more and more dependant on exogenous sources. Eventually, the patient will become dependent on insulin for life. Lastly, there are many complications of ddiabetes mellitus. Some are well controlled by drugs, others are not.

Traditional Chinese Medicine Approach: Many herbs effectively treat both diabetes and its complications. For diabetes, herbs have shown marked effect to stimulate the endocrine system, increase production of insulin from the pancreas, and control blood glucose. Furthermore, many herbs are effective to alleviate symptoms of diabetes, such as thirst, hunger, frequent urination, and other manifestations of *xiao ke* (wasting and thirsting) syndrome. Lastly, as described in this monograph, many other formulas may be used as adjuncts to successfully treat complications of diabetes. However, herbal therapy has its limitations. Because herbs work primarily by stimulating the pancreas to produce insulin, it is only effective for type II diabetes. Therefore, for type I diabetic patients, herbs should be used to manage complications, but not to treat diabetes itself.

Summation: For type I diabetic patients, insulin must be used for diabetes, and both drugs and herbs may be used to treat complications. For type II diabetes patients, both drugs and herbs may be used to treat both the disease and complications. Optimal treatment requires integration of both medicines and selection of the most effective agents with least side effects.

CASE STUDIES

A 45-year-old female with type I diabetes mellitus presented with night sweats and aching feet with a blood sugar level of 200 to 300 mg/dL. The practitioner diagnosed her condition as Kidney yin deficiency. Within one week of taking *Equilibrium*, the patient's blood sugar level dropped so drastically that she needed to ingest some sugar in order to elevate her blood sugar level. Her condition stabilized during the second week of treatment at which point her blood sugar level reading was around 160 mg/dL. Surprisingly, her night sweats also subsided.

S.T., Morgan Hill, California

J.K., a 45-year-old female, was 5' 3" and weighed 160 pounds. She had urinary tract infections once or twice each month within the last 12 months. Her other symptoms and signs included constant thirst, increased fluid intake, and increased frequency and volume of urination. She was diagnosed with diabetes mellitus after testing positive for high levels of blood glucose. She was prescribed *Equilibrium*, 4 capsules three times daily before meals. Two weeks after the initial treatment, she reported significant improvement of her signs and symptoms. Two months after the initial treatment, her blood glucose levels were within the ideal range. She did not have any urinary tract infections during these two months. She continues to take *Equilibrium*, 4 capsules three times daily before meals.

J.C., Diamond Bar, California

A 45-year-old female with type I diabetes mellitus presented with malaise, fatigue, night sweats, hot flashes and low back pain. Other signs and symptoms included abdominal bloating, red eyes, weak nails and a pale complexion. She was diagnosed with hepatitis C. The practitioner prescribed *Liver DTX* (3 capsules three times daily) and *Equilibrium* (3 capsules three times daily). The treatment regimen also integrated a pancreatic homeopathic (10 drops 6 times a day) as well as another homeopathic prescription, Hepan Comp (1 drop three times daily). Two and a half months later, the patient was able to cease her insulin intake. Once viral load reached normal range, she discontinued taking all her prescribed pharmaceuticals. There was a total reversal of her clinical picture.

I.B., Miami, Florida

A 49-year-old male computer analyst presented with chronic skin lesions over his entire body. Visual inspection of his body exposed scars from past lesions as well as fresh, red, edematous sores especially on the lower extremities. The severity of his lesions appeared to fluctuate. He also complained of pain in both legs and right arm, which were all indicative of peripheral neuropathy. He was diagnosed with type I diabetes mellitus and had a history of kidney problems. The patient was also reported to be overweight. His tongue was dusky with purple veins on the underside. His tongue coating was scanty and his pulse was deep, weak, thready, and slippery. The practitioner diagnosed the patient's condition as Liver and Kidney yin deficiencies, qi deficiency, damp-heat in the skin, and qi and blood stagnation. Along with acupuncture, the patient started a combination of *Equilibrium* and *Silerex* at one-third the dose since he was on a large variety of other herbal treatment. After one week, no improvement of his lesions was noted and fluctuations of his blood sugar levels were minimal. After the second week, the herbal dose was increased by two-thirds the recommended dose. The patient's lesions slightly improved along with the blood sugar levels. The severity of the arm and leg pain also decreased. His pulses were also noticeably stronger. The practitioner concluded that some of the symptoms might have been due to other medications, which were taken concurrently by the patient. Nevertheless, the practitioner hypothesized that by clearing the skin condition, the patient would eventually decrease use of other skin medications.

N.M., Torrance, CA

A.G., a 60-year-old male, was 6' 1" and weighed 280 pounds. He was always hungry and ate two or three bowls of rice with every meal. He noticed that his cuts or scratches required a longer period of time to heal, sometimes up to one month. His diagnoses were diabetes mellitus and high cholesterol. He was given *Equilibrium*, 4 capsules three times daily for his diabetes; and *Cholisma*, 4 capsules three times daily for his cholesterol. After taking the herbs for three months, his blood glucose levels were within the ideal range and his cholesterol level dropped from 260 to 220 mg/dL. His weight also dropped from 280 to 255 pounds. He ate less and did not feel constantly hungry. He continues to take both *Equilibrium* and *Cholisma*.

J.C., Diamond Bar, California

[1] Yen, ZH. et al. American Ginseng (xi yang shen), *Chinese Herbology*, Zhiyin Publishing Company, pg. 738, 1998.
[2] Zhang, XP. Treatment Of Endocrine Disorders With Herbs. Presentation given by Professor Zhang at the Seminar hosted by California Association of Acupuncture and Oriental Medicine. July 1998
[3] Yeung, HC. *Handbook of Chinese Herbs*. Institute of Chinese Medicine, 1996.
[4] Bensky, D. et al. *Chinese Herbal Medicine Materia Medica*. Eastland Press, 1993.

FORMULAS

FLEX (CD) ™

(Cold/Deficiency)

CLINICAL APPLICATIONS

- ☙ Chronic arthritis or arthralgia that worsens during cold and rainy seasons [1]
- ☙ Chronic low back pain and sciatica with underlying deficiencies [2,3]
- ☙ Degenerative disorders with weakness of the lower back and knees with reduced mobility
- ☙ General aches and pains characterized by cold manifestations [4]
- ☙ Fibromyalgia characterized by cold or numbness

WESTERN THERAPEUTIC ACTIONS

- ☙ Analgesic function to relieve pain [2,3,4]
- ☙ Antirheumatic function to treat connective tissue disorders [2,3]
- ☙ Strengthens soft connective tissues to speed up recovery [2,3]

CHINESE THERAPEUTIC ACTIONS

- ☙ Expels wind, cold and damp
- ☙ Warms channels and collaterals; disperses painful obstruction
- ☙ Tonifies Kidney yin and yang
- ☙ Invigorates the blood circulation and relieves pain

DOSAGE

Take 3 to 4 capsules three times daily with a glass of warm water. The dosage may be increased up to 6 capsules every six hours as needed for pain.

INGREDIENTS

Bai Shao (Radix Paeoniae Alba)
Cao Wu (Radix Aconiti Kusnezoffii)
Chuan Niu Xi (Radix Cyathulae)
Chuan Wu (Radix Aconiti Preparata)
Chuan Xiong (Rhizoma Ligustici Chuanxiong)
Dang Gui Wei (Extremitas Radicis Angelicae Sinensis)
Du Huo (Radix Angelicae Pubescentis)
Du Zhong (Cortex Eucommiae)
Fang Feng (Radix Saposhnikoviae)

Ji Xue Teng (Caulis Spatholobi)
Qian Nian Jian (Rhizoma Homalomenae)
Qin Jiao (Radix Gentianae Macrophyllae)
Ren Shen (Radix Ginseng)
Sang Ji Sheng (Herba Taxilli)
Sheng Di Huang (Radix Rehmanniae)
Wei Ling Xian (Radix Clematidis)
Wu Jia Pi (Cortex Acanthopanacis)
Yan Hu Suo (Rhizoma Corydalis)

FORMULA EXPLANATION

Flex (CD) is formulated specifically to treat musculoskeletal disorders characterized by cold and damp. It contains herbs with functions to eliminate cold and damp, tonify Kidney yin and yang, warm up channels and collaterals, activate qi and blood circulation, and relieve pain.

Du Huo (Radix Angelicae Pubescentis), *Qin Jiao* (Radix Gentianae Macrophyllae) and *Fang Feng* (Radix Saposhnikoviae) have antirheumatic, anti-inflammatory, and analgesic functions. They expel wind, dampness and cold from the lower back and remove painful obstruction. *Du Zhong* (Cortex Eucommiae), *Sheng Di Huang* (Radix Rehmanniae), *Chuan Niu Xi* (Radix Cyathulae), and *Sang Ji Sheng* (Herba Taxilli) replenish the vital essence of the Liver and the Kidney that are responsible for strengthening the bones, sinews and the muscles of the lower back and

FORMULAS

FLEX (CD) ™

(Cold/Deficiency)

knees. *Bai Shao* (Radix Paeoniae Alba) has analgesic, antispasmodic and anti-inflammatory effects. *Wei Ling Xian* (Radix Clematidis), *Yan Hu Suo* (Rhizoma Corydalis), *Dang Gui Wei* (Extremitas Radicis Angelicae Sinensis), *Chuan Xiong* (Rhizoma Ligustici Chuanxiong), *Qian Nian Jian* (Rhizoma Homalomenae), *Wu Jia Pi* (Cortex Acanthopanacis) and *Ji Xue Teng* (Caulis Spatholobi) increase qi and blood circulation to the extremities to relax the muscles and the tendons. *Ren Shen* (Radix Ginseng) and *Wu Jia Pi* (Cortex Acanthopanacis) tonify qi and address the underlying deficiency. *Chuan Wu* (Radix Aconiti Preparata) and *Cao Wu* (Radix Aconiti Kusnezoffii) restore Kidney yang, dispel cold, and warm up the channels and collaterals to relieve pain.

SUPPLEMENTARY FORMULAS

- For neck and shoulder, combine with *Neck & Shoulder (Acute)* or *Neck & Shoulder (Chronic)*.
- For upper back pain, add *Back Support (Upper)*.
- For lower back pain, add *Back Support (Acute)* or *Back Support (Chronic)*.
- For herniated disk in the back and swelling and inflammation, add *Back Support (HD)*.
- For pain in the arms, add *Arm Support*.
- For knee pain, add *Knee & Ankle (Acute)* or *Knee & Ankle (Chronic)*.
- For spasms and cramps, combine with *Flex (SC)*.
- For bone fractures, injuries, and bruises, combine with *Traumanex*.
- For post-stroke numbness and atrophy, use *Neuro Plus*.
- For bone spurs, add *Flex (Spur)*.
- For prevention and treatment of osteoporosis, add *Osteo 8*.
- For degeneration of muscles, ligaments, tendons and ligaments, add *Flex (MLT)*.
- To potentiate the effect to relieve pain, add *Herbal Analgesic*.
- For arthritic pain with inflammation, swelling, redness and pain, use *Flex (Heat)* instead of *Flex (CD)*.

NUTRITION

- Sulfur helps the absorption of calcium, and adequate intake and absorption of calcium is essential for the repair and the rebuilding of bones, tendons, cartilage, and connective tissues. Patients are encouraged to consume foods high in sulfur such as asparagus, eggs, fresh garlic, and onions.
- Histidine, an amino acid, is responsible for removing the high levels of copper and iron found in arthritic patients. Patients are encouraged to consume foods high in histidine such as rice, wheat and rye.
- Fresh pineapples are recommended as they contain bromelain, an enzyme that is excellent in reducing inflammation.
- Patients with gout should increase their intake of cherries and strawberries. Both of them are excellent in neutralizing uric acid.
- Foods that contain purines or uric acid, such as meat, anchovies, herring, meat gravies and broths, mushrooms, mussels, sardines, sweetbreads, and fried foods, should be avoided. Alcohol also increases the production of uric acid and should also be avoided.
- Increase the intake of water, as it helps to flush out uric acid.
- Avoid cold beverages, uncooked foods, ice cream, caffeine, sugar, tomatoes, milk, dairy products and red meat.
- Intake of sour food, drinks or fruits (citrus) should be decreased as its nature constricts and may contribute to further stagnation in the channels and collaterals
- Fish oil may help alleviate pain associated with rheumatoid arthritis. It can be taken in conjunction with the herbs.

FLEX (CD) ™

The Tao of Nutrition by Ni and McNease
- Recommendations: garlic, green onions, pepper, black beans, sesame seeds, chicken, lamb, mustard greens, ginger, and a small amount of rice wine (if individual does not have hypertension). Rub garlic, ginger or rice wine on painful areas.
- Avoid cold foods, raw foods, and cold weather elements.
- For more information, please refer to *The Tao of Nutrition* by Dr. Maoshing Ni and Cathy McNease.

LIFESTYLE INSTRUCTIONS

- Weight loss is strongly recommended in individuals who are overweight. This lessens the pressure on the joints, which can then help in relieving pain.
- Exercise is recommended. However, sports such as swimming or skiing that exposure affects joints to cold and dampness should be avoided.
- Ice packs should never be used in patients with joint pain due to coldness and pain. Use heat pads instead.

CAUTIONS

- Side effects of this herbal formula may include nausea, vomiting, stomach discomfort and irritability. Discontinue using this formula if these adverse reactions occur.
- Do not use this formula if the patient presents with heat signs such as redness, burning or inflammation of the joints that worsens with heat.
- This formula is contraindicated during pregnancy and nursing.
- Patients who are on anticoagulant or antiplatelet therapies, such as Coumadin (Warfarin), should use this formula with caution as there may be a slightly higher risk of bleeding and bruising.
- Patients who wear a pacemaker, take anti-arrhythmic drugs or cardiac glycosides such as Lanoxin (Digoxin), and those with pre-existing cardiovascular problems should not take this formula. *Chuan Wu* (Radix Aconiti Preparata) and *Cao Wu* (Radix Aconiti Kusnezoffii) may interact with these drugs by affecting the rhythm and potentiating the contractile strength of the heart.

ACUPUNCTURE POINTS

Traditional Points:
- Moxa and needle *ah shi* points.

Balance Method by Dr. Richard Tan:
- Use Dr. Tan's Balance Method accordingly as determined by where the pain is (use mirror or image system).
- For additional information on the Balance Method, please refer to *Dr. Tan's Strategy of Twelve Magical Points* by Dr. Richard Tan.

Ear Points:
- Related joints, Adrenal Glands. Embed magnetic ear balls and switch ear every three days.

Auricular Acupuncture by Dr. Li-Chun Huang:
- Arthritis of finger: Finger (front and back of ear).
  - Supplementary points: Lesser Occipital Nerve. Bleed Ear Apex.
- For additional information on the location and explanation of these points, please refer to *Auricular Treatment Formula and Prescriptions* by Dr. Li-Chun Huang.

FLEX (CD) ™

(Cold/Deficiency)

MODERN RESEARCH

Flex (CD) is an empirical herbal formula for treating general aches and pains with cold manifestations. ***Flex (CD)*** contains herbs that have shown strong analgesic, antirheumatic, and anti-inflammatory functions.

Du Huo (Radix Angelicae Pubescentis) and *Sang Ji Sheng* (Herba Taxilli) are two herbs commonly used together. These two herbs have antirheumatic and anti-inflammatory functions and are especially effective in treating general body aches and pains.[1,2] In addition, *Du Huo* (Radix Angelicae Pubescentis) has strong analgesic functions that work on the central nervous system to relieve pain. [3,4]

Qin Jiao (Radix Gentianae Macrophyllae) and *Wei Ling Xian* (Radix Clematidis) eliminate wind and damp, and are commonly used for their antirheumatic properties. According to research, *Qin Jiao* (Radix Gentianae Macrophyllae) is found to have anti-inflammatory activities similar to salicylic acid.[2]

Bai Shao (Radix Paeoniae Alba) demonstrates muscle-relaxant activity to relieve spasms and cramps of the skeletal and intestinal muscles. Clinically, *Bai Shao* (Radix Paeoniae Alba) is used to relieve leg cramps, muscle spasm, and general aches and pain. Furthermore, *Bai Shao* (Radix Paeoniae Alba) also has analgesic and anti-inflammatory effects.[1,2,3]

Yan Hu Suo (Rhizoma Corydalis), containing corydaline, exerts strong anti-inflammatory activity and is effective in both the acute and chronic phases of inflammation.[5] *Yan Hu Suo* (Rhizoma Corydalis) also possesses strong analgesic properties that act directly on the central nervous system.[6] Due to this action, *Yan Hu Suo* (Rhizoma Corydalis) works synergistically with acupuncture to relieve pain. It was demonstrated in a research study that when combined with *Yan Hu Suo* (Rhizoma Corydalis), the analgesic effect of electro-acupuncture increased significantly when compared to a control group that received electro-acupuncture only.[7] Furthermore, *Yan Hu Suo* (Rhizoma Corydalis) has been used as a local anesthetic for surgery. In a study with 105 patients who received *Yan Hu Suo* (Rhizoma Corydalis) as an anesthetic prior to surgery, 98 patients (93.4%) showed satisfactory results while 6 patients (5.7%) experienced mild pain.[8]

Cao Wu (Radix Aconiti Kusnezoffii) and *Chuan Wu* (Radix Aconiti Preparata) have excellent analgesic and anti-inflammatory properties and are commonly used to treat a wide variety of aches and pains. It was demonstrated in one study of 225 patients with low back pain that the use of *Chuan Wu* (Radix Aconiti Preparata) is up to 87.4% effective in relieving pain when used on a daily basis for 10 to 15 days.[9] In another study, *Chuan Wu* (Radix Aconiti Preparata) and *Zhang Nao* (Camphora) were used topically to treat frozen shoulder. The herbs were applied topically on a daily basis for an average duration of 7 days. Out of 35 patients, 22 reported significant improvement, 8 reported moderate improvement, 4 reported slight improvement, and 1 reported no effect. [10]

PHARMACEUTICAL DRUGS & CHINESE MEDICINE: A COMPARATIVE ANALYSIS

Western Medical Approach: pain is a basic bodily sensation induced by a noxious stimulus that causes physical discomfort (as pricking, throbbing, or aching). Pain may be of acute or chronic state, and may be of nociceptive, neuropathic, or psychogenic type.

Non-steroidal anti-inflammatory agents (NSAID), such as Motrin (Ibuprofen), Naprosyn (Naproxen) and Voltaren (Diclofenac) are very frequently used to treat mild to moderate pain characterized by inflammation and swelling. Clinical applications include headache, arthritis, dysmenorrhea, and general aches and pain. Though effective, they may cause such serious side effects as gastric ulcer, duodenal ulcer, gastrointestinal bleeding, tinnitus, blurred vision, dizziness and headache. Furthermore, the newer NSAID's, also known as Cox-2 inhibitors [such as Celebrex (Celecoxib)], are associated with significantly higher risk of cardiovascular events, including heart attack and stroke. In fact, these side effects are so serious that two Cox-2 inhibitors have already been withdrawn from the market

FLEX (CD) ™
(Cold/Deficiency)

[Vioxx (Rofecoxib) and Bextra (Valdecoxib)]. In brief, it is important to remember that while drugs offer reliable and potent symptomatic pain relief, they should be used only if and when needed. Frequent use and abuse leads to unnecessary side effects and complications.

Traditional Chinese Medicine Approach: Treatment of pain is a sophisticated balance of art and science. Proper treatment of pain requires a careful evaluation of the type of disharmony (excess or deficiency, cold or heat, exterior or interior), characteristics (qi and/or blood stagnations), and locations (upper body, lower body, extremities, or internal organs). Furthermore, optimal treatment requires integrative use of herbs, acupuncture and *Tui-Na* therapies. All these therapies work together to tonify the underlying deficiencies, strengthen the body, and facilitate recovery from chronic pain. TCM pain management targets both the symptom and the cause of pain, and as such, often achieves immediate and long-term success. Furthermore, TCM pain management is often associated with few or no side effects.

Summation: For treatment of mild to severe pain due to various causes, TCM pain management offers similar treatment effects with significantly fewer side effects.

CASE STUDIES

P.M., an 89-year-old male, presented with chronic back pain and sciatica for the past four months. He also experienced two other episodes of the same type of pain, once after sitting outside in cold weather for a football game and the other at the funeral for his wife. The pain was in both legs and knees, down the sides of the legs and into the buttocks. Right leg pain was worse than the left. Knee pain was bilateral. Pitting edema on both ankles was noticed. His blood pressure was 130/80 mmHg and the heart rate was 80 beats per minute. Trigger points were felt at the left quadratus lumborum and glute, L3, and L4 areas. In general, he was a very healthy and active 89 year old. The diagnoses were *bi zheng* (painful obstruction syndrome) due to cold, Kidney qi deficiency, and qi and blood stagnation on the Gallbladder channel. *Flex (CD)* was prescribed at 4 capsules twice a day. He had a total of 3 acupuncture visits and felt 90% better. He then planned a European walking vacation so he can get better even faster to avoid seeing a physical therapist.

M.H., West Palm Beach, Florida

C.M., a 48-year-old female, presented with joint pain (hands, feet, knees) that worsened in cold and rainy weather, reporting a family history of arthritis and osteoporosis. She also suffered from tendonitis of both forearms. She had decreased range of motion, with calcification of joints in fingers. Her western diagnosis was rheumatoid arthritis; the TCM diagnosis was cold and damp obstruction. *Osteo 8* and *Flex (CD)* were prescribed at four capsules each, twice daily. Within one day, the symptoms began improving. After one week, joints and tendons were not stiff, and almost pain free. During the winter (the season in which her condition usually deteriorated), the symptoms even improved. The patient reported later that if she stopped taking the herbs, the symptoms returned.

C.D., Phoenix, Oregon

A 73-year-old female daycare worker presented with constant pain in the low back, right hip and right knee due to osteoarthritis. Her pain was aggravated especially after any type of activity or prolonged sitting. Sharp pain was also elicited upon walking. Other signs and symptoms included fatigue, dizziness, and an intermittent high blood pressure. Her tongue body appeared red with a scanty tongue coating. Her left pulse was irregular, hesitant and thready at the Liver and Kidney positions. The right pulse was choppy, irregular, and weak at the Spleen position. The practitioner diagnosed her condition as Kidney and Liver yin deficiency, qi and blood stagnation, and damp-cold *bi zheng* (painful obstruction syndrome) in the joints. Along with acupuncture treatment, the patient was instructed to take *Flex (CD)* at 3 spoonfuls, two times a day. The patient experienced a reduction in joint pain by almost 30%.

N.M., Torrance, CA

FLEX (CD) ™
(Cold/Deficiency)

A 63-year-old female homemaker presented with sciatica-like pain in the lumbar and left sacral region, which was worse in the evening and cold to the touch. The patient also reported swelling in her left ankle, which was also cold upon palpation and had been the source of her chronic pain for almost a year. She mentioned that her cold symptoms were relieved by warmth. A disc herniation was also diagnosed at her L3 to L4 lumbar level. Her tongue was thin, red with a thick tongue coat especially at the base. The pulse was tight and deep. The practitioner diagnosed this case as Liver and Kidney yin deficiency, Kidney yang deficiency and wind-damp *bi zheng* (painful obstruction syndrome). The patient was given *Flex (CD)* at 3 capsules three times daily. A significant decrease in pain level was quite evident during the initial treatment. Although the patient did experience minor indigestion in the beginning, the side effect resolved after only a short while. After taking three bottles of *Flex (CD)*, the patient felt her pain was manageable enough that she was able to return to exercising in order to prevent further relapse.

J.T., Kingsport, Tennessee

[1] Bensky, D. et al. *Chinese Herbal Medicine Formulas & Strategies*. Eastland Press. 1990
[2] Yeung, HC. *Handbook of Chinese Herbs*. Institute of Chinese Medicine. 1996
[3] Bensky, D. et al. *Chinese Herbal Medicine Materia Medica*. Eastland Press. 1993
[4] Liao, JF. Evaluation with receptor binding assay on the water extracts of ten CNS-active Chinese herbal drugs. Proceedings of the National Science Council, Republic of China – Part B, *Life Sciences*. Jul. 1995; 19(3):151-8,
[5] Kubo, M. et al. Anti-inflammatory activities of methanolic extract and alkaloidal components from corydalis tuber. *Biol Pharm Bull*.; February 1994; 17(2):262-5
[6] Zhu, XZ. Development of natural products as drugs acting on central nervous system. *Memorias do Instituto Oswaldo Cruz*. 1991; 86 2:173-5
[7] Hu, J. et al. Effect of some drugs on electroacupuncture analgesia and cytosolic free Ca2+ concentration of mice brain. *Chen Tzu Yen Chiu*; 1994; 19(1):55-8
[8] Use of corydalis (yan hu suo) injectables for surgical anesthesia. Tangshang Medical Hospital Second Branch. *Hebei Xin Yi Yao* (Medical Journal of Hebei); 1973 ; 4:34
[9] Military Hospital Unit #64. Effectiveness of aconite wu tou (chuan wu) in treating low back pain, a report with 225 patients. *New Journal of Medicine and Pharmacology*. 1975; 4:45
[10] Zhang, HT. et al. Treatment of frozen shoulders with aconite wu tou (chuan wu) and camphor (zhang nao). *Shanghai Journal of Medicine and Pharmacolog*. 1987; 1:29

FORMULAS

FLEX (GT) ™

CLINICAL APPLICATIONS

- Gout
- Gouty arthritis

WESTERN THERAPEUTIC ACTIONS

- Decrease the absorption and increase the elimination of uric acid and other unwanted substances
- Analgesic effect to relieve pain
- Anti-inflammatory effect to reduce swelling and inflammation
- Antipyretic effect to relieve burning sensations and reduce inflammation

CHINESE THERAPEUTIC ACTIONS

- Strengthens the Spleen and Stomach
- Drains damp-heat
- Opens the channels and collaterals
- Relieves pain

DOSAGE

Take 4 capsules three times daily. The herbal therapy should begin immediately upon the notice of the first warning signs. The dosage may be doubled on day one and two of herbal therapy to achieve faster onset of action. If necessary, this formula may be taken at reduced dosages for maintainance and prevention.

INGREDIENTS

Cang Zhu (Rhizoma Atractylodis)
Che Qian Zi (Semen Plantaginis)
Chi Shao (Radix Paeoniae Rubrae)
He Zi (Fructus Chebulae)
Huang Bai (Cortex Phellodendri)
Ji Xue Teng (Caulis Spatholobi)
Jin Qian Cao (Herba Lysimachiae)

Sheng Di Huang (Radix Rehmanniae)
Shi Gao (Gypsum Fibrosum)
Wu Bei Zi (Galla Chinensis)
Yi Yi Ren (Semen Coicis)
Ze Xie (Rhizoma Alismatis)
Zhi Mu (Radix Anemarrhenae)

FORMULA EXPLANATION

According to traditional Chinese medicine, gout is generally considered as a *bi zheng* (painful obstruction syndrome) characterized by damp-heat. The presence of damp-heat begins with inability of Spleen and Stomach to adequately transform and transport food, followed by accumulation of damp-heat blocking the channels and collaterals leading to severe pain. This correlates with the western medicine concept of gout, which starts with improper diet followed by excessive accumulation of uric acid. Therefore, optimal treatment requires use of herbs to strengthen the Spleen and Stomach, drain damp-heat, open the channels and collaterals, and relieve pain.

In this formula, *Cang Zhu* (Rhizoma Atractylodis) and *Yi Yi Ren* (Semen Coicis) strengthen the Spleen and Stomach to resolve dampness and swelling. *Jin Qian Cao* (Herba Lysimachiae), *Ze Xie* (Rhizoma Alismatis) and *Che Qian Zi* (Semen Plantaginis) drain damp-heat and help expel uric acid from the body through urination. *Shi Gao* (Gypsum Fibrosum), *Zhi Mu* (Radix Anemarrhenae), *Huang Bai* (Cortex Phellodendri) and *Sheng Di Huang* (Radix Rehmanniae) clear heat and sedate fire. Together they reduce the inflammation and burning sensation. *Ji Xue Teng* (Caulis Spatholobi) opens the channels and collaterals. *Chi Shao* (Radix Paeoniae Rubrae) activates blood circulation and relieves pain. Lastly, *He Zi* (Fructus Chebulae) and *Wu Bei Zi* (Galla Chinensis) are two astringent herbs that reduce swelling and inflammation.

In summary, **Flex (GT)** is a comprehensive formula that targets both the cause and the symptoms of gout. It incorporates herbs to strengthen the Spleen and Stomach, drain damp-heat, open the channels and collaterals, and relieve pain.

SUPPLEMENTARY FORMULAS

- For severe pain, combine with **Herbal Analgesic**.
- For gout in individuals with obesity, use with **Herbalite** to reduce body weight.
- For gout in individuals with diabetes, use with **Equilibrium** to control blood glucose levels.
- For gout in individuals with hyperlipidemia, use with **Cholisma** to reduce cholesterol and triglyceride levels.
- For gout in individuals with obesity and high cholesterol, add **Cholisma (ES)**.
- For gout with kidney stones, add **Dissolve (KS)**.
- With hypertension, add **Gastrodia Complex** or **Gentiana Complex**.

NUTRITION

- *Hai Zao* (Sargassum) and *Kun Bu* (Thallus Laminariae seu Eckloniae) are helpful, as they contain protein and vital minerals to reduce uric acid levels in the blood.
- Adequate amounts of vitamin C and bioflavonoids (3,000 to 5,000 mg daily) should be taken, as they help to reduce uric acid levels in the blood.
- Essential fatty acids are beneficial for gout, as they are needed to repair tissues and healing of joint disorders.
- Since gout attack is caused by excessive deposit of uric acid in the joints, increased intake of food rich in uric acid will increase the risk of gout attacks. Purine-rich food should be avoided, including meat, soup (bone broth), gravies, meat extracts, seafood (anchovies, fish roes, herring, sardine, mussels), shellfish, internal organ meats (liver and kidneys), beer and other alcoholic beverages, spinach, asparagus, mushrooms, and cauliflower.
- Patients with gout should increase their intake of cherries, blueberries and strawberries, all of which are excellent in neutralizing uric acid.
- It is important to always consume an adequate amount of distilled water, and avoid tap water whenever possible. This will help flush out the uric acid crystals.
- After an attack of gout, it is recommended to eat only raw fruits and vegetables for about 1 to 2 weeks.

CAUTIONS

- This formula should not be used in cases of deficiency and cold.
- Heat packs should not be used in patients with gout, as it is a condition characterized by heat.

ACUPUNCTURE POINTS

Traditional Points:
- Needle *ah shi* points using the sedating technique (counter-clock wise).

Balance Method by Dr. Richard Tan:
- Use Dr. Tan's Balance Method accordingly as determined by where the pain is (use mirror or image system). If the pain is in the toes, needle around the thumb. If the pain is in the knees, needle the elbow. Needle the *ah shi* points.
- For additional information on the Balance Method, please refer to *Dr. Tan's Strategy of Twelve Magical Points* by Dr. Richard Tan.

FORMULAS

FLEX (GT) ™

Auricular Acupuncture Dr. by Li-Chun Huang:

❧ Points selection: Corresponding Points (to the area of pain), *San Jiao*, Endocrine, Kidney, Liver, Spleen, and Coronary Vascular Subcortex. Bleed Ear Apex.

❧ For additional information on the location and explanation of these points, please refer to *Auricular Treatment Formula and Prescriptions* by Dr. Li-Chun Huang.

MODERN RESEARCH

Gout is a form of arthritis that is characterized by sudden, severe attacks of pain, tenderness, redness, warmth and swelling (inflammation) in some joints. Gout usually affects the large toe, but it can affect other joints in the leg (knee, ankle, and foot) and sometimes also joints in the arm (hand, wrist, and elbow). Gout is caused in part by excessive intake of food rich in uric acid, or decreased excretion of uric acid through the kidneys. As uric acid deposits in the joints, it causes severe pain known as gout.

Flex (GT) is a comprehensive formula that treats various aspects of gout. It incorporates herbs that decrease the absorption and increase the elimination of uric acid and other unwanted substances. Furthermore, it contains herbs with analgesic effect to relieve pain, anti-inflammatory effect to reduce swelling and inflammation, and antipyretic effect to relieve burning sensations and reduce inflammation.

Jin Qian Cao (Herba Lysimachiae) and *Ze Xie* (Rhizoma Alismatis) have a remarkable diuretic effect that flush out unwanted substances from the body. *Jin Qian Cao* (Herba Lysimachiae) is one of the most effective herbs to dissolve and flush out gallstones, kidney stones, and bladder stones.[1,2] *Ze Xie* (Rhizoma Alismatis) is effective in eliminating excessive amount of electrolytes, cholesterols, and triglycerides from the blood.[3,4]

He Zi (Fructus Chebulae) and *Wu Bei Zi* (Galla Chinensis) are astringent herbs with binding effects that help decrease the absorption of fatty foods and uric acids.[5]

Shi Gao (Gypsum Fibrosum), *Zhi Mu* (Radix Anemarrhenae), and *Sheng Di Huang* (Radix Rehmanniae) have excellent antipyretic and anti-inflammatory effects to reduce swelling and inflammation.[6,7,8] Use of *Shi Gao* (Gypsum Fibrosum) was associated with over 80% rate of effectiveness for treating osteoarthrosis deformans endemica;[9] use of *Zhi Mu* (Radix Anemarrhenae) was linked with 71.4% rate of effectiveness for treating acute rheumatism;[10] and use of *Sheng Di Huang* (Radix Rehmanniae) had good results in treating rheumatoid arthritis.[11]

Lastly, *Yi Yi Ren* (Semen Coicis) has analgesic and antipyretic properties, and it helps to relieve pain and reduce the burning sensations.[12]

In summary, *Flex (GT)* is a formula specifically designed to treat gout by decreasing plasma levels of uric acid, reducing swelling and inflammation, and relieving pain.

PHARMACEUTICAL DRUGS & CHINESE MEDICINE: A COMPARATIVE ANALYSIS

Gout is a form of arthritis that is characterized by sudden, severe attacks of pain, tenderness, redness, warmth and swelling (inflammation) in some joints. Gout is caused in part by excessive intake of food rich in uric acid, or decreased excretion of uric acid through the kidneys. As uric acid deposits in the joints, they cause severe pain known as gout.

Western Medical Approach: acute gout may be treated with colchicine, but use of this drug is not recommended as it may cause severe bone marrow suppression and possibly death. Non-steroidal anti-inflammatory agents (NSAID), such as Indocin (Indomethacin), Motrin (Ibuprofen), and Naprosyn (Naproxen) are very frequently used to treat mild to moderate pain characterized by inflammation and swelling. However, they may cause such serious side effects as gastric ulcer, duodenal ulcer, gastrointestinal bleeding, tinnitus, blurred vision, dizziness and headache. In short, drug treatment of gout is limited and less than satisfactory.

Traditional Chinese Medicine Approach: Treatment of gout must focus on treating the symptom and the cause. In this formula, many herbs with strong analgesic effect treat pain. Furthermore, many herbs with draining effect flush out excess uric acid. Though herbs are not as potent as the drugs, they offer both short- and long-term improvement for treatment of gout.

Summation: It is important to remember that optimal treatment lies not in use of drugs or herbs, but in commitment to make diet and lifestyle changes. Long-term success can be accomplished only if changes are made to decrease intake and increase elimination of uric acid.

[1] *Zhong Yi Za Zhi* (Journal of Chinese Medicine), 1958; 11:749
[2] *Guang Xi Zhong Yi Yao* (Guangxi Chinese Medicine and Herbology), 1990; 13(6):40
[3] *Sheng Yao Xue Za Zhi* (Journal of Raw Herbology), 1982; 36(2):150
[4] *Zhong Hua Yi Xue Za Zhi* (Chinese Journal of Medicine), 1976; 11:693
[5] Chen, J. *The Herbal Safety Course*, National Alliance Conference, 2002
[6] *Zhong Yao Xue* (Chinese Herbology), 1998, 115:119
[7] *Zhong Hua Wai Ke Za Zhi* (Chinese Journal of External Medicine), 1960; 4:366
[8] *Zhong Yao Yao Li Yu Ying Yong* (Pharmacology and Applications of Chinese Herbs), 1983: 400
[9] *Shan Xi Yi Yao* (Shanxi Medicine and Herbology), 1973; 4:17
[10] *Ji Lin Zhong Yi Yao* (Jilin Chinese Medicine and Herbology), 1992; (1):16
[11] *Tian Jing Yi Xue Za Zhi* (Journal of Tianjing Medicine and Herbology), 1966; 3:209
[12] *Zhong Yao Xue* (Chinese Herbology), 1998; 337-339

FORMULAS

FLEX (Heat) ™

CLINICAL APPLICATIONS

- ❧ Acute muscle aches and pain with heat manifestations, such as swelling, burning sensation and inflammation
- ❧ Acute arthritis, arthralgia or gout with redness and swelling
- ❧ Fibromyalgia with heat manifestations
- ❧ Rheumatic heat disorders

WESTERN THERAPEUTIC ACTIONS

- ❧ Strong analgesic function to relieve pain [3]
- ❧ Anti-inflammatory effect to reduce inflammation and swelling [1,2]
- ❧ Antirheumatic function to treat disorders of the connective tissue such as joints, muscles, bursae, tendons and fibrous tissues [1,2]

CHINESE THERAPEUTIC ACTIONS

- ❧ Expels wind and heat
- ❧ Disperses *bi zheng* (painful obstruction syndrome)
- ❧ Clears damp-heat and reduces swelling
- ❧ Alleviates pain

DOSAGE

Take 3 to 4 capsules three times daily. Dosage may be increased up to 5 to 6 capsules every four to six hours as needed. For quick and maximum effectiveness, take the herbs on an empty stomach with warm water.

INGREDIENTS

Cang Zhu (Rhizoma Atractylodis)
Dang Gui Wei (Extremitas Radicis Angelicae Sinensis)
Du Huo (Radix Angelicae Pubescentis)
Fen Fang Ji (Radix Stephaniae Tetandrae)
Huang Bai (Cortex Phellodendri)
Lu Lu Tong (Fructus Liquidambaris)
Luo Shi Teng (Caulis Trachelospermi)
Qiang Huo (Rhizoma et Radix Notopterygii)

Qin Jiao (Radix Gentianae Macrophyllae)
Sang Zhi (Ramulus Mori)
Shi Gao (Gypsum Fibrosum)
Wei Ling Xian (Radix Clematidis)
Wu Jia Pi (Cortex Acanthopanacis)
Xi Xian Cao (Herba Siegesbeckiae)
Yi Yi Ren (Semen Coicis)
Zhi Mu (Radix Anemarrhenae)

FORMULA EXPLANATION

Flex (Heat) is formulated specifically to treat musculoskeletal disorders characterized by heat. It contains herbs with functions to eliminate wind, heat and damp, remove painful obstructions, and relieve pain.

Cang Zhu (Rhizoma Atractylodis) dries dampness and *Huang Bai* (Cortex Phellodendri) clears damp-heat in the lower parts of the body. These two herbs have an excellent effect to treat pain in the lower half of the body, as in the classic formula *Er Miao San* (Two-Marvel Powder). *Qiang Huo* (Rhizoma et Radix Notopterygii), *Du Huo* (Radix Angelicae Pubescentis), and *Sang Zhi* (Ramulus Mori) have antirheumatic, anti-inflammatory, and analgesic functions. They remove painful obstruction by expelling wind, damp and heat in the upper and lower body. *Shi Gao* (Gypsum Fibrosum) and *Zhi Mu* (Radix Anemarrhenae) have anti-inflammatory functions to clear heat and reduce painful swelling sensation of the joints. *Yi Yi Ren* (Semen Coicis) and *Fen Fang Ji* (Radix Stephaniae Tetandrae) are

FLEX (Heat) ™

diuretics that reduce swelling of the joints. *Wei Ling Xian* (Radix Clematidis), *Luo Shi Teng* (Caulis Trachelospermi) and *Dang Gui Wei* (Extremitas Radicis Angelicae Sinensis) have Antirheumatic and blood-invigorating effects to clear the channels and collaterals therefore enhancing the flexibility and integrity of the joints. *Xi Xian Cao* (Herba Siegesbeckiae), *Lu Lu Tong* (Fructus Liquidambaris), and *Qin Jiao* (Radix Gentianae Macrophyllae) dredge the channels and scour residual blood stagnation. They are often used in wind disorders including paralysis or hemiplegia. *Wu Jia Pi* (Cortex Acanthopanacis) strengthens sinews and bones and helps relieve chronic pain.

SUPPLEMENTARY FORMULAS

- To potentiate the effect to relieve pain, add **Herbal Analgesic**.
- With excess heat, add **Gardenia Complex**.
- For severe pain with severe blood stagnation, add **Circulation (SJ)**.
- For gout, use **Flex (GT)** instead.
- For neck and shoulder pain, add **Neck & Shoulder (Acute)** or **Neck & Shoulder (Chronic)**.
- For upper back pain, add **Back Support (Upper)**.
- For lower back pain, add **Back Support (Acute)** or **Back Support (Chronic)**.
- For herniated disk in the back with swelling and inflammation, add **Back Support (HD)**.
- For knee pain, add **Knee & Ankle (Acute)** or **Knee & Ankle (Chronic)**.
- For spasms and cramps, combine with **Flex (SC)**.
- For bone fractures, injuries, and bruises, combine with **Traumanex**
- For bone spurs, add **Flex (Spur)**.
- For post-stroke numbness and atrophy, use **Neuro Plus**.
- For osteoporosis, add **Osteo 8**.
- For degeneration of muscles, ligaments, tendons and ligaments, add **Flex (MLT)**.
- For arthritic pain that worsens during cold and rainy weather, use **Flex (CD)** instead of **Flex (Heat)**.

NUTRITION

- Sulfur helps the absorption of calcium, and adequate intake and absorption of calcium is essential for the repair and the rebuilding of bones, tendons, cartilage, and connective tissues. Patients are encouraged to consume foods high in sulfur such as asparagus, eggs, fresh garlic, and onions.
- Histidine, an amino acid, is responsible for removing the high levels of copper and iron found in arthritic patients. Patients are encouraged to consume foods high in histidine such as rice, wheat and rye.
- Fresh pineapples are recommended as they contain bromelain, an enzyme that is excellent in reducing inflammation.
- Avoid spicy food, caffeine, citrus fruits, sugar, milk, dairy products and red meat.
- Fish oil may help alleviate pain associated with rheumatoid arthritis. It can be taken in conjunction with the herbs.
- Decrease the intake of sour foods, drinks or fruits (citrus) as their nature constricts and may contribute to further stagnation in the channels and collaterals.

LIFESTYLE INSTRUCTIONS

- For obese patients, weight loss is suggested as it lessens the pressure on the joints, which can then help in relieving pain.
- Heat packs should not be used in patients with joint pain due to heat.

FLEX (Heat) ™

CLINICAL NOTES

❧ *Flex (Heat)* can be combined with *Traumanex* in the early stages of sports injury when there is severe pain with inflammation, swelling and redness. Begin treating the patient immediately for maximum effectiveness.

❧ Internal hemorrhage must be ruled out first prior to treating patients with head injuries.

❧ The use of ice packs is recommended to reduce redness, swelling and inflammation.

CAUTIONS

❧ Patients who are on anticoagulant or antiplatelet therapies, such as Coumadin (Warfarin), should use this formula with caution, as there may be a slightly higher risk of bleeding and bruising.

❧ This formula is contraindicated during pregnancy and nursing.

ACUPUNCTURE POINTS

Traditional Points:
1. Needle *ah shi* points.
2. *Taichong* (LR 3), *Xingjian* (LR 2), *Zusanli* (ST 36), and *Geshu* (BL 17).

Balance Method by Dr. Richard Tan:
❧ Use Dr. Tan's Balance Method accordingly as determined by where the pain is (use mirror or image system).
❧ For additional information on the Balance Method, please refer to *Dr. Tan's Strategy of Twelve Magical Points* by Dr. Richard Tan.

Ear Points:
Related joints, Adrenal Glands. Embed magnetic ear balls and switch ears every three days.

Auricular Acupuncture by Dr. Li-Chun Huang:
❧ Arthritis of finger: Finger (front and back of ear).
  ▪ Supplementary points: Lesser Occipital Nerve. Bleed Ear Apex
❧ Rheumatic Arthritis: Corresponding Points (to the area of pain), Allergic Area, Adrenal Gland, and Endocrine. Bleed Ear Apex
  ▪ Supplementary points: Kidney, Liver, Spleen, Sanjiao
❧ For additional information on the location and explanation of these points, please refer to *Auricular Treatment Formula and Prescriptions* by Dr. Li-Chun Huang.

MODERN RESEARCH

Flex (Heat) is formulated with herbs that have antirheumatic, anti-inflammatory, analgesic, and antipyretic functions.

Cang Zhu (Rhizoma Atractylodis), *Fen Fang Ji* (Radix Stephaniae Tetandrae), *Qiang Huo* (Rhizoma et Radix Notopterygii), and *Du Huo* (Radix Angelicae Pubescentis) all have antirheumatic and anti-inflammatory functions to relieve acute inflammation and swelling.[1,2] In addition, *Du Huo* (Radix Angelicae Pubescentis) has a strong analgesic function which works on the central nervous system to relieve pain. [1,3]

Fen Fang Ji (Radix Stephaniae Tetandrae) is an excellent herb for treating muscular disorders with redness, swelling and inflammation. In a clinical study on the treatment of *bi zheng* (painful obstruction syndrome), 120 patients were given *Fen Fang Ji* (Radix Stephaniae Tetandrae) tincture two to three times daily for three to six cycles of treatment.

FLEX (Heat) ™

Each cycle of treatment is ten days, with three to six days between the cycles with no intake of herbs. It was concluded at the end of the study that *Fen Fang Ji* (Radix Stephaniae Tetandrae) was 93.3% effective in treating heat type of *bi zheng* (painful obstruction syndrome).[4]

Many herbs in **Flex (Heat)** have antipyretic functions to relieve fever and swelling associated with external or sports injuries. Herbs with strong antipyretic functions include *Shi Gao* (Gypsum Fibrosum), *Zhi Mu* (Radix Anemarrhenae), and *Huang Bai* (Cortex Phellodendri).[1,2]

PHARMACEUTICAL DRUGS & CHINESE MEDICINE: A COMPARATIVE ANALYSIS

Western Medical Approach: Pain is a basic bodily sensation induced by a noxious stimulus that causes physical discomfort (as pricking, throbbing, or aching). Pain may be of acute or chronic state, and may be of nociceptive, neuropathic, or psychogenic type.

Non-steroidal anti-inflammatory agents (NSAID), such as Motrin (Ibuprofen), Naprosyn (Naproxen) and Voltaren (Diclofenac) are very frequently used to treat mild to moderate pain characterized by inflammation and swelling. Clinical applications include headache, arthritis, dysmenorrhea, and general aches and pain. Though effective, they may cause such serious side effects as gastric ulcer, duodenal ulcer, gastrointestinal bleeding, tinnitus, blurred vision, dizziness and headache. Furthermore, the newer NSAID's, also known as Cox-2 inhibitors [such as Celebrex (Celecoxib)], are associated with significantly higher risk of cardiovascular events, including heart attack and stroke. In fact, these side effects are so serious that two Cox-2 inhibitors have already been withdrawn from the market [Vioxx (Rofecoxib) and Bextra (Valdecoxib)]. In brief, it is important to remember that while drugs offer reliable and potent symptomatic pain relief, they should be used only if and when needed. Frequent use and abuse leads to unnecessary side effects and complications.

Traditional Chinese Medicine Approach: Treatment of pain is a sophisticated balance of art and science. Proper treatment of pain requires a careful evaluation of the type of disharmony (excess or deficiency, cold or heat, exterior or interior), characteristics (qi and/or blood stagnations), and locations (upper body, lower body, extremities, or internal organs). Furthermore, optimal treatment requires integrative use of herbs, acupuncture and *Tui-Na* therapies. All these therapies work together to tonify the underlying deficiencies, strengthen the body, and facilitate recovery from chronic pain. TCM pain management targets both the symptoms and the causes of pain, and as such, often achieves immediate and long-term success. Furthermore, TCM pain management is often associated with few or no side effects.

Summation: For treatment of mild to severe pain due to various causes, TCM pain management offers similar treatment effects with significantly fewer side effects.

CASE STUDIES

E.K., a 54-year-old female, presented with severe, burning, sacral pain. MRI evaluation revealed a bulging lumbar disk. The patient stated she had previously been managing her chronic low back pain but that this was the first time she had had the burning sensation. The TCM diagnosis was heat in the lower *jiao*. The patient reported that taking **Flex (Heat)** at four capsules, four times daily, took away the burning sensation but did not completely resolve the pain. She then used this formula time from to time, when the burning sensation came back.

M.C., Sarasota, Florida

A female broker presented with pain, heat and swelling in her joints that would flare up and subside intermittently. Limited range of motion was also present along with joint rigidity. The pain and swelling was felt especially in the 4th finger bilaterally and occasionally on either ankles. There was a butterfly rash (yin deficiency) on her face. Other

FORMULAS

FLEX (Heat) ™

symptoms included hot flashes and night sweats. The practitioner diagnosed the condition as *bi zheng* (painful obstruction syndrome) due to wind-damp-heat with underlying Kidney yin deficiency. The patient was given *Flex (Heat)* to treat the pain, and *Zhi Bai Di Huang Wan* (Anemarrhena Phellodendron and Rehmannia Formula) to nourish yin. The patient had been treated with various medications previously and found that *Flex (Heat)* produced the best results. Past treatments for her condition also showed diminished efficacy after a period of 4 to 6 months. With *Flex (Heat)* she was able to continue treatment for almost a year while still maintaining its therapeutic value. The practitioners noted that *Flex (Heat)* was a very effective formula for inflammatory joint conditions.

T.W., Santa Monica, California

[1] Bensky, D. et al. *Chinese Herbal Medicine Materia Medica*. Eastland Press. 1993
[2] Yeung, HC. *Handbook of Chinese Herbs*. Institute of Chinese Medicine. 1996
[3] Liao, JF. Evaluation with receptor binding assay on the water extracts of ten CNS-active Chinese herbal drugs. Proceedings of the National Science Council, Republic of China – Part B, *Life Sciences*. Jul. 1995; 19(3):151-8
[4] Sun, DH. Treatment of heat type of painful obstruction (Bi) syndrome with stephania (fang ji) in 120 patients. *Shangdong Journal of Traditional Chinese Medicine*. 1987; 6:21

FORMULAS

FLEX (MLT) ™

CLINICAL APPLICATIONS

- Atrophy and wasting of muscles, ligaments and tendons
- Cartilage damages from chronic wear and tear
- Decreased range of motion and mobility of the joints
- Rehabilitation from chronic or late-stages of musculoskeletal injuries
- Prevention against wear and tear or breakdown of cartilage and soft tissue surrounding joints
- Individuals engaging in repetitive motions who wish to maintain healthy joints and connective tissue

WESTERN THERAPEUTIC ACTIONS

- Adaptogenic effect to facilitate rehabilitation
- Anti-inflammatory effect to reduce swelling and inflammation
- Analgesic effect to relieve pain
- Muscle-relaxant effect to relieve spasms and cramps
- Aids in cartilage formation and repair

CHINESE THERAPEUTIC ACTIONS

- Tonifies qi and blood
- Activates qi and blood circulation
- Nourishes yin
- Dispels wind-damp
- Strengthens muscles, tendons, ligaments, and bones

DOSAGE

Take 4 to 6 capsules three times daily. This formula should be taken during the mid-to-late stages of recovery and rehabilitation. It should not be taken during the acute phases of injuries, where there may be bleeding and bruises.

INGREDIENTS

Bai Shao (Radix Paeoniae Alba)
Chu Shi Zi (Fructus Broussonetiae)
Chuan Niu Xi (Radix Cyathulae)
Dang Gui (Radicis Angelicae Sinensis)
Dang Shen (Radix Codonopsis)

He Shou Wu (Radix Polygoni Multiflori)
Qian Nian Jian (Rhizoma Homalomenae)
Sheng Di Huang (Radix Rehmanniae)
Wu Jia Pi (Cortex Acanthopanacis)
Xu Duan (Radix Dipsaci)

FORMULA EXPLANATION

Flex (MLT) is designed specifically to treat chronic or mid-to-late stages of musculoskeletal injuries, with atrophy of the soft tissues (muscles, tendons, ligaments, and cartilage), decreased mobility of the joints, cartilage degeneration, and generalized weakness and pain. This formula contains herbs to tonify blood, activate blood circulation, nourish yin, and dispel wind-damp.

In this formula, many herbs are used to tonify the underlying deficiencies. Dang Shen (Radix Codonopsis) tonifies qi. Dang Gui (Radicis Angelicae Sinensis), Sheng Di Huang (Radix Rehmanniae), and Bai Shao (Radix Paeoniae Alba) nourish blood and yin. Healthy joints depend on healthy surrounding cartilage and soft tissue. Because there is no blood supply to the cartilage, it gets nutrition and oxygen from the surrounding joint fluids. Therefore, adequate blood supply to the surrounding areas of the cartilage will ensure a healthy joint. Dang Gui (Radicis Angelicae Sinensis) tonifies blood and promotes blood circulation to generate new tissues. Chuan Niu Xi (Radix Cyathulae)

FORMULAS

tonifies the Liver and Kidney, strengthens tendons and bones, and helps *Dang Gui* (Radicis Angelicae Sinensis) move blood. Together, they stimulate soft tissue (tendons, ligaments and cartilage) growth and restoration. Furthermore, *Wu Jia Pi* (Cortex Acanthopanacis), *Qian Nian Jian* (Rhizoma Homalomenae), and *Xu Duan* (Radix Dipsaci) dispel wind-damp, strengthen bones and tendons and relieve pain. *Chu Shi Zi* (Fructus Broussonetiae) and *He Shou Wu* (Radix Polygoni Multiflori) tonify Liver and Kidney to strengthen muscles, tendons, cartilage, and ligaments. The yin tonics of this formula, *Bai Shao* (Radix Paeoniae Alba), *He Shou Wu* (Radix Polygoni Multiflori), and *Chuan Niu Xi* (Radix Cyathulae) prevent the narrowing of the space between joints, especially in the vertebrae or the knee joint due to degeneration.

In summary, *Flex (MLT)* works to support connective tissues around the joints. It contains herbs that tonify the underlying deficiencies and facilitate healing and recovery. It treats chronic or mid-to-late stages of musculoskeletal injuries with soft tissue degeneration as it encourages repair and restoration.

SUPPLEMENTARY FORMULAS

- ☙ For recovery from chronic neck and shoulder injuries, combine with *Neck & Shoulder (Chronic)*.
- ☙ For recovery from chronic low back pain, combine with *Back Support (Chronic)*.
- ☙ For individuals with severe weakness and deficiencies, combine with *Imperial Tonic*.
- ☙ For recovery from chronic arm (shoulder, elbow and wrist) injuries, combine with *Arm Support*.
- ☙ For recovery from chronic knee and ankle injuries, combine with *Knee & Ankle (Chronic)*.
- ☙ With osteoarthritis, add *Osteo 8* and *Flex (Heat)* or *Flex (CD)*.
- ☙ With bone spur, add *Flex (Spur)*.

NUTRITION

- ☙ Sea cucumber is very beneficial, because it is a rich source of lubricating compounds that are needed in all connective tissues, especially joints and joint fluids. Gelatin is also recommended.
- ☙ It is important to consume an adequate amount of multiple vitamins and minerals, as they are essential to prevent bone loss and promote bone growth.
- ☙ Glucosamine sulfate and chondroitin sulfate are great nutritional supports. They are important for the formation of bones, tendons, ligaments, and cartilages.

LIFESTYLE INSTRUCTION

- ☙ While it is important to relax and rest during the recovery process of injuries, it is also important not to stay completely bed-ridden. Gentle exercises will not only facilitate recovery, but will also prevent muscle atrophy and muscle wasting.

CLINICAL NOTES

- ☙ Cold packs should be used during the first 24 to 48 hours of acute injuries to reduce swelling and inflammation. On the other hand, hot packs should be used for chronic injuries to promote blood circulation and enhance healing in the affected area.
- ☙ This formula should be taken during the mid-to-late stages of recovery and rehabilitation.

CAUTIONS

- ☙ This formula should *not* be taken during the acute phases of injuries with bleeding and bruises, as there are many tonic or warm herbs that may worsen the condition.

FLEX (MLT) ™

◐ *Dang Gui* (Radicis Angelicae Sinensis) may enhance the overall effectiveness of Coumadin (Warfarin), an anticoagulant drug. Patients who take anticoagulant or antiplatelet medications should *not* take this herbal formula without supervision by a licensed health care practitioner.

ACUPUNCTURE POINTS

Balance Method by Dr. Richard Tan:
◐ Left side: *Ququan* (LR 8), *Rangu* (KI 2), *Dazhong* (KI 4), *Fuliu* (KI 7), *Neiguan* (PC 6), and *Tongli* (HT 5).
◐ Right side: *Waiguan* (TH 5), *Yangxi* (LI 5), *Zusanli* (ST 36), and *Yanglingquan* (GB 34).
◐ For additional information on the Balance Method, please refer to *Acupuncture 1, 2, 3* by Dr. Richard Tan.

MODERN RESEARCH

Flex (MLT) is an excellent formula for rehabilitation of patients who suffer from chronic musculoskeletal injuries. After acute injuries (such as broken bones, bone fracture, and tear of muscles, tendons or ligaments), patients are often asked to rest for an extended amount of time. As a result, lack of movement on a long-term basis often contributes to atrophy of the soft tissues (muscles, tendons, ligaments, and cartilage), decreased mobility of the joints, and generalized weakness and pain. This formula is designed specifically to treat this condition, and it contains herbs with adaptogenic effects to facilitate rehabilitation, anti-inflammatory effects to reduce swelling and inflammation, analgesic effects to relieve pain, and muscle-relaxant effects to relieve spasms and cramps.

Flex (MLT) uses many herbs with adaptogenic effect to facilitate both mental and physical aspects of rehabilitation. *Dang Shen* (Radix Codonopsis) has a regulatory effect on the central nervous system to help with adaptation to various stressful environments.[1] *Wu Jia Pi* (Cortex Acanthopanacis) enhances physical adaptation by increasing endurance and performance.[2]

Many herbs in this formula have marked analgesic and anti-inflammatory effects to relieve pain, and reduce swelling and inflammation. For example, *Dang Gui* (Radicis Angelicae Sinensis) has a marked analgesic and anti-inflammatory effect, with potency similar to or stronger than that of acetylsalicylic acid.[3,4] *Wu Jia Pi* (Cortex Acanthopanacis) also has excellent analgesic and anti-inflammatory effects, with duration of action lasting up to five hours.[5,6] *Bai Shao* (Radix Paeoniae Alba) and *Sheng Di Huang* (Radix Rehmanniae) have anti-inflammatory and antipyretic effects to reduce inflammation and swelling and relieve burning sensations in the affected areas.[7,8] Clinically, these herbs have been used with great success to treat a wide variety of musculoskeletal conditions, including but not limited to muscle wasting, muscle atrophy, chronic soft tissue injuries, and various types of pain.[9,10] Lastly, *Bai Shao* (Radix Paeoniae Alba) has an excellent muscle-relaxant effect to relieve spasms, cramps, and muscle stiffness.[11] This efficacy has been demonstrated in both smooth and skeletal muscles.

In summary, *Flex (MLT)* is an excellent formula for chronic or mid-to-late stages of musculoskeletal injuries. With chronic injuries, degeneration of the soft tissues (muscles, tendons, ligaments, and cartilage) leads to decreased range of motion and mobility of the joints. With mid-to-late stages of musculoskeletal injuries, muscle wasting and muscle atrophy due to lack of exercise and physical movement is the main concern. This formula is developed specifically to address all of these conditions by using herbs that compliment the rehabilitation process and complete the recovery from these illnesses.

PHARMACEUTICAL DRUGS & CHINESE MEDICINE: A COMPARATIVE ANALYSIS

Western Medical Approach: Pain is a basic bodily sensation induced by a noxious stimulus that causes physical discomfort (as pricking, throbbing, or aching). Pain may be of acute or chronic state, and may be of nociceptive, neuropathic, or psychogenic type.

FORMULAS

FLEX (MLT) ™

Western medicine excels in treatment of acute pain. There are many drugs with potent and reliable analgesic effects. Furthermore, many drugs are available as injection for immediate pain relief. However, these drugs treat the symptom of pain but do not alter the underlying disease. Furthermore, long-term use of these drugs for chronic pain are likely to cause more side effects, and complicate the condition further. In short, while drugs are effective for treating acute pain, they should be used sparingly to manage chronic pain.

Traditional Chinese Medicine Approach: Treatment of pain is a sophisticated balance of art and science. Proper treatment of pain requires a careful evaluation of the type of disharmony (excess or deficiency, cold or heat, exterior or interior), characteristics (qi and/or blood stagnations), and locations (upper body, lower body, extremities, or internal organs). Furthermore, optimal treatment requires integrative use of herbs, acupuncture and *Tui-Na* therapies. All these therapies work together to tonify the underlying deficiencies, strengthen the body, and facilitate recovery from chronic pain. TCM pain management targets both the symptom and the cause of pain, and as such, often achieves immediate and long-term success. Furthermore, TCM pain management is often associated with few or no side effects.

Summation: For treatment of mild to severe pain due to various causes, TCM pain management offers similar treatment effects with significantly fewer side effects.

[1] *Zhong Yao Tong Bao* (Journal of Chinese Herbology), 1986; 11(8):53
[2] *Zhong Cao Yao* (Chinese Herbal Medicine), 1987; 18(3):28
[3] *Xin Yi Yao Xue Za Zhi* (New Journal of Medicine and Herbology), 1975; (6):34
[4] *Yao Xue Za Zhi* (Journal of Medicinals), 1971; (91):1098
[5] *Zhong Guo Yao Li Xue Tong Bao* (Journal of Chinese Herbal Pharmacology), 1986; 2(2):21
[6] *Zhong Cheng Yao Yan Jiu* (Research of Chinese Patent Medicine), 1984; 10:22
[7] *Zhong Yao Yao Li Yu Ying Yong* (Pharmacology and Applications of Chinese Herbs), 1983; 400
[8] *Zhong Yao Zhi* (Chinese Herbology Journal), 1993; 183
[9] *Xin Yi Yao Xue Za Zhi* (New Journal of Medicine and Herbology), 1976; 12:26
[10] *Shang Hai Zhong Yi Yao Za Zhi* (Shanghai Journal of Chinese Medicine and Herbology), 1983; 4:14
[11] *Zhong Yi Za Zhi* (Journal of Chinese Medicine), 1983; 11:9

FORMULAS

FLEX (NP) ™

CLINICAL APPLICATIONS

- Nerve pain from peripheral neuropathy, polyneuropathy, and diabetic neuropathy
- Neuralgia, trigeminal neuralgia
- *Wei* (atrophy) syndrome
- Peripheral vascular disease
- General pain, numbness, tingling, swelling, and muscle wasting, especially in the extremities

WESTERN THERAPEUTIC ACTIONS

- Analgesic function to relieve pain
- Restores sensory loss
- Improves peripheral blood circulation
- Treats causes of peripheral neuropathy, such as increased pressure, trauma, infection, and buildup of drugs and toxic agents

CHINESE THERAPEUTIC ACTIONS

- Invigorates blood circulation
- Relieves pain
- Opens channels and collaterals

DOSAGE

Take 3 to 4 capsules three times daily on an empty stomach, with warm water. Dosage may be increased to 6 to 8 capsules three times daily, if necessary.

INGREDIENTS

Bai Shao (Radix Paeoniae Alba)	*Lu Lu Tong* (Fructus Liquidambaris)
Chuan Niu Xi (Radix Cyathulae)	*Mo Gu Xiao* (Caulis Hyptis Capitatae)
Chuan Xiong (Rhizoma Ligustici Chuanxiong)	*Mo Yao* (Myrrha)
Da Huang (Radix et Rhizoma Rhei)	*Mu Dan Pi* (Cortex Moutan)
Da Zao (Fructus Jujubae)	*Mu Xiang* (Radix Aucklandiae)
Dang Gui (Radicis Angelicae Sinensis)	*Qiang Huo* (Rhizoma et Radix Notopterygii)
Dang Gui Wei (Extremitas Radicis Angelicae Sinensis)	*Qin Jiao* (Radix Gentianae Macrophyllae)
Er Cha (Catechu)	*Ru Xiang* (Gummi Olibanum)
Fu Ling (Poria)	*Sheng Ma* (Rhizoma Cimicifugae)
Gan Cao (Radix Glycyrrhizae)	*Tao Ren* (Semen Persicae)
Hong Hua (Flos Carthami)	*Xue Jie* (Sanguis Draconis)
Huang Jin Gui (Caulis Vanieriae)	*Yan Hu Suo* (Rhizoma Corydalis)
Liu Zhi Huang (Herba Solidaginis)	

FORMULA EXPLANATION

According to traditional Chinese medicine, peripheral neuropathy, polyneuropathy, diabetic neuropathy, distal polyneuropathy, neuralgia, and fibromyalgia have various etiologies. However, they all share one common factor – pain due to blood stagnation. Therefore, *Flex (NP)* is formulated to treat nerve pain by activating blood circulation and eliminating blood stagnation.

FLEX (NP) ™

Tao Ren (Semen Persicae), and *Hong Hua* (Flos Carthami) are often paired together to synergistically invigorate blood circulation and remove blood stagnation. *Ru Xiang* (Gummi Olibanum), *Mo Yao* (Myrrha), *Chuan Niu Xi* (Radix Cyathulae), and *Yan Hu Suo* (Rhizoma Corydalis) together invigorate blood circulation and relieve pain. *Er Cha* (Catechu), and *Xue Jie* (Sanguis Draconis) promote the generation of new tissues. *Mu Dan Pi* (Cortex Moutan) moves blood and clears heat associated with local inflammation due to blood stagnation. *Dang Gui* (Radicis Angelicae Sinensis), *Dang Gui Wei* (Extremitas Radicis Angelicae Sinensis), *Chuan Xiong* (Rhizoma Ligustici Chuanxiong), and *Lu Lu Tong* (Fructus Liquidambaris) open the channels and collaterals to relieve pain by invigorating blood circulation to the extremities. *Fu Ling* (Poria) is used to strengthen the middle *jiao* to promote absorption of the herbs.

Da Huang (Radix et Rhizoma Rhei) clears heat, removes blood stasis and helps with blood circulation. *Bai Shao* (Radix Paeoniae Alba) softens the Liver and benefits the tendons and sinews to relieve tightness, numbness, tingling and pain. *Mu Xiang* (Radix Aucklandiae) invigorates qi circulation in the channels to assist the overall pain-relieving effects of this formula.

Qin Jiao (Radix Gentianae Macrophyllae), *Qiang Huo* (Rhizoma et Radix Notopterygii), *Huang Jin Gui* (Caulis Vanieriae), *Mo Gu Xiao* (Caulis Hyptis Capitatae), and *Liu Zhi Huang* (Herba Solidaginis) are used to relieve pain in the joints and extremities. *Da Zao* (Fructus Jujubae), and *Gan Cao* (Radix Glycyrrhizae) are used to harmonize the formula and the middle *jiao*.

SUPPLEMENTARY FORMULAS

- For neuropathy due to chronic exposure to harmful toxins and chemicals, add **Herbal DTX**.
- For diabetic neuropathy, use with **Equilibrium**.
- To potentiate the effect to relieve pain, add **Herbal Analgesic**.
- For nerve pain in the neck and shoulder area, add **Neck & Shoulder (Acute)** or **Neck & Shoulder (Chronic)**.
- For nerve pain in the upper back, add **Back Support (Upper)**.
- For nerve pain in the lower back, add **Back Support (Acute)** or **Back Support (Chronic)**.
- For nerve pain in the back from herniated disk, add **Back Support (HD)**.
- For nerve pain in the arm (shoulder, elbow and wrist), add **Arm Support**.
- For nerve pain in the knees, add **Knee & Ankle (Acute)** or **Knee & Ankle (Chronic)**.
- For nerve pain with chronic musculoskeletal disorder with damaged soft tissues (muscles, tendons, ligaments), add **Flex (MLT)**.
- For degeneration of muscles, ligaments, tendons and cartilage, add **Flex (MLT)**.
- For *wei* (atrophy) syndrome, add **Flex (MLT)**.
- With excess heat, add **Gardenia Complex**.
- With severe blood stagnation, add **Circulation (SJ)**.
- For lymphedema, add **Resolve (AI)**.

NUTRITION

- Nutritional balance is essential in the treatment and prevention of neuropathy. It is important to make sure that there is adequate intake of various nutrients in a well-balanced diet. If necessary, supplement the diet with vitamins and minerals.
- Increase the intake of foods that contain thiamine (vitamin B1), such as whole grains and green vegetables, to maintain nerve health. Do not consume white sugar and white-flour products, as they deplete the body of B vitamins.

FORMULAS

FLEX (NP) ™

LIFESTYLE INSTRUCTIONS

- ❂ Tight control over blood glucose levels is essential in patients with diabetic neuropathy. Diet, exercise, and herbal treatment will be extremely beneficial in maintaining normal blood glucose levels.
- ❂ Avoid unnecessary exposure to toxic agents or intake of harmful drugs.
- ❂ Nerve pain can be relieved with light massage using a solution of apple cider vinegar water, which is made by mixing ½ cup apple cider vinegar with 2 cups of warm water.
- ❂ Application of hot wraps for half an hour is also effective to relieve pain.

CLINICAL NOTES

- ❂ It is essential to identify and eliminate the cause(s) of neuropathy, especially if it is induced by drugs or toxic agents. Without elimination of the offending agent, treatment will offer only symptomatic relief.
- ❂ Neuropathy due to nutritional deficiency must be identified and treated accordingly. Adequate intake of vitamin B complex is beneficial. Though it is uncommon in the developed countries, patients with polyneuropathy due to nutritional deficiency should be put on vitamin B supplementation.
- ❂ Neuropathy due to metabolic disorders, such as diabetic neuropathy, must be identified, and the root cause treated accordingly. Blood glucose levels must be monitored to ensure that the patient's levels stay within acceptable range.
- ❂ Acupuncture is sometimes more effective than herbs in cases of neuropathy. *See* Acupuncture Points for treatment protocols.

CAUTIONS

- ❂ This formula is contraindicated during pregnancy and nursing.
- ❂ Patients who are on anticoagulant or antiplatelet therapies, such as Coumadin (Warfarin), should use this formula with caution, as there may be a slightly higher risk of bleeding and bruising.

ACUPUNCTURE POINTS

Traditional Points:
- ❂ *Hua Tou Jia Ji* and local *ah shi* points.
- ❂ *Hegu* (LI 4), *Shenshu* (BL 23), *Pishu* (BL 20), *Sanyinjiao* (SP 6), and *Taichong* (LR 3).

Balance Method by Dr. Richard Tan:
- ❂ Use Dr. Tan's Balance Method accordingly as determined by where the pain is (use mirror or image system).
- ❂ For additional information on the Balance Method, please refer to *Dr. Tan's Strategy of Twelve Magical Points* by Dr. Richard Tan.

Ear Points:
- ❂ Affected area, Adrenal Gland, and Lung. Embed magnetic balls and switch ears every five days.

Auricular Acupuncture by Dr. Li-Chun Huang:
- ❂ Intercostal neuralgia: Intercostal Area, Large Auricular Nerve, and Corresponding points (to the area affected).
  - ▪ Supplementary points: Liver, Gallbladder, Chest, Occiput
- ❂ Diabetes mellitus: Diabetes Point, Pancreas, Ear Center, Pituitary, Thalamus, *San Jiao*, and Endocrine.
  - ▪ For numbness in the extremities, add Lesser Occipital Nerve, Large Auricular Nerve
- ❂ For additional information on the location and explanation of these points, please refer to *Auricular Treatment Formula and Prescriptions* by Dr. Li-Chun Huang.

FORMULAS

FLEX (NP) ™

MODERN RESEARCH

Neuropathy is defined as a functional disturbance or pathological change in the peripheral nervous system.[1] Symptoms of neuropathy include sensory loss, muscle weakness and atrophy, and pain. Etiologies of neuropathy include trauma, infection by micro-organisms, drugs, nutritional deficiency, metabolic disorders, malignancy, and unknown causes. [2] Due to the wide range of causes, treatment varies. Herbal treatment of neuropathy focuses on relieving symptoms (pain) and the cause (poor circulation, increased cellular pressure, trauma, infection, and others).

Pain is one of the main symptoms associated with neuropathy. Many herbs in this formula have excellent properties to treat pain and reduce inflammation. For example, *Dang Gui* (Radicis Angelicae Sinensis), *Bai Shao* (Radix Paeoniae Alba), *Gan Cao* (Radix Glycyrrhizae), and *Qiang Huo* (Rhizoma et Radix Notopterygii) are used to alleviate pain.[3,4,5,6,7,8] *Mu Dan Pi* (Cortex Moutan), and *Qin Jiao* (Radix Gentianae Macrophyllae) are used to reduce inflammation.[9,10,11] More specifically, nerve-related pain, such as trigeminal pain, responds remarkably to such herbs as *Chuan Xiong* (Rhizoma Ligustici Chuanxiong), *Bai Shao* (Radix Paeoniae Alba), and *Gan Cao* (Radix Glycyrrhizae).[12,13] And injury-related pain, such as pain of the extremities, responds equally well to the paired herbs of *Ru Xiang* (Gummi Olibanum), *Mo Yao* (Myrrha), *Yan Hu Suo* (Rhizoma Corydalis), *Bai Shao* (Radix Paeoniae Alba), and *Gan Cao* (Radix Glycyrrhizae).[14,15]

Poor circulation is a significant factor contributing to neuropathy and hindering recovery. *Tao Ren* (Semen Persicae), *Hong Hua* (Flos Carthami), *Chuan Xiong* (Rhizoma Ligustici Chuanxiong), and *Mu Dan Pi* (Cortex Moutan) have pronounced influence on improving blood circulation, increasing microcirculation to peripheral parts of the body, eliminating blood stasis, and facilitating recovery. [16,17,18,19]

Increased cellular pressure is another contributor to neuropathy. *Mu Dan Pi* (Cortex Moutan) is used to reduce swelling and pressure in the periphery of the body by inhibiting prostaglandin synthesis and decreasing permeability of the blood vessels. [20,21]

Trauma is another cause of neuropathy. *Ru Xiang* (Gummi Olibanum), *Mo Yao* (Myrrha), and *Yan Hu Suo* (Rhizoma Corydalis) are commonly used in treatment of trauma and sports injuries.[22] *Tao Ren* (Semen Persicae) facilitates recovery from injuries.[23] Other injuries, such as frostbite, that damage both nerves and soft tissue, can be treated with *Dang Gui* (Radicis Angelicae Sinensis), *Gan Cao* (Radix Glycyrrhizae), and other herbs.[24,25]

Infection and its complications also contribute to neuropathy. There are many herbs with remarkable antibiotic properties. *Er Cha* (Catechu) has an inhibitory effect *in vitro* against *Staphylococcus aureus, Pseudomonas aeruginosa, Corynebacterium diphtheriae, Bacillus proteus, Bacillus dysenteriae,* and *Salmonella typhi*.[26] *Xue Jie* (Sanguis Draconis) has an inhibitory effect on various pathogenic fungi and dermatophytes.[27] *Mu Dan Pi* (Cortex Moutan) exerts inhibitory action against *Staphylococcus aureus, beta-hemolytic Streptococcus, Bacillus subtilis,* E. *coli, Shigella dysenteriae, Pseudomonas aeruginosa, Bacillus proteus, Diplococcus pneumoniae,* and *Vibrio cholerae*.[28]

Drugs and toxic agents are two of the main causes of neuropathy. While elimination of these offending agents is the best solution, sometimes drugs cannot be discontinued, or toxicity develops and becomes deposited deep in the body. To remedy these situations, *Gan Cao* (Radix Glycyrrhizae) is prescribed to treat various kinds of poisoning. It is one of the most effective detoxifying herbs for treatment of physiological insults, including drug poisoning (chloral hydrate, urethane, cocaine, picrotoxin, caffeine, pilocarpine, nicotine, barbiturates, mercury and lead), food poisoning (tetrodotoxin, snake, and mushrooms), and others (enterotoxin, herbicides, pesticides). The exact mechanism of this action is unclear, but it is thought that it is related to the regulatory effect of *Gan Cao* (Radix Glycyrrhizae) on the endocrine or hepatic systems.[29]

FLEX (NP) ™

In summary, *Flex (NP)* is an effective formula for treatment of nerve pain. It contains herbs that relieve the symptoms and the cause, and achieves both short- and long-term improvements.

PHARMACEUTICAL DRUGS & CHINESE MEDICINE: A COMPARATIVE ANALYSIS

Western Medical Approach: Pain is a basic bodily sensation induced by a noxious stimulus that causes physical discomfort (as pricking, throbbing, or aching). Pain may be of acute or chronic state, and may be of nociceptive, neuropathic, or psychogenic type. For neuropathic pain of acute or chronic origins, the drugs of choice include antiseizure [Dilantin (Phenytoin) and Neurontin (Gabapentin)] and antidepressant drugs [Elavil (Amitriptyline)]. Though effective, these drugs are associated with numerous and significant side effects. Antiseizure drugs cause side effects such as bleeding, burning sensations, clumsiness or unsteadiness, confusion, irregular eye movements, blurred or double vision, swollen glands in neck or underarms, slurred speech, delusions, dementia, bone malformations, and many others. Antidepressant drugs cause blurred vision, confusion or delirium, hallucinations, constipation (especially in the elderly), problems in urinating, decreased sexual ability, difficulty in speaking or swallowing, eye pain, fainting, fast or irregular heartbeat, loss of balance control, mask-like face, nervousness or restlessness, slowed movements, stiffness of arms and legs, and shortness of breath or troubled breathing. In short, these drugs should be prescribed only when benefits significantly outweigh the risks. Furthermore, use of these drugs must be monitored carefully to avoid developing serious side effects and complications.

Traditional Chinese Medicine Approach: Treatment of pain is a sophisticated balance of art and science. Proper treatment of pain requires a careful evaluation of the type of disharmony (excess or deficiency, cold or heat, exterior or interior), characteristics (qi and/or blood stagnations), and locations (upper body, lower body, extremities, or internal organs). Furthermore, optimal treatment requires integrative use of herbs, acupuncture and *Tui-Na* therapies. All these therapies work together to tonify the underlying deficiencies, strengthen the body, and facilitate recovery from chronic pain. TCM pain management targets both the symptom and the cause of pain, and as such, often achieves immediate and long-term success. Furthermore, TCM pain management is often associated with few or no side effects.

Summation: For treatment of mild to severe pain due to neuropathic causes, TCM pain management offers similar treatment effects to those of pharmaceuticals, with significantly fewer side effects.

CASE STUDIES

A 36-year-old diabetic (Type 1) female presented with severe neuropathy of her hands along with chronic fungal and bacterial infections, sores all over her lower limbs, feet numbness, severe fatigue, malaise and weakness. Besides her diabetes, she also was diagnosed with kidney failure as well as immune deficiency due to immuno-suppressants. She had a kidney transplant as a result of her kidney failure. The TCM practitioner diagnosed her condition as severe Kidney *jing* (essence) deficiency with underlying Spleen qi deficiency, damp-heat, and qi and blood stagnation. Her circulation was severely impaired along with noticeable signs of wasting and thirsting. The patient prescribed an herbal combination of *Flex (NP)* (3 to 4 capsules three times daily) and a customized special formula to tonify her Spleen qi, move the blood, and circulate the qi. The patient experienced relief from her hand pain within 2 to 3 days. Although stinging sensations still persisted, the pain was less in occurrence and intensity. Her sores and warts displayed signs of improvement as well as becoming less visible.

A.R., Encinitas, California

M.F., a 57-year-old female, presented with pain in the leg and big toe with pressure, metallic taste, absence of thirst, heat sensations except in the hands and feet, and upper body sweating. She had been exposed to toxic chemicals and pesticides for six months. The TCM diagnosis was yin deficiency with heat, damp-heat and toxic heat accumulation, and *bi zheng* (painful obstruction syndrome) of the legs. After six weeks of taking *Liver DTX*, *Balance (Heat)* and

FLEX (NP) ™

Flex (NP), she experienced less leg pain, decreased sweating, subsiding heat sensations, and warmer hands. The patient still had a metallic taste in the mouth. The patient was also advised to increase her intake of carrot juice and cucumbers.

M.C., Sarasota, Florida

[1] *Dorland's Illustrated Medical Dictionary 28th Edition*. W.B. Saunders Company, 1994.
[2] Berkow, R. *The Merck Manual of Diagnosis and Therapy 16th Edition*. 1992.
[3] *Xin Yi Yao Xue Za Zhi (New Journal of Medicine and Herbology)*, 1975; (6):34
[4] *Gui Yang Yi Xue Yuan Xue Bao (Journal of Guiyang Medical University)*, 1959; 113
[5] *Zhong Yao Xue (Chinese Herbology)*, 1998; 380:382
[6] *Zhong Yao Xue (Chinese Herbology)*, 1998; 386:387
[7] *Shang Hai Zhong Yi Yao Za Zhi (Shanghai Journal of Chinese Medicine and Herbology)* 1983; 4:14
[8] *Zhong Cao Yao (Chinese Herbal Medicine)*, 1991; 22(1):28
[9] *Sheng Yao Xue Za Zhi (Journal of Raw Herbology)*, 1979; 33(3):178
[10] *Chang Yong Zhong Yao Cheng Fen Yu Yao Li Shou Ce (A Handbook of the Composition and Pharmacology of Common Chinese Drugs)*, 1994; 1479:1482
[11] *Yao Xue Xue Bao (Journal of Herbology)*, 1982; 17(1):12
[12] *He Bei Zhong Yi Za Zhi (Hebei Journal of Chinese Medicine)*, 1982; 4:34
[13] *Zhong Yi Za Zhi (Journal of Chinese Medicine)*, 1983;11:9
[14] *He Nan Zhong Yi Xue Yuan Xue Bao (Journal of University of Henan School of Medicine)*, 1980; 3:38
[15] *Yun Nan Zhong Yi (Yunnan Journal of Traditional Chinese Medicine)*, 1990; 4:15
[16] *Zhong Guo Zhong Yi Yao Xue Bao (Chinese Journal of Chinese Medicine and Herbology)*, 1985; 7:45
[17] *Zhong Yao Yao Li Yu Ying Yong (Pharmacology and Applications of Chinese Herbs)*, 1989; (2):40
[18] *Zhong Yao Xue (Chinese Herbology)*, 1989; 535:539
[19] *Guo Wai Yi Xue Zhong Yi Zhong Yao Fen Ce (Monograph of Chinese Herbology from Foreign Medicine)*, 1983; (3):5,1984;(5):54
[20] *Sheng Yao Xue Za Zhi (Journal of Raw Herbology)*, 1979; 33(3):178
[21] *Zhong Guo Yao Ke Da Xue Xue Bao (Journal of University of Chinese Herbology)*, 1990; 21(4):222
[22] *He Nan Zhong Yi Xue Yuan Xue Bao (Journal of University of Henan School of Medicine)*, 1980; 3:38
[23] *Shang Hai Zhong Yi Yao Za Zhi (Shanghai Journal of Chinese Medicine and Herbology)*, 1985; 7:45
[24] *Zhong Hua Yi Xue Za Zhi (Chinese Journal of Medicine)*, 1956; 10:978
[25] *Xin Zhong Yi (New Chinese Medicine)*, 1980
[26] *Zhong Cao Yao Xue (Study of Chinese Herbal Medicine)*, 1976; 431
[27] *Zhong Yao Xue (Chinese Herbology)*, 1998; 987:988
[28] *Zhong Yao Cai (Study of Chinese Herbal Material)*, 1991; 14(2):41
[29] *Zhong Yao Tong Bao (Journal of Chinese Herbology)*, 1986; 11(10):55

FORMULAS

FLEX (SC) ™

(Spasms and Cramps)

CLINICAL APPLICATIONS

- Spasms and cramps of skeletal muscles in the extremities
- Spasms and cramps of the smooth muscles in the internal organs
- External injuries with muscle sprain and strain
- Muscle tightness and stiffness due to repetitive movements

WESTERN THERAPEUTIC ACTIONS

- Muscle-relaxant effect to treat muscle spasms and cramps [2,5,7,8,9]
- Anti-inflammatory function to reduce inflammation and swelling [2,9]
- Analgesic effect to relieve pain [1,23,,6,9]

CHINESE THERAPEUTIC ACTIONS

- Tonifies Liver yin and Liver blood
- Relieves spasms and cramps
- Tonifies the blood
- Warms the meridians and unblocks stagnation
- Invigorates blood circulation

DOSAGE

Take 3 to 4 capsules every four to six hours as needed for muscle spasms and cramps. The dosage may be increased up to 5 to 6 capsules every two to four hours if necessary. For maximum effectiveness, take *Flex (SC)* on an empty stomach with a tall glass of warm water.

INGREDIENTS

Bai Shao (Radix Paeoniae Alba)
Dang Gui Wei (Extremitas Radicis Angelicae Sinensis)

Gan Cao (Radix Glycyrrhizae)
Hua Jiao (Pericarpium Zanthoxyli)

FORMULA EXPLANATION

Flex (SC) is formulated to relieve muscle spasms and cramps. According to traditional Chinese medicine, the etiology of muscle spasms and cramps is Liver yin and Liver blood deficiencies. Effective treatment, therefore, must focus on nourishing Liver yin and Liver blood deficiencies, activating qi and blood circulation, and removing stagnation.

Bai Shao (Radix Paeoniae Alba) tonifies Liver yin and Liver blood to relieve spasms and cramps. Paeoniflorin, the active constituent in *Bai Shao* (Radix Paeoniae Alba), has strong analgesic, antispasmodic and anti-inflammatory effects. Together with the harmonizing function of *Gan Cao* (Radix Glycyrrhizae), they nourish and relax the tendons and smooth muscles. *Hua Jiao* (Pericarpium Zanthoxyli) and *Dang Gui Wei* (Extremitas Radicis Angelicae Sinensis) are used to warm and invigorate qi and blood circulation in the peripheral channels and collaterals.

SUPPLEMENTARY FORMULAS

- To enhance the analgesic effect, add *Herbal Analgesic*.
- For neck and shoulder pain, combine with *Neck & Shoulder (Acute)* or *Neck & Shoulder (Chronic)*.

FORMULAS

FLEX (SC) ™

(Spasms and Cramps)

- For upper back pain, combine with **Back Support (Upper)**.
- For lower back pain, combine with **Back Support (Acute)** or **Back Support (Chronic)**.
- For pain in the arm (shoulder, elbow and wrist), add **Arm Support**.
- For knee pain, combine with **Knee & Ankle (Acute)** or **Knee & Ankle (Chronic)**.
- For chronic musculoskeletal disorder with damaged soft tissues (muscles, tendons, ligaments, and cartilage), add **Flex (MLT)**.
- For arthritis with inflammation, swelling, redness and pain, combine with **Flex (Heat)**.
- For arthritic pain that worsens during cold and rainy weather, combine with **Flex (CD)**.
- For bone fractures, injuries, and bruises, combine with **Traumanex**.
- To improve blood circulation to the extremities, combine with **Flex (NP)**.
- For bone spurs, add **Flex (Spur)**.
- For osteoporosis, add **Osteo 8**.
- For severe blood stagnation, add **Circulation (SJ)**.
- For dryness and thirst, add **Nourish (Fluids)**.

NUTRITION

- Drink large amounts of water throughout the day (steam-distilled) to hydrate the muscles and flush out toxins residing in the muscles.
- To prevent muscle cramps and spasms, eat plenty of fruits and vegetables, especially those high in potassium such as bananas and oranges.
- Avoid foods that increase the acidity of the body, such as red meat, baked goods, sweet foods, and processed foods.
- Increase the intake of foods rich in alkaline minerals, such as fresh raw vegetables, alfalfa sprouts, and seaweed.

LIFESTYLE INSTRUCTIONS

- Cigarette smoking and alcohol intake should be avoided as they dry out yin and may cause more cramping.
- Warm baths relax the tense muscles and relieve spasms and cramps.
- Avoid tight shoes and clothing, which impair normal circulation of blood to peripheral parts of the body.
- Stretch for at least 30 minutes daily, especially before exercising.

CAUTIONS

- Patients who are on anticoagulant or antiplatelet therapies, such as Coumadin (Warfarin), should use this formula with caution as there may be a slightly higher risk of bleeding and bruising.
- This formula should not be taken long term in patients who have hypertension, as prolonged use of *Gan Cao* (Radix Glycyrrhizae) may be associated with water retention.

ACUPUNCTURE POINTS

Traditional Points:
- *Shousanli* (LI 10), *Waiguan* (TH 5), and *Zusanli* (ST 36).
- *Zhigou* (TH 6), *Zusanli* (ST 36), *Zhongwan* (CV 12), *Neiguan* (PC 6), *Guanyuan* (CV 4), *Taichong* (LR 3), and *Shenque* (CV 8)

Balance Method by Dr. Richard Tan:
- Use Dr. Tan's Balance Method accordingly as determined by where the pain is (use mirror or image system).

FORMULAS

FLEX (SC) ™

(Spasms and Cramps)

❧ For additional information on the Balance Method, please refer to *Dr. Tan's Strategy of Twelve Magical Points* by Dr. Richard Tan.

Auricular Acupuncture by Dr. Li-Chun Huang:
❧ Calf Cramps: Calf
  ▪ Supplementary points: Popliteal Fossa, Lesser Occipital Nerve, Liver, Spleen, and Coronary Vascular Subcortex.
❧ For additional information on the location and explanation of these points, please refer to *Auricular Treatment Formula and Prescriptions* by Dr. Li-Chun Huang.

MODERN RESEARCH

Flex (SC) is formulated based on a classic Chinese herbal formula, *Shao Yao Gan Cao Tang* (Peony and Licorice Decoction), which has been used for thousands of years to treat spasms and cramps of skeletal and intestinal muscles. Modern research has confirmed the ingredients of *Flex (SC)* to have excellent spasmolytic, anti-inflammatory, and analgesic effects.

Bai Shao (Radix Paeoniae Alba) and *Gan Cao* (Radix Glycyrrhizae) are commonly combined to relieve muscle spasms and cramps. Clinically, they may be used for musculoskeletal spasms and cramps associated with external or sports injuries. The combination is effective in treating both skeletal and smooth muscles. [1,2] They may also be used for smooth-muscle cramps, such as abdominal and intestinal cramps or dysmenorrhea. [3]

Bai Shao (Radix Paeoniae Alba) and *Gan Cao* (Radix Glycyrrhizae) have been used in many studies for treatment of musculoskeletal disorders: 30 out of 42 patients reported relief of trigeminal pain; [4] 11 out of 11 patients experienced reduction of muscle spasms and twitching in the facial region; [5] and out of 33 elderly patients with pain in the lower back and legs, 12 patients reported significant improvement, 16 reported moderate improvement, 4 reported slight improvement, and 1 reported no effect. [6]

For treatment of smooth muscle disorders, the combination of *Bai Shao* (Radix Paeoniae Alba) and *Gan Cao* (Radix Glycyrrhizae) relieved abdominal pain and cramps due to intestinal parasites in 11 out of 11 patients; [7] and in 185 patients with epigastric and abdominal pain, 139 patients reported significant improvement, 41 reported moderate improvement, and 5 reported no effect. [8] Lastly, *Bai Shao* (Radix Paeoniae Alba) has tranquilizing and analgesic effects to relieve pain. [9]

PHARMACEUTICAL DRUGS & CHINESE MEDICINE: A COMPARATIVE ANALYSIS

Western Medical Approach: Spasms and cramps are common musculoskeletal complaints that can be treated effectively with both drug and herbal therapies. In western medicine, muscle relaxants, such as Soma (Carisoprodol) and Flexeril (Cyclobenzaprine) are generally prescribed for spasms and cramps. These drugs are only mild to moderate in potency. However, they are also relatively safe, with relatively mild side effects such as blurred or double vision, dizziness, lightheadedness, and drowsiness.

Traditional Chinese Medicine Approach: Herbs that nourish yin and replenish fluids are most effective to relax the muscles. These herbs are also of mild to moderate potency, and are associated with few or no side effects.

Summation: drugs and herbs have comparable effect to treat spasms and cramps, and both are associated with few side effects. In addition to drug or herbal therapies, one can incorporate non-medicine modalities to enhance overall effectiveness, such as drinking water, stretching affected muscles, and taking potassium and calcium supplements.

FORMULAS

FLEX (SC) ™

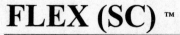

(Spasms and Cramps)

CASE STUDIES

E.B., a 79-year-old female, presented with stiffness of the middle and ring finger on the right hand. She was unable to close her hand and make a fist, nor was she also able to extend her fingers. The range of motion was greatly reduced, and she was unable to sculpt. The patient refused to see a medical doctor. The previous CTS surgery in 1983 left a small scar in the palm of her hand. The tendons of the palm were very tight, ropy in quality, enlarged and swollen. The palms were red, the skin was dry and the nails were brittle. She also complained of dry mouth and throat at night. The western diagnoses were contraction of the palmar fascia and Dupuytren's Contracture. The TCM diagnoses were *bi zheng* (painful obstruction syndrome), Liver and Kidney yin deficiencies and blood stagnation. Acupuncture, micro-current, massage, and *Flex (SC)* were all part of the treatment regime that helped her gain 90% range of motion within one week. She was almost able to close her hands and make a fist. The palm was less red and the swelling decreased. The patient was thrilled.

M. H., West Palm Beach, Florida

A 44-year-old female presented with upper back spasm. The patient stated, "It feels like creepy crawlers." In addition to her upper back dysfunction, floaters were also present with bright lights disturbing her eyes. The practitioner diagnosed her condition as Liver qi stagnation with Liver yin deficiency. After taking *Flex (SC)*, the patient was calmer; more relaxed and had fewer moods swings. Consequently, she was not as irritable and had less muscle spasms in her mid back. She also slept much better.

D.M., Raton, New Mexico

L.P., a 77-year-old female, presented with severe pain in the left wrist and right rib cage after a fall. She had numbness of the wrist and palm where she landed on the cement. The patient showed bruises on the right eye. The right wrist was painful to light movement and palpation. There were tender points on the right subclavicular area. There were no visible contusions on the right rib cage. The diagnoses were qi and blood stagnation with soft tissue damage. *Traumanex, Neck & Shoulder (Acute)* and *Flex (SC)* were prescribed at 2 capsules of each formula three times daily. The patient reported daily lowering of pain levels. Numbness was reduced to a light tingling after 2 days. She reported continuous and steady improvement each day. She was instructed to reduce the dosage to 2 capsules of each formula twice a day when the pain subsided. After the swelling was reduced, the patient was referred to a chiropractor for cervical and occipital adjustments.

M. H., West Palm Beach, Florida

D.D., a 41-year-old nurse, presented with a work-related injury. She had severe back pain that was the result of a fall from lifting a patient. She said she heard a popping sound in her back when she fell. MRI confirmed her diagnosis of lumbar herniated disc. She was 9 weeks post-injury and had scheduled for steroid epidurals. She refused injections and came to our clinic for 'safe and non-invasive care.' Her blood pressure was 140/80 mmHg and the heart rate was 80 beats per minute. The TCM diagnoses include qi and blood stagnation and soft tissue damage. *Back Support (Acute)*, *Flex (SC)* and *Traumanex* were prescribed at 3 capsules each three times a day. After the herbs, the patient was able to reduce Vicodin (APAP/Hydrocodone) use from 2 to 0.5 tablets per day, and none at all on some days. She had increased blood pressure from stress over the injury, which was up to 170/110 mmHg. After the herbs and massage, the blood pressure came down to normal and is staying down. She had received no additional physical therapy. She did remarkably well in a short period of time.

M.H., West Palm Beach, Florida

FLEX (SC) ™

(Spasms and Cramps)

[1] Bensky, D. et al. *Chinese Herbal Medicine Materia Medica*. Eastland Press. 1993
[2] Tan, H. et al. Chemical components of decoction of radix paeoniae and radix glycyrrhizae. *Chung-Kuo Chung Yao Tsao Chih* – China Journal of Chinese Materia Medica. Sept. 1995; 20(9):550-1,576
[3] Bensky, D. et al. *Chinese Herbal Medicine Formulas and Strategies*. Eastland Press. 1990
[4] Huang, DD. *Journal of Traditional Chinese Medicine*. 1983; 11:9
[5] Luo, DP. *Hunan Journal of Traditional Chinese Medicine*. 1989; 2:7
[6] Chen, Hong. *Yunnan Journal of Traditional Chinese Medicine*. 1990; 4:15
[7] Zhang, RB. *Jiangxu Journal of Traditional Chinese Medicine*. 1966; 5:38-39
[8] You, JH. *Guanxi Journal of Chinese Herbology*. 1987; 5:5-6
[9] Yeung, HC. *Handbook of Chinese Herbs*. Institute of Chinese Medicine. 1996

FORMULAS

FLEX (Spur) ™

CLINICAL APPLICATIONS

- ❧ Bone spurs with pain
- ❧ Joint stiffness
- ❧ Calcification of joints

WESTERN THERAPEUTIC ACTIONS

- ❧ Analgesic action to relieve pain [1]
- ❧ Anti-inflammatory influence to reduce inflammation [2]
- ❧ Analgesic effect to alleviate visceral and musculo-skeletal pain [3,4]
- ❧ Relieves pain associated with bone spurs

CHINESE THERAPEUTIC ACTIONS

- ❧ Invigorates blood circulation and breaks up blood stagnation
- ❧ Relieves pain
- ❧ Dispels phlegm

DOSAGE

Take 3 to 4 capsules three times daily as needed to relieve pain. For maximum effectiveness, take the herbs on an empty stomach with two tall glasses of warm water.

INGREDIENTS

Bai Zhi (Radix Angelicae Dahuricae)
Chen Pi (Pericarpium Citri Reticulatae)
Da Ding Huang (Caulis Euonymi)
Dang Gui (Radicis Angelicae Sinensis)
Fang Feng (Radix Saposhnikoviae)
Gan Cao (Radix Glycyrrhizae)
Huang Jin Gui (Caulis Vanieriae)
Jin Yin Hua (Flos Lonicerae)
Liu Zhi Huang (Herba Solidaginis)

Mo Gu Xiao (Caulis Hyptis Capitatae)
Mo Yao (Myrrha)
Po Bu Zi Ye (Folium Cordia Dichotoma)
Ru Xiang (Gummi Olibanum)
Tong Cao (Medulla Tetrapanacis)
Zao Jiao (Fructus Gleditsiae)
Zao Jiao Ci (Spina Gleditsiae)
Zhe Bei Mu (Bulbus Fritillariae Thunbergii)

FORMULA EXPLANATION

Flex (Spur) is formulated to relieve pain due to bone spurs and joint stiffness arising from overuse. According to theories in traditional Chinese medicine, bone spurs form as the result of repetitive use and are diagnosed as stagnation of blood and phlegm.

Po Bu Zi Ye (Folium Cordia Dichotoma) regulates qi circulation to relieve pain. Unbeknownst to most practitioners, it is one of the most effective herbs in the Chinese *Materia Medica* for treating bone spurs. *Mo Gu Xiao* (Caulis Hyptis Capitatae), *Liu Zhi Huang* (Herba Solidaginis), and *Huang Jin Gui* (Caulis Vanieriae) have anti-inflammatory and analgesic effects and are often used to treat acute pain associated with traumatic injuries or sprains and strains. *Da Ding Huang* (Caulis Euonymi) further reduces inflammation and relieves pain. *Ru Xiang* (Gummi Olibanum), *Mo Yao* (Myrrha), and *Dang Gui* (Radicis Angelicae Sinensis) have potent effects to move blood, disperse blood stagnation and relieve pain. *Jin Yin Hua* (Flos Lonicerae), *Bai Zhi* (Radix Angelicae Dahuricae), *Zhe*

FLEX (SC)™

(Spurs and Tumor)

Bensky, David et al. *Chinese Herbal Medicine: Materia Medica*. Irvine: Eastland Press, 1993.
Tan, H. et al. *Chen entregistration its et dose a hen oradis gaa moo sea ane ratez Gyynimo use of Chinese Materia Mezik*. Apul. 1995, 7906:1162.
Hsu, H.Y. et al. *Chinese Me pea Mantique*. Palagias and Trung gwa: Instituted Press, 1986.
Huang, K.C. *The Pharmacology of Chinese Herbs*. Boca Rato: CRC Press, 1993.
Huang, D.: Joursa of Traditional Chinese Medicine. 1988: 11:9.
Luo, Di. *Jvosm Journal of Traditional Chinese Medicine*. 1987: 7:12.
Chen, Hong Xuanng Journal Of Traditional Chinese Medicine, 1998: 4:9.
Zhang, RH. *Aingana Joetsal of Traiotiget Chinese Medicine*. 1995: 3:8.
Yu, TH. Qveum Joumal et Chinese Herbology. 1987: 5:56.
Yang, HC. *Handbook of Chinese Mesteria Medica*. Xi'an: Hastc of Chine Mediche, 1970.

FLEX (Spur) ™

Bei Mu (Bulbus Fritillariae Thunbergii), *Zao Jiao* (Fructus Gleditsiae), and *Zao Jiao Ci* (Spina Gleditsiae) break up phlegm that is obstructing the channels and joints, to restore proper qi and blood circulation. *Chen Pi* (Pericarpium Citri Reticulatae) regulates qi, while *Fang Feng* (Radix Saposhnikoviae) disperses wind and releases pain lodged in peripheral levels of the body. *Tong Cao* (Medulla Tetrapanacis) drains accumulation of damp and phlegm out of the body via urination. Lastly, *Gan Cao* (Radix Glycyrrhizae) relieves pain and harmonizes the entire formula.

In summary, *Flex (Spur)* is an effective formula with both immediate and long-term therapeutic effects.

SUPPLEMENTARY FORMULAS

- For bone spurs in the neck and shoulder, add *Neck & Shoulder (Acute)*.
- For bone spurs in the upper back, add *Back Support (Upper)*.
- For bone spurs in the lower back, add *Back Support (Acute)*.
- For bone spurs in the back with herniated disks, add *Back Support (HD)*.
- For bone spurs in the arm (shoulder, elbow or wrist), add *Arm Support*.
- For bone spurs in the knees, add *Knee & Ankle (Acute)*.
- For arthritis, add *Flex (Heat)* or *Flex (CD)*.
- For bone spurs with nerve pain, combine with *Flex (NP)*.
- For severe pain, add *Herbal Analgesic*.
- For degeneration of muscles, tendons, ligaments and cartilage, add *Flex (MLT)*.
- For severe blood stagnation, add *Circulation (SJ)*.
- With excess heat, add *Gardenia Complex*.

NUTRITION

- Patients are encouraged to increase intake of vinegar.
- Discourage the intake of bamboo and acidic fruit, such as oranges or grapefruit.
- Minimize the consumption of seafood and red meat to avoid creating additional deposits of uric acid.

LIFESTYLE INSTRUCTIONS

- Rest is essential to the recovery of bone spurs. If possible, discontinue repetitive movement and overuse of the joint where the bone spur is located.
- Slow stretching exercises of the affected area are effective to reduce or diminish pain.
- Initially in the first 24 hours, use of an ice pack to reduce swelling and inflammation. However, long-term use of ice pack is not recommended, as it may cause more stagnation.

CLINICAL NOTES

- The primary purpose of *Flex (Spur)* is to relieve pain related to bone spurs. However, it can be taken as a supplemental formula to relieve pain. Some patients may experience immediate relief, while others may require as much as half a year for relief of the pain. Adequate rest of affected joints is essential to a complete recovery.
- According to clinical experience, patients taking *Flex (Spur)* generally have an all-or-none response for treating bone spurs. Most patients will experience varying degrees of relief from pain and inflammation. Up to 20 to 30% will experience long-term resolution of pain. However, it is possible that some patients who will not notice any change. Evaluation of patients' condition should be done every 1 to 2 months to determine the progress of the patient and the efficacy of the formula.
- *Flex (Spur)* has been used with good success to treat animals with joint pain.

FORMULAS

FLEX (Spur) ™

- According to Dr. Luo Jun-Qing, a *Tui-Na* master from China, patients who suffer from bone spur of the knee should not over-exercise their knee. Mild to moderate movements such as that in *Tai Chi Chuan* and walking should suffice.

- In addition to taking *Flex (Spur)* orally, herbs should also be applied topically to enhance the overall treatment. The topical preparation is made by cooking herbs in water and filtering out the herb residue. Use the herbal decoction topically by soaking a towel in the decoction while hot, and apply the decoction-soaked towel to the affected area while warm. The towel should be re-soaked in the decoction as needed to keep warm, for a total duration of 30 minutes. Perform this procedure twice per day. One herbal formula that has been used with good results contains the following herbs: *Dang Gui* (Radicis Angelicae Sinensis) 15g, *Chi Shao* (Radix Paeoniae Rubrae) 15g, *Chuan Xiong* (Rhizoma Ligustici Chuanxiong) 12g, *Hong Hua* (Flos Carthami) 12g, *Dan Nan Xing* (Arisaema cum Bile) 12g, *Bai Jie Zi* (Semen Sinapis) 15g, *Ji Xue Teng* (Caulis Spatholobi) 20g, *Wei Ling Xian* (Radix Clematidis) 15g, *Ru Xiang* (Gummi Olibanum) 15g, *Mo Yao* (Myrrha) 15g, *Gui Zhi* (Ramulus Cinnamomi) 15g and *Du Huo* (Radix Angelicae Pubescentis) 15g.

Pulse Diagnosis by Dr. Jimmy Wei-Yen Chang:

- Thick and forceful pulse proximal to the right *chi* indicates spur or soft tissue damage to the upper *jiao*, and on the left *chi* indicates lower *jiao*. This pulse feels like a toothpick underneath the skin.

- Note: Dr. Chang takes the pulse in slightly different positions. He places his index finger directly over the wrist crease, and his middle and ring fingers alongside to locate *cun*, *guan* and *chi* positions. For additional information and explanation, please refer to *Pulsynergy* by Dr. Jimmy Wei-Yen Chang and Marcus Brinkman.

CAUTIONS

- This formula is contraindicated during pregnancy and nursing.

- Though there are no known side effects or adverse reactions, it is prudent to not recommend this formula for infants or young children, as the long-term impact on the growth of teeth and the skeleton is unclear.

- Patients who are on anticoagulant or antiplatelet therapies, such as Coumadin (Warfarin), should use this formula with caution, as there may be a slightly higher risk of bleeding and bruising.

ACUPUNCTURE POINTS

Traditional Points:

- For bone spurs in the neck: *Dazhui* (GV 14), *Fengchi* (GB 20), and *Jianjing* (GB 21). With numbness and pain in the arms, add *Jianyu* (LI 15), *Quchi* (LI 11), and *Hegu* (LI 4).

- For bone spurs in the back: *Yaoyangguan* (GV 3), *shu* (transport) points on the back, and *ah shi* points on the affected areas.

- For sciatica with bone spurs: *Huantiao* (GB 30), *Yanglingquan* (GB 34), and *Quchi* (LI 11).

- For bone spurs of the knees: *Xiyan*, *Heding*, and *Zusanli* (ST 36).

- Technique: use even method. Leave the needle in place for 30 minutes. Perform one acupuncture treatment daily or every other day, for 12 treatments per course of treatment prior to evaluation.

Balance Method by Dr. Richard Tan:

- Treatment depends on the individual presentation and the location of the spur.

- For additional information on the Balance Method, please refer to *Dr. Tan's Strategy of Twelve Magical Points* by Dr. Richard Tan.

FORMULAS

FLEX (Spur) ™

MODERN RESEARCH

Flex (Spur) is formulated by Dr. Jimmy Wei-Yen Chang with herbs that treat bone spurs, relieve pain, and reduce swelling. *Flex (Spur)* has helped many patients with bone spurs to relieve pain and improve range of movement.

Po Bu Zi Ye (Folium Cordia Dichotoma), *Mo Gu Xiao* (Caulis Hyptis Capitatae), *Liu Zhi Huang* (Herba Solidaginis), *Huang Jin Gui* (Caulis Vanieriae), and *Da Ding Huang* (Caulis Euonymi) are five herbs commonly used to treat various types of musculo-skeletal pain. As an indigenous herb in Taiwan that was not recorded in the *Materia Medica* in China, *Po Bu Zi Ye* (Folium Cordia Dichotoma) is an herb that has been used traditionally for treatment of "sharp pain of the heel." This traditional use has been expanded as *Po Bu Zi Ye* (Folium Cordia Dichotoma) is now recognized by many experts as the chief and most effective herb for treating bone spurs affecting various parts of the body. *Mo Gu Xiao* (Caulis Hyptis Capitatae), *Liu Zhi Huang* (Herba Solidaginis), *Huang Jin Gui* (Caulis Vanieriae), and *Da Ding Huang* (Caulis Euonymi) are also from Taiwan. These four herbs are commonly used together to treat acute pain and inflammation.[1]

Ru Xiang (Gummi Olibanum) and *Mo Yao* (Myrrha) are two herbs with long recognized efficacy in treating injuries and relieving pain. According to various *in vitro* and *in vivo* studies, the combination of these two herbs demonstrated pronounced analgesic effects.[2] Clinical applications include chest pain, colicky or sharp pain,[3] and the pain of acute sprain of the lower back and legs.[4]

Chen Pi (Pericarpium Citri Reticulatae) and *Dang Gui* (Radicis Angelicae Sinensis) are added to improve blood and energy circulation.

In conclusion, there are very few treatments available for bone spurs. *Flex (Spur)* offers a much-needed treatment option for those who suffer from this disorder.

PHARMACEUTICAL DRUGS & CHINESE MEDICINE: A COMPARATIVE ANALYSIS

Western Medical Approach: Pain is a basic bodily sensation induced by a noxious stimulus that causes physical discomfort (as pricking, throbbing, or aching). Pain may be of acute or chronic state, and may be of nociceptive, neuropathic, or psychogenic type. For neuropathic pain due to bone spurs, drugs such as antiseizure [Dilantin (Phenytoin) and Neurontin (Gabapentin)] and antidepressant drugs [Elavil (Amitriptyline)] are prescribed. Though effective, these drugs are associated with numerous and significant side effects. Antiseizure drugs cause side effects such as bleeding, burning sensations, clumsiness or unsteadiness, confusion, irregular eye movements, blurred or double vision, swollen glands in neck or underarms, slurred speech, delusions, dementia, bone malformations, and many others. Antidepressant drugs cause blurred vision, confusion or delirium, hallucinations, constipation (especially in the elderly), problems in urinating, decreased sexual ability, difficulty in speaking or swallowing, eye pain, fainting, fast or irregular heartbeat, loss of balance control, mask-like face, nervousness or restlessness, slowed movements, stiffness of arms and legs, and shortness of breath or troubled breathing. In short, these drugs should be prescribed only when benefits significantly outweigh the risks. Furthermore, use of these drugs must be monitored carefully to avoid developing serious side effects and complications. Lastly, these drugs treat the symptom (pain) and not the cause (bone spurs). When the pain becomes intolerable, or if drugs cause too many side effects, the only other option is surgery.

Traditional Chinese Medicine Approach: Bone spurs are caused by repetitive use of, or recurrent injuries to, the affected joint(s). Bone spurs are diagnosed as blood and phlegm stagnation, and are treated with herbs that activate blood circulation, resolve phlegm, and relieve pain. Clinically, herbal treatment of bone spurs has been shown to be relatively effective, though the required duration of treatment must be longer than 1 to 2 months.

FORMULAS

FLEX (Spur) ™

Summation: Treatment of bone spurs is a challenge to both drug and herbal medicine. While drugs do not treat bone spurs, they do offer potent and effective means to control pain. On the other hand, herbs are relatively effective to treat pain and resolve spurs, but may require a prolonged period of treatment. In light of limited options, herbs should definitely be tried before consideration of surgery.

[1] Chen, J. and Chen, T. Chinese Medical Herbology and Pharmacology, Art of Medicine Press, 2004
[2] Zhong Yao Xue (Chinese Herbology), 1998; 539
[3] Zhong Yao Xue (Chinese Herbology), 1998; 540
[4] He Nan Zhong Yi Xue Yuan Xue Bao (Journal of University of Henan School of Medicine), 1980; 3:38

FORMULAS

GARDENIA COMPLEX ™

CLINICAL APPLICATIONS

- Any excess conditions characterized by heat, fire and toxins
- Excess fire in all three *jiaos*
- Infectious diseases with fever
- Inflammatory conditions with swelling, inflammation, burning sensations and pain
- Diseases with high blood pressure and fast heart rate

WESTERN THERAPEUTIC ACTIONS

- Antipyretic effect to reduce body temperature
- Antibiotic effect to treat infection
- Anti-inflammatory and analgesic effects to reduce swelling and relieve pain
- Antihypertensive effect to reduce blood pressure
- Hepatoprotective effect to treat hepatitis and liver cirrhosis
- Cholagogic effect to treat jaundice
- Gastrointestinal effect to decrease production and secretion of stomach acid

CHINESE THERAPEUTIC ACTIONS

- Clears heat
- Purges fire
- Eliminates toxins

DOSAGE

Take 3 to 4 capsules three times daily. Dosage can be increased up to 6 to 8 capsules three times daily in acute cases. This formula should not be taken for more than 2 months continuously.

INGREDIENTS

Bian Xu (Herba Polygoni Avicularis)
Chai Hu (Radix Bupleuri)
Che Qian Zi (Semen Plantaginis)
Dang Gui (Radicis Angelicae Sinensis)
Fu Ling (Poria)
Gan Cao (Radix Glycyrrhizae)
Geng Mi (Semen Oryzae)
Huang Bai (Cortex Phellodendri)
Huang Qin (Radix Scutellariae)
Long Dan Cao (Radix Gentianae)

Mu Dan Pi (Cortex Moutan)
Shan Yao (Rhizoma Dioscoreae)
Shan Zhu Yu (Fructus Corni)
Sheng Di Huang (Radix Rehmanniae)
Shi Gao (Gypsum Fibrosum)
Shu Di Huang (Radix Rehmanniae Preparata)
Ze Xie (Rhizoma Alismatis)
Zhi Mu (Radix Anemarrhenae)
Zhi Zi (Fructus Gardeniae)

FORMULA EXPLANATION

Gardenia Complex is designed for conditions manifesting in excess heat/fire in the body. This formula purges fire, drains damp-heat and clears toxic-heat from the *zang fu* organs that are most susceptible to heat invasion, namely the Heart, Liver and Stomach.

Zhi Zi (Fructus Gardeniae) clears heat in all three *jiaos*. *Shi Gao* (Gypsum Fibrosum), *Zhi Mu* (Radix Anemarrhenae), and *Geng Mi* (Semen Oryzae) represent the effect of the classic formula *Bai Hu Tang* (White Tiger Decoction) to drain *yangming* Stomach fire. *Chai Hu* (Radix Bupleuri) is a channel-guiding herb to the Liver to

GARDENIA COMPLEX ™

enhance *Long Dan Cao* (Radix Gentianae) and *Huang Qin* (Radix Scutellariae) in sedating Liver fire. *Mu Dan Pi* (Cortex Moutan) and *Huang Bai* (Cortex Phellodendri) are added to clear deficiency heat from the Kidney. *Sheng Di Huang* (Radix Rehmanniae), *Shu Di Huang* (Radix Rehmanniae Preparata), and *Dang Gui* (Radicis Angelicae Sinensis) are added to tonify the blood and prevent the harsh herbs from damaging Liver blood. *Che Qian Zi* (Semen Plantaginis), *Ze Xie* (Rhizoma Alismatis), *Bian Xu* (Herba Polygoni Avicularis), and *Fu Ling* (Poria) drain dampness and eliminate heat through urination. *Shan Zhu Yu* (Fructus Corni) nourishes Kidney yin to prevent the herbs that drain dampness from damaging the yin. *Shan Yao* (Rhizoma Dioscoreae) with *Gan Cao* (Radix Glycyrrhizae) protect the middle *jiao* from the harsh heat-clearing herbs and harmonize the formula.

In summary, *Gardenia Complex* is an excellent formula to clear excess fire and heat in the body affecting various *zang fu* organs such as the Heart, Liver and Stomach. *Gardenia Complex* can also be used with another formula to enhance the overall effect to clear excess fire and heat.

SUPPLEMENTARY FORMULAS

- With lung infection, combine with **Respitrol (Heat)** or **Poria XPT**.
- With acid reflux, stomach ulcer, or duodenal ulcer, combine with **GI Care**.
- With stomach or intestinal infection, combine with **GI Care II**.
- With urinary tract infection or infection of the lower *jiao*, combine with **V-Statin**.
- With hypertension, combine with **Gastrodia Complex** or **Gentiana Complex**.
- With psychological disorder or emotional instability with excess nature, combine with **Calm** or **Calm (ES)**.
- With liver and gallbladder disorders such as hepatitis, liver cirrhosis, and jaundice, add **Liver DTX**.
- With coronary artery disease, add **Circulation**.
- With *re bi* (heat painful obstruction), add **Flex (Heat)**.
- With constipation, add **Gentle Lax (Excess)**.
- With kidney stone, add **Dissolve (KS)**.
- With unknown swelling or hard lesions, add **Resolve (AI)**.

NUTRITION

- Avoid hot, spicy, and fried foods, which aggravate an excess conditions of heat and fire. Foods that are hot in nature such as pepper and lamb should be avoided.
- Foods that are cold in nature may be helpful in expelling fire in the body. These include cucumber, tomatoes, cactus, celery, tofu, etc.

LIFESTYLE INSTRUCTIONS

- Avoid stress and stressful situations whenever possible.
- Refrain from alcoholic beverages and cigarette smoking.

CLINICAL NOTES

- *Gardenia Complex* and *Herbal ABX* are two formulas with strong and broad-spectrum of heat-clearing effects.
  - *Gardenia Complex* is designed to purge heat in the organs due to internal imbalances or improper dietary intake such as excessive spicy or greasy food or lifestyle (lack of sleep, excessive smoking, etc).
  - *Herbal ABX* clears heat and detoxifies, and is best for infection that is contracted from outside sources, such as influenza or urinary tract infection.
  - Therefore, although both formulas clear heat, their use should still be distinguished.

GARDENIA COMPLEX ™

Pulse Diagnosis by Dr. Jimmy Wei-Yen Chang:
- Forceful and thick on all three positions.
- Note: Dr. Chang takes the pulse in slightly different positions. He places his index finger directly over the wrist crease, and his middle and ring fingers alongside to locate *cun*, *guan* and *chi* positions. For additional information and explanation, please refer to *Pulsynergy* by Dr. Jimmy Wei-Yen Chang and Marcus Brinkman.

CAUTIONS

- This formula is contraindicated in patients who have generalized weakness and deficiency. It is also contraindicated during pregnancy and nursing.
- *Dang Gui* (Radicis Angelicae Sinensis) may enhance the overall effectiveness of Coumadin (Warfarin), an anticoagulant drug. Patients who take anticoagulant or antiplatelet medications should **not** take this herbal formula without supervision by a licensed health care practitioner.

ACUPUNCTURE POINTS

Traditional Points:
- *Quchi* (LI 11), *Hegu* (LI 4), *Neiguan* (PC 6), *Shousanli* (LI 10), *Zusanli* (ST 36), *Yanglingquan* (GB 34), and *Sanyinjiao* (SP 6).
- Bleed *Shaoshang* (LU 11), *Quchi* (LI 11), *Weizhong* (BL 40), and *Shixuan*.
- *Gua Sha* can be performed all along the Urinary Bladder channel and medial sides of *Weizhong* (BL 40) until bruises are apparent may be helpful. (Note: *Gua Sha* is the act of scraping the skin with a small board or with a coin after applying oil on the skin).
- *Dazhui* (GV 14), *Quchi* (LI 11), *Hegu* (LI 4), *Yuji* (LU 10), *Waiguan* (TH 5), *Zhongchong* (PC 9), *Waiguan* (TH 5), and *Xiangu* (ST 43).

Balance Method by Dr. Richard Tan:
- Needle *Yemen* (TH 2) and *Yuji* (LU 10) bilaterally. Bleed *Zhongchong* (PC 9) and the back of the ears.

Ear Acupuncture:
- *Shenmen*, Adrenals, Apex of the Ear. Use strong stimulation and remove the needles after 15 minutes.

Auricular Acupuncture by Li-Chun Huang:
- Common cold: Lung, Internal Nose, and Throat (Larynx, Pharynx).
  - For fever, bleed Ear Apex and Helix 1-6
  - For dizziness, add Dizziness Area
  - For pain and soreness all over the body, add Liver, Spleen; bleed Helix 4
  - For cough, add Trachea, Bronchus, Stop Asthma

MODERN RESEARCH

From traditional Chinese medicine perspectives, *Gardenia Complex* is designed to treat all excess conditions, including presentations of heat, fire, and toxins in various *zang fu* organs. From western medical perspectives, these disorders are often characterized by inflammation, pain, and hyperactivity of various organ systems, such as cardiovascular, hepatic, gastrointestinal, etc. As such, this formula has an extremely broad range of action, and may be used to treat many disorders.

Fever is one of the most typical symptoms of heat, and may be treated effectively with heat-clearing herbs in this formula. Many herbs in this formula have an excellent antipyretic effect to reduce fever and lower body temperature, such as *Shi Gao* (Gypsum Fibrosum),[1] *Zhi Mu* (Radix Anemarrhenae),[2] and *Huang Qin* (Radix Scutellariae).[3]

GARDENIA COMPLEX ™

Infection is another common presentation of heat, fire and toxins. This formula contains many herbs with marked antibiotic effect to treat many types of infections, such as bacterial, viral, and fungal infections. Among herbs with marked antibiotic effects are *Zhi Zi* (Fructus Gardeniae),[4] *Zhi Mu* (Radix Anemarrhenae),[5,6] *Chai Hu* (Radix Bupleuri),[7] *Mu Dan Pi* (Cortex Moutan),[8] *Huang Qin* (Radix Scutellariae),[9] *Long Dan Cao* (Radix Gentianae),[10] and *Shan Zhu Yu* (Fructus Corni).[11] In terms of clinical applications, these herbs have been used to treat various types of infections throughout the body, including, but not limited to, diseases such as common cold and influenza,[12] infectious hepatitis,[13] pneumonia,[14] bronchitis,[15] and encephalitis.[16]

Inflammatory conditions with swelling, inflammation, burning sensations and pain are also presentations of heat and fire. Many herbs in this formula have marked anti-inflammatory effect to treat such conditions, such as *Chai Hu* (Radix Bupleuri),[17] *Sheng Di Huang* (Radix Rehmanniae),[18] *Shan Zhu Yu* (Fructus Corni),[19] *Huang Qin* (Radix Scutellariae),[20] and *Mu Dan Pi* (Cortex Moutan).[21] Clinically, these herbs have been used with great success to treat various inflammatory conditions, including but not limited to, lymphadenitis, cellulitis, and erysipelas.[22] Furthermore, many of these herbs also have an analgesic effect to relieve pain, such as *Chai Hu* (Radix Bupleuri) and *Zhi Zi* (Fructus Gardeniae), which are beneficial for treatment of arthritis and rheumatism.[23,24,25]

Certain **cardiovascular diseases** are also considered excess in nature, such as hypertension and coronary artery disease. Many herbs in this formula have a marked antihypertensive effect, such as *Huang Qin* (Radix Scutellariae),[26] *Huang Bai* (Cortex Phellodendri),[27] *Mu Dan Pi* (Cortex Moutan),[28] and *Zhi Zi* (Fructus Gardeniae).[29] Though their mechanisms of action differ, they have all been shown to reduce blood pressure. According to one study, use of *Huang Qin* (Radix Scutellariae) three times daily was effective in treating 51 patients with hypertension.[30] According to another study, administration of *Mu Dan Pi* (Cortex Moutan) effectively lowered blood pressure within 5 days among 20 patients with hypertension.[31] Furthermore, *Mu Dan Pi* (Cortex Moutan) and *Zhi Zi* (Fructus Gardeniae) have cardiovascular effects to increase blood perfusion to the coronary arteries, decrease cardiac output and decrease load on the left ventricle.[32,33] These actions offer a protective effect against ischemia of the heart and coronary artery disorders.[34]

Liver and **gallbladder disorders**, such as hepatitis, liver cirrhosis, and jaundice, are often diagnosed as damp-heat in traditional Chinese medicine. This formula incorporates many herbs with marked effect to treat these types of disorders. Pharmacologically, *Zhi Zi* (Fructus Gardeniae) and *Huang Qin* (Radix Scutellariae) are two herbs with excellent hepatoprotective effect.[35,36] Clinically, *Zhi Zi* (Fructus Gardeniae), *Huang Qin* (Radix Scutellariae), *Chai Hu* (Radix Bupleuri), and *Long Dan Cao* (Radix Gentianae) have all been used with great success to treat hepatitis and liver cirrhosis.[37,38,39,40] Furthermore, *Zhi Zi* (Fructus Gardeniae), *Chai Hu* (Radix Bupleuri), *Long Dan Cao* (Radix Gentianae), and *Huang Qin* (Radix Scutellariae) all have a cholagogic effect to stimulate the production of bile, enhance contraction of the gallbladder, increase excretion of bile into the intestines, and may be used to treat jaundice.[41,42,43]

Hyperactivity of the central nervous system is another presentation of excess, and may be treated with herbs in this formula. *Zhi Zi* (Fructus Gardeniae) has an inhibitory effect on the central nervous system to decrease spontaneous activity, increase sleeping time, and decrease body temperature.[44] *Chai Hu* (Radix Bupleuri) has a sedative effect and prolongs sleeping time induced by barbiturates.[45]

Hyperacidity of the stomach is also a presentation of heat and fire rising upwards and damaging the surrounding area. Hyperacidity of the stomach may present in such diseases as acid reflux, belching, stomach ulcer, duodenal ulcer, and gastrointestinal bleeding. In this formula, *Zhi Zi* (Fructus Gardeniae) is the herb that has the effect to decrease the secretion of gastric acid and increase pH in the stomach.[46]

In conclusion, *Gardenia Complex* has an extremely broad range of action, and may be used to treat many disorders characterized by fever, infection, inflammation, pain, and hyperactivity of various organ systems, such as the cardiovascular, hepatic, and gastrointestinal systems.

GARDENIA COMPLEX™

ADDITIONAL INFORMATION

Using Blood Pressure + Heart Rate for *Ba Gang Bian Zheng* (Eight Principle Differentiation)

Dr. Jimmy Wei-Yen Chang, author of *Pulsynergy* and creator of this formula, explains that excess heat can be defined by the objective findings of fast heart rate and high blood pressure. This formula is designed for any condition with the finding of high blood pressure and fast heart rate. The following is an article written by Dr. Chang entitled: "Interpreting Blood Pressure and Heart Rate Readings by Eight Principle Diagnostic Standards."

Whether approached by a seasoned practitioner or a novice, there are always cases that are difficult to differentiate and diagnose based on the classic *Ba Gang Bian Zheng* (Eight Principle Differentiation). When a patient presents complex symptoms, it is not always easy to sort out the tangle to come up with a confident, simple diagnosis and herbal prescription. Maybe the patient is taking one or more pharmaceuticals that complicate the clinical presentation, so that it is difficult to know which symptoms are true and which ones are side effects of the drug(s). Alternatively, maybe the patient is just not telling their entire history or complaints for one reason or another.

Conversely, maybe the difficulty in reaching a diagnosis is because the patient is describing too many symptoms, whether related to the chief complaint or not. In other cases, contradictory elements are in play, such as when a patient exhibits all excess signs but states that he or she suffers from chronic fatigue syndrome. On the other hand, maybe they feel cold, but their pulse is forceful and rapid, and their tongue is extremely red, with a definite yellow coating. One way or another, subjective complaints from patients may not always point to an immediate correct diagnosis.

One objective way to find out exactly whether the patient is truly suffering from deficiency, excess, heat or cold is to measure the blood pressure and the heart rate. Dr. Jimmy Wei-Yen Chang uses this method daily on all of his patients and has confirmed its practical usefulness through thousands of cases in his 20 years of practice. Below is a brief summary of the patterns representing the most commonly seen complex types in the clinic.

Type 1: Systolic (High) + Diastolic (High) + Heart Rate (Fast) = Excess Heat
Patients with both high blood pressure and a fast heart rate are, without exception, suffer from an excess heat condition. Please note that these patients may complain that they are tired and depressed. However, if they have high blood pressure and a fast heart rate, tonic herbs should *never* be used, despite the fact that the patient complains of tiredness. The diagnosis is excess fire, which should be addressed with heat-clearing herbs.

Type 2: Systolic (Low) + Diastolic (Low) + Heart Rate (Slow) = Yang Deficiency
Patients who have low blood pressure and a slow heart rate are experiencing deficiency, mostly qi or yang deficiency. These deficiencies are best helped by tonic herbs; never give these patients purging and sedating herbs.

Type 3: Systolic (High) + Diastolic (Normal) + Heart Rate (Slow) = Deficiency Heat + Blood Stasis
Patients who belong to this category usually suffer from blood stasis, which may be the result of an old injury or surgery. The heart rate is slow because of blood stasis and obstruction of the flow. In turn, systolic pressure is increased, as the body attempts to maintain balance. The increased pressure and lack of flow result in heat from deficiency. Carefully selecting appropriate blood-moving and stasis-resolving herbs with herbs to clear deficiency heat will be the most helpful strategy for treating these patients.

Type 4: Systolic (Low) + Diastolic (Low) + Heart Rate (Fast) = Yin Deficiency Heat
The last group might appear to reflect heat because of the rapid heart rate, but the low blood pressure tells a different story: the insufficient quantities of blood and yin in circulation require a rapid heart rate to maintain positive circulation. This is similar to a car engine running with insufficient oil: eventually, heat begins to build up from the deficiency of lubricating yin. These patients are suffering from yin deficiency heat, and must be treated with herbs that tonify yin and sedate the deficiency heat.

FORMULAS

GARDENIA COMPLEX ™

Summary:

	Systolic Pressure	Diastolic Pressure	Heart rate	Diagnosis	Herbs
Type 1	High	High	Fast	Excess Heat	Heat-Clearing Herbs
Type 2	Low	Low	Slow	Yang Deficiency	Tonic Herbs
Type 3	High	Normal	Slow	Deficient heat + Blood stasis	Blood moving herbs + Deficiency heat-clearing herbs
Type 4	Low	Low	Fast	Yin deficiency heat	Tonify yin and sedate deficiency heat

This approach provides a guideline to follow when confronted with a confusing presentation in the patient. Tongue and pulse diagnoses should be combined with this approach to reach an accurate diagnostic conclusion. Here is an example of a recent case that was addressed using this method:

A 45-year-old female states that she suffers from chronic fatigue syndrome, is extremely tired, and has no energy even for driving or simple activities. She complains of how stressful life is, how depressed she feels, and states that everything in life is "just not right." Tonic herbs might be the first approach that comes to mind. However, the objective findings of her blood pressure (170/120 mmHg) and heart rate (110 beats per minute) suggest otherwise. It is important to look at the tongue and take the pulse to arrive at an accurate diagnosis. If the tongue is red and the pulse rapid, then the patient's complaint of tiredness and fatigue can be ruled out. In this particular case, it would be important to avoid using a warming, drying tonic formula like *Vitality* or *Venus*. Heat-clearing formulas like *Gardenia Complex* and *Herbal ABX* would appropriately provide sedation for this patient. Although it seems wrong on the surface of things to use a sedating formula for someone identifying herself as having chronic fatigue syndrome, this would be the correct and effective approach.

Please remember that this is a guideline to follow when the presentation of the illness is complicated and confusing. It is important to gather all the details (signs, symptoms, tongue diagnosis, pulse diagnosis, and objective readings of blood pressure and heart rate) so the diagnosis will be accurate.

PHARMACEUTICAL DRUGS & CHINESE MEDICINE: A COMPARATIVE ANALYSIS

One striking difference between western and traditional Chinese medicine is that western medicine focuses and excels in crisis management, while traditional Chinese medicine emphasizes and shines in holistic and preventative treatments. Therefore, in emergencies, such as gun shot wounds or surgery, western medicine is generally the treatment of choice. However, for treatment of chronic idiopathic illness of unknown origins, where all lab tests are normal and a clear diagnosis cannot be made, traditional Chinese medicine is distinctly superior.

In cases of general presentations of inflammation, increased metabolism and elevated body temperature, where there are definite signs and symptoms of illness but not a clear diagnosis, western medicine offers few treatment options. Under these circumstances, traditional Chinese medicine is beneficial as it excels in regulating imbalances and alleviating associated signs and symptoms. Therefore, herbal therapy should definitely be employed to prevent deterioration of this condition, and to restore optimal health. Because this formula has a broad spectrum of therapeutic effect [including antipyretic, antibiotic, and anti-inflammatory effects], it treats a wide variety of disorders. If a specific imbalance can be identified, treatment is most effective if this formula is combined with another formula that targets the identified imbalance.

[1] *Zhong Yao Xue* (Chinese Herbology), 1998; 115:119
[2] *Zhong Yao Xue* (Chinese Herbology), 1998; 115:119
[3] *Zhong Hua Yi Xue Za Zhi* (Chinese Journal of Medicine), 1956; 42(10):964
[4] *Zhong Yao Zhi* (Chinese Herbology Journal), 1984; 578
[5] *Zhong Yao Xue* (Chinese Herbology), 1998; 115:119
[6] *Yao Xue Qing Bao Tong Xun* (Journal of Herbal Information), 1987; 5(4):62

FORMULAS

GARDENIA COMPLEX™

[7] *Zhong Yao Xue* (Chinese Herbology), 1998; 103:106

[8] *Zhong Yao Cai* (Study of Chinese Herbal Material), 1991; 14(2):41

[9] *Zhong Yao Xue* (Chinese Herbology), 1988; 137:140

[10] *Zhong Yao Da Ci Dian* (Dictionary of Chinese Herbs), 1977; 2032

[11] *CA*, 1953; 47:12652g

[12] *Zhong Yi Za Zhi* (Journal of Chinese Medicine), 1985; 12:13

[13] *Xin Yi Yao Xue Za Zhi* (New Journal of Medicine and Herbology), 1974; 2:18

[14] *Zhong Yao Xue* (Chinese Herbology), 1998; 105

[15] *Zhong Guo Zhong Xi Yi Jie He Za Zhi* (Chinese Journal of Integrative Chinese and Western Medicine), 1984; 4:222

[16] *Xin Yi Xue* (New Medicine), 1972; 8:11

[17] *Zhong Yao Yao Li Yu Ying Yong* (Pharmacology and Applications of Chinese Herbs), 1983; 888

[18] *Zhong Yao Yao Li Yu Ying Yong* (Pharmacology and Applications of Chinese Herbs), 1983; 400

[19] *Chang Yong Zhong Yao Cheng Fen Yu Yao Li Shou Ce* (A Handbook of the Composition and Pharmacology of Common Chinese Drugs), 1994; 368:376

[20] *Chem Pharm Bull*, 1984; 32(7):2724

[21] *Sheng Yao Xue Za Zhi* (Journal of Raw Herbology), 1979; 33(3):178

[22] *Zhong Hua Wai Ke Za Zhi* (Chinese Journal of External Medicine), 1960; 4:366

[23] *Si Chuan Zhong Yi* (Sichuan Chinese Medicine), 1988; 9:11

[24] *Shen Yang Yi Xue Yuan Xue Bao* (Journal of Shenyang University of Medicine), 1984; 1(3):214

[25] *Ji Lin Zhong Yi Yao* (Jilin Chinese Medicine and Herbology), 1992; (1):16

[26] *Zhong Yao Xue* (Chinese Herbology), 1988; 137:140

[27] *Zhong Guo Yao Li Xue Tong Bao* (Journal of Chinese Herbal Pharmacology), 1989; 10(5):385

[28] *Guo Wai Yi Xue Zhong Yi Zhong Yao Fen Ce* (Monograph of Chinese Herbology from Foreign Medicine), 1983; (3):5,1984;(5):54

[29] *Zhong Yao Yao Li Yu Ying Yong* (Pharmacology and Applications of Chinese Herbs), 1983; 934

[30] *Shang Hai Zhong Yi Yao Za Zhi* (Shanghai Journal of Chinese Medicine and Herbology), 1956; 1:24

[31] *Liao Ning Yi Xue Za Zhi* (Liaoning Journal of Medicine), 1960; (7):48

[32] *Guo Wai Yi Xue Zhong Yi Zhong Yao Fen Ce* (Monograph of Chinese Herbology from Foreign Medicine), 1983; (3):5,1984;(5):54

[33] *Shan Xi Yi Yao Za Zhi* (Shanxi Journal of Medicine and Herbology), 1984; 13(4):359

[34] *Zhong Ji Yi Kan* (Medium Medical Journal); 4:19

[35] *Yun Nan Yi Yao* (Yunan Medicine and Herbology), 1991; 12(5):304

[36] *Ri Ben Yao Wu Xue Za Zhi* (Japan Journal of Pharmacology), 1957; 53(6):215

[37] *Xin Yi Yao Xue Za Zhi* (New Journal of Medicine and Herbology), 1974; 2:18

[38] *Xin Yi Yao Xue Za Zhi* (New Journal of Medicine and Herbology), 1974; 2:18

[39] *Shang Hai Zhong Yi Yao Za Zhi* (Shanghai Journal of Chinese Medicine and Herbology), 1965; 4:4

[40] *Zhong Hua Nei Ke Za Zhi* (Chinese Journal of Internal Medicine), 1978; 2:127

[41] *Zhong Yao Yao Li Yu Ying Yong* (Pharmacology and Applications of Chinese Herbs), 1983; 934

[42] *Zhong Yi Yao Xue Bao* (Report of Chinese Medicine and Herbology), 1988; (1):45

[43] *Ri Ben Yao Wu Xue Za Zhi* (Japan Journal of Pharmacology), 1957; 53(6):215

[44] *Jiang Su Yi Yao* (Jiangsu Journal of Medicine and Herbology), 1976; (1):28

[45] *Zhong Yao Yao Li Yu Ying Yong* (Pharmacology and Applications of Chinese Herbs), 1983; 888

[46] *Zhong Yao Yao Li Yu Ying Yong* (Pharmacology and Applications of Chinese Herbs), 1983; 934

FORMULAS

GASTRODIA COMPLEX ™

CLINICAL APPLICATIONS

- Hypertension (deficient types) with dizziness, blurred vision, headache, and/or generalized weakness
- Seizures and convulsions in hypertensive patients
- Prevention of stroke in hypertensive patients
- Prevention of angina and myocardial infarction in hypertensive patients

WESTERN THERAPEUTIC FUNCTIONS

- Antihypertensive effect to lower blood pressure [8,10,11,12]
- Vasodilator to increase blood perfusion to cardiac muscles [1,2,9]
- Anticonvulsant effect to treat seizures and convulsions [3,4,5]
- Anti-oxidant, antispasmodic, and anti-arrhythmic effects [14,15]

CHINESE THERAPEUTIC FUNCTIONS

- Extinguishes Liver wind
- Calms Liver yang
- Clears heat
- Nourishes Liver and Kidney yin

DOSAGE

Take 3 to 4 capsules three times daily with warm water on an empty stomach.

INGREDIENTS

Cha Chi Huang (Herba Stellariae Aquaticae)
Chuan Niu Xi (Radix Cyathulae)
Dan Shen (Radix Salviae Miltiorrhizae)
Ge Gen (Radix Puerariae)
Gou Qi Zi (Fructus Lycii)
Gou Teng (Ramulus Uncariae cum Uncis)
Jue Ming Zi (Semen Cassiae)

Sha Yuan Zi (Semen Astragali Complanati)
Shan Zhu Yu (Fructus Corni)
Sheng Di Huang (Radix Rehmanniae)
Shi Jue Ming (Concha Haliotidis)
Tian Ma (Rhizoma Gastrodiae)
Xia Ku Cao (Spica Prunellae)
Zhen Zhu Mu (Concha Margaritaferae)

FORMULA EXPLANATION

Gastrodia Complex is designed to extinguish Liver wind, calm Liver yang, and nourish Liver and Kidney yin. The main clinical applications of *Gastrodia Complex* are hypertension and headache. It can also be used in hypertensive patients to reduce the risks of seizure, convulsion, stroke, angina, and myocardial infarction.

Tian Ma (Rhizoma Gastrodiae), *Gou Teng* (Ramulus Uncariae cum Uncis), *Zhen Zhu Mu* (Concha Margaritaferae), and *Shi Jue Ming* (Concha Haliotidis) are the chief herbs used to calm or anchor Liver yang and extinguish the wind. Together they function to lower the blood pressure and relieve headache and dizziness caused by hypertension. *Cha Chi Huang* (Herba Stellariae Aquaticae), *Xia Ku Cao* (Spica Prunellae), and *Jue Ming Zi* (Semen Cassiae) have antihypertensive effects, which can clear red, painful, or swollen eyes associated with hypertension. *Sha Yuan Zi* (Semen Astragali Complanati) and *Gou Qi Zi* (Fructus Lycii) are used to alleviate visual problems associated with hypertension. *Sheng Di Huang* (Radix Rehmanniae) and *Shan Zhu Yu* (Fructus Corni) tonify the Liver and Kidney yin to prevent Liver yang rising. *Dan Shen* (Radix Salviae Miltiorrhizae) improves micro-circulation, myocardial

GASTRODIA COMPLEX ™

contraction, and heart rate. *Ge Gen* (Radix Puerariae) dilates blood vessels to lower blood pressure. It also relieves neck and occipital stiffness and tension commonly associated with hypertension. *Chuan Niu Xi* (Radix Cyathulae) directs the blood downward and gives this formula a descending property.

SUPPLEMENTARY FORMULAS

- For high cholesterol and triglycerides, add *Cholisma*.
- For high cholesterol and triglycerides in individuals with fatty liver and obesity, add *Cholisma (ES)*.
- For headache, add *Corydalin*.
- For migraine, add *Migratrol*.
- For hypertension with edema and water accumulation, combine with *Herbal DRX*.
- For high blood pressure and fast heart rate due to excess heat, add *Gardenia Complex*.
- For deviation of the eyes and mouth in post-stroke or Bell's palsy patients, add *Symmetry*.
- For coronary heart disorders, combine with *Circulation*.
- For cardiovascular and circulatory disorders throughout the entire body, or for stubborn hypertension with blood stagnation, combine with *Circulation (SJ)*.
- For qi and blood deficiencies, combine with a small amount of *Imperial Tonic*.
- For constipation, combine with *Gentle Lax (Excess)* or *Gentle Lax (Deficient)*.
- For insomnia due to stress and anxiety in individuals with underlying deficiencies, combine with *Calm ZZZ*.
- For stress and anxiety, combine with *Calm (ES)*.
- For insomnia due to anemia, generalized weakness or excessive worrying, combine with *Schisandra ZZZ*.
- To treat stroke complications, use *Neuro Plus*.
- For trigeminal neuralgia or hemiplegia in hypertensive patients, combine with *Flex (NP)*.
- With Kidney yin deficiency, add *Nourish*.

NUTRITION

- Eliminate salt from the diet in cases of hypertension. Avoid MSG, baking soda, meat, fat, aged foods, alcohol, diet soft drinks, preservatives, sugar substitutes, meat tenderizers, and soy sauce. Over-the-counter medications that contain ibuprofen, such as Advil or Motrin, should not be used. Increase the intake of fresh fruits and vegetables.
- Aspartame should also be avoided, since a high level may increase blood pressure.
- Increase the intake of fresh, raw vegetables and fruits to control blood pressure. Nuts and seeds should be consumed daily for source of protein.
- Vitamin C and bioflavonoids help to reduce blood pressure by stabilizing the blood vessel walls.
- Garlic is effective to lower blood pressure and thin the blood.

The Tao of Nutrition by Ni and McNease
- Hypertension
  - Recommendations: celery, spinach, garlic, bananas, sunflower seeds, honey, tofu, mung beans, bamboo shoots, seaweed, vinegar, tomatoes, water chestnuts, corn, apples, persimmons, peas, buckwheat, jellyfish, watermelon, hawthorn berries, eggplant, plums, mushrooms, lemons, lotus root, chrysanthemums, and cassia seeds.
  - Recommendations: Steam or bake jellyfish about 12 minutes, add vinegar, soy sauce, and sesame oil; take daily for about 2 months.
  - Recommendations: Make tea from chrysanthemum flowers and cassia seeds and drink daily.
  - Recommendations: Take black or white mushrooms and cook soup daily.
  - Avoid smoking, alcohol, spicy foods, coffee, caffeine, all stimulants, fatty or fried foods, salty foods, stress, constipation, potatoes, strong emotions, pork, and overeating.

FORMULAS

GASTRODIA COMPLEX ™

- Headache
  - Recommendations: chrysanthemum flowers, mint, green onions, oyster shells, pearl barley, carrots, prunes, buckwheat, peach kernels, and green tea.
  - Avoid spicy food, lack of sleep, alcohol, smoking, excess stimulation, eye strain, and stress.
- For more information, please refer to *The Tao of Nutrition* by Dr. Maoshing Ni and Cathy McNease.

LIFESTYLE INSTRUCTIONS

- Normal bowel and urinary functions help to reduce blood pressure. Diuretics and stool softeners should be taken as needed.
- Maintain a positive attitude and outlook. Control emotions and reduce stress. Emotional fluctuations should be reduced whenever possible.
- Individuals who are aware of circumstances or activities that trigger tension and hypertensive responses need to initiate patterns in their lives that help them avoid or reduce the impact of those triggers.
- Stop alcohol consumption and cigarette smoking.
- Weight loss is highly recommended to help lower blood pressure.
- Exercises such as swimming and brisk walking are excellent for hypertension.
- Practice of meditation, *Tai Chi Chuan*, and yoga are beneficial to relax, reduce stress, and lower blood pressure.

CLINICAL NOTE

- Western medicine classifies hypertension into two types: "red" and "pale" high blood pressure. "Red" high blood pressure corresponds with TCM diagnosis of "excess," and generally occurs in energetic and stressed individuals with marked redness and vascularized skin. "Pale" high blood pressure corresponds with the TCM diagnosis of "deficiency," and generally occurs in individuals with compromised kidneys, glands, or metabolism.

CAUTIONS

- Some patients may experience mild stomach discomfort, which may be alleviated by reducing the dosage of herbs or taking the herbs with food.
- Herbal treatment is ineffective for malignant hypertension and some secondary hypertension, such as renal stenosis or pheochromocytoma. Refer the patients to a medical doctor as surgical intervention may be necessary.
- If untreated, hypertension can lead to various complications such as myocardial infarction, cerebral hemorrhage, renal failure, and premature death from these or other developments. Effective treatment must include both lifestyle changes and herbal therapy.
- Patients who are on anticoagulant or antiplatelet therapies, such as Coumadin (Warfarin), should use this formula with caution, as there may be a slightly higher risk of bleeding and bruising.

ACUPUNCTURE POINTS

Traditional Points:
- *Baihui* (GV 20), *Zusanli* (ST 36), *Renying* (ST 9), *Taichong* (LR 3), and *Renying* (ST 9).
- *Taichong* (LR 3), *Xingjian* (LR 2), *Fenglong* (ST 40), *Ganshu* (BL 18), *Yongquan* (KI 1), and *Zusanli* (ST 36).

Balance Method by Dr. Richard Tan:
- Left side: *Xuanzhong* (GB 39), *Fenglong* (ST 40), *Chengshan* (BL 57), *Lieque* (LU 7), and *Tongli* (HT 5).
- Right side: *Taichong* (LR 3), *Rangu* (KI 2), *Gongsun* (SP 4), *Waiguan* (TH 5), and *Binao* (LI 14).

FORMULAS

GASTRODIA COMPLEX ™

- ☙ Left and right side can be alternated from treatment to treatment.
- ☙ For additional information on the Balance Method, please refer to *Dr. Tan's Strategy of Twelve Magical Points* by Dr. Richard Tan.

Ear Points:
- ☙ Depression groove in the back of the ear to lower blood pressure, Prostate Gland. Use magnetic ear seeds. Switch ear every five days. Advise patient to massage the points until he/she feels a hot or distended sensation.
- ☙ Adrenal gland, bleed the depression groove in the back of the ear to lower blood pressure, Heart, *Shenmen*, Endocrine, Taiyang, Liver, Kidney. Select four or five points for each treatment, which lasts three days. Ten treatments equal one treatment course. Rest for 1 week in between treatment courses.

Auricular Acupuncture by Dr. Li-Chun Huang:
- ☙ Hypertension: Decrease Blood Pressure Point, *Shenmen*, Kidney, Liver, Heart, Occiput, Forehead, Sympathetic, and Coronary Vascular Subcortex. Bleed Ear Apex.
- ☙ For additional information on the location and explanation of these points, please refer to *Auricular Treatment Formula and Prescriptions* by Dr. Li-Chun Huang.

MODERN RESEARCH

Gastrodia Complex is formulated based on one of the most commonly used traditional formulas that lowers Liver yang. It is now frequently used to treat hypertension, cerebrovascular disease, and other complications related to hypertension.

Tian Ma (Rhizoma Gastrodiae) has been demonstrated through various studies to have positive cardiovascular effects. It increases the amount of blood flow to the cardiac muscle and increases resistance to hypoxia.[1] Additionally, by increasing blood flow to the cardiac muscle, *Tian Ma* (Rhizoma Gastrodiae) decreases the risks of myocardial ischemia and myocardial infarct. It was demonstrated in a study that *Tian Ma* (Rhizoma Gastrodiae) reduced the size of myocardial ischemia and myocardial infarct by 23.5% and 34.5%, respectively.[2] Furthermore, *Tian Ma* (Rhizoma Gastrodiae) has been shown to have a positive effect in the treatment of seizures, cranial-cerebral injury, cervical spondylosis and cerebrovascular diseases.[3,4] *Tian Ma* (Rhizoma Gastrodiae) is also used to treat convulsions. In comparison with phenobarbital, *Tian Ma* (Rhizoma Gastrodiae) has a similar anticonvulsant effect and a longer duration of action.[5] The pharmacological effect of *Tian Ma* (Rhizoma Gastrodiae) is attributed mostly to its antioxidant and free-radical scavenging activities.[6,7]

Gou Teng (Ramulus Uncariae cum Uncis) also has profound influences on the cardiovascular system. *Gou Teng* (Ramulus Uncariae cum Uncis) has been studied extensively in various clinical trials for its antihypertensive effects.[8] One study showed *Gou Teng* (Ramulus Uncariae cum Uncis) to be a potent and long-lasting vasodilator by relaxing the aorta and thereby reducing blood pressure.[9] More specifically, the vasodilative effects of *Gou Teng* (Ramulus Uncariae cum Uncis) were attributed to its alpha-adrenoceptor blocking and calcium channel blocking activities.[10,11,12] Clinically, administration of *Gou Teng* (Ramulus Uncariae cum Uncis) lowers both systolic and diastolic blood pressure as well as lowering the heart rate.[13] *Gou Teng* (Ramulus Uncariae cum Uncis) also demonstrates antispasmodic, antiarrhythmic and anticonvulsant effects.[14,15]

PHARMACEUTICAL DRUGS & CHINESE MEDICINE: A COMPARATIVE ANALYSIS

Western Medical Approach: Hypertension is one of the most common disorders in developed countries. In western medicine, many different categories of drugs may be used to treat hypertension, including but not limited to diuretics [Lasix (Furosemide) and hydrochlorothiazide], beta-blockers [Tenormin (Atenolol) and Inderal (Propranolol)], calcium channel blockers [Procardia (Nifedipine) and Calan (Verapamil)], ACE inhibitors [Vasotec (Enalapril)] and

FORMULAS

GASTRODIA COMPLEX ™

Capoten (Captopril)], and vasodilators [hydralazine and minoxidil]. All these drugs have benefits and risks, and may be given individually or in combinations to control blood pressure. The main advantage of drug therapy is its potency to suppress blood pressure. The main disadvantages, however, are that the drugs cause a great number of side effects, and they do not change the underlying constitution of the patient. Therefore, while they are effective to suppress blood pressure, they must be used continually and cannot be stopped. Discontinuing use of drugs often leads to rebound hypertension.

Traditional Chinese Medicine Approach: Hypertension may be characterized by both excess and deficiency. Excess refers to Liver yang rising, and deficiency refers to Liver and Kidney yin deficiencies. Both conditions may be treated effectively with herbal medicine. The main advantage of using herbs is the effective ability to change the fundamental constitution of the body, thereby achieving long-term efficacy to reduce blood pressure, even after the herbs are discontinued. The main disadvantage, however, is that herbs are less immediately potent than drugs for treatment of hypertensive crisis, or secondary hypertension, thus should not be used in lieu of drugs in these cases.

Summation: Both drugs and herbs are effective to treat hypertension, and they have their distinct advantages and disadvantages. In addition to choosing either drugs or herbal therapy, it is also important to make diet and lifestyle changes to ensure successful long-term management of hypertension.

CASE STUDIES

A 45-year-old male presented with headache, high blood pressure, and high cholesterol. The patient was diagnosed with Liver yang rising with stagnation of qi and blood. *Cholisma* and *Gastrodia Complex* were prescribed for the patients with positive results reported by the physician.

R.C., MD, Ph.D., New York, New York

J.L., a 86-year-old male, presented with hypertension, insomnia, anxiety and high cholesterol. His blood pressure was 180/90 mmHg and the heart rate was 60 beats per minute. The blood pressure was higher in the morning (180-190/90-95 mmHg) than in the evening (170-180/85-90 mmHg). The TCM diagnosis was damp-heat accumulation. *Gastrodia Complex* at 4.5 grams a day and *Cholisma* at 1.5 grams a day were prescribed. This patient also received acupuncture. After six weeks of treatment, both morning and evening blood pressure were down to an average of 147/80 mmHg.

W.F., Bloomfield, New Jersey

S.O., a 51-year-old female patient, presented with extremely painful migraine headaches four to six times a month for three years. The pain developed during a time of intense involvement with a job that required serious focus and long hours. The pain was pounding and throbbing at her temples and behind her eyes. Her head itself felt "big" and each headache was accompanied by photosensitivity and occasionally nosebleeds and nausea. The patient didn't want to take any pharmaceutical drugs so she "rode out" the headaches by sleeping all day. Objective findings included sogginess and softness with palpation at the vertex where one would expect to feel only bone hardness of the skull. Blood pressure was 128/78 mmHg with a heart rate of 76 to 80 beats per minute. Tongue was red and peeled, especially at the sides. Pulse was wiry/floating and the left side was very thin. The patient appeared debilitated. Her diagnosis according to traditional Chinese medicine was Liver yang rising with Liver and Kidney yin deficiencies. The practitioner felt her episodic stress-related migraine headaches probably were due to poor regulation of blood vessel dilation/constriction in the head. *Gastrodia Complex* was prescribed at 4 capsules three times a day. After six weeks of herbal treatment, the patient reported that her headaches diminished in ferocity. During the next four weeks, the patient reported only one headache and it lasted only a few hours instead of putting her to bed for the entire day. Over the months that the patient continued the treatment, headaches became a rare event and she felt stronger overall.

H.H., San Francisco, California

GASTRODIA COMPLEX ™

A 39-year-old female presented with elevated blood pressure, palpitations, hot flashes, anxiety, and swelling in her neck, with a heart rate of 92 beats per minute. The Western diagnosis was hyperthyroidism; the TCM diagnosis was Liver and Kidney yin deficiencies. After she began taking *Thyrodex*, the patient experienced diminished hot flashes and anxiety. Her blood pressure remained unchanged but the goiter diminished in size. After *Gastrodia Complex* was added to the herbal treatment, the patient noticed improvement after just one bottle.

P.W., Paulet, Vermont

A 47-year-old female acupuncturist presented with one-sided severely debilitating migraines, which occurred particularly during the weekends. The TCM diagnosis was Kidney yin deficiency leading to Liver yang rising. A dose of *Corydalin* relieved the pain especially when the drug Imitrex (Sumatriptan) was unsuccessful. Within two weeks of taking *Corydalin*, she was free from headaches. She supplemented her treatment with *Gastrodia Complex* in addition to acupuncture treatments. She has experienced no migraine episodes for more than six months, and continues using the herbal combination of *Corydalin* and *Gastrodia Complex*.

D.W., Hashbrouck Heights, New Jersey

[1] Huang, JH. Comparison studies on pharmacological properties of injection gastrodia elata, gastrodin-free fraction and gastrodin. *Acta Academiae Medicinae Sinicae*. 11(2):147-50, Apr. 1989

[2] Luo, H. et al. Effects of tian-ma injection on myocardial ischemia and lipid peroxidation in rabbits. *Journal of West China University of Medical Sciences*. 23(1):53-6, Mar. 1992

[3] Wu, HQ. et al. The effect of vanillin on the fully amygdala-kindled seizures in the rat. *Acta Pharmaceutica Sinica*. 24(7):482-6, 1989

[4] Lu, SL. et al. The development of nao li shen and its clinical application. *J Pharm Pharmacol* 1997 Nov;49(11):1162-4.

[5] Bensky D, et al. *Chinese Herbal Medicine Materia Medica*. Eastland Press. 1993

[6] Liu, J and Mori, A. antioxidant and free radical scavenging activities of gastrodia elata bl. and uncaria rhynchophylla (Miq) Jacks. *Neuropharmacology*. 31(12):1287-98, Dec. 1992

[7] Antioxidant and pro-oxidant activities of p-hydroxybenzyl alcohol and vanillin: effects on free radical brain peroxidation and degradation of benzoate deoxyribose. *Neuropharmacology*, 32(7):659-69, Jul. 1993

[8] Aisaka, K. et al. Hypotensive action of 3-alpha-dihydrocadambine, an indol alkaloid glycoside of uncaria hooks. *Planta Med*, (5):424-7 Oct. 1985

[9] Kuramochi, T. et al. Gou-Teng (from uncaria rhynchophylla miquel)-induced endothelium-dependent and –independent relaxation in the isolated rat aorta. *Life Science*, 54(26):2061-9 1994

[10] Ozaki, Y. Vasodilative effects of indole alkaloids obtained from domestic plants uncaria rhynchophylla miq. and amsonia elliptica roem. et schult. *Nippon Yakurigaku Zasshi*, 95(2):47-54 Feb. 1990

[11] Horie, S. et al. Effects of hirsutine and antihypertensive indol alkaloid from uncaria rhynchophylla on intracellular calcium in rat throacic aorta. *Life Science*, 50(7):491-8 1992

[12] Yano, S. et al. Calcium channel blocking effects of hirsutine and indol alkaloid from uncaria genus in the isolated rat aorta. *Planta Med*, 57(5):403-5 Oct. 1991

[13] Mok, SJ. et al. Cardiovascular responses in the normotensive rat produced by intravenous injection of gambirine isolated from uncariae bl. ex korth.

[14] Ozaki, Y. Pharmacological studies of indol alkaloids obtained from domestic plants, uncaria rhynchophylla miq. and amsonia elliptica roem. et schult. *Nippon Yakurigaku Zassi*, 94(1):17-26 Jul. 1989

[15] Mimaki, Y. et al. Anti-convulsant effects of choto-san and chotoko (uncariae uncis cum ramulus) in mice, and identification of the active principles. *Yakugaku Zasshi*; 117(12):1011-21. Dec 1997

FORMULAS

GENTIANA COMPLEX ™

CLINICAL APPLICATIONS

- ❧ Hypertension (excess types) with anger, flushed face and throbbing headache
- ❧ Viral infection, such as genital herpes
- ❧ Bacterial or fungal infections, such as urinary tract infection, vaginal infection, yeast infection, herpes infection, boils, carbuncles, acute cystitis, urethritis, and related discomforts or dysfunctions
- ❧ Liver and gallbladder disorders, such as acute icteric hepatitis, acute cholecystitis, and more
- ❧ Hangovers with headache and gastrointestinal discomfort

WESTERN THERAPEUTIC ACTIONS

- ❧ Antihypertensive effect to lower blood pressure Error! Bookmark not defined. [1,2,9]
- ❧ Antibiotic, antibacterial, antiviral and antifungal effects for a variety of infections [2,3,5,6,9]
- ❧ Anti-inflammatory properties to treat inflammation of the internal organs and soft tissue [2,9]

CHINESE THERAPEUTIC ACTIONS

- ❧ Drains damp-heat from the Liver and the Gallbladder channels
- ❧ Sedates excess fire
- ❧ Nourishes yin

DOSAGE

Take 4 capsules three times daily. For treatment of infections and inflammation of internal organs, the dosage may be increased to 6 to 8 capsules three to four times daily. Treatment is most effective if herbal therapy begins immediately with the first sign of outbreak and continues throughout the entire course of infection. Advise the patients to take the herbs with meals if they experience stomach discomfort.

INGREDIENTS

Che Qian Zi (Semen Plantaginis)
Da Huang (Radix et Rhizoma Rhei)
Dan Shen (Radix Salviae Miltiorrhizae)
Ge Gen (Radix Puerariae)
Hua Shi (Talcum)
Huai Niu Xi (Radix Achyranthis Bidentatae)
Huang Bai (Cortex Phellodendri)

Huang Qin (Radix Scutellariae)
Long Dan Cao (Radix Gentianae)
Sheng Di Huang (Radix Rehmanniae)
Shi Jue Ming (Concha Haliotidis)
Ze Xie (Rhizoma Alismatis)
Zhen Zhu Mu (Concha Margaritaferae)
Zhi Zi (Fructus Gardeniae)

FORMULA EXPLANATION

Gentiana Complex is formulated to treat damp-heat in the Liver and the Gallbladder channels. Clinical applications of Gentiana Complex include hypertension, hepatic disorders, gallbladder disorders, hangovers, and bacterial, viral or fungal infections. Hypertension is the manifestation of Liver yang rising; hepatic and gallbladder disorders are manifestations of damp-heat in the Liver and Gallbladder; hangover are a manifestation of damp-heat affecting the Liver, Spleen and Stomach; and bacterial, viral or fungal infections are manifestations of damp-heat in the affected area.

Shi Jue Ming (Concha Haliotidis) and Zhen Zhu Mu (Concha Margaritaferae) descend and anchor the rising Liver yang to treat dizziness and headache. Da Huang (Radix et Rhizoma Rhei) eliminates damp-heat and purges toxic

GENTIANA COMPLEX ™

fire. The active ingredient puerarin in *Ge Gen* (Radix Puerariae) has been found to effectively relieve neck stiffness, pain, headache and dizziness associated with hypertension. *Dan Shen* (Radix Salviae Miltiorrhizae) adjusts the heart rate and improves micro-circulation and myocardial contraction.

Damp-heat is considered to be the cause of various bacterial, viral and fungal infections in traditional Chinese medicine. A large quantity of *Long Dan Cao* (Radix Gentianae) is used in this formula to drain damp-heat in the Liver channel and the lower *jiao*, to treat herpes, urinary tract infection, cystitis and other infections. *Huang Qin* (Radix Scutellariae), *Huang Bai* (Cortex Phellodendri) and *Zhi Zi* (Fructus Gardeniae) clear heat and drain dampness. *Ze Xie* (Rhizoma Alismatis), *Che Qian Zi* (Semen Plantaginis), *Hua Shi* (Talcum) and *Huai Niu Xi* (Radix Achyranthis Bidentatae) eliminate damp-heat in the lower *jiao* and drain the damp-heat out of the body through urination. *Sheng Di Huang* (Radix Rehmanniae) protects the Liver from the strong sedative nature of the rest of the herbs in this formula.

SUPPLEMENTARY FORMULAS

- For high cholesterol and triglycerides, add *Cholisma*.
- For high cholesterol and triglycerides in individuals with fatty liver and obesity, add *Cholisma (ES)*.
- For icteric hepatitis, acute cholecystitis or liver cirrhosis, combine with *Liver DTX*.
- For coronary heart disorders, combine with *Circulation*.
- For cardiovascular and circulatory disorders throughout the entire body, combine with *Circulation (SJ)*.
- For hypertension with edema and water accumulation, combine with *Herbal DRX*.
- For headache, add *Corydalin*.
- For migraine, add *Migratrol*.
- To treat shingles, herpetic lesions, and post-herpetic pain, add *Dermatrol (HZ)*.
- For increased thirst and constipation, combine with *Gentle Lax (Excess)*.
- To enhance the antibiotic effect, combine with *Herbal ABX*.
- To treat ear infection, combine with *Herbal ENT*.
- For insomnia and stress in patients with underlying deficiency, add *Calm ZZZ*.
- For cholecystitis or gallstones, combine with *Dissolve (GS)*.
- For high blood pressure and fast heart rate due to excess fire, add *Gardenia Complex*.
- For severe blood stagnation, add *Circulation (SJ)*.
- To prevent herpes attacks, use *Nourish* and *Immune* + when the patient is asymptomatic.

NUTRITION

- Increase the intake of fresh fruits and vegetables. Increase the intake of fresh, raw vegetables and fruits to control blood pressure. Nuts and seeds should be consumed daily as a source of protein. Vitamin C and bioflavonoids help to reduce blood pressure by stabilizing the blood vessel walls. Garlic is also effective to lower blood pressure and thin the blood.
- Patients with hypertension should minimize intake of salt from the diet. Avoid MSG, baking soda, meat, fat, aged foods, alcohol, diet soft drinks, preservatives, sugar substitutes, meat tenderizers, and soy sauce. Aspartame should also be avoided, since a high level may increase blood pressure. Over-the-counter medications, such as Advil (Ibuprofen) or Motrin (Ibuprofen), should not be used because they may increase the blood pressure.
- Individuals with cystitis should increase the intake of cranberries or cranberry juice. Cranberry produces hippuric acid in the urine that prohibits the growth of bacteria, thus preventing bacteria from adhering to the lining of the bladder. Juices that contain a large percentage of high-fructose syrup, sugar or sweeteners, on the other hand, should be avoided as they provide nutrients for bacterial growth.

GENTIANA COMPLEX ™

❧ Patients should drink plenty of fluids, as it helps to flush out the bacteria in the bladder. Women are encouraged to empty the bladder before and after intercourse, and wash the genitalia thoroughly.

❧ Individuals with hangovers should drink plenty of water to keep their body properly hydrated.

The Tao of Nutrition by Ni and McNease

❧ Hypertension
- Recommendations: celery, spinach, garlic, bananas, sunflower seeds, honey, tofu, mung beans, bamboo shoots, seaweed, vinegar, tomatoes, water chestnuts, corn, apples, persimmons, peas, buckwheat, jellyfish, watermelon, hawthorn berries, eggplant, plums, mushrooms, lemons, lotus root, chrysanthemums, and cassia seeds.
- Recommendations: Steam or bake jellyfish about 12 minutes, add vinegar, soy sauce, and sesame oil; take daily for about 2 months.
- Recommendations: Make tea from chrysanthemum flowers and cassia seeds and drink daily.
- Recommendations: Take black or white mushrooms and cook soup daily.
- Avoid smoking, alcohol, spicy foods, coffee, caffeine, all stimulants, fatty or fried foods, salty foods, stress, constipation, potatoes, strong emotions, pork, and overeating.

❧ Candida yeast infection
- Recommendations: dandelions, beet tops, carrot tops, barley, garlic, rice vinegar, mung beans, citrus fruits.
- Avoid sugar, excessive fruits, yeast-containing foods, processed foods, cheese, fermented foods, soy sauce, smoking, alcohol, caffeine, and constipation.

❧ Chronic bladder infections
- Recommendations: watermelon, pears, carrots, celery, corn, mung beans, corn-silk, squash, wheat, water chestnuts, barley, red beans, millet, oranges, cantaloupe, grapes, strawberries, lotus roots, loquats, and plenty of water.
- Avoid heavy proteins, meat, dairy products, onions, scallions, ginger, black pepper, and alcohol.

❧ For more information, please refer to *The Tao of Nutrition* by Dr. Maoshing Ni and Cathy McNease.

LIFESTYLE INSTRUCTIONS

❧ Weight loss is highly recommended to help lower blood pressure.

❧ Normal bowel and urinary functions help to reduce blood pressure. Diuretics and stool softeners should be taken as needed.

❧ Maintain a positive attitude and outlook. Control emotions and reduce stress. Emotional fluctuations should be reduced whenever possible.

❧ Stop alcohol consumption and cigarette smoking.

❧ Exercise such as swimming and brisk walking are excellent exercises for hypertension.

❧ Individuals with herpes should stay away from heat, over-exertion, stress, spicy and greasy foods, alcohol, coffee, or anything else that may trigger an attack. Patients should keep the infected area clean and dry in order to promote healing and avoid secondary infections. It is also recommended that patients abstain from sex during the outbreak period. Avoid citrus fruits and juices while the virus is active.

❧ For leukorrhea, yogurt and sour products should be included in the diet.

❧ Cotton underwear, instead of nylon, is recommended to promote air circulation in the genital region.

❧ Ointments containing cortisone or petroleum jelly should not be used on genital sores as they need air to heal. Cortisone inhibits the immune system and can encourage the virus to grow.[9]

❧ Advise the patient to wipe from front to back after a bowel movement to avoid infection.

❧ Strengthening the immune system is the key to preventing another herpes attack. *See* Supplementary Formulas for appropriate formula.

❧ Practice of meditation, *Tai Chi Chuan*, and yoga are also beneficial to relax, reduce stress, and lower blood pressure.

FORMULAS

GENTIANA COMPLEX ™

CLINICAL NOTES

❧ Western medicine classifies hypertension into two types: "red" and "pale" high blood pressure. "Red" high blood pressure corresponds with The TCM diagnosis of "excess," and generally occurs in energetic and stressed individuals with marked redness and vascularized skin. "Pale" high blood pressure corresponds with The TCM diagnosis of "deficiency," and generally occurs in individuals with compromised kidneys, glands, or metabolism.

❧ *Gentiana Complex* may be applied topically for treatment of genital herpes. Break open the capsules and apply the powder directly onto the lesion. Or, mix the powder with water to make a paste and apply to the lesions.

❧ From a TCM perspective, *Gentiana Complex* has a broader effect to treat damp-heat in the Liver and Gallbladder channel. *V-Statin* has a localized effect to treat damp-heat in the genital area.

❧ *V-Statin* and *Gentiana Complex* are very similar in treating damp-heat of the lower *jiao*. *Gentiana Complex* has an additional function to treat hypertension. Therefore, in patients who have normal blood pressure or low blood pressure suffering from damp-heat of the lower *jiao*, *V-Statin* would be more a more appropriate formula to use. In patients who have both hypertension (Liver yang rising) and also damp-heat in the lower *jiao*, *Gentiana Complex* should be used.

CAUTIONS

❧ Herbal treatment is ineffective for malignant hypertension and some secondary hypertension, such as renal stenosis or pheochromocytoma. Refer the patient to a medical doctor, as surgical intervention may be necessary.

❧ *Gentiana Complex* should be taken for approximately one to two weeks when treating viral, bacterial or fungal infection. Once the infection subsides, the patient should be placed on a maintenance regimen using *Nourish* to prevent future attacks.

❧ *Gentiana Complex* is contraindicated for long-term use when treating viral, bacterial or fungal infection. This formula is designed to treat only the acute conditions, and should not be used for long-term or prophylactic treatments.

❧ Some patients may experience mild stomach discomfort or loose stool, which may be alleviated by reducing the dosage of herbs or taking the herbs with food.

❧ This formula is contraindicated during pregnancy and nursing.

❧ Patients who are on anticoagulant or antiplatelet therapies, such as Coumadin (Warfarin), should use this formula with caution, as there may be a slightly higher risk of bleeding and bruising.

ACUPUNCTURE POINTS

Traditional Points:
❧ *Quchi* (LI 11), *Hegu* (LI 4), *Taichong* (LR 3), and *Renying* (ST 9).
❧ *Taichong* (LR 3), *Qihai* (CV 6), *Zhongwan* (CV 12), *Fenglong* (ST 40), *Geshu* (BL 17), *Renzhong* (GV 26), *Ganshu* (BL 18), *Pishu* (BL 20), and *Danshu* (BL 19).

Balance Method bu Dr. Richard Tan:
❧ Left side: Bleed *Dadun* (LR 1), Needle *Taichong* (LR 3), and *Hegu* (LI 4).
❧ Right side: Needle *Neiguan* (PC 6) and *Zulinqi* (GB 41). Bleed *Zhongchong* (PC 9).
❧ Left and right side can be alternated from treatment to treatment.
❧ For additional information on the Balance Method, please refer to *Dr. Tan's Strategy of Twelve Magical Points* by Dr. Richard Tan.

GENTIANA COMPLEX ™

Ear Points:

- For hypertension: Depression groove in the back of the ear to lower blood pressure, Prostate Gland. Use magnetic ear seeds. Switch ear every five days. Patient should be advised to massage the points until he/she feels a hot or distended sensation.
- For hypertension: Adrenal gland, bleed the depression groove in the back of the ear to lower blood pressure, Heart, *Shenmen*, Endocrine, *Taiyang*, Liver, Kidney. Select four or five points for each treatment, which lasts three days. Ten treatments equal one treatment course. Rest for one week in between treatment courses.
- Eczema of the rectum: Rectum, Anus, Spleen, Lung, and Adrenal Gland. Embed steel balls or ear needle and switch ears every three to five days. Instruct the patient to massage the points three to four times daily for two minutes each time.

Auricular Acupuncture by Dr. Li-Chun Huang:

- Hypertension: Decrease Blood Pressure Point, *Shenmen*, Kidney, Liver, Heart, Occiput, Forehead, Sympathetic, and Coronary Vascular Subcortex. Bleed Ear Apex.
- For additional information on the location and explanation of these points, please refer to *Auricular Treatment Formula and Prescriptions* by Dr. Li-Chun Huang.

MODERN RESEARCH

Gentiana Complex is formulated based on one of the most frequently used Chinese herbal formulas that drain damp-heat from the Liver and Gallbladder channels. Historically, it had a wide range of clinical applications including, but not limited to, hypertension, migraine headaches, eczema, intercostal neuralgia, gallstones, conjunctivitis, corneal ulcers, acute glaucoma, central retinitis, suppurative otitis media, herpes zoster, herpes simplex, cystitis, pelvic inflammatory disease and hyperthyroidism.[1] Because *Gentiana Complex* has a wide range of clinical applications, its ingredients also have a wide variety of therapeutic functions.

Long Dan Cao (Radix Gentianae) has demonstrated excellent antibiotic effects. It has been found to be active against many common pathogenic bacteria and malarial parasites.[2] It also has specific antifungal activity and inhibits the growth of human pathogenic yeast such as *Candida albicans*.[3] In addition, *Long Dan Cao* (Radix Gentianae) exhibits antibiotic effects to kill bacteria and antipyretic effects to lower fever.[4]

Huang Qin (Radix Scutellariae) also has a wide range of therapeutic actions. It has a broad-spectrum of antimicrobial effects against *Staphylococcus*, *Pseudomonas*, *Streptococcus* and *Neisseria*.[2] It also showed clear antifungal activities, especially against *Candida albicans*, *Cryptococcus neoformans* and *Pityrosporum ovale*.[5] Furthermore, it can be used to treat viral infections. One study shows that *Huang Qin* (Radix Scutellariae) starts to suppress the replication of influenza viruses within 6 to 12 hours.[6] Another study shows that *Huang Qin* (Radix Scutellariae) starts to reduce replication of influenza viruses within 4 to 12 hours in a dose-dependent manner.[7] In addition to its broad antibiotic effects, *Huang Qin* (Radix Scutellariae) also has excellent anti-inflammatory activities. One study concluded that the effectiveness of *Huang Qin* (Radix Scutellariae) is comparable to indomethacin, one of the strongest non-steroidal anti-inflammatory drugs.[8]

Zhi Zi (Fructus Gardeniae) has a wide range of therapeutic effects including antihypertensive, antibiotic and anti-inflammatory.[2] It was found to have long-lasting effects in lowering the blood pressure, antibiotic effects against pathogenic tinea and other fungal organisms, and anti-inflammatory effects in treating soft tissue injuries.[2,9]

PHARMACEUTICAL DRUGS & CHINESE MEDICINE: A COMPARATIVE ANALYSIS

Western Medical Approach: Hypertension is one of the most common disorders in developed countries. In western medicine, many different categories of drugs may be used to treat hypertension, including but not limited to diuretics

GENTIANA COMPLEX ™

[Lasix (Furosemide) and hydrochlorothiazide], beta-blockers [Tenormin (Atenolol) and Inderal (Propranolol)], calcium channel blockers [Procardia (Nifedipine) and Calan (Verapamil)], ACE inhibitors [Vasotec (Enalapril)] and Capoten (Captopril)], and vasodilators [hydralazine and minoxidil]. All these drugs have benefits and risks, and may be given individually or in combinations to control blood pressure. The main advantage of drug therapy is its potency to suppress blood pressure. The main disadvantages, however, are that the drugs cause a great number of side effects, and they do not change the underlying constitution of the patient. Therefore, while they are effective to suppress blood pressure, they must be used continually and cannot be stopped. Discontinuing use of drugs often leads to rebound hypertension.

Traditional Chinese Medicine Approach: Hypertension may be characterized by both excess and deficiency. Excess refers to Liver yang rising, and deficiency refers to Liver and Kidney yin deficiencies. Both conditions may be treated effectively with herbal medicine. The main advantage of using herbs is the effective ability to change the fundamental constitution of the body, thereby achieving long-term efficacy to reduce blood pressure, even after the herbs are discontinued. The main disadvantage, however, is that herbs are less immediately potent than drugs for treatment of hypertensive crisis, and should not be used in lieu of drugs for these cases or for individuals with secondary hypertension.

Summation: Both drugs and herbs are effective to treat hypertension, and they have their distinct advantages and disadvantages. In addition to choosing either drugs or herbal therapy, it is also important to make diet and lifestyle changes to ensure successful long-term management of hypertension.

CASE STUDIES

A 27-year-old female with a history of genital warts due to HPV (Human Papilloma Virus) presented with small growths around the perineum. The patient reported this as the third or fourth outbreak. After six rounds of *Gentiana Complex,* three capsules, three times daily, the patient reported that the genital warts were completely resolved. Furthermore, the patient did not suffer from another outbreak for nine years following this treatment.

C.L., Chino Hills, California

L.L., a 56-year-old female, presented with frustration, anger and sadness over losing her home in the hurricanes. She was unable to move through these emotions. She was also diagnosed with hypertension, high cholesterol, and post-traumatic stress syndrome recently, and refused to take medications. Her blood pressure was 138/78 mmHg and her heart rate was 82 beats per minute. She also suffered from headaches in the temporal region and the vertex. Other symptoms included twitching of the eyes, agitation, red eyes, and a scalloped tongue with thick yellow tongue coating. TCM diagnoses were damp-heat in the Liver and Gallbladder, Kidney yin deficiency, and excess fire and wind rising. She was prescribed the following formulas: *Calm (ES)* at 1 to 3 capsules, as needed, *Cholisma* at 4 capsules twice daily, and *Gentiana Complex* at 5 capsules twice daily. The patient gained control of her emotions immediately after taking *Calm (ES)*. Blood pressure gradually reduced over time to 120/72 mmHg. The practitioner commented that the combination of these formulas are phenomenal.

M.H., West Palm Beach, Florida

A 27-year-old female health care provider presented with genital herpes. The affected area in the genital region was itchy, red and swollen with thick white discharge. She was also having menstrual pain. Her pulse was slippery, deep and strong. Her tongue was pale purple with a red tip, and the sides were swollen with scalloped edges. The practitioner diagnosed the condition as damp-heat in the Liver and Liver qi stagnation. After taking *Nourish* and *Gentiana Complex*, there was a decrease in symptoms. Symptoms flared up when the patient stopped using the formulas.

B.H., Pearl City, Hawaii

FORMULAS

GENTIANA COMPLEX ™

A 36-year-old female patient presented with a yeast infection characterized by vaginal itching for two days. The TCM diagnosis was damp-heat in the lower *jiao*. *Gentiana Complex* was prescribed at three capsules, three times daily. Within a couple of doses, the patient reported that both the vaginal discharge and itching were resolved.

C.L., Chino Hills, California

A.T., a 34-year-old female, had a history of oral herpes outbreaks that usually lasted 2 to 3 weeks. She presented with tingling sensations of the lips, progressing to burning sensations, with eruption of fever blisters. The TCM diagnosis was damp-heat in the middle *jiao* with Stomach fire. *Gentiana Complex* was prescribed at three capsules, three times daily. After one or two doses, the patient reported the symptoms were relieved without further exacerbation of fever blisters. Furthermore, there was no return of or spread of lesions to other areas of the lips. *Gentiana Complex* was discontinued after only three days.

C.L., Chino Hills, California

A 41-year-old female presented with headaches that had been persistent for almost two weeks. She noted that her headache was more localized to the top of her head. Aside from the headaches, she also reported having large amounts of yellowish, foul-smelling, vaginal discharge. The practitioner diagnosed her condition as damp-heat in the lower *jiao* with underlying excess Liver fire. Within two weeks of taking *Gentiana Complex*, the fetid discharge had stopped along with the headaches. Although the patient experienced some diarrhea during the first three days of treatment, her condition improved overall.

T.G., Albuquerque, New Mexico

E.P., a 32-year-old female, presented with a 2½-year history of vertigo, associated with insomnia, palpitations, anxiety and nausea. She also suffered from irritable bowel syndrome with alternating diarrhea and constipation. She had an unsteady gait and was unable to drive. For the Western diagnosis of anxiety disorder, the TCM diagnosis was Liver fire. Initially, *Calm* and *Gentiana Complex* were prescribed at two capsules each, three times daily, but then the dosage was increased to three capsules of each, three times daily. After three weeks, the signs and symptoms of irritable bowel syndrome were resolved, and *Gentiana Complex* was discontinued. On the sixth treatment, the patient reported all symptoms improved. However, work-related stress anxiety remained. On the 15th visit, *Calm* was changed to *Schisandra ZZZ* to help with her insomnia. After taking this formula for nine days, the patient reported much improvement in her sleeping patterns, from 5 to 6 hours of interrupted sleep to 6 to 7 hours of uninterrupted sleep. The patient was treated with acupuncture five times throughout the course of herbal treatment.

C.L., Chino Hills, California

[1] Bensky, D. et al. *Chinese Herbal Medicine Formulas and Strategies*. Eastland Press. 1990
[2] Bensky, D. et al. *Chinese Herbal Medicine Materia Medica*. Eastland Press. 1993
[3] Tan, RX. et al. *Phytochemistry*. July 1996
[4] Hsu, HY. et al. *Oriental Materia Medica A Concise Guide*. Oriental Healing Arts Institute. 1986
[5] Yang, D. et al. Anti-fungal activity in vitro of scutellaria baicalensis. *Ann Pharm Fr*; 1995; 53(3):138-41
[6] Nagai, T. et al. Antiviral activity of plant flavonoid, 5,7,4-trihydroxy-8-methoxyflavone, from scutellaria baicalensis against influenza A (H3N2) and B viruses. *Biol Pharm Bull*; Feb 1995; 18(2):195-9.
[7] Nagai, T. et al. Mode of action of the anti-influenza virus activity of plant flavonoid, 5,7,4-trihydroxy-8-methoxyflavone, from the roots of scutellaria baicalensis. *Antiviral Res*; Jan 1995; 26(1):11-25.
[8] *Chem Pharm Bull*, 1984; 32(7):2724
[9] Yao, Q. et al. Screening studies on anti-inflammatory function of traditional Chinese herb gardenia jasminoides ellis and its possibility in treating soft tissue injuries in animals. *Chung Kuo Chung Yao Tsa Chih*, Aug. 1991; 16(8):489-93' 513
[9] Gottlieb, W, *The Doctor's Book of Home Remedies*. 1990, p. 301

GENTLE LAX (Deficient) ™

CLINICAL APPLICATIONS

- Constipation
- Deficient, chronic or habitual constipation with red tongue, pale or sallow face
- Constipation in postpartum, postsurgical, or convalescing individuals
- Mild colon cleanser

WESTERN THERAPEUTIC ACTIONS

- Emollient effect to lubricate the bowel and moisten the intestines [1,2]
- Laxative effect to relieve mild to moderate constipation [1,2]
- Treats chronic constipation associated with hemorrhoids by reducing inflammation and dilating the varicose veins [1,2]

CHINESE THERAPEUTIC ACTIONS

- Moistens the intestines
- Unblocks the bowels
- Drains heat
- Nourishes yin and blood

DOSAGE

Take 4 capsules three times daily on an empty stomach with warm water. Individuals with sensitive gastrointestinal tracts should decrease the dosage and increase the dosing frequency to avoid stomach discomfort. For example, instead of taking 4 capsules three times daily, take 2 capsules four or five times daily.

INGREDIENTS

Bai Shao (Radix Paeoniae Alba)
Bai Zi Ren (Semen Platycladi)
Da Huang (Radix et Rhizoma Rhei)
Dang Gui Wei (Extremitas Radicis Angelicae Sinensis)
He Shou Wu (Radix Polygoni Multiflori)
Hou Po (Cortex Magnoliae Officinalis)
Jue Ming Zi (Semen Cassiae)

Mai Men Dong (Radix Ophiopogonis)
Tao Ren (Semen Persicae)
Xing Ren (Semen Armeniacae Amarum)
Xuan Shen (Radix Scrophulariae)
Yu Li Ren (Semen Pruni)
Zhi Shi (Fructus Aurantii Immaturus)

FORMULA EXPLANATION

Gentle Lax (Deficient) is a mild formula suitable for deficient-type constipation. Deficient-type constipation is defined as chronic or habitual constipation, constipation in geriatric patients, or constipation in patients with red tongue, pale or sallow face, and general signs and symptoms of weakness.

Yu Li Ren (Semen Pruni) and *Bai Zi Ren* (Semen Platycladi) moisten the intestines and unblock the bowels. *Xing Ren* (Semen Armeniacae Amarum) and *Tao Ren* (Semen Persicae) lubricate the large intestine and direct qi downward. *Zhi Shi* (Fructus Aurantii Immaturus) and *Hou Po* (Cortex Magnoliae Officinalis) dissipate stagnation and reduce distention and bloating. *Xuan Shen* (Radix Scrophulariae) and *Mai Men Dong* (Radix Ophiopogonis) clear heat, cool the blood and nourish the yin. *Bai Shao* (Radix Paeoniae Alba) nourishes blood and relieves pain, which may be associated with constipation. *Da Huang* (Radix et Rhizoma Rhei) is a purgative that clears toxic heat

GENTLE LAX (Deficient) ™

lodged in the intestines. *Jue Ming Zi* (Semen Cassiae) moistens the intestines and facilitates the passage of stools. *Dang Gui Wei* (Extremitas Radicis Angelicae Sinensis) and *He Shou Wu* (Radix Polygoni Multiflori) enrich blood and act as gentle laxatives by moistening the desiccated intestines.

SUPPLEMENTARY FORMULAS

- ❧ For constipation due to stress, add **Calm**.
- ❧ For insomnia due to disturbed *shen* (spirit), combine with **Calm (ES)**.
- ❧ For gastrointestinal disorders such as acid reflux or ulcers, use **GI Care** instead.
- ❧ For irritable bowel syndrome (IBS), use **GI Harmony**.
- ❧ For ulcerative colitis, use **GI Care (UC)** instead.
- ❧ For hemorrhoids and pain, add **GI Care (HMR)** and **Herbal Analgesic**.
- ❧ To tonify blood, combine with **Schisandra ZZZ**.
- ❧ For dry, brittle hair, combine with **Polygonum 14**.
- ❧ For constipation due to neurodegenerative disorders, Alzheimer's, Parkinson's and stroke, use **Neuro Plus**.
- ❧ With excess fire, add **Gardenia Complex**.
- ❧ For rectal bleeding, add **Notoginseng 9**.
- ❧ For severe blood stagnation, add **Circulation (SJ)**.
- ❧ For constipation in postpartum women with deficiency, add **Imperial Tonic**.
- ❧ For constipation and postpartum depression, add **Shine**.

NUTRITION

- ❧ Eat plenty of foods with high fiber, such as fresh fruits, green leafy vegetables, cabbage, peas, sweet potatoes, and whole grains.
- ❧ Avoid fried foods. Follow a low-fat diet.
- ❧ Drink plenty of water, at least 8 glasses per day.
- ❧ Avoid fatty and spicy foods that may irritate the mucous membranes of the intestines.
- ❧ Prunes or prune juice are very effective to regulate bowels and relieve mild cases of constipation.
- ❧ A combination of wild honey with fresh grapefruit will also relieve dry stool or constipation.
- ❧ Black sesame with wild honey is a helpful combination to soften stool and facilitate bowel movement.

The Tao of Nutrition by Ni and McNease
- ❧ Recommendations: bananas, apples, walnuts, figs, spinach, peaches, pears, pine nuts, sesame seeds, mulberries, grapefruit, yams, honey, apricot kernel, milk, yogurt, alfalfa sprouts, beets, cabbage, bok-choy, cauliflower, and potato.
- ❧ Avoid stress, tension, spicy foods, fried foods, and meat.
- ❧ For more information, please refer to *The Tao of Nutrition* by Dr. Maoshing Ni and Cathy McNease.

LIFESTYLE INSTRUCTIONS

- ❧ Avoid stress whenever possible.
- ❧ Exercise regularly to increase peristalsis of the intestines. Walking is one of the best exercises as it massages the intestines to regulate the bowels.
- ❧ Do not suppress the urge to relieve bowels. Suppressing the urge is one of the main causes of chronic constipation. Empty the bowel whenever there is a desire, especially in the morning when the digestive system is most active.
- ❧ Massaging the abdomen along the directional flow of the large intestine will also help.
- ❧ Patients with hemorrhoids should not lift anything heavy.

FORMULAS

GENTLE LAX (Deficient) ™

CAUTIONS

❦ Individuals with a sensitive gastrointestinal tract should take this formula with caution, as it may be irritating to the stomach and intestinal mucosa. Those who experience stomach discomfort should reduce the dosage and take the herbs with food.

❦ This formula is contraindicated during pregnancy and nursing.

❦ Patients who are on anticoagulant or antiplatelet therapies, such as Coumadin (Warfarin), should use this formula with caution, as there may be a slightly higher risk of bleeding and bruising.

ACUPUNCTURE POINTS

Traditional Points:

❦ *Zhigou* (TH 6) and *Zhaohai* (KI 6).

❦ *Qihai* (CV 6), *Zhongwan* (CV 12), *Geshu* (BL 17), *Renzhong* (GV 26), *Zhigou* (TH 6), *Tianshu* (ST 25), *Taichong* (LR 3), *Zusanli* (ST 36), and *Dachangshu* (BL 25)

Balance Method by Dr. Richard Tan:

❦ Left side: *Waiguan* (TH 5), *Zhigou* (TH 6), *Zhaohai* (KI 6), and *Hegu* (LI 4).

❦ Right side: *Zusanli* (ST 36), *Shangjuxu* (ST 37), and *Kongzui* (LU 6) or *ah shi* points nearby.

❦ Left and right side can be alternated from treatment to treatment.

❦ For additional information on the Balance Method, please refer to *Dr. Tan's Strategy of Twelve Magical Points* by Dr. Richard Tan.

Ear Points:

❦ Large Intestine, Colon, Rectum, and Sympathetic. Tape magnetic balls onto the points and switch ears every three days. If both ears are taped at the same time, rest 1 day in between the three-day treatments.

❦ Large Intestine, Rectum. Strong stimulation is necessary twice or three times daily. Leave the needles in for one hour. Embed ear seeds in Spleen, Large Intestine and Rectum. Switch ear every week.

Auricular Acupuncture by Dr. Li-Chun Huang:

❦ Constipation: Large Intestine, Sigmoid, Liver, Spleen, Lung, *San Jiao*, and Digestive Subcortex.

❦ For additional information on the location and explanation of these points, please refer to *Auricular Treatment Formula and Prescriptions* by Dr. Li-Chun Huang.

MODERN RESEARCH

Gentle Lax (Deficient) is composed of herbs with mild laxative functions to promote regular bowel movements in individuals who have chronic or habitual constipation.

Da Huang (Radix et Rhizoma Rhei) is a purgative that generally induces bowel movement within 6 to 8 hours after oral ingestion. It works mainly on the transverse and descending colon as it inhibits the re-absorption of water and causes the evacuation of the stool.[1,2] In addition, it increases peristalsis of the large intestine without interfering with absorption of nutrients in the small intestines.[3]

Bai Zi Ren (Semen Platycladi) also has laxative effects, as its fatty oil content stimulates the mucosa and increases peristalsis of the intestines.[1] *He Shou Wu* (Radix Polygoni Multiflori), containing emodin and rhein as two active ingredients, also has mild laxative effects.[1] *Da Huang* (Radix et Rhizoma Rhei) and *He Shou Wu* (Radix Polygoni Multiflori) are used in small dosages to promote normal bowel movement without causing paradoxical diarrhea.

FORMULAS

GENTLE LAX (Deficient) ™

PHARMACEUTICAL DRUGS & CHINESE MEDICINE: A COMPARATIVE ANALYSIS

Western Medical Approach: Constipation is a very common problem that may be treated effectively using western and traditional Chinese medicine. In western medicine, bulking agents (bran, psyllium and methylcellulose) are the gentlest and safest. These drugs are not habit forming, and may be used safely on a long-term basis. However, they act slowly and are not very strong. Laxatives (docusate and mineral oil) soften the stool by increasing the implementation of intestinal water. However, these drugs must be used carefully, as they interfere with absorption of nutrients and other drugs. Lastly, cathartics (senna, cascara, and bisacodyl) are used for severe cases of constipation by increasing intestinal peristalsis and intraluminal fluids. However, these drugs should only be used on a short-term basis, as prolonged use will cause "lazy bowel" syndrome and serious fluid and electrolyte imbalance.

Traditional Chinese Medicine Approach: Constipation may be treated with great success. Those with mild to moderate constipation are usually treated with herbs that moisten the intestines and regulate bowel movement. Those with moderate to severe constipation are generally treated with herbs that purge the intestines and induce bowel movement. These formulas should be used as needed, and discontinued when desired effects are achieved. Herbal formulas that contain *Da Huang* (Radix et Rhizoma Rhei) should be taken with meals, as it may irritate the stomach if taken on an empty stomach. Prolonged use of formula with *Da Huang* (Radix et Rhizoma Rhei) is not recommended, as it may increase the risk of habitual constipation and fluid and electrolyte imbalance.

Summation: Both drugs and herbs are equally effective in treating constipation. Both modalities of medicines should be used sparingly, and when needed, as prolonged use may cause side effects. Once bowel movement is induced, herbal therapy may be initiated to change the fundamental constitution of the body in those with habitual constipation. Lastly, diet and lifestyle adjustments are also needed to ensure regular bowel movement.

CASE STUDIES

A 32-year-old female presented with chronic constipation, which started since her early teens. Her bowel movements had occurred every three to four days. The practitioner diagnosed her condition as Spleen qi deficiency. After taking *Gentle Lax (Deficient)*, her bowel movements became daily and regular. She noted that using *Gentle Lax (deficient)* did not cause a feeling of fullness. After two months, her bowel movements have maintained a regular and daily schedule.

S.T., San Jose, California

A 49-year-old female teacher presented with constipation with gas as her chief complaint. Other signs and symptoms included bloating, low back pain, stress, anger, irritability and fatigue. Her overall condition was indicative of irritable bowel syndrome. The practitioner attributed the patient's constipation and gas to Liver qi stagnation. The patient was previously treated with a combination of *Xiao Yao San* (Rambling Powder) and *Ma Zi Ren Wan* (Hemp Seed Pill) with little success. Once the practitioner substituted *Gentle Lax (Deficient)* and *GI Care*, the patient's chief complaint abated. Her stress level lessened as well.

D.M., Raton, New Mexico

F.L., a 53-year-old female patient, presented with recent history of TIA (transient ischemic attack). Objective findings included right-sided pulling and numbness of the face with difficulty smiling and closing the right eye, as well as drooping of facial muscles on the right side when smiling, and partial facial flaccidity. Treatment using three capsules of *Circulation,* three times daily, was successful: no recurring episodes were noted during subsequent follow-up visits. This patient also had constipation with hard, difficult to move stools, abdominal pain, and cramps with bloating. All these gastrointestinal symptoms were resolved with *Gentle Lax (Deficient)* taken at four capsules, three times daily.

C.L., Chino Hills, California

GENTLE LAX (Deficient) ™

J.N., a 68-year-old male patient, presented with constipation and bloating. His blood pressure was 176/86 mmHg and the heart rate was 54 beats per minute. The practitioner diagnosed him with constipation and bloating due to blood deficiency, dryness and from side effects of the high blood pressure medications. *Gentle Lax (Deficient)* was prescribed at 2 grams three times daily. Acupuncture was also given to balance the system. Patient reported that the formula helped him go to the bathroom daily and that it took less effort to pass stools.

W.F., Bloomfield, New Jersey

[1] Yeung, HC. *Handbook of Chinese Herbs*. Institute of Chinese Medicine. 1996
[2] Bensky, D. et al. *Chinese Herbal Medicine Materia Medica*. Eastland Press. 1993
[3] Yang, ZH. et al. *Chinese Herbology*. Zhi Yin Publishing Company. 1990.

FORMULAS

GENTLE LAX (Excess) ™

CLINICAL APPLICATIONS

- Constipation
- Excess types of constipation with red tongue, yellow tongue coat and red face
- Food stagnation or indigestion with abdominal distention and pain

WESTERN THERAPEUTIC ACTIONS

- Strong laxative effect which treats moderate-to-severe constipation [1,2]
- Emollient effect which lubricates the bowel and promotes normal peristalsis of intestines [1,2]
- Treats constipation with hemorrhoids by reducing inflammation and dilating the varicose veins [1,2]
- Increases intestinal peristalsis and removes food stagnation [3]

CHINESE THERAPEUTIC ACTIONS

- Relieves constipation
- Disperses lower abdominal distention and pain
- Purges stagnant heat accumulation

DOSAGE

Take 3 to 4 capsules three times daily with warm water. To avoid stomach discomfort for individuals with sensitive gastrointestinal tract, take the herbs with meals, or decrease dosage and increase frequency of intake. The recommended starting dosage is 2 capsules four times daily.

INGREDIENTS

Bai Shao (Radix Paeoniae Alba)
Da Huang (Radix et Rhizoma Rhei)
Fan Xie Ye (Folium Sennae)
Hou Po (Cortex Magnoliae Officinalis)

Mang Xiao (Natrii Sulfas)
Tao Ren (Semen Persicae)
Zhi Shi (Fructus Aurantii Immaturus)

FORMULA EXPLANATION

Gentle Lax (Excess) is an herbal formula designed to treat patients with excess type constipation. Excess type constipation is defined as acute constipation, constipation in young adults, constipation with abdominal distention or pain, or constipation in patients with a red tongue, red face, and yellow tongue coat.

Da Huang (Radix et Rhizoma Rhei) is a strong purgative that clears heat and detoxifies. *Mang Xiao* (Natrii Sulfas) softens and facilitates the passage of stool. *Zhi Shi* (Fructus Aurantii Immaturus) and *Hou Po* (Cortex Magnoliae Officinalis) dissipate stagnation and reduce distention. *Bai Shao* (Radix Paeoniae Alba) nourishes blood and relieves abdominal or intestinal pain, which may be associated with constipation. *Fan Xie Ye* (Folium Sennae) and *Tao Ren* (Semen Persicae) are emollients used to lubricate the large intestine to facilitate the passage of stool.

SUPPLEMENTARY FORMULAS

- For constipation due to stress, add *Calm*.
- For insomnia due to disturbed *shen* (spirit), combine with *Calm (ES)*.
- For gastrointestinal disorders such as acid reflux or ulcers, use *GI Care* instead.

GENTLE LAX (Excess) ™

- For irritable bowel syndrome (IBS), use with *GI Harmony*.
- For ulcerative colitis, use *GI Care (UC)* instead.
- For hemorrhoids and pain, add *GI Care (HMR)* and *Herbal Analgesic*.
- For hemorrhoid bleeding, add *GI Care (HMR)* and *Notoginseng 9*.
- For hypertension, add *Gastrodia Complex*.
- To help with detoxification, add *Liver DTX*.
- For constipation due to neuro-degenerative disorders such as Alzheimer's disease, Parkinson's disease or stroke, use with *Neuro Plus*.
- With excess fire, add *Gardenia Complex*.
- For severe blood stagnation, add *Circulation (SJ)*.

NUTRITION

- Eat plenty of foods with high fiber, such as fresh fruits, green leafy vegetables, cabbage, peas, sweet potatoes, and whole grains.
- Avoid fried foods. Follow a low-fat diet.
- Drink plenty of water, at least 8 glasses per day.
- Avoid fatty and spicy foods, which may irritate the mucous membranes of the intestines.
- A combination of honey with grapefruit will also relieve dry stool or constipation.
- Prunes or prune juice are very effective to regulate bowels and relieve mild cases of constipation.
- Long-term use of laxatives wipes out the normal flora of the intestines and leads to frequent constipation and/or secondary infections. Therefore, if purgatives are to be used for a prolonged period of time, acidophilus should also be used to replace the "good" intestinal flora.

The Tao of Nutrition by Ni and McNease
- Recommendations: bananas, apples, walnuts, figs, spinach, peaches, pears, pine nuts, sesame seeds, mulberries, grapefruit, yams, honey, apricot kernel, milk, yogurt, alfalfa sprouts, beets, cabbage, bok-choy, cauliflower, and potato.
- Avoid stress, tension, spicy foods, fried foods, and meat.
- For more information, please refer to *The Tao of Nutrition* by Dr. Maoshing Ni and Cathy McNease.

LIFESTYLE INSTRUCTIONS

- Avoid stress whenever possible.
- Exercise regularly to increase peristalsis of the intestines. Walking is one of the best exercises as it massages the intestines to regulate the bowels.
- Do not suppress the urge to relieve bowels. Suppressing the urge is one of the main causes of chronic constipation. Empty the bowel whenever there is a desire, especially in the morning when the digestive system is most active.
- Massaging the abdomen along the directional flow of the large intestine will also help.
- Patients with hemorrhoids should not lift anything heavy.

CAUTIONS

- This is a strong herbal formula that should be reserved for those with severe constipation. Stop taking the herbs when the desired effect is achieved. Long-term use of *Gentle Lax (Excess)* is not recommended as it may cause diarrhea and dehydration. *Gentle Lax (Deficient)* is the herbal formula of choice if the patient has chronic or habitual constipation.

GENTLE LAX (Excess) ™

   ❧ *Gentle Lax (Excess)* may be irritating to the intestinal mucosa. Patients should take this formula with caution by starting with a lower dosage or taking it with food.

   ❧ Patients with intestinal obstruction should be referred to a medical doctor for immediate help. Surgical intervention may be necessary in some cases.

   ❧ Patients with hemorrhoids should only take *Gentle Lax (Excess)* to relieve constipation. Should more bleeding occur, stop taking the formula immediately and switch to *Notoginseng 9* instead.

   ❧ This formula is contraindicated during pregnancy and nursing.

ACUPUNCTURE POINTS

Traditional Points:
   ❧ *Tianshu* (ST 25) and *Shangjuxu* (ST 37).
   ❧ *Tianshu* (ST 25), *Dachangshu* (BL 25), *Zusanli* (ST 36), *Hegu* (LI 4), *Zhigou* (TH 6), *Taichong* (LR 3), and *Xingjian* (LR 2).

Balance Method by Dr. Richard Tan:
   ❧ Left side: *Waiguan* (TH 5), *Zhigou* (TH 6), *Zhaohai* (KI 6), and *Quchi* (LI 11).
   ❧ Right side: *Shangjuxu* (ST 37), *Tiaokou* (ST 38), *Kongzui* (LU 6) or *ah shi* points nearby, *Quze* (PC 3).
   ❧ Left and right side can be alternated from treatment to treatment.
   ❧ For additional information on the Balance Method, please refer to *Dr. Tan's Strategy of Twelve Magical Points* by Dr. Richard Tan.

Ear Points:
   ❧ Large Intestine, Colon, Rectum, Sympathetic. Tape magnetic balls onto the points and switch ears every three days. If both ears are taped at the same time, rest one day in between the three-day treatments.
   ❧ Large Intestine, Rectum. Strong stimulation is necessary twice or three times daily. Leave the needles in for one hour. Embed ears seeds in Spleen, Large Intestine and Rectum. Switch ear every week.

Auricular Acupuncture by Dr. Li-Chun Huang:
   ❧ Constipation: Large Intestine, Sigmoid, Liver, Spleen, Lung, *San Jiao*, and Digestive Subcortex.
   ❧ For additional information on the location and explanation of these points, please refer to *Auricular Treatment Formula and Prescriptions* by Dr. Li-Chun Huang.

MODERN RESEARCH

Gentle Lax (Excess) is composed of herbs with moderate-to-strong laxative functions to promote regular bowel movements in individuals who have acute or stubborn constipation. *Da Huang* (Radix et Rhizoma Rhei) is a strong purgative that generally induces a bowel movement within 6 to 8 hours after oral ingestion. It works mainly on the transverse and descending colon as it inhibits the re-absorption of water and causes evacuation of the stool.[1,2] In addition, it increases peristalsis of the large intestine without interfering with absorption of nutrients in the small intestine.[3]

Mang Xiao (Natrii Sulfas) is commonly used with *Da Huang* (Radix et Rhizoma Rhei) in cases of severe constipation. *Mang Xiao* (Natrii Sulfas) treats constipation via osmosis. It is not absorbed systemically; instead, it remains in the intestines, increases the water content, and stimulates peristalsis. *Mang Xiao* (Natrii Sulfas) works best when it is taken with plenty of extra fluid.[2]

GENTLE LAX (Excess) ™

Fan Xie Ye (Folium Sennae) also has laxative effects as it increases peristalsis of the intestines.[1] Lastly, *Hou Po* (Cortex Magnoliae Officinalis) has an excitatory effect on the smooth muscles of the gastrointestinal tract. It promotes strong, forceful, and rhythmic peristalsis. [1]

PHARMACEUTICAL DRUGS & CHINESE MEDICINE: A COMPARATIVE ANALYSIS

Western Medical Approach: Constipation is a very common problem that may be treated effectively using western and traditional Chinese medicine. In western medicine, bulking agents (bran, psyllium and methylcellulose) are the gentlest and safest. These drugs are not habit forming, and may be used safely on a long-term basis. However, they act slowly and are not very strong. Laxatives (docusate and mineral oil) soften stool by increasing the implementation of intestinal water. However, these drugs must be used carefully, as they interfere with absorption of nutrients and other drugs. Lastly, cathartics (senna, cascara, and bisacodyl) are used for severe cases of constipation by increasing intestinal peristalsis and intraluminal fluids. However, these drugs should only be used on a short-term basis, as prolonged use will cause "lazy bowel" syndrome and serious fluid and electrolyte imbalance.

Traditional Chinese Medicine Approach: Constipation may be treated with great success. Those with mild to moderate constipation are usually treated with herbs that moisten the intestines and regulate bowel movement. Those with moderate to severe constipation are generally treated herbs that purge the intestines and induce bowel movement. These formulas should be used as needed, and discontinued when the desired effects have been achieved. Herbal formulas that contain *Da Huang* (Radix et Rhizoma Rhei) should be taken with meals, as it may irritate the stomach if taken on an empty stomach. Prolonged use of formulas with *Da Huang* (Radix et Rhizoma Rhei) are not recommended, as this may increase the risk of habitual constipation and fluid and electrolyte imbalance.

Summation: Both drugs and herbs are equally effective in treating constipation. Both modalities of medicines should be used sparingly, and when needed, as prolonged use may cause side effects. Once bowel movement is induced, herbal therapy may be initiated to change the fundamental constitution of the body in those with habitual constipation. Lastly, diet and lifestyle adjustments are also needed to ensure regular bowel movement.

CASE STUDIES

A 63-year-old retired male presented with lower abdominal pain, abdominal swelling, foul-smelling flatulence and constipation persistent for almost three days. His diet consisted of large amounts of chili. His tongue body appeared red with a thick, white, dry, tongue coating. His pulse was noted to be deep, "rolling," and wiry. Pain was elicited upon abdominal palpation. The practitioner diagnosed his condition as excess heat in the Large Intestine. Bowel movement was induced after three doses of *Gentle Lax (Excess)*. The herbal treatment was continued for another week with smaller doses. The patient soon experienced a daily bowel movement activity.

T.G., Albuquerque, New Mexico

A 50-year-old female patient presented with bowel obstruction and constipation that had persisted for five or six days. On a scale of severity of 1 to 10, with one being minimal or no severity, the patient described her condition as 10+. The TCM diagnosis was qi deficiency with internal heat. After beginning to take four capsules of *Gentle Lax (Excess)* four times daily, she had a bowel movement the next day. Dosage was then reduced to three capsules, three times daily until bowel functioning normalized.

M.C., Sarasota, Florida

[1] Yeung, HC. *Handbook of Chinese Herbs*. Institute of Chinese Medicine. 1996
[2] Bensky, D. et al. *Chinese Herbal Medicine Materia Medica*. Eastland Press. 1993
[3] Yang, ZH. et al. *Chinese Herbology*. Zhi Yin Publishing Company. 1990.

FORMULAS

GI CARE ™

CLINICAL APPLICATIONS

- Gastric or duodenal ulcers
- Stress ulcers
- Gastritis
- Acid reflux with heartburn, foul breath, bitter taste in the mouth, indigestion
- Generalized gastrointestinal (GI) disorders, such as nausea, vomiting, indigestion, belching, bloating, epigastric fullness, bloating, food sensitivities and others.

WESTERN THERAPEUTIC ACTIONS

- Restores normal gastrointestinal functions [1]
- Promotes smooth and complete digestion [1]
- Antacid effect which relieves heartburn and treats ulcers [1,6]
- Antispasmodic effect to stop pain and relieve intestinal cramps [1]
- Antibiotic effect against *Helicobacter pylori* [6]

CHINESE THERAPEUTIC ACTIONS

- Quells Stomach fire
- Spreads Liver qi stagnation and relieves pain
- Strengthens middle *jiao* to promote digestion

DOSAGE

Take 4 capsules three times daily on an empty stomach one to two hours before meals. For maximum effect, advise the patient to lie down for 10 minutes following ingestion of *GI Care*.

INGREDIENTS

Bai Hua She She Cao (Herba Oldenlandia)
Bai Shao (Radix Paeoniae Alba)
Chai Hu (Radix Bupleuri)
Di Yu (Radix Sanguisorbae)
Hai Piao Xiao (Endoconcha Sepiae)
Huang Lian (Rhizoma Coptidis)
Huang Qi (Radix Astragali)
Huang Qin (Radix Scutellariae)

Pu Gong Ying (Herba Taraxaci)
Sha Ren (Fructus Amomi)
Shen Qu (Massa Fermentata)
Wu Bei Zi (Galla Chinensis)
Wu Zhu Yu (Fructus Evodiae)
Xiang Fu (Rhizoma Cyperi)
Yan Hu Suo (Rhizoma Corydalis)
Zhe Bei Mu (Bulbus Fritillariae Thunbergii)

FORMULA EXPLANATION

Gastrointestinal disorders are often associated with emotional stress. According to the Five-Element Theory of traditional Chinese medicine, these conditions have excess fire lodging in the Liver and the Stomach, and the symptoms are typical of "wood overacting on earth."

Huang Lian (Rhizoma Coptidis) drains fire from the Stomach and the Liver. *Wu Zhu Yu* (Fructus Evodiae) directs the Stomach qi downward to treat vomiting, nausea and acid regurgitation. *Hai Piao Xiao* (Endoconcha Sepiae), *Bai Shao* (Radix Paeoniae Alba), and *Zhe Bei Mu* (Bulbus Fritillariae Thunbergii) are used to neutralize excessive stomach acid and ease heartburn. *Yan Hu Suo* (Rhizoma Corydalis) has anti-ulceration effects as well as strong analgesic effects similar to those of morphine and codeine. *Huang Qin* (Radix Scutellariae), *Bai Hua She She Cao* (Herba Oldenlandia), and *Pu Gong Ying* (Herba Taraxaci) have antibacterial effects that clear heat and detoxify. *Huang Qin* (Radix Scutellariae) has also been shown through research to be effective against *Helicobacter pylori*, a bacteria known to cause gastric ulcers. *Huang Qi* (Radix Astragali) tonifies the Spleen, augments the qi and is essential in rebuilding the gastrointestinal system. *Sha Ren* (Fructus Amomi) promotes the movement of qi, strengthens the Stomach and helps with gastrointestinal symptoms such as abdominal distention, pain, nausea, and diarrhea. *Di Yu* (Radix Sanguisorbae) and *Wu Bei Zi* (Galla Chinensis) provide a coating for the stomach and are used to stop bleeding, generate flesh and expedite the recovery of peptic and duodenal ulcers. *Shen Qu* (Massa Fermentata) aids digestion. *Chai Hu* (Radix Bupleuri) and *Xiang Fu* (Rhizoma Cyperi) spread the constrained Liver qi and relieve abdominal pain and distention.

SUPPLEMENTARY FORMULAS

- For irritability, nervousness, and/or anxiety, add **Calm**.
- For severe restlessness and stress, add **Calm (ES)**.
- For restlessness, stress, and insomnia with underlying deficiency, add **Calm ZZZ**.
- For irritable bowel syndrome (IBS), use **GI Harmony**.
- For excess fire, add **Gardenia Complex**.
- For bleeding, add **Notoginseng 9**.
- For ulcerative colitis, use **GI Care (UC)** instead.
- To tonify the constitution of the body and nourish blood, combine with **Schisandra ZZZ** or **Imperial Tonic**.
- For constipation, combine with **Gentle Lax (Excess) or Gentle Lax (Deficient)**.
- For hemorrhoids, add **GI Care (HMR)**.
- For nausea, vomiting and poor appetite due to chemotherapy, use **C/R Support** instead.
- For excess appetite, obesity, combine with **Herbalite**.
- For gallbladder disorders such as cholecystitis or gallstones, combine with **Dissolve (GS)**.
- For hepatic disorders such as hepatitis or liver cirrhosis, combine with **Liver DTX**.

NUTRITION

- Drinking a large amount of water often helps when the first sign of heartburn appears.
- Increase the intake of papayas and pineapples as they contain bromelain, a digestive enzyme that helps with indigestion. Acidophilus is also helpful for digestion. Avoid lentils, peanuts and soybeans because they contain enzyme inhibitors.
- Avoid fried, spicy or greasy foods, refined sugar, tea, coffee, caffeine, salt, chocolate, strong spices, and carbonated drinks. Stay away from sour and acidic food and fruits.
- For ulcers, intake of vitamin K, found in green leafy vegetables, should be increased as it helps with the healing process.
- Individuals who cannot tolerate raw vegetables can drink vegetable and fruit juices instead.
- Avoid consumption of alcohol completely. Stop smoking cigarettes or avoid exposure to second-hand smoke whenever possible.
- Plan regular meals and chew slowly and thoroughly.

The Tao of Nutrition by Ni and McNease
- Peptic ulcers
  - Recommendations: potatoes, honey, cabbage, ginger, figs, papayas, squid bone, peanut oil, kale, and persimmons. Drink fig juice.
  - Avoid spicy foods, hot foods, stimulants, shellfish, coffee, smoking, alcohol, fried foods, and stress.
- For more information, please refer to *The Tao of Nutrition* by Dr. Maoshing Ni and Cathy McNease.

GI CARE ™

LIFESTYLE INSTRUCTIONS

☙ Avoid stress as it may trigger stomach discomfort. Do not eat when angry, overly tired or stressed, and always chew food thoroughly.

☙ Non-steroidal-anti-inflammatory drugs, such as aspirin and ibuprofen, should not be ingested as they are very irritating to the stomach.

☙ Infection in the oral region, emotional disturbance, and diet may trigger gastritis and should be controlled.

☙ Keep the digestive tract warm at all times. Whenever possible, place a hot compress or a hot-water bottle on the stomach.

☙ Use of antacids may suppress the symptoms of ulcer, but do not treat the cause. Do not rely on or use antacid excessively.

CLINICAL NOTES

☙ When treating gastric or duodenal ulcers, it is imperative to rule out atrophic gastritis. Ulcers and atrophic gastritis share many similar signs and symptoms. The underlying etiologies, however, are completely different. Ulcers are caused by an excessive secretion of gastric acid and must be treated by neutralizing or reducing the acid secretion. Conversely, atrophic gastritis is caused by decreased (or, lack of secretion) of gastric acid and must be treated by increasing the production of gastric acid. If untreated, atrophic gastric may lead to gastric carcinoma.

☙ Patients with ulcers induced by the use of non-steroidal anti-inflammatory drugs are often asymptomatic. These drugs cause peptic ulcers and gastrointestinal bleeding, but they mask these symptoms because they also have pain-relieving effects. Therefore, those who use these drugs on regular basis should be checked to rule out gastric or duodenal ulcers.

Pulse Diagnosis by Dr. Jimmy Wei-Yen Chang:
☙ Floating and forceful pulse on the right *guan* position.
☙ Note: Dr. Chang takes the pulse in slightly different positions. He places his index finger directly over the wrist crease, and his middle and ring fingers alongside to locate *cun*, *guan* and *chi* positions. For additional information and explanation, please refer to *Pulsynergy* by Dr. Jimmy Wei-Yen Chang and Marcus Brinkman.

CAUTIONS

☙ *GI Care* should not be used to treat patients with atrophic gastritis with decreased or lack of secretion of stomach acid. *GI Care* contains herbs that neutralize and stop the secretion of stomach acid and may worsen the condition.

☙ Patients with cholecystitis and cholelithiasis are often mis-diagnosed as having gastrointestinal problems. Correct diagnosis is critical in the overall success of the treatment.

ACUPUNCTURE POINTS

Traditional Points:
☙ *Xiangu* (ST 43), *Zhongwan* (CV 12), and *Liangqiu* (ST 34).
☙ *Zhongwan* (CV 12), *Weishu* (BL 21), *Pishu* (BL 20), *Hegu* (LI 4), *Zusanli* (ST 36), *Shenque* (CV 8), *Neiguan* (PC 6), and *Gongsun* (SP 4).

Balance Method by Dr. Richard Tan:
☙ Left side: *Waiguan* (TH 5), *Hegu* (LI 4), *Yinlingquan* (SP 9), and *Liangqiu* (ST 34).
☙ Right side: *Liangqiu* (ST 34), *Xuehai* (SP 10), and *Neiguan* (PC 6), *Lieque* (LU7).

FORMULAS

GI CARE ™

- Left and right side can be alternated from treatment to treatment.
- For additional information on the Balance Method, please refer to *Dr. Tan's Strategy of Twelve Magical Points* by Dr. Richard Tan.

Ear Points:
- Stomach, Adrenal Gland, Prostate Gland, Duodenum. Use ear seeds.
- Nausea, vomiting: Stomach, Liver, Spleen, and *Shenmen*. Needle once a day for three to five days. For severe cases, needle two or three times daily. These points can also be used for morning sickness during pregnancy. However, ear seeds with mild massage are recommended.

Auricular Acupuncture by Dr. Li-Chun Huang:
- Gastritis: Stomach, Spleen, and Digestive Subcortex.
  - For superficial gastritis, add Sympathetic.
  - For atrophic gastritis, add Pancreas and Endocrine.
  - For disharmony between the Liver and Stomach, add Stomach, Abdominal Distention Area, and *San Jiao*.
- Gastric and duodenum ulcers: Stomach, Spleen, Duodenum, Sympathetic, and Digestive Subcortex.
  - For disharmony between the Liver and Stomach, add Liver and *San Jiao*.
  - For insufficiency of Stomach yin, add Pancreas and Endocrine.
  - For gastric ulcer and duodenal ulcer due to abdominal pain, add Groove of Stomach and Intestine, and Duodenum Ball of Posterior.
  - For gastric ulcer and duodenal ulcer due to insomnia, add Neurasthenia Point, and Neurasthenia Area.
- For additional information on the location and explanation of these points, please refer to *Auricular Treatment Formula and Prescriptions* by Dr. Li-Chun Huang.

MODERN RESEARCH

GI Care is formulated with herbs that promote regular function of the gastrointestinal tract. Ingredients in *GI Care* have demonstrated anti-ulcer, antacid, antispasmodic and antidiarrheal activities.

One active ingredient of *Bai Shao* (Radix Paeoniae Alba), paeoniflorin, has strong antispasmodic effects on the smooth muscle to relieve intestinal cramps. It has an anti-inflammatory effect and protective function against stress ulcers.[1]

Hai Piao Xiao (Endoconcha Sepiae) is an excellent antacid. It has been demonstrated through clinical trials that *Hai Piao Xiao* (Endoconcha Sepiae) effectively treats duodenal ulcers. In a study consisting of over 40 patients with bleeding ulcers, the use of *Hai Piao Xiao* (Endoconcha Sepiae) and others stopped bleeding within 3 to 7 days. In another study, 29 out of 31 patients with perforated ulcers were cured using the same herbs.[1]

Wu Zhu Yu (Fructus Evodiae) has been used to treat various gastrointestinal disorders. Clinical trials have demonstrated the internal use of *Wu Zhu Yu* (Fructus Evodiae) to effectively treat diarrhea, and the external use of *Wu Zhu Yu* (Fructus Evodiae) to effectively treat irritable bowel syndrome. [1,2]

Huang Qin (Radix Scutellariae) also has a wide range of antibiotic actions against pathogenic bacteria, virus, and fungus.[1,3,4,5] Most importantly, *Huang Qin* (Radix Scutellariae) has excellent properties in treating *Helicobacter pylori*, a pathogen responsible for chronic and recurrent ulcers in up to 59.6% of the ulcer patients. In one study, it was reported that *Huang Qin* (Radix Scutellariae) has an effective rate of 80 to 85.7% in controlling ulcers due to *Helicobacter pylori*.[6]

FORMULAS

GI CARE ™

PHARMACEUTICAL DRUGS & CHINESE MEDICINE: A COMPARATIVE ANALYSIS

Western Medical Approach: Gastrointestinal conditions, such as gastric or duodenal ulcers, stress ulcers, gastritis and heartburn, are extremely common complaints in developed countries. As a result, many new drugs have been developed in recent years to treat these conditions. Antacids (such as Maalox and Mylanta) neutralize stomach acid, have a quick onset of action but only a short duration. Histamine-2 antagonists [such as Zantac (Ranitidine) and Tagamet (Cimetidine)] have potent effect and medium duration of action and are well tolerated in most cases. However, they inhibit liver metabolism, and may cause drug-drug and drug-herb interactions and must be monitored carefully. Proton-pump inhibitors [such as Prilosec (Omeprazole) and Protonix (Pantoprazole)] have potent and irreversible effect to inhibit production of stomach acid. Unfortunately, prolonged use may cause atrophic gastritis, and in laboratory studies, stomach cancer in animal subjects. In brief, though these drugs are effects to reduce stomach acid and treat several gastrointestinal conditions, they must be prescribed and monitored carefully.

Traditional Chinese Medicine Approach: These gastrointestinal disorders may be treated effectively with herbs. According to numerous clinical studies, herbs neutralize stomach acid, decrease production and secretion of stomach acid, relieve pain, kill *H. pylori*, and in severe cases of bleeding ulcers, stop bleeding. Furthermore, herbs are also effective to treat drug- and stress-induced gastrointestinal disorders, two of the main causes. In short, by targeting both symptoms and causes, herbs achieve short- and long-term success to treat many gastrointestinal disorders. However, herbs do have their limitations. In cases of severe peptic ulcers, herbs are not as potent as, and do not last as long as, proton-pump inhibitors. Furthermore, acute cases of profuse gastrointestinal bleeding are medical emergencies, and require immediate medical intervention. Use of herbs is not recommended in these two scenarios.

CASE STUDIES

A 54-year-old female clerk presented with belching, esophageal reflux and acid regurgitation. Sleep was disturbed due to relentless nighttime cough with thick and sticky phlegm. At times, the patient would also experience vomiting. Her medical doctor prescribed Prilosec (Omeprazole), but the patient preferred not to take pharmaceuticals if possible. The patient was given *GI Care*, 4 capsules daily. Within 2 weeks, the patient was able to refrain from Prilosec (Omeprazole) and continued with just *GI Care*. Subsequently, the patient experienced no discomfort, slept well and has had no acid reflux. She was no longer expelling phlegm or mucus. Four months later, she was still taking *GI Care* and doing fine. The practitioner's intention was to slowly reduce her dosage and monitor her symptoms.

J.Y., Vancouver, Washington

J.R., a 17-year-old female, presents with various gastrointestinal complaints including nausea, epigastric fullness with sensations of "pulling or tightness," abdominal pain that is "annoying and dull," intermittent abdominal pain, and alternating diarrhea and constipation. The TCM diagnosis was Liver qi stagnation with Stomach fire rising. The practitioner prescribed *GI Care*. After one month of care, including three acupuncture treatments and steady herbal therapy, the patient reported improvement in the abdominal pain, to the point that it is now minimal, with increased periods of relief between exacerbations. Furthermore, the nausea resolved and bowel movements became normal. [Note: The practitioner commented that the patient improved although she was not totally compliant, and forget to take the herbs once in a while.]

C.L., Chino Hills, California

A 45-year-old female presented with stomach sensitivity that worsened with stress. The Western diagnosis was acid reflux; the TCM diagnosis was Liver qi stagnation with heat. After beginning to take *GI Care,* the patient reported it to be a gentle formula that helped her be free of stomach pain for two years. Due to financial reasons, the patient stopped coming in for acupuncture but remained on *GI Care* consistently.

M.C., Sarasota, Florida

FORMULAS

GI CARE ™

[1] Bensky, D. et al. *Chinese Herbal Medicine Materia Medica*. Eastland Press. 1993

[2] Yu, LL. et al. Effect of the crude extract of evodiae fructus on the intestinal transit in mice. *Planta Med*, Aug 1994; 60(4):308-12

[3] Yang, D. et al. Antifungal activity in vitro of scutellaria baicalensis. *Ann Pharm Fr*; 1995; 53(3):138-41.

[4] Nagai, T. et al. Antiviral activity of plant flavonoid, 5,7,4-trihydroxy-8-methoxyflavone, from scutellaria baicalensis against influenza A (H3N2) and B viruses. *Biol Pharm Bull*; Feb 1995; 18(2):195-9.

[5] Nagai, T. et al. Mode of action of the anti-influenza virus activity of plant flavonoid, 5,7,4-trihydroxy-8-methoxyflavone, from the roots of scutellaria baicalensis. *Antiviral Res*; Jan 1995; 26(1):11-25.

[6] Zhang, L. et al. Relation between Helicobacter pylori and pathogenesis of chronic atrophic gastritis and the research of its prevention and treatment. *Chung Kuo Chung His Chieh Ho Tsa Chih*, Sep. 1992; 12(9):521-3' 515-6

FORMULAS

GI CARE II ™

CLINICAL APPLICATIONS

- All excess type diarrhea characterized by heat and dampness
- Gastroenteritis, enteritis, dysentery or food poisoning: expressed by foul-smelling stools with burning sensations of the anus, abdominal discomfort, pain, borborygmus, possibly nausea, vomiting and a feeling of incomplete defecation.
- Traveler's diarrhea
- Gastrointestinal disorders with damp-heat
- Monosodium Glutamate (MSG) poisoning

WESTERN THERAPEUTIC ACTIONS

- Treats diarrhea, dysentery, enteritis, stomach flu, and other intestinal disorders [2,3,4,5]
- Treats acute diarrhea due to infection [7,8,9,10,11,12,13,14]
- Treats acute diarrhea due to drug or food poisoning [15,16,17]
- Treats acute diarrhea with mucus or blood present in the stool [28,29]
- Alleviates the signs and symptoms of acute diarrhea, such as nausea, vomiting, abdominal pain, intestinal cramps and spasms, and fever [18,19,20,21,22,23,24,25,26,27]

CHINESE THERAPEUTIC ACTIONS

- Dispels damp-heat in the intestine
- Binds the intestine and stops diarrhea
- Promotes digestion and relieves pain

DOSAGE

Take 3 to 4 capsules three times daily on an empty stomach, with warm water. Dosage may be increased to 6 to 8 capsules three times daily, if necessary. Herbs should be taken for at least seven days in cases of acute infection to completely expel the pathogens.

INGREDIENTS

Bai Shao (Radix Paeoniae Alba)
Bai Zhi (Radix Angelicae Dahuricae)
Bai Zhu (Rhizoma Atractylodis Macrocephalae)
Chen Pi (Pericarpium Citri Reticulatae)
Chi Shi Zhi (Halloysitum Rubrum)
Da Huang (Radix et Rhizoma Rhei)
Da Zao (Fructus Jujubae)
Dang Gui (Radicis Angelicae Sinensis)
Fu Ling (Poria)
Gan Cao (Radix Glycyrrhizae)
Ge Gen (Radix Puerariae)
Hou Po (Cortex Magnoliae Officinalis)

Huang Lian (Rhizoma Coptidis)
Huang Qin (Radix Scutellariae)
Huo Xiang (Herba Agastache)
Jie Geng (Radix Platycodonis)
Mu Xiang (Radix Aucklandiae)
Qing Pi (Pericarpium Citri Reticulatae Viride)
Rou Gui (Cortex Cinnamomi)
Shen Qu (Massa Fermentata)
Sheng Jiang (Rhizoma Zingiberis Recens)
Wu Bei Zi (Galla Chinensis)
Zhi Ke (Fructus Aurantii)
Zi Su Ye (Folium Perillae)

FORMULAS

GI CARE II ™

FORMULA EXPLANATION

This herbal prescription is formulated specifically to treat diarrhea, dysentery, enteritis, and other intestinal disorders. According to traditional Chinese medicine, such conditions are often characterized by damp-heat in the intestines, leading to such symptoms as pain, nausea, vomiting, abdominal pain, fever, urgency, tenesmus, burning sensation of the anus after defecation, and diarrhea with or without the presence of mucus or blood. Therefore, this formula uses herbs to dispel damp-heat in the intestines, promote digestion, relieve pain, and bind the intestines to stop diarrhea.

Ge Gen (Radix Puerariae) raises the yang qi of the Spleen to stop diarrhea. It generates fluids to replenish the loss of water due to diarrhea. With its ability to relieve the exterior, it also works for patients with intestinal flu or traveler's diarrhea. *Ge Gen* (Radix Puerariae) works synergistically with *Bai Shao* (Radix Paeoniae Alba) and *Gan Cao* (Radix Glycyrrhizae) to relieve abdominal and intestinal pain, spasms and tenesmus associated with diarrhea or dysentery.

Huang Qin (Radix Scutellariae) and *Huang Lian* (Rhizoma Coptidis) clear damp-heat in the intestines to relieve burning sensations, feelings of incomplete defecation and frequent urges to defecate. This pair of herbs also relieves pain by reducing inflammation and infection. *Rou Gui* (Cortex Cinnamomi) and *Dang Gui* (Radicis Angelicae Sinensis) are used to moderate the heat-clearing effect to prevent damages to the Spleen and Stomach.

Chi Shi Zhi (Halloysitum Rubrum) and *Wu Bei Zi* (Galla Chinensis) are astringents used symptomatically to bind the intestines for relief of diarrhea. *Chi Shi Zhi* (Halloysitum Rubrum) replenishes trace minerals and electrolytes that are lost with diarrhea. It adheres to the intestinal walls to stop possible bleeding and promote the healing of chronic ulcerations. *Wu Bei Zi* (Galla Chinensis), sticky by nature, patches ulcerations to repair the intestinal walls.

Mu Xiang (Radix Aucklandiae), *Hou Po* (Cortex Magnoliae Officinalis), *Chen Pi* (Pericarpium Citri Reticulatae), *Qing Pi* (Pericarpium Citri Reticulatae Viride), and *Zhi Ke* (Fructus Aurantii) promote the movement of qi and help eliminate stagnation, turbidity, bloating and gas in the intestines. *Da Huang* (Radix et Rhizoma Rhei), *Mu Xiang* (Radix Aucklandiae) and *Hou Po* (Cortex Magnoliae Officinalis) dispel turbidity and remove the bacteria causing the infection or inflammation. With their descending and purgative functions, they prevent the retention of pathogenic factors in the intestines. A small amount of processed *Da Huang* (Radix et Rhizoma Rhei) is used in this formula to completely purge damp-heat.

Jie Geng (Radix Platycodonis) raises the qi of both the Lung and Large Intestine, two organs connected by their *zang fu* relationship. It is commonly used to treat diarrhea and tenesmus, due to its function of lifting the sunken qi. *Bai Zhi* (Radix Angelicae Dahuricae) dispels pus and has an ascending effect to help *Jie Geng* (Radix Platycodonis) lift the sunken qi to treat diarrhea and tenesmus.

Chen Pi (Pericarpium Citri Reticulatae), *Sheng Jiang* (Rhizoma Zingiberis Recens), *Da Zao* (Fructus Jujubae), and *Shen Qu* (Massa Fermentata) harmonize the middle *jiao* to relieve possible nausea and vomiting. *Huo Xiang* (Herba Agastache) and *Zi Su Ye* (Folium Perillae) are both fragrant and wake the Spleen. They are used to harmonize the middle *jiao*, dispel dampness, and relieve vomiting and nausea. Finally, *Fu Ling* (Poria) and *Bai Zhu* (Rhizoma Atractylodis Macrocephalae) strengthen the Spleen to relieve diarrhea.

SUPPLEMENTARY FORMULAS

- For excessive burning sensations in the anus, pus-filled pockets of infection or abscess, fever or inflammation, use with **Herbal ABX**.
- For irritable bowel syndrome (IBS) with bloating and gas, use with **GI Harmony**.
- With stress, add **Calm** or **Calm ES**.

FORMULAS

GI CARE II ™

- For irritable bowel syndrome with constipation, use with *GI Harmony* and *Gentle Lax (Deficient)* instead.
- For intestinal and abdominal cramping and pain, use with *Flex (SC)*.
- In monosodium glutamate (MSG) poisoning, use with *Herbal DTX*.
- For ulcerative colitis, add *GI Care (UC)*.
- For hemorrhoids, add *GI Care (HMR)*.
- For excess heat, add *Gardenia Complex*.
- For dryness and thirst, add *Nourish (Fluids)*.
- For bleeding, add *Notoginseng 9*.

NUTRITION

- Patients with diarrhea should keep taking in plenty of pure water and appropriate foods to prevent dehydration and malnutrition.
- During the recovery phase of diarrhea, eat foods that are easy to digest early in the meal, such as soup, yogurt, toast, and porridge, and cooked fruits and vegetables.
- Avoid foods that may trigger diarrhea or are hard to digest, such as sorbitol, dairy products, spicy food, alcohol, and caffeine.
- Avoid eating raw, cold or unsanitary food and beverages.
- Use a separate chopping board to prepare raw food and fruits, to prevent contamination with other foods.
- Do not eat foods with refined sugar during the recovery phase, especially if the diarrhea is caused by bacterial infection.

The Tao of Nutrition by Ni and McNease
- Diarrhea
  - Recommendations: garlic, blueberries, raspberry leaves, lotus seeds, burned rice, yams, sweet potatoes, fresh fig leaves, peas, buckwheat, and guava peel.
  - Avoid cold, raw foods, most fruits, juices, and overeating.
- For more information, please refer to *The Tao of Nutrition* by Dr. Maoshing Ni and Cathy McNease.

LIFESTYLE INSTRUCTIONS

- Remind patients of the importance of washing their hands prior to eating.
- Patients with intestinal disturbance due to stress should engage in regular exercise, adequate rest, and normal sleep patterns. Practicing meditation exercises at least twice daily will also be beneficial. Get away from the daily routine to do something enjoyable to relieve stress whenever possible.
- Relax, rest and drink plenty of water until the condition clears up.

CLINICAL NOTES

- Diarrhea is a symptom, not a disease. Therefore, if it persists after taking this formula for 1 to 2 weeks, have a stool sample examined microscopically for cells, mucus, fat, blood, infectious organisms and other substances to determine the exact cause.
- Patients taking *GI Care II* for colitis or traveler's diarrhea should continue taking the formula for an additional 2 to 3 days after all the symptoms have subsided. This is to ensure that all the pathogenic factors are cleared out from the intestines in order to prevent development of chronic colitis in the future. To strengthen the Spleen afterwards, *GI Tonic* should be administered for three to five days.
- *GI Care II* is a great formula to bring during traveling to prevent or treat traveler's diarrhea and other gastrointestinal infections.

GI CARE II ™

Pulse Diagnosis by Dr. Jimmy Wei-Yen Chang:
- Floating and forceful pulse on the right *guan* position.
- Note: Dr. Chang takes the pulse in slightly different positions. He places his index finger directly over the wrist crease, and his middle and ring fingers alongside to locate *cun*, *guan* and *chi* positions. For additional information and explanation, please refer to *Pulsynergy* by Dr. Jimmy Wei-Yen Chang and Marcus Brinkman.

CAUTIONS

- This formula is contraindicated for patients who have diarrhea caused by deficiency and cold, Spleen qi deficiency, or Spleen and Kidney yang deficiencies.
- This formula is contraindicated for patients who are pregnant or nursing.
- Patients who are on anticoagulant or antiplatelet therapies, such as Coumadin (Warfarin), should use this formula with caution as there may be a slightly higher risk of bleeding and bruising.

ACUPUNCTURE POINTS

Traditional Points:
- Bleed vein next to *Zusanli* (ST 36). Needle *Tianshu* (ST 25), *Shangjuxu* (ST 37), and *Xiajuxu* (ST 39).
- Needle *Shangjuxu* (ST 37), *Tianshu* (ST 25), *Zusanli* (ST 36), *Shangwan* (CV 13), and *Guanyuan* (CV 4).

Balance Method by Dr. Richard Tan:
- Left side: *Liangqiu* (ST34), *Zusanli* (ST 36), *Shangjuxu* (ST 37), *Tiaokou* (ST 38), *Ximen* (PC 4), *Neiguan* (PC 6) or *ah shi* points nearby, and Large Intestine on the left ear.
- Right side: *Taibai* (SP 3), *Gongsun* (SP 4), *Xuehai* (SP 10), *Hegu* (LI 4), *Quchi* (LI 11), *Shousanli* (LI 10) or *ah shi* points nearby, and Small Intestine on the right side.
- Left and right side can be alternated from treatment to treatment.
- For additional information on the Balance Method, please refer to *Dr. Tan's Strategy of Twelve Magical Points* by Dr. Richard Tan.

Ear Points:
- Stomach, Small Intestine, Large Intestine, and Spleen. Use ear seeds.
- Stomach, Large Intestine, lower part of the Rectum, and Spleen. Use three needles on different parts of the Large Intestine. Large Intestine and Stomach are the main points. Strength of stimulation should be determined by the patient's constitution and tolerance. Both needles and seeds can be used. Strong stimulation is necessary if ear seeds are selected. If diarrhea is severe, points should be massaged every two to four hours. After symptoms subside, needle every other day or twice a week. Ten days equals one treatment course.

Auricular Acupuncture by Dr. Li-Chun Huang:
- Diarrhea: Sympathetic, Lower *Jiao*, Large Intestine, Rectum, Spleen, *Shenmen*, Occiput, and Digestive Subcortex.
- For additional information on the location and explanation of these points, please refer to *Auricular Treatment Formula and Prescriptions* by Dr. Li-Chun Huang.

MODERN RESEARCH

GI Care II has been specifically formulated for the treatment of acute diarrhea with signs and symptoms such as nausea, vomiting, abdominal pain, fever, and diarrhea, with or without the presence of mucus or blood. According to western medicine, the most common causes of acute diarrhea are infection, drugs, and toxins.[1] The purpose of this formula is to simultaneously address both the causes and symptoms of diarrhea, for immediate relief and recovery.

FORMULAS

GI CARE II ™

The herbs in this formula have shown excellent effectiveness, in laboratory and clinical research, for treatment of diarrhea due to various causes, including (but not limited to) infection, dysentery, and enteritis. *Huang Lian* (Rhizoma Coptidis), individually or in an herbal formula, exhibited excellent clinical results in treating over 1,000 patients with bacterial dysentery. The treatments showed marked effectiveness in a short course of treatment with low incidence of side-effects.[2,3] Diarrhea can be addressed with many herbs, such as *Fu Ling* (Poria) and *Bai Zhu* (Rhizoma Atractylodis Macrocephalae). In a clinical study, 93 infants with diarrhea were treated with *Fu Ling* (Poria) three times daily. Complete recovery was documented in 79 cases, improvement in 8 cases, and no effect in 6 cases.[4] In another study, 320 infants with diarrhea responded well to treatment with 3 to 4 grams of an herbal powder that contained *Bai Zhu* (Rhizoma Atractylodis Macrocephalae) and other herbs.[5]

Infection is one of the most common causes of acute diarrhea. In this formula, many herbs with marked antibiotic properties are used to eradicate the offending micro-organisms. Use of multiple herbs within this herbal formula is necessary because this strategy will not only increase the antibiotic effect, it will also decrease the risk of developing bacterial and viral resistance.[6] Herbs with antibiotic effects include *Bai Shao* (Radix Paeoniae Alba), *Huang Qin* (Radix Scutellariae), *Huang Lian* (Rhizoma Coptidis), *Hou Po* (Cortex Magnoliae Officinalis), and *Fu Ling* (Poria).[7,8,9,10,11,12,13] Of these herbs, *Huang Qin* (Radix Scutellariae) and *Huang Lian* (Rhizoma Coptidis) are the most potent and have the widest spectrum of antibiotic properties. In fact, their effectiveness is comparable to antibiotics such as ampicillin, amoxicillin, methicillin and cefotaxime.[14]

Another common reason for acute diarrhea is drug or food poisoning. Ideally, the offending agent should be eliminated to remove the cause of the diarrhea. However, if discontinuation of the implicated drug is not possible; or if the poisonous food has already been absorbed, herbs should be used to remove the buildup of drugs and/or minimize toxicity. *Gan Cao* (Radix Glycyrrhizae) is one of the best herbs to treat poisoning from toxic agents, including, but not limited to, drug poisoning (chloral hydrate, urethane, cocaine, picrotoxin, caffeine, pilocarpine, nicotine, barbiturates, mercury and lead), food poisoning (tetrodotoxin, snake, and mushrooms), and others (enterotoxin, herbicides, pesticides). The exact mechanism of this action is unclear, but it is thought to be related to the regulatory effect of *Gan Cao* (Radix Glycyrrhizae) on the endocrine and/or hepatic systems.[15,16,17]

In addition to eliminating the causes of acute diarrhea, it is also necessary to prescribe herbs to alleviate the symptoms. Use of *Sheng Jiang* (Rhizoma Zingiberis Recens) has been demonstrated by many studies to be one of safest and most effective ways to relieve nausea and vomiting.[18] Abdominal pain may be relieved with herbs that have analgesic and antispasmodic effects. *Gan Cao* (Radix Glycyrrhizae) relieves pain; additional herbs that relieve spasms and cramps of the intestines include *Ge Gen* (Radix Puerariae), *Bai Shao* (Radix Paeoniae Alba), and *Bai Zhi* (Radix Angelicae Dahuricae).[19,20,21,22] According to one clinical trial, these herbs are so effective that 241 out of 254 patients (94.8%) with intestinal spasms showed significant improvement within 3 to 6 days of beginning herbal treatment.[23] To reduce fever and inflammation associated with acute diarrhea, *Ge Gen* (Radix Puerariae), *Bai Shao* (Radix Paeoniae Alba), *Huang Qin* (Radix Scutellariae), and *Zi Su Ye* (Folium Perillae) are added for their demonstrated antipyretic and anti-inflammatory effects.[24,25,26,27]

Diarrhea is sometimes accompanied by mucus or blood in the stool, which can be treated with *Da Huang* (Radix et Rhizoma Rhei) and *Wu Bei Zi* (Galla Chinensis). *Da Huang* (Radix et Rhizoma Rhei), if processed appropriately, has strong properties for treatment of hemorrhagic necrotic enteritis. In this disease syndrome, most patients who take *Da Huang* (Radix et Rhizoma Rhei) report lessened pain and diminished levels of blood in the stool within 2 to 6 doses.[28] Similarly, according to one clinical study on gastrointestinal bleeding, the use of *Wu Bei Zi* (Galla Chinensis) was over 90% effective in stopping bleeding in 33 patients within nine days.[29]

GI CARE II ™

PHARMACEUTICAL DRUGS & CHINESE MEDICINE: A COMPARATIVE ANALYSIS

Western Medical Approach: Gastrointestinal disorders, such as food poisoning, traveler's diarrhea, dysentery, gastroenteritis, and enteritis, are generally caused by ingestion of a foreign substance that causes symptoms such as nausea, vomiting, diarrhea with foul-smelling stools with burning sensations of the anus, and abdominal pain and discomfort. In western medicine, these conditions are often treated symptomatically. For example, diarrhea is usually treated with antidiarrheal drugs, such as Lomotil (Diphenoxylate) and Imodium (Loperamide). Nausea and vomiting are treated with injection of antiemetics, such as Thorazine (Chlorpromazine). Lastly, for gastrointestinal infections, antibiotics are used to kill the micro-organism. Overall, these gastrointestinal disorders are acute problems that require immediate and aggressive treatments. While drugs are effective to treat the symptoms and the cause, they are likely to consume and weaken the body, therefore requiring a prolonged period of time for complete recovery.

Traditional Chinese Medicine Approach: From traditional Chinese medicine perspectives, these gastrointestinal disorders are considered to be damp-heat in the intestines. The herbs that treat damp-heat are effective to address both the symptoms and the cause. As described above, these herbs have been shown to have antiemetic effect to treat nausea and vomiting, antidiarrheal effect to stop diarrhea, analgesic effect to relieve pain, muscle-relaxant effect to alleviate spasms and cramps, and antibiotic effect to kill the pathogens. In addition to having marked therapeutic effects, these herbs are gentle and are well tolerated by those individuals who are already under a tremendous amount of stress. In short, herbal treatment offer immediate relieve, and facilitate long-term recovery from these gastrointestinal disorders.

Summation: Drugs and herbs are both effective to treat gastrointestinal disorders by addressing both symptoms and cause. In addition to these treatments, it is extremely important to make sure patients receive plenty of rest and fluids, as excessive vomiting and diarrhea may lead to dehydration. Fluids can be replenished orally in most cases, or intravenously in severe cases. Furthermore, because these gastrointestinal disorders are consuming and depleting in nature, it is important to use herbs to strengthen the body and supplement deficiencies once the patients begin the recovery process.

CASE STUDY

A 35-years-old male with a history of digestive problems presented with severe abdominal pain, nausea, and vomiting after eating sushi during dinner. This condition was immediately diagnosed as food poisoning due to damp-heat in the intestines. *GI Care II* was prescribed at 4 grams three times daily until the symptoms resolve. One hour after taking the first dose, the patient felt much better with decreased abdominal pain. After the second dose, all symptoms were completely resolved.

J.C., Diamond Bar, California

[1] Fauci, A. et al. *Harrison's Principles of Internal Medicine, 14th Edition*. McGraw-Hill Health Professions Division. 1998.
[2] *Zhong Hua Nei Ke Za Zhi* (Chinese Journal of Internal Medicine), 1976; 4: 219
[3] *Si Chuan Yi Xue Yuan Xue Bao* (Journal of Sichuan School of Medicine), 1959; 1: 102
[4] *Bei Jing Zhong Yi* (Beijing Chinese Medicine), 1985; 5:31
[5] *Shan Dong Zhong Yi Za Zhi* (Shandong Journal of Chinese Medicine), 1982; 2:107
[6] *Zhong Yao Xue* (Chinese Herbology), 1988; 140:144
[7] *Xin Zhong Yi* (New Chinese Medicine), 1989; 21(3):51
[8] *Zhong Yao Xue* (Chinese Herbology), 1988; 137:140
[9] *Zhong Yao Xue* (Chinese Herbology), 1988, 140:144
[10] *Planta med*, 1982; 44(2):100
[11] *Yao Jian Gong Zuo Tong Xun* (Journal of Herbal Preparations), 1980; 10(4):209
[12] *Xin Hua Ben Cao Gang Mu* (New Chinese Materia Medica), 1988; 58
[13] *Zhong Yao Da Ci Dian* (Dictionary of Chinese Herbs), 1977; 1596
[14] *J Pharm Pharmacol* 2000 Mar; 52(3):361-6
[15] *Zhong Yao Tong Bao* (Journal of Chinese Herbology), 1986; 11(10):55

FORMULAS

GI CARE II ™

[16] *Xin Zhong Yi* (New Chinese Medicine), 1985; 2:34
[17] *Xin Zhong Yi* (New Chinese Medicine), 1978; 1:36
[18] *Xin Zhong Yi* (New Chinese Medicine), 1986; 12:24
[19] *Zhong Yao Xue* (Chinese Herbology), 1998; 101:103
[20] *Zhong Yao Zhi* (Chinese Herbology Journal), 1993; 358
[21] *Zhong Yao Yao Li Yu Ying Yong* (Pharmacology and Applications of Chinese Herbs), 1983; 796
[22] *Zhi Wu Yao You Xiao Cheng Fen Shou Ce* (Manual of Plant Medicinals and Their Active Constituents), 1986; 624,603,197
[23] *Zhong Hua Wai Ke Za Zhi* (Chinese Journal of External Medicine), 1960; 4:354
[24] *Zhong Yao Xue* (Chinese Herbology), 1998; 101:103
[25] *Zhong Yao Zhi* (Chinese Herbology Journal), 1993:183
[26] *Zhong Hua Yi Xue Za Zhi* (Chinese Journal of Medicine), 1956; 42(10):964
[27] *Planta Med*, 1985; (6):4
[28] *Fu Jian Zhong Yi Yao* (Fujian Chinese Medicine and Herbology), 1985; 1:36
[29] *Zhe Jiang Zhong Yi Xue Yuan Xue Bao* (Journal of Zhejiang University of Chinese Medicine), 1987; 6:20

GI CARE (HMR) ™

(Hemorrhoids)

CLINICAL APPLICATIONS

❧ Hemorrhoids (internal or external)
❧ Hemorrhoids with or without swelling, inflammation or bleeding

WESTERN THERAPEUTIC ACTIONS

❧ Anti-inflammatory effect to reduce the swelling and inflammation of hemorrhoid tissues
❧ Hemostatic effect to stop rectal bleeding
❧ Mild laxative effect to relieve constipation

CHINESE THERAPEUTIC ACTIONS

❧ Clears damp-heat and eliminates toxic-heat from the intestines
❧ Stops bleeding
❧ Regulates bowel movements

DOSAGE

Take 4 capsules three times daily on an empty stomach with warm water.

INGREDIENTS

Chun Gen Pi (Cortex Ailanthi)
Dang Gui (Radicis Angelicae Sinensis)
Di Yu (Radix Sanguisorbae) (charred)
He Zi (Fructus Chebulae)
Huai Hua (Flos Sophorae) (charred)
Huang Qin (Radix Scutellariae)

Jin Yin Hua (Flos Lonicerae)
Lian Qiao (Fructus Forsythiae)
Pu Gong Ying (Herba Taraxaci)
Wu Bei Zi (Galla Chinensis)
Xian He Cao (Herba Agrimoniae)
Yu Li Ren (Semen Pruni)

FORMULA EXPLANATION

GI Care (HMR) is designed as a first-line therapy to treat various presentations of hemorrhoids, including internal and external hemorrhoids, and with or without swelling, inflammation and bleeding. In traditional Chinese medicine, hemorrhoids are generally considered as a condition characterized by damp-heat and toxic-heat attacking the intestines, leading to signs and symptoms such as enlarged and protruding tissues in the rectum, constipation, rectal bleeding, and others.

In this formula, *Jin Yin Hua* (Flos Lonicerae), *Lian Qiao* (Fructus Forsythiae), *Pu Gong Ying* (Herba Taraxaci), and *Huang Qin* (Radix Scutellariae) clear damp-heat and eliminate toxic-heat from the intestines. Charred *Huai Hua* (Flos Sophorae), charred *Di Yu* (Radix Sanguisorbae), *Chun Gen Pi* (Cortex Ailanthi) and *Xian He Cao* (Herba Agrimoniae) clear heat, cool the blood, and stop rectal bleeding. *Dang Gui* (Radicis Angelicae Sinensis) tonifies blood and replenishes blood lost through rectal bleeding. It also moves blood to treat the blood clots around the anus that are associated with hemorrhoidal condition. *Yu Li Ren* (Semen Pruni) moistens the intestines and relieves diarrhea. *He Zi* (Fructus Chebulae) and *Wu Bei Zi* (Galla Chinensis) have astringent effect to reduce inflammation of swollen hemorrhoid tissues. Overall, *GI Care (HMR)* is an excellent formula that treats various presentations of hemorrhoids, including internal or external hemorrhoids, with or without swelling, inflammation or bleeding.

SUPPLEMENTARY FORMULAS

❧ With mild to moderate constipation, combine with *Gentle Lax (Deficient)*.
❧ With moderate to severe constipation, combine with *Gentle Lax (Excess)*.

FORMULAS

GI CARE (HMR) ™

(Hemorrhoids)

- With severe and profuse bleeding, combine with *Notoginseng 9*.
- For hemorrhoids in individuals with extreme weakness and deficiency, use with *Imperial Tonic*.
- With blood deficiency, add *Schisandra ZZZ*.
- With ulcerative colitis, add *GI Care (UC)*.
- With irritable bowel syndrome, add *GI Harmony*.

NUTRITION

- It is very beneficial to eat foods that are high in fiber to ensure regular bowel movements, such as wheat bran, fresh fruits, and nearly all vegetables. A diet high in fiber is one of the most important factors for the prevention and treatment of hemorrhoids.
- It is important to make sure the diet contains an adequate amount of vitamins and minerals, as many of them are essential for blood clotting and coagulation. Vitamins and minerals that are especially important are vitamin B complex, vitamin C, vitamin K, and calcium.
- Foods that should be avoided include fats, animal products, coffee, alcohol, pepper, mustard, and things that are spicy or pungent. These foods are generally harder to digest, and are more likely to irritate the digestive system. Alcohol consumption may worsen the pain and cause further bleeding.
- Advise the patient to increase water intake.
- A folk remedy that may be helpful in treating hemorrhoids involves eating one fresh cucumber (not peeled with ends removed) each morning and evening.
- Another folk remedy states to eat two to three pieces of banana (riper the better) with wild honey daily. Treatment course is 30 to 50 days.

The Tao of Nutrition by Ni and McNease
- Hemorrhoid
    - Recommendations: sea cucumber, black fungus, water chestnut, buckwheat, tangerines, figs, plums, fish, prunes, guavas, bamboo shoots, mung beans, winter melon, black sesame seeds, persimmons, bananas, squash, cucumbers, taro, tofu, and cooling foods.
    - Avoid stimulating foods, spicy foods, alcohol, smoking, constipation, stress, lack of exercise, and standing or sitting too long.
- For more information, please refer to *The Tao of Nutrition* by Dr. Maoshing Ni and Cathy McNease.

LIFESTYLE INSTRUCTIONS

- It is important to maintain normal and soft bowel movements on a regular basis, as straining for bowel movement will often worsen hemorrhoids. Empty the bowels as soon as the urge to defecate occurs, to avoid unnecessary straining. Bowel movements should take no more than three to five minutes. Refrain from reading on the toilet.
- Avoid excessive wiping after a bowel movement. Avoid using rough toilet paper, since it may cause more irritation and bleeding. Use soft and moist toilet paper or baby wipes.
- Regular walking helps to stimulate peristalsis and promote normal bowel movements.
- Soak in a sitz bath with hot water for 20 minutes each night to focus blood circulation in the area of the anus. This helps clear the blue, ballooned veins. It also helps disperse the blood clots that cause the firm, tender mass in the anal area.
- Prolonged sitting or standing is not recommended as it may aggravate the condition. Rest face down on a bed whenever possible in times of flare-ups.
- Sit on soft cushions or surfaces whenever possible. Avoid sitting on hard surfaces, which increases pressure upon the hemorrhoidal blood vessels and tissues. Also, when it is necessary to sit for a long period of time, always try to leave the seat for 5 minutes each hour or shift the buttocks often from side to side to help relieve the constant rectal pressure.
- Patients should learn to exhale and not hold their breath when straining or lifting heavy objects.

FORMULAS

GI CARE (HMR) ™

(Hemorrhoids)

CAUTIONS

- This formula is contraindicated during pregnancy.
- Individuals with bleeding hemorrhoids should **not** take drugs with anticoagulant or antiplatelet effects, such as aspirin, Motrin (Ibuprofen), Advil (Ibuprofen), and Aleve (Naproxen). These drugs may encourage or cause more bleeding.
- *Dang Gui* (Radicis Angelicae Sinensis) may enhance the overall effectiveness of Coumadin (Warfarin), an anticoagulant drug. Patients who take anticoagulant or antiplatelet medications should **not** take this herbal formula without supervision by a licensed health care practitioner.

ACUPUNCTURE POINTS

Traditional Points:
- *Changqiang* (GV 1), *Chengshan* (BL 57), *Sanyinjiao* (SP 6), *Kunlun* (BL 60), *Huiyang* (BL 35), *Erbai*, *Taichong* (LR 3), *Ciliao* (BL 32), *Fuliu* (KI 7), *Yaoyangguan* (GV 3), *Weizhong* (BL 40), *Qihai* (CV 6), *Dachangshu* (BL 25), and *Shangqiu* (SP 5).

Balance Method by Dr. Richard Tan:
- Needle *Chengjiang* (CV 24) Bleed *Weizhong* (BL 40).
- *Huagai* (CV 20), *Shuiquan* (KI 5), and *Qiuxu* (GB 40).
- For additional information on the Balance Method, please refer to *Dr. Tan's Strategy of Twelve Magical Points* by Dr. Richard Tan.

Ear Points:
- Large Intestine, Rectum, Spleen, Adrenals, and Subcortex.

Auricular Acupuncture by Dr. Li-Chun Huang:
- Hemorrhoid: Anus, Rectum, Spleen, Large Intestine, Diaphragm, Pituitary, and Adrenal Gland.
- For additional information on the location and explanation of these points, please refer to *Auricular Treatment Formula and Prescriptions* by Dr. Li-Chun Huang.

MODERN RESEARCH

GI Care (HMR) is a formula developed specifically to treat hemorrhoids. It contains many herbs with a marked anti-inflammatory effect to reduce the swelling and inflammation of hemorrhoid tissues, hemostatic effect to stop rectal bleeding, and mild laxative effect to relieve constipation.

Jin Yin Hua (Flos Lonicerae), *Lian Qiao* (Fructus Forsythiae), *Di Yu* (Radix Sanguisorbae), and *Huang Qin* (Radix Scutellariae) are four herbs in this formula that have an anti-inflammatory effects to reduce the swelling and inflammation of hemorrhoidal tissues. [1,2,3] The mechanism of this action has been attributed in part to the decreased permeability of the blood vessels and subsequent reduction of swelling and inflammation.[4] Bleeding is a typical symptom that occurs after a bowel movement, producing blood-streaked stools or blood on the toilet paper. Therefore, this formula uses several herbs with marked hemostatic function to stop bleeding, such as *Huai Hua* (Flos Sophorae), *Di Yu* (Radix Sanguisorbae), *Chun Gen Pi* (Cortex Ailanthi), and *Xian He Cao* (Herba Agrimoniae). The mechanism of their hemostatic effect has been attributed in part to the increased number and activities of platelets.[5] More specifically, *Huai Hua* (Flos Sophorae) and *Di Yu* (Radix Sanguisorbae) have marked hemostatic effect to stop bleeding, and have been shown to reduce time of bleeding by as much as 31.9 to 45.5% when ingested orally.[6,7] For clinical applications, use of *Di Yu* (Radix Sanguisorbae) and *Xian He Cao* (Herba Agrimoniae) has been shown to effectively treat gastrointestinal bleeding,[8,9] while *Chun Gen Pi* (Cortex Ailanthi) has an excellent effect to stop bleeding among patients with hematochezia due to various causes.[10] Lastly, individuals with hemorrhoids often have

FORMULAS

GI CARE (HMR) ™

(Hemorrhoids)

constipation, and straining during a bowel movement will often make hemorrhoids worse. Therefore, this formula uses two herbs to lubricate the intestines and restore normal bowel movement. *Dang Gui* (Radicis Angelicae Sinensis) and *Yu Li Ren* (Semen Pruni) both have mild to moderate laxative effects to increase intestinal peristalsis and promote bowel movement.[11]

In summary, *GI Care (HMR)* is an excellent formula to treat hemorrhoids as it contains herbs that address both the causes and the complications of hemorrhoids.

PHARMACEUTICAL DRUGS & CHINESE MEDICINE: A COMPARATIVE ANALYSIS

Western Medical Approach: Hemorrhoids are swollen tissues located in the wall of the rectum and anus that contain veins. In western medicine, hemorrhoids are generally not treated except with use of over-the-counter (OTC) stool softeners and soothing agents. These methods offer only temporary and symptomatic relief. In more severe cases, invasive treatments may be performed, such as injection sclerotherapy, rubber-band ligation, laser destruction, infrared photocoagulation, and surgical hemorrhoidectomy. In other words, there are few options between mild OTC drugs that offer only temporary and symptomatic relief, and serious invasive treatments that completely eradicate body tissues.

Traditional Chinese Medicine Approach: Herbs offer effective treatment options for various presentations of hemorrhoids, including internal and/or external hemorrhoids, with or without swelling, inflammation or bleeding, and in both acute, chronic conditions. As described above, herbs have been shown to have mild laxative effect to relieve constipation, anti-inflammatory effect to reduce the swelling and inflammation of hemorrhoid tissues, and hemostatic effect to stop rectal bleeding. Therefore, not only are the herbs beneficial, they provide additional treatment options not available in western medicine.

Summation: The therapeutic benefits of herbs should be explored for treatment of hemorrhoids, as they offer great relief with few or no side effects. When necessary, and only in the most severe cases of hemorrhoids that do not respond to any other therapies, should the patient consider invasive treatment options.

CASE STUDY

A 65-year-old woman has a 7 to 8 year history of constipation and occasional rectal bleeding. In the last 10 days, the passing of stools has become increasingly more difficult, with severe pain and straining, and accompanied by rectal bleeding of bright red blood. The tongue coat was yellow and greasy, and the pulse was wiry and fine. The patient was diagnosed with damp-heat and toxic-heat in the intestines, with stagnation of qi and blood. After taking *GI Care (HMR)* for 7 days, the patient reported complete recovery with normal bowel movement, absence of bleeding, and resolution of hemorrhoids.

Anonymous

---

[1] *Shan Xi Yi Kan* (Shanxi Journal of Medicine), 1960; (10):22
[2] *Ke Yan Tong Xun* (Journal of Science and Research), 1982; (3):35
[3] *Chem Pharm Bull*, 1984; 32(7):2724
[4] *Ke Yan Tong Xun* (Journal of Science and Research), 1982; (3):35
[5] *Zhong Yao Yao Li Yu Ying Yong* (Pharmacology and Applications of Chinese Herbs), 1983; 323
[6] *Guang Xi Zhong Yi Yao* (Guangxi Chinese Medicine and Herbology), 1990; 13(1):44
[7] *Zhong Yao Yao Li Yu Ying Yong* (Pharmacology and Applications of Chinese Herbs), 1983; 406
[8] *Zhe Jiang Zhong Yi Xue Yuan Xue Bao* (Journal of Zhejiang University of Chinese Medicine), 1985; 9(4):26
[9] *Shang Hai Zhong Yi Yao Za Zhi* (Shanghai Journal of Chinese Medicine and Herbology), 1979; 4:28
[10] *An Hui Zhong Yi Xue Yuan Xue Bao* (Journal of Anhui University School of Medicine); 1985; 2:62
[11] *Zhong Yao Tong Bao* (Journal of Chinese Herbology), 1988; 13(8):43

GI CARE (UC) ™

(Ulcerative Colitis)

CLINICAL APPLICATIONS

- Ulcerative colitis
- Crohn's disease
- Chronic diarrhea with mucus, pus and blood, feeling of incomplete evacuation and abdominal cramps

WESTERN THERAPEUTIC ACTIONS

- Anti-inflammatory effect to reduce swelling and inflammation [2]
- Antibiotic effect to treat infection [3,4,5,6,7,8,9,10,11]
- Promotes normal digestion and absorption of nutrients [12,13]
- Relieves diarrhea [14,15]
- Alleviates abdominal spasms and cramps [16]
- Eliminates irritating toxins [17,18]

CHINESE THERAPEUTIC ACTIONS

- Dispels damp-heat in the intestines
- Relieves diarrhea
- Disperses stagnation and detoxifies
- Tonifies yin

DOSAGE

Take 3 to 4 capsules three times daily on an empty stomach with warm water. Dosage may be increased up to 8 to 10 capsules three times daily in acute conditions for no more than 4 days or until symptoms subside. After relief of symptoms the dosage then can be reduced to 3 to 4 capsules daily. For prevention or maintenance, take 2 capsules daily.

INGREDIENTS

Bai Shao (Radix Paeoniae Alba)
Chi Shi Zhi (Halloysitum Rubrum)
Chun Gen Pi (Cortex Ailanthi)
Dong Gua Zi (Semen Benincasae)
Fang Feng (Radix Saposhnikoviae)
Hou Po (Cortex Magnoliae Officinalis)
Huang Lian (Rhizoma Coptidis)
Ma Chi Xian (Herba Portulacae)

Mai Ya (Fructus Hordei Germinatus)
Nan Sha Shen (Radix Adenophorae)
Shan Yao (Rhizoma Dioscoreae)
Shan Zha (Fructus Crataegi)
Shi Liu Pi (Pericarpium Granati)
Wu Bei Zi (Galla Chinensis)
Yi Yi Ren (Semen Coicis)

FORMULA EXPLANATION

According to traditional Chinese medicine, ulcerative colitis is diagnosed as a disorder characterized by the disharmony between the Spleen/Stomach and the Liver. Liver qi stagnation overacts on the Spleen and Stomach to impair the normal transformation and transportation of food. Over a long period of time, this dampness combines with heat to lodge in the Large Intestine to cause diarrhea with inflammation. Because of prolonged diarrhea and loss of fluids, yin also become deficient.

FORMULAS

GI CARE (UC) ™

(Ulcerative Colitis)

The treatment principles of *GI Care (UC)* are based on the traditional formulas *Shao Yao San* (Peony Combination) and *Da Huang Mu Dan Pi Tang* (Rhubarb and Moutan Combination) but without the draining effects from the purgative herbs such as *Da Huang* (Radix et Rhizoma Rhei) and *Mang Xiao* (Natrii Sulfas).

Nan Sha Shen (Radix Adenophorae) nourishes yin and dries up dampness. *Shan Yao* (Rhizoma Dioscoreae) nourishes the Spleen yin and relieves diarrhea. *Mai Ya* (Fructus Hordei Germinatus) and *Shan Zha* (Fructus Crataegi) promote digestion and stop bleeding. *Ma Chi Xian* (Herba Portulacae) and *Huang Lian* (Rhizoma Coptidis) dispel damp-heat in the intestines to relieve intestinal irritations. *Chi Shi Zhi* (Halloysitum Rubrum), *Chun Gen Pi* (Cortex Ailanthi), *Shi Liu Pi* (Pericarpium Granati) and *Wu Bei Zi* (Galla Chinensis) are used to bind the intestines to stop diarrhea, dispel pus, stop bleeding and generate new tissue. *Yi Yi Ren* (Semen Coicis) and *Dong Gua Zi* (Semen Benincasae) are traditionally used to treat intestinal abscess and are used here to dispel pus and mucus present in the stool. They both enter the Lung, which is connected to the Large Intestine via the *zang fu* relationship. These two herbs help to dry up dampness and enhance the ability of the Lung to metabolize water and prevent further accumulation of dampness, especially in the Large Intestine. *Fang Feng* (Radix Saposhnikoviae) is used to stop diarrhea and relieve pain. Together with *Bai Shao* (Radix Paeoniae Alba), these two herbs relieve abdominal and intestinal spasms, cramps, and pain. *Hou Po* (Cortex Magnoliae Officinalis) regulates qi in the abdomen to relieve bloating, distension and pain.

GI Care (UC) effectively treats ulcerative colitis and Crohn's disease by targeting both the cause and the symptoms. Herbs are used to treat the underlying cause of disharmony between the Spleen/Stomach and the Liver, and accumulation of damp-heat in the intestines. In addition, herbs are used to symptomatically relieve diarrhea, treat intestinal abscess, dispel pus, and alleviate pain and distention.

SUPPLEMENTARY FORMULAS

- ☙ With bleeding, add *Notoginseng 9*.
- ☙ For chronic diarrhea with qi deficiency manifesting in weight loss, malaise, fatigue and poor appetite, add *GI Tonic*. This formula should be taken to tonify the Spleen qi when the symptoms are in remission or under control.
- ☙ For chronic diarrhea with overall weakness and deficiency, add *Imperial Tonic*.
- ☙ For burning diarrhea with tenesmus, add *GI Care II*.
- ☙ For stress related ulcerative colitis, add *Calm* or *Calm ES*.
- ☙ For hemorrhoids, add *GI Care (HMR)*.
- ☙ For low-grade fever or night fever, add *Balance (Heat)*.
- ☙ For excess heat or fever, add *Gardenia Complex*.
- ☙ For bloating, add *GI Harmony*.
- ☙ For perirectal abscesses, fever, add *Resolve (AI)* and *Herbal ABX*.
- ☙ For intestinal spasms or abdominal cramping, add *Flex (SC)*.
- ☙ With anemia, add *Schisandra ZZZ*.
- ☙ For constipation, add *Gentle Lax (Deficient)*.

NUTRITION

- ☙ Avoid raw fruits, vegetables, spicy food, alcohol and others that may be stimulating to the mucosal lining of the intestines. High roughage foods such as raw fruits or vegetables sometimes worsen intestinal obstruction and colic and may need to be avoided. Alcohol and canned products should be avoided, as they may be irritating to the stomach and the intestine.
- ☙ Avoid drinking cold beverages or eating cold foods.

GI CARE (UC) ™

☙ Some patients may notice improvement of symptoms if they drink less or no milk. Dairy products in general tend to create dampness and therefore should be consumed less. Milk, cheese and other dairy products should be avoided, especially if patients are lactose intolerance.

☙ Oral iron supplements may be necessary if there is anemia due to chronic loss of blood from diarrhea. If the patient has a sensitive stomach and cannot tolerate regular oral iron supplements, sustained release iron products are recommended.

☙ In addition to avoiding certain foods (e.g. alcohol, dairy, and other irritants), it is equally important to make sure that patients have adequate calorie and fluid intake, as malnutrition and dehydration are common problems associated with ulcerative colitis.

☙ Increased intake of acidophilus and fresh yams are highly recommended to build the intestinal flora.

The Tao of Nutrition by Ni and McNease
☙ Diarrhea
  ▪ Recommendations: garlic, blueberries, raspberry leaves, lotus seeds, burned rice, yams, sweet potatoes, fresh fig leaves, peas, buckwheat, and guava peel.
  ▪ Avoid cold, raw foods, most fruits, juices, and overeating.
☙ For more information, please refer to *The Tao of Nutrition* by Dr. Maoshing Ni and Cathy McNease.

LIFESTYLE INSTRUCTIONS

☙ Avoid the use of certain drugs and chemicals that cause and/or aggravate ulcerative colitis. The list of offending drugs and/or chemicals may be different for every patient.

☙ Certain over-the-counter or prescription antidiarrheal drugs may worsen the condition and create a toxic mega colon. These drugs should not be taken unless supervised by a qualified health care provider.

☙ Bed rest and relaxation are helpful for short- and long-term recovery.

CLINICAL NOTES

☙ *GI Care (UC)* and *GI Care II* are two formulas that can be used to treat inflammation of the bowel.
  ▪ *GI Care (UC)* is designed more for patients suffering from chronic ulcerative colitis without the active infection. Therefore, it contains many herbs that would generate new tissue and repair the normal flora of the intestines.
  ▪ *GI Care II* is designed more for an active infection and inflammation of the intestines due to improper food intake. Because bacteria lodged in the intestines need to be purged out, purgative herbs such as *Da Huang* (Radix et Rhizoma Rhei) are used.

CAUTIONS

☙ This formula is contraindicated during pregnancy and nursing.
☙ This formula is contraindicated in cases of diarrhea due to Spleen qi deficiency or Kidney yang deficiency.
☙ While the use of herbs is effective in treating mild to moderate ulcerative colitis, it may not be appropriate for treating certain complications, such as toxic colitis, toxic mega colon, massive hemorrhage, free perforation, or fulminating toxic colitis. Surgical intervention may be necessary for such complications, but will require permanent ileostomy in addition to a physical and emotional burden.

FORMULAS

GI CARE (UC) ™

(Ulcerative Colitis)

ACUPUNCTURE POINTS

Traditional Points:

✪ *Zusanli* (ST 36), *Dadun* (LR 1), *Daimai* (GB 26), *Weizhong* (BL 40), *Huangshu* (KI 16), *Guilai* (ST 29), *Fushe* (SP 13), *Tianshu* (ST 25), *Sanyinjiao* (SP 6), and *Yinlingquan* (SP 9).

Balance Method by Dr. Richard Tan:

✪ Left side: *Zhongfeng* (LR 4), *Gongsun* (SP 4), *Yinlingquan* (SP 9), *Hegu* (LI 4), and *Lingku*.

✪ Right side: *Lieque* (LU 7), *Kongzui* (LU 6), *Neiguan* (PC 6), *Zusanli* (ST 36), *Tiaokou* (ST 38) or *ah shi* points nearby.

✪ Left and right side can be alternated from treatment to treatment.

✪ Ear points: *Shenmen* and Intestine.

✪ Note: *Lingku* is one of Master Tong's points on both hands. *Lingku* is located in the depression just distal to the junction of the first and second metacarpal bones, approximately 0.5 *cun* proximal to *Hegu* (LI 4), on the *yangming* line.

✪ For additional information on the Balance Method, please refer to *Twelve and Twelve in Acupuncture* and *Twenty-Four More in Acupuncture* by Dr. Richard Tan.

Ear Points:

✪ Main points: Large Intestine, Small Intestine, and Sympathetic.

✪ Adjunct points: Spleen, Rectum, *San Jiao*, and Endocrine.

MODERN RESEARCH

Ulcerative colitis is a chronic, non-specific, idiopathic, inflammatory and ulcerative disease of the colon and the rectum. It has no known etiology. Possible risk factors include immunological factors, infectious agents (such as bacteria, virus or amoeba), dietary factors (including chemicals and drugs), and psychosomatic factors. Ulcerative colitis usually occurs between ages 15 to 30, or between 50 to 70. Clinical presentations of ulcerative colitis vary greatly depending on the extent and severity of the illness. The initial presentation begins with gradual onset of diarrhea with mucus and blood. There are symptomatic and asymptomatic intervals of diarrhea. Patients may also experience tenesmus and left lower quadrant pain and cramps. [1] Optimal treatment requires use of herbs to address the cause, the symptoms, and the complications.

In treating ulcerative colitis, many herbs are used with marked effect to treat inflammation of the gastrointestinal tract. According to one clinical study, 100 patients with inflammation of the gastrointestinal tract were treated with *Huang Lian* (Rhizoma Coptidis) and *Bai Dou Kou* (Fructus Amomi Rotundus), 2 to 3 grams per dose for 4 to 6 doses per day, with all patients reporting improvement. [2]

Since infection is one of the main causes of ulcerative colitis, this formula uses many herbs with marked antibiotic effects. Herbs in this formula have shown marked antibacterial, antiviral and antifungal effects. Examples of such herbs include *Bai Shao* (Radix Paeoniae Alba),[3] *Hou Po* (Cortex Magnoliae Officinalis),[4] *Ma Chi Xian* (Herba Portulacae),[5] *Huang Lian* (Rhizoma Coptidis),[6,7] and *Shi Liu Pi* (Pericarpium Granati).[8] In fact, many herbs have been used successfully specifically for treatment of infection and inflammation of the gastrointestinal tract. In one study, *Shan Zha* (Fructus Crataegi) was used to treat 100 patients with acute bacterial enteritis with satisfactory results. [9] In another study, use of *Ma Chi Xian* (Herba Portulacae) was 83.62% effective in treating 403 patients with chronic bacterial dysentery, and 89.12% effective in treating 331 patients with acute bacterial dysentery. [10] Lastly, use of *Huang Lian* (Rhizoma Coptidis), individually or in an herbal formula, is associated with excellent clinical results in treating over 1,000 patients with bacterial dysentery. The treatments showed marked effectiveness, short duration of treatment, and low incidence of side effects. [11]

GI CARE (UC) ™

(Ulcerative Colitis)

GI Care (UC) employs such herbs as *Shan Yao* (Rhizoma Dioscoreae), *Mai Ya* (Fructus Hordei Germinatus) and *Shan Zha* (Fructus Crataegi) to promote normal digestion and absorption, and reduce the stress of the intestines. *Shan Yao* (Rhizoma Dioscoreae) is used to treat indigestion and reduce the stress of the intestines. In one study, it was found that use of *Shan Yao* (Rhizoma Dioscoreae) and other herbs were effective in treating 101 infants with indigestion and related complications.[12] *Mai Ya* (Fructus Hordei Germinatus) improves digestion by increasing gastric emptying time and intestinal peristalsis. Lastly, *Shan Zha* (Fructus Crataegi) facilitates digestion and absorption by inducing the production of gastric acid.[13]

In addition to treating the cause, herbs that address the symptoms of ulcerative colitis are incorporated. *Shan Yao* (Rhizoma Dioscoreae) and *Shan Zha* (Fructus Crataegi) consolidate the stool and treat diarrhea.[14,15] *Bai Shao* (Radix Paeoniae Alba) has an antispasmodic effect to relieve intestinal spasms and cramps.[16]

Lastly, herbs are added to eliminate toxins, which may irritate the bowel causing inflammation of the intestines. *Fang Feng* (Radix Saposhnikoviae) has been shown to facilitate the elimination of heavy metals.[17] *Chi Shi Zhi* (Halloysitum Rubrum) is effective in eliminating various offending agents, including but not limited to phosphorus, mercury, and bacterial endotoxin.[18]

In summary, *GI Care (UC)* is a carefully crafted formula with many herbs that treat the cause and the symptoms of ulcerative colitis. *GI Care (UC)* contains herbs that reduce the inflammation of the gastrointestinal tract, treat the infection, promote normal digestion and absorption, relieve diarrhea, alleviate abdominal spasms and cramps, and eliminate irritating toxins.

PHARMACEUTICAL DRUGS & CHINESE MEDICINE: A COMPARATIVE ANALYSIS

Western Medical Approach: Ulcerative colitis is a chronic, non-specific, idiopathic, inflammatory and ulcerative disease of the colon and rectum.[19] Because western medicine recognizes no known etiology, drug treatments are focused primarily to treat symptoms. Three classes of drugs used to treat ulcerative colitis include antidiarrheals, 5-Aminosalicylates, and corticosteroids. Antidiarrheal agents [such as Lomotil (Diphenoxylate) and Imodium (Loperamide)] stop diarrhea, but may cause dizziness, drowsiness, sedation, and in some cases, dependence with long-term use. 5-Aminosalicylates [such as Azulfidine (Sulfasalazine), Dipentum (Olsalazine) and Pentasa (Mesalamine)] suppress low-grade inflammation, but are not used often because of side effects such as anorexia, dyspepsia, nausea and vomiting. Lastly, oral or IV corticosteroids are used to suppress moderate to severe cases of ulcerative colitis. However, long-term use of corticosteroids has numerous side effects, including but not limited to osteoporosis, glucose intolerance, cataract formation, fluid retention, dependence and muscle wasting. Finally, surgical colectomy is performed in severe and emergency cases of massive hemorrhage, free perforation, or fulminating toxic colitis. The disadvantages of surgery include permanent ileostomy, possible sexual dysfunction in males, and physical and emotional burden.

Traditional Chinese Medicine Approach: Use of acupuncture and herbs is effective to treat inflammatory conditions of the colon, including both ulcerative colitis, Crohn's disease, and traveler's diarrhea. While acupuncture and herbal treatments are effective for both prevention and treatment, they do have limitations. Certain complications of ulcerative colitis are considered medical emergencies, and should not be treated with acupuncture and herbs. Complications such as toxic colitis or toxic megacolon require immediate hospitalization. Furthermore, serious complications such as massive hemorrhage, free perforation, or fulminating toxic colitis require immediate surgical intervention.

FORMULAS

GI CARE (UC) ™

(Ulcerative Colitis)

CASE STUDY

A 49-year-old female has chronic ulcerative colitis as well as epigastric and abdominal pain and bloody stool. In the past 12 months, the patient has been treated with various herbs and drugs. The patient stated that while the treatments were effective, bloody stools returned as soon as the treatment was discontinued. The patient had 2 to 3 bowel movements per day and was constantly tired. The tongue was dark purple with thick greasy yellow coat. The pulse was deep and slippery. The diagnosis was accumulation of damp-heat and toxins in the Large Intestine. After taking *GI Care (UC)* for 30 days, the patient reported significant improvement of all symptoms. Furthermore, her bowel movement returned to normal without blood. In the follow-up session one year later, the patient noted that she has remained healthy and without a relapse of her original chief complaint.

Y.L., Hebei, China

[1] Beers, M. and Berkow, R. *The Merck Manual of Diagnosis and Therapy 17th Edition*. 1999.
[2] *Si Chuan Yi Xue Yuan Xue Bao* (Journal of Sichuan School of Medicine), 1959; 1:102
[3] *Xin Zhong Yi* (New Chinese Medicine), 1989; 21(3):51
[4] *Yao Jian Gong Zuo Tong Xun* (Journal of Herbal Preparations), 1980; 10(4):209
[5] *Ji Lin Zhong Yi Yao* (Jilin Chinese Medicine and Herbology), 1985; 3:28
[6] *Zhong Guo Yi Yao Bao* (Chinese Journal of Medicine and Medicinals), 1958; 44(9):888
[7] *Zhong Xi Yi Jie He Za Zhi* (Journal of Integrated Chinese and Western Medicine), 1989; 9(8):494)
[8] *Zhong Cao Yao Xue* (Study of Chinese Herbal Medicine), 1976; 694
[9] *Xin Yi Xue* (New Medicine), 1975; 2:111
[10] *Fu Jian Zhong Yi Yao* (Fujian Chinese Medicine and Herbology), 1959; 6:1
[11] *Zhong Hua Nei Ke Za Zhi* (Chinese Journal of Internal Medicine), 1976; 4:219
[12] *Zhong Yi Za Zhi* (Journal of Chinese Medicine), 1984; 5:9
[13] *Ying Yang Xue Bao* (Report of Nutrition), 1984; 6(2):109
[14] *Hu Nan Yi Yao Za Zhi* (Hunan Journal of Medicine and Herbology), 1982; 4:17
[15] *Yun Nan Zhong Yao Zhi* (Yunan Journal of Chinese Herbal Medicine), 1973; 3:31
[16] *Zhong Yi Za Zhi* (Journal of Chinese Medicine), 1985; 6:50
[17] *Xin Yi Yao Tong Xun* (Journal of New Medicine and Herbology), 1973; 7:6
[18] *Chang Yong Zhong Yao Xian Dai Yan Jiu Yu Lin Chuang* (Recent Study & Clinical Application of Common Traditional Chinese Medicine), 1995; 679:680
[19] Berkow, Robert. The Merck Manual of Diagnosis and Therapy 16th Edition. Merck & Co., Inc. 1992

FORMULAS

GI HARMONY ™

CLINICAL APPLICATIONS

- Irritable bowel syndrome (IBS)
- Other bowel disorders, such as diverticulitis, mucous colitis, nervous bowel, irritable colon, and spastic colon
- Alternating diarrhea and constipation with abdominal bloating, pain, flatulence and a feeling of incomplete evacuation, and straining and urgency of bowel movements

WESTERN THERAPEUTIC ACTIONS

- Soothes the irritation of the gastrointestinal tract caused by drugs, chemicals, and certain foods [1,2,3]
- Relieves diarrhea and constipation [4,5,6,7,8,9,10,11]
- Regulates gastrointestinal function [12,13,14,15]
- Relieves pain, spasms and cramps [16,17,18,19]
- Relieves bloating, flatulence and inflammation [20,21,22]

CHINESE THERAPEUTIC ACTIONS

- Tonifies the Spleen
- Regulates Liver qi
- Stops diarrhea
- Clears damp-heat

DOSAGE

Take 3 to 4 capsules three times daily with warm water. Dosage can be increased up to 8 to 10 capsules three times daily in acute cases until symptoms subside. For maximum effectiveness, take the herbs on an empty stomach.

INGREDIENTS

Bai Shao (Radix Paeoniae Alba)
Bai Zhi (Radix Angelicae Dahuricae)
Bai Zhu (Rhizoma Atractylodis Macrocephalae)
Bo He (Herba Menthae)
Chai Hu (Radix Bupleuri)
Che Qian Zi (Semen Plantaginis)
Chen Pi (Pericarpium Citri Reticulatae)
Dang Gui (Radicis Angelicae Sinensis)
Dang Shen (Radix Codonopsis)
Fang Feng (Radix Saposhnikoviae)
Fu Ling (Poria)

Hou Po (Cortex Magnoliae Officinalis)
Huang Bai (Cortex Phellodendri)
Huang Lian (Rhizoma Coptidis)
Huo Xiang (Herba Agastache)
Mu Xiang (Radix Aucklandiae)
Pao Jiang (Rhizoma Zingiberis Preparatum)
Qin Pi (Cortex Fraxini)
Wu Wei Zi (Fructus Schisandrae Chinensis)
Yi Yi Ren (Semen Coicis)
Yin Chen Hao (Herba Artemisiae Scopariae)
Zhi Gan Cao (Radix Glycyrrhizae Preparata)

FORMULA EXPLANATION

According to traditional Chinese medicine, irritable bowel syndrome (IBS) is a condition caused by Spleen qi deficiency and Liver qi stagnation. Symptoms associated with IBS are closely related to stress. Gastrointestinal symptoms such as loose stool, mucus in the stool, pain, incomplete evacuation and bloating are all results of Liver overacting on the Spleen and Stomach. Similarly, many other bowel disorders exhibit similar signs and symptoms described above. *GI Harmony* focuses on tonifying the Spleen, spreading the Liver qi to relieve bloating and pain, reducing inflammation in the intestines by dispelling damp-heat and harmonizing the Stomach.

FORMULAS

GI HARMONY ™

Dang Shen (Radix Codonopsis), *Bai Zhu* (Rhizoma Atractylodis Macrocephalae), *Fu Ling* (Poria), and *Yi Yi Ren* (Semen Coicis) tonify the Spleen and dispel dampness. Dampness in the body is manifested by presence of mucus in the stool. Dampness in the intestines also causes feelings of incomplete evacuation. The above herbs are used to strengthen Spleen qi and avoid the conditions characterized by Wood overacting on the Earth element. *Huo Xiang* (Herba Agastache), *Fang Feng* (Radix Saposhnikoviae), and *Wu Wei Zi* (Fructus Schisandrae Chinensis) are used to stop diarrhea. *Chai Hu* (Radix Bupleuri), *Hou Po* (Cortex Magnoliae Officinalis), *Chen Pi* (Pericarpium Citri Reticulatae), *Bo He* (Herba Menthae), and *Mu Xiang* (Radix Aucklandiae) are qi-regulating herbs used to relieve bloating, pain, gas and stress. *Bai Shao* (Radix Paeoniae Alba) and *Dang Gui* (Radicis Angelicae Sinensis) nourish blood to soften the Liver and relieve cramps. To reduce the inflammation in the intestines, heat-clearing herbs, such as *Huang Bai* (Cortex Phellodendri), *Huang Lian* (Rhizoma Coptidis), *Yin Chen Hao* (Herba Artemisiae Scopariae), *Che Qian Zi* (Semen Plantaginis), and *Qin Pi* (Cortex Fraxini), are used. *Yin Chen Hao* (Herba Artemisiae Scopariae) also increases the production of bile to help digestion. *Che Qian Zi* (Semen Plantaginis) also dispels water through urination to consolidate stool. *Pao Jiang* (Rhizoma Zingiberis Preparatum) and *Zhi Gan Cao* (Radix Glycyrrhizae Preparata) are used to harmonize the middle *jiao*. Finally, *Bai Zhi* (Radix Angelicae Dahuricae) enters the Stomach and the Spleen channels to stop diarrhea, eliminate pus, and relieve pain.

GI Harmony is a comprehensive formula that addresses many aspects of irritable bowel syndrome and other bowel disorders. *GI Harmony* treats the cause of the disorder by tonifying the Spleen and spreading Liver qi stagnation. Furthermore, *GI Harmony* treats the symptoms by relieving bloating and flatulence, regulating bowel movement, and alleviating abdominal pain.

SUPPLEMENTARY FORMULAS

- For bowel irritation due to stress, add *Calm*.
- For irritable bowel with insomnia due to *shen* (spirit) disturbance in patients with excess, add *Calm (ES)*.
- For irritable bowel with insomnia due to stress in patients with deficiency, add *Calm ZZZ*.
- For irritable bowel associated with accumulation of toxins in the body, add *Herbal DTX*.
- For constipation, add *Gentle Lax (Deficient)*.
- For hemorrhoids, add *GI Care (HMR)*.
- For diverticulitis, add *Resolve (AI)*.
- For peptic ulcer, add *GI Care*.
- For burning diarrhea or dysentery, add *GI Care II*.
- For fatigue or weakness, add *Imperial Tonic*.
- For excess fire, add *Gardenia Complex*.
- For bleeding, add *Notoginseng 9*.

CAUTIONS

- Patients who are on anticoagulant or antiplatelet therapies, such as Coumadin (Warfarin), should use this formula with caution, as there may be a slightly higher risk of bleeding and bruising.
- This formula is contraindicated during pregnancy and nursing.

ACUPUNCTURE POINTS

Traditional Points:
- *Dachangshu* (BL 25), *Tianshu* (ST 25), *Zhongji* (CV 3), and *Shenque* (CV 8).

GI HARMONY ™

Balance Method by Dr. Richard Tan:
- Left side: *Zhongfeng* (LR 4), *Gongsun* (SP 4), *Sanyinjiao* (SP 6), *Yinlingquan* (SP 9), *Hegu* (LI 4), and *Lingku*.
- Right side: *Lieque* (LU 7), *Kongzui* (LU 6), *Neiguan* (PC 6), *Liangqiu* (ST 34), *Zusanli* (ST 36), *Tiaokou* (ST 38) or any *ah shi* points nearby, Ear *Shenmen* and Intestine.
- Left and right side can be alternated from treatment to treatment.
- Ear points: *Shenmen* and Intestine.
- Note: *Lingku* is one of Master Tong's points on both hands. *Lingku* is located in the depression just distal to the junction of the first and second metacarpal bones, approximately 0.5 *cun* proximal to *Hegu* (LI 4), on the *yangming* line.
- For additional information on the Balance Method, please refer to *Twelve and Twelve in Acupuncture* and *Twenty-Four More in Acupuncture* by Dr. Richard Tan.

NUTRITION

- Diet is essential to complete recovery. Foods that are associated with gas production should not be consumed, such as onions, soda, beans, cabbage, brussels sprouts, cauliflower and broccoli. Also avoid the intake of milk, as some patients may be lactose intolerant.
- Foods that are spicy, acidic or that are stimulating to the lining of the intestine should also be avoided whenever possible.
- Stop smoking and reduce the intake of coffee, as they may irritate the bowel.

The Tao of Nutrition by Ni and McNease
- Diarrhea
  - Recommendations: garlic, blueberries, raspberry leaves, lotus seeds, burned rice, yams, sweet potatoes, fresh fig leaves, peas, buckwheat, and guava peel.
  - Avoid cold, raw foods, most fruits, juices, and overeating.
- For more information, please refer to *The Tao of Nutrition* by Dr. Maoshing Ni and Cathy McNease.

LIFESTYLE INSTRUCTIONS

- Stress is a major factor in patients suffering from IBS. A relaxed or positive outlook on life is very important to recovery. Patients should be advised to learn to become more relaxed.
- Application of a heat pad to the abdomen may help with relieving pain associated with bloating and distension. Light abdominal massage in circular motions clockwise and then counter-clock wise starting from small circles gradually becoming bigger may also help relieve distension, discomfort and pain. A five-minute abdominal massage is recommended daily. Patients should be advised to pass gas whenever needed to relieve qi stagnation.

CLINICAL NOTES

- Patients should take **Calm** to continually relieve Liver qi stagnation, especially if they have a stressful lifestyle or career. **GI Harmony** and **Calm** can be taken at an equal portions for patients who have IBS and are constantly stressed.
- Female patients suffering from IBS are likely to note aggravation of symptoms before each menstrual cycle. **Calm** is recommended with **GI Harmony** for maximum effect.

MODERN RESEARCH

Irritable bowel syndrome (IBS) is a motility disorder involving the entire gastrointestinal tract causing varying degrees of abdominal pain, constipation and/or diarrhea and abdominal bloating. In addition, patients often notice a

FORMULAS

change in the pattern of bowel movement, mucus in the stool, and sensation of incomplete evacuation after defecation. Though the exact cause is unknown, it has been found that emotional factors, diet, drugs, or hormones often precipitate or aggravate the condition. Optimal treatment, therefore, must focus on alleviating the gastrointestinal symptoms and eliminating the factors that trigger the bowel irritation.

Since the bowel irritation may be associated with intake of certain foods and/or drugs, herbs are added to detoxify the offending substances. Administration of *Dan Shen* (Radix Salviae Miltiorrhizae) showed marked protective effect against irritation of the gastrointestinal tract as caused by aspirin and non-steroidal-anti-inflammatory drugs.[1] In addition, glycyrrhizin, one of the main constituents of *Gan Cao* (Radix Glycyrrhizae), has a remarkable detoxifying effect to treat various kinds of poisonings, including but not limited to drug poisoning (chloral hydrate, urethane, cocaine, picrotoxin, caffeine, pilocarpine, nicotine, barbiturates, mercury and lead), food poisoning (tetrodotoxin, snake, and mushrooms), and others (enterotoxin, herbicides, pesticides).[2] Finally, *Gan Cao* (Radix Glycyrrhizae) is also effective for treatment of food poisoning.[3]

Because irritable bowel syndrome is a disorder characterized by alternation of diarrhea and constipation, *Bai Zhu* (Rhizoma Atractylodis Macrocephalae) is one of the most important herbs in treatment. *Bai Zhu* (Rhizoma Atractylodis Macrocephalae) is well known for its regulating and dual effect on the gastrointestinal tract. It treats diarrhea at low doses and constipation at high doses. With this dual effect, it is the ideal herb for cases where there is alternation of diarrhea and constipation.[4]

Many other herbs in *GI Harmony* have a marked effects to influence the gastrointestinal tract. Herbs that treat diarrhea include *Bai Zhu* (Rhizoma Atractylodis Macrocephalae), *Wu Wei Zi* (Fructus Schisandrae Chinensis), *Che Qian Zi* (Semen Plantaginis), *Huang Bai* (Cortex Phellodendri) and *Huang Lian* (Rhizoma Coptidis). In one study, 320 infants with diarrhea were treated with an herbal powder containing *Bai Zhu* (Rhizoma Atractylodis Macrocephalae) three times daily before meals with good results.[5] In another study, 63 out of 69 infants with diarrhea showed complete recovery within 1 to 2 days following treatment using an herbal decoction containing 30 grams of *Che Qian Zi* (Semen Plantaginis) and a small amount of sugar.[6] Furthermore, in a clinical study, 93 infants with diarrhea were treated with *Fu Ling* (Poria) with good symptomatic relief and a shortened duration of diarrhea.[7] In addition to diarrhea, many herbs in *GI Harmony* are also effective for treating dysentery, such as *Wu Wei Zi* (Fructus Schisandrae Chinensis), *Che Qian Zi* (Semen Plantaginis), *Huang Bai* (Cortex Phellodendri), and *Huang Lian* (Rhizoma Coptidis).[8,9] Specifically with *Huang Bai* (Cortex Phellodendri), 40 patients with chronic bacterial dysentery were treated twice daily for 7 days with marked results in all patients.[10] Lastly, the use of *Huang Lian* (Rhizoma Coptidis) is associated with excellent clinical results in treating over 1,000 patients with bacterial dysentery. The treatments showed marked effectiveness, short duration of treatment, and low incidence of side effects.[11] In short, *GI Harmony* contains many herbs with well-documented results to treat diarrhea.

Many of the herbs in *GI Harmony* have a general regulatory effect on the gastrointestinal tract. For example, *Dang Shen* (Radix Codonopsis) has marked preventative and treatment effects on peptic ulcers. It increases gastric emptying time, decreases severity of ulceration, and increases the amount of prostaglandin in the stomach.[12] Deoxyschizandrin, one ingredient of *Wu Wei Zi* (Fructus Schisandrae Chinensis), inhibits the secretion of gastric acid in rats, and has shown beneficial effects in treatment of gastric ulcer.[13] *Hou Po* (Cortex Magnoliae Officinalis) has an inhibitory effect on the gastrointestinal system, leading to decreased secretion of gastric acid.[14] Many components of *Gan Cao* (Radix Glycyrrhizae) have shown protective and treatment effect in peptic ulcer. The mechanisms of action include inhibition of gastric acid secretion, binding and deactivation of gastric acid, and promotion of recovery from ulceration.[15]

Many herbs in *GI Harmony* have an antispasmodic effect to alleviate pain and relieve spasms and cramps of the intestines. *Gan Cao* (Radix Glycyrrhizae) has an inhibitory influence on smooth muscle to stop spasms and cramps of the intestines.[16] In one clinical trial, 241 out of 254 patients (94.8%) with intestinal spasms showed a significant

FORMULAS

improvement after receiving 10 to 15 ml of extract of *Gan Cao* (Radix Glycyrrhizae) three times daily for 3 to 6 days.[17] Furthermore, various components of *Bai Zhi* (Radix Angelicae Dahuricae) have demonstrated a marked muscle-relaxant effect to treat muscle spasms and cramps.[18,19]

Lastly, there are many herbs in **GI Harmony** that provides symptomatic relief for irritable bowel syndrome. For example, use of *Hou Po* (Cortex Magnoliae Officinalis) was associated with decreased incidence of intestinal bloating.[20] Administration of *Mu Xiang* (Radix Aucklandiae) was 100% effective in 29 patients in reducing flatulence due to indigestion, acute gastroenteritis, gastric nervosa, and post-surgical complications.[21] Lastly, an herbal formula composed of 80% *Huang Lian* (Rhizoma Coptidis) was effective in treating 100 patients with inflammatory bowel condition, such as acute gastroenteritis or enteritis.[22]

In summary, **GI Harmony** contains herbs with marked effectiveness to address causes and symptoms of irritable bowel syndrome. **GI Harmony** neutralizes the irritation caused by toxic and offending agents (such as drugs and chemicals), regulates the bowel movement, and relieves pain and distention.

PHARMACEUTICAL DRUGS & CHINESE MEDICINE: A COMPARATIVE ANALYSIS

Western Medical Approach: Irritable bowel syndrome (IBS) is a motility disorder that affects the entire gastrointestinal tract. This disorder has no known anatomic cause. Therefore, most drug treatments focus on relieving symptoms. Anticholinergic drugs [such as Pro-Banthine (Propantheline)], tranquilizers [such as Librium (Chlordiazepoxide)], and sedatives [such as phenobarbital] are frequently given to relieve gastrointestinal symptoms and to calm the patients. Those with depression are treated with antidepressants, and ones with diarrhea are treated with antidiarrheals. While this discussion of drug treatment is an over simplification, it nonetheless illustrates that these drugs only treat symptoms, and not the cause, of irritable bowel syndrome. Therefore, though they offer short-term effectiveness, symptoms often flare up again once the drugs are discontinued.

Traditional Chinese Medicine Approach: Use of acupuncture and herbs is effective to treat various gastrointestinal disorders, including but not limited to irritable bowel syndrome, diverticulitis, mucous colitis, nervous bowel, irritable colon, and spastic colon. Not only do they control the symptoms, they often change the underlying constitution of the body to achieve long-term results. In fact, most patients remain symptom free for at least several months after the herbs are discontinued.

Summation: It is important to remember that stress and diet are two main factors that trigger irritable bowel syndrome. In addition to considering drugs or herbal treatment, it is important to follow the guidelines described above, and make diet and lifestyle changes. Only then will treatment successfully ensure short- and long-term effectiveness, and minimize frequency and severity of irritable bowel syndrome.

CASE STUDIES

P.Q., a 42-year-old female, presented with acid reflux and a 20-year history of irritable bowel syndrome. She had been on Xanax (Alprazolam), Nexium (Esomeprazole) and other western medications. After only four days of taking **GI Harmony** at four capsules, three times daily, the patient saw improvement. She is now successfully off all western medications. The doctor commented that this formula is a "miracle in a bottle."

H.C., Stephens City, Virginia

G.M., a 42-year-old female, presented with pain in the lower *jiao*, extreme fatigue, constipation, depression, poor concentration, pain with diarrhea, palpitations and night sweats. The Western diagnosis was chronic fatigue syndrome [as the doctors couldn't find anything specific wrong]; the TCM diagnosis was yin deficiency with deficiency heat. After taking **Balance (Heat)**, **GI Harmony** and **Gentle Lax (Deficient)**, the patient reported little to no night sweats within three weeks. Her bowels normalized, and the GI tract pain was much better. She stated that she felt she could now smile and face the day.

M.C., Sarasota, Florida

[1] *Zhong Yao Yao Li Yu Lin Chuang* (Pharmacology and Clinical Applications of Chinese Herbs), 1991; 14(5):47
[2] *Zhong Yao Tong Bao* (Journal of Chinese Herbology), 1986; 11(10):55
[3] *Xin Zhong Yi* (New Chinese Medicine), 1978; 1:36
[4] *Chang Yong Zhong Yao Cheng Fen Yu Yao Li Shou Ce* (A Handbook of the Composition and Pharmacology of Common Chinese Drugs), 1994; 739:742
[5] *Shan Dong Zhong Yi Za Zhi* (Shandong Journal of Chinese Medicine), 1982; 2:107
[6] *Zhong Xi Yi Jie He Za Zhi* (Journal of Integrated Chinese and Western Medicine), 1987; 11:697
[7] *Bei Jing Zhong Yi* (Beijing Chinese Medicine), 1985; 5:31
[8] *Tian Jing Yi Xue Za Zhi* (Journal of Tianjing Medicine and Herbology), 1965; 4:338
[9] *Zhong Hua Nei Ke Za Zhi* (Chinese Journal of Internal Medicine), 1960; 4:351
[10] *Zhong Yi Za Zhi* (Journal of Chinese Medicine), 1959; 8:23
[11] *Zhong Hua Nei Ke Za Zhi* (Chinese Journal of Internal Medicine), 1976; 4:219
[12] *Zhong Yao Yao Li Yu Lin Chuang* (Pharmacology and Clinical Applications of Chinese Herbs), 1990; 6(6):9
[13] *Ri Ben Yao Li Xue Za Zhi* (Japanese Journal of Herbology), 1986; 87(3):209
[14] *Guo Wai Yi Yao Zhi Wu Yao Fen Ce* (Monograph of Foreign Botanical Medicine), 1988; 10(1):43
[15] *Zhong Yao Zhi* (Chinese Herbology Journal), 1993; 358
[16] *Zhong Yao Zhi* (Chinese Herbology Journal), 1993; 358
[17] *Zhong Hua Wai Ke Za Zhi* (Chinese Journal of External Medicine), 1960; 4:354
[18] *Zhong Yao Yao Li Yu Ying Yong* (Pharmacology and Applications of Chinese Herbs), 1983; 796
[19] *Zhi Wu Yao You Xiao Cheng Fen Shou Ce* (Manual of Plant Medicinals and Their Active Constituents), 1986; 624, 603, 197
[20] *Xin Yi Yao Xue Za Zhi* (New Journal of Medicine and Herbology), 1973; 4:25
[21] *Yun Nan Zhong Yao Zhi* (Yunan Journal of Chinese Herbal Medicine), 1979; 3:37
[22] *Si Chuan Yi Xue Yuan Xue Bao* (Journal of Sichuan School of Medicine), 1959; 1:102

GI TONIC ™

CLINICAL APPLICATIONS

- ☯ General weakness and deficiency of the digestive system: loose stool or diarrhea, poor appetite, anorexia, fatigue, borborygmus, bloating, weight loss, sallow complexion, weak pulse, and scalloped tongue
- ☯ Spleen qi deficiency with inflammatory bowel condition with diarrhea: irritable bowel syndrome, ulcerative colitis or Crohn's disease
- ☯ Spleen qi deficiency causing various gastrointestinal disorders: diarrhea, superficial gastritis, inflammatory condition of the intestines, chronic inflammatory bowel disease, and chronic colitis
- ☯ Malnutrition in children or those with poor appetites and loose stools

WESTERN THERAPEUTIC ACTIONS

- ☯ General gastrointestinal effect to relieve diarrhea [1,2,3,4,5]
- ☯ Anti-inflammatory effect to treat gastritis, gastric ulcer and duodenal ulcer [6,7,8]
- ☯ Anti-inflammatory effect to treat inflammatory bowel syndrome [9]

CHINESE THERAPEUTIC ACTIONS

- ☯ Tonifies Spleen qi
- ☯ Stops diarrhea
- ☯ Promotes digestion
- ☯ Dispels dampness and stagnation

DOSAGE

Take 2 to 4 capsules three times daily on an empty stomach, one hour before or two hours after meals. The formula can be used to treat diarrhea symptomatically. However, to achieve long-term and lasting effect, *GI Tonic* should be taken continuously for 3 to 6 months to change the constitution of the Spleen and the Stomach.

INGREDIENTS

Bai Zhu (Rhizoma Atractylodis Macrocephalae)
Bian Dou (Semen Lablab Album)
Fu Ling (Poria)
Gan Cao (Radix Glycyrrhizae)
Huang Qi (Radix Astragali)
Jie Geng (Radix Platycodonis)

Lian Zi (Semen Nelumbinis)
Ren Shen (Radix Ginseng)
Sha Ren (Fructus Amomi)
Shan Yao (Rhizoma Dioscoreae)
Yi Yi Ren (Semen Coicis)

FORMULA EXPLANATION

GI Tonic is designed to treat Spleen deficiency leading to symptoms of diarrhea, loose stool, poor appetite, fatigue, borborygmus, bloating and other gastrointestinal disorders. In traditional Chinese medicine, the main function of the Spleen is to extract qi from the food and turn it into energy. When the Spleen and the Stomach are deficient, they will not be able to carry out the normal digestive functions. As a result, food may travel quickly out of the body without being digested or absorbed. A weak digestive system would directly result in low appetite. Lack of nutrients would cause weak extremities, weight loss and sallow facial appearance. Deficiency of the Spleen may cause accumulation of dampness, which may obstruct the qi flow and cause fullness in the chest.

FORMULAS

GI TONIC ™

GI Tonic contains many herbs to strengthen the Spleen and dispel dampness to restore normal digestive functions. *Ren Shen* (Radix Ginseng) and *Huang Qi* (Radix Astragali) tonify the *yuan* (source) *qi* and Spleen qi to relieve weakness and fatigue. They also have a strong effect to increase energy and vitality. *Bai Zhu* (Rhizoma Atractylodis Macrocephalae) and *Fu Ling* (Poria) strengthen the Spleen, dispel dampness and relieve diarrhea. As they strengthen the Spleen, they also help increase appetite as well. *Shan Yao* (Rhizoma Dioscoreae), *Bian Dou* (Semen Lablab Album) and *Lian Zi* (Semen Nelumbinis) tonify both qi and Spleen yin. They are also slightly astringent in taste, and therefore have stabilizing and binding effect to relieve diarrhea or loose stool. *Yi Yi Ren* (Semen Coicis) dispels dampness, promotes urination and expels excess fluid retention in the body. *Sha Ren* (Fructus Amomi) is aromatic as it dries up dampness and stops diarrhea. It also regulates qi to relieve bloating and borborygmus. *Jie Geng* (Radix Platycodonis) raises qi and prevents prolapse that may be caused by diarrhea. *Gan Cao* (Radix Glycyrrhizae) is used to harmonize the middle *jiao* and also the entire formula.

In short, *GI Tonic* contains herbs with great effect to tonify Spleen qi, stop diarrhea, promote digestion, and dispel dampness and stagnation. It is an excellent formula to treat digestive disorder characterized by generalized weakness and deficiency.

SUPPLEMENTARY FORMULAS

- For early morning diarrhea with coldness, add *Kidney Tonic (Yang)*.
- Diarrhea or dysentery due to infection of the gastrointestinal tract, use *GI Care II* and *Herbal ABX*.
- For inflammatory bowel syndrome or ulcerative colitis caused by damp-heat in the intestines, use *GI Care (UC)*.
- For constipation with irritable bowel syndrome, add *Gentle Lax (Deficient)* and *GI Harmony*.
- For hemorrhoids, add *GI Care (HMR)*.
- For irritable bowel syndrome with irritability and stress, add *Calm* and *GI Harmony*.
- For extreme fatigue and deficiency in qi, blood, yin and yang, add *Imperial Tonic*.
- For an immediate boost of energy, add *Vibrant*.
- For depression, add *Shine*.
- For hepatitis, add *Liver DTX*.
- For bleeding, add *Notoginseng 9*.

NUTRITION

- Good nutrition is essential to complete recovery.
- Avoid cold, raw, greasy, fried food, sweets or alcohol. Also avoid foods that are hard to digest. Do not eat fresh fruits or vegetables on an empty stomach as they are too cold. All the above may irritate the stomach and cause poor digestion.
- Avoid dairy products if the patient is lactose intolerant.
- Ginger, scallions and garlic are recommended for daily intake.
- Increase intake of vinegar in the diet. It helps to stop diarrhea.

The Tao of Nutrition by Ni and McNease
- Diarrhea
  - Recommendations: garlic, blueberries, raspberry leaves, lotus seeds, burned rice, yams, sweet potatoes, fresh fig leaves, peas, buckwheat, and guava peel.
  - Avoid cold, raw foods, most fruits, juices, and overeating.
- For more information, please refer to *The Tao of Nutrition* by Dr. Maoshing Ni and Cathy McNease.

GI TONIC ™

LIFESTYLE INSTRUCTIONS

- Sanitation of food is important to prevent further damage to the digestive system.
- Do not sit directly on wet cement or marble floors, to prevent attack of damp cold.
- A positive outlook on life is important. Worrying and thinking too much consume Spleen qi.
- Individuals suffering from irritable bowel syndrome with alternating spells of constipation and diarrhea should stay away from stress as it may aggravate the symptoms.

CLINICAL NOTES

- *GI Tonic* may be used on a short-term basis (1 to 2 weeks) to treat diarrhea symptomatically, or on a long-term basis (3 to 6 months) to treat chronic gastrointestinal disorders.
- *GI Tonic* is beneficial for patients suffering from all kinds of gastrointestinal disorders involving Spleen qi deficiency. By strengthening the Spleen, it increases the production of post-natal qi and improves the wellness of the patients.

CAUTIONS

- This formula is contraindicated in cases of interior heat accumulation, exterior wind-cold, or exterior wind-heat.
- This formula should not be used by itself in cases of with diarrhea due to damp-heat in the intestines, with such symptoms as burning sensations in the anus, tenesmus and foul-smelling stool. This condition is an indication of infection, and must be treated first with herbs that clear damp-heat from the intestines.

ACUPUNCTURE POINTS

Traditional Points:
- *Pishu* (BL 20), *Shenshu* (BL 23), *Zhongwan* (CV 12), *Tianshu* (ST 25), *Shangjuxu* (ST 37), *Yinlingquan* (SP 9), *Guanyuan* (CV 4), and *Mingmen* (GV 4).

Balance Method by Dr. Richard Tan:
- Left side: *Zusanli* (ST 36), *Shangjuxu* (ST 37), *Neiguan* (PC 6), *Xuehai* (SP 10).
- Right side: *Hegu* (LI 4), *Waiguan* (TH 5), *Yinlingquan* (SP 9), *Liangqiu* (ST 34).
- Left and right side can be alternated from treatment to treatment.
- To read more about Dr. Tan's theories behind acupuncture, see his book *Dr. Tan's Strategy of Twelve Magic Points*.

Ear Points:
- Large Intestine, Small Intestine, Lung, and Spleen.

MODERN RESEARCH

GI Tonic is an herbal formula designed to restore normal function of the gastrointestinal tract. Clinically, it is used to treat such disorders as diarrhea, inflammatory bowel condition, gastritis, and colitis. Furthermore, it is also effective in relieving anorexia and malnutrition secondary to gastrointestinal disorders. *GI Tonic* is an effective formula to address both the causes and the symptoms of gastrointestinal problems. *GI Tonic* contains herbs that have been shown through clinical studies to have pronounced effectiveness in the treatment of diarrhea, superficial gastritis, and inflammatory condition of the intestines.

FORMULAS

GI TONIC ™

In one clinical study, 95 patients with chronic diarrhea were treated using this formula with an overall effective rate of 71.6%.[1] In another study, 42 children with diarrhea due to deficiency of the Spleen were treated, resulting in improvement in all cases.[2] The individual herbs in this formula have also shown great promise for treatment of gastrointestinal conditions. For example, 93 infants with diarrhea were treated with *Fu Ling* (Poria) with complete recovery in 79 cases, improvement in 8 cases, and no effect in 6 cases (93.4% effective rate).[3] In another study, 320 infants with diarrhea were treated three times daily with *Bai Zhu* (Rhizoma Atractylodis Macrocephalae) and *Shan Yao* (Rhizoma Dioscoreae) with good results.[4] Furthermore, 10 children diagnosed with Spleen deficiency according to traditional Chinese medicine were treated with a decoction of *Ren Shen* (Radix Ginseng) twice daily for 7 to 14 days. At the end of the study, it was reported that all had an increase in appetite, cessation of spontaneous perspiration, increase in body weight, and improvement of facial complexion.[5]

Herbs in *GI Tonic* have also shown marked effect for treatment of superficial gastritis. In one study, 32 patients were treated with complete recovery in 15 cases (46.8%), marked effect in 9 cases (28.1%), moderate effect in 7 cases (21.8%), and no effect in 1 case. The overall effective rate was 96.7%.[6] In another study, 43 patients with gastric or duodenal ulcer were treated successfully using *Sha Ren* (Fructus Amomi) in powder form. The study reported significant improvement in such symptoms as epigastric pain, abdominal distention, and acid reflux.[7] Furthermore, many components of *Gan Cao* (Radix Glycyrrhizae) have shown protective and treatment effect in patients with peptic ulcer. The mechanisms of action include inhibition of gastric acid secretion, binding and deactivation of the gastric acid, and promotion of recovery from ulceration.[8] Lastly, administration of *Huang Qi* (Radix Astragali) for one month is also associated with marked effect for treatment of peptic ulcer disease.

Patients with inflammatory bowel condition also responded well to herbs in *GI Tonic*. In one study, 24 patients with chronic inflammatory bowel disease were treated for an average of 36.2 days with complete recovery in 19 cases, improvement in 4 cases, and no effect in 1 case. In another study, patients with colitis due to deficiency of the Spleen with accumulation of dampness were treated with satisfactory results. Out of 60 patients, 38 reported complete recovery, 14 reported marked improvement, 6 reported slight improvement, and 2 reported no effect. The overall effective rate was 97%.[9]

In conclusion, *GI Tonic* is essential for the treatment of various gastrointestinal disorders, including but not limited to diarrhea, inflammatory bowel condition, colitis, superficial gastritis, and inflammatory condition of the intestines. *GI Tonic* contains herbs that will address both the cause and the symptoms of such gastrointestinal problems, thereby providing both immediate and long-term relief.

PHARMACEUTICAL DRUGS & CHINESE MEDICINE: A COMPARATIVE ANALYSIS

One striking difference between western and traditional Chinese medicine is that western medicine focuses and excels in crisis management, while traditional Chinese medicine emphasizes and shines in holistic and preventative treatments. Therefore, in emergencies, such as gun shot wounds or surgery, western medicine is generally the treatment of choice. However, for treatment of chronic idiopathic illness of unknown origins, where all lab tests are normal and a clear diagnosis cannot be made, traditional Chinese medicine is distinctly superior.

In cases of chronic energetic and digestive disorders, where all tests are normal but there are still general and non-diagnostic signs and symptoms, western medicine offers few treatment options since there is not a clear diagnosis. On the other hand, traditional Chinese medicine is beneficial as it excels in maintainance and preventative therapies. Herbs can be used to regulate imbalances and alleviate associated signs and symptoms. Therefore, herbal therapy should definitely be employed to prevent deterioration of this condition, and to restore optimal health.

GI TONIC ™

CASE STUDY

A 25-years-old female with a long-term history of digestive problems presented with indigestion and diarrhea. She stated that she experienced abdominal pain and diarrhea whenever she eats food that is slightly unclean or spoiled. In addition, she has poor appetite and indigestion. She has a skinny appearance and an aversion to cold. The diagnosis was diarrhea due to deficiency of the Spleen and Stomach. She started taking *GI Tonic*, and began to improve within one week. She continued to take the herbs for one month to strengthen the underlining deficiency.

J.C., Diamond Bar, California

[1] *Xin Yi Yao Xue Za Zhi* (New Journal of Medicine and Herbology), 1979; 3:129
[2] *Jiang Xi Zhong Yi Yao* (Jiangxi Chinese Medicine and Herbology), 1959; 4:36
[3] *Bei Jing Zhong Yi* (Beijing Chinese Medicine), 1985; 5:31
[4] *Shan Dong Zhong Yi Za Zhi* (Shandong Journal of Chinese Medicine), 1982; 2:107
[5] *Chong Qing Yi Yao* (Chongching Medicine and Herbology), 1984; 6:41
[6] *Zhong Yi Fang Ji Xian Dai Yan Jiu* (Modern Study of Medical Formulae in Traditional Chinese Medicine), 1997; 507
[7] *Fu Jian Zhong Yi Yao* (Fujian Chinese Medicine and Herbology), 1983; (6):36
[8] *Zhong Yao Zhi* (Chinese Herbology Journal), 1993; 358
[9] *Shan Dong Zhong Yi Za Zhi* (Shandong Journal of Chinese Medicine), 1991; 10(6):24)

FORMULAS

HERBAL ABX ™

(Antibiotics)

CLINICAL APPLICATIONS

☙ All types of infection, with or without fever, inflammation, redness and swelling
☙ All excess conditions presenting with fire, heat, damp-heat, or toxic heat
☙ Conditions with red tongue, yellow or greasy yellow tongue coating or forceful, rapid pulse
☙ This combination is used as an adjunct formula to clear heat

WESTERN THERAPEUTIC ACTIONS

☙ Antibacterial effects [1,2,3,4,5,6,7,8,9,13,14,15,16]
☙ Antiviral effects [10,12]
☙ Antifungal effects [10,11]
☙ Broad spectrum antibiotic functions [2,10]

CHINESE THERAPEUTIC ACTIONS

☙ Clears fire, damp-heat and toxic heat
☙ Reduces swelling and redness

DOSAGE

Take 3 to 4 capsules three times daily on an empty stomach, with warm water. Dosage may be increased to 6 to 8 capsules three times daily, if necessary. The herbs should be taken with meals for those with a sensitive stomach.

INGREDIENTS

Cha Chi Huang (Herba Stellariae Aquaticae)
Da Qing Ye (Folium Isatidis)
Feng Wei Cao (Herba Pteris)
Hu Yao Huang (Herba Leucas Mollissimae)
Huang Lian (Rhizoma Coptidis)
Liu Zhi Huang (Herba Solidaginis)

Pao Zai Cao (Herba Physalis Angulatae)
Pu Gong Ying (Herba Taraxaci)
Shu Wei Huang (Herba Rostellulariae)
Xian Feng Cao (Herba Bidentis)
Ya She Huang (Herba Lippiae)

FORMULA EXPLANATION

Herbal ABX is designed specifically as an antibiotic formula for treatment of infections. According to traditional Chinese medicine, infection is often characterized by the presentation of fire, damp-heat and/or toxic heat attacking various parts of the body. Therefore, treatment requires use of herbs that eliminate the offending pathogens. Furthermore, it is important to also treat the complications of infection, such as swelling, inflammation, and fever.

Many herbs in this formula focus on eliminating the fire, damp-heat or toxic heat causes of infection. *Huang Lian* (Rhizoma Coptidis) clears heat, sedates fire, and eliminates toxic heat. *Da Qing Ye* (Folium Isatidis) clears heat, eliminates toxins and cools the blood. *Pu Gong Ying* (Herba Taraxaci) enters the Liver, detoxifies and helps promote the Liver's function to clear toxins. *Xian Feng Cao* (Herba Bidentis) reduces inflammation, clears heat, reduces swelling, drains pus and promotes urination. *Feng Wei Cao* (Herba Pteris) clears heat, drains dampness, reduces inflammation, cools the blood and detoxifies. *Shu Wei Huang* (Herba Rostellulariae) invigorates the blood and reduces inflammation. *Ya She Huang* (Herba Lippiae) regulates menstruation and reduces inflammation. *Liu Zhi Huang* (Herba Solidaginis) relieves pain, reduces inflammation, swelling, detoxifies, and regulates menstruation. *Hu Yao Huang* (Herba Leucas Mollissimae) clears heat, eliminates toxins, invigorates blood circulation and promotes

HERBAL ABX ™

diuresis. *Cha Chi Huang* (Herba Stellariae Aquaticae) clears heat, detoxifies, invigorates blood and reduces swelling. *Pao Zai Cao* (Herba Physalis Angulatae) reduces inflammation, detoxifies, and promotes diuresis.

SPECIFIC INDICATIONS

Herbal ABX is used to treat respiratory tract infections, gastrointestinal infections, hepatic disorders, reproductive system infections, sexually-transmitted diseases, urinary tract infections, and other infectious disease.

Respiratory tract infections: *Da Qing Ye* (Folium Isatidis), *Feng Wei Cao* (Herba Pteris), *Ya She Huang* (Herba Lippiae), *Pao Zai Cao* (Herba Physalis Angulatae) and *Shu Wei Huang* (Herba Rostellulariae) treat respiratory infections. Clinical presentations include common cold, influenza, bacterial or viral infections, bronchitis, pneumonia, encephalitis, upper respiratory tract infection, fever, sore and swollen throat, laryngitis, middle-ear infections, oral sores, parotitis, rhinitis, sinusitis, pharyngitis, and cough with yellow sputum.

Gastrointestinal infections: *Huang Lian* (Rhizoma Coptidis), *Hu Yao Huang* (Herba Leucas Mollissimae), *Pao Zai Cao* (Herba Physalis Angulatae), *Cha Chi Huang* (Herba Stellariae Aquaticae), *Feng Wei Cao* (Herba Pteris), and *Pu Gong Ying* (Herba Taraxaci) clear fire and damp-heat in the digestive tract. These toxins cause gastritis, peptic ulcers, duodenal ulcers, esophagitis, gastroenteritis, pancreatitis, enteritis, dysentery, colitis, diarrhea, ulcerative colitis, Crohn's disease, irritable bowel syndrome, acute and chronic appendicitis, hemorrhoids, vomiting, foul breath, swollen or bleeding gums and abdominal pain.

Hepatic disorders: *Huang Lian* (Rhizoma Coptidis), *Da Qing Ye* (Folium Isatidis), *Pu Gong Ying* (Herba Taraxaci), *Hu Yao Huang* (Herba Leucas Mollissimae), *Cha Chi Huang* (Herba Stellariae Aquaticae), *Xian Feng Cao* (Herba Bidentis), and *Liu Zhi Huang* (Herba Solidaginis) enter the Liver channel to treat Liver fire. Manifestations of Liver fire include hepatitis, cholecystitis, jaundice, erysipelas, herpes zoster, fibrocystic breast disorder, migraine, acid reflux, conjunctivitis, a bitter taste in the mouth, tinnitus, irritability, and hypochondriac pain.

Reproductive system infections: *Pao Zai Cao* (Herba Physalis Angulatae), *Ya She Huang* (Herba Lippiae), *Cha Chi Huang* (Herba Stellariae Aquaticae), *Hu Yao Huang* (Herba Leucas Mollissimae), and *Feng Wei Cao* (Herba Pteris) treat inflammation or infections of the reproductive organs. In women, symptoms include vaginitis, foul-smelling yellow or white leukorrhea, inflammation of the pelvis, ovaries, uterus, fallopian tubes, inflammation or infection following abortion or delivery, lower abdominal pain, genital itching, cervicitis, hypermenorrhea, yeast infections, prolapse of the uterus with inflammation and infection. In men, disorders include prostatitis, genital itching, and orchitis.

Sexually-transmitted diseases (STDs): This formula is a useful adjunct formula to clear toxic or damp-heat associated with STDs such as gonorrhea, genital herpes, trichomoniasis, candidiasis, chancroid lesions, HIV and crab lice (*Phthirus pubis).*

Urinary tract infections (UTI): *Huang Lian* (Rhizoma Coptidis), *Ya She Huang* (Herba Lippiae), *Shu Wei Huang* (Herba Rostellulariae), *Pao Zai Cao* (Herba Physalis Angulatae), *Hu Yao Huang* (Herba Leucas Mollissimae), *Xian Feng Cao* (Herba Bidentis), and *Cha Chi Huang* (Herba Stellariae Aquaticae) treat infection of the urinary system manifesting in dysuria and frequent urges to urinate. In such cases, the urine is mostly yellow and turbid. Disorders include nephritis, cystitis, UTI and kidney stones.

Other: This formula is effective for treatment of cellulitis, sores, carbuncles, hypertension, environmental poisoning, pericarditis, arteritis, gout, paronychia, phlebitis, toxic insect bites, hordeolum, keratitis, trachomata, ear infection, perichondritis, aural eczematoid dermatitis, conjunctivitis and external otitis.

HERBAL ABX ™

(Antibiotics)

In summary, *Herbal ABX* consists of a wide array of herbs with marked antibiotic properties, beneficial for the treatment of various infections.

SUPPLEMENTARY FORMULAS

- ❧ For infection of the ear, nose and throat, add *Herbal ENT*.
- ❧ For common cold or influenza with sore throat, combine with *Lonicera Complex*.
- ❧ For sinus infections, use with *Magnolia Clear Sinus* or *Pueraria Clear Sinus*.
- ❧ For genital infections, use with *Gentiana Complex* or *V-Statin*.
- ❧ For shingles, use with *Dermatrol (HZ)*.
- ❧ For respiratory tract infections, add *Respitrol (Heat)* or *Respitrol (Cold)*.
- ❧ For cough, add *Respitrol (CF)*.
- ❧ For yellow phlegm due to respiratory tract infections, use with *Poria XPT*.
- ❧ For gastric or duodenal ulcers with *H. pylori* infection, use with *GI Care*.
- ❧ For hepatitis, add *Liver DTX*.
- ❧ For chronic nephritis or nephritic syndrome, add *Kidney DTX*.
- ❧ For chemical or heavy metal poisoning, add *Herbal DTX*.
- ❧ For gallstones, combine with *Dissolve (GS)*.
- ❧ For kidney or bladder stones, use with *Dissolve (KS)*.
- ❧ For infection from external injuries or surgeries, use with *Traumanex*.
- ❧ For unknown condition with blood stagnation, add *Circulation (SJ)*.
- ❧ For bleeding, use *Notoginseng 9*.
- ❧ For high blood pressure and fast heart rate due to excess fire, add *Gardenia Complex*.
- ❧ For inflammation and swelling, add *Resolve (AI)*.
- ❧ This formula can be combined with other herbal formulas to enhance its heat clearing, fire purging and detoxifying actions.

NUTRITION

- ❧ Avoid spicy, fried or greasy foods.
- ❧ Be sure to include foods and beverages that are cool or cold in nature. Among these are watermelon, lotus nodes, melon, seaweed, cranberries, celery, cucumber, cactus and wintermelon.
- ❧ Drink plenty of water and urinate often.
- ❧ Increase supplementation with Vitamin C and B complex.

CLINICAL NOTES

- ❧ In individuals with constipation, purgative herbs such as *Gentle Lax (Excess)* should be used first before selecting an appropriate formula.
- ❧ *Herbal ABX* should be taken for at least 7 to 10 days to ensure complete eradication of micro-organisms. Early discontinuation may increase the risk of subsequent resistance by the micro-organisms.
- ❧ Many herbs in *Herbal ABX* are indigenous herbs from Taiwan. Because of their geographic isolation, they maintain potent antibiotic effect without any tolerance or resistance of micro-organisms. Therefore, for infections that do not respond to antibiotic drugs or classic herbal formulas, *Herbal ABX* will often provide excellent clinical results.
- ❧ If the condition does not improve after 7 to 10 days, modification of the formula may be necessary.
- ❧ This herbal combination is designed as a supplementary formula for treatment of various infections. In traditional Chinese medicine, such infectious diseases are characterized by heat, fire, damp-heat or toxic heat with elevated temperatures and/or inflammation.

☯ In gynecological disorders, this formula should be continued for two or three days more, after the symptoms subside.

☯ There is no evidence thus far that use of clearing herbs may permit secondary infections to arise (as is the case with antibiotics). However, those who have recurrent infections may take acidophilus prophylactically, especially if they have a history of repeated antibiotic usage.

☯ When boils or cysts break and are draining, keep the local area clean to prevent the spread of infection to other parts of the body. After handling a boil, hands should be washed thoroughly, as staph bacteria may infect other areas or cause food poisoning.

☯ Use of a yin tonic formula, such as **Nourish**, is recommended after the use of antibiotics to restore the normal balance of yin and yang in the body.

Pulse Diagnosis by Dr. Jimmy Wei-Yen Chang:

☯ Superficial, thick and forceful on any position.

☯ Note: Dr. Chang takes the pulse in slightly different positions. He places his index finger directly over the wrist crease, and his middle and ring fingers alongside to locate *cun*, *guan* and *chi* positions. For additional information and explanation, please refer to *Pulsynergy* by Dr. Jimmy Wei-Yen Chang and Marcus Brinkman.

CAUTIONS

☯ This formula is contraindicated in cases of deficiency and coldness. Use with caution for those who have weak digestive systems.

☯ This formula is contraindicated during pregnancy and nursing.

☯ Because antibiotic therapy may decrease the absorption of birth control pills by interfering with the normal flora in the intestines, women should use additional prophylactics if they are on antibiotic therapy and birth control pills concurrently.

ACUPUNCTURE POINTS

Traditional Points:

☯ *Hegu* (LI 4), *Zusanli* (ST 36), *Quchi* (LI 11), *Neiguan* (PC 6), *Shousanli* (LI 10), *Yanglingquan* (GB 34), and *Sanyinjiao* (SP 6).

Balance Method by Dr. Richard Tan:

☯ Left side: *Quchi* (LI 11), *Hegu* (LI 4), and *Yinlingquan* (SP 9).

☯ Right side: *Zusanli* (ST 36) and *Chize* (LU 5).

☯ Left and right side can be alternated from treatment to treatment.

☯ For additional information on the Balance Method, please refer to *Dr. Tan's Strategy of Twelve Magical Points* by Dr. Richard Tan.

Ear Points:

☯ Chronic middle ear infection: Eustachian Tube, Middle Ear, Mastoid Process, and Kidney.

☯ Acute conjunctivitis: Bleed protruding vein in the back of the ear once a day. Needle for 30 minutes the following points: Eyes, *Shenmen*, and apex of tragus.

☯ Acute tonsillitis: Bleed the protruding vein in the back of the ear, and apex of the tragus once a day. Needle and strongly stimulate the Throat, Pharynx and Tonsil.

FORMULAS

HERBAL ABX ™

(Antibiotics)

MODERN RESEARCH

Herbal ABX contains herbs with marked antibiotic properties, including antibacterial, antiviral and antifungal effects. This formula incorporates multiple herbs for two reasons. First, the use of multiple herbs within one formula has been shown to increase the antibiotic action more than ten-fold. Second, using a single herb in isolation is often ineffective and increases the risk of contributing to bacterial and viral resistance.[1] Given these facts, it is both wise and necessary to combine herbs with different properties to ensure effectiveness in treating the infection and to minimize the potential risks of resistance and mutation by the micro-organisms.

Da Qing Ye (Folium Isatidis) has broad-spectrum antibacterial, antiviral and antifungal applications. It is effective against *Staphylococcus aureus, alpha-hemolytic streptococcus, Diplococcus meningitidis, Salmonella typhi, E. coli, Corynebacterium diphtheriae, Bacillus dysenteriae*, and *leptospirosis*.[2] The effectiveness of *Da Qing Ye* (Folium Isatidis) is reflected in numerous clinical research reports. In one study, 168 children with upper respiratory infections were treated, with great results.[3] In another study, 51 children between the ages of one and thirteen were treated for encephalitis B, with marked effectiveness.[4]

Pu Gong Ying (Herba Taraxaci) has a bactericidal effect *in vitro* against *Staphylococcus aureus, beta-hemolytic streptococcus, Diplococcus pneumoniae, Diplococcus meningitidis, Corynebacterium diphtheriae, Pseudomonas aeruginosa, Bacillus dysenteriae* and *Salmonella typhi*.[5] Clinical research has shown this herb to be 83% effective against acute tonsillitis,[6] and 98% effective for sore throat.[7] Similar successes were reported using *Pu Gong Ying* (Herba Taraxaci) for topical treatment of parotitis or of burn patients with concurrent infection(s).[8,9]

Huang Lian (Rhizoma Coptidis) is one of the most commonly used and effective herbs for many infections. It has potent, broad-spectrum antibacterial action against *Bacillus dysenteriae, Mycobacterium tuberculosis, Salmonella typhi, E. coli, Vibrio cholerae, Bacillus proteus, Pseudomonas aeruginosa, Diplococcus meningitidis, Staphylococcus aureus, beta-hemolytic streptococcus, Diplococcus pneumoniae, Corynebacterium diphtheriae, Bordetella pertussis, Bacillus anthracis*, and *Leptospira*. In addition to its antibacterial properties, *Huang Lian* (Rhizoma Coptidis) has antifungal and antiviral actions.[10] It is effective against numerous pathogenic fungi and dermatophytes.[11] *Huang Lian* (Rhizoma Coptidis) inhibits influenza and hepatitis viruses.[12] This herb showed excellent results in treating bacterial dysentery in over 1000 patients, with short course of treatment and low incidence of side effects.[13] It was shown to be effective in treating acute gastroenteritis or enteritis in over 100 patients.[14] Good results were reported when a constituent of *Huang Lian* (Rhizoma Coptidis) was used to treat over 100 patients suffering from pulmonary tuberculosis.[15] *Huang Lian* (Rhizoma Coptidis) is also effective when used topically in treating suppurative otitis media.[16]

PHARMACEUTICAL DRUGS & CHINESE MEDICINE: A COMPARATIVE ANALYSIS

Western Medical Approach: Discovery of antibiotic drugs is one of the major breakthroughs in modern medicine. It enables doctors to effectively treat many different types of infections. Unfortunately, decades of abuse and misuse have led to growing problems of bacterial mutation and resistance. At this moment, many of these "super bugs" can only be treated with the newest and most potent antibiotic drugs, and unfortunately, many of them have potent side effects as well. Due to the number of antibiotic drugs, and the various species of micro-organisms, it is beyond the scope of this monograph to discuss the benefits and risks of each individual drug. As a category, antibiotic drugs are extremely effective against most types of bacterial infections. The key points are to select the correct antibiotic drug with least potential side effects, and make sure that the patient finishes the entire course of therapy.

Traditional Chinese Medicine Approach: Herbs are also extremely effective for treatment of various infections. In fact, most modern pharmaceutical drugs were originally derived from natural sources, including penicillin [the oldest antibiotic] and gentimicin [one of the most potent]. One of the main benefits of using herbs is their wide spectrum of antibiotic effect, with indications for bacterial, viral and fungal infections. Furthermore, most of these herbs are extremely safe, and do not have the same harsh side effects as drugs.

Summation: Both drugs and herbs are effective to treat mild to moderate cases of bacterial infections. However, drugs are most effective and more appropriate for life-threatening infections, such as meningitis or encephalitis, because drugs are more immediately potent and can be prescribed with more laboratory precision (via cultures and sensitivity tests). On the other hand, use of herbs is far more effective than drugs for treating certain viral infections, such as the common cold and influenza, as drugs are essentially ineffective for these conditions. Most importantly, herbs are much gentler to the body and safer than drugs. In other words, herbs treat infection without damaging the patient's underlying constitution. This allows the patient to recover faster, and become more resistant to secondary or re-current infections.

CASE STUDIES

A 35-year-old female presented with an ear infection with pain. The patient was given 10 days of antibiotics with no relief. After antibiotic therapy, she continued to have a slight fever and body aches. Her medical doctor diagnosed her with an ear infection, but upon examination, not much fluid was observed. The practitioner diagnosed the patient's condition as phlegm heat in the Lung and *San Jiao*. After taking *Herbal ABX*, her ear pain, congestion and infection all cleared up. The practitioner has found *Herbal ABX* quite effective in treating other patients for ear infections.

M.K., Sherman Oaks, California

A 42-year-old midwife presented with sinus infection (for 10 days) with yellow green discharge, increased pressure and pain in the sinus cavity and the ears, and severe pain. Upon examination, it was found that there was also lymph node swelling and pain. The TCM diagnosis was phlegm heat in the Lung and toxic heat in the throat. The patient was instructed to take *Pueraria Clear Sinus* (4 capsules three times daily) and *Herbal ABX* (4 capsules three times daily). Within one day, the patient responded that there was a lot less pain and marked decrease in swelling. She continued to improve with each dose and stated that she felt "all better" by the third day. The practitioner commented the formulas were "very amazing and powerful."

M.N., Knoxville, Tennessee

B.F., a 55-year-old male, presented with cough, thick nasal discharge, headache and fatigue. The tongue was pale, flabby and slightly purple. The pulse was slow. He was diagnosed with common cold and wind-cold invasion. *Magnolia Clear Sinus*, *Respitrol (Cold)* and *Herbal ABX* were prescribed. The patient reported that the sinus cleared in three days.

B.F., Newport Beach, California

H.M., a 59-year-old female, presented with seasonal nasal allergies, rhinitis, stuffy sinuses and profuse, clear, nasal mucus. She was allergic to mold and mildew. *Herbal ABX* and *Magnolia Clear Sinus* were prescribed. They brought about relief after 10 days, when the patient would usually be battling the symptoms for months and would have to take antibiotics.

H.C., Stephens City, Virginia

The owner brought in a male cat that had oozing sores and ulcers filled with yellow pus that started after a fight with another cat. The TCM diagnosis was toxic damp-heat at the skin level. *Herbal ABX* was prescribed topically. The cat licked it off, so it worked internally as well. After one day, the condition became much better as the sores began drying up. After three days, the cat was 90% better. After five days, all sores healed completely.

M.C., Sarasota, Florida

HERBAL ABX ™

(Antibiotics)

[1] *Zhong Yao Xue* (Chinese Herbology), 1988; 140:144
[2] *Zhong Yao Xue* (Chinese Herbology), 1998; 174:175
[3] *Fu Jian Zhong Yi Yao* (Fujian Chinese Medicine and Herbology), 1965; 4:14
[4] *Fu Jian Zhong Yi Yao* (Fujian Chinese Medicine and Herbology), 1965; 4:11
[5] *Zhong Yi Yao Xue Bao* (Report of Chinese Medicine and Herbology), 1991; (1):41
[6] *Xin Yi Yao Xue Za Zhi* (New Journal of Medicine and Herbology), 1977; 8:8
[7] *Liao Ning Zhong Yi Za Zhi* (Liaoning Journal of Chinese Medicine), 1988; 9:27
[8] *Xin Yi Xue* (New Medicine), 1972; 10:49
[9] *Zhong Xi Yi Jie He Za Zhi* (Journal of Integrated Chinese and Western Medicine), 1987; 5:301
[10] *Zhong Yao Xue* (Chinese Herbology), 1988, 140:144
[11] *Zhong Hua Yi Xue Za Zhi* (Chinese Journal of Medicine), 1958; 44(9):888
[12] *Zhong Xi Yi Jie He Za Zhi* (Journal of Integrated Chinese and Western Medicine), 1989; 9(8):494
[13] *Zhong Hua Nei Ke Za Zhi* (Chinese Journal of Internal Medicine), 1976; 4:219
[14] *Si Chuan Yi Xue Yuan Xue Bao* (Journal of Sichuan School of Medicine), 1959; 1:102
[15] *Zhe Jiang Zhong Yi Za Zhi* (Zhejiang Journal of Chinese Medicine), 1964; 10:51
[16] *Zhong Hua Er Bi Hou Ke Za Zhi* (Chinese Journal of ENT), 1954; 4:272

HERBAL ANALGESIC ™

CLINICAL APPLICATIONS

☯ Pain management: dull, sharp, fixed or moving, numbing, stabbing, cramping.
☯ Pain of skeletal and smooth muscles
☯ This is an extra-strength formula to be used in conjunction with other formulas to relieve severe pain

WESTERN THERAPEUTIC ACTIONS

☯ Potent analgesic effect to relieve pain
☯ Strong anti-inflammatory effect to reduce swelling and inflammation
☯ Anesthetic effect to relieve pain

CHINESE THERAPEUTIC ACTIONS

☯ Invigorates blood circulation
☯ Relieves pain

DOSAGE

When taken alone, the recommended dosage is 3 to 4 capsules three times daily as needed to relieve pain. For severe pain, dosage can be increased to 7 to 8 capsules every 4 to 6 hours as needed to relieve pain. As an adjunct with other formulas to relieve pain, the recommended dose is 2 to 3 capsules in addition to the regular dose of the base formula. Take the herbs on an empty stomach with two tall glasses of warm water. This formula should be discontinued when the desired effects are achieved.

INGREDIENTS

Dang Gui (Radicis Angelicae Sinensis)
Mo Yao (Myrrha)
Ru Xiang (Gummi Olibanum)

Sheng Ma (Rhizoma Cimicifugae)
Yan Hu Suo (Rhizoma Corydalis)

FORMULA EXPLANATION

"Where there is pain, there is stagnation. When stagnation is cleared, so will the pain." For practitioners of traditional Chinese medicine, this is one of the most important fundamental principles for treatment of pain. *Herbal Analgesic* is designed as an adjunct formula to relieve severe pain. It can be used alone, or with any other formulas for any pain in the body.

Yan Hu Suo (Rhizoma Corydalis) is the strongest and the most effective herb in the entire Chinese herbal pharmacopoeia to relieve pain. It enters both *xue* (blood) and *qi* (energy) levels to effectively invigorate blood circulation, regulate qi and relieve pain in the chest, abdomen and limbs. It is effective to relieve pain of the visceral organs and the musculoskeletal system. To enhance the analgesic effect of *Yan Hu Suo* (Rhizoma Corydalis), *Ru Xiang* (Gummi Olibanum) and *Mo Yao* (Myrrha) are added to *Herbal Analgesic*. This pair of herbs is often used together synergistically to relieve a wide range of pain that may be caused by qi or blood stagnation, trauma or arthritic syndrome. *Dang Gui* (Radicis Angelicae Sinensis) tonifies blood and moves blood. Finally, *Sheng Ma* (Rhizoma Cimicifugae) is used as a channel-guiding herb. It moves upwards and outwards and has a dispersing nature, which helps break up stagnation and relieve pain.

FORMULAS

HERBAL ANALGESIC ™

In short, *Herbal Analgesic* is an extremely effective formula to relieve pain. It can be used individually, or in combination with another formula for pain at a specific location.

SUPPLEMENTARY FORMULAS

- For headache, add *Corydalin* or *Migratrol*.
- For pain in the neck and shoulder area, add *Neck & Shoulder (Acute)* or *Neck & Shoulder (Chronic)*.
- For pain in the arm (shoulder, elbow and wrist), add *Arm Support*.
- For pain in the upper back, add *Back Support (Upper)*.
- For pain in the lower back, add *Back Support (Acute)* or *Back Support (Chronic)*.
- For pain in the back from herniated disk, add *Back Support (HD)*.
- For pain in the knees, add *Knee & Ankle (Acute)* or *Knee & Ankle (Chronic)*.
- For gout, add *Flex (GT)*.
- For pain with chronic musculoskeletal disorder with damaged soft tissues (muscles, tendons, ligaments and cartilage), add *Flex (MLT)*.
- For arthritic syndrome or fibromyalgia due to coldness, add *Flex (CD)*.
- For arthritic syndrome or fibromyalgia due to heat, add *Flex (Heat)*.
- For spasms and cramps or fibromyalgia with stiffness, add *Flex (SC)*.
- For neuropathy, add *Flex (NP)*.
- For bone spurs, add *Flex (Spur)*.
- For dysmenorrhea, add *Mense-Ease*.
- For pain due to gallstones, use *Dissolve (GS)*.
- For pain due to kidney stones, use *Dissolve (KS)*.
- For external or trauma injuries, use with *Traumanex*.
- For post-surgical care, *Traumanex* or *Herbal ABX* can be added to invigorate blood circulation or relieve pain and prevent infection.
- For pain in the gastric region, add *GI Care*.
- For pain or bloating due to irritable bowel syndrome, add *GI Harmony*.
- For abdominal pain due to food poisoning or traveler's diarrhea, add *GI Care II*.
- For pain due to ulcerative colitis, add *GI Care (UC)*.
- For hemorrhoids, add *GI Care (HMR)*.
- For painful menstruation, add *Mense-Ease*.
- For pain due to endometriosis, uterine fibroids, ovarian cysts or mass, add *Resolve (Lower)*.
- For fibrocystic breast disorder, add *Resolve (Upper)*.
- For unknown pain with blood stagnation, add *Circulation (SJ)*.
- For pain due to Bell's Palsy or TMJ (temporo-mandibular joint) pain, add *Symmetry*.

NUTRITION

- If pain is due to "cold," avoid cold or raw food, vegetables, salads, drinks and exposure to cold weather or surface. Avoid taking cold showers or swimming in cold water. Fruits that are cold in nature such as watermelon and pear should not be consumed. Foods that are warm or hot in nature such as lamb, pepper, onions and scallions are recommended.
- If pain is due to "heat," avoid eating spicy food. Increase the intake of vegetables or fruits that are cold in nature such as watermelon and cucumber.
- If pain is due to "dampness," avoid eating greasy, fatty or fried food. Dairy products are not recommended.
- Increase the intake of minerals such as calcium and magnesium, which calm the nerves and reduce sensitivity to pain.

HERBAL ANALGESIC ™

LIFESTYLE INSTRUCTIONS

☯ Proper diet and exercise are extremely important in preventing recurrent pain syndrome. Chronic pain is often the result of occupations that require repetitive use of the same joints or repeated injuries to the same area. Strong efforts should be made to eliminate or improve such working conditions.

☯ Exercise is always helpful in keeping qi and blood circulating properly in the body.

☯ Other therapies that are effective for pain management include massage, relaxation techniques, deep breathing, and heat/cold therapy.

CLINICAL NOTES

☯ *Herbal Analgesic* is an excellent formula to treat both internal and external injuries leading to pain of the body and the extremities. The diagnosis for such conditions is often qi and blood stagnation. Therefore, *Herbal Analgesic* can be used safely and effectively to relieve pain.

☯ If the pain is located in the trunk of the body, such as in the chest or abdominal regions, additional examination is necessary to diagnose the underlying cause of the pain. While *Herbal Analgesic* is still effective to relieve pain, it will not address the underlying illness and may delay the treatment. For example, patients with kidney stones may have tremendous pain in the lower back. Though it is important to relieve pain, it is even more important to the address kidney stones. In other words, while it is important to treat pain in acute cases, it is also important to identify the underlying cause so the overall treatment will not be delayed.

☯ *Herbal Analgesic* will begin to show effectiveness within 30 minutes. It can be used in conjunction with acupuncture treatment for synergistic analgesic effect.

☯ Pain from cancer is often severe and excruciating, which may not be relieved effectively by herbs. Under these circumstances, narcotic drugs should be used for pain management. *CA Support* and *C/R Support* may be used as adjunct treatments.

CAUTIONS

☯ This formula should be discontinued one week prior to surgery.

☯ This formula is contraindicated during pregnancy and nursing.

☯ Patients who are on anticoagulant or antiplatelet therapies, such as Coumadin (Warfarin), should use this formula with caution, as there may be a slightly higher risk of bleeding and bruising.

☯ This formula is designed for short-term symptomatic treatment of pain. It is not recommended for long-term use. The longest patients should be on this formula is two months.

ACUPUNCTURE POINTS

Traditional Points:

☯ *Ah shi* points; *Taibai* (SP 3), *Neiguan* (PC 6), *Waiguan* (TH 5), and *Hegu* (LI 4).

☯ *Hegu* (LI 4), *Neiguan* (PC 6), *Ximen* (PC 4), *Sanyangluo* (TH 8), *Guangming* (GB 37) with local points:

- Head: *Quanliao* (SI 18), *Yifeng* (TH 17), *Guangming* (GB 37), *Hegu* (LI 4), *Lieque* (LU 7), and *Jinmen* (BL 63).
- Neck: *Hegu* (LI 4), *Neiguan* (PC 6), and *Futu* (ST 32).
- Chest/Thoracic: *Hegu* (LI 4), *Neiguan* (PC 6), and *Ximen* (PC 4).
- Abdomen: *Zusanli* (ST 36), *Shangjuxu* (ST 37), *Hegu* (LI 4), *Neiguan* (PC 6), *Taichong* (LR 3), and *Yinlingquan* (SP 9).
- Lower limbs: *Huantiao* (GB 30), *Chengshan* (BL 57), and *Sanyinjiao* (SP 6).

HERBAL ANALGESIC ™

Balance Method by Dr. Richard Tan:

- Left side: *Fengchi* (GB 20), *Zhongchong* (PC 9), *Shaochong* (HT 9), *Shaoshang* (LU 11), *Zusanli* (ST 36), *Weizhong* (BL 40), *Yanglingquan* (GB 34), and ear *Shenmen*.
- Right side: *Fengchi* (GB 20), *Hegu* (LI 4), *Houxi* (SI 3), *Zhongzhu* (TH 3), *Taixi* (KI 3), *Zhongfeng* (LR 4), *Sanyinjiao* (SP 6), *Yintang* (Extra 1), and ear *Shenmen*.
- For additional information on the Balance Method, please refer to *Dr. Tan's Strategy of Twelve Magical Points* by Dr. Richard Tan.

MODERN RESEARCH

Herbal Analgesic is formulated specifically for relieving pain throughout the body. It contains ingredients that have shown exceptional analgesic and anti-inflammatory effects. Clinical applications include treatment of various aches and pains, swelling, inflammation, and external injuries.

Yan Hu Suo (Rhizoma Corydalis) is one of the strongest and most potent herbs for treatment of pain. Its effects are well documented in both historical references and modern research studies. Classical texts have stated that *Yan Hu Suo* (Rhizoma Corydalis) may be used to treat chest and hypochondriac pain, epigastric and abdominal pain, hernial pain, amenorrhea or menstrual pain, and pain of the extremities. According to laboratory studies, the extract of *Yan Hu Suo* (Rhizoma Corydalis) was found to be effective in both acute and chronic phases of inflammation. The mechanism of its anti-inflammatory effect was attributed to its effect to inhibit the release of histamine and formation of edema.[1] Furthermore, it has a strong analgesic effect. With adjustment in dosage, the potency of *Yan Hu Suo* (Rhizoma Corydalis) has been compared to that of morphine. In fact, the analgesic effect of *Yan Hu Suo* (Rhizoma Corydalis) is so strong and reliable that it has been used with satisfactory anesthetic effect in 98 out of 105 patients (93.4%) who underwent surgery.[2] The analgesic effect can be potentiated further with concurrent acupuncture therapy. In one research study, it was demonstrated that the analgesic effect is increased significantly with concurrent treatments using *Yan Hu Suo* (Rhizoma Corydalis) and electro-acupuncture, when compared to a control group, which received electro-acupuncture only.[3] Overall, it is well understood that *Yan Hu Suo* (Rhizoma Corydalis) has a marked effect to treat pain. Though the maximum analgesic effect of *Yan Hu Suo* (Rhizoma Corydalis) is not as strong as morphine, it has been determined that the herb is much safer, with significantly less side effects, less risk of tolerance, and no evidence of physical dependence even with long-term use. [4]

Ru Xiang (Gummi Olibanum) and *Mo Yao* (Myrrha) are added to the formula to specifically enhance the effect of *Yan Hu Suo* (Rhizoma Corydalis) to treat acute trauma and injuries. These two herbs have an excellent effect to treat injuries and relieve pain. According to various studies, the combination of these two herbs has demonstrated marked *in vitro* and *in vivo* analgesic effects.[5] The clinical applications include chest pain, colicky or sharp pain,[6] and pain due to acute sprain of the lower back and legs. [7]

Lastly, *Dang Gui* (Radicis Angelicae Sinensis) and *Sheng Ma* (Rhizoma Cimicifugae) are added for their synergistic effects. *Sheng Ma* (Rhizoma Cimicifugae) functions as a guiding herb, as it has the effects to reach the far ends of the body, such as the extremities. *Dang Gui* (Radicis Angelicae Sinensis) has excellent effects to improve blood circulation to relieve pain, and is commonly used to treat migraine,[8] pain of the low back and legs,[9] menstrual pain,[10] herpetic neuralgia,[11] and various conditions characterized by inflammation and pain.[12] In fact, various research has indicated that the anti-inflammatory effect of *Dang Gui* (Radicis Angelicae Sinensis) is approximately 1.1 times stronger than aspirin and the analgesic effect is approximately 1.7 times stronger.[13]

In summary, *Herbal Analgesic* contains herbs with marked analgesic and anti-inflammatory effects. Furthermore, there are herbs in the formula that potentiate the overall effect by improving peripheral circulation, and guiding the effect of the herbs specifically to the affected area. *Herbal Analgesic* can be used to treat various types of pain of the extremities.

HERBAL ANALGESIC ™

PHARMACEUTICAL DRUGS & CHINESE MEDICINE: A COMPARATIVE ANALYSIS

Western Medical Approach: Pain is a basic bodily sensation induced by a noxious stimulus that causes physical discomfort (as pricking, throbbing, or aching). Pain may be of acute or chronic state, and may be of nociceptive, neuropathic, or psychogenic type. Two classes of drugs commonly used to treat pain include non-steroidal anti-inflammatory agents (NSAID) and opioid analgesics. NSAID's [such as Motrin (Ibuprofen) and Voltaren (Diclofenac)] are generally used for mild to moderate pain, and are most effective to reduce inflammation and swelling. Though effective, they may cause such serious side effects as gastric ulcer, duodenal ulcer, gastrointestinal bleeding, tinnitus, blurred vision, dizziness and headache. Furthermore, the newer NSAID's, also known as Cox-2 inhibitors [such as Celebrex (Celecoxib)], are associated with significantly higher risk of cardiovascular events, including heart attack and stroke. Opioid analgesics [such as Vicodin (APAP/Hydrocodone) and morphine] are usually used for severe to excruciating pain. While they may be the most potent agents for pain, they also have the most serious risks and side effects, including but not limited to dizziness, lightheadedness, drowsiness, upset stomach, vomiting, constipation, stomach pain, rash, difficult urination, and respiratory depression resulting in difficult breathing. Furthermore, long-term use of these drugs leads to tolerance and addiction. In brief, it is important to remember that while drugs offer reliable and potent symptomatic pain relief, they should be used only if and when needed. Frequent use and abuse leads to unnecessary side effects and complications.

Traditional Chinese Medicine Approach: Treatment of pain is a sophisticated balance of art and science. Proper treatment of pain requires a careful evaluation of the type of disharmony (excess or deficiency, cold or heat, exterior or interior), characteristics (qi and/or blood stagnations), and locations (upper body, lower body, extremities, or internal organs). Furthermore, optimal treatment requires integrative use of herbs, acupuncture and *Tui-Na* therapies. All these therapies work together to tonify underlying deficiencies, strengthen the body, and facilitate recovery from chronic pain. TCM pain management targets both the symptoms and the causes of pain, and as such, often achieves immediate and long-term success. Furthermore, TCM pain management is often associated with few or no side effects.

Summation: For treatment of mild to severe pain due to various causes, TCM pain management offers similar treatment effects with significantly fewer side effects. However, as with any therapeutic modality, it is important to recognize the limitations of TCM pain management. In some cases, such as excruciating cancer pain in terminally ill patients, drugs are simply superior to herbs. Under these circumstances, immediate, potent and consistently reliable pain relief is the main objective, and this can be accomplished more effectively with drugs such as intravenous injection of morphine. Herbs should be used to support the underlying constitution of the body, and to alleviate the side effects of the drugs.

CASE STUDY

At a seminar in Providence, Rhode Island, a question was raised as whether *Yan Hu Suo* (Rhizoma Corydalis) would cause a person treated with this herb to test positive in a drug screen (as do a number of analgesic substances). A very small study was conducted in a laboratory at the Rhode Island Clinical Research Center: two people taking 6 capsules of **Corydalin** were screened for drugs 3 hours later. Both were completely negative in the seven drug panels. A solution of 5% *Yan Hu Suo* (Rhizoma Corydalis) powdered extract (freed from excessive carbohydrate) was also tested in the drug-screening test, again with negative results. It was concluded by the researchers that a person being treated for pain with the usual dosage of **Corydalin** would not risk testing positive for opiates, benzodiazepines, barbiturates, etc. [Note: *Yan Hu Suo* (Rhizoma Corydalis) is the main ingredient that is present in both **Corydalin** and **Herbal Analgesic**.]

D.W., Hadley, MA

---

[1] *Biol Pharm Bull*, Feb 1994; 17(2):262-5
[2] *He Bei Xin Yi Yao* (Hebei New Medicine and Herbology), 1973; 4:34

FORMULAS

HERBAL ANALGESIC ™

[3] *Chen Tzu Yen Chiu* (Acupuncture Research), 1994;19(1):55-8
[4] *Zhong Yao Yao Li Yu Ying Yong* (Pharmacology and Applications of Chinese Herbs), 1983; 447
[5] *Zhong Yao Xue* (Chinese Herbology), 1998; 539
[6] *Zhong Yao Xue* (Chinese Herbology), 1998; 540
[7] *He Nan Zhong Yi Xue Yuan Xue Bao* (Journal of University of Henan School of Medicine), 1980; 3:38
[8] *Yao Xue Za Zhi* (Journal of Medicinals), 1971; (91):1098
[9] *Xin Zhong Yi* (New Chinese Medicine), 1980; 2:34
[10] *Zhong Hua Yi Xue Za Zhi* (Chinese Journal of Medicine), 1961; 5:317
[11] *Zhong Hua Yi Xue Za Zhi* (Chinese Journal of Medicine), 1961; 5:318
[12] *Xin Yi Yao Xue Za Zhi* (New Journal of Medicine and Herbology), 1975; (6):34
[13] *Yao Xue Za Zhi* (Journal of Medicinals), 1971; (91):1098

FORMULAS

HERBAL DRX ™

(Diuretics)

CLINICAL APPLICATIONS

☯ Edema and generalized water accumulation
☯ Feeling of heaviness or sluggishness in the body, preference to lay down or sleep all day
☯ *Tan yin* (phlegm retention) syndrome
☯ Swelling due to water accumulation

WESTERN THERAPEUTIC ACTIONS

☯ Diuretic effect to eliminate water and treat edema

CHINESE THERAPEUTIC ACTIONS

☯ Strengthens the Spleen
☯ Resolves dampness
☯ Promotes urination and treats edema

DOSAGE

Take 3 to 4 capsules three times daily. For maximum effectiveness, take the herbs on an empty stomach.

INGREDIENTS

Bai Zhu (Rhizoma Atractylodis Macrocephalae)
Chen Pi (Pericarpium Citri Reticulatae)
Chi Fu Ling (Poria Rubrae)
Fu Ling (Poria)
He Zi (Fructus Chebulae)
Hua Shi (Talcum)

Mu Xiang (Radix Aucklandiae)
Sheng Jiang Pi (Pericarpium Zingiberis Recens)
Wu Bei Zi (Galla Chinensis)
Yi Yi Ren (Semen Coicis)
Ze Xie (Rhizoma Alismatis)
Zhu Ling (Polyporus)

FORMULA EXPLANATION

Herbal DRX is designed specifically to treat edema, water retention and swelling. It treats the cause of edema by strengthening the Spleen and resolving dampness. It treats the symptoms of edema by clearing damp-heat and draining water through urination.

In this formula, *Fu Ling* (Poria), *Bai Zhu* (Rhizoma Atractylodis Macrocephalae), and *Yi Yi Ren* (Semen Coicis) strengthen the Spleen to resolve dampness. *Fu Ling* (Poria), *Zhu Ling* (Polyporus), *Ze Xie* (Rhizoma Alismatis), and *Sheng Jiang Pi* (Pericarpium Zingiberis Recens) resolve dampness, regulate water circulation, and drain water accumulation. *Sheng Jiang Pi* (Pericarpium Zingiberis Recens) is especially good for water trapped in the superficial parts of the skin. *Hua Shi* (Talcum) and *Chi Shao* (Radix Paeoniae Rubrae) clear damp-heat to promote normal urination. *Mu Xiang* (Radix Aucklandiae) and *Chen Pi* (Pericarpium Citri Reticulatae) activate qi circulation, which is often stagnant in cases of water and damp accumulation. Lastly, *Wu Bei Zi* (Galla Chinensis) and *He Zi* (Fructus Chebulae) are astringent herbs that reduce swelling, and constrict and push the excess fluids out of the body.

In summary, *Herbal DRX* is an excellent formula to treat both the cause and symptoms of edema. This formula may be used individually, or in combination with others to treat the cause and/or complications of edema.

FORMULAS

HERBAL DRX ™

(Diuretics)

SUPPLEMENTARY FORMULAS

- For deficient types of hypertension with edema, add *Gastrodia Complex*.
- For excess types of hypertension with edema, add *Gentiana Complex*.
- For dysuria due to prostate enlargement with edema, add *Saw Palmetto Complex*.
- For obesity with edema, add *Herbalite*.
- For Spleen deficiency with edema, add *GI Tonic*.
- For high cholesterol with excessive dampness, add *Cholisma*.
- For gallstones, add *Dissolve (GS)*.
- For kidney stones, add *Dissolve (KS)*
- For women with coldness and deficiency and water retention, add *Balance (Cold)*.
- For cysts or fibroids in the uterus or ovaries, add *Resolve (Lower)*.
- For fibroids in the breast with excessive dampness, add *Resolve (Upper)*.
- For excessive dampness in conditions such as dysuria, vaginitis, yellow vaginal discharge, add *V-Statin*.
- For yang deficiency type of edema with coldness and possible low back pain, add *Zhen Wu Tang (True Warrior Decoction)*

NUTRITION

- Avoid drinking ice, cold beverages or eating cold or raw foods.
- Avoid citrus and other foods that are cold in nature such as watermelon, salads, tomatoes and cucumbers.
- Avoid eating fried, greasy or food high in fat content.
- Reduce the intake of dairy and sugar.
- A low-sodium diet is recommended, as sodium may cause fluid retention.
- Consume an adequate amount of vitamin B complex, which helps to reduce water retention.
- Consume a sufficient amount of free-form amino acid complex, as edema is sometimes caused by inadequate protein assimilation.
- Increase the consumption of foods that have natural diuretic effects, such as *Lu Dou* (Semen Phaseoli Radiati) and *Yi Yi Ren* (Semen Coicis).

The Tao of Nutrition by Ni and McNease
- Edema and swelling
  - Recommendations: red (azuki) beans, corn, ginger skin, winter melon, winter melon skin, squash, apples, mulberries, peaches, tangerines, coconuts, seaweeds, fish, celery, green onions, garlic, bamboo shoots, spinach, water chestnuts, millet, wheat, black beans, pearl barley, carrots, watermelon, oats, and beef.
  - Avoid rich foods, salty foods, lamb, stimulating foods, wine, garlic, pepper, shellfish, fatty foods, and greasy foods.
- For more information, please refer to *The Tao of Nutrition* by Dr. Maoshing Ni and Cathy McNease.

LIFESTYLE INSTRUCTIONS

- Individuals with swelling and edema of legs and feet should sit with their legs up as much as possible. Wearing support hose will also reduce swelling in the legs.
- Exercise daily to help push fluids away from the legs and lower body.
- Avoid exposure to the rain. Do not engage in water sport activities while under treatment.

CLINICAL NOTES

- In comparison with pharmaceutical drugs, diuretic herbs have a moderate potency and a slower onset of action. Therefore, most patients will experience noticeable diuretic effect only after 2 to 4 weeks. This formula is designed as a long-term therapy for treatment and prevention of edema-related disorders. Acute conditions, such as acute nephritis with edema, should be treated with other methods and formulas.

- ☙ In addition to eliminating excessive water, some herbs in this formula have also shown marked effect to reduce blood pressure, blood glucose levels, and cholesterol levels, improve kidney functions, etc.
- ☙ Severity of water retention can be easily checked by pressing the first metacarpal-phalangeal joint against the patient's shin bone [around the area of *Ligou* (LR 5)]. The deeper the indentation and the longer it stays without bouncing back, the more severe the condition is.

Pulse Diagnosis by Dr. Jimmy Wei-Yen Chang:

- ☙ Deep pulse on all three positions on both hands.
- ☙ Note: Dr. Chang takes the pulse in slightly different positions. He places his index finger directly over the wrist crease, and his middle and ring fingers alongside to locate *cun*, *guan* and *chi* positions. For additional information and explanation, please refer to *Pulsynergy* by Dr. Jimmy Wei-Yen Chang and Marcus Brinkman.

CAUTIONS

- ☙ This is an excellent formula to eliminate accumulation of water and treat edema. However, in addition to elimination excessive water, diuretic herbs may lead to elimination of some electrolytes. Therefore, if the formula is to be taken for more than 2 weeks, it is important to receive supplementation of additional electrolytes to prevent imbalance. Symptoms of electrolyte imbalance include muscle spasms and cramps. Common supplements include bananas, orange juice, multivitamins and minerals, and sports drinks.
- ☙ Concurrent use of diuretic herbs and diuretic drugs is not recommended as they have the same functions to eliminate water and electrolytes. Concurrent use may contribute to dehydration and electrolyte imbalance.
- ☙ This formula is contraindicated during pregnancy.

ACUPUNCTURE POINTS

Traditional Points:

- ☙ *Lieque* (LU 7), *Hegu* (LI 4), *Piani* (LI 6), *Yinlingquan* (SP 9), *Weiyang* (BL 39), *Pishu* (BL 20), *Shenshu* (BL 23), *Shuifen* (CV 9), *Ciliao* (BL 32), *Guanyuan* (CV 4), *Shangqiu* (SP 5), and *Fenglong* (ST 40).

Balance Method by Dr. Richard Tan:

- ☙ Left side: Needle *Hegu* (LI 4), and *Yinlingquan* (SP 9).
- ☙ Right side: Needle *Chize* (LU 5), and *Fenglong* (ST 40).
- ☙ Alternate sides in between treatments.
- ☙ For additional information on the Balance Method, please refer to *Dr. Tan's Strategy of Twelve Magical Points* by Dr. Richard Tan.

MODERN RESEARCH

Herbal DRX is formulated with many herbs that offer tremendous benefit to treat edema and its causes and/or complications. Most herbs have direct diuretic functions to eliminate the accumulation of water.

According to one study, use of *Fu Ling* (Poria) was associated with marked diuretic effect and a significant increase in urine output.[1] According to another study, use of *Fu Ling* (Poria) in an herbal formula was associated with marked effectiveness in treating 23 of 30 patients with edema.[2] *Zhu Ling* (Polyporus) and *Ze Xie* (Rhizoma Alismatis) also have a marked diuretic effect, and they increase the excretion of water, sodium, chloride, and potassium.[3,4] *Bai Zhu* (Rhizoma Atractylodis Macrocephalae) is also used frequently for its diuretic effect to treat of edema. The mechanism of action for this herb has been attributed to the inhibition of sodium re-absorption leading

HERBAL DRX ™

(Diuretics)

to increased diuresis.[5] Lastly, the use of *Shi Gao* (Gypsum Fibrosum) in an herbal formula has been shown to promote normal urination among 10 patients with urinary tract infection and dysuria.[6]

In summary, *Herbal DRX* contains many herbs that offer tremendous benefit for the treatment and prevention of edema and its complications. Most herbs have direct diuretic functions to eliminate the accumulation of water.

PHARMACEUTICAL DRUGS & CHINESE MEDICINE: A COMPARATIVE ANALYSIS

Western Medical Approach: Water accumulation, as in edema, is a symptom that occurs in various diseases, such as hypertension, congestive heart failure, and nephropathy. This condition is usually treated in part with diuretic drugs, such as Lasix (Furosemide), Aldactone (Spironolactone), and Dyazide (HCTZ/Triamterene). While these drugs all have excellent diuretic effect to eliminate water, their risks include dizziness, vertigo, orthostatic hypotension, electrolyte imbalance, and in severe cases, agranulocytosis, leukopenia and thrombopenia. Furthermore, long-term use of these drugs may increase plasma levels of glucose and cholesterol level, thereby complicating overall management of cardiovascular and circulatory disorders. In short, diuretic drugs must be used carefully, as there are many potential side effects and adverse reactions.

Traditional Chinese Medicine Approach: Water accumulation is treated with herbs that treat both symptom and cause. Diuretic herbs, known as herbs that regulate water and resolve dampness, have excellent effect to facilitate elimination of water through urination. Furthermore, herbs are also used to strengthen the body and increase its own ability to regulate water circulation in and out of the body. Thus, use of herbs is effective and achieves both short- and long-term benefits.

Summation: Drugs and herbs are both effective to drain water and treat edema. Drugs are more potent, and in severe cases, have stronger and immediate onset of effect (especially with intravenous use). However, diuretic drugs should be used and monitored carefully to ensure safe and effective use. Herbs, on the other hand, are gentle and effective. Though they are not as potent, they exert consistent and moderate diuretic effect over the course of therapy. Furthermore, herbs have much better safety profile in comparison with drugs. In conclusion, selection of optimal treatment depends on the severity of the condition and the patient's risk tolerance.

---

[1] *Chang Yong Zhong Yao Cheng Fen Yu Yao Li Shou Ce* (A Handbook of the Composition and Pharmacology of Common Chinese Drugs), 1994; 1383:1391
[2] *Shang Hai Zhong Yi Yao Za Zhi* (Shanghai Journal of Chinese Medicine and Herbology), 1986; 8:25
[3] *Yao Xue Xue Bao* (Journal of Herbology), 1964; 11(12):815
[4] *Sheng Yao Xue Za Zhi* (Journal of Raw Herbology), 1982; 36(2):150
[5] *Zhong Hua Yi Xue Za Zhi* (Chinese Journal of Medicine), 1961; 47(1):7
[6] *Liao Ning Yi Yao* (Liaoning Medicine and Herbology), 1976; (2):69

HERBAL DTX ™

(Detoxification)

CLINICAL APPLICATIONS

- ❧ Chemical poisoning (insecticide, pesticide, herbicide, artificial hormones and preservatives, chemical compounds, chemical solvents, plastics, cleaning products, pollutants, detergents, paint thinner, nail polish remover, new carpet fibers and any other products that may contain toxic fumes or fragrance)
- ❧ Heavy metal poisoning in water, food and the environment (lead, arsenic, mercury)
- ❧ Air pollution (gas exhaust, fumes, perfumes, air freshener, burned plastic, and other airborne toxins)
- ❧ Drug overdose and/or poisoning
- ❧ This formula is designed for long-term use to alleviate symptoms associated with chronic poisoning. It is not suitable to treat acute conditions.

WESTERN THERAPEUTIC ACTIONS

- ❧ General detoxification effect [1]
- ❧ Treats overdose and poisoning by drugs [6,7]
- ❧ Treats herbicide and pesticide poisoning [6,7,8]
- ❧ Treats heavy metal poisoning [9]
- ❧ Treats overdose and poisoning of food and plants [2,3,4,5,6,7]
- ❧ Protects the liver and treats hepatitis and liver cirrhosis [10,11,12,13,14,15,16,17]
- ❧ Protects the kidney and treats nephritis and renal impairment [18,19,20,21,22]

CHINESE THERAPEUTIC ACTIONS

- ❧ Clears heat and eliminates toxins
- ❧ Expels toxins through urine and stool
- ❧ Nourishes yin
- ❧ Tonifies Kidney and Heart

DOSAGE

Take 3 to 4 capsules three times daily with a large glass of water for 6 to 12 months for optimal effect. This formula is ineffective if taken only for a short period of time. Do not use this formula to treat acute poisoning.

INGREDIENTS

Bai Mao Gen (Rhizoma Imperatae)
Da Huang (Radix et Rhizoma Rhei)
Dan Shen (Radix Salviae Miltiorrhizae)
Fang Feng (Radix Saposhnikoviae)

Gan Cao (Radix Glycyrrhizae)
Gou Qi Zi (Fructus Lycii)
Lian Qiao (Fructus Forsythiae)
Lu Dou (Semen Phaseoli Radiati)

FORMULA EXPLANATION

Herbal DTX is designed to treat various symptoms related to different kinds of poisonings such as by drugs, chemicals or heavy metals. Patients may exhibit symptoms of heat sensation, low-grade fever or high fever, thirst, dry mouth, headache, nasal congestion, allergy, irritability, nausea, vomiting, turbid urination or disorientation.

The key to treatment of poisoning is to accelerate the elimination of toxins in the body and protect the organs at the same time. *Lu Dou* (Semen Phaseoli Radiati) is sweet and cold, and clears heat and eliminates toxins. *Gan Cao* (Radix Glycyrrhizae) is sweet and neutral, and is the most essential harmonizing herb to detoxify various

HERBAL DTX ™

(Detoxification)

substances. *Dan Shen* (Radix Salviae Miltiorrhizae) is bitter and slightly cold, and has great effect to invigorate blood and cleanse the toxicity from the blood. It also clears heat, reduces irritability and tranquilizes the Heart. *Bai Mao Gen* (Rhizoma Imperatae) is cold in property and clears heat and promotes the expelling of toxicity through urination. It also prevents potential bleeding and protects the Kidney. *Lian Qiao* (Fructus Forsythiae) clears heat, detoxifies and further helps *Bai Mao Gen* (Rhizoma Imperatae) to dispel toxins through the Kidney. *Gou Qi Zi* (Fructus Lycii) is sweet, and it is mainly used for nourishing the Stomach yin and generating body fluids. It has a unique effect to create a protective layer in the stomach to prevent the absorption of toxins from the digestive tract. *Da Huang* (Radix et Rhizoma Rhei) is a purgative herb that detoxifies and purges heat simultaneously by invigorating blood circulation and purging downwards. *Fang Feng* (Radix Saposhnikoviae) dispels internal Liver wind and is used to relieve stiffness, discomfort and pain in the muscles associated with poisoning.

Herbal DTX is an excellent formula for the prevention and treatment of overdose and accumulation of harmful chemicals and toxins. *Herbal DTX* eliminates toxins through urination and defecation, invigorates blood circulation to accelerate recovery, and strengthens the body to increase its natural defensive ability.

SUPPLEMENTARY FORMULAS

- For liver damage or hepatitis due to poisoning, or to enhance the immediate effect, add *Liver DTX*.
- For kidney damage or nephritis due to poisoning, add *Kidney DTX*.
- To enhance the detoxifying function, add *Herbal ABX*.
- For general signs and symptoms of heat and excess conditions, add *Gardenia Complex*.
- For headaches, add *Corydalin* or *Migratrol*.
- For toxicity manifesting in skin rashes or unexplainable itching of the skin, add *Silerex* or *Dermatrol (PS)*.
- For mild nasal congestion and post-nasal drip, add *Magnolia Clear Sinus*.
- For severe nasal obstruction with yellow and sticky discharge, add *Pueraria Clear Sinus*.
- For difficulty breathing and feeling of chest tightness, add *Respitrol (Heat)* or *Respitrol (Deficient)*.
- For excess perspiration or fatigue, add *Immune +*.
- For diarrhea with weakness, add *GI Tonic* or *GI Care II*.
- *Zhu Dan* (Fel Porcus) and *Tu Fu Ling* (Rhizoma Smilacis Glabrae) can be added to detoxify poison in difficult cases. Dosage of *Tu Fu Ling* (Rhizoma Smilacis Glabrae) can be used up to 6 grams a day in addition to *Herbal DTX* to achieve desired effect.
- For unknown causes or strange symptoms of blood stagnation, add *Circulation (SJ)*.

NUTRITION

- Organic products are highly recommended for patients who are suffering from poisoning.
- Take lactobacillus acidophilus supplement to restore normal balance of intestinal flora.
- Drink plenty of water throughout the day to help flush out toxins.
- Avoid preserved foods such as ham, canned food, peanut butter, etc.

LIFESTYLE INSTRUCTIONS

- Exposure to the offending toxins should be avoided as much as possible. Do not drink tap water if it contains high levels of heavy metals. Avoid eating foods that contain preservatives, artificial hormones, herbicides and pesticides. Minimize outdoor activities if the air quality is poor, in order to avoid inhalation of air pollutants. Avoid all products that may contain artificial scents and flavor. Lastly, individuals with hypersensitivity should avoid the use and inhalation of certain chemicals, such as hair spray and perfumes.

HERBAL DTX ™

(Detoxification)

❧ The work environment should also be considered when determining the cause of poisoning. Chronic poisoning is sometimes related to the work environment.

❧ Taking deep breaths for ten minutes each day can enhance the elimination process of toxins in the body.

CLINICAL NOTES

❧ *Herbal DTX* should be used continuously for at least three months for optimal results.

❧ Because of its effect to eliminate the accumulation of toxins and enhance the functions of the liver and kidney, *Herbal DTX* is a good formula for individuals who have hypersensitivity to certain toxins, chemicals, and environmental factors. *Herbal DTX* contains herbs that will enhance the body's natural ability to break down and eliminate the buildup of toxins in the body. *Herbal DTX* is a gentle formula that gradually and continuously remove toxins from the body. It should be taken persistently for 6 to 12 months for optimal effect.

❧ General actions for acute poisoning are as follows:
1. For inhaled poison, open the doors and windows and get the person fresh air as quickly as possible.
2. For poison on the skin, remove the contaminated clothing and flood the skin with water for at least 10 minutes.
3. For poison in the eye, flood the affected eye(s) with lukewarm water poured from a glass 2 or 3 inches from the eye(s) and repeat for 15 minutes.
4. For swallowed poison, give a glass of water (2 to 8 ounces) immediately unless the person is unconscious, having convulsions, or cannot swallow. For more information, please contact the National Poison Control System at (800) 222-1222.

CAUTIONS

❧ Patients with an acute overdose or poisoning should be treated in an emergency room or urgent care center. Call 911, or contact the local poison control center for additional instructions.

❧ Patients with hematuria (blood in the urine) should be treated with extreme caution because this symptom may indicate the possibility of significant damage to the kidney.

❧ Patients who are disorientated or having a seizure/convulsion associated with poisoning should consult their medical doctor immediately.

❧ Patients with a sensitive stomach should take this formula with food. If stomach upset still occurs, reduce the dosage and increase the frequency.

❧ Patients who are on anti-coagulant or anti-platelet therapies, such as Coumadin (Warfarin), should use this formula with caution, as there may be a slightly higher risk of bleeding and bruising.

ACUPUNCTURE POINTS

Traditional Points:
❧ Unconsciousness:
- Needle with strong stimulation *Renzhong* (GV 26), *Yongquan* (KI 1), *Hegu* (LI 4), *Suliao* (GV 25), and *Baihui* (GV 20).
- Apply moxa to *Shenque* (CV 8) and *Qihai* (CV 6).

Balance Method by Dr. Richard Tan:
❧ Left side: *Dadun* (LR 1), *Yinbai* (SP 1), *Yongquan* (KI 1), *Hegu* (LI 4), *Zhongzhu* (TH 3), and *Houxi* (SI 3).
❧ Right side: *Daling* (PC 7), *Lieque* (LU 7), *Lingdao* (HT 4), *Zusanli* (ST 36), *Yanglingquan* (GB 34), and *Xialiao* (BL 34).
❧ Left and right side can be alternated from treatment to treatment.

HERBAL DTX ™

(Detoxification)

☯ For additional information on the Balance Method, please refer to *Dr. Tan's Strategy of Twelve Magical Points* by Dr. Richard Tan.

MODERN RESEARCH

Herbal DTX is designed to treat various kinds of chronic poisoning reactions, including but not limited to such toxins as environmental toxins, chemical compounds, heavy metals, and drugs. Such toxins are present in our everyday lives, including but not limited to insecticides, pesticides, herbicides, preservatives, gas exhaust, artificial hormones, heavy metals, air and water pollution. Acute poisonings are easy to diagnose, and are usually treated by physicians in the emergency room or urgent care center. Chronic poisonings, however, are far more difficult to diagnose as the signs and symptoms are often vague and non-conclusive. Chronic poisoning usually occurs following long-term exposure to toxic agents and their gradual accumulation in the body. Eventually, the accumulation of toxins will begin to interfere with the normal functions of the body to create various illnesses and diseases. Furthermore, since the liver and kidney are the two organs that are primarily responsible for metabolizing and eliminating foreign substances, it is extremely important to ensure that these organs are functioning properly. Individuals with chronic poisoning often have damaged liver and kidney functions. Therefore, optimal treatment must address both detoxification of the offending agent and healing of these two organs.

Gan Cao (Radix Glycyrrhizae) is one of the most commonly used herbs for treatment of overdose and poisoning reactions. It has been proposed that *Gan Cao* (Radix Glycyrrhizae) should be used as the first agent in cases where the identity of the ingested poison or the specific antidote is unknown.[1] Research and clinical reports have all confirmed *Gan Cao* (Radix Glycyrrhizae) has a marked effect to reduce the toxicity of numerous agents, such as toxic foods and plants.[2,3] More recently, it was reported that the use of *Gan Cao* (Radix Glycyrrhizae) showed satisfactory results in treating 454 patients with various types of food poisoning.[4] In another report, 20 out of 22 patients with mushroom poisoning had complete recovery after being treated with an herbal decoction of *Gan Cao* (Radix Glycyrrhizae).[5] Furthermore, glycyrrhizin, generally considered one of the main constituents of *Gan Cao* (Radix Glycyrrhizae), has a marked detoxifying effect to treat various kinds of poisonings, including but not limited to drug poisoning (chloral hydrate, urethane, cocaine, picrotoxin, caffeine, pilocarpine, nicotine, barbiturates, mercury and lead), food poisoning (tetrodotoxin, snake, and mushrooms), and others (herbicides, pesticides, enterotoxin).[6,7] In addition to *Gan Cao* (Radix Glycyrrhizae), *Lu Dou* (Semen Phaseoli Radiati) has been used to treat cases of pesticide poisoning with complete recovery after only three doses.[8]

Herbal DTX also contains herbs that are effective for treating heavy metal poisoning. In one report, 278 patients were treated for arsenic poisoning with an herbal decoction twice daily consisting of *Fang Feng* (Radix Saposhnikoviae), *Lu Dou* (Semen Phaseoli Radiati), *Gan Cao* (Radix Glycyrrhizae) and sugar. At the end of the 28-day treatment, 155 patients (55.76%) reported a significant improvement in subjective signs and symptoms, with normal levels of arsenic found through urinalysis.[9]

Herbal DTX contains many herbs with marked hepatoprotective effect, and can be used to treat various disorders related to the liver. Such herbs include *Gan Cao* (Radix Glycyrrhizae), *Dan Shen* (Radix Salviae Miltiorrhizae) and *Da Huang* (Radix et Rhizoma Rhei). In one report, 330 patients with hepatitis B were treated with glycyrrhizin with 77% effectiveness. The study reported that glycyrrhizin reduced the damage and death of the liver cells, reduced inflammatory reaction, promoted the regeneration of liver cells, and decreased in risk of liver cirrhosis and necrosis.[10] The mechanism of action of *Gan Cao* (Radix Glycyrrhizae) was attributed to the increase of enzyme cytochrome P-450 in the liver, which is responsible for the protective effect of the herb on the liver against chemical- or tetrachloride-induced liver damage and liver cancer.[11] In addition, *Dan Shen* (Radix Salviae Miltiorrhizae) is another herb with marked benefit to protect the liver and treat hepatitis. Administration of *Dan Shen* (Radix Salviae Miltiorrhizae) is associated with a marked hepatoprotective effect against carbon tetrachloride by lowering liver enzyme levels.[12] The hepatoprotective function of *Dan Shen* (Radix Salviae Miltiorrhizae) is due in part to its effect to improve blood circulation and promote regeneration of new liver cells.[13] Clinically, the use of *Dan Shen* (Radix Salviae Miltiorrhizae) was found to be 81.7% effective in treating acute viral hepatitis.[14] It was also used with great success in treating patients with chronic hepatitis.[15] Lastly, *Da Huang* (Radix et Rhizoma Rhei) can also be used to treat hepatitis and acute icteric hepatitis. *Da Huang* (Radix et Rhizoma Rhei) has an a hepatoprotective effect by reducing the extent of liver damage (necrosis of hepatocytes), especially by carbon tetrachloride.[16] According to one study, 80 cases of acute icteric hepatitis were treated with a large dosage of *Da Huang* (Radix et Rhizoma Rhei) with 95% effective rate based on symptomatic evaluation and improvement of liver function.[17]

In addition, many herbs in **Herbal DTX** have remarkable effects to protect the kidney and treat kidney related disorders, including but not limited to acute and chronic nephritis. According to one study, an herbal formula with *Lian Qiao* (Fructus Forsythiae) was found to have good success in treating 8 patients with acute nephritis and 1 patient with tuberculosis of the kidney.[18] In another study, 11 children with acute nephritis were treated with an herbal decoction containing *Bai Mao Gen* (Rhizoma Imperatae) for 32 to 59 doses with marked reduction in edema, lowered blood pressure, absence of protein and blood cells, and normalization of urine. Out of 11 patients, there was complete recovery in 9 and moderate improvement in 2 patients.[19] Furthermore, intravenous infusion of a *Dan Shen* (Radix Salviae Miltiorrhizae) preparation for 14 days was determined to be 62.5 to 80% effective for treating chronic nephritis of varying degrees of severity.[20] Lastly, patients with general kidney impairment also respond well to herbs in **Herbal DTX**. Decoction of *Da Huang* (Radix et Rhizoma Rhei) is effective in reducing blood urea nitrogen and creatinine as demonstrated in both *in vitro* and *in vivo* studies.[21] In one clinical study, an herbal formula with *Da Huang* (Radix et Rhizoma Rhei) and others was effective in treating 20 patients with various degrees of renal impairment by reducing the blood urea nitrogen and creatinine levels significantly.[22]

In summary, **Herbal DTX** contains many herbs that have been used successfully to treat overdose and poisoning by many substances, as stated in the paragraphs above. Furthermore, herbs in **Herbal DTX** prevent and treat disorders of the liver and kidney caused by the accumulation of foreign and toxic substances. By restoring the normal functions of the liver and kidney, **Herbal DTX** ensures the healing and recovery of toxic reactions.

PHARMACEUTICAL DRUGS & CHINESE MEDICINE: A COMPARATIVE ANALYSIS

One striking difference between western and traditional Chinese medicine is that western medicine focuses and excels in crisis management, while traditional Chinese medicine emphasizes and shines in holistic and preventative treatments. Therefore, in emergencies, such as gun shot wounds or surgery, western medicine is generally the treatment of choice. However, for treatment of chronic idiopathic illness of unknown origins, where all lab tests are normal and a clear diagnosis cannot be made, traditional Chinese medicine is distinctly superior.

In cases of chronic poisoning (from chemicals, heavy metals, and various environmental toxins), there are often many vague, non-specific, non-diagnostic signs and symptoms accompanied by normal laboratory tests. Under these circumstances, western medicine struggles to determine the exact diagnosis and corresponding treatments. On the other hand, traditional Chinese medicine is beneficial as it excels in regulating imbalances and alleviating associated signs and symptoms. This formula is extremely beneficial because many herbs in this formula have been shown to have marked effect to detoxify various types of toxins, and to protect and restore normal functions of internal organs (liver and kidneys). This, however, is a gradual process that requires long-term commitment. Herbs should be taken continuously for 6 to 12 months for optimal success. By treating both symptoms and cause, herbal therapy effectively prevents deterioration and restores optimal health.

CASE STUDY

This formula has been used with great success in China for treatment of drug overdose (sedatives and hypnotics), accidental ingestion of rat poison, and adverse reactions associated with *Shang Lu* (Radix Phytolaccae). This

HERBAL DTX ™

(Detoxification)

formula has been used with excellent results by itself, in combination with drug treatment, or following gastric lavage.

W.C., Shanxi, China.

[1] *Jin Gui Yao Lue* (Essentials from the Golden Cabinet) by Zhang Zhong-Jing in Eastern Han
[2] *Shang Hai Zhong Yi Yao Za Zhi* (Shanghai Journal of Chinese Medicine and Herbology), 1964; 8:22
[3] *Fu Jian Zhong Yi Yao* (Fujian Chinese Medicine and Herbology), 1965; 4:44
[4] *Xin Zhong Yi* (New Chinese Medicine), 1985; 2:34
[5] *Xin Zhong Yi* (New Chinese Medicine), 1978; 1:36
[6] *Zhong Yao Tong Bao* (Journal of Chinese Herbology), 1986; 11(10):54
[7] *Zhong Yao Tong Bao* (Journal of Chinese Herbology), 1986; 11(10):55
[8] *Zhe Jiang Zhong Yi Za Zhi* (Zhejiang Journal of Chinese Medicine), 1965; 7:7
[9] *Xin Yi Xue* (New Medicine), 1973; 7:6
[10] *Zhong Yao Tong Bao* (Journal of Chinese Herbology), 1987; 9:60
[11] *Zhong Yao Tong Bao* (Journal of Chinese Herbology), 1986; 11(10):55
[12] *Zhong Yi Za Zhi* (Journal of Chinese Medicine), 1982; (1):67
[13] *Zhong Xi Yi Jie He Za Zhi* (Journal of Integrated Chinese and Western Medicine), 1983; 3(3):180
[14] *Shan Xi Zhong Yi* (Shanxi Chinese Medicine), 1980; 6:15
[15] *Zhong Xi Yi Jie He Za Zhi* (Journal of Integrated Chinese and Western Medicine), 1984; 2:86
[16] *Zhong Guo Zhong Yao Za Zhi* (People's Republic of China Journal of Chinese Herbology), 1989; 14(10):46
[17] *Zhong Xi Yi Jie He Za Zhi* (Journal of Integrated Chinese and Western Medicine), 1983; 1:19
[18] *Jiang Xi Yi Yao* (Jiangxi Medicine and Herbology), 1961; 7:18
[19] *Guang Dong Yi Xue* (Guangdong Medicine), 1965; 3:28
[20] *Shang Hai Yi Yao Za Zhi* (Shanghai Journal of Medicine and Herbology), 1981; 1:17
[21] *Chang Yong Zhong Yao Xian Dai Yan Jiu Yu Lin Chuang* (Recent Study & Clinical Application of Common Traditional Chinese Medicine), 1995; 181:190
[22] *Zhong Yi Za Zhi* (Journal of Chinese Medicine), 1981; 9:21

FORMULAS

HERBAL ENT ™

(Ear, Nose, Throat)

CLINICAL APPLICATIONS

- Infection and inflammation in the upper parts of the body, including ears, nose, and throat (ENT)
- Ear infection: suppurative otitis media
- Nose infection: sinus infection, sinusitis, and rhinitis
- Throat infection: infectious parotitis, tonsillitis, streptococcal pharyngitis, strep throat, severe sore throat, bad breath, and mouth ulcers
- Lung infection: common cold, chronic bronchitis, pulmonary abscess, and pulmonary tuberculosis
- Infectious mononucleosis, erysipelas, infectious parotitis, and mumps

WESTERN THERAPEUTIC ACTIONS

- Antibiotic effect to treat infection
- Anti-inflammatory effect to reduce swelling, relieve inflammation and alleviate pain
- Antipyretic effect to reduce fever

CHINESE THERAPEUTIC ACTIONS

- Clears heat in the head and the upper *jiao*
- Eliminates toxins

DOSAGE

Take 3 to 4 capsules three times daily on an empty stomach, with warm water. Dosage may be increased to 6 to 8 capsules three times daily, if necessary. The herbs should be taken with meals for those with a sensitive stomach.

INGREDIENTS

Ban Lan Gen (Radix Isatidis)
Bo He (Herba Menthae)
Chai Hu (Radix Bupleuri)
Chen Pi (Pericarpium Citri Reticulatae)
Gan Cao (Radix Glycyrrhizae)
Huang Lian (Rhizoma Coptidis)
Huang Qin (Radix Scutellariae)

Jie Geng (Radix Platycodonis)
Lian Qiao (Fructus Forsythiae)
Ma Bo (Lasiosphaera seu Calvatia)
Niu Bang Zi (Fructus Arctii)
Xuan Shen (Radix Scrophulariae)
Zhe Bei Mu (Bulbus Fritillariae Thunbergii)

FORMULA EXPLANATION

Herbal ENT is designed to treat wind, heat and toxin invasion to the head region, leading to symptoms such as severe sore throat, redness and swelling of the face and head, difficulties opening the eyes, swollen glands, ear infection and thirst. It contains herbs with actions to clear heat and eliminate toxins.

Huang Qin (Radix Scutellariae) and *Huang Lian* (Rhizoma Coptidis), the chief herbs of this formula, are used to clear heat in the head and eliminate toxins. *Niu Bang Zi* (Fructus Arctii), *Lian Qiao* (Fructus Forsythiae), and *Bo He* (Herba Menthae) disperse the accumulation of the wind-heat factor in the head. They are all crucial herbs in the treatment of sore throat. *Xuan Shen* (Radix Scrophulariae), *Ma Bo* (Lasiosphaera seu Calvatia) and *Ban Lan Gen* (Radix Isatidis) clear heat and eliminate toxins. *Ma Bo* (Lasiosphaera seu Calvatia) is especially effective for severe sore throat with difficulty to swallow. *Jie Geng* (Radix Platycodonis), *Zhe Bei Mu* (Bulbus Fritillariae Thunbergii) and *Gan Cao* (Radix Glycyrrhizae) have the synergistic effect to soothe sore throat, thus helping the heat-clearing herbs. *Xuan Shen* (Radix Scrophulariae), besides benefiting the throat, also prevents the heat-clearing dampness-drying herbs from

FORMULAS

HERBAL ENT ™

(Ear, Nose, Throat)

injuring the yin. *Chen Pi* (Pericarpium Citri Reticulatae) descends Lung qi, relieves cough and eliminates phlegm. Finally, besides dispersing the wind-heat factor, *Chai Hu* (Radix Bupleuri), acts as a guiding herb to bring the other herbs upward to the head region, where the condition is most critical.

SUPPLEMENTARY FORMULAS

- For common cold or influenza with sore throat, combine with *Lonicera Complex*.
- For sinus infections, use with *Magnolia Clear Sinus* or *Pueraria Clear Sinus*.
- For respiratory tract infections, add *Respitrol (Heat)* or *Respitrol (Cold)*.
- For yellow or greenish phlegm due to respiratory tract infections, use with *Poria XPT*.
- For headache, add *Corydalin*.
- To enhance the antibiotic effect to treat infection, add *Herbal ABX*.
- With severe infectious mononucleosis with swollen lymph nodes, add *Resolve (AI)*.
- With severe suppurative otitis media, add *Gentiana Complex*.
- For high fever and excess heat in the body, add *Gardenia Complex*.
- For constipation, add *Gentle Lax (Excess)*.

NUTRITION

- Avoid spicy, fried or greasy foods.
- Food or beverages that are cool or cold in nature should be consumed. Among these are watermelon, lotus nodes, melon, seaweed, cranberries, celery, cucumber, cactus and winter melon.
- Drink plenty of water and urinate often.
- Increase supplementation with vitamin C and B complex.

The Tao of Nutrition by Ni and McNease
- Chronic sinusitis or rhinitis
  - Recommendations: ginger, green onions, magnolia flower, bananas, garlic, black mushrooms, chrysanthemum flowers, mulberry leaves, and apricot kernel.
  - Avoid extremes of exposure to weather elements, coffee, smoking, stress, picking the nose, polluted air and smog.
- Sore throat
  - Recommendations: carrots, olives, daikon, celery, seaweed, licorice, Chinese prunes, cilantro, and mint. Drink a lot of water and gargle with warm salt water.
  - Avoid alcohol, smoking, pollution, sleeping with the mouth open, stimulating or spicy foods, and fatty foods.
- For more information, please refer to *The Tao of Nutrition* by Dr. Maoshing Ni and Cathy McNease.

LIFESTYLE INSTRUCTIONS

- It is important to build up a strong immune system. When not suffering from an infection, exercise regularly, take a short cold shower following a hot shower, and ingest tonic herbs to enhance the immune system.
- Adequate rest is essential for recovery. Stay away from wind by putting on more clothing. Individuals with infection should rest and recover in a separate room, to prevent spreading germs to other people. Ventilate the patient's room frequently – but make sure the patient is kept warm.
- Stop smoking and drinking, which weaken the immune system.
- Steam inhalation heals the throat, nasal passages, and bronchial tubes. During the acute phase, inhale the steam vapor for 15 minutes three times daily. During the chronic phase, inhale the steam vapor for 15 minutes before going to bed.

HERBAL ENT ™

CLINICAL NOTES

- If the condition does not improve after 7 days, modification of the formula may be necessary.
- There is no evidence thus far that use of heat-clearing herbs may permit secondary infections to arise (as is the case with antibiotic drugs). However, those who have recurrent infections may take acidophilus prophylactically, especially if they have a history of repeated antibiotic drug usage.
- This formula is stronger than **Lonicera Complex** in the treatment of wind-heat invasion. It is used in cases where there is severe sore throat accompanied with other wind-heat symptoms.

CAUTIONS

- This formula is contraindicated during pregnancy and nursing.
- This formula should be used with caution in those with loose stool or diarrhea caused by Spleen qi deficiency. Take this formula after meals in patients who have a weak digestive system.
- Use this formula with caution in cases of yang and qi deficiencies.

ACUPUNCTURE POINTS

Traditional Points:
- Middle ear infection: *Fengchi* (GB 20), *Yifeng* (TH 17), *Tinggong* (SI 19), *Hegu* (LI 4), *Waiguan* (TH 5), *Zulinqi* (GB 41), *Shenshu* (BL 23), and *Quchi* (LI 11).
- Sinus infection:
  - *Feishu* (BL 13), *Hegu* (LI 4), *Quchi* (LI 11), *Shangyang* (LI 1), and *Lingtai* (GV 10).
  - *Shaoshang* (LU 11), *Quchi* (LI 11), and *Yingxiang* (LI 20).
- Sore Throat:
  - *Tinghui* (GB 2), *Yifeng* (TH 17), *Jiache* (ST 6), *Hegu* (LI 4), *Lieque* (LU 7), *Fenglong* (ST 40), *Jiexi* (ST 41), *Shaoshang* (LU 11), and *Jiaosun* (TH 20).
  - *Shaoshang* (LU 11), *Hegu* (LI 4), *Neiting* (ST 44), and *Tianrong* (SI 17).

Balance Method by Dr. Richard Tan:
- Left side: *Tianjing* (TH 10), *Quchi* (LI 11), *ah shi* points from *Yinxi* (HT 6) to *Shenmen* (HT 7), *Yingu* (KI 10), *Ququan* (LR 8), and *Yinlingquan* (SP 9).
- Right side: *Quze* (PC 3), *Shaofu* (HT 8), *ah shi* points from *Taiyuan* (LU 9) to *Yuji* (LU 10), *Yanglingquan* (GB 34), *Zusanli* (ST 36), and *Weizhong* (BL 40).
- For additional information on the Balance Method, please refer to *Dr. Tan's Strategy of Twelve Magical Points* by Dr. Richard Tan.

Ear Acupuncture:
- Kidney, Inner Ear, Endocrine, and Outer Ear. Bleed any distended veins on the back of the ear.

Auricular Acupuncture by Dr. Li-Chun Huang:
- Otitis media: Internal Ear, External Ear, Temple, Sanjiao, Endocrine, Spleen, and Adrenal Gland. Bleed Ear Apex.
- Tonsillitis: Tonsil, Throat, Larynx, and Teeth. Bleed Ear Apex.
- Acute laryngeal pharyngitis: Pharynx, Larynx, Mouth, Sanjiao, Endocrine, Larynx, Teeth, and Trachea. Bleed Ear Apex.
- Chronic laryngeal pharyngitis: Larynx, Pharynx, Lung, Larynx, Teeth, Trachea, Spleen, *San Jiao*, and Endocrine.
- For additional information on the location and explanation of these points, please refer to *Auricular Treatment Formula and Prescriptions* by Dr. Li-Chun Huang.

HERBAL ENT ™

(Ear, Nose, Throat)

MODERN RESEARCH

Herbal ENT contains many herbs with wide-spectrums of antibiotic effect to treat a wide variety of infectious disorders. Furthermore, it also contains several herbs that address the related symptoms of infection that affect the upper parts of the body, such as fever, swelling, inflammation, and pain.

Many herbs in this formula have excellent antibiotic effects, including but not limited to *Huang Qin* (Radix Scutellariae),[1] *Huang Lian* (Rhizoma Coptidis),[2] *Xuan Shen* (Radix Scrophulariae),[3] *Lian Qiao* (Fructus Forsythiae),[4] *Chai Hu* (Radix Bupleuri),[5] *Ban Lan Gen* (Radix Isatidis),[6] and *Niu Bang Zi* (Fructus Arctii).[7] Among these herbs, *Huang Qin* (Radix Scutellariae) and *Huang Lian* (Rhizoma Coptidis) are generally considered as the most potent herbal antibiotics, as they are effective against micro-organisms such as *Bacillus anthracis, Bacillus dysenteriae, Bacillus proteus,* beta-hemolytic streptococcus, *Bordetella pertussis, Corynebacterium diphtheriae, Diplococcus meningitidis, Diplococcus pneumoniae, E. coli, Mycobacterium tuberculosis, Pseudomonas aeruginosa, Salmonella typhi, Staphylococcus aureus, Vibrio cholerae,* and various species of influenza viruses, pathogenic fungi and dermatophytes.[8,9] Furthermore, these herbs have also shown effectiveness against beta-lactam-resistant *Staphylococcus aureus* and methicillin-resistant *Staphylococcus aureus* (MRSA).[10]

With addition to treating the infection, *Herbal ENT* also contains many herbs that treat the related symptoms of infection. *Huang Qin* (Radix Scutellariae), *Huang Lian* (Rhizoma Coptidis), *Chen Pi* (Pericarpium Citri Reticulatae), *Jie Geng* (Radix Platycodonis) and *Lian Qiao* (Fructus Forsythiae) all have anti-inflammatory effects to reduce swelling, relieve inflammation, and alleviate pain.[11,12,13,14,15] *Huang Qin* (Radix Scutellariae) and *Huang Lian* (Rhizoma Coptidis) also have antipyretic effects to reduce fever.[16,17]

In regards to clinical applications, herbs in this formula have been used effectively to treat disorders such as epidemic encephalitis,[18] pulmonary tuberculosis,[19] suppurative otitis media,[20] chronic bronchitis,[21] tonsillitis,[22] pulmonary abscess,[23] common cold,[24] cough,[25] upper respiratory tract infection,[26] encephalitis B,[27] epidemic hemorrhagic fever,[28] infectious parotitis,[29] respiratory tract infection,[30] and myocarditis.[31]

Overall, *Herbal ENT* is an excellent herbal antibiotic formula that treats infection and inflammation in the upper parts of the body. Clinically, it may be used for bacterial, viral or fungal infections. Its indications include treatment of ear, nose, throat and lung infections.

PHARMACEUTICAL DRUGS & CHINESE MEDICINE: A COMPARATIVE ANALYSIS

Western Medical Approach: Discovery of antibiotic drugs is one of the major breakthroughs in modern medicine. It enables doctors to effectively treat many different types of infections. Unfortunately, decades of abuse and misuse have led to growing problems of bacterial mutation and resistance. At this moment, many of these "super bugs" can only be treated with the newest and most potent antibiotic drugs, and unfortunately, many of them have potent side effects as well. Due to the number of antibiotic drugs, and the various species of micro-organisms, it is beyond the scope of this monograph to discuss the benefits and risks of each individual drugs. As a category, antibiotic drugs are extremely effective against most types of bacterial infections. The key points are to select the correct antibiotic drug with least potential side effects, and make sure that the patient finishes the entire course of therapy.

Traditional Chinese Medicine Approach: Herbs are also extremely effective for treatment of various infections. In fact, most modern pharmaceutical drugs were originally derived from natural sources, including penicillin [the oldest antibiotic] and gentimicin [one of the most potent]. One of the main benefits of using herbs is their wide spectrum of antibiotic effect, with indications for bacterial, viral and fungal infections. Furthermore, most of these herbs are extremely safe, and do not have the same harsh side effects as drugs.

Summation: Both drugs and herbs are effective to treat mild to moderate cases of bacterial infections. However, drugs are most effective and more appropriate for life-threatening infections, such as meningitis or encephalitis,

FORMULAS

HERBAL ENT ™

because drugs are more immediately potent and can be prescribed with more laboratory precision (with culture and sensitivity tests). On the other hand, use of herbs is far more effective than drugs for treating certain viral infections, such as the common cold and influenza, as drugs are essentially ineffective for these conditions. Most importantly, herbs are much gentler to the body and safer than drugs. In other words, herbs treat infection without damaging the underlying constitution of the patient. This allows the patient to recover faster, and become more resistant to secondary or re-current infections.

[1] *Zhong Yao Xue* (Chinese Herbology), 1988; 137:140
[2] *Zhong Yao Xue* (Chinese Herbology), 1988; 140:144
[3] *Zhong Yao Yao Li Yu Ying Yong* (Pharmacology and Applications of Chinese Herbs), 1983; 370
[4] *Shan Xi Xin Yi Yao* (New Medicine and Herbology of Shanxi), 1980; 9(11):51
[5] *Zhong Yao Xue* (Chinese Herbology), 1998; 103:106
[6] *Zhong Cheng Yao Yan Jiu* (Research of Chinese Patent Medicine), 1987; 12:9
[7] *Zhong Yao Zhi* (Chinese Herbology Journal), 1984; 250
[8] *J Pharm Pharmacol* 2000 Mar; 52(3):361-6
[9] *Zhong Hua Yi Xue Za Zhi* (Chinese Journal of Medicine), 1958; 44(9):888
[10] *J Pharm Pharmacol* 2000 Mar; 52(3):361-6
[11] *Chem Pharm Bull*, 1984; 32(7):2724
[12] *Yao Xue Za Zhi* (Journal of Medicinals), 1981; 101(10):883
[13] *Zhong Yao Yao Li Yu Ying Yong* (Pharmacology and Applications of Chinese Herbs), 1983; 567
[14] *Zhong Yao Yao Li Yu Ying Yong* (Pharmacology and Applications of Chinese Herbs), 1983; 866
[15] *Ke Yan Tong Xun* (Journal of Science and Research), 1982; (3):35
[16] *Zhong Hua Yi Xue Za Zhi* (Chinese Journal of Medicine), 1956; 42(10):964
[17] *Zhong Guo Bing Li Sheng Li Za Zhi* (Chinese Journal of Pathology and Biology), 1991; 7(3):264
[18] *Zhong Yi Za Zhi* (Journal of Chinese Medicine), 1960; 6:20
[19] *Zhe Jiang Zhong Yi Za Zhi* (Zhejiang Journal of Chinese Medicine), 1964; 10:51
[20] *Zhong Hua Er Ke Za Zhi* (Chinese Journal of Pediatrics), 1954; 4:272
[21] *Zhe Jiang Zhong Yi Za Zhi* (Zhejiang Journal of Chinese Medicine), 1985; 1:18
[22] *Yun Nan Zhong Yi Xue Yuan Xue Bao* (Journal of Yunnan University School of Medicine), 1983; 1:20
[23] *Jiang Su Zhong Yi Za Zhi* (Jiangsu Journal of Chinese Medicine), 1981; 3:35
[24] *Zhong Yi Za Zhi* (Journal of Chinese Medicine), 1985; 12:13
[25] *Zhong Yao Xue* (Chinese Herbology), 1998; 105
[26] *Zhong Yi Za Zhi* (Journal of Chinese Medicine), 1983; 24(11):19
[27] *Xian Dai Shi Yong Yao Xue* (Practical Applications of Modern Herbal Medicine), 221
[28] *Shan Xi Zhong Yi* (Shanxi Chinese Medicine), 1984; 3:16
[29] *Zhong Yi Za Zhi* (Journal of Chinese Medicine), 1958; 7:463
[30] *Guang Xi Zhong Yi Yao* (Guangxi Chinese Medicine and Herbology), 1989; (1):5
[31] *Zhong Guo Zhong Xi Yi Jie He Za Zhi* (Chinese Journal of Integrative Chinese and Western Medicine), 1993; 13(4):244

FORMULAS

HERBALITE ™

CLINICAL APPLICATIONS

- ❧ Obesity with excess appetite and constant craving for food
- ❧ Weight gain

WESTERN THERAPEUTIC ACTIONS

- ❧ Increases energy level and promotes a sense of well-being [1,10,13,14,15,16]
- ❧ Speeds up body metabolism to burn off excess fat and body weight [10,13]
- ❧ Suppresses appetite to decrease unnecessary food intake [11,12]
- ❧ Mild diuretic effect to eliminate water accumulation

CHINESE THERAPEUTIC ACTIONS

- ❧ Clears Stomach heat
- ❧ Cleanses the bowels
- ❧ Detoxifies residual toxins

DOSAGE

Take 3 to 4 capsules on an empty stomach half an hour before meals with a large glass of water. Avoid eating any food or snacks after dinner and for the last 3 to 4 hours before bedtime.

INGREDIENTS

Bai Shao (Radix Paeoniae Alba)
Chai Hu (Radix Bupleuri)
Ci Wu Jia (Radix et Caulis Acanthopanacis Senticosi)
Da Huang (Radix et Rhizoma Rhei)
Da Zao (Fructus Jujubae)
He Ye (Folium Nelumbinis)
Huang Qi (Radix Astragali)

Huang Qin (Radix Scutellariae)
Ji Xue Cao (Herba Centellae)
Lu Cha (Folium Camellia Sinensis)
Sheng Jiang (Rhizoma Zingiberis Recens)
Zao Jiao (Fructus Gleditsiae)
Zhi Shi (Fructus Aurantii Immaturus)

FORMULA EXPLANATION

Herbalite is an herbal formula specifically designed for gradual yet effective weight loss. *Herbalite* contains herbs that suppress appetite, increase body metabolism, and speed up the breakdown of fatty tissues.

Chai Hu (Radix Bupleuri), the principle herb of this formula, is used with *Huang Qin* (Radix Scutellariae) to harmonize the *shaoyang* and clear heat from the Gallbladder (*shaoyang*). *Da Huang* (Radix et Rhizoma Rhei) and *Zhi Shi* (Fructus Aurantii Immaturus) purge heat from the Stomach (*yangming*). *Da Huang* (Radix et Rhizoma Rhei) and *Zhi Shi* (Fructus Aurantii Immaturus) also activate the qi circulation to dispel hardened stools. *Bai Shao* (Radix Paeoniae Alba) combines with *Da Huang* (Radix et Rhizoma Rhei) to relieve abdominal pain due to constipation. *Bai Shao* (Radix Paeoniae Alba) harmonizes qi and blood to help relieve depression and fidgeting. *He Ye* (Folium Nelumbinis) dissolve and eliminate dampness. *Da Zao* (Fructus Jujubae) and *Sheng Jiang* (Rhizoma Zingiberis Recens) harmonize all of the herbs in this formula. *Zao Jiao* (Fructus Gleditsiae) dries dampness and helps to break down fat through its function to dissipate phlegm stagnation. *Ci Wu Jia* (Radix et Caulis Acanthopanacis Senticosi) and *Huang Qi* (Radix Astragali) are used for their adaptogenic effects and to enhance overall well being. Finally, *Lu*

HERBALITE ™

Cha (Folium Camellia Sinensis) and *Ji Xue Cao* (Herba Centellae) are added to increase the basal body metabolism and to burn excess fat.

SUPPLEMENTARY FORMULAS

- For high cholesterol levels, add *Cholisma*.
- For high cholesterol levels and fatty liver, add *Cholisma (ES)*.
- For edema and water accumulation, add *Herbal DRX*.
- With constipation, combine with *Gentle Lax (Excess)* or *Gentle Lax (Deficient)*.
- For hypertension, add *Gastrodia Complex* or *Gentiana Complex*.
- With diabetes, combine with *Equilibrium*.
- To boost energy and raise the level of awareness, add *Vibrant* or *Imperial Tonic*.
- For excess fire in the body, add *Gardenia Complex*.

NUTRITION

- Include in the diet more complex carbohydrates, such as tofu, potatoes, sesame seeds, beans, brown rice and whole grains.
- Consume large quantities of fresh fruits and vegetables.
- Drink six to eight glasses of water on a daily basis.
- Drink tea (especially *pu-er*, green, *oolong*, and black tea) as it helps to flush the oils from the intestines.
- Decrease the consumption of red meat, fatty foods, processed or fried foods, soda, pastries, pies, doughnuts, candy, etc.
- Eat small, frequent meals throughout the day instead of a few large ones. Eat slowly and chew thoroughly.

LIFESTYLE INSTRUCTIONS

- The importance of a regular exercise routine cannot be over-emphasized. Exercise will stimulate the glands, improve energy levels, normalize metabolic functions, reduce fat and burn calories.
- The following exercise can also be done in the shower to help weight loss: While in the shower, use a luffa to massage the body in circular motion starting from the toes to the heart, then the fingers to the heart. It is preferable to follow the channels while massaging to achieve maximum effect. Spend extra time to massage those places with the most fat deposits. Metabolism at those places where fat accumulates is usually slower and the surrounding muscles are not used as much. Therefore, massaging will enhance circulation to the area to help break up the stagnation. After the shower, drink one glass of water and soak in a tub with water that is warmer than 42°C (108°F). A high temperature bath stimulates the sympathetic nervous system and increases metabolism in a short period of time to help invigorate the body. However, this temperature is not suitable for long periods of soaking. One should not soak until he or she is dizzy. Finally, rinse off with cold water for at least 20 to 30 seconds to help tighten up muscle tone. [Note: For individuals who have *wei* (defensive) *qi* deficiency or those who catch colds frequently, it is not recommended to start this cold water rinsing regimen, as extreme changes in water temperature from high to low may trigger them to catch a cold. It is better to gradually lower the temperature, starting from warm then to cold water so the body can become accustomed to the change. Once the pores are conditioned to open and close with this temperature change, the body will become less susceptible to catching a cold.]

CLINICAL NOTES

- *Herbalite* is designed to help with weight loss safely and gradually. Individuals who take *Herbalite* lose an average of one pound per week.

HERBALITE ™

- Do not to lose weight drastically. Rapid weight loss may be hazardous and is more likely to lead to rebound weight gain.
- It is extremely important to change the dietary and exercise habits to avoid rebound weight gain.

CAUTIONS

- *Lu Cha* (Folium Camellia Sinensis), commonly known as green tea, contains a small amount of caffeine as its natural ingredient.
- This formula is contraindicated during pregnancy and nursing.
- Discontinue *Herbalite* once the desired effect is achieved.

ACUPUNCTURE POINTS

Traditional Points:
- *Shenmen* (HT 7), *Liangqiu* (ST 34), *Gongsun* (SP 4), *Tianshu* (ST 25), *Daling* (PC 7), *Qihai* (CV 6), and *Guanyuan* (CV 4).

Balance Method by Dr. Richard Tan:
- Left side: *Waiguan* (TH 5), *Hegu* (LI 4) and *Yinlingquan* (SP 9).
- Right side: *Zusanli* (ST 36) and *Neiguan* (PC 6).
- Left and right side can be alternated from treatment to treatment.
- For additional information on the Balance Method, please refer to *Dr. Tan's Strategy of Twelve Magical Points* by Dr. Richard Tan.

Ear Points:
- Stomach, Small Intestine, Kidney, and Hypothalamus.
- Embed ear seeds and massage the points for two to three minutes thirty minutes before meals to decrease his/her appetite. Replace ear seeds once a week, and continue for five weeks per course of treatment. Rest for one to two weeks in between courses of treatments.
- The most effective ear seeds for weight loss are *Bai Jie Zi* (Semen Sinapis) and *Wang Bu Liu Xing* (Semen Vaccariae).

Auricular Acupuncture by Dr. Li-Chun Huang:
- Treating obesity by regulating endocrine function: Pituitary and Endocrine.
  - Strengthen exciting of the human body: Forehead and Exciting Point.
  - Heighten satiety: Hunger Point and Thalamus.
  - Promote Excretion: *San Jiao*, Kidney, Large Intestine and Lung.
- Treating obesity by reducing fat deposit: Abdomen, Buttock, and corresponding points of fat deposits.
- For additional information on the location and explanation of these points, please refer to *Auricular Treatment Formula and Prescriptions* by Dr. Li-Chun Huang.

MODERN RESEARCH

Herbalite is designed to help with weight loss safely and gradually. *Herbalite* contains herbs that suppress the appetite to reduce unnecessary food intake, increase body metabolism to burn off excess fat, enhance energy levels to promote a sense of well being, and eliminate water accumulation.

Lu Cha (Folium Camellia Sinensis), commonly known as green tea, has a wide range of functions and is commonly used for different clinical applications. *Lu Cha* (Folium Camellia Sinensis) is an effective central nervous system stimulant and increases body metabolism and boosts energy level.[1] *Lu Cha* (Folium Camellia Sinensis) has a cancer-protective function as it inhibits the formation of cancer-inducing compounds and suppresses the mutation of bone marrow cells.[2,3] In addition to its cancer-protective effect, the use of *Lu Cha* (Folium Camellia Sinensis) also reduces cholesterol levels. Overall, the use of *Lu Cha* (Folium Camellia Sinensis) prolongs life span, contributes to longevity, and protects against life-threatening diseases.[4,5]

Huang Qi (Radix Astragali) is one of the most frequently used Chinese herbs and is historically used for its function to tonify *wei* (defensive) *qi*. In terms of Western medicine, modern research has confirmed repeatedly that *Huang Qi* (Radix Astragali) increases both specific and non-specific immunity.[6,7,8] In one clinical study with 115 leucopenic patients, it was found that the use of *Huang Qi* (Radix Astragali) is associated with an "obvious rise of the white blood cell (WBC) count" with a dose-dependent relationship.[9]

Ci Wu Jia (Radix et Caulis Acanthopanacis Senticosi) has been used for centuries in both Russia and China for its "adaptogenic" effect to normalize high or low blood pressure, stimulate the immune system and increase work productivity. Clinical effects of *Ci Wu Jia* (Radix et Caulis Acanthopanacis Senticosi) include an increase in energy level, protection against toxins and free radicals, and treatment of atherosclerosis.[10] One study demonstrated that *Ci Wu Jia* (Radix et Caulis Acanthopanacis Senticosi) reduces plasma sugar level and may be beneficial in treating diabetes.[11,12] Another study showed *Ci Wu Jia* (Radix et Caulis Acanthopanacis Senticosi) to effectively increase human physical working capacity.[13]

Ji Xue Cao (Herba Centellae) also has an adaptogenic effect, and is commonly used to address both mental and physical conditions. Numerous studies have demonstrated its effectiveness to improve memory, overcome stress, fatigue, mental confusion,[14] and deterioration in mental function.[15,16]

PHARMACEUTICAL DRUGS & CHINESE MEDICINE: A COMPARATIVE ANALYSIS

Western Medical Approach: Obesity is a increasingly common health problem that has few treatment options available. Due to diet and lifestyle changes, many people in developed countries now struggle continual weight gain. Furthermore, there are few or no drug treatments available. Many older drugs, such as "fen-phen" (fenfluramine and phentermine) and dexfenfluramine, are now rarely used or withdrawn from the market because of serious and potentially life-threatening side effects, such as cardiac valvular dysfunction. Currently, there are only two drugs approved by the Food and Drug Administration for long-term weight loss, and they both have serious side effects. Xenical (Orlistat) reduces body weight by blocking absorption of fat in the digestive tract. Because it interferes with the normal absorption process, this drug is known to cause many gastrointestinal side effects, such as fecal incontinence, fecal urgency, flatulence with discharge, increased defecation, oily evacuation, oily rectal leakage, steatorrhea, and projectile diarrhea. Meridia (Sibutramine) is a stimulant agent that causes weight loss by increasing metabolism and suppressing appetite. Similar to many other stimulant weight-loss drugs, use of Meridia (Sibutramine) may cause anorexia, anxiety, constipation, dizziness, headache, insomnia, irritability, nervousness, rhinitis, xerostomia, hypertension, congestive heart failure, arrhythmias, seizure and stroke.

Traditional Chinese Medicine Approach: Obesity may be treated with herbs that suppress appetite, increase energy and metabolism, and eliminate accumulation of dampness and water. Use of herbs has been shown to be effective to slowly and steadily lower body weight. Based on clinical experience and case studies, most individuals lose an average of 1 pound per week while taking this herbal formula. Therefore, this formula is considered a gentle formula that needs to be taken on a long-term basis for optimal results. For those who are grossly overweight and have immediate health risks, use of this formula is inappropriate and not recommended, as it will not cause instantaneous weight loss. Lastly, it is extremely important to remember there is no magic bullet for weight loss. Without commitment to changing diet and lifestyles, use of either drugs or herbs will have limited effectiveness. The practitioners and patients must work together to achieve significant and sustainable clinical results.

HERBALITE ™

CASE STUDIES

A 53-year-old female business owner presented with low energy, muscle pain and low back pain. The patient was 45 pounds overweight. Pain was felt in her lumbar area upon palpation. The pulse was slow and the tongue was pale and swollen with a thin white coat. The practitioner diagnosed the condition as Kidney yang deficiency, qi deficiency and Liver yang excess. The practitioner also suspected a possibility of hypothyroidism, which had yet to be confirmed by lab tests. The patient was treated with *Herbalite*, acupuncture, and diet modification. She then lost 43 pounds in 4 months and her energy level increased dramatically. The pain in her low back has also disappeared. *Herbalite* appeared to suppress her food cravings, increase her energy and improve her psychological status. The patient became more energetic, radiant, and positive.

T.S., East Providence, Rhode Island

A 58-year-old female was concerned about her voracious appetite, stress and inability to lose weight. The practitioner felt that the patient's overeating was directly caused by the patient's stress and her tendency to worry too much. The patient had problems with over-consumption of caffeine and sweets, which lead to her poor digestion and sluggish metabolism. Her diagnosis was Liver qi stagnation, Spleen qi deficiency and Kidney yin deficiency. After taking *Herbalite*, the patient reported losing 7 lbs in the first two weeks. She felt that her excessive appetite tapered down considerably, especially at night. With *Herbalite*, she reported a reduction for sweet cravings and a break from her detrimental eating cycle that was driven by emotions and stress.

S.A., Santa Fe, New Mexico

A 30-year-old female who worked in a computer company wanted to lose 10 pounds within 1 month. She was 5' 1" and weighed 125 pounds. She was instructed to take *Herbalite* (4 capsules three times daily on an empty stomach), along with recommendations to control her diet and engage in moderate exercise. On follow-up visits, she lost 6 pounds after 2 weeks, and a total of 11 pounds after 4 weeks. The patient was able to keep the weight off in a subsequent visit 3 months later.

J.C., Diamond Bar, California

A 39-year-old female came in complaining of weight gain and an increased hunger sensation. The practitioner diagnosed the condition as Spleen qi deficiency. After taking *Herbalite*, the patient noted a reduction in appetite.

M.B., Bend, Oregon

A long history of battling weight gain had plagued a 34-year-old female teacher consequently causing her to feel low in energy along with bouts of depression. Diagnosis according to traditional Chinese medicine was damp and phlegm stagnation. Tongue analysis showed a "puffy" tongue body with a thick coating. The pulse was described as "rolling." Although she had encountered difficulties in losing weight in the past, she was able to loose 10 pounds in 3 months by using *Herbalite*.

Anonymous

A 32-year-old female computer technician who had gained almost 20 pounds within a year was diagnosed with damp and phlegm stagnation. Objective findings included a pale tongue body with teeth marks, a "rolling" pulse, low energy, and slow metabolism. Weight loss from taking *Herbalite* gradually appeared after two weeks of the initial intake of the formula. Within six months of *Herbalite* treatment, she had lost another 40 pounds, had increased energy level, and felt better about herself.

T.G., Albuquerque, NM

HERBALITE ™

A 49-year-old perimenopausal female presented with cold extremities, easily fatigued, and weight gain. The practitioner diagnosed her condition as yang deficiency. After a little more than a week of taking *Herbalite*, the patient lost 5 pounds. Along with the weight loss, she also felt more energized, had reduced appetite and felt warm sensations in her extremities. Dietary modifications, fluid intake, and exercise such as yoga were also implemented into her treatment protocol.

W.E., San Diego, California

D.K, a 33-year-old female, came to the office for weight loss. She had two children, ages 3 years and 1 year, and had not managed to drop the weight she had gained during her pregnancies. She was getting married in two months and wanted to be thinner for her wedding. Her weight-loss goal was 15 to 20 pounds. She did not feel that she had very good eating habits - she ate large portions and craved sweets. The patient said she was frequently irritable and exhausted. She also complained of constipation. Her blood pressure was 110/90 mmHg and her heart rate was 66 to 68 beats per minute. Her diagnosis according to traditional Chinese medicine was dampness in the Spleen with Liver qi stagnation. *Herbalite* was prescribed at 4 capsules three times a day. The patient took six bottles altogether. The first four bottles were without *Da Huang* (Radix et Rhizoma Rhei) since the patient was still nursing. The patient reported losing five pounds. She stated that *Herbalite* regulated her appetite sufficiently that she was able to be satisfied with smaller portions at meals. She also reduced her sugar consumption and increased her fiber intake. The client said that she took the herbs faithfully but she admitted that unless she greatly modified her diet and instituted an exercise regime, it was unlikely that she would succeed in meeting her weight loss goal. D.K was happy to report that *Herbalite* also relieved her constipation.

H.H., San Francisco, California

P.Z., a 61-year-old male patient, presented with obesity. He was 288 pounds and stated that he overate his whole life. Besides obesity, he also suffered from hypertension and high cholesterol and triglycerides levels. His blood pressure was 140/88 mmHg and his heart rate was 84 beats per minute. The diagnosis according to traditional Chinese medicine was damp accumulation. *Herbalite* was prescribed at 4 capsules three times daily. He lost a total of 66 pounds in approximately 10 months. Patient was also given acupuncture treatment.

W.F., Bloomfield, New Jersey

[1] Olin, R. et al. *The Lawrence Review of Natural Products by Facts and Comparison*. Green Tea. May 1993
[2] Wang, H. and Wu, Y. Inhibitory effect of Chinese tea on N-nitrosation in vitro and in vivo. *IARC Sci Publ*;105:546. 1991
[3] Imanishi, H. et al. Tea tannin components modify the induction of sister-chromatid exchanges and chromosome aberrations in mutagen-treated cultured mammalian cells and mice. *Mutat Res*; 259(1):79. 1991
[4] Uchida, S. et al. Radioprotective effects of (-)-epigallocatechin 3-0-gallate (green tea tannin) in mice. *Life Sci*; 50(2):147; 1992
[5] Sadakata, S. et al. Mortality among female practitioners of Chanoyu (Japanese "tea-ceremony"). *Tohoku J Exp Med*;166(4):475. 1992
[6] Chu, DT. et al. Immunotherapy with Chinese medicinal herbs. I. Immune restoration of local xenogenetic graft-versus-host reaction in cancer patients by fractionated astragalus membranaceus in vitro. *Journal of Clinical & Laboratory Immunology*. 25(3):119-23, Mar. 1988
[7] Sun, Y. et al. Immune restoration and/or augmentation of local graft versus host reaction by traditional Chinese medicinal herbs. *Cancer*. 52(1):70-3, July 1. 1983
[8] Sun, Y. et al. Preliminary observations on the effects of the Chinese medicinal herbs astragalus membranaceus and Ligustrum lucidum on lymphocyte blastogenic responses. *Journal of Biological Response Mopdifiers*. 2(3):227-37, 1983
[9] Weng, XS. *Chung Juo Chung Hsia I Chieh Ho Tsa Chih* August 1995
[10] Sprecher, E. Eleutherococcus Senticosus on the Way to Being a Phytopharmacon. *Pharma Ztg*; 134:9. 1989
[11] Hinino, H. et al. Isolation and Hypoglycemic Activity of Eleutherans A, B, C, D, E, F, and G: Glycans of Eleutherococcus senticosus roots. *J Nat Prod*; 49(2):293. 1986
[12] Molokovskii, DS. et al. The Action of Adaptogenic Plant Preparations in Experimental Alloxan Diabetes. *Probl Endokrinol*; 35(6):82. 1989
[13] Asano, K. et al. Effect of Eleutherococcus Senticosus Extract on Human Physical Working Capacity. *Planta Med*; 48(3):175. 1986
[14] Bartram, T. *Encyclopedia of Herbal Medicine 1st edition*. Dorest, England: Grace Publishers. 1995
[15] Kapoor, LD. *CRC Handbook of Ayurvedic Medicinal Plants*. Boca Raton, FL: CRC Press. 1990
[16] Murray, M. Centella asiatica (Gotu Kola) Monograph *American Journal of Natural Medicine*. Volume 3, No. 6 Jul/Aug:22-26 1996

FORMULAS

IMMUNE + ™

CLINICAL APPLICATIONS

❧ Weak or compromised immune system
❧ Frequent bacterial or viral infections, such as common colds and/or influenza
❧ Prolonged recovery period from bacterial or viral infections
❧ Cancer patients with weakened immune systems from radiation or chemotherapy treatment
❧ HIV/AIDS patients with weakened immune systems [7]
❧ Individuals with no significant complaints, but desire to enhance their immunity

WESTERN THERAPEUTIC ACTIONS

❧ Enhances the immune system: increases white blood cell count [1,2,3,8,9,10,11,14,15,16]
❧ Anticancer activity: inhibits the growth of cancer cells. Use as an immune supportive therapy for patients receiving radiation or chemotherapy. [5,6,8,12,13]
❧ Inhibits the growth of harmful bacteria [7]
❧ Boosts energy and vitality

CHINESE THERAPEUTIC ACTIONS

❧ Consolidates the *wei* (defensive) *qi* and dispels lingering pathogenic factors
❧ Tonifies normal qi and strengthens the body
❧ Tonifies the Lung, Spleen, and Kidney

DOSAGE

Treatment dosage: take 4 capsules three times daily. Maintenance dosage: take 2 capsules daily to enhance the immune system and prevent viral or bacterial infections.

INGREDIENTS

Bai Zhu (Rhizoma Atractylodis Macrocephalae)
Dong Chong Xia Cao (Cordyceps)
Fang Feng (Radix Saposhnikoviae)

Huang Qi (Radix Astragali)
Ling Zhi (Ganoderma)
Wu Wei Zi (Fructus Schisandrae Chinensis)

FORMULA EXPLANATION

According to traditional Chinese medicine, *wei* (defensive) *qi* is located at the exterior surface of the body and provides the initial protection against foreign or pathogenic factors. When *wei* (defensive) *qi* is strong, pathogenic factors cannot penetrate the body. When it is weak, a wide variety of infections occur. Therefore, prevention of infections relies on normal functioning of *wei* (defensive) *qi*.

Huang Qi (Radix Astragali) is the chief herb in this formula. It fortifies the Lung, strengthens the *wei* (defensive) *qi* and indirectly protects against external pathogenic factors. Its anticancer effects increase the content of cAMP and inhibit the growth of tumor cells. *Ling Zhi* (Ganoderma) increases white blood cells and inhibits the growth of various viruses and bacteria. *Ling Zhi* (Ganoderma) has also been traditionally used to tonify blood and vital energy, which are essential in rebuilding the underlying constitution. *Dong Chong Xia Cao* (Cordyceps) has been used traditionally for chronically debilitated patients. It is an excellent herb to tonify Kidney yin and yang and improve overall bodily constitution. *Bai Zhu* (Rhizoma Atractylodis Macrocephalae) strengthens the Spleen, and *Wu Wei Zi* (Fructus Schisandrae Chinensis) closes the skin pores to stop sweating and prevent exterior attack of wind. *Fang*

IMMUNE + ™

Feng (Radix Saposhnikoviae) circulates in the peripheral channels of the body and expels lingering pathogenic factors.

SUPPLEMENTARY FORMULAS

- ☯ To minimize the side effects of chemotherapy and radiation treatment, combine with *C/R Support*.
- ☯ For end-stage cancer or cancer patients who are too weak to receive chemotherapy or radiation, add *CA Support*.
- ☯ *Cordyceps 3* can be added to enhance the anticancer effect of *Immune +*.
- ☯ To tonify constitutional qi, blood, yin and yang, combine with *Imperial Tonic*.
- ☯ For a quick boost of energy and awareness, use *Vibrant*.
- ☯ To improve memory, add *Enhance Memory*.
- ☯ During the initial stages of cold and flu with sore throat, fever and/or headache, use *Lonicera Complex* instead of *Immune +*.
- ☯ During the secondary stage of pathogenic invasion with Lung heat, use *Respitrol (Heat)* instead of *Immune +*.
- ☯ For cold and flu with sneezing, clear nasal discharge, and chills, use *Respitrol (Cold)* instead of *Immune +*.
- ☯ For cold and flu with profuse, yellow phlegm, and cough, use *Poria XPT* instead of *Immune +*.
- ☯ For allergic conditions, sinus infection, and yellow nasal discharge, use *Pueraria Clear Sinus* instead of *Immune +*. Patients may resume taking *Immune +* after flu symptoms subside.
- ☯ For allergic conditions, sinus headache, nasal obstruction, with or without white or clear nasal discharge, use *Magnolia Clear Sinus* instead of *Immune +*. Patients may continue taking *Immune +* after flu symptoms subside.
- ☯ For weaker, older patients who have asthma attacks, wheezing or dyspnea, use *Respitrol (Deficient)* instead.
- ☯ For cough, add *Respitrol (CF)*.
- ☯ For all types of infection, use *Herbal ABX* instead of *Immune +*.
- ☯ For inflammation with swelling, add *Resolve (AI)*.
- ☯ With dryness and thirst, add *Nourish (Fluids)*.
- ☯ With Kidney yin deficiency, add *Kidney Tonic (Yin)*.
- ☯ With Kidney yang deficiency, add *Kidney Tonic (Yang)*.

NUTRITION

- ☯ Vitamins A, C, E and zinc are essential in promoting a healthy immune system.
- ☯ Drink plenty of fluids to ensure that the lymphatic system drains freely and circulates smoothly.
- ☯ Foods that are helpful to strengthen the body and fight infection include garlic, citrus fruits and green vegetables.
- ☯ Limit the intake of sweet foods and refined white sugar: they impair the body's ability to kill bacteria.

The Tao of Nutrition by Ni and McNease
- ☯ AIDS
  - Recommendations: Make brown rice porridge with pearl barley, mung beans, yams and lotus seeds.
  - Avoid dairy, alcohol, sugar, coffee, fatty or fried foods, overly spicy foods, cold or raw foods, tomato, eggplant, bell peppers, and shellfish.
- ☯ Cancer
  - Recommendations: Blend shitake or ganoderma mushrooms and white fungus, boil and drink the soup three times a day.
  - Recommendations: Boil together mung beans, pearl barley, azuki beans, and figs. This makes a delicious dessert that will aid appetite and sustain energy level.

IMMUNE + ™

- Avoid meat, chicken, coffee, cinnamon, anise, pepper, dairy products, spicy foods (except garlic), high fat foods, cooked oils, chemical additives, moldy foods, smoking, constipation, stress, and all irritations.
- For more information, please refer to *The Tao of Nutrition* by Dr. Maoshing Ni and Cathy McNease.

LIFESTYLE INSTRUCTIONS

- Avoid over-exertion both mentally and physically, either of which can suppress the immune system.
- Wear appropriate clothing on cold, damp or windy days, and to avoid becoming chilled or over-heated.
- Rest is essential in the recovery of a weak immune system or as protection against catching a cold.
- The skin is the largest organ of the body, and the first defense against pathogenic factors. Exercises that stimulate the skin will strengthen the immune system. Engage in such exercises as cold-water stepping, dew walking, dry brushing, and swimming in cold water. However, transition into these activities slowly to avoid catching a cold from sudden exposure.
- Regular exercise and adequate sleep (at least 8 hours) are essential to maintaining a strong immune system.

CLINICAL NOTES

- *Immune +* should *not* be used alone to treat infections since it does not have any antibiotic properties.
- *Immune +* can be taken on a long-term basis to enhance the immune system in a normal or immuno-deficient person.
- *Immune +* is safe to use for children experiencing recurrent respiratory infections.

CAUTIONS

- The main focus of this herbal formula is to enhance the immune system, not to treat infection. Patients with an active infection must be treated with other formulas accordingly.
- This formula is contraindicated for individuals who are on immune suppressant drugs (i.e. cyclosporin) after receiving an organ transplant. *Immune +* contains many herbs that enhance both specific and non-specific immunity, and may increase the risk of organ rejection.

ACUPUNCTURE POINTS

Traditional Points:
- *Zusanli* (ST 36), *Sanyinjiao* (SP 6), *Fengchi* (GB 20), *Fengmen* (BL 12), and *Hegu* (LI 4).
- *Qihai* (CV 6), *Pishu* (BL 20), *Zhongwan* (CV 12), *Zusanli* (ST 36), *Hegu* (LI 4), and *Weishu* (BL 21).

Balance Method by Dr. Richard Tan:
- Left side: *Hegu* (LI 4) and *Xuehai* (SP 10).
- Right side: *Chize* (LU 5), *Lieque* (LU 7), and *Zusanli* (ST 36).
- Left and right side can be alternated from treatment to treatment.
- For additional information on the Balance Method, please refer to *Dr. Tan's Strategy of Twelve Magical Points* by Dr. Richard Tan.

Ear Points:
- Nose, Spleen, and Bone Marrow.

Auricular Acupuncture by Dr. Li-Chun Huang:
- Preventing common cold: Spleen, Lung, Endocrine, Allergic Area, and Adrenal Gland. Bleed Ear Apex.

IMMUNE + ™

☙ For additional information on the location and explanation of these points, please refer to *Auricular Treatment Formula and Prescriptions* by Dr. Li-Chun Huang.

MODERN RESEARCH

Immune + is an excellent formula to enhance specific and non-specific immunity, as confirmed by various independent research.

Huang Qi (Radix Astragali) is one of the most frequently used Chinese herbs and has been used historically for its ability to tonify the *wei* (defensive) *qi*. In allopathic medical terms, modern research has confirmed repeatedly that *Huang Qi* (Radix Astragali) increases both specific and non-specific immunity.[1,2,3] In a clinical trial of 115 leucopenic patients, it was found that the use of *Huang Qi* (Radix Astragali) is associated with an "obvious rise of the white blood cell (WBC) count" with a dose-dependent relationship.[4] In addition, *Huang Qi* (Radix Astragali) works well with concurrent drug therapy in enhancing the overall effectiveness of the treatment. *Huang Qi* (Radix Astragali) potentiates the antitumor effect of chemotherapy drugs,[5] while reversing drug-induced immune suppression.[6] Lastly, *Huang Qi* (Radix Astragali) also demonstrates anticancer activity as it increases the content of cAMP and inhibits the growth of tumor cells.[7]

Ling Zhi (Ganoderma) has a wide range of therapeutic effects in the treatment of cancer. It has been demonstrated in various clinical studies that *Ling Zhi* (Ganoderma) enhances the immune system. The specific effects of *Ling Zhi* (Ganoderma) include an increase in monocytes, macrophages and T lymphocytes.[8,9,10,11] In addition, it also increases the production of cytokine, interleukin, tumor necrosis factor and interferon.[8] Furthermore, *Ling Zhi* (Ganoderma) has a broad spectrum of antibacterial activities and inhibits the growth of *pneumococci*, *streptococci* (type A), *staphylococci*, *E. coli*, *B. dysenteriae, pseudomonas*, and others.[7]

Dong Chong Xia Cao (Cordyceps) is another herb that has antitumor and immunomodulatory functions. *Dong Chong Xia Cao* (Cordyceps) was found to significantly inhibit the proliferation of cancer cells;[12] and in some instances, the growth inhibition rate of the cancer cells reached 78 to 83%.[13] In addition to antitumor activities, *Dong Chong Xia Cao* (Cordyceps) enhances overall immunity by increasing the number of lymphocytes and natural killer cells and the production of interleukin, interferon and tumor necrosis factor.[14,15,16,17,18]

Wu Wei Zi (Fructus Schisandrae Chinensis) has a wide range of functions and clinical applications. In addition to its classical function as a general tonic, it is also used to protect the liver, regulate the nervous system and the digestive tract, and enhance the body's ability to adapt to stress. *Wu Wei Zi* (Fructus Schisandrae Chinensis) possesses pronounced liver-protectant effect by increasing blood flow to the liver and increasing regeneration of liver cells.[19] It stimulates the nervous system to increase reflex responses and improve mental alertness and treat memory loss.[20] In addition, it helps the body adapt to stress by balancing body fluids, improving sexual stamina, and improving failing senses.[21]

PHARMACEUTICAL DRUGS & CHINESE MEDICINE: A COMPARATIVE ANALYSIS

One striking difference between western and traditional Chinese medicine is that western medicine focuses and excels in crisis management, while traditional Chinese medicine emphasizes and shines in holistic and preventative treatments. Therefore, in emergencies, such as gun shot wounds or surgery, western medicine is generally the treatment of choice. However, for treatment of chronic idiopathic illness of unknown origins, where all lab tests are normal and a clear diagnosis cannot be made, traditional Chinese medicine is distinctly superior.

In cases of chronic immunodeficiency, even when confirmed with distinct symptoms (frequent and prolonged infections) and laboratory diagnosis (decreased white blood cells count), western medicine has no drug treatment available. Though there is one drug available for acute immunosuppression, it is only indicated for treatment of bone marrow suppression in cancer patients receiving chemotherapy and radiation. In other words, patients with compromised immune system have few or no options for drug treatments. On the other hand, traditional Chinese medicine is beneficial as it excels in maintainance and preventative therapies. Herbs can be used to regulate imbalances and alleviate associated signs and symptoms. In this case, many herbs have been shown via *in vitro* and *in vivo* studies to have remarkable effect to boost both specific and non-specific immune systems. Therefore, herbal therapy should definitely be employed to restore optimal health and prevent contraction of infections.

CASE STUDIES

M.M., a 31-year-old male patient, presented with chronic cough and allergies after hurricanes last year. The patient also worked in a bar that had mold damage. He was placed on a leave of absence from work to recover and then placed on antibiotics. Other findings included pale face, low voice, and dark circles under the eyes, blue nail beds, weakness and lack of motivation. Western diagnosis was compromised immune system with lingering pathogenic factors. The TCM diagnosis was Lung qi, Spleen qi and *wei* (defensive) *qi* deficiencies. *Immune* + was prescribed at 6 capsules twice daily. After taking the herbs, the patient reported he regained his strength and had gone back to work after 2 months of acupuncture and herbs. He caught another cold during the two-month treatment period but was able to recover quickly.

M.H., West Palm Beach, Florida

A 20-year-old female student presented with a history of recurrent viral or bacterial infection since starting college. Other objective findings included lack of sleep, high stress, strep throat, bladder infection, and susceptibility to the flu. She was diagnosed as having qi deficiency and a weakened immune system. Within six months of taking *Immune* +, her signs and symptoms decreased by 50%. The patient has noticed a marked decrease in recurrence of infection and sickness.

T.G., Albuquerque, New Mexico

A 66-year-old female reported repeated episodes of respiratory infection that turned into asthma and bronchitis. The patient reported that she had allergy shots from her medical doctor because she could not take different drugs as they would give her irregular heartbeat. She could not take *Ma Huang* (Herba Ephedrae) or any other stimulants. Her blood pressure was 110/78 mmHg and her heart rate was 66 beats per minute. The diagnosis according to traditional Chinese medicine was *wei* (defensive) qi deficiency. *Immune* + was prescribed and after three months of treatment, the patient reported significantly less attacks of asthma. She was also advised to eat more vegetables and decrease the intake of dairy and gluten products.

D.W., Los Angeles, California

A 36-year-old female presented with fatigue, anxiety and low immune function. She said she catches cold easily and frequently. Her pulse was weak and thready, and her tongue was purple. She was pale, with dark circles under her eyes. The TCM diagnosis was Lung and Kidney qi deficiencies. The patient was instructed to take *Immune* +. After 2 months of *Immune* + and acupuncture treatment (every other week), the patient has not fallen ill from contact with her family and friends. She said prior to the treatments, she "would always get sick from others."

M.B., Bend, Oregon

S.C., a 42-year-old female, was over-worked and under constant stress. She wanted to enhance her immune system, as her health was compromised by stress and exhaustion. She was prescribed *Immune* + at two capsules, three times daily. During seven months of taking the herbs, she had no illnesses or symptoms.

C.L., Chino Hills, California

S.W. suffered from tiredness, restless sleep, and occasional, recurrent nasal congestion during allergy season. She was diagnosed with Kidney yin, yang, and *wei* (defensive) *qi* deficiencies. **Immune** + along with **Vibrant** were prescribed. **Immune** + was prescribed to build the *wei* (defensive) *qi* while **Vibrant** was used to sustain and build her Kidney yin and yang over time. The patient greatly commented on the positive results from **Vibrant** to increase her daily energy level and positive outlook.

J.P., Naples, Florida

A 59-year-old male physician presented with extreme fever (over 104°F), extreme difficulty breathing, pain in the chest, shortness of breath aggravated by exertion, unsteady walk, dizziness, and inability to speak more than one word per breath. His tongue was pale with red tip and body, and his was rapid and superficial. The diagnosis was phlegm heat in the Lung. The patient was treated with **Poria XPT** (6 capsules four times daily) and **Immune** + (6 capsules four times daily), along with other homeopathics and drugs (Combivent (Albuterol/Ipratropium) and aspirin). The patient had a definite response to the herbs. The respiration became much easier, energy level and sense of vitality enhanced, and cough was no longer productive. The practitioner commented that "While all protocols employed resulted in benefit – it is without question that the herbal formulas generated imminent benefit and long term recuperation."

I.B.J., Miami, Florida.

A 54-year-old property manager presented with chronic sinus congestion and headache. Food allergies included E-95 panel to dairy, egg white, kidney beans and lima beans. The practitioner's diagnosis was Lung qi deficiency with excess damp. The patient stated that symptoms of sinus congestion and headaches would subside upon taking **Immune** +. Subsequently, he continued to use **Immune** + during allergy seasons, more in the fall, but as needed throughout the year.

Anonymous

[1] Chu, DT. et al. Immunotherapy with Chinese medicinal herbs. I. Immune restoration of local xenogenetic graft-versus-host reaction in cancer patients by fractionated astragalus membranaceus in vitro. *Journal of Clinical & Laboratory Immunology*. 25(3):119-23, Mar. 1988

[2] Sun, Y. et al. Immune restoration and/or augmentation of local graft versus host reaction by traditional Chinese medicinal herbs. *Cancer*. 52(1):70-3, July 1, 1983

[3] Sun, Y. et al. Preliminary observations on the effects of the Chinese medicinal herbs Astragalus membranaceus and Ganoderma lucidum on lymphocyte blastogenic responses. *Journal of Biological Response Mopdifiers*. 2(3):227-37, 1983

[4] Weng, XS. *Chung Juo Chung Hsia I Chieh Ho Tsa Chih*, August 1995

[5] Chu, DT. et al. Fractionated extract of astragalus membranaceus, a Chinese medicinal herb, potentiates LAK cell cytotoxicity generated by a low dose of recombinant interleukin-2. *Journal of Clinical & Laboratory Immunology*. 26(4):183-7, Aug. 1988

[6] Chu, DT. et al. Immunotherapy with Chinese medicinal herbs. II. Reversal of cyclophosphamide-induced immune suppression by administration of fractionated astragalus membranaceus in vivo. *Journal of Clinical & Laboratory Immunology*. 25(3):125-9, Mar. 1988

[7] Yeung, HC. *Handbook of Chinese Herbs*. Institute of Chinese Medicine. 1996

[8] Wang, SY. et al. The anti-tumor effect of ganoderma lucidum is mediated by cytokines released from activated macrophages and T-lymphocytes. *International Journal of Cancer*. 70(6):699-705, Mar 17, 1997

[9] Van der Hem, LG. et al. Ling Zhi-8: studies of a new immunomodulating agent. *Transplantation*. 60(5):438-43, Sep 15, 1995

[10] Haak-Frendscho, M. et al. Ling Zhi-8: a novel T-cell mitogen induces cytokine production and upregulation of ICAM-1 expression. *Cellular Immunology*. 150(1):101-13, Aug. 1993

[11] Tanaka, S. et al. Complete amino acid sequence of a novel immunomodulatory protein, ling zhi-9. An immuno-modulator from a fungus, ganoderma lucidum, having similar effect to immunoglobulin variable regions.

[12] Kuo, YC. et al. Growth inhibitors against tumor cells in Cordyceps sinensis other than cordycepin and polysaccharides. *Cancer Investigation*. 12(6):611-5,1994.

[13] Chen, YJ. et al. Effect of Cordyceps sinensis on the proliferation and differentiation of human leukemic U937 cells. *Life Sciences*. 60(25):2349-59, 1997

[14] Kuo, YC. et al. Cordyceps sinensis as an immunomodulatory agent. *American Journal of Chinese Medicine*. 24(2):111-25, 1996

[15] Guan, YJ. et al. Effect of Cordyceps sinensis on T-lymphocyte subsets in chronic renal failure. *Chung-Kuo Chung His I Chieh Ho Tsa Chih*. 12(6):338-9,323, Jun. 1992

[16] Liu, C. et al. Effects of Cordyceps sinensis (CS) on in vitro natural killer cells. *Chung-Kuo Chung His I Chieh Ho Tsa Chih*. 12(5):267-9,259, May, 1992

[17] Xu, RH. et al. Effects of cordyceps sinensis on natural killer activity and colony formation of B16 melanoma. *Chinese Medical Journal*. 105(2):97-101, Feb. 1992

FORMULAS

IMMUNE + ™

[18] Liu, P. et al. Influence of Cordyceps sinensis (Berk.) Sacc. and rat serum containing same medicine on IL-1, IFN and TNF produced by rat Kupffer's cells *Chung Kuo Chung Yao Tsa Chih*; 21(6):367-9, 384, Jun 1996
[19] Takeda, S. et al. *Nippon Yakurigaku Zasshi*. 88(4): 321-30. 1986
[20] Chevallier, A. *Encyclopedia of Medicinal Plants*. New York, NY: DK Publishing. 1996
[21] Chevallier, A. *Encyclopedia of Medicinal Plants*. New York, NY: DK Publishing. 1996

IMPERIAL TONIC ™

CLINICAL APPLICATIONS

- Chronic fatigue syndrome: constant tiredness, low energy, lack of interest, etc.
- General tonic: increases both mental and physical functions, enhances academic and sports performance
- Recovery enhancement: speeds up recovery from any event that contributes to mental or physical exhaustion, such as surgery, severe illness, childbirth, etc.
- Anemia with dizziness, fatigue, lack of energy or poor appetite
- Anti-aging: enhances longevity, promotes general wellness and increases energy level

WESTERN THERAPEUTIC ACTIONS

- Adaptogenic function to enhance both mental and physical functions [5]
- Enhances basal metabolic rate and increases the overall energy level [6]
- Boosts the immune system, increases the number of white blood cells [1,2,3,4,7]
- Treats anemia by increasing the number and function of red blood cells

CHINESE THERAPEUTIC ACTIONS

- Tonifies qi, blood, yin and yang
- Strengthens the overall constitution of the body

DOSAGE

The dosage for long-term administration is 2 to 4 capsules three times daily. The dosage may be increased up to 5 to 6 capsules three times daily for short-term use, for its adaptogenic effect or recovery enhancement.

INGREDIENTS

Bai Shao (Radix Paeoniae Alba)
Bai Zhu (Rhizoma Atractylodis Macrocephalae)
Chuan Xiong (Rhizoma Ligustici Chuanxiong)
Da Zao (Fructus Jujubae)
Dang Gui (Radicis Angelicae Sinensis)
Fu Ling (Poria)
Gui Xin (Cortex Rasus Cinnamomi)

Huang Qi (Radix Astragali)
Shan Yao (Rhizoma Dioscoreae)
Sheng Jiang (Rhizoma Zingiberis Recens)
Shu Di Huang (Radix Rehmanniae Preparata)
Wu Wei Zi (Fructus Schisandrae Chinensis)
Xi Yang Shen (Radix Panacis Quinquefolii)
Zhi Gan Cao (Radix Glycyrrhizae Preparata)

FORMULA EXPLANATION

Imperial Tonic is one of the most comprehensive and most effective herbal formulas. It treats both specific and general constitutional disorders. *Imperial Tonic* contains herbs that tonify yin, yang, qi and blood. Clinically, it can be used to treat chronic fatigue syndrome, anemia, post-surgical recovery, postpartum recovery, and many other conditions. It can also be used in healthy individuals to increase mental and physical functions, improve academic and sports performances, enhance longevity, and promote general wellness.

Huang Qi (Radix Astragali) strengthens the immune system and *Xi Yang Shen* (Radix Panacis Quinquefolii) tonifies the *yuan* (source) *qi* of the body. *Bai Zhu* (Rhizoma Atractylodis Macrocephalae) and *Fu Ling* (Poria) strengthen the Spleen and promote absorption of nutrients from food. They work together to strengthen qi and the immune system. *Shu Di Huang* (Radix Rehmanniae Preparata) tonifies the Liver and Kidney yin. *Dang Gui* (Radicis Angelicae Sinensis), *Bai Shao* (Radix Paeoniae Alba), and *Chuan Xiong* (Rhizoma Ligustici Chuanxiong) nourish and

FORMULAS

IMPERIAL TONIC ™

invigorate the blood. *Shan Yao* (Rhizoma Dioscoreae) tonifies the Spleen, the Lung, and the Kidney. *Gui Xin* (Cortex Rasus Cinnamomi) tonifies Kidney yang. *Wu Wei Zi* (Fructus Schisandrae Chinensis) has astringent and binding effects to prevent leakage of *jing* (essence). *Zhi Gan Cao* (Radix Glycyrrhizae Preparata), *Sheng Jiang* (Rhizoma Zingiberis Recens), and *Da Zao* (Fructus Jujubae) harmonize the gastrointestinal tract.

SUPPLEMENTARY FORMULAS

- ❧ To boost energy and awareness, use *Vibrant*.
- ❧ To increase immunity, use *Immune +*.
- ❧ For brittle, dry hair or scalp, or hair loss, combine with *Polygonum 14*.
- ❧ For decreased sexual activity, low sex drive, and other sexual dysfunction in men and women, use *Vitality*.
- ❧ For insomnia and anemia, combine with *Schisandra ZZZ*.
- ❧ For menopause with hot flashes, mood swings, and excessive perspiration, combine *Balance (Heat)* with *Nourish*.
- ❧ For supportive cancer therapy and to decrease the side effects of chemotherapy including nausea, vomiting, poor appetite, and fatigue, use with *C/R Support*.
- ❧ For supportive therapy in patients with cancer who are too weak to receive chemotherapy or radiation, add *CA Support*.
- ❧ *Cordyceps 3* can be added to enhance the overall anti-aging effect.
- ❧ To enhance memory, add *Enhance Memory*.
- ❧ To prevent osteoporosis, add *Osteo 8*.
- ❧ To increase the shape and size of breasts, or to increase libido, use with *Venus*.
- ❧ To strengthen the Spleen and the Stomach, add *GI Tonic*.
- ❧ For stress and anxiety, add *Calm*.
- ❧ For stress, anxiety and insomnia with underlying deficiency, add *Calm ZZZ*.
- ❧ For severe stress and anxiety, add *Calm ES*.
- ❧ For Kidney yang deficiency, add *Kidney Tonic (Yang)*.
- ❧ For Kidney yin deficiency, add *Kidney Tonic (Yin)*.
- ❧ For male infertility, add *Vital Essence*.
- ❧ For female infertility, add *Blossom (Phase 1-4)*.

NUTRITION

- ❧ Increase the consumption of fresh fruits, vegetables, grains, seeds and nuts.
- ❧ Eat more fish and fish oils, onions, garlic, olives, olive oil, herbs, spices, soy products, tofu, yogurt, and fiber.
- ❧ Sea vegetables, such as kelp and seaweeds, replenish the body with minerals like magnesium, potassium, calcium, iodine and iron.
- ❧ Ensure adequate intake of vitamin B complex to process and utilize energy.
- ❧ Decrease intake of red meat, alcohol, fats, caffeine, and highly processed foods.
- ❧ Avoid the use of stimulants, such as coffee, caffeine, and high-sugar products.
- ❧ Food allergies or chemical hypersensitivity can drain energy and cause fatigue. Tests should be done to confirm or rule out allergy and/or hypersensitivity.

The Tao of Nutrition by Ni and McNease
- ❧ Chronic fatigue syndrome
  - ▪ Recommendations: winter melon, pumpkin, pumpkin seed, yam, sweet potato, lima bean, black bean, soy bean, strawberry, watermelon, pineapple, chestnut, papaya, figs, garlic, onions, and pearl barley.

IMPERIAL TONIC ™

- Avoid dairy products, alcohol, coffee, sugar, fatty or fried foods, overly spicy foods, cold and raw foods, tomato, eggplant, bell pepper, and shellfish.
- For more information, please refer to *The Tao of Nutrition* by Dr. Maoshing Ni and Cathy McNease.

LIFESTYLE INSTRUCTIONS

- Regular exercise and adequate rest are essential to optimal health.
- Take a hot bath for about 20 minutes prior to bedtime to relax. Sea salt or Epsom salt can be added to the bath water.
- Engage in activities such as *Tai Chi Chuan*, walking, or meditation that allow calmness of mind without creating stagnation or excessive fatigue.
- Avoid exposure to heavy metal, such as lead, cadmium, aluminum, copper and arsenic, which can all suppress the immune system and cause fatigue.

CLINICAL NOTES

- *Imperial Tonic* is an excellent postpartum tonic. Women lose a tremendous amount of *jing* (essence) and blood after labor. The concept of replenishing the Kidney *jing* (essence) is not prevalent in the West. As a result, many women age faster than they should and suffer from low back pain or symptoms of Kidney yin or *jing* (essence) deficiency later in their lives. This is a great formula to use for one month starting one or two weeks after delivery. It helps to replenish qi, blood, yin and yang that were lost due to labor. It is commonly taken for a month after labor.
- Important Note: Before tonifying with *Imperial Tonic*, *Traumanex* should be used for 3 to 5 days (3 days for natural birth, 5 days for Cesarean) to clear out residual blood stagnation and to relieve pain. This will prevent future gynecological complications due to blood stagnation in the pelvis. *Herbal ABX* can also be used if there is infection present.

Pulse Diagnosis by Dr. Jimmy Wei-Yen Chang:
- Weak on all three positions on both hands.
- Note: Dr. Chang takes the pulse in slightly different positions. He places his index finger directly over the wrist crease, and his middle and ring fingers alongside to locate *cun*, *guan* and *chi* positions. For additional information and explanation, please refer to *Pulsynergy* by Dr. Jimmy Wei-Yen Chang and Marcus Brinkman.

CAUTIONS

- This formula is contraindicated in patients who are on immune suppressant drugs (i.e. cyclosporin) after receiving an organ transplant. *Imperial Tonic* contains many herbs that enhance both specific and non-specific immunity and may increase the risk of organ rejection.
- Patients who are on anticoagulant or antiplatelet therapies, such as Coumadin (Warfarin), should use this formula with caution as there may be a slightly higher risk of bleeding and bruising.
- *Imperial Tonic* is safe for long-term use. However, because it is a warm formula, it should be reduced in dosage or discontinued if it causes side effects characterized by heat, such as dry mouth, thirst, nosebleeds, and others.
- This formula is contraindicated in cases of infection, inflammation, and other excess conditions.

ACUPUNCTURE POINTS

Traditional Points:
- *Zusanli* (ST 36), *Guanyuan* (CV 4), *Qihai* (CV 6), *Mingmen* (GV 4), and *Shenshu* (BL 23).
- *Qihai* (CV 6), *Zhongwan* (CV 12), *Neiguan* (PC 6), *Gongsun* (SP 4), *Zusanli* (ST 36), and *Geshu* (BL 17).

IMPERIAL TONIC ™

Balance Method by Dr. Richard Tan:

- Left side: *Hegu* (LI 4), *Zusanli* (ST 36), *Taixi* (KI 3), and *Yinlingquan* (SP 9).
- Right side: *Lieque* (LU 7), *Tongli* (HT 5), and *Zusanli* (ST 36).
- Left and right side can be alternated from treatment to treatment.
- For additional information on the Balance Method, please refer to *Dr. Tan's Strategy of Twelve Magical Points* by Dr. Richard Tan.

Auricular Acupuncture by Dr. Li-Chun Huang:

- Fatigue: Sympathetic, Kidney, Liver, Spleen, Speed Recovered Fatigue, *San Jiao*, Anxious, Nervous Subcortex, and Thyroid. Bleed Ear Apex.
- For additional information on the location and explanation of these points, please refer to *Auricular Treatment Formula and Prescriptions* by Dr. Li-Chun Huang.

MODERN RESEARCH

Imperial Tonic is an herbal formula specifically designed to treat chronic degenerative illnesses. It contains herbs with adaptogenic functions to enhance both mental and physical performances. It boosts energy levels and increases the basal metabolic rate. It enhances the immune system to strengthen both specific and non-specific immunity.

Huang Qi (Radix Astragali) is one of the most frequently used Chinese herbs and has historically been used for its function to tonify the *wei* (defensive) *qi*. In terms of Western medicine, studies have shown repeatedly that *Huang Qi* (Radix Astragali) increases both specific and non-specific immunity.[1,2,3] In one clinical study with 115 leucopenic patients, it was found that the use of *Huang Qi* (Radix Astragali) is associated with an "obvious rise of the white blood cell (WBC) count" in a dose-dependent relationship.[4]

Xi Yang Shen (Radix Panacis Quinquefolii), also known as American ginseng, is perhaps the most recognized herb in the herbal health care market. Common applications of this herb include a general strengthening effect, adaptogenic effects against stress, and enhancement of both mental and physical performance.[5] The general strengthening or adaptogenic effects include a general increase in resistance to the noxious effects of physical, chemical or biological stress.[6] *Xi Yang Shen* (Radix Panacis Quinquefolii) may also enhance both mental and physical performance as demonstrated by human and animal studies. These studies illustrated that *Xi Yang Shen* (Radix Panacis Quinquefolii) can prevent stress-induced ulcers, stimulate the proliferation of liver cells, increase natural killer cell activities, and enhance the secretion of interferons.[7]

Shu Di Huang (Radix Rehmanniae Preparata), *Dang Gui* (Radicis Angelicae Sinensis), *Bai Shao* (Radix Paeoniae Alba), and *Chuan Xiong* (Rhizoma Ligustici Chuanxiong) are four herbs commonly used together to tonify blood. Clinical applications of these herbs include anemia with weakness, dizziness, blurred vision, and lusterless complexion of the skin and nails.[8]

Wu Wei Zi (Fructus Schisandrae Chinensis) has a wide range of functions and clinical applications. In addition to its classical function as a general tonic, it is also used to protect the liver, regulate the nervous system and the digestive tract, and enhance the body's ability to adapt to stress. *Wu Wei Zi* (Fructus Schisandrae Chinensis) possesses pronounced liver-protectant effect by increasing blood flow to the liver and increasing regeneration of liver cells.[9] It stimulates the nervous system to increase reflex responses, improve mental alertness, and treat memory loss.[10] In addition, it helps the body adapt to stress by balancing body fluids, improving sexual stamina, and improving failing senses.[10]

IMPERIAL TONIC ™

PHARMACEUTICAL DRUGS & CHINESE MEDICINE: A COMPARATIVE ANALYSIS

One striking difference between western and traditional Chinese medicine is that western medicine focuses and excels in crisis management, while traditional Chinese medicine emphasizes and shines in holistic and preventative treatments. Therefore, in emergencies, such as gun shot wounds or surgery, western medicine is generally the treatment of choice. However, for treatment of chronic idiopathic illness of unknown origins, where all lab tests are normal and a clear diagnosis cannot be made, traditional Chinese medicine is distinctly superior.

In cases of chronic energetic disorders, where all tests are normal but there are still general and non-diagnostic signs and symptoms, western medicine offers few treatment options since there is not a clear diagnosis. On the other hand, traditional Chinese medicine is beneficial as it excels in maintainance and preventative therapies. Herbs can be used to regulate imbalances and alleviate associated signs and symptoms. Therefore, herbal therapy should definitely be employed to prevent deterioration and to restore optimal health.

CASE STUDIES

A tired and exhausted patient presented with general aches and pain in the neck and low back. There was also a history of poor sleep and digestion with no constipation. The practitioner felt the patient had over-worked herself throughout the years and that the condition was due to "wear and tear." The diagnosis was qi and blood deficiencies with underlying yin and yang deficiencies. *Imperial Tonic, Schisandra ZZZ* and *Bu Zhong Yi Qi Tang* (Tonify the Middle and Augment the Qi Decoction) were given along with acupuncture and massage therapy. The treatment was concluded to be quite effective.

S.C., La Crescenta, California

A 44-year-old female with hepatitis C, necrosis of the liver, and diabetes (insulin-dependent) was treated with interferon, Rebetron (Ribavirin and Interferon alpha 2B), Zantac (Ranitidine), Prozac (Fluoxetine) and insulin. Her clinical manifestations included pain in the liver region, fatigue, insomnia, blurred vision, constipation, melancholy, frontal headache, dizziness, tremors, abdominal bloating, and a pale complexion. Her tongue was maroon in color, and the pulse was slippery. The diagnosis for this patient was dampness in the Liver and Gallbladder, with Liver overacting on the Spleen and the Stomach, hence disrupting the transformation and transportation of the digestive system. The patient was treated with two herbal formulas (*Liver DTX* and *Imperial Tonic*) and two homeopathic formulas (sarcode liver formula and oral insulin). The treatment also included acupuncture involving meridian treatment and extraordinary vessel treatment. After three weeks, the patient had significant improvements in her vitality, complexion, appetite, sleep, attitude and energy level. A dramatic reduction of her abdominal pain was also noted. Her insulin use was reduced by approximately 25%.

I.B., Miami, Florida

A 35-year-old female complained of the following symptoms: bedwetting, fatigue, low back pain, abdominal pain, loss of appetite and depression. The doctor diagnosed her with Kidney *jing* (essence), yin and yang deficiencies. *Imperial Tonic* and *Vibrant* were prescribed. The patient reported that bedwetting, depression and pain went away and the energy level went from 2 to 10. As an added and unexpected joy for her, the patient stated she also lost 10 pounds even though she had been eating more.

S.C., Santa Monica, California

R.D., a 54-year-old male patient, presented with the complaints of always being sick for long periods of time, always cold, weak and tired. Western diagnosis was chronic fatigue syndrome and immune dysfunction. His blood pressure was 110/70 mmHg and his heart rate was 66 beats per minute. The diagnosis was yang and qi deficiencies. *Imperial Tonic* was prescribed at 2 grams three times a day. After taking the herbs, the patient reported that he first

FORMULAS

began to feel more energy and a better sense of well being. He also noticed that he wasn't as sick as often and it did not last as long as before. The patient also received acupuncture treatment. The result of both the herbs and the acupuncture was evident within a few weeks.

W.F., Bloomfield, New Jersey

A 44-year-old, 215-pound male patient presented with excessive night sweats to the point he had to change his clothes twice every night. His blood pressure was 115/78 mmHg and his heart rate was 70 beats per minute. The patient also complained of pain in the big toe. The diagnosis was *wei* (defensive) *qi* and Lung qi deficiencies. *Sheng Mai San* (Generate the Pulse Powder) and ***Imperial Tonic*** were prescribed and the sweating stopped after using half a bottle of each formula.

H.K.C., Studio City, California

M.M., a 41-year-old female, complained of fatigue, malaise, cognitive problems, headache, slightly blurred vision, irritable bowel syndrome, muscle pain and constipation. The Western diagnosis was chronic fatigue syndrome; the TCM diagnosis was qi, blood and yin deficiencies. ***Imperial Tonic*** was prescribed, two capsules, three times daily. She took the herbs for nine weeks, and noted continual improvement, a significant decrease of fatigue and malaise, and an overall good constitution.

C.L., Chino Hills, California

---

[1] Chu, DT. et al. Immunotherapy with Chinese medicinal herbs: immune restoration of local xenogenetic graft-versus-host reaction in cancer patients by fractionated astragalus membranaceus in vitro. *Journal of Clinical & Laboratory Immunology*. 25(3):119-23, Mar. 1988
[2] Sun, Y. et al. Immune restoration and/or augmentation of local graft versus host reaction by traditional Chinese medicinal herbs. *Cancer*. 52(1):70-3, July 1, 1983
[3] Sun, Y. et al. Preliminary observations on the effects of the Chinese medicinal herbs astragalus membranaceus and Ganoderma lucidum on lymphocyte blastogenic responses. *Journal of Biological Response Modifiers*. 2(3):227-37, 1983
[4] Weng, XS. *Chung Juo Chung Hsia. I Chieh Ho Tsa Chih*. August 1995
[5] Olin, B, et al. Ginseng. *The Lawrence Review of Natural Products by Facts and Comparison*. Sep 1990
[6] Brekhman, II. *Dardymov IV*, Lloydia 32:46, 1969
[7] Singh, VK. et al. *Planta Medica* 50:462, 1984
[8] Bensky, D. et al. *Chinese Herbal Medicine Formulas & Strategies*. Eastland Press. 1990
[9] Takeda, S. et al. *Nippon Yakurigaku Zasshi*. 88(4): 321-30. 1986
[10] Chevallier, A. *Encyclopedia of Medicinal Plants*. New York, NY: DK Publishing. 1996

FORMULAS

KIDNEY DTX ™

(Detoxification)

CLINICAL APPLICATIONS

- Chronic nephritis
- Chronic nephrotic syndrome
- Proteinuria
- Kidney disease with such symptoms as edema, soreness of the lower back, fatigue, emaciation, flabby tongue, greasy tongue coating, deep, thready or wiry pulse.
- This formula is *not* recommended for acute kidney disorders.

WESTERN THERAPEUTIC ACTIONS

- Restores the normal filtration and excretion functions of the kidney [1,2,3,4,5,6,7]
- Reduces the presence of protein in the urine [1,5]
- Regulates water circulation to eliminate edema [8,9,10]

CHINESE THERAPEUTIC ACTIONS

- Dispels dampness
- Tonifies Kidney yin
- Tonifies qi

DOSAGE

Take 3 to 4 capsules three times daily with warm water. For maximum effectiveness, take the herbs on an empty stomach. This formula is safe for long-term use.

INGREDIENTS

Bai Mao Gen (Rhizoma Imperatae)
Du Zhong (Cortex Eucommiae)
Fu Ling (Poria)
Huang Bai (Cortex Phellodendri)
Huang Qi (Radix Astragali)

Jin Ying Zi (Fructus Rosae Laevigatae)
Lu Han Cao (Herba Pyrolae)
Mu Li (Concha Ostreae)
Shan Zhu Yu (Fructus Corni)
Shi Wei (Folium Pyrrosiae)

FORMULA EXPLANATION

Chronic nephritis or chronic nephrotic syndrome in traditional Chinese medicine is considered a complicated disease as it involves both excess and deficiency. The excess refers to the clinical manifestation of the illness, which is the accumulation of dampness and turbidity in the lower *jiao*. The deficiency refers to the underlying cause, which are Kidney qi and yin deficiencies. Most patients are extremely Kidney deficient. Since Kidney is the organ that stores *jing* (essence), deficiency of the Kidney leads to its inability to retain the *jing* (essence). As a result, the *jing* (essence) is leaked out from the body in the form of serum protein, albumin, immunoglobulins, red blood cells, blood and trace minerals.

To treat patients with chronic nephritis or nephrotic syndrome, **Kidney DTX** uses herbs to tonify the deficiency and drain the excess. *Huang Qi* (Radix Astragali) tonifies qi and regulates water metabolism in the body to reduce edema. *Shan Zhu Yu* (Fructus Corni) is sour, which consolidates Kidney *jing* (essence). It also has an excellent effect to tonify Kidney yin and *jing* (essence). *Du Zhong* (Cortex Eucommiae) tonifies the Kidney yang and strengthens the back to relieve soreness. *Shi Wei* (Folium Pyrrosiae) dispels dampness and stops bleeding in the urine. *Lu Han*

FORMULAS

KIDNEY DTX ™

(Detoxification)

Cao (Herba Pyrolae) further helps to stop bleeding. *Huang Bai* (Cortex Phellodendri) clears deficiency heat from the Kidney and reduces chronic inflammation. *Fu Ling* (Poria) and *Bai Mao Gen* (Rhizoma Imperatae) dispel dampness and promote urination to relieve edema. *Bai Mao Gen* (Rhizoma Imperatae) is frequently used for *lin zheng* (dysuria syndrome) to relieve blood in the urine. *Fu Ling* (Poria) and *Bai Mao Gen* (Rhizoma Imperatae) also help *Huang Bai* (Cortex Phellodendri) to clear damp-heat in the lower *jiao* to dispel creatinine and blood urea nitrogen in the blood. *Mu Li* (Concha Ostreae) and *Jin Ying Zi* (Fructus Rosae Laevigatae) are astringent herbs used to prevent loss of Kidney *jing* (essence) through the urine. They also help to keep protein in the body and prevent the loss of protein and red blood cells through urine.

Kidney DTX is an excellent formula to treat kidney disorder because it tonifies without causing stagnation and sedates without injuring the body's constitution. Furthermore, it contains herbs to treat the cause and the symptoms of the illness, thereby offering both immediate and long-term therapeutic benefits.

SUPPLEMENTARY FORMULAS

- For accumulation of environmental pollutant, chemical compounds, and other toxins in the body, add *Herbal DTX*.
- For edema and water accumulation, add *Herbal DRX*.
- For unknown cause of symptoms with blood stagnation in patients with excess condition, add *Circulation (SJ)*.
- For excess fire in the body, add *Gardenia Complex*.
- For *wei* (defensive) *qi* deficiency and frequent infections, add *Immune +*.
- For dry mouth, deficiency heat symptoms, tinnitus or dizziness, add *Nourish* or *Nourish (Fluids)*.
- For Kidney yang deficiency with frequent urination especially at night, soreness, weakness and coldness of the lower back and knees, add *Kidney Tonic (Yang)*.
- For Spleen qi deficiency with poor appetite, add *GI Tonic*.
- For high blood pressure, add *Gastrodia Complex*.
- To reduce cholesterol, *Cholisma* or *Cholisma (ES)* can be added.
- For fever, headache, nausea, add *Herbal ABX*.
- With compromised liver function, add *Liver DTX*.
- With bleeding, add *Notoginseng 9*.

NUTRITION

- Intake of salt should be restricted to 1 to 2 grams per day, as excessive presence of salt will increase the severity of edema.
- Diet with restricted protein is recommended to reduce proteinuria and lower the stress on the kidneys. A high protein diet is discouraged since it accelerates the deterioration of kidney disease by increasing the intraglomerular pressure and urinary protein excretion.
- Vitamin D supplementation is encouraged in patients with clinical or biochemical evidence of vitamin D deficiency.
- Lotus nodes are recommended to be included in the diet.
- Avoid smoking and drinking. Do not eat sour and spicy foods.

The Tao of Nutrition by Ni and McNease
- Nephritis (acute)
  - Recommendations: black beans, mung beans, azuki beans, pearl barley, garlic, carp, winter melon, watermelon, watermelon rind, corn-silk, sweet rice, lotus root, and water chestnuts.
  - Avoid stimulating (sour, spicy, salty) foods, alcohol, caffeine, smoking, overworking, and high protein foods.

KIDNEY DTX ™

(Detoxification)

- Nephritis (chronic)
  - Recommendations: ginger, Chinese black dates, sweet rice, soybeans, winter melon, carp, yams, mung beans, and black beans.
  - Avoid stimulating (sour, spicy, salty) foods, alcohol, caffeine, smoking, overworking, and high protein foods.
- For more information, please refer to *The Tao of Nutrition* by Dr. Maoshing Ni and Cathy McNease.

LIFESTYLE INSTRUCTIONS

- Adequate rest is essential to recovery. Strenuous exercise increases the stress of the kidneys and accelerates their deterioration.
- To minimize stress on the kidneys, encourage elimination of toxins through lung, skin and bowel. Practice breathing exercises, ensure regular bowel movements, and take hot baths.

CLINICAL NOTES

- To effectively treat kidney disorder, it is extremely important to identify and eliminate the cause(s). It is important to make sure disease conditions that are known to increase the risk and acceleration of kidney disorders are well controlled, such as diabetes and lupus. Furthermore, certain drugs, toxins and heavy metals are known to cause kidney damage, and must be avoided as well. Examples of drugs include certain antibiotics, analgesics, and anti-epileptics. Examples of environmental toxins include chemical solvents, biological agents, herbicides and pesticides. Examples of heavy metals include lead and cadmium. Avoidance of such factors will significantly improve both short- and long-term prognosis.
- Though the use of herbs can treat kidney disorders and restore the normal kidney functions, this formula is **not** recommended for acute renal diseases.
- It is prudent to monitor progress objectively with urine analysis. Such laboratory tests will confirm the effectiveness of the treatment and assist in the long-term treatment strategy.

CAUTIONS

- *Kidney DTX* is **not** suitable for acute nephritis. Such conditions should be referred to a medical doctor for immediate treatment.
- This formula is contraindicated during pregnancy and nursing.

ACUPUNCTURE POINTS

Traditional Points:
- *Sanyinjiao* (SP 6), *Zhigou* (TH 6), *Shuifen* (CV 9), *Guanyuan* (CV 4), *Feishu* (BL 13), *Hegu* (LI 4), *Zhongji* (CV 3), *Yinlingquan* (SP 9), and *Zusanli* (ST 36).

Balance Method:
- Left side: *Shenmen* (HT 7), *Lingdao* (HT 4), *Chize* (LU 5), *Feiyang* (BL 58), and *Weizhong* (BL 40).
- Right side: *Zhubin* (KI 9), *Yingu* (KI 10), *Taichong* (LR 3), *Sanyangluo* (TH 8), Kidney point on the ear, and *Lingku*.
- Left and right side can be alternated from treatment to treatment.
- Note: *Lingku* is one of Master Tong's points on both hands. *Lingku* is located in the depression just distal to the junction of the first and second metacarpal bones, approximately 0.5 *cun* proximal to *Hegu* (LI 4), on the *yangming* line.

KIDNEY DTX ™

(Detoxification)

❧ For additional information on the Balance Method, please refer to *Twelve and Twelve in Acupuncture* and *Twenty-Four More in Acupuncture* by Dr. Richard Tan.

Ear Points:
❧ Kidney and surrounding tender points. Leave needles in for four to six hours. Needle once a day for seven days. Stop all diuretic medications while under ear acupuncture therapy.

Auricular Acupuncture by Dr. Li-Chun Huang:
❧ Nephritis: Points selection: Kidney, Nephritis Point, Endocrine, Adrenal Gland, Sympathetic, Spleen, San Jiao, Allergic Area, and Coronary Vascular Subcortex. Bleed Ear Apex.
❧ Pyelonephritis: Points selection: Kidney, Bladder, Urethra, Spleen, Sanjiao, Adrenal Gland, Endocrine, Allergic Area; bleed Ear Apex
❧ For additional information on the location and explanation of these points, please refer to *Auricular Treatment Formula and Prescriptions* by Dr. Li-Chun Huang.

MODERN RESEARCH

Kidney DTX is a carefully crafted formula that treats chronic and generalized kidney disorders in which the filtering and excretion functions are compromised. Compromised kidney function is often evident with the presence of protein, blood cells, and fat in the urine. In addition, chronic nephritis or chronic nephrotic syndrome will also cause edema, especially in the lower parts of the body. The causes for such kidney disorders vary and may include conditions such as diabetes, lupus, use of certain drugs, exposure to certain toxins, and chronic heavy metal poisoning. Therefore, optimal treatment requires comprehensive herbal therapy with appropriate adjustments in both lifestyle and dietary habits.

Kidney DTX is a comprehensive formula with many herbs that address all aspects of chronic and generalized kidney disorders. Herbs in *Kidney DTX* have been shown to restore normal functions of the kidneys, reduce protein in the urine, promote normal urination, and eliminate edema.

Huang Qi (Radix Astragali) is used as the main herb in this formula, as it has a remarkable effect to treat kidney related disorders, such as proteinuria and nephritis. According to one study, the oral use of *Huang Qi* (Radix Astragali) was found to decrease the amount of protein present in urine.[1] Furthermore, clinical studies have also shown that *Huang Qi* (Radix Astragali) is effective in treating nephritis and glomerulonephritis by increasing the volume of urine and elimination of chloride and ammonia.[2,3] In one clinical trial, use of *Huang Qi* (Radix Astragali) twice daily for 15 to 90 days was effective in treating 16 out of 20 patients with nephritis. Most patients also reported symptomatic improvement as well as a decrease of protein in the urine.[4] Furthermore, in another clinical study with 56 patients with chronic glomerulonephritis, use of *Huang Qi* (Radix Astragali) by intramuscular injection for one month had a 61.7% effective rate in improving the function of the kidneys and reducing the amount of protein in the urine.[5] All these clinical results clearly indicate that the use of *Huang Qi* (Radix Astragali) is effective in treating kidney disorders.

In addition to *Huang Qi* (Radix Astragali), *Bai Mao Gen* (Rhizoma Imperatae) and *Lu Han Cao* (Herba Pyrolae) also have excellent effects in treating general kidney disorders. According to one clinical trial, 11 children with acute nephritis were treated with an herbal decoction of *Bai Mao Gen* (Rhizoma Imperatae) for 32 to 59 doses with marked reduction in edema, lowered blood pressure, absence of protein and blood cells in the urine, and normalization of urine. Out of 11 patients who participated in the clinical trial, there was complete recovery in 9 patients and moderate improvement in 2 patients.[6] Furthermore, in one other study, it was found that the combination of *Huang Qi* (Radix Astragali) and *Lu Han Cao* (Herba Pyrolae) was effective in preventing drug-induced kidney and ear damages.[7]

KIDNEY DTX ™

(Detoxification)

Kidney DTX also employs herbs with marked diuretic effect since edema is a common complication of kidney disorder. *Bai Mao Gen* (Rhizoma Imperatae) has been shown to have a marked diuretic effect, especially if taken continuously for 5 to 10 days.[8] *Fu Ling* (Poria) also has a marked diuretic effect by increasing the urine output.[9] In one clinical study, 30 patients with edema were treated with a preparation of *Fu Ling* (Poria) three times daily for 7 days, with marked effectiveness in 23 cases and moderate effects in 7 cases.[10]

In summary, *Kidney DTX* is formulated with many herbs that have a marked effects to treat kidney disorders, such as chronic nephritis and chronic nephrotic syndrome. These herbs have been shown to regulate water circulation, eliminate edema, reduce the presence of protein in the urine, and restore the normal filtration and excretion function of the kidney.

PHARMACEUTICAL DRUGS & CHINESE MEDICINE: A COMPARATIVE ANALYSIS

Western Medical Approach: Kidney diseases, such as nephritis, nephrotic syndrome and kidney failure, are serious and extremely complicated diseases. There are many potential causes of kidney diseases, and therefore, treatments vary depending on the exact etiology and prognosis. If the conditions continue to deteriorate, kidney dialysis, and eventually kidney transplant may become necessary. Kidney dialysis and transplant are generally considered to be the last options, but they do prolong life and offer additional hope.

Traditional Chinese Medicine Approach: Treatment of kidney diseases is also a very challenging and complicated matter. However, many herbs have been shown to have marked effect to relieve stress for the kidney by promoting elimination of water and other unwanted substances. Furthermore, certain herbs have been shown to restore normal functions of the kidney, thereby offering hope of a life free from kidney dialysis and kidney transplant. However, herbs are generally only effective for early- to mid-stage of kidney diseases, and only for those with mild to moderate severity. Furthermore, herbs are more suitable for chronic kidney diseases, and not recommended for acute kidney failure. Nonetheless, for patient on kidney dialysis who have no options other than kidney transplant, use of herbal therapy offer one additional hope and option.

Summation: Kidney diseases are very challenging for both western and traditional Chinese medicine. Both drugs and herbs offer hope to reverse the illness, especially in early stages of kidney diseases with mild to moderate severity. If the patient is already on kidney dialysis, it may still be worthwhile to explore herbal therapy, as there is a small possibility of recovery. When all else fail, kidney transplant is the final option.

CASE STUDIES

A 40-year-old female presented with slow mental functions. She answered questions slowly, and reported hot flashes, acid reflux after eating spicy foods, and a history of alcoholism and smoking. Objective findings revealed that her ankles were slightly swollen. The TCM diagnosis was toxic damp-heat accumulation with yin deficiency. *Herbal DTX* was prescribed for one month with *Wu Pi Yin* (Five-Peel Decoction) and *Jia Wei Xiao Yao San* (Augmented Rambling Powder). After one month, the swelling in her legs was down and the woman felt less brain fog. She wanted to drink more water and less alcohol. After six months of herbal, acupuncture and homeopathic treatment, she felt better all around.

M.C., Sarasota, Florida

A 51-years-old male had chronic recurrent nephritis for 6 years. In the past 6 months, the patient reported frequent urination at night (4 to 5 times), soreness and pain of the lower back, tinnitus in both ears, fatigue, pale red and flabby tongue with teethmarks, white greasy tongue coat, and deep thready pulse. Objective tests confirmed the presence of protein (++) in the urine. The patient was diagnosed as qi and yin deficiencies of the Kidney with accumulation of dampness. After 50 days of herbal treatment, the patient reported a reduction of urination at night

FORMULAS

KIDNEY DTX ™

(Detoxification)

from 4 to 5 times down to 1 to 2 times, improvement of low back pain, reduction of tinnitus in the ears, and increased energy levels. Furthermore, urine analysis was negative for protein in three consecutive tests. The treatment was concluded to be effective.

W.J., Zhejiang, China

[1] *Chinese Convention on Biophysiology, 2nd Annual Convention,* 1963; 63
[2] *Zhong Hua Nei Ke Xue Za Zhi* (Journal of Chinese Internal Medicine), 1986; 25(4):222
[3] *Jiang Su Yi Xue* (Jiangsu Medical Journal), 1989; 15(1):12
[4] *Hei Long Jiang Zhong Yi Yao* (Heilongjiang Chinese Medicine and Herbology), 1982; 1:39
[5] *Zhong Xi Yi Jie He Za Zhi* (Journal of Integrated Chinese and Western Medicine), 1987; 7:403
[6] *Guang Dong Yi Xue* (Guangdong Medicine), 1965; 3:28
[7] Xuan, W., Dong, M., and Dong, M. *Annals of Otology, Rhinology and Laryngology*, May 1995; vol. 104(5): 374-80)
[8] *Ren Min Wei Sheng Chu Ban She* (Journal of People's Public Health), 1983; 327
[9] *Chang Yong Zhong Yao Cheng Fen Yu Yao Li Shou Ce* (A Handbook of the Composition and Pharmacology of Common Chinese Drugs), 1994; 1383:1391
[10] *Shang Hai Zhong Yi Yao Za Zhi* (Shanghai Journal of Chinese Medicine and Herbology), 1986; 8:25

KIDNEY TONIC (Yang) ™

CLINICAL APPLICATIONS

☯ Kidney yang deficiency with diminished *ming men* (life gate) fire
☯ Clinical signs and symptoms: low energy and lethargy, aversion to cold, cold extremities, intolerance to cold, urinary incontinence, loose stools, diarrhea, early morning diarrhea, weakness of the lower back and knees, and edema of the legs.
☯ Clinical applications: infertility, impotence, spermatorrhea, frequent urination, incontinence, nephrotic syndrome, chronic nephritis, diabetes mellitus, bronchial asthma, sciatica, lumbago, and hypertrophic myelitis.

WESTERN THERAPEUTIC ACTIONS

☯ Improves urinary functions
☯ Alleviates musculoskeletal aches and pains
☯ Treats kidney disorders
☯ Adaptogenic effect to alleviate mental stress and physical stress
☯ Antiaging functions to stop premature or accelerated aging

CHINESE THERAPEUTIC ACTIONS

☯ Warms and tonifies Kidney yang
☯ Replenishes *jing* (essence) and tonifies blood

DOSAGE

Take 3 to 4 capsules three times daily. Dosage can be increased up to 6 to 8 capsules three times daily as needed to treat more severe symptoms.

INGREDIENTS

Dang Gui (Radicis Angelicae Sinensis)
Du Zhong (Cortex Eucommiae)
Fu Zi (Radix Aconiti Lateralis Praeparata)
Jiu Cai Zi (Semen Allii Tuberosi)
Lu Jiao Shuang (Cornu Cervi Degelatinatium)
Rou Gui (Cortex Cinnamomi)

Shan Yao (Rhizoma Dioscoreae)
Shan Zhu Yu (Fructus Corni)
Shu Di Huang (Radix Rehmanniae Preparata)
Suo Yang (Herba Cynomorii)
Tu Si Zi (Semen Cuscutae)
*Zhi Gan Cao (*Radix Glycyrrhizae Preparata)

FORMULA EXPLANATION

Kidney Tonic (Yang) is designed to treat Kidney yang deficiency. Chronic illness may consume the yang qi of the body, causing low energy and lethargy. Deficiency of the Kidney yang may lead to internal coldness, resulting in aversion to cold and cold extremities. In males, Kidney yang deficiency often leads to sexual and reproductive disorders, such as impotence, premature ejaculation, spermatorrhea, and low sperm count. Kidney yang deficiency can also cause deficiency of the urinary function of the body, leading to frequent urination and urinary incontinence. Kidney yang deficiency may impair its functions to regulate water metabolism, leading to edema of the lower legs and loose stool. Because the kidney is located in the low back, Kidney deficiency may cause weakness of the lower back and knees.

Kidney Tonic (Yang) uses *Rou Gui* (Cortex Cinnamomi), *Fu Zi* (Radix Aconiti Lateralis Praeparata), *Suo Yang* (Herba Cynomorii), *Jiu Cai Zi* (Semen Allii Tuberosi), and *Lu Jiao Shuang* (Cornu Cervi Degelatinatium) warm the Kidney yang and raise the *ming men* (life gate) fire. *Du Zhong* (Cortex Eucommiae) enhances the Kidney to treat

FORMULAS

KIDNEY TONIC (Yang) ™

low back pain and soreness associated with yang deficiency. According to the yin-yang theory of mutual dependence, in order to effectively tonify the Kidney yang, the Kidney yin also needs to be nourished. Therefore, this formula also uses *Shu Di Huang* (Radix Rehmanniae Preparata), *Shan Zhu Yu* (Fructus Corni), *Shan Yao* (Rhizoma Dioscoreae), and *Tu Si Zi* (Semen Cuscutae) to nourish the yin and replenish *jing* (essence). *Dang Gui* (Radicis Angelicae Sinensis) tonifies blood and nourishes the Liver. *Zhi Gan Cao* (Radix Glycyrrhizae Preparata) harmonizes the entire formula.

SUPPLEMENTARY FORMULAS

- For diarrhea due to Spleen qi and Kidney yang deficiency, add *GI Tonic*.
- For extreme low energy, add *Imperial Tonic*.
- For impotence or spermatorrhea, add *Vitality*.
- For male infertility, add *Vital Essence*.
- For female infertility, add *Blossom (Phase 1-4)*.
- For edema, add *Herbal DRX*.
- For hypothyroidism, add *Thyro-forte*.
- For back pain, add *Back Support (Chronic)*.
- For low adrenal functions, add *Adrenoplex*.
- For asthma, add *Cordyceps 3* or *Respitrol (Deficient)*.

NUTRITION

- Foods that are warming are recommended. Those ones include fennel, cardamon, pepper and lamb.
- Avoid food, fruits and beverages that are raw, cold or icy. Those foods include salad, sushi, ice or cold beverages, grapefruit, cucumbers, tomatoes, watermelon, cactus, etc.

The Tao of Nutrition by Ni and McNease
- Recommendations: warming foods, chicken, lamb, scallions, sesame seeds, fish, baked tofu, soybeans, walnuts, eggs, lentils, black beans, lotus seeds, a little wine, ginger, and cinnamon bark tea.
- Avoid cold foods, cold fruits, and raw foods.
- For more information, please refer to *The Tao of Nutrition* by Dr. Maoshing Ni and Cathy McNease.

LIFESTYLE INSTRUCTIONS

- Avoid exposure to the cold, such as water sports or exposure to cold and windy weather.

CLINICAL NOTES

- This formula is relatively warm. It should be taken as needed to treat Kidney yang deficient conditions. However, once the desired effect is achieved, the dose should be lowered or the formula may be discontinued.

Pulse Diagnosis by Dr. Jimmy Wei-Yen Chang:
- Deep and weak pulse on the right *chi* indicates urinary dysfunction due to Kidney yang deficiency. Weak pulse on the left *chi* indicates reproductive dysfunction due to Kidney yang deficiency.
- Note: Dr. Chang takes the pulse in slightly different positions. He places his index finger directly over the wrist crease, and his middle and ring fingers alongside to locate *cun*, *guan* and *chi* positions. For additional information and explanation, please refer to *Pulsynergy* by Dr. Jimmy Wei-Yen Chang and Marcus Brinkman.

KIDNEY TONIC (Yang) ™

CAUTIONS

- This formula is contraindicated in cases of Kidney deficient with dampness accumulation.
- *Dang Gui* (Radicis Angelicae Sinensis) may enhance the overall effectiveness of Coumadin (Warfarin), an anticoagulant drug. Patients who take anticoagulant or antiplatelet medications should ***not*** take this herbal formula without supervision by a licensed health care practitioner.
- Patients who wear a pacemaker, or individuals who take anti-arrhythmic drugs or cardiac glycosides such as Lanoxin (Digoxin), should not take this formula. *Fu Zi* (Radix Aconiti Lateralis Praeparata) may interact with these drugs by affecting the rhythm and potentiating the contractile strength of the heart.

ACUPUNCTURE POINTS

Traditional Points:
- *Shenshu* (BL 23), *Taixi* (KI 3), *Ganshu* (BL 18), *Pishu* (BL 20), *Geshu* (BL 17), *Guanyuan* (CV 4), *Qihai* (CV 6), and *Mingmen* (GV 4).

Balance Method by Dr. Richard Tan:
- Bilateral *Rangu* (KI 2), *Dazhong* (KI 4), and *Fuliu* (KI 7).
- For additional information on the Balance Method, please refer to *Dr. Tan's Strategy of Twelve Magical Points* by Dr. Richard Tan.

Auricular Acupuncture by Dr. Li-Chun Huang:
- Enuresis: Bladder, Urethra, Ear Center, and Pituitary.
  - For nocturia, add Forehead, Exciting Point
  - For enuresis due to trauma of spinal cord, add Lumbosacral Vertebral
- Urinary incontinence of: Urethra, Occiput, Lumbosacral, Liver Pituitary, Bladder, and Nervous Subcortex.
- For additional information on the location and explanation of these points, please refer to *Auricular Treatment Formula and Prescriptions* by Dr. Li-Chun Huang.

MODERN RESEARCH

Kidney Tonic (Yang) is formulated specifically to tonify Kidney yang and raise *ming men* (life gate) fire. From the western perspective, this formula improves urinary functions, treats kidney disorders, and alleviates musculoskeletal aches and pains. Furthermore, this formula contains many herbs with general adaptogenic and antiaging functions.

Kidney Tonic (Yang) contains many herbs that strongly improve urinary functions and treat kidney disorders. According to one study, use of these herbs, and others, was effective in treating frequent urination in elderly patients characterized by Kidney yang deficiency with great success. Of 64 patients who received herbal therapy for three weeks, 17 had complete recovery, 21 showed significant improvement, 21 showed slight improvement, and 5 showed no change.[1] According to another study, use of these herbs showed beneficial results to treat six patients with nephrotic syndrome unresponsive to drug treatment (steroids). Improvements included resolution of symptoms and reduction of protein in the urine.[2]

Many herbs in this formula have functions to tonify yang and raise *ming men* (life gate) fire to relieve pain and treat musculoskeletal disorders. One report stated that *Dang Gui* (Radicis Angelicae Sinensis) has marked analgesic and anti-inflammatory effects to relieve pain and reduce inflammation.[3] One study showed that use of *Dang Gui* (Radicis Angelicae Sinensis) and others via injection was associated with a 97% rate of effectiveness to relieve low back and leg pain.[4] According to another study, use of *Rou Gui* (Cortex Cinnamomi) was associated with a 98% rate of effectiveness to treat low back pain.[5] Additionally, two studies showed that sciatica could be treated effectively using many herbs in this formula.[6,7]

FORMULAS

KIDNEY TONIC (Yang) ™

Lastly, in addition to specific effects, many herbs in this formula have general adaptogenic and antiaging effects to alleviate mental stress, physical stress, and premature aging.[8,9]

PHARMACEUTICAL DRUGS & CHINESE MEDICINE: A COMPARATIVE ANALYSIS

One striking difference between western and traditional Chinese medicine is that western medicine focuses and excels in crisis management, while traditional Chinese medicine emphasizes and shines in holistic and preventative treatments. Therefore, in emergencies, such as gun shot wounds or surgery, western medicine is generally the treatment of choice. However, for treatment of chronic idiopathic illness of unknown origins, where all lab tests are normal and a clear diagnosis cannot be made, traditional Chinese medicine is distinctly superior.

In traditional Chinese medicine, Kidney yang is responsible for energetics and proper functioning of the body, including growth, maturation, and aging processes. Therefore, a decline in Kidney yang leads to symptoms such as low energy and lethargy, aversion to cold, cold extremities, intolerance to cold, urinary incontinence, loose stools, diarrhea, early morning diarrhea, weakness of the lower back and knees, and edema of the legs. Specific indications include infertility, impotence, spermatorrhea, frequent urination, incontinence, and many others. In short, Kidney yang regulates many systems in the body, including but not limited to urinary, sexual and reproductive systems. Proper use of Kidney yang tonics ensures optimal health and prevents deterioration of these conditions.

Western medicine, on the other hand, considers many of these symptoms to be non-specific and non-diagnostic. Furthermore, laboratory tests are generally normal, despite the patients still having various signs and symptoms. Under these circumstances, western medicine struggles to identify a specific diagnosis and treatments. As a result, these conditions continue to deteriorate, becoming increasingly debilitating on daily basis.

---

[1] *Xin Zhong Yi* (New Chinese Medicine), 1997; 1:48
[2] *Shen De Yan Jiu* (Research of Kidney), 1981; 93
[3] *Yao Xue Za Zhi* (Journal of Medicinals), 1971; (91):1098
[4] *Xin Zhong Yi* (New Chinese Medicine), 1980; 2:34
[5] *Zhong Xi Yi Jie He Za Zhi* (Journal of Integrated Chinese and Western Medicine), 1984; 2:115
[6] *Si Chuan Zhong Yi* (Sichuan Chinese Medicine), 1985; 11:51
[7] *Zhong Yao Xue* (Chinese Herbology), 1998; 797:799
[8] *Zhong Yao Yao Li Yu Lin Chuang* (Pharmacology and Clinical Applications of Chinese Herbs), 1990; 6(4):6
[9] *Tong Ji Yi Ke Da Xue Xue Bao* (Journal of Tongji University of Medicine), 1989; (3):198

FORMULAS

KIDNEY TONIC (Yin) ™

CLINICAL APPLICATIONS

- Kidney yin deficiency with depletion of the marrow and *jing* (essence)
- Clinical signs and symptoms: dizziness, vertigo, weakness of knees, soreness of the lower back, night and/or spontaneous sweating, spermatorrhea and/or nocturnal emission, tinnitus, dribbling of urine, thirst with desire to drink, dry mouth and throat, mirror-like tongue surface with little coating
- Clinical applications: male sexual dysfunction (spermatorrhea and nocturnal emission), infertility due to premature ovarian failure, uterine bleeding, amenorrhea, multiple neuritis, and polyneuritis

WESTERN THERAPEUTIC ACTIONS

- Treats sexual and reproductive disorders
- Improves sensory and nerve functions
- Adaptogenic effect to alleviate mental stress and physical stress
- Antiaging functions to stop premature aging

CHINESE THERAPEUTIC ACTIONS

- Nourishes yin
- Tonifies the Kidney

DOSAGE

Take 3 to 4 capsules three times daily. Dosage can be increased up to 6 to 8 capsules three times daily to treat more severe symptoms.

INGREDIENTS

Fu Ling (Poria)
Gan Cao (Radix Glycyrrhizae)
Gou Qi Zi (Fructus Lycii)
Gui Ban Jiao (Gelatinum Plastrum Testudinis)
Huai Niu Xi (Radix Achyranthis Bidentatae)
Huang Jing (Rhizoma Polygonati)

Lu Jiao Shuang (Cornu Cervi Degelatinatium)
Nu Zhen Zi (Fructus Ligustri Lucidi)
Shan Yao (Rhizoma Dioscoreae)
Shan Zhu Yu (Fructus Corni)
Shu Di Huang (Radix Rehmanniae Preparata)
Tu Si Zi (Semen Cuscutae)

FORMULA EXPLANATION

Kidney Tonic (Yin) is designed to tonify the Kidney yin and replenish the marrow and *jing* (essence). Since the brain is the sea of marrow, deficiency of the marrow may lead to dizziness and vertigo. Deficiency of the Kidney often causes deficiency of the lower body, leading to weak knees and sore back. Night sweating, dry mouth and throat, and thirst indicate general yin deficiency and lack of body fluids. Nocturnal emission and spermatorrhea are the result of deficiency fire causing the *jing* (essence) to leak out. Mirror-like tongue surface with little coating indicates severe yin deficiency.

Kidney Tonic (Yin) uses *Shu Di Huang* (Radix Rehmanniae Preparata) to tonify the Kidney and replenish the Kidney yin. *Gou Qi Zi* (Fructus Lycii) tonifies *jing* (essence) and improves vision to relieve dizziness. *Shan Zhu Yu* (Fructus Corni) has a sour taste, and astringes the yin and body fluids to prevent further depletion. *Gui Ban Jiao* (Gelatinum Plastrum Testudinis) and *Lu Jiao Shuang* (Cornu Cervi Degelatinatium) are two animal substances that have a very strong effect to nourish the Kidney and tonify the *jing* (essence). *Tu Si Zi* (Semen Cuscutae) combines with *Huai Niu Xi* (Radix Achyranthis Bidentatae) to tonify the Kidney and strengthen the lower body to relieve sore

KIDNEY TONIC (Yin) ™

back and weak knees. *Shan Yao* (Rhizoma Dioscoreae) tonifies the Kidney and strengthens the Spleen. *Nu Zhen Zi* (Fructus Ligustri Lucidi) and *Huang Jing* (Rhizoma Polygonati) further replenish Kidney yin while *Fu Ling* (Poria) strengthens the Spleen to help with absorption of the tonics. Finally, *Gan Cao* (Radix Glycyrrhizae) harmonizes the entire formula.

SUPPLEMENTARY FORMULAS

- For hot flashes, tidal fever and steaming bone sensations, add *Balance (Heat)*.
- For thirst and dryness, add *Nourish (Fluids)*.
- For qi deficiency, add *Imperial Tonic*.
- For dry cough with scanty sputum, add *Respitrol (CF)*.
- For dry stool, add *Gentle Lax (Deficient)*.
- For infertility, add *Blossom (Phase 1-4)*.
- For dizziness, vertigo or high blood pressure, add *Gastrodia Complex*.
- For osteoporosis, add *Osteo 8*.
- For degeneration of soft tissue (muscles, tendons, ligaments and cartilage), add *Flex (MLT)*
- For weakness and soreness of the back, add *Back Support (Chronic)*.
- For weakness and soreness of the knees, add *Knee Support (Chronic)*.
- For hair loss, add *Polygonum 14*.

NUTRITION

- Any type of melon (watermelon, winter melon, and cantaloupe), roots (radishes, yam, and squash), honey, grains are all recommended.
- Avoid spicy or pungent foods, as they dry out the yin.

The Tao of Nutrition by Ni and McNease
- Recommendations: cooling foods, mulberries, apples, peaches, pears, fresh vegetables, mung beans, most beans, soybeans, tofu, soy sprouts, and chrysanthemum flowers.
- Avoid hot foods, spicy foods, smoking, alcohol, stress, and strong emotions.
- For more information, please refer to *The Tao of Nutrition* by Dr. Maoshing Ni and Cathy McNease.

CLINICAL NOTE

- This formula is heavy and full of nutrients to nourish the yin aspect of the body. For that reason, it is to be used for treatment purposes and stopped once desired effect is achieved. To consolidate the effect, switch to a lighter yin tonic formula such as *Nourish* for better result.

CAUTIONS

- This formula is contraindicated in cases of excess, stagnation or fire, inflammation and infection.
- Patients with weak digestion should take this formula with caution as the yin tonic herbs may cause stagnation in the middle *jiao* and create bloating sensation.
- This formula is not recommended for prolonged use (more than 2 months). Switching to lighter yin tonic formulas such as *Nourish (Fluids)* or *Nourish* is recommended.

ACUPUNCTURE POINTS

Traditional Points:
- *Shenshu* (BL 23), *Taixi* (KI 3), *Guanyuan* (CV 4), *Sanyinjiao* (SP 6), *Qihai* (CV 6), and *Zhishi* (BL 52).

KIDNEY TONIC (Yin) ™

Balance Method by Dr. Richard Tan:
- ❧ Bilateral *Rangu* (KI 2), *Dazhong* (KI 4), and *Fuliu* (KI 7).
- ❧ For additional information on the Balance Method, please refer to *Dr. Tan's Strategy of Twelve Magical Points* by Dr. Richard Tan.

Auricular Acupuncture by Dr. Li-Chun Huang:
- ❧ Frequent micturition: Urethra, Prostate, Pituitary, Internal Urethra (for female patients), and Occiput.
  - ▪ For inflammation due to frequent micturition, bleed Ear Apex.
  - ▪ For frequent micturition due to nervous, add Nervous Subcortex and *Shenmen*.
- ❧ Tinnitus: Internal Ear, Temple (Auditory Center), and *San Jiao*.
  - ▪ For tinnitus due to excess, add Gallbladder, Liver; bleed Ear Apex
  - ▪ For tinnitus due to deficiency, add Kidney
- ❧ For additional information on the location and explanation of these points, please refer to *Auricular Treatment Formula and Prescriptions* by Dr. Li-Chun Huang.

MODERN RESEARCH

Kidney Tonic (Yin) is formulated specifically to tonify Kidney yin and replenish marrow and *jing* (essence). From the western perspectives, this formula treats sexual and reproductive disorders, and improves sensory and nerve functions. Furthermore, this formula contains many herbs with general adaptogenic and antiaging functions.

Many herbs in this formula have been used with great success to treat various sexual dysfunctions. For example, *Shu Di Huang* (Radix Rehmanniae Preparata), *Shan Yao* (Rhizoma Dioscoreae), *Shan Zhu Yu* (Fructus Corni), *Tu Si Zi* (Semen Cuscutae) and others were found to effectively treat seven men with sexual dysfunction and decreased levels of testosterone. The herbal therapy effectively reversed signs and symptoms of sexual dysfunction, and raised the plasma testosterone level to normal.[1]

This formula also addresses reproductive disorders, including male and female infertility. For male infertility, the herbs effectively increased sperm count and improved sperm motility among 33 of 42 men within approximately two months. In follow-up visits two years after the initial treatment, all 33 men were successful in having children.[2] For female infertility, the herbs were used successfully to treat infertility caused by premature ovarian failure and secondary amenorrhea.[3]

Furthermore, this formula also treats menstrual disorders, such as amenorrhea and uterine bleeding. According to one study, use of these herbs for two to three months was successful in treating 9 of 14 patients with amenorrhea due to Kidney yin deficiency.[4] For uterine bleeding, one study reported significant improvement in 17 of 22 patients using these herbs to treat uterine bleeding characterized by Kidney yin and/or yang deficiency.[5] According to another study, use of these Kidney yin tonic herbs was associated with complete recovery in 38 of 45 patients with uterine bleeding.[6]

In addition to tonifying Kidney yin, this formula also replenishes the marrow and *jing* (essence) to treat sensory and nerve disorders. For sensory disorder, use of *Huang Jing* (Rhizoma Polygonati) enhanced auditory function and improved hearing in 100 patients with deafness.[7] For nerve disorders, use of many herbs in this formula has been shown to treat multiple neuritis,[8] polyneuritis,[9] and retrogressive myelitis.[10]

Lastly, in addition to specific effects, many herbs in this formula have general adaptogenic and antiaging effect to alleviate mental stress, physical stress, and premature aging.[11,12]

FORMULAS

KIDNEY TONIC (Yin) ™

PHARMACEUTICAL DRUGS & CHINESE MEDICINE: A COMPARATIVE ANALYSIS

One striking difference between western and traditional Chinese medicine is that western medicine focuses and excels in crisis management, while traditional Chinese medicine emphasizes and shines in holistic and preventative treatments. Therefore, in emergencies, such as gun shot wounds or surgery, western medicine is generally the treatment of choice. However, for treatment of chronic idiopathic illness of unknown origins, where all lab tests are normal and a clear diagnosis cannot be made, traditional Chinese medicine is distinctly superior.

In traditional Chinese medicine, Kidney yin provides the substance needed for normal growth and functioning of the body. Therefore, a decline in Kidney yin leads to symptoms such as dizziness, vertigo, weakness of knees, soreness of the lower back, night and/or spontaneous sweating, spermatorrhea and/or nocturnal emission, tinnitus, dribbling of urine, thirst with desire to drink, dry mouth and throat, mirror-like tongue surface with little coating. Clinical applications include male sexual dysfunction (spermatorrhea and nocturnal emission), infertility due to premature ovarian failure, uterine bleeding, and amenorrhea. In short, Kidney yin affects many systems in the body, including the sexual and reproductive systems. Proper use of Kidney yin tonics ensures optimal health and prevents deterioration of these conditions.

Western medicine, on the other hand, considers many of these symptoms to be non-specific and non-diagnostic. Furthermore, laboratory tests are generally normal, despite the patients still having various signs and symptoms. Under these circumstances, western medicine struggles to identify a specific diagnosis and treatments. As a result, these conditions continue to deteriorate, becoming increasingly debilitating on daily basis.

---

[1] *Nan Jing Yi Xue Yuan Xue Bao* (Journal of Nanjing University of Medicine), 1988, 4:331

[2] *Xin Zhong Yi* (New Chinese Medicine), 1988; 2:20

[3] Chao SL. Huang LW. Yen HR. Pregnancy in premature ovarian failure after therapy using Chinese herbal medicine. Chang Gung Medical Journal. 26(6):449-52, 2003 Jun.

[4] *Zhong Yi Za Zhi* (Journal of Chinese Medicine), 1984; 7:35

[5] *Zhong Xi Yi Jie He Za Zhi* (Journal of Integrated Chinese and Western Medicine), 1984; 8:496

[6] *Hu Nan Zhong Yi Za Zhi* (Hunan Journal of Chinese Medicine), 1997; 3:57

[7] *Zhong Xi Yi Jie He Za Zhi* (Journal of Integrated Chinese and Western Medicine), 1982; 1:19

[8] *Zhong Hua Ren Min Gong He Guo Yao Dian* (Chinese Herbal Pharmacopoeia by People's Republic of China), 1995; 348

[9] *Zhong Yi Yao Xue Bao* (Report of Chinese Medicine and Herbology), 1993; 6:34

[10] *Liao Ning Zhong Yi Za Zhi* (Liaoning Journal of Chinese Medicine), 1982; 3:40

[11] *Zhong Yao Yao Li Du Li Yu Lin Chuang* (Pharmacology, Toxicology and Clinical Applications of Chinese Herbs), 1990; 6(3):28

[12] *Chang Yong Zhong Yao Cheng Fen Yu Yao Li Shou Ce* (A Handbook of the Composition and Pharmacology of Common Chinese Drugs), 1994; 1563:1564

KNEE & ANKLE (Acute) ™

CLINICAL APPLICATIONS

- Acute swelling, inflammation, sprain and strain and pain of the knees from external or trauma injuries
- Acute injury with damage to the soft tissues of the knees: anterior cruciate ligament (ACL), posterior cruciate ligament (PCL), medial collateral ligament (MCL), and lateral collateral ligament (LCL)
- Acute injury with damage of the soft tissues of the ankle: anterior talofibular ligament, calcaneofibular ligament, posterior talofibular ligament, posterior tibiofibular ligament, tibiocalcaneal ligament, anterior tibiotalar ligament, tibionavicular ligament.
- Acute injury with damage to the bones of the knees: bone fracture, dislocation of kneecap
- Acute cartilage injuries, meniscal tear, articular cartilage damage
- Soreness of the knee from repeated pressure and use of the knees, tendonitis, bursitis, sprain and strain, patellar tendonitis

WESTERN THERAPEUTIC ACTIONS

- Anti-inflammatory effect to reduce swelling and inflammation
- Analgesic effect to relieve pain

CHINESE THERAPEUTIC ACTIONS

- Clears heat
- Activates blood circulation
- Eliminates blood stasis
- Drains fluids

DOSAGE

Take 3 to 4 capsules three times daily. Dosage may be increased up to 5 to 6 capsules every four to six hours as needed. For quick and maximum effectiveness, take the herbs on an empty stomach with warm water.

INGREDIENTS

Chi Shao (Radix Paeoniae Rubrae)
Chuan Xiong (Rhizoma Ligustici Chuanxiong)
Da Huang (Radix et Rhizoma Rhei)
Dang Gui (Radicis Angelicae Sinensis)
Du Huo (Radix Angelicae Pubescentis)
Gan Cao (Radix Glycyrrhizae)
Hong Hua (Flos Carthami)
Huai Niu Xi (Radix Achyranthis Bidentatae)
Mo Yao (Myrrha)
Mu Gua (Fructus Chaenomelis)

Mu Xiang (Radix Aucklandiae)
Ru Xiang (Gummi Olibanum)
San Qi (Radix Notoginseng)
Sheng Di Huang (Radix Rehmanniae)
Su Mu (Lignum Sappan)
Tao Ren (Semen Persicae)
Wu Yao (Radix Linderae)
Xu Duan (Radix Dipsaci)
Ze Lan (Herba Lycopi)

FORMULA EXPLANATION

Knee & Ankle (Acute) is designed to treat disorders of the knee and ankle characterized by swelling, inflammation and pain. It contains herbs that activate qi and blood circulation, eliminate qi and blood stasis, clear heat, and reduce swelling and inflammation.

In this formula, many herbs are used to activate qi and blood circulation. *Dang Gui* (Radicis Angelicae Sinensis), *Sheng Di Huang* (Radix Rehmanniae) and *Chuan Xiong* (Rhizoma Ligustici Chuanxiong) are used to tonify blood

FORMULAS

and activate blood circulation. *Gan Cao* (Radix Glycyrrhizae), *Mu Xiang* (Radix Aucklandiae) and *Wu Yao* (Radix Linderae) tonify qi and activate qi circulation. Furthermore, *San Qi* (Radix Notoginseng), *Ze Lan* (Herba Lycopi), *Tao Ren* (Semen Persicae), *Chi Shao* (Radix Paeoniae Rubrae) and *Hong Hua* (Flos Carthami) activate blood circulation and eliminate blood stasis to treat pain. *Ze Lan* (Herba Lycopi) also has the effect to drain swelling associated with the inflammatory stage in acute pain conditions. *Su Mu* (Lignum Sappan), *Xu Duan* (Radix Dipsaci) and *Du Huo* (Radix Angelicae Pubescentis) open peripheral channels and collaterals to relieve pain. *Mu Gua* (Fructus Chaenomelis) relaxes the muscles to treat cramps, spasms, and stiffness. It helps repair damaged tendons and ligaments. *Da Huang* (Radix et Rhizoma Rhei) drains swelling and inflammation that often occur with acute physical injuries. It is one of the most commonly used herbs for acute trauma. Together, *Ru Xiang* (Gummi Olibanum) and *Mo Yao* (Myrrha) are used as a pair to dramatically reduce pain associated with external and trauma injuries. *Huai Niu Xi* (Radix Achyranthis Bidentatae) and *Du Huo* (Radix Angelicae Pubescentis) act as channel-guiding herbs to direct the effect of the formula to the lower extremities and increase blood circulation to the area of the knees. Lastly, *Gan Cao* (Radix Glycyrrhizae) tonifies qi and harmonizes the formula.

In summary, *Knee & Ankle (Acute)* is an excellent formula to treat acute injuries of the knees and ankles with accompanying swelling, inflammation and pain.

SUPPLEMENTARY FORMULAS

- For severe pain, combine with *Herbal Analgesic*.
- For knee and ankle disorder with heat manifestations or *re bi* (heat painful obstruction), combine with *Flex (Heat)*.
- For knee and ankle disorder with cold and damp manifestations or *zhuo bi* (fixed painful obstruction), combine with *Flex (CD)*.
- For knee and ankle disorders caused by acute injury or trauma or fracture of bones, use *Traumanex*.
- For ligament injury of the knee and ankle, add *Flex (MLT)*.
- For knee and ankle disorders characterized by atrophy and degeneration, use *Osteo 8*.
- For bone spurs, add *Flex (Spur)*.

NUTRITION

- Sulfur helps the absorption of calcium. Adequate intake and absorption of calcium is essential for the repair and the rebuilding of bones, tendons, cartilage, and connective tissues. Consume foods high in sulfur such as asparagus, eggs, fresh garlic, and onions.
- Histidine, an amino acid, is responsible for removing the high levels of copper and iron found in arthritic patients. Consume foods high in histidine, such as rice, wheat and rye.
- Fresh pineapples are recommended as they contain bromelain, an enzyme that is excellent in reducing inflammation.
- Avoid spicy food, caffeine, citrus fruits, sugar, milk, dairy products and red meat.
- Fish oil may help alleviate pain associated with rheumatoid arthritis. It can be taken in conjunction with the herbs.
- Decrease the intake of sour foods, drinks or fruits (citrus), as their nature constricts and may contribute to further stagnation in the channels and collaterals.

LIFESTYLE INSTRUCTIONS

- For obese patients, weight loss is suggested as it lessens the pressure on the joints, which can then help in relieving pain.
- Patients who are active in sports should take time off to rest the knee in order to gain full recovery.

KNEE & ANKLE (Acute) ™

ꙮ Patients with meniscus and ligament injuries are encouraged to rest and move the knee as little as possible to prevent recurrent injuries. Full movement or sports should not be performed until the knee is completely healed. Jumping or sudden landing are contraindicated.

ꙮ The above principles also apply to the ankles, too.

CLINICAL NOTES

ꙮ *Knee & Ankle (Acute)* is most effective for knee disorders due to acute external or trauma injuries with swelling, inflammation and pain. These types of acute physical injury often affect both the bones and the soft tissues. Clinical applications of this formula include disorders of the bones (bone fracture, dislocation, or meniscus injury of the knees) and surrounding soft tissue damage [anterior cruciate ligament (ACL), posterior cruciate ligament (PCL), medial collateral ligament (MCL), and lateral collateral ligament (LCL)]. Anterior drawer test and posterior drawer test can also be performed to determine whether the ACL or the PCL is damaged.

ꙮ Patients with chronic knee disorders, such as with repetitive wear and tear of the joint leading to atrophy and degeneration, should be treated with *Knee & Ankle (Chronic)*.

ꙮ According to Dr. Jun-Qing Luo, a *Tui-Na* master from China, 70 to 80% of MCL and LCL damage involve a posterior shift of those ligaments. Treatment involves resetting the soft tissue in an upward motion towards the patella. The MCL/LCL should never be stroked downwards toward the popliteal fossa. Treating ACL and PCL injuries does not require excessive force, twisting or pulling motion. He also does not recommend using *Tui-Na* treatment during the acute inflammation stage of knee disorders. However, if left untreated, tendons and ligaments may adhere and make treatment more difficult and painful. According to Dr. Luo Jun-Qing, ligament and meniscus injuries are better treated with *Tui-Na* and herbs instead of surgery.

ꙮ According to Dr. Jun-Qing Luo's experience, many times, patients will seek your help after their medical doctor confirmed that there is nothing wrong. However, patients still feel knee pain or discomfort. In such cases, many times the cause is a minor ligament injury. In some cases, knee pain may not reflect where the problem is. It may be caused by problems elsewhere, such as in the greater trochanter causing radiating pain to the knee, the tensor fasciae latae and the iliotibial band, with physical structural changes to compensate for these imbalances that leads to the knee pain. Accurate diagnosis is essential to prescribing the correct formula.

ꙮ Because the meniscus is a cartilage and receives very little blood supply, it is important to increase blood supply to the knees so that the surrounding soft tissues receives adequate supply of fresh blood and oxygen to facilitate healing. If blood stagnation is not removed, recovery time will be prolonged and adhesion is more likely to develop. Following this principle, blood-invigorating herbs are used extensively in this formula.

ꙮ This formula is an adjunct formula to acupuncture treatment. Optimal results will occur with acupuncture, electro-stimulation and herbs are all included in the treatment regime.

CAUTIONS

ꙮ This formula is contraindicated during pregnancy and while nursing.

ꙮ This formula is *not* as effective for knee disorders due to osteoarthritis or rheumatoid arthritis. Osteoarthritis should be treated with *Osteo 8* and *Knee & Ankle (Chronic)*. Rheumatoid arthritis of the knees may be treated with *Flex (Heat)*.

ꙮ *Dang Gui* (Radicis Angelicae Sinensis) may enhance the overall effectiveness of Coumadin (Warfarin), an anticoagulant drug. Patients who take anticoagulant or antiplatelet medications should *not* take this herbal formula without supervision by a licensed health care practitioner.

KNEE & ANKLE (Acute) ™

ACUPUNCTURE POINTS

Traditional Points:
❧ *Xiyan*, *Liangqiu* (ST 34), *Xiyangguan* (GB 33), *Jiexi* (ST 41), *Kunlun* (BL 60), *Qiuxu* (GB 40) and any *ah shi* points.

Balance Method by Dr. Richard Tan:
❧ *Ah shi* points around *Quchi* (LI 11), *Chize* (LU 5) and *Shaohai* (HT 3). Needle the side that is more tender upon palpation. If the pain is deep on the knee, needle the elbow for up to 1.5 to 2 *cun* if necessary.

❧ For additional information on the Balance Method, please refer to *Twelve and Twelve in Acupuncture*, *Twenty-Four More in Acupuncture*, *Dr. Tan's Strategy of Twelve Magical Points*, and *Acupuncture 1, 2, 3* by Dr. Richard Tan.

Ear Points:
❧ Select the respective points on the ear for the pain in addition to Subcortex, *Shenmen*, and Adrenals.

Auricular Acupuncture by Dr. Li-Chun Huang:
❧ Knee pain: Knee Joint.
- For external knee joint pain, add External Knee
- For internal knee joint pain, add Internal Knee Joint

❧ For additional information on the location and explanation of these points, please refer to *Auricular Treatment Formula and Prescriptions* by Dr. Li-Chun Huang.

MODERN RESEARCH

Knee & Ankle (Acute) is most effective for knee and ankle disorders due to acute external or trauma injuries with swelling, inflammation and pain. Pharmacological effects of this formula include analgesic mechanisms to relieve pain, anti-inflammatory actions to reduce swelling, and antispasmodic properties to alleviate spasms and cramps.

Huai Niu Xi (Radix Achyranthis Bidentatae) has marked analgesic and anti-inflammatory effects. These effects have been demonstrated via various routes of administration, including oral, intravenous, intraperitoneal, and subcutaneous.[1] *Dang Gui* (Radicis Angelicae Sinensis) has marked analgesic and anti-inflammatory effects, with potency similar or stronger than that of acetylsalicylic acid.[2,3]

Ru Xiang (Gummi Olibanum) and *Mo Yao* (Myrrha) have synergistic analgesic effects,[4] and are commonly used together to treat various manifestations of pain, such as chest pain, colicky or sharp pain, and severe pain from acute sprain of the lower back and legs.[5,6] *Chuan Xiong* (Rhizoma Ligustici Chuanxiong) has excellent effects in treating various presentations of pain, including but not limited to headache,[7] angina,[8] and trigeminal nerve pain.[9] Additional herbs with analgesic effects to relieve pain include *Du Huo* (Radix Angelicae Pubescentis) and *Huai Niu Xi* (Radix Achyranthis Bidentatae).[10,11]

Sheng Di Huang (Radix Rehmanniae) has marked effectiveness in reducing inflammation and swelling,[12] and has been used with great success to treat rheumatoid arthritis.[13] Other herbs with anti-inflammatory effect to reduce swelling and inflammation include *Su Mu* (Lignum Sappan) and *Tao Ren* (Semen Persicae).[14,15]

Gan Cao (Radix Glycyrrhizae) has both anti-inflammatory and antispasmodic effects, and may be used to reduce swelling, decrease inflammation, and treat spasms and cramps.[16,17]

In conclusion, ***Knee & Ankle (Acute)*** is an excellent formula to use during the first days and weeks of an acute knee injury to relieve pain, reduce swelling and inflammation, and alleviate spasms and cramps.

KNEE & ANKLE (Acute) ™

PHARMACEUTICAL DRUGS & CHINESE MEDICINE: A COMPARATIVE ANALYSIS

Western Medical Approach: Pain is a basic bodily sensation induced by a noxious stimulus that causes physical discomfort (as pricking, throbbing, or aching). Pain may be of acute or chronic states. For acute pain of the legs (including knees and ankles), two classes of drugs commonly used for treatment include non-steroidal anti-inflammatory agents (NSAID) and opioid analgesics. NSAID's [such as Motrin (Ibuprofen) and Voltaren (Diclofenac)] are generally used for mild to moderate pain, and are most effective to reduce inflammation and swelling. Though effective, they may cause such serious side effects as gastric ulcer, duodenal ulcer, gastrointestinal bleeding, tinnitus, blurred vision, dizziness and headache. Furthermore, the newer NSAID's, also known as Cox-2 inhibitors [such as Celebrex (Celecoxib)], are associated with significantly higher risk of cardiovascular events, including heart attack and stroke. Opioid analgesics [such as Vicodin (APAP/Hydrocodone) and morphine] are usually used for severe to excruciating pain. While they may be the most potent agents for pain, they also have the most serious risks and side effects, including but not limited to dizziness, lightheadedness, drowsiness, upset stomach, vomiting, constipation, stomach pain, rash, difficult urination, and respiratory depression resulting in difficult breathing. Furthermore, long-term use of these drugs leads to tolerance and addiction. In brief, it is important to remember that while drugs offer reliable and potent symptomatic pain relief, they should be used only if and when needed. Frequent use and abuse leads to unnecessary side effects and complications.

Traditional Chinese Medicine Approach: Treatment of pain is a sophisticated balance of art and science. Proper treatment of pain requires a careful evaluation of the type of disharmony (excess or deficiency, cold or heat, exterior or interior), characteristics (qi and/or blood stagnations), and locations (upper body, lower body, extremities, or internal organs). Furthermore, optimal treatment requires integrative use of herbs, acupuncture and *Tui-Na* therapies. All these therapies work together to tonify the underlying deficiencies, strengthen the body, and facilitate recovery from chronic pain. TCM pain management targets both the symptoms and causes of pain, and as such, often achieves immediate and long-term success. Furthermore, TCM pain management is often associated with few or no side effects.

Summation: For treatment of mild to severe pain due to various causes, TCM pain management offers similar treatment effects with significantly fewer side effects.

---

[1] *Zhong Yao Tong Bao* (Journal of Chinese Herbology), 1988; 13(7):43
[2] *Xin Yi Yao Xue Za Zhi* (New Journal of Medicine and Herbology), 1975; (6):34
[3] *Yao Xue Za Zhi* (Journal of Medicinals), 1971; (91):1098
[4] *Zhong Yao Xue* (Chinese Herbology), 1998; 539:540
[5] *He Nan Zhong Yi Xue Yuan Xue Bao* (Journal of University of Henan School of Medicine), 1980; 3:38
[6] *Zhong Yao Xue* (Chinese Herbology), 1998; 539:540
[7] *Shan Xi Zhong Yi Za Zhi* (Shanxi Journal Chinese Medicine), 1985; 10:447
[8] *Chong Qing Yi Yao* (Chongching Medicine and Herbology), 1978; 1:23
[9] *He Bei Zhong Yi Za Zhi* (Hebei Journal of Chinese Medicine), 1982; 4:34
[10] *Zhong Yao Yao Li Yu Ying Yong* (Pharmacology and Applications of Chinese Herbs), 1983; 796
[11] *Zhong Yao Tong Bao* (Journal of Chinese Herbology), 1988; 13(7):43
[12] *Zhong Yao Yao Li Yu Ying Yong* (Pharmacology and Applications of Chinese Herbs), 1983: 400
[13] *Tian Jing Yi Xue Za Zhi* (Journal of Tianjing Medicine and Herbology), 1966; 3:209
[14] *Zhi Wu Yao You Xiao Cheng Fen Shou Ce* (Manual of Plant Medicinals and Their Active Constituents), 1986; 137
[15] *Zhong Yao Tong Bao* (Journal of Chinese Herbology), 1986; 11(11):37
[16] *Zhong Cao Yao* (Chinese Herbal Medicine), 1991; 22(10):452
[17] *Zhong Yao Zhi* (Chinese Herbology Journal), 1993; 358

FORMULAS

KNEE & ANKLE (Chronic) ™

CLINICAL APPLICATIONS

- ❧ Chronic knee and ankle disorders with atrophy and degeneration of the soft tissues (muscles, tendons and ligaments)
- ❧ Chronic knee and ankle disorders with weakness, stiffness, decreased range of motion and mobility of the joints
- ❧ Chronic knee and ankle pain that was not addressed properly in the acute phase of injury
- ❧ Sprain, partial rupture, stretch or tear of ankle ligaments leading to instability and frequent re-injuries.

WESTERN THERAPEUTIC ACTIONS

- ❧ Anti-inflammatory effect to reduce swelling and inflammation
- ❧ Analgesic effect to relieve pain
- ❧ Muscle-relaxant effect to relieve spasms and cramps

CHINESE THERAPEUTIC ACTIONS

- ❧ Tonifies qi, blood and yin
- ❧ Activates qi and blood circulation and removes qi and blood stagnation
- ❧ Opens channels and collaterals of the lower limb to relieve pain

DOSAGE

Take 4 to 6 capsules three times daily. This formula is most effective if taken during recovery and rehabilitation of chronic knee and ankle disorders. It should not be taken during the acute phases of injuries, where there is still bleeding, inflammation and bruising.

INGREDIENTS

Bai Shao (Radix Paeoniae Alba)
Bai Zhu (Rhizoma Atractylodis Macrocephalae)
Chuan Niu Xi (Radix Cyathulae)
Da Zao (Fructus Jujubae)
Dan Shen (Radix Salviae Miltiorrhizae)
Dang Gui (Radicis Angelicae Sinensis)
Dang Shen (Radix Codonopsis)
Du Zhong (Cortex Eucommiae)
Fu Ling (Poria)
Gan Cao (Radix Glycyrrhizae)
Huang Bai (Cortex Phellodendri)

Ji Xue Teng (Caulis Spatholobi)
Mu Dan Pi (Cortex Moutan)
Qian Nian Jian (Rhizoma Homalomenae)
Shan Yao (Rhizoma Dioscoreae)
Shen Jin Cao (Herba Lycopodii)
Sheng Di Huang (Radix Rehmanniae)
Sheng Jiang (Rhizoma Zingiberis Recens)
Shu Di Huang (Radix Rehmanniae Preparata)
Wu Jia Pi (Cortex Acanthopanacis)
Ze Xie (Rhizoma Alismatis)
Zhi Mu (Radix Anemarrhenae)

FORMULA EXPLANATION

Knee & Ankle (Chronic) is designed to treat chronic degenerative knee disorders with swelling, inflammation and pain. This formula incorporates tonic herbs to address the chronic and degenerative nature of illness. Furthermore, it contains herbs that activate qi and blood stagnation, clears heat to reduce swelling and inflammation, and opens the channels and collaterals to relieve pain.

Dang Gui (Radicis Angelicae Sinensis), *Sheng Di Huang* (Radix Rehmanniae), *Shu Di Huang* (Radix Rehmanniae Preparata), and *Dan Shen* (Radix Salviae Miltiorrhizae) tonify blood, activate blood circulation, and disperse blood stagnation. *Dang Shen* (Radix Codonopsis), *Bai Zhu* (Rhizoma Atractylodis Macrocephalae), and *Gan Cao* (Radix Glycyrrhizae) tonify qi. *Bai Shao* (Radix Paeoniae Alba) and *Shan Yao* (Rhizoma Dioscoreae) nourish yin to relieve

KNEE & ANKLE (Chronic) ™

chronic *bi zheng* (painful obstruction syndrome) with underlying Kidney deficiencies. *Mu Dan Pi* (Cortex Moutan), *Zhi Mu* (Radix Anemarrhenae), and *Huang Bai* (Cortex Phellodendri) clear deficiency heat to reduce chronic swelling and inflammation. *Ze Xie* (Rhizoma Alismatis) and *Fu Ling* (Poria) eliminate water accumulation and reduce swelling. *Chuan Niu Xi* (Radix Cyathulae) dispels stagnation and opens the channels and collaterals. As many patients experience pain or worsening of condition prior to rainy days, antirheumatic herbs should be used. *Wu Jia Pi* (Cortex Acanthopanacis), *Qian Nian Jian* (Rhizoma Homalomenae), *Du Zhong* (Cortex Eucommiae) and *Shen Jin Cao* (Herba Lycopodii) dispel wind-damp to treat *bi zheng* (painful obstruction syndrome). *Shen Jin Cao* (Herba Lycopodii) also has the effect to relieve stiffness. *Sheng Jiang* (Rhizoma Zingiberis Recens), *Da Zao* (Fructus Jujubae) and *Gan Cao* (Radix Glycyrrhizae) harmonize all the herbs in the formula. *Ji Xue Teng* (Caulis Spatholobi) moves blood, opens channels and collaterals, and enhances flexibility. Lastly, *Chuan Niu Xi* (Radix Cyathulae) also acts as a channel-guiding herb to direct the therapeutic qualities of the formula to the affected area in the lower extremities.

Overall, *Knee & Ankle (Chronic)* is a well-balanced formula that addresses chronic and degenerative aspects of chronic knee disorders.

SUPPLEMENTARY FORMULAS

- For acute injuries with severe pain, combine with *Knee & Ankle (Acute)* or *Herbal Analgesic*.
- For ligament injuries or degeneration of soft tissue, add *Flex (MLT)*.
- For knee disorders with manifestations of heat or *re bi* (heat painful obstruction), combine with *Flex (Heat)*.
- For knee disorders with manifestations of cold and damp or *zhuo bi* (fixed painful obstruction), combine with *Flex (CD)*.
- For bone spurs, add *Flex (Spur)*.
- For osteoarthritis of the knee, add *Osteo 8*.
- For acute pain in the lower back, combine with *Back Support (Acute)*.
- For chronic pain in the lower back, combine with *Back Support (Chronic)*.
- For spasms and cramps in the legs, combine with *Flex (SC)*.

NUTRITION

- Glucosamine sulfate and chondroitin sulfate are well recognized for their nutritional support, as they are important for the formation of bones, tendons, ligaments and cartilages.
- Sea cucumber is very beneficial, as it contains a rich source of compounds that are needed in all connective tissues, especially synovial joints and joint fluids.
- It is important to consume an adequate amount of various vitamins and minerals, as they are essential to prevent bone loss and promote bone growth.

LIFESTYLE INSTRUCTIONS

- It is important to engage in gentle exercises daily. This will not only facilitate recovery, but will also prevent muscle atrophy and muscle wasting.
- Avoid activities with high impact or high risk of injuries.

CLINICAL NOTES

- This formula is an excellent adjunct formula to acupuncture treatment. Optimal results will occur when acupuncture, electro-stimulation and herbs are all included in the treatment regimen.

FORMULAS

KNEE & ANKLE (Chronic) ™

- Patients with acute physical injuries of the knees or ankles, such as external injuries or trauma with actual damage to the soft tissues (muscles, tendons and ligaments), should be treated with *Traumanex*, *Knee & Ankle (Acute)* or *Herbal Analgesic*.
- Patients with arthritis should avoid vigorous exercise of the knee. Mild exercise, such as *Tai Chi Chuan* and walking, are recommended.
- This formula is most effective when taken during the recovery and rehabilitation phases of treatment. Strengthening exercises, such as *Tai Chi Chuan*, ensure recovery of the integrity of the knee and ankle ligaments.
- In cases where acute sprain and strain of the knees and ankles are not treated properly, the ligaments and joints will become unstable and re-injury may occur more frequently. *Knee & Ankle (Chronic)* can ensure the repair of minor tears of the ligaments and can facilitate complete recovery to prevent the future possibility of re-injury.

CAUTIONS

- This formula should *not* be used alone in patients with acute physical injuries of the knees, such as external injuries or trauma with actual damage to the soft tissues (muscles, tendons and ligaments).
- This formula should *not* be used alone in patients with inflammatory knee disorders, such as rheumatoid arthritis, bursitis, synovitis and tenosynovitis.
- *Dan Shen* (Radix Salviae Miltiorrhizae) and *Dang Gui* (Radicis Angelicae Sinensis) may enhance the overall effectiveness of Coumadin (Warfarin), an anticoagulant drug. Patients who take anticoagulant or antiplatelet medications should *not* take this herbal formula without supervision by a licensed health care practitioner.

ACUPUNCTURE POINTS

Traditional Points:
- *Xiyan*, *Liangqiu* (ST 34), *Xiyangguan* (GB 33), *Jiexi* (ST 41), *Kunlun* (BL 60), *Qiuxu* (GB 40) and relevant *ah shi* points.

Balance Method by Dr. Richard Tan:
- *Ah shi* points around *Quchi* (LI 11), *Chize* (LU 5) and *Shaohai* (HT 3). Needle the side that is more tender upon palpation. If the pain is deep in the knee, needle the elbow for up to 1.5 to 2 *cun* if necessary.
- For additional information on the Balance Method, please refer to *Twelve and Twelve in Acupuncture*, *Twenty-Four More in Acupuncture*, *Dr. Tan's Strategy of Twelve Magical Points*, and *Acupuncture 1, 2, 3* by Dr. Richard Tan.

Ear Points:
- Select the respective points on the ear for the pain in addition to Subcortex, *Shenmen*, and Adrenals.

Auricular Acupuncture by Dr. Li-Chun Huang:
- Knee pain: Knee Joint
  - For external knee joint pain, add External Knee
  - For internal knee joint pain, add Internal Knee Joint
- For additional information on the location and explanation of these points, please refer to *Auricular Treatment Formula and Prescriptions* by Dr. Li-Chun Huang.

MODERN RESEARCH

Knee & Ankle (Chronic) is an excellent formula for rehabilitation from chronic knee or ankle disorders, such as repetitive knee injuries or long-term wear and tear of the joint. As a result, the chronic nature of this condition may eventually contribute to atrophy and degeneration of the knee joints, accompanied by decreased mobility of the

FORMULAS

joints, and generalized weakness and pain. This formula is designed specifically to treat this condition, as it contains herbs with adaptogenic effect to facilitate rehabilitation, anti-inflammatory effects to reduce swelling and inflammation, analgesic effects to relieve pain, and muscle-relaxant effects to relieve spasms and cramps.

Knee & Ankle (Chronic) uses many herbs with adaptogenic effects to facilitate both mental and physical aspects of rehabilitation. *Dang Shen* (Radix Codonopsis) has a regulatory effect on the central nervous system to help with adaptation to various stressful environments.[1] *Wu Jia Pi* (Cortex Acanthopanacis) enhances physical adaptation by increasing endurance and performance.[2]

Many herbs in this formula also have marked analgesic and anti-inflammatory effects to relieve pain, and reduce swelling and inflammation. For example, *Dang Gui* (Radicis Angelicae Sinensis) has marked analgesic and anti-inflammatory effects, with potency similar or stronger than that of acetylsalicylic acid.[3,4] *Wu Jia Pi* (Cortex Acanthopanacis) also has excellent analgesic and anti-inflammatory effects with the duration of action lasting up to five hours.[5,6] *Bai Shao* (Radix Paeoniae Alba) and *Sheng Di Huang* (Radix Rehmanniae) have anti-inflammatory and antipyretic effects, and are helpful to reduce inflammation and swelling, as well as relieve burning sensations in affected areas.[7,8] *Mu Dan Pi* (Cortex Moutan) and *Du Zhong* (Cortex Eucommiae) have demonstrated strong anti-inflammatory actions.[9] Pharmacologically, the mechanisms behind the anti-inflammatory effects of these herbs vary, but most have been attributed primarily to the inhibition of prostaglandin synthesis and decreased permeability of the blood vessels.[10] Alternatively, mechanisms involve stimulation of the endocrine system and consequent secretion of steroids from the adrenal cortex.[11] Clinically, these herbs have been used with great success to treat a wide variety of musculoskeletal conditions, including but not limited to muscle wasting, muscle atrophy, chronic soft tissue injuries, and various types of pain.[12,13]

Bai Shao (Radix Paeoniae Alba) has excellent muscle-relaxant effect to relieve spasms, cramp and muscle stiffness.[14] This efficacy has been demonstrated in both smooth and skeletal muscles. In addition, *Bai Shao* (Radix Paeoniae Alba) and *Gan Cao* (Radix Glycyrrhizae) are effective in treating neuralgia.[15] Furthermore, *Bai Shao* (Radix Paeoniae Alba) and *Gan Cao* (Radix Glycyrrhizae) have shown marked effectiveness to treat pain of the entire body, especially in the lower back and legs.[16]

In summary, *Knee & Ankle (Chronic)* is an excellent formula for chronic knee and ankle disorders. Degeneration of soft tissues (muscles, tendons and ligaments) is often seen in chronic knee and ankle disorders that lead to decreased range of motion and mobility of the joints. With late-stage musculoskeletal injuries, muscle wasting and atrophy are present due to lack of exercise and physical movement. This formula is developed specifically to address all of these conditions by using herbs that compliment the rehabilitation process and complete the recovery from these injuries.

PHARMACEUTICAL DRUGS & CHINESE MEDICINE: A COMPARATIVE ANALYSIS

Western Medical Approach: Pain is a basic bodily sensation induced by a noxious stimulus that causes physical discomfort (as pricking, throbbing, or aching). Pain may be of acute or chronic state, and may be of nociceptive, neuropathic, or psychogenic type. For acute pain, use of non-steroidal anti-inflammatory agents (NSAID) and opioid analgesics offer immediate and reliable effects to relieve pain. Though these drugs have serious side effects, short-term use can be justified because the benefits often outweigh the risks. For chronic pain, on the other hand, use of NSAID's and opioid analgesics are usually not the desired treatment options, as they symptomatically relieve pain, but do not change the underlying course of illness. Unfortunately, the convenience of these drugs contributes to the vicious cycle of pain, followed by continuous and repetitive use of drugs to symptomatically relieve pain. When the effect of the drugs dissipates, patients are often left with nothing but more pain and more complications from side effects. Therefore, it is important to understand that while these drugs may be beneficial for acute pain, they do not adequately address most cases of chronic pain. Additional treatment modalities must be incorporated to ensure effective and complete recovery from chronic pain conditions. [Note: Common side effects of NSAID's include gastric ulcer, duodenal ulcer, gastrointestinal bleeding, tinnitus, blurred vision, dizziness and headache. Serious side effects of newer NSAID's, also known as Cox-2 inhibitors [such as Celebrex (Celecoxib)], include significantly

KNEE & ANKLE (Chronic) ™

higher risk of cardiovascular events, including heart attack and stroke. Side effects of opioid analgesics [such as Vicodin (APAP/Hydrocodone) and morphine] include dizziness, lightheadedness, drowsiness, upset stomach, vomiting, constipation, stomach pain, rash, difficult urination, and respiratory depression resulting in difficult breathing. Furthermore, long-term use of these drugs leads to tolerance and addiction.]

Traditional Chinese Medicine Approach: Treatment of chronic pain is a sophisticated balance of art and science. Proper treatment of pain requires a careful evaluation of the type of disharmony (excess or deficiency, cold or heat, exterior or interior), characteristics (qi and/or blood stagnations), and locations (upper body, lower body, extremities, or internal organs). Furthermore, optimal treatment requires integrative use of herbs, acupuncture and *Tui-Na* therapies. All these therapies work together to tonify the underlying deficiencies, strengthen the body, and facilitate recovery from chronic pain. TCM pain management targets both the symptom and the cause of pain, and as such, often achieves immediate and long-term success. Furthermore, TCM pain management is often associated with few or no side effects.

Summation: For treatment of mild to severe pain due to various causes, TCM pain management offers similar treatment effects with significantly fewer side effects. Though TCM therapies may not be as potent as drugs for acute pain management, they are often superior [better effects with fewer side effects] for chronic pain management.

---

[1] *Zhong Yao Tong Bao* (Journal of Chinese Herbology), 1986; 11(8):53
[2] *Zhong Cao Yao* (Chinese Herbal Medicine), 1987; 18(3):28
[3] *Xin Yi Yao Xue Za Zhi* (New Journal of Medicine and Herbology), 1975; (6):34
[4] *Yao Xue Za Zhi* (Journal of Medicinals), 1971; (91):1098
[5] *Zhong Guo Yao Li Xue Tong Bao* (Journal of Chinese Herbal Pharmacology), 1986; 2(2):21
[6] *Zhong Cheng Yao Yan Jiu* (Research of Chinese Patent Medicine), 1984; 10:22
[7] *Zhong Yao Yao Li Yu Ying Yong* (Pharmacology and Applications of Chinese Herbs), 1983: 400
[8] *Zhong Yao Zhi* (Chinese Herbology Journal), 1993; 183
[9] *Sheng Yao Xue Za Zhi* (Journal of Raw Herbology), 1979; 33(3):178
[10] *Zhong Guo Yao Ke Da Xue Xue Bao* (Journal of University of Chinese Herbology), 1990; 21(4):222
[11] *Zhong Cao Yao* (Chinese Herbal Medicine), 1983; 14(8):27
[12] *Xin Yi Yao Xue Za Zhi* (New Journal of Medicine and Herbology), 1976; 12:26
[13] *Shang Hai Zhong Yi Yao Za Zhi* (Shanghai Journal of Chinese Medicine and Herbology), 1983; 4:14
[14] *Zhong Yi Za Zhi* (Journal of Chinese Medicine), 1983; 11:9
[15] *Zhong Yi Za Zhi* (Journal of Chinese Medicine), 1983; 11:9
[16] *Yun Nan Zhong Yi* (Yunnan Journal of Traditional Chinese Medicine), 1990; 4:15

LIVER DTX ™

(Detoxification)

CLINICAL APPLICATIONS

☯ Liver damage with high levels of SGPT and SGOT [12]
☯ Liver detoxification: enhances the normal metabolic and detoxification functions of the liver [1]
☯ Hepatitis: treats hepatitis with or without jaundice, repairs liver cell damage [2,3,4,5,6]
☯ Liver cirrhosis from excessive alcohol intake [6,21]
☯ Addiction: detoxifies liver during alcohol, drug or smoking cessation [8]
☯ Cholecystitis with increased liver enzymes, possibly with liver impairment [6,7]

WESTERN THERAPEUTIC ACTIONS

☯ Enhances the liver function by increasing the regeneration of liver cells [1]
☯ Protects the liver from damage due to foreign chemicals and substances, medications, and alcohol [13,14,16,17]
☯ Treats liver cirrhosis by preventing and repairing liver damage [6]
☯ Anti-oxidant effects to neutralize free radicals and prevent cell damage [11]
☯ Lowers elevated levels of hepatic enzymes [12]

CHINESE THERAPEUTIC ACTIONS

☯ Clears heat and eliminates toxins
☯ Spreads the Liver qi
☯ Drains dampness
☯ Tonifies deficiency

DOSAGE

Take 3 to 4 capsules three times daily on an empty stomach with warm water.

INGREDIENTS

Bai Shao (Radix Paeoniae Alba)
Chai Hu (Radix Bupleuri)
Da Huang (Radix et Rhizoma Rhei)
Fu Ling (Poria)
Ge Hua (Flos Puerariae)
Hu Zhang (Rhizoma Polygoni Cuspidati)
Huang Qin (Radix Scutellariae)
Ma Bian Cao (Herba Verbenae)

Pu Tao Zi (Semen Vitis Vinifera)
Qing Pi (Pericarpium Citri Reticulatae Viride)
Silybum marianum (Milk Thistle)
Wu Wei Zi (Fructus Schisandrae Chinensis)
Yin Chen Hao (Herba Artemisiae Scopariae)
Yu Jin (Radix Curcumae)
Zhi Zi (Fructus Gardeniae)

FORMULA EXPLANATION

According to traditional Chinese medicine, hepatic disorders are characterized by damp-heat or toxic heat in the Liver. *Liver DTX* is formulated to eliminate damp-heat, clear toxic heat, and regulate Liver qi. Clinical applications of *Liver DTX* include hepatitis, liver cirrhosis, and cholecystitis. It can also be used to protect the liver and lower liver enzymes secondary to the use of drugs and alcohol, and subsequent to viral infections.

To detoxify the liver, the treatment protocol is to strengthen the liver function. Capillarisin, one of the active ingredients of *Yin Chen Hao* (Herba Artemisiae Scopariae), increases the secretion of bile, bile salts and bilirubin. It increases the regeneration of liver cells and is an indispensable herb when treating jaundice or cholecystitis. *Chai Hu*

LIVER DTX ™

(Detoxification)

(Radix Bupleuri) is a channel-guiding herb and is also extremely effective in protecting the liver cells from denaturalization and necrosis. It is often used to decrease the SGOT and SGPT in patients with fatty liver or chronic hepatitis.[7] *Ge Hua* (Flos Puerariae) relieves alcohol poisoning. *Hu Zhang* (Rhizoma Polygoni Cuspidati), *Zhi Zi* (Fructus Gardeniae), *Huang Qin* (Radix Scutellariae) and *Da Huang* (Radix et Rhizoma Rhei) clear heat, detoxify and improve the liver function. *Bai Shao* (Radix Paeoniae Alba) nourishes the Liver blood and qi. *Ma Bian Cao* (Herba Verbenae) enters the Liver channel to clear heat and detoxify. *Fu Ling* (Poria) strengthens the Spleen and promotes the excretion of toxins through urination. *Yu Jin* (Radix Curcumae) benefits the Gallbladder and the Liver in treating viral hepatitis. It also invigorates blood circulation to promote generation of new liver cells. *Qing Pi* (Pericarpium Citri Reticulatae Viride) spreads the stagnant Liver qi and relieves constraint. *Wu Wei Zi* (Fructus Schisandrae Chinensis) improves the Liver function in patients with hepatitis. Both *Pu Tao Zi* (Semen Vitis Vinifera) and *Silybum marianum* (Milk Thistle) have excellent hepatoprotective and anti-oxidant functions.

SUPPLEMENTARY FORMULAS

- ✪ For cholecystitis or gallstones with elevated liver enzymes, combine with *Dissolve GS*.
- ✪ *Gentiana Complex* may be combined with *Liver DTX* for a synergistic effect to treat hepatic disorders.
- ✪ To enhance the overall heat-clearing and detoxifying effects, add *Herbal ABX*.
- ✪ For excess fire signs and symptoms throughout the body, add *Gardenia Complex*.
- ✪ For dark complexion and blood stagnation, add *Circulation (SJ)*.
- ✪ For fatty liver, add *Cholisma (ES)*.
- ✪ For compromised kidney function, use *Kidney DTX*.
- ✪ To cleanse the colon, add *Gentle Lax (Deficient)*.
- ✪ For stomach discomfort, heartburn, and/or acid reflux, add *GI Care*.
- ✪ To enhance the immune system, add *Immune +*.
- ✪ For nervousness, irritability, and stress, combine with *Calm* or *Calm ES*.
- ✪ For a quick burst of energy and awareness, combine with *Vibrant*.
- ✪ To tonify the underlying deficiencies of qi, blood, yin and yang, use *Imperial Tonic*.
- ✪ For heavy metal, chemical or environmental poisoning, add *Herbal DTX*.

NUTRITION

- ✪ Patients with liver cirrhosis should increase the intake of vitamin K found in such foods as green leafy vegetables, almonds, bananas, kelp, prunes, raisins, rice, wheat bran, and seeds. They should increase their intake of vegetables, especially artichokes, carrots, and beets. Water intake should be increased.
- ✪ Artichokes contain cynarin, a substance that stimulates the bile flow and regulates the liver.
- ✪ Patients with hepatitis should avoid alcohol, sugar, fat, raw fish, shellfish and highly-processed foods with chemicals or food additives. Fat, butter, margarine, cheese, fish, fowl, meat, salt, soft drinks, sugar, tea, cod liver oil, vitamin A, spicy, and fried foods should be eliminated from the diet. Also avoid over-eating, cigarette smoking, alcohol, coffee, and drugs.
- ✪ Patients with jaundice should *not* consume alcohol, raw or undercooked fish, meat or poultry.

The Tao of Nutrition by Ni and McNease
- ✪ Hepatitis
  - ▪ Recommendations: rice, barley, millet, azuki beans, pearl barley, squash, cucumber, grapefruit, dandelion greens, beet greens, pears, water chestnut, carrot, cabbage, spinach, celery, winter melon, rice vinegar, pineapple, and lotus root.
  - ▪ Avoid dairy products, alcohol, coffee, sugar, fatty and fried foods, overly spicy foods, cold and raw foods, tomato, eggplant, bell peppers, and shellfish.
- ✪ For more information, please refer to *The Tao of Nutrition* by Dr. Maoshing Ni and Cathy McNease.

FORMULAS

LIVER DTX ™
(Detoxification)

LIFESTYLE INSTRUCTIONS

- Avoid physical and mental stress and exhaustion whenever possible. Maintain a cheerful and positive outlook and avoid dramatic emotional swings.
- Avoid exposure to toxins whenever possible, including but not limited to chemicals, heavy metals, herbicides, pesticides, environmental pollutants, etc.
- Physical stimulation to the back by scratching or intense massage will stimulate the liver to increase activity.

CLINICAL NOTES

- Lab exams are extremely useful in diagnosis, treatment and prognosis assessment for patients with liver dysfunction. Understanding the implications of laboratory tests empowers health care practitioners to effectively treat hepatic and gallbladder disorders.
- Elevation of liver enzymes is common in hepatitis. Though western medicine has treatments for lowering liver enzymes, the results are sometimes unsatisfactory, especially in chronic hepatitis B. Therefore, herbs that clear heat, remove damp, strengthen the Spleen and regulate the Liver are used to normalize liver enzyme levels. In addition, small dosages of blood-activating and stasis-removing herbs can be used together for their synergistic effect. Patients should continue to take herbs for a period of time after liver enzyme levels return to normal to prevent rebound increase of liver enzymes.
- Liver cirrhosis is a common complication of chronic hepatitis infection. To reduce the risk of developing cirrhosis of the liver in chronic hepatitis, use large dosages of *Dan Shen* (Radix Salviae Miltiorrhizae) with regular dosages of *Hong Hua* (Flos Carthami). Addition of *Bie Jia* (Carapax Trionycis) to the herbal formula will further reduce the risk of developing liver cirrhosis.
- The five main reasons hepatitis B patients remain chronic carriers of the hepatitis B virus:
  1. Enhanced or suppressed immunity. Patients with irregular immune systems are less likely to become negative on the HBV exam. Indications of irregular immune system include high or low levels of IgG, IgM and IgA.
  2. Frequent infection of the oral region indicates a suppressed immunity. This can be treated with *Ye Ju Hua* (Flos Chrysanthemi Indici) and *Gan Cao* (Radix Glycyrrhizae).
  3. Seasonal factors. The treatment of hepatitis is less effective in spring and summer. In spring, there is a higher incidence of Liver qi damaging the yin. In summer, the damp-heat in the environment may increase dampness and heat inside the body. Thus, the ideal seasons to treat hepatitis B are autumn and winter. To enhance the overall effectiveness of the treatment, *Yi Guan Jian* (Linking Decoction) can be added in autumn and *Liu Yi San* (Six-to-One Powder) can be added in summer.
  4. Increase in liver enzymes such as SGPT and SGOT.
  5. Dietary restrictions. Patients should reduce their intake of alcohol, hot and spicy food, and any other foods that worsen the condition.

CAUTIONS

- *Liver DTX* is contraindicated during pregnancy and nursing. It should be used with caution in cases of qi and yang deficiencies.
- Do *not* use this formula to treat acute liver failure – such conditions must be sent to the emergency room for immediate medical care.
- Decrease the dosage to 2 capsules twice a day if there is loose stool after taking the herbs.
- Patients who are on anticoagulant or antiplatelet therapies, such as Coumadin (Warfarin), should use this formula with caution as there may be a slightly higher risk of bleeding and bruising.

LIVER DTX ™

(Detoxification)

ACUPUNCTURE POINTS

Traditional Points:
- *Taichong* (LR 3), *Xingjian* (LR 2), *Ganshu* (BL 18), and *Zusanli* (ST 36).
- *Xingjian* (LR 2), *Taichong* (LR 3), *Fenglong* (ST 40), *Sanyinjiao* (SP 6), *Ganshu* (BL 18), and *Danshu* (BL 19).

Balance Method by Dr. Richard Tan:
- Left side: *Hegu* (LI 4), *Zhizheng* (SI 7), *Ligou* (LR 5), *Ququan* (LR 8), and *Ganmen,* and Liver and Pancreas on the ear.
- Right Side: *Neiguan* (PC 6), *Ximen* (PC 4) or *ah shi* points nearby, *Yanglingquan* (GB 34), *Zusanli* (ST 36) or *ah shi* points nearby, and Liver and Pancreas on the ear.
- Left and right side can be alternated from treatment to treatment.
- For additional information on the Balance Method, please refer to *Dr. Tan's Strategy of Twelve Magical Points* by Dr. Richard Tan.

Ear Points:
- To detoxify the Liver. Use three needles on the Liver or embed needles on the Liver point.
- To quit cigarette smoking: Mouth, Bronchi, Lung, Pituitary Gland, *Shenmen*, and Subcortex. Switch ear every five days. Instruct the patient to massage the points for 1 to 2 minutes when smoking urges occur.

Auricular Acupuncture by Dr. Li-Chun Huang:
- Hepatitis: Liver, Gall Bladder, Rib Rim, Spleen, Sanjiao, Endocrine, Abdominal Distention Area, Digestive Subcortex, Ear Center, and Hepatitis.
- Addiction
  - Smoking addiction: Sympathetic, *Shenmen*, Mouth, and Lower Lung.
  - Alcohol addiction: Sympathetic, *Shenmen*, Drunk Point, Liver, Nervous Subcortex, and Anxious Point.
  - Drug addiction: Sympathetic, *Shenmen*, Kidney, Liver, Lower Lung, Anxious Point, Nervous Subcortex
- For additional information on the location and explanation of these points, please refer to *Auricular Treatment Formula and Prescriptions* by Dr. Li-Chun Huang.

MODERN RESEARCH

Liver DTX is formulated with herbs that enhance the normal metabolic and detoxification functions of the liver.[1] Clinical applications of *Liver DTX* include hepatitis with or without jaundice,[2,3,4,5,6] cholecystitis with increased liver enzymes and possible liver impairment,[6,7] liver cirrhosis from excessive alcohol intake,[6] and detoxification of the liver during alcohol, drug or smoking cessation.[8] Ingredients in *Liver DTX* have demonstrated functions that increase the regeneration of liver cells,[9] protect the liver from damage by foreign chemicals and substances,[1] prevent and repair liver damage,[10] neutralize free radicals thereby preventing damage to liver cells with their anti-oxidant effect,[11] and lowering elevated levels of hepatic enzymes.[12]

Silybum marianum, also known as milk thistle, is one of the main ingredients in *Liver DTX*. The use of *Silybum marianum* can be traced back over 2,000 years to a Greek reference when Pliny the Elder (A.D. 23-79) first noted it had an excellent effect to "carry off bile."[13] The active ingredient of *Silybum marianum* is silymarin, which has been found to have hepatoprotective and anti-oxidant effects.[1] Silymarin protects the liver by changing the outer liver cell membrane and preventing the entrance of toxins into the liver cells.[13,14] Specific indications for silymarin include cirrhosis and hepatitis. Silymarin was found to be effective in treating alcoholic cirrhosis as concluded by a 41-month double-blind study of 170 patients.[12] Silymarin also improved liver function in 20 patients with chronic active hepatitis.[15]

FORMULAS

LIVER DTX ™

(Detoxification)

Pu Tao Zi (Semen Vitis Vinifera), also known as grape seed extract, also showed promising hepatoprotective activity,[16] as illustrated by one study that determined *Pu Tao Zi* (Semen Vitis Vinifera) to have hepatoprotective activity against foreign chemicals such as carbon tetrachloride.[17]

Wu Wei Zi (Fructus Schisandrae Chinensis) has a wide range of functions and clinical applications. In addition to its use as a liver protectant, it has such uses as a general tonic, nervous system effects, GI therapy, adaptogenic properties and others. *Wu Wei Zi* (Fructus Schisandrae Chinensis) possesses pronounced hepatoprotective effect by protecting the hepatocyte plasma membrane and preventing the entry of toxic substances.[18] Furthermore, it repairs liver damages by increasing blood flow to the liver and increasing regeneration of liver cells. [19] In addition to its hepatoprotective effect, *Wu Wei Zi* (Fructus Schisandrae Chinensis) stimulates the nervous system to increase reflex responses and improve mental alertness to treat memory loss. [20] It also helps the body to adapt to stress by balancing body fluids and improving failing senses. [20]

Lastly, a study on *Ge Gen* (Radix Puerariae) and *Ge Hua* (Flos Puerariae) illustrated that this herb can treat alcohol abuse and overdose safely and effectively. The antidipsotropic activity of *Ge Hua* (Flos Puerariae) has been used in China for more than a millennium.[21]

PHARMACEUTICAL DRUGS & CHINESE MEDICINE: A COMPARATIVE ANALYSIS

Western Medical Approach: Liver diseases, such as hepatitis and liver cirrhosis, are serious and very complicated diseases. In western medicine, these conditions are usually treated with interferon. These drugs, however, have limited success, but are extremely expensive and create significant number of serious side effects, including dizziness, confusion, coma, arrhythmia, heart failure, leukopenia, thrombocytopenia, and many others. In severe and life threatening cases, such as liver cirrhosis and liver cancer, surgery may be perform.

Traditional Chinese Medicine Approach: In traditional Chinese medicine, treatment of liver disorders is also a very challenging and complicated matter. These conditions are usually treated with herbs that drain damp-heat from the Liver. Pharmacologically, these herbs have hepatoprotective effects that remove toxins from the liver, prevent the entrance of toxins into the liver cells, and increase blood circulation to the liver to facilitate recovery. In most cases, herbs are most effective in early stage of liver disorder characterized by increased liver enzymes. Immediate and aggressive treatment with herbs generally lowers liver enzyme levels and reverses the illness. Once the disease progresses into various stages of hepatitis and/or liver cirrhosis, customized treatments should be considered for maximum effectiveness.

Summation: Liver diseases, such as hepatitis and liver cirrhosis, are serious and very complicated diseases that are challenging to both western and traditional Chinese medicines. Herbal treatment is generally more effective for early stages of liver disease, and ones with mild to moderate severity. Drug treatment, such as with interferon, are generally not utilized unless there is moderate to severe liver disease, because the risks of side effects are generally greater than the potential benefits. Unfortunately, severe cases of liver diseases are extremely difficult to manage for both western medicine and traditional Chinese medicine. Under these circumstance, customized treatment with careful supervision is most effective.

CASE STUDIES

A 41-year-old male complained of occasional bouts of irritability. He had elevated liver enzymes, elevated HCT and was positive for Hepatitis C. The practitioner diagnosed his condition as damp-heat in the Liver and Gallbladder. After taking **Liver DTX**, the liver enzyme levels tested within normal limits. The patient's medical doctor, after recognizing all supporting evidence, encouraged the herbal treatment wholeheartedly.

P.C., Stanwood, Washington

FORMULAS

LIVER DTX ™

(Detoxification)

M.C., a 49-year-old highly-stressed executive, presented elevated SGPT, LDL and cholesterol levels. He stated he frequently checked his blood pressure and it ranged from 135-148/85-91 mmHg. He was never diagnosed with hypertension but had an upcoming insurance physical and wanted to lower his blood pressure naturally [without using drugs]. He also complained of low-grade temporal headaches, pressured feeling in the head, neck and shoulder tension. His blood pressure at the time of examination was 148/94 mmHg and his heart rate was 72 beats per minute. He worried excessively, in part because his son was diagnosed with brain tumor ten years ago. He also suffered from insomnia, and fist clenching that lasted throughout the day. He said that his stress caused numbness and tension on his left shoulder and rhomboid area. The TCM diagnoses were Liver qi stagnation and Spleen qi deficiency. *Cholisma* at 4 capsules three times daily and *Liver DTX* at 5 capsules at night were prescribed. He reported after taking the herbs, he passed his insurance exam. Blood pressure has stayed down at 120/72 mmHg. His stress was manageable and there were no more headaches. Energy level was also excellent. His cholesterol levels had also dropped from 216 to 186 mg/dL. The practitioner reported that the patient is now a believer of herbs.

M.H., West Palm Beach, Florida

A 45-year-old female with insulin-dependent diabetes presented with malaise, fatigue, night sweats, hot flashes and low back pain. She also had abdominal bloating, red eyes, weak nails and a pale complexion. She was diagnosed with hepatitis C. The practitioner prescribed *Liver DTX* (3 capsules three times daily) and *Equilibrium* (3 capsules three times daily). Also given was a pancreatic homeopathic remedy (10 drops 6 times a day) and another homeopathic remedy, Hepan Comp (1 drop three times daily). Two and a half months later, the patient discontinued her insulin use. Her viral load was almost within the normal range and she decided to discontinue all pharmaceuticals. There was a total reversal of her clinical picture.

I.B., Miami, Florida

A 68-year-old retired male complained of diminishing vision. In turn, he became frustrated with the fact that he was no longer able to play tennis as well as before or competitively. Other visual dysfunctions included a reduction in visual field and the inability to track objects. The practitioner diagnosed the patient's condition as Liver qi stagnation and Liver fire with underlying Liver yin deficiency. The practitioner suspected blood leakage into the post-retinal layer, which would have been indicative of a detached retina. The patient was given *Liver DTX*. Along with the herbal treatment, the practitioner also stressed the importance of diet, especially devoid of alcohol and sugar. Although the patient was not completely compliant with the treatment, his visual compromise stabilized and the deterioration stopped. The practitioner observed a reversal of the patient's symptoms and anticipated an encouraging prognosis.

T.W., Santa Monica, California

J.J., a 45-year-old male, presented with tiredness, aching joints, occasional jaundice, bleeding gums and nose, thirst, foul and sticky bowel movements, short-temper, irritability, disturbed sleep, dry eyes and floaters. His tongue was red, quivering and the tip was red. His pulse was wiry on both sides. Blood pressure was 125/80 mmHg and the heart rate was 72 beats per minute. Western medical diagnosis was Hepatitis C. The TCM diagnosis was damp-heat in the Liver, Liver blood deficiency and Liver overacting on the Spleen. *Liver DTX* combined with *Huang Bai* (Cortex Phellodendri) were prescribed totaling at 12 grams a day. Omega-3 fatty acids were also recommended at 1 tablespoon per day. Patient had a very recent liver profile done before the treatment. Within three weeks of acupuncture and herbal treatments, his total liver profile (by a new blood test) imbalances were reduced by over 66%. He felt amazingly better. No bloating or hypochondrial pain. Digestion was much improved, as well as energy and well-being. Proper dietary recommendations were also implemented. The practitioner reported that he consistently found the *Liver DTX* to be an amazing and very powerful formula, especially with hepatitis.

M.N., Knoxville, Tennessee

LIVER DTX ™

(Detoxification)

A 44-year-old female with hepatitis C, necrosis of the liver, and diabetes (insulin-dependent) was treated with interferon, Rebetron (Ribavirin and Interferon alpha 2B), Zantac (Ranitidine), Prozac (Fluoxetine) and insulin. Her clinical manifestations included pain in the liver region, fatigue, insomnia, blurred vision, constipation, melancholy, frontal headache, dizziness, tremors, abdominal bloating, and a pale complexion. Her tongue was maroon in color, and the pulse was slippery. The diagnosis for this patient was dampness in the Liver and Gallbladder, with Liver overacting on the Spleen and the Stomach, hence disrupting the transformation and transportation of the digestive system. The patient was treated with two herbal formulas (*Liver DTX* and *Imperial Tonic*) and two homeopathic formulas (sarcode liver formula and oral insulin). The treatment also included acupuncture involving meridian treatment and extraordinary vessel treatment. After three weeks, the patient had significant improvements in her vitality, complexion, appetite, sleep, attitude and energy level. A dramatic reduction of her abdominal pain was also noted. Her insulin use was reduced by approximately 25%.

I.B., Miami, Florida

A 22-year-old female presented with high triglycerides and high ALT. The patient appeared thin and pale. Her limbs were always cold and she was easily agitated. Her blood pressure was 115/70 mmHg and the heart rate was 72 beats per minute. The TCM diagnosis was yang deficiency with heat in the Liver. *Liver DTX* at 3 capsules three times a day was prescribed with *Cholisma* at 2 capsules twice a day. She also received acupuncture. After six weeks, her liver enzymes and triglycerides levels returned to normal.

W.F., Bloomfield, New Jersey

M.C., a 49-year-old male, presented with elevated SGPT levels (72, normal 0-40) but his medical doctor told him it was normal. At age 8, this patient suffered from a blood disorder called "Fatty Bone Marrow" with no hemoglobins. He was treated but the results were reported to be moderate in effectiveness. There was negative history for any liver disorders. His blood pressure was 120/72 mmHg and his heart rate was 62 beats per minute. The TCM diagnoses were Spleen qi deficiency and Liver qi stagnation. He was instructed to take 5 capsules of *Liver DTX* at bedtime for three months. After the herbs, the SGOT level reduced to 21 and the SGPT level to 32. The patient was thrilled.

M.H., West Palm Beach, Florida

A 36-year-old female patient presented with severe hangover from excessive alcohol consumption. Clinical signs and symptoms included nausea, vomiting, anorexia, frontal headache, diarrhea, and extreme weakness and fatigue. Her tongue was pale and flabby, with a moist, greasy tongue coating. Her face was pale and puffy, with dark, sunken eyes. The Western diagnosis was acute alcohol intoxication; the TCM diagnosis was damp-heat in the Liver and Gallbladder, with qi deficiency. *Liver DTX* was prescribed at four capsules every four to six hours for one day. Within two hours after taking the first dose, the patient reported that she felt 98% improvement, and said that she had regained her strength and appetite. She stated that her headache, nausea, vomiting and diarrhea had all diminished. She took the second dose, ate a large meal, and recovered from alcohol intoxication.

C.L., Chino Hills, California

M.F., a 57-year-old female, presented with pain in the leg and big toe with pressure, metallic taste, absence of thirst, heat sensations except in the hands and feet, and upper body sweating. She had been exposed to toxic chemicals and pesticides for six months. The TCM diagnosis was yin deficiency with heat, damp-heat and toxic heat accumulation, and *bi zheng* (painful obstruction syndrome) of the legs. After six weeks of taking *Liver DTX*, *Balance (Heat)* and *Flex (NP)*, she experienced less leg pain, decreased sweating, subsiding heat sensations, and warmer hands. The patient still had a metallic taste in the mouth. The patient also increased her intake of carrot juice and cucumbers.

M.C., Sarasota, Florida

FORMULAS

LIVER DTX ™

(Detoxification)

[1] Olin, B. et al. *The Lawrence Reviews of Natural Products by Facts and Comparisons*. Milk Thistle, January 1997

[2] Magliulo, E. et al. *Med Klin*; 73: 1060-65. 1978

[3] Cavalieri, S. *Gazz Med Ital*; 133: 628. 1974

[4] Trinchet, J. et al. *Gastroenterol Clin Biol*; 13 (2): 120-4. 1989

[5] Rumyatseva, Z. *Vrach Delo*; (5): 15-19. 1991

[6] Bensky, D. et al. *Chinese Herbal Medicine Formulas & Strategies*. Eastland Press. 1990

[7] Bensky, D. et al. *Chinese Herbal Medicine Materia Medica*. Eastland Press. 1993

[8] Condrault, JL. et al. *Planta Medica*; 29:247. 1980

[9] Sonnenbichler, J. et al. Proceedings of the International Bioflavonoid Symposium (Munich, Frg); 477. 1981

[10] Muzes, G. et al. *Orv Hetil*; 131 (16): 863-6. 1990

[11] Rui, Y. *Mem Inst Oswaldo Cruz*; 86 (Suppl) 2: 79-85. 1991

[12] Lang, I. et al. *Acta Med Hung*; 45 (3-4): 287-95. 1988

[13] Foster, S. Milk Thistle-Silybum Marianum, Botanical Series No. 305, Am. Botanical Council, Austin TX 1991; 3-7

[14] Floersheim, GL. *Medical Toxicology*; 2:1. 1987

[15] Rumyantseva, Z. *Vrach Delo*; (5): 15-19. 1991

[16] Olin, B, et al. *The Lawrence Reviews of Natural Products by Facts and Comparisons*. Grape Seed. Sep 1995

[17] Oshima, Y. et al. Dietary grape seed tannins: effects of nutritional balance on some enzymatic activities along the crypt-villus axis of rat small intestine. *Ann Nutr Metab*; 38(2):75. 1994

[18] Nagai, H. et al. *Planta Medica*. 55(1):13-17. 1989.

[19] Takeda, S. et al. *Nippon Yakurigaku Zasshi*. 88(4):321-30. 1986

[20] Chevallier, A. *Encyclopedia of Medicinal Plants*. New York, NY: DK Publishing. 1996

[21] Keung, WM. and Vallee, BL. Kudzu root: an ancient Chinese source of modern antidipsotropic agent. *Phytochemistry*. 47(4):499-506, Feb. 1998

FORMULAS

LONICERA COMPLEX ™

CLINICAL APPLICATIONS

- Viral infections: common cold, influenza, measles, oral herpes, cold sores, and fever blisters
- Bacterial infections: bronchitis, pneumonia
- Mild throat infections: sore throat

WESTERN THERAPEUTIC ACTIONS

- Herbal antibiotic: treats both viral and bacterial infections [1,2,3,5,6]
- Antiviral properties: reduces the severity and duration of viral infections [1,3,10]
- Antibacterial properties: reduces the severity and duration of bacterial infections [1,2,4,9]
- Enhances the immune system [1,8]

CHINESE THERAPEUTIC ACTIONS

- Clears wind-heat
- Eliminates fire and heat toxins from the upper *jiao*
- Benefits the throat

DOSAGE

For treatment of viral or bacterial infections, take 4 capsules three times daily on an empty stomach with warm water. Begin herbal treatment with the first sign of viral or bacterial infection and continue for one to two weeks or until symptoms resolve. To shorten the duration of infection, take 6 capsules four times daily until symptoms resolve.

INGREDIENTS

Ban Lan Gen (Radix Isatidis)
Bo He (Herba Menthae)
Da Qing Ye (Folium Isatidis)
Dan Dou Chi (Semen Sojae Praeparatum)
Dan Zhu Ye (Herba Lophatheri)
Echinacea Angustifolia
Gan Cao (Radix Glycyrrhizae)
Jie Geng (Radix Platycodonis)
Jin Yin Hua (Flos Lonicerae)

Jing Jie (Herba Schizonepetae)
Lian Qiao (Fructus Forsythiae)
Lu Gen (Rhizoma Phragmitis)
Lysine
Niu Bang Zi (Fructus Arctii)
Pu Gong Ying (Herba Taraxaci)
Ye Ju Hua (Flos Chrysanthemi Indici)
Zi Hua Di Ding (Herba Violae)

FORMULA EXPLANATION

Lonicera Complex is an herbal formula designed to treat the early stages of bacterial or viral infections. It contains herbs with antibacterial and antiviral functions to treat infections such common cold, influenza, oral herpes, pneumonia, bronchitis, chicken pox, measles, tonsillitis, and pharyngitis.

Lian Qiao (Fructus Forsythiae) and *Jin Yin Hua* (Flos Lonicerae) are the principle herbs in this formula. They have a broad spectrum of antibacterial and antiviral functions. *Jing Jie* (Herba Schizonepetae), *Dan Dou Chi* (Semen Sojae Praeparatum) and *Bo He* (Herba Menthae) relieve exterior pathogenic wind. *Niu Bang Zi* (Fructus Arctii) and *Ban Lan Gen* (Radix Isatidis) clear heat and treat acute tonsillitis. *Dan Zhu Ye* (Herba Lophatheri) and *Lu Gen* (Rhizoma Phragmitis) clear heat, generate body fluids and relieve thirst. *Ye Ju Hua* (Flos

LONICERA COMPLEX ™

Chrysanthemi Indici), *Da Qing Ye* (Folium Isatidis), *Pu Gong Ying* (Herba Taraxaci), *Zi Hua Di Ding* (Herba Violae), and echinacea are antibacterial and antiviral herbs which clear toxic heat and treat infections. *Jie Geng* (Radix Platycodonis) dispels phlegm, lysine reduces the duration of oral herpes outbreaks, and *Gan Cao* (Radix Glycyrrhizae) harmonizes the formula.

SUPPLEMENTARY FORMULAS

- To enhance the overall antibiotic function, add *Herbal ABX*.
- To treat infection of ear, nose and throat, add *Herbal ENT*.
- To treat cough, add *Respitrol (CF)*.
- For respiratory infection with sore throat, fever, dyspnea, chest discomfort, use *Respitrol (Heat)*.
- To treat cold type respiratory disorders with chills, clear nasal discharge, sneezing, nasal congestion, use *Respitrol (Cold)*.
- For respiratory infection in patients with deficiency, add *Respitrol (Deficient)*.
- For upper respiratory infection with profuse, yellow, thick sputum, combine with *Poria XPT*.
- For sinusitis or rhinitis with yellow nasal discharge, use *Pueraria Clear Sinus*.
- For sinusitis or rhinitis with clear nasal discharge, use *Magnolia Clear Sinus*.
- For tonsillitis with swelling, add *Resolve (AI)*.
- For stomach flu with diarrhea, add *GI Care II*.
- *Immune* + can be used on a regular basis to strengthen the immune system and prevent bacterial or viral infections. However, *Immune* + should only be used after symptoms of cold and flu have completely subsided.
- For headache, add *Corydalin* or *Migratrol*.
- For high fever, add *Gardenia Complex*.
- For chicken pox with severe itching, add *Silerex*.
- For shingles, add *Dermatrol (HZ)*.

NUTRITION

- For treatment of common cold or influenza, always drink plenty of water, juice, soup, and tea as they can help flush out the body and prevent dehydration. At least 6 to 8 glasses of water per day is recommended.
- Vitamin C is well recognized for its effect to prevent and treat common colds and influenza. Foods high in vitamin C, such as oranges, are strongly recommended.
- Vitamin A, a vital nutrient for the mucous membranes throughout the respiratory system, should also be consumed in adequate quantity. Foods rich in vitamin A include raw fruits and vegetables, such as carrots.
- To avoid infection, a diet high in garlic and onions is recommended as these two foods contain natural antibiotic effect.
- Phlegm-producing foods such as sweets, dairy products, and heavy or greasy foods are not recommended.

The Tao of Nutrition by Ni and McNease
- Common cold (wind-heat)
  - Recommendations: mint, cabbage, chrysanthemum flowers, burdock root, cilantro, dandelion, apples, appears, and bitter melon. Drink plenty of fluids and lots of rest
  - Avoid shellfish, meats, vinegar, drafts, hot foods.
- Oral herpes or mouth sores
  - Recommendations: mung beans, daikon, carrots, lotus root, persimmon caps, mint, and honeysuckle flower.
  - Avoid spicy foods, stimulating foods, smoking, stress, alcohol, coffee, and chocolate.

LONICERA COMPLEX ™

❧ Sore throat
  ▪ Recommendations: carrots, olives, daikon, celery, seaweed, licorice, Chinese prunes, cilantro, and mint. Drink a lot of water and gargle with warm salt water.
  ▪ Avoid alcohol, smoking, pollution, sleeping with the mouth open, stimulating or spicy foods, and fatty foods.
❧ For more information, please refer to *The Tao of Nutrition* by Dr. Maoshing Ni and Cathy McNease.

LIFESTYLE INSTRUCTIONS

❧ Adequate rest is essential for recovery. Avoid exposure to wind by putting on more clothing. Covering the head and neck area is especially important. Fluctuation of temperature increases the risk of bacterial and viral infection. Installation of an air purifier is recommended for patients who repeatedly catch infectious respiratory disorders.
❧ Patients should be advised to stop smoking and drinking.
❧ It is recommended to take a hot shower or bath after taking the herbs to promote the diaphoretic function. Warm temperature burns up and destroys the viruses. Low body temperature decreases resistance to viruses and bacteria.
❧ Steam inhalation heals the throat, nasal passages, and bronchial tubes. During the acute phase, inhale the steam vapor for 15 minutes three times daily. During the chronic phase, inhale the steam vapor for 15 minutes before going to bed.
❧ It is important to build up a strong immune system prior to the cold and flu season. Regular exercise, short cold shower following a hot shower, and ingestion of tonic herbs are all beneficial to strengthen the body and its immune system.
❧ Individuals with an infection should rest and recover in a separate room to prevent spreading germs to other people. Ventilate the room frequently – but make sure the patient is kept warm.
❧ Patients with oral herpes should stay away from heat, UV rays, over-exertion, stress, spicy or greasy foods, seafood, or anything that may trigger an attack. Conversely, they are advised to eat plenty of vegetables or fruits that are cold in nature (cucumber, pear, watermelon, tomatoes) and yogurt. Replacement of toothbrush is also recommended as some herpes virus may linger on the bristles.

CLINICAL NOTES

❧ To enhance immunity in patients who are susceptible to catching colds, take *Immune* + at a low dose (1 to 2 capsules a day) prior to the flu season.
❧ *Lonicera Complex* is derived from classic formula *Yin Qiao San* (Honeysuckle and Forsythia Powder). However, the classic formula has two major limitations. First, it is more specific for viral infections. Second, because of the long-term use, many pathogens have developed resistance to the formula. Therefore, *Lonicera Complex* is formulated with additional herbs to treat both viral and bacterial infections, and to boost the overall antibiotic effect of the formula. For patients with infections that do not respond to the classic formulas, *Lonicera Complex* will often provide good clinical results.
❧ For prevention of viral or bacterial infections, take *Immune* + on an empty stomach with warm water .

CAUTIONS

❧ *Lonicera Complex* is designed for patients with wind-heat attacks. Should the patient experience wind-cold symptoms such as clear nasal discharge, headache, or chills, use *Respitrol (Cold)* instead.
❧ Patients with encephalitis or menigitis should be sent to the emergency room for immediate medical treatment. Warning signs and symptoms of encephalitis or menigitis include fever, headache, stiff neck, sore throat, vomiting, and mental confusion. In addition to soreness, the stiffness is also characterized by

FORMULAS

severe pain with gentle taps to the neck, and extreme stiffness and immobility when the patient tries to lower the chin to the chest.

ACUPUNCTURE POINTS

Traditional Points:
- *Quchi* (LI 11), *Fengchi* (GB 20), *Chize* (LU 5), *Hegu* (LI 4), and *Dazhui* (GV 14).

Balance Method by Dr. Richard Tan:
- Left side: *Yuji* (LU 10), *Taiyuan* (LU 9), *Hegu* (LI 4), and *Yangxi* (LI 5).
- Right Side: *Yuji* (LU 10), *Taiyuan* (LU 9), *Hegu* (LI 4), *Yangxi* (LI 5), *Taichong* (LR 3), and *Neiting* (ST 44).
- Left and right side can be alternated from treatment to treatment.
- For additional information on the Balance Method, please refer to *Dr. Tan's Strategy of Twelve Magical Points* by Dr. Richard Tan.

Ear Points:
- Nose, Pharynx, Bronchi, and Adrenal Gland. Needle for thirty minutes or embed needles on the points and switch ears every three days. Patient should be advised to press on the points three times daily for one to two minutes each time.
- Acute tonsillitis: Bleed the protruding vein in the back of the ear, and apex of the tragus once a day. Needle and strongly stimulate the Throat, Pharynx and Tonsils.

Auricular Acupuncture by Dr. Li-Chun Huang:
- Common cold: Lung, Internal Nose, Throat (Larynx, Pharynx)
  - For fever, bleed Ear Apex and Helix 1-6
  - For dizziness, add Dizziness Area
  - For pain and soreness all over the body, add Liver, Spleen; bleed Helix 4
  - For cough, add Trachea, Bronchus, Stop Asthma
- Recurrent ulcerative stomatitis: Corresponding points (to the area of pain), Lower Palate, Upper Palate, Tongue, *San Jiao*, Mouth, Spleen, and Allergic Area. Bleed Ear Apex.
- For additional information on the location and explanation of these points, please refer to *Auricular Treatment Formula and Prescriptions* by Dr. Li-Chun Huang.

MODERN RESEARCH

Lonicera Complex is an excellent formula to treat mild to moderate cases of bacterial and viral infections. It consists of herbs that have antibacterial and antiviral activities as verified by the following studies.

Jin Yin Hua (Flos Lonicerae) is one of the most effective herbal antibiotics in the Chinese pharmacopoeia. It has a wide spectrum of antibacterial and antiviral activities. Its antibacterial activities include a strong inhibitory effect against *salmonella, pseudomonas, staphylococcus* and *streptococcus*.[1] In a research study, *Jin Yin Hua* (Flos Lonicerae) was found to inhibit the growth of up to 73.9% of common oral pathogens.[2] In addition, it has a strong inhibitory effect against the influenza and HIV viruses.[1,3]

Lian Qiao (Fructus Forsythiae) has a wide spectrum of antibacterial activities similar to *Jin Yin Hua* (Flos Lonicerae). It is most effective for treating infections due to *Shigella dysenteriae, Staphylococcus aureus, streptococcus, pneumococcus,* and other species.[1,4]

FORMULAS

LONICERA COMPLEX ™

Echinacea is an herb indigenous to the central United States and has been used since the 1800's for its anti-infectious properties.[5] Echinacea enhances the immune response by stimulating phagocytosis, increasing cellular respiratory activity, and increasing the mobility of leukocytes.[6] In addition, echinacea induces macrophages to produce tumor necrosis factors, and increases the production of interleukin and interferon. This makes echinacea extremely valuable in treating tumors and infectious diseases particularly in immuno-compromised patients.[7]

Ban Lan Gen (Radix Isatidis) and *Da Qing Ye* (Folium Isatidis) are derived from different parts of the same plant and have immuno-stimulating and antimicrobial activities. It was demonstrated in one research study that *Ban Lan Gen* (Radix Isatidis) and *Da Qing Ye* (Folium Isatidis) enhance humoral and cellular immune functions by increasing the number of white blood cells and lymphocytes in blood circulation.[8] Another study showed that they are helpful in treating patients with chronic lung infections, such as *Pseudomonas aeruginosa* infection in patients with cystic fibrosis of the lungs.[9] Lastly, lysine is used for its effect to suppress recurrent herpes simplex infection.[10]

PHARMACEUTICAL DRUGS & CHINESE MEDICINE: A COMPARATIVE ANALYSIS

Western Medical Approach: Discovery of antibiotic drugs is one of the major breakthroughs in modern medicine. It enables doctors to effectively treat many different types of infections. Unfortunately, decades of abuse and misuse have led to growing problems of bacterial mutation and resistance. One of the key problems is the use of these antibacterial drugs to treat viral infections. These drugs are offer nothing but placebo effect, as they are completely useless in treating virus infection. Despite all the advances in western medicine, there is still no cure for the common cold, and the best treatment is still rest and water.

Traditional Chinese Medicine Approach: Herbs are also extremely effective for treatment of various infections. In fact, most modern pharmaceutical drugs were originally derived from natural sources, including penicillin [the oldest antibiotic] and gentimicin [one of the most potent]. One of the main benefits of using herbs is their wide spectrum of antibiotic effect, with indications for bacterial, viral and fungal infections. Furthermore, most of these herbs are extremely safe, and do not have the same harsh side effects as drugs.

Summation: Those who have a viral infection, such as common cold or influenza, should not be treated with antibiotic drugs since they are useless. Other drugs may be used, but only for symptomatic control. On the other hand, use of herbs is very effective, as they suppress replication of the virus, and reduce the duration of the infections. Furthermore, additional herbs may be prescribed to address the symptoms, such as nasal congestion, sore throat, cough, etc. Most importantly, herbs are much gentler to the body and safer than the drugs. In other words, use of herbs treats infection without damaging the underlying constitution of the patient. This allows the patient to recover faster, and become more resistant to secondary or re-current infections.

CASE STUDIES

F.L. is a 53-year-old female with a history of oral herpes that often began with tingling sensations of the lips that progressed to burning sensations and eruption of fever blisters lasting two to three weeks. Occasionally, an outbreak was associated with eruption of additional lesions. The patient was given specific instructions to begin taking *Lonicera Complex* at the initial onset of symptoms, at three capsules, three times daily. During a follow-up visit, the patient reported that *Lonicera Complex* was extremely effective—it stopped the exacerbation of oral blisters, there was no return of lesions, and no spread of lesions to other areas. The affected area on the lips simply changed to a small painless scab that healed quickly.

C.L., Chino Hills, California

LONICERA COMPLEX ™

A 33-year-old female presented with localized burning pain on her upper lip. The patient had a history of cold sores due to herpes simplex I. At the time, the practitioner classified the condition as wind-heat invasion. Once any signs of a cold sore outbreak could be sensed, *Lonicera Complex* was taken immediately. In addition to the herbal formula, a topical application of *San Huang Xie Xin Tang* (Three-Yellow Decoction to Sedate the Epigastrium) was supplemented. Unlike the previous resolution time of 14 days or longer, the cold sore disappeared within a total of 5 days, which was a significant improvement in recovery time. On a follow-up visit several months later, the patient noticed warning signs of a cold sore, and began taking *Lonicera Complex* without delay. After the *Lonicera Complex* treatment, the cold sore never presented itself. The practitioner concluded that the herbal formula was quite effective for prevention of cold sores.

S.A., Santa Fe, New Mexico

A robustly healthy female presented with flu symptoms. She had a sore throat and yellow mucus. The practitioner diagnosed her condition as wind-heat. In conjunction with acupuncture treatment, the practitioner also had the patient utilize a vaporizer for steaming her face. *Lonicera Complex* and *Pueraria Clear Sinus* worked quite effectively after taking them for 3 to 4 days at larger dosages. The practitioner also noted that *Pu Ji Xiao Du Yin* (Universal Benefit Decoction to Eliminate Toxin) could be used if the condition were more severe and had presence of heat and toxins.

S.C., La Crescenta, California

A 53-year-old female presented with a common cold. She had the typical cold symptoms such as headaches, sore throat, fever and a stiff neck. The practitioner diagnosed the condition as an upper respiratory tract infection due to wind-heat attack. *Lonicera Complex* was instantly administered. The following morning, her symptoms reduced dramatically. Within four days, almost all symptoms had abated. The practitioner stated that *Lonicera Complex* was quite effective in the treatment of common cold conditions.

S.K., Beverly Hills, California

A 28-year-old female on a one-day course of antibiotic treatment was recovering from strep throat. She had chills, fever and a sore throat. She was diagnosed with wind-heat invasion, which was indicative of her feverish complexion, red throat and rapid pulse. The practitioner recommended *Lonicera Complex*. Within one day, the patient felt her sore throat and pain reduced. By the end of the 5th day, her symptoms were totally diminished.

S.A., Santa Fe, New Mexico

M.M., a 41-year-old female, presented with sinus infection and frontal pain, sore throat, post-nasal drip and fatigue. The TCM diagnosis was wind-heat invasion. Within one or two days of beginning to take three capsules of *Lonicera Complex*, three times daily, the patient reported most symptoms resolved. This patient now uses *Lonicera Complex* whenever she feels early signs of infection. She reports that this stops the progress of symptoms.

C.L., Chino Hills, California

[1] Bensky, D. et al. *Chinese Herbal Medicine Materia Medica*. Eastland Press. 1993
[2] Sun, Y. et al. Antimicrobial properties of flos lonicerae against oral pathogens. *China Journal of Chinese Material Medica*. 21(4):242-3 *Inside Backcover*, Apr. 1996
[3] Chang, CW. et al. *Antiviral Res*. August 1995
[4] Yeung, HC. Handbook of Chinese Herbs. *Institute of Chinese Medicine*. 1996
[5] Tyler, VE. *The New Honest Herbal*. Philadelphia: GF Stickley Co., 1987
[6] Bauer, VR. et al. Immunologic in vivo and in vitro studies on echinacea extracts. Arzneimittelforschung;38(2):276. 1988

LONICERA COMPLEX ™

[7] Steinmuller, C. et al. Polysaccharides isolated from plant cell cultures of echinacea purpurea enhance the resistance of immuno-suppressed mice against systemic infections with Candida albicans and Listeria monocytogenes. *Int J Immunopharmacol*; 15(5):605. 1993

[8] Xu, YM and Lu, PC. Experimental studies on immuno-stimulatory effects of the Isatis indigotica polysaccharide. *Chung his I Chieh Ho Tsa Chih*, 11(6):357-9' 325-6 Jun. 1991

[9] Song, Z. et al. Effects of Chinese medicinal herbs on a rat model of chronic pseudomonas aeruginosa lung infection.

[10] Flodin, NW. *Journal of American Collective Nutrition*. February 1997

FORMULAS

LPS SUPPORT ™

CLINICAL APPLICATIONS

- Systemic lupus erythematosus (SLE), lupus
- Lupus with inflammation in joints, tendons, and other connective tissues and organs
- Lupus with arthritis, mouth sores, skin rash, facial rash, hair loss, depression, fever and/or sunlight sensitivity, extreme fatigue, joint pain, muscle pain and weakness, anemia, malar flush, headache, general malaise, and in severe cases, destruction of vital organs. Some people will show only a few symptoms, some may have them all.

WESTERN THERAPEUTIC ACTIONS

- Inhibits and suppresses the growth and multiplications of cells
- Anti-inflammatory effect to reduce swelling and inflammation

CHINESE THERAPEUTIC ACTIONS

- Clears heat
- Eliminates toxins
- Nourishes yin, tonifies blood, and promotes generation of body fluids

DOSAGE

Take 4 to 6 capsules three times daily. For acute recurrences, the dosage may be increased to 6 capsules four times daily.

INGREDIENTS

Bai Hua She She Cao (Herba Oldenlandia)
Ban Zhi Lian (Herba Scutellariae Barbatae)
Chi Shao (Radix Paeoniae Rubrae)
Han Lian Cao (Herba Ecliptae)
Hong Hua (Flos Carthami)
Ji Xiang Teng (Caulis Paederiae)
Jin Yin Hua (Flos Lonicerae)
Lian Qiao (Fructus Forsythiae)

Mu Dan Pi (Cortex Moutan)
Sheng Di Huang (Radix Rehmanniae)
Tao Ren (Semen Persicae)
Xuan Shen (Radix Scrophulariae)
Ye Ju Hua (Flos Chrysanthemi Indici)
Zhi Mu (Radix Anemarrhenae)
Zi Cao Gen (Radix Lithospermi)

FORMULA EXPLANATION

From traditional Chinese medicine perspective, lupus is a condition characterized by both excess and deficiency. Excess represents the inflammatory conditions of the body, with such symptoms as arthritis, mouth sores, skin rash, facial rash, and sunlight sensitivity. Deficiency represents the fundamental and underlying weakness, such as anemia, and dysfunction of the kidney, nerves or brain.

Most young girls suffering from lupus will show signs of excess heat in the blood level. Middle-aged women with lupus exhibit symptoms of chronic low-grade fever with exacerbation of symptoms upon exertion and tidal fever, flushed cheeks, petechiae spots on the skin, leg and heel pain, weakness of the limbs, night sweats, hair loss and thready and rapid pulse. Therefore, optimal treatment of lupus requires use of herbs to treat both the excess and the deficiency.

Sheng Di Huang (Radix Rehmanniae), *Chi Shao* (Radix Paeoniae Rubrae), *Mu Dan Pi* (Cortex Moutan), *Zhi Mu* (Radix Anemarrhenae) and *Xuan Shen* (Radix Scrophulariae) clear heat and cool the blood to treat the fever, mouth

FORMULAS

sores and skin lesions. *Jin Yin Hua* (Flos Lonicerae), *Lian Qiao* (Fructus Forsythiae), *Zi Cao Gen* (Radix Lithospermi), *Ye Ju Hua* (Flos Chrysanthemi Indici), *Bai Hua She She Cao* (Herba Oldenlandia) and *Ban Zhi Lian* (Herba Scutellariae Barbatae) are added to clear heat, eliminate toxins and relieve inflammation. *Tao Ren* (Semen Persicae) and *Hong Hua* (Flos Carthami) activate blood circulation and eliminate blood stasis to relieve pain, and deliver the formula to the affected parts of the body. To nourish yin, tonify blood and promote the generation of body fluids, herbs such as *Sheng Di Huang* (Radix Rehmanniae), *Han Lian Cao* (Herba Ecliptae), *Xuan Shen* (Radix Scrophulariae), and *Mu Dan Pi* (Cortex Moutan) are used. *Ji Xiang Teng* (Caulis Paederiae) is used to relieve pain. By nourishing the body, symptoms of extreme fatigue, joint pain, muscle aches, anemia, and general malaise can be alleviated.

Overall, *LPS Support* is a balanced formula to address both the excess and the deficient aspects of lupus. However, lupus is a complicated disorder with a wide variety of symptoms and severities. Therefore, additional formulas are often needed to address related symptoms and complications, as stated in the Supplementary Formulas section.

SUPPLEMENTARY FORMULAS

- With facial or skin rash, combine with *Silerex* or *Dermatrol (PS)*.
- With mouth sores, use *Lonicera Complex* as a mouthwash and gargle with it for 5 minutes three times daily.
- With arthritis, combine with *Flex (Heat)* or *Flex (CD)*.
- With nerve dysfunction, combine with *Flex (NP)*.
- With kidney dysfunction or scanty yellow urination, combine with *Kidney DTX*.
- With low white or red blood cell count, combine with *Imperial Tonic*.
- With exterior wind-heat condition, add *Lonicera Complex*.
- With cough, add *Respitrol (CF)*.
- With constipation, add *Gentle Lax (Excess)* or *Gentle Lax (Deficient)*.
- With high fever, add *Gardenia Complex*.
- With thirst, add *Nourish (Fluids)*.
- With Kidney yin deficiency manifesting chronic low-grade fever, flushed cheeks, body pain, purpura, add *Balance (Heat)* and *Nourish*.
- With intermittent pulse, palpitation, anemia and pale complexion, add *Schisandra ZZZ*.
- In extreme severe cases where there is also yang deficiency, add *Kidney Tonic (Yang)*.
- With back pain, add *Back Support (Acute)*.
- With signs of mania, delirious speech, twitching of muscles, add *Zhen Gan Xi Feng Tang* (Sedate the Liver and Extinguish Wind Decoction) or *Da Ding Feng Zhu* (Major Arrest Wind Pearl).
- With jaundice, add *Yin Chen Hao Tang* (Artemisia Scoparia Decoction).

NUTRITION

- Adequate intake of calcium and magnesium is important, as they are necessary for pH balance and protection against bone loss.
- L-cysteine, L-methionine and L-lysine are important in skin formation and cellular protection and preservation.
- Diet low in fat, salt and animal protein is less stressful to the kidneys. It also keeps the immune system from becoming overly reactive.
- Foods that contain sulfur, such as eggs, garlic and onions are essential for the repair and rebuilding of bones, cartilages and connective tissues.
- Avoid caffeine, citrus fruits, salt, tobacco and foods that contain sugar.
- Raw, cold, greasy and salty foods are contraindicated.
- Barley, mung bean, mushrooms, lotus nodes, honey, soybean and duck are recommended.

FORMULAS

LPS SUPPORT ™

LIFESTYLE INSTRUCTIONS

- Get an adequate amount of rest and exercise regularly to promote muscle tone and fitness.
- Use hypoallergenic soaps, lotions and cosmetics.

CLINICAL NOTES

- Lupus may develop after taking certain prescription medications. Symptoms generally disappear after the drug is discontinued.
- According to New England Journal of Medicine, up to 10% of lupus cases are related to drug reactions. Therefore, drugs that are most likely to cause lupus should be avoided, such as Apresoline (Hydralazine) and Procan (Procainamide). Certain birth control pills may also cause lupus to flare-up.

CAUTION

- The main emphasis of this formula is to use herbs to clear heat, eliminate toxins, and control the autoimmune and inflammatory conditions of lupus. Therefore, it contains many bitter and cold herbs, which may consume qi and yin. If the patient shows more signs and symptoms of such deficiencies, additional herbs and formulas should be given to strengthen the underlying constitutions. *See* Supplementary Formula section for details.

ACUPUNCTURE POINTS

Balance Method by Dr. Richard Tan:
Treatment plan one:
- Right side: *Hegu* (LI 4), *Houxi* (SI 3), *Zhongzhu* (TH 3), *Sanyinjiao* (SP 6), *Zhongfeng* (LR 4), and *Taixi* (KI 3).
- Left side: *Shaoshang* (LU 11), *Zhongchong* (PC 9), *Shaochong* (HT 9), *Zusanli* (ST 36), *Yanglingquan* (GB 34), and *Weizhong* (BL 40).

Treatment plan two:
- Right side: *Shaoshang* (LU 11), *Zhongchong* (PC 9), *Shaochong* (HT 9), *Zusanli* (ST 36), *Yanglingquan* (GB 34), and *Weizhong* (BL 40).
- Left side: *Hegu* (LI 4), *Houxi* (SI 3), *Zhongzhu* (TH 3), *Sanyinjiao* (SP 6), *Zhongfeng* (LR 4), and *Sanjian* (LI 3).
- For additional information on the Balance Method, please refer to *Dr. Tan's Strategy of Twelve Magical Points* by Dr. Richard Tan.

Auricular Acupuncture by Dr. Li-Chun Huang:
- Lupus erythematosus: Corresponding point (to the affected area), Kidney, Liver, Spleen, Lung, Endocrine, Allergic Area, *San Jiao*, and Adrenal Gland. Bleed Ear Apex.
- For additional information on the location and explanation of these points, please refer to *Auricular Treatment Formula and Prescriptions* by Dr. Li-Chun Huang.

MODERN RESEARCH

Systemic lupus erythematosus (SLE), simply referred to as lupus, is a complicated autoimmune disorder that results in episodes of inflammation in joints, tendons, and other connective tissues and organs. It is complicated because the symptoms and their severity can differ drastically from person to person, ranging from mild to disabling to fatal. This formula contains many herbs with various actions: some address the autoimmune aspect of lupus by suppressing the multiplication of cells; others alleviate the symptoms of inflammation, rash, and dysfunction of the organs.

LPS SUPPORT ™

LPS Support incorporates many herbs that inhibit and suppress the growth and multiplication of cells to address the autoimmune aspect of lupus. Herbs with this therapeutic effect include *Zi Cao Gen* (Radix Lithospermi),[1] *Bai Hua She She Cao* (Herba Oldenlandia),[2] and *Ban Zhi Lian* (Herba Scutellariae Barbatae).[3] By controlling the autoimmune aspect of lupus, these herbs help to control the underlying cause of the illness.

LPS Support also uses many herbs specifically to control the inflammatory symptoms of lupus. Many herbs in this formula have marked anti-inflammatory effect, including but not limited to *Sheng Di Huang* (Radix Rehmanniae),[4] *Zi Cao Gen* (Radix Lithospermi),[5] *Mu Dan Pi* (Cortex Moutan),[6] *Tao Ren* (Semen Persicae),[7] and *Jin Yin Hua* (Flos Lonicerae).[8] The exact mechanisms of these herbs differ, but have been attributed in part to inhibition of prostaglandin synthesis and subsequent reduction of swelling and inflammation.[9,10]

With regards to clinical applications, many herbs in this formula have shown excellent results to treat related symptoms and illnesses of lupus, including but not limited to arthritis, skin disorders, and dysfunction of the internal organs. According to one study, use of *Zi Cao Gen* (Radix Lithospermi) in one formula has been associated with 71.4% rate of effectiveness to treat 56 patients with acute-onset rheumatism.[11] Use of *Sheng Di Huang* (Radix Rehmanniae) was effective in treating 23 patients with rheumatoid arthritis.[12] For skin disorders, numerous herbs have been used for multiple indications, such as *Sheng Di Huang* (Radix Rehmanniae) for rashes and urticaria,[13] and *Zi Cao Gen* (Radix Lithospermi) for psoriasis and measles.[14,15] Lastly, use of *Lian Qiao* (Fructus Forsythiae) in herbal formulas has been shown to be effective to treat nephropathy.[16]

In summary, lupus is a complicated disorder, as it is an autoimmune disorder that affects multiple areas of the body, leading to different symptoms of various severities. *LPS Support* integrates principles of traditional Chinese medicine and western medicine, to address both the cause and the main symptoms of lupus.

PHARMACEUTICAL DRUGS & CHINESE MEDICINE: A COMPARATIVE ANALYSIS

Systemic lupus erythematosus (SLE) is an illness that poses great challenge for both western and traditional Chinese medicines. It is quite challenging to manage lupus because the cause of the disease has not yet been clearly identified, and the illness may be complicated by its effect on tissues and organs in the body.

Western Medical Approach: Drug treatments for lupus focus mainly on relieving the symptoms. Mild to moderate lupus is managed by use of non-steroidal anti-inflammatory agents (NSAID) to relieve pain and reduce inflammation. These drugs, however, may cause such serious side effects as gastric ulcer, duodenal ulcer, gastrointestinal bleeding, tinnitus, blurred vision, dizziness and headache. Severe lupus is treated with corticosteroids, such as prednisone and immunosuppressant drugs. Both of these medications, however, have very serious side effects and must be use with extreme caution.

Traditional Chinese Medicine Approach: Heat-clearing herbs manage both the symptoms and the cause of lupus. These herbs have been shown to have analgesic effect to relieve pain and anti-inflammatory effect to reduce swelling and inflammation. Furthermore, certain herbs are also effective to suppress the immune system and help to control the auto-immune aspect of lupus.

Summation: Lupus is a challenging illness that has no cure, but may be managed with drugs and/or herbs. Drugs effectively suppress symptoms, but do not change the progress of illness or the underlying condition of the patients. Herbs help to manage symptoms and control the underlying cause of the illness. Both options should be explored to identify the most effective treatment.

[1] *Zhong Xi Yi Jie He Za Zhi* (Journal of Integrated Chinese and Western Medicine), 1990; 10(7):422
[2] *Zhong Yao Xue* (Chinese Herbology), 1998; 204
[3] *Ren Min Wei Sheng Chu Ban She* (Journal of People's Public Health), 1988; 302
[4] *Zhong Yao Yao Li Yu Ying Yong* (Pharmacology and Applications of Chinese Herbs), 1983; 400

FORMULAS

LPS SUPPORT ™

[5] *Zhong Yao Xue* (Chinese Herbology), 1998; 164:167

[6] *Sheng Yao Xue Za Zhi* (Journal of Raw Herbology), 1979; 33(3):178

[7] *Zhong Yao Tong Bao* (Journal of Chinese Herbology), 1986; 11(11):37

[8] *Shan Xi Yi Kan* (Shanxi Journal of Medicine), 1960; (10):22

[9] *Ke Yan Tong Xun* (Journal of Science and Research), 1982; (3):35

[10] *Zhong Guo Yao Ke Da Xue Xue Bao* (Journal of University of Chinese Herbology), 1990; 21(4):222

[11] *Ji Lin Zhong Yi Yao* (Jilin Chinese Medicine and Herbology), 1992; (1):16

[12] *Tian Jing Yi Xue Za Zhi* (Journal of Tianjing Medicine and Herbology), 1966; 3:209

[13] *Tian Jing Yi Xue Za Zhi* (Journal of Tianjing Medicine and Herbology), 1966; 3:209

[14] *Zhong Hua Pi Fu Ke Xue Za Zhi* (Chinese Journal of Dermatology), 1981; 1:40

[15] *Zhong Yao Xue* (Chinese Herbology), 1998; 164:167

[16] *Jiang Xi Yi Yao* (Jiangxi Medicine and Herbology), 1961; 7:18

MAGNOLIA CLEAR SINUS ™

CLINICAL APPLICATIONS

- ❧ Sinusitis and/or rhinitis
- ❧ Sinus pain and headache
- ❧ Seasonal allergies, especially in the winter and spring
- ❧ General nasal problems, such as stuffy nose, sneezing, loss of smell, clear watery nasal discharge, etc.

WESTERN THERAPEUTIC ACTIONS

- ❧ Constricts the vessels in the nasal mucosa to treat sinusitis and rhinitis [1,2]
- ❧ Reduces nasal mucous secretions
- ❧ Desensitizes the patients from allergens to prevent seasonal allergies [1,2]

CHINESE THERAPEUTIC ACTIONS

- ❧ Unblocks nasal congestion and disperses wind-cold
- ❧ Transforms congested fluids
- ❧ Warms the Lung

DOSAGE

For treatment of sinusitis or rhinitis, take 4 to 6 capsules with warm water three times daily between meals. For prevention, begin taking 3 capsules three times daily just prior to the start of allergy season.

INGREDIENTS

Bai Zhi (Radix Angelicae Dahuricae)
Cang Er Zi (Fructus Xanthii)
Che Qian Cao (Herba Plantaginis)
Chuan Xiong (Rhizoma Ligustici Chuanxiong)
Fang Feng (Radix Saposhnikoviae)
Gan Cao (Radix Glycyrrhizae)
Gan Jiang (Rhizoma Zingiberis)
Gao Ben (Rhizoma Ligustici)

Jie Geng (Radix Platycodonis)
Jing Jie (Herba Schizonepetae)
Lu Cha (Folium Camellia Sinensis)
Sheng Ma (Rhizoma Cimicifugae)
Wu Wei Zi (Fructus Schisandrae Chinensis)
Xin Yi Hua (Flos Magnoliae)
Zhi Shi (Fructus Aurantii Immaturus)

FORMULA EXPLANATION

Magnolia Clear Sinus is formulated to treat allergies, sinusitis or rhinitis due to wind-cold and fluid congestion. Clinically, patients will have a stuffy nose, clear watery discharge, sneezing, loss of smell and headache.

Xin Yi Hua (Flos Magnoliae) unblocks nasal congestion and treats loss of smell with its pungent, dispersing and warming properties. *Cang Er Zi* (Fructus Xanthii) helps *Xin Yi Hua* (Flos Magnoliae) to relieve allergy symptoms of sneezing, white watery nasal discharge, and/or nasal obstruction. *Bai Zhi* (Radix Angelicae Dahuricae), *Gao Ben* (Rhizoma Ligustici), and *Chuan Xiong* (Rhizoma Ligustici Chuanxiong) are used to alleviate sinus pain and headache. *Gan Jiang* (Rhizoma Zingiberis) warms the interior, transforms congested fluids and dispels nasal congestion. *Jing Jie* (Herba Schizonepetae) and *Fang Feng* (Radix Saposhnikoviae) expel lingering pathogenic factors and prevent allergies from turning into a cold or triggering an asthma attack. With its ascending property, *Sheng Ma* (Rhizoma Cimicifugae) is used as a guiding herb. *Che Qian Cao* (Herba Plantaginis) drains nasal obstruction and postnasal drip caused by dampness and water congestion through diuresis. *Zhi Shi* (Fructus Aurantii

FORMULAS

MAGNOLIA CLEAR SINUS ™

Immaturus) unblocks sinus congestion by regulating qi, while *Jie Geng* (Radix Platycodonis) dispels phlegm, expands the chest, and relieves constipation. To counter-balance the strong dispersing property of this formula, a small amount of *Wu Wei Zi* (Fructus Schisandrae Chinensis) is added to prevent the leakage of Lung qi. *Lu Cha* (Folium Camellia Sinensis) is used to relieve sinus headaches commonly associated with sinus congestion. Lastly, *Gan Cao* (Radix Glycyrrhizae) harmonizes the formula.

SUPPLEMENTARY FORMULAS

- For infection of the ear, nose and throat, add **Herbal ENT**.
- With cough, add **Respitrol (CF)**.
- To treat cold-type respiratory disorders with chills, clear nasal discharge, sneezing, or congestion, combine with **Respitrol (Cold)**.
- For respiratory infection due to heat with yellow post-nasal discharge, add **Respitrol (Heat)**.
- For nasal obstruction due to sinus infection, add **Herbal ABX**.
- For nasal symptoms associated with environmental or toxic poisoning, add **Herbal DTX**.
- For sinus congestion with sinus headache, add **Corydalin**.
- To strengthen the overall constitution, use **Imperial Tonic**.
- For sinusitis or rhinitis with yellow nasal discharge, use **Pueraria Clear Sinus**.
- To enhance immunity against allergies, take **Immune** + at a low dose (1 to 2 capsules a day) during non-allergy seasons.

NUTRITION

- Reduce or eliminate intake of dairy foods, as they increase mucus production.
- Drink plenty of distilled water throughout the day to help drainage.
- Make sure the diet is adequate in supplies of vitamin A and C. Vitamin A is essential for healthy mucous lining of the respiratory tract. Vitamin C is well recognized for its effect to prevent and treat infection.

The Tao of Nutrition by Ni and McNease
- Allergy
  - Recommendations: Drink beet top tea as a water source.
  - Avoid wheat, citrus fruits, chocolate, shellfish, dairy products, eggs, potatoes, polluted meats, and polluted air.
- Chronic sinusitis
  - Recommendations: ginger, green onions, magnolia flower, bananas, garlic, black mushrooms, chrysanthemum flowers, mulberry leaves, and apricot kernel.
  - Avoid extremes of exposure to weather elements, coffee, smoking, stress, picking the nose, polluted air and smog.
- For more information, please refer to *The Tao of Nutrition* by Dr. Maoshing Ni and Cathy McNease.

LIFESTYLE INSTRUCTIONS

- Avoid allergens that may trigger sinusitis and rhinitis whenever possible.
- Application of a saline solution to the nose three to four times daily helps to reduce nasal congestion.
- Strengthen the immune system by exercising, reducing worry and stress, and developing a normal sleep habit.
- Steam inhalation is helpful to drain sinus infection. Nasal septum flush with cold saline water is helpful to desensitize the nose to temperature and common allergens. Repeatedly perform nasal flush for 1 to 2 minutes every morning.

MAGNOLIA CLEAR SINUS ™

FORMULAS

CLINICAL NOTES

- Approximately 25% of all sinusitis are related to food allergies. Therefore, it is extremely important to identify and avoid the allergy. Common allergens include milk, wheat, eggs, citrus fruits, corn and peanuts.
- *Magnolia Clear Sinus* is most effective for sinusitis and rhinitis due to seasonal allergies. *Pueraria Clear Sinus* is more effective for sinus infections.

CAUTION

- This formula is contraindicated during pregnancy and nursing.

ACUPUNCTURE POINTS

Traditional Points:
- *Yingxiang* (LI 20), *Yintang* (Extra 1), *Fengchi* (GB 20), and *Zusanli* (ST 36).
- *Lieque* (LU 7), *Hegu* (LI 4), *Yingxiang* (LI 20), *Fengchi* (GB 20), and *Zanzhu* (BL 2).

Balance Method by Dr. Richard Tan:
- Left side: *Zusanli* (ST 36), *Gongsun* (SP 4), *Yinlingquan* (SP 9), *Sanjian* (LI 3), and *Quchi* (LI 11).
- Right side: *Jiexi* (ST 41), *Chize* (LU 5), and *Taiyuan* (LU 9).
- Left and right side can be alternated from treatment to treatment.
- For additional information on the Balance Method, please refer to *Dr. Tan's Strategy of Twelve Magical Points* and *Acupuncture 1, 2, 3* by Dr. Richard Tan.

Ear Points:
- Nose, Adrenal Gland, and Prostate Gland. Tape ear seeds and switch ear every three days.

Auricular Acupuncture by Dr. Li-Chun Huang:
- Allergic rhinitis: Internal Nose, External Nose, Adrenal Gland, Endocrine, Allergic Area, Spleen, Lung, and Sympathetic. Bleed Ear Apex.
- Sinusitis: Upper Jaw, Upper Palate, Forehead, Internal Nose, External Ear, Sanjiao, Lung, Endocrine, and Adrenal Gland.
- Chronic rhinitis: Internal Nose, External Ear, Lower Lung, Allergic Area, and Adrenal Gland.
- For additional information on the location and explanation of these points, please refer to *Auricular Treatment Formula and Prescriptions* by Dr. Li-Chun Huang.

MODERN RESEARCH

Magnolia Clear Sinus is formulated to treat sinusitis or rhinitis due to seasonal allergies. The ingredients in this formula have been shown to constrict the blood vessels in the nose, stop nasal discharge, and relieve sinus headaches.

Xin Yi Hua (Flos Magnoliae) is one of the most effective herbs for treating nasal disorders. It constricts the blood vessels of the nasal mucosa and is used for treating stuffy nose, rhinitis and sinusitis.[1] It reduces nasal secretions and treats runny nose and nasal discharge.[2] In a clinical study on the effectiveness of *Xin Yi Hua* (Flos Magnoliae) in treating sinusitis or rhinitis, patients were given the herb orally once to twice daily. Out of 120 patients, 114 patients (95%) reported positive effect.[3] In another study, *Xin Yi Hua* (Flos Magnoliae) was given as an injectable to treat sinusitis and rhinitis. The injections were given once or twice daily, either subcutaneously close to the nose or intramuscularly. Out of 2450 patients, 17.3% reported complete recovery, 28.65% reported significant improvement, 28.5% reported moderate improvement, 46.7% reported slight improvement, and 7.5% reported no change.[4]

PHARMACEUTICAL DRUGS & CHINESE MEDICINE: A COMPARATIVE ANALYSIS

Western Medical Approach: Sinusitis and rhinitis are two common nasal disorders. In western medicine, these two conditions are primarily treated with vasoconstrictive drugs that promote drainage, such as pseudoephedrine. Though effective, it is a strong stimulant and may cause many side effects, such as nervousness, restlessness, dizziness, difficulty sleeping, upset stomach, difficulty breathing, fast or irregular heartbeat, muscle weakness, palpitations, tremors, and hallucinations. In addition to vasoconstrictive drugs, antihistamines, such as Claritin (Loratadine), may be used to address allergic sinusitis and rhinitis. The main advantage of these two medications is that they are relatively effective, and reasonably safe, so long as they are used correctly.

Traditional Chinese Medicine Approach: Sinusitis and rhinitis are effectively treated with herbs that drain the sinus cavity, reduce nasal mucous secretions, and desensitize allergenic reactions. These herbs may be given before, during, and after episodes of sinusitis and rhinitis. These herbs are very effective, and do not have the stimulating side effects that drugs have.

Summation: In addition to using drugs or herbs to treat sinusitis and rhinitis, it is also important to identify the cause, especially in individuals with allergic sinusitis and rhinitis. Whenever possible, avoid or minimize exposure to these allergens. It is important to remember that drugs and herbs do not cure allergy, they are only effective as preventative and symptomatic treatments.

CASE STUDIES

A 41-year-old male actor presented with chronic sinus infection and nasal congestion. Surgical procedure to scrape and drain the sinus cavity was done with post-surgical care required. The practitioner suspected that the patient's work environment exposed him to smoke particles that irritated the sinus cavity. The practitioner diagnosed the patient's condition as Lung qi deficiency with compromised *wei* (defensive) *qi*. He was given *Magnolia Clear Sinus* to address the sinus cavity irritation and keep it clear of mucus. In conjunction with the herbs, acupuncture treatment was employed as well. The results were quite effective. The patient was free of breathing difficulty and mucus drainage discomfort. The practitioner noted that *Magnolia Clear Sinus* also benefited other patients with similar conditions.

T.W., Santa Monica, California

A 50-year-old female patient presented with itchy and watery eyes. She had clear phlegm, headaches and wheezing. The patient was treated with Ventolin (Albuterol) for wheezing, and Claritin (Loratadine) for allergy. The practitioner diagnosed this as seasonal, allergic rhinitis due to phlegm-cold. The treatment protocol included both acupuncture and herbs. During the allergy season, acupuncture treatment was given every two weeks. In addition, the patient took *Magnolia Clear Sinus*, 4 caps three times daily for 10 days. After taking *Magnolia Clear Sinus*, the patient no longer complained of wheezing and sneezing, and the headaches were less severe. The practitioner noted that the patient responded quite well with *Magnolia Clear Sinus*, especially during allergic attacks with asthma.

M.K., Sherman Oaks, California

B.F., a 55-year-old male, presented with cough, thick nasal discharge, headache and fatigue. The tongue was pale, flabby and slightly purple. The pulse was slow. He was diagnosed with common cold and wind-cold invasion. *Magnolia Clear Sinus*, *Respitrol (Cold)* and *Herbal ABX* were prescribed. The patient reported that the sinus cleared in three days.

B.F., Newport Beach, California

MAGNOLIA CLEAR SINUS ™

A 54-year-old female property manager presented with chronic sinus congestion and headaches. She had food allergies to dairy, egg whites, kidney beans and lima beans. The practitioner diagnosed the case as Lung qi deficiency with excess damp. After taking *Magnolia Clear Sinus*, the patient commented that the herbs were effective in treating headache and nasal congestion. The patient continued to take *Magnolia Clear Sinus* intermittently throughout the year, but more so during the fall season.

T.W., Santa Monica, California

A 41-year-old female presented with sinus pressure and swelling around the right eye. A one-inch diameter growth on the neck and a cyst-like lump on the right side of the head were also noted. Other symptoms included extreme fatigue, overall body pain, and frequent coldness. The practitioner diagnosed her condition as cold damp nasal congestion and wind-cold attack. Within one month of taking *Magnolia Clear Sinus*, the eye swelling abated and the sinus pressure was reduced to almost 90%. The lump on the neck decreased to 20% the original size while the cyst on the head desiccated. Overall body pain diminished, energy level increased, and cold sensations stopped. Her sleep pattern was also much improved. Prior to the herbal treatment with *Magnolia Clear Sinus*, the patient spent almost four months going to different specialists only to come up with no results. In addition to taking *Magnolia Clear Sinus*, the treatment protocol included acupuncture as well as a diet devoid of any cold, raw foods.

S.T., Morgan Hill, California

J.C., a 34-year-old female, presented chronic allergic rhinitis with itchy, stuffy, runny nose, itchy eyes and aversion to wind. These symptoms started in her childhood and worsened during the morning and allergy seasons. Her blood pressure was 125/85 mmHg and her heart rate was 78 beats per minute. Her tongue was pink with normal thin white coating. Her pulse was moderate and slightly slippery. The diagnosis was Lung qi deficiency with underlying Kidney and Spleen deficiencies. *Magnolia Clear Sinus* was prescribed. After taking the herbs, the patient reported 70% decrease in allergy symptoms. She said she was able to wake up with clear nasal passage. Santa Ana winds still triggered the symptoms, but *Magnolia Clear Sinus* keeps it under control.

J.C., Whittier, California

I.L., a 35-year-old male with a history of seasonal allergies, presented with sinus congestion and orbital pain that had lasted two months. The TCM diagnosis was wind-cold invasion. After taking three capsules of *Magnolia Clear Sinus* three times daily for five days, the patient reported mild relief of symptoms, and complete resolution of symptoms after one week. Furthermore, the condition did not return in the three months following completion of this herbal regimen.

C.L., Chino Hills, California

H.M., a 59-year-old female, presented with seasonal nasal allergies, rhinitis, stuffy sinuses and profuse, clear, nasal mucus. She was allergic to mold and mildew. *Herbal ABX* and *Magnolia Clear Sinus* were prescribed. They brought about relief after 10 days, when the patient would usually be battling the symptoms for months and would have to take antibiotics.

H.C., Stephens City, Virginia

---

[1] Yeung, HC. *Handbook of Chinese Herbs.* Institute of Chinese Medicine. 1996
[2] Bensky, D. et al. *Chinese Herbal Medicine Materia Medica.* Eastland Press. 1993
[3] Ren, Y. effectiveness of magnolia flower (xin yi hua) in treating sinusitis or rhinitis, a report of 120 patients. *Journal of Chinese Herbal Medicine.* 5:45. 1985.
[4] Gou, DJ. Treatment of sinusitis and rhinitis with injection of magnolia flower (xin yi hua), a report of 2450 patients. *Journal of Modern Medicine.* 1:12. 1981

FORMULAS

MENOTROL ™

CLINICAL APPLICATIONS

- Infertility
- Amenorrhea
- Polycystic ovarian disease
- Irregular, delayed or scanty menstruation
- Conditions above should be accompanied by dark purple tongue and cold signs and symptoms

WESTERN THERAPEUTIC ACTIONS

- Restores normal menstruation by removing physical obstructions [4,5,6,7,8]
- Restores normal menstruation by regulating the hormones [16,17,18,19]
- Relieves pain [9,10,11,12,13,14,15]

CHINESE THERAPEUTIC ACTIONS

- Warms the *ming men* (life gate) fire, tonifies Kidney yang
- Nourishes the womb and the *chong* (thoroughfare) and *ren* (conception) channels
- Invigorates blood circulation in the lower *jiao* and the womb
- Tonifies Liver blood
- Tonifies *yuan* (source) *qi*

DOSAGE

Take 3 to 4 capsules three times daily on an empty stomach with warm water. Dosage may be increased to 6 to 8 capsules three times daily if necessary. The minimum period for treatment with this formula is one to three months. For treatment of infertility, advise the patients to stop taking the herbs immediately once pregnancy is confirmed.

INGREDIENTS

Bai Shao (Radix Paeoniae Alba)
Chai Hu (Radix Bupleuri)
Chi Shao (Radix Paeoniae Rubrae)
Chuan Niu Xi (Radix Cyathulae)
Chuan Xiong (Rhizoma Ligustici Chuanxiong)
Dang Gui (Radicis Angelicae Sinensis)
Fu Ling (Poria)
Fu Zi (Radix Aconiti Lateralis Praeparata)
Gan Cao (Radix Glycyrrhizae)
Gan Jiang (Rhizoma Zingiberis)
Gui Zhi (Ramulus Cinnamomi)
Hong Hua (Flos Carthami)
Mai Men Dong (Radix Ophiopogonis)
Mo Yao (Myrrha)
Mu Dan Pi (Cortex Moutan)

Pu Huang (Pollen Typhae)
Ren Shen (Radix Ginseng)
Rou Gui (Cortex Cinnamomi)
Shan Yao (Rhizoma Dioscoreae)
Shan Zhu Yu (Fructus Corni)
Sheng Di Huang (Radix Rehmanniae)
Sheng Jiang (Rhizoma Zingiberis Recens)
Shu Di Huang (Radix Rehmanniae Preparata)
Tao Ren (Semen Persicae)
Wu Zhu Yu (Fructus Evodiae)
Xiao Hui Xiang (Fructus Foeniculi)
Yan Hu Suo (Rhizoma Corydalis)
Ze Xie (Rhizoma Alismatis)
Zhi Ke (Fructus Aurantii)

MENOTROL ™

FORMULA EXPLANATION

Menotrol is designed to treat amenorrhea, infertility and other gynecological disorders with underlying Kidney yang deficiency and blood stagnation. In addition, *Menotrol* also addresses such conditions as irregular menstrual cycles, delayed menstruation, spotting or scanty menstruation, weakness and soreness of the low back and knees, coldness of the extremities, accompanied by a pale purplish tongue.

If the Kidney is deficient, reproductive function will be impaired. This results in symptoms such as amenorrhea, irregular menstruation, vaginal dryness, infertility, decreased libido, habitual miscarriage, hair loss and fatigue. The Kidney also controls the "Sea of Marrow," that is, the brain, where the hypothalamus and pituitary gland are located. Kidney deficiency can be correlated with the inability of the hypothalamus to signal the pituitary gland to release hormones that cause ovaries to release eggs. In other words, the normal menstrual cycle will be disturbed. Therefore, optimal treatment requires use of herbs that tonify Kidney yang, yin, and *jing* (essence).

Fu Zi (Radix Aconiti Lateralis Praeparata) and *Rou Gui* (Cortex Cinnamomi) restore depleted Kidney yang, augment *ming men* (life gate) fire, and warm and open the channels, to treat obstruction due to coldness. *Gan Jiang* (Rhizoma Zingiberis) enhances the warming action and decreases the toxicity of *Fu Zi* (Radix Aconiti Lateralis Praeparata). *Xiao Hui Xiang* (Fructus Foeniculi) and *Wu Zhu Yu* (Fructus Evodiae) are used to warm the Liver channel where it circulates around the genital organs.

Chi Shao (Radix Paeoniae Rubrae), *Gui Zhi* (Ramulus Cinnamomi), *Mu Dan Pi* (Cortex Moutan), *Tao Ren* (Semen Persicae), *Hong Hua* (Flos Carthami), *Chuan Niu Xi* (Radix Cyathulae), *Pu Huang* (Pollen Typhae), *Mo Yao* (Myrrha), *Yan Hu Suo* (Rhizoma Corydalis) and *Chuan Xiong* (Rhizoma Ligustici Chuanxiong) are indispensable herbs for treating any obstetric/gynecologic disorders involving blood stagnation. Together, they invigorate blood circulation, dispel blood stasis, clear blood clots and relieve pain that may be caused by blood stagnation. The use of these herbs follows the same principles as the famous formulas *Gui Zhi Fu Ling Wan* (Cinnamon Twig and Poria Pill) and *Shao Fu Zhu Yu Tang* (Drive Out Blood Stasis in the Lower Abdomen Decoction).

The *chong* (thoroughfare) channel is known as "the sea of all twelve channels," and as "the sea of blood." The *ren* (conception) channel is known as "the sea of all yin channels." Therefore, in order to regulate menstruation and treat infertility, the *chong* (thoroughfare) and *ren* (conception) channels must be nourished. *Dang Gui* (Radicis Angelicae Sinensis), *Bai Shao* (Radix Paeoniae Alba) and *Shu Di Huang* (Radix Rehmanniae Preparata), the chief ingredients in *Si Wu Tang* (Four-Substance Decoction), are used to tonify blood. In addition, *Shan Zhu Yu* (Fructus Corni), *Shan Yao* (Rhizoma Dioscoreae) and *Sheng Di Huang* (Radix Rehmanniae) tonify Liver blood, replenish Kidney *jing* (essence) and nourish the *chong* (thoroughfare) and *ren* (conception) channels. Other tonic herbs here include *Ren Shen* (Radix Ginseng) to tonify the *yuan* (source) *qi*, *Mai Men Dong* (Radix Ophiopogonis) to nourish yin, and *Fu Ling* (Poria) to strengthen the Spleen.

Zhi Ke (Fructus Aurantii) and *Chai Hu* (Radix Bupleuri) are used to regulate Liver qi to ensure smooth flow. They are used to enhance the effectiveness of the blood invigorating herbs and also to prevent stagnation that may be caused by the tonic herbs. *Sheng Jiang* (Rhizoma Zingiberis Recens) and *Gan Cao* (Radix Glycyrrhizae) are used to harmonize the formula.

SUPPLEMENTARY FORMULAS

- For female infertility, add *Blossom (Phase 1-4)*.
- For polycystic ovaries, endometriosis or fibroids, combine with *Resolve (Lower)*.
- For severe Kidney yang deficiency, add *Kidney Tonic (Yang)*.
- For severe Kidney yin deficiency, add *Kidney Tonic (Yin)*.

MENOTROL ™

- For lower abdominal pain, use with *Mense-Ease*.
- For menopause, use with *Balance (Heat)*.
- For fatigue and overall weakness, use with *Imperial Tonic*.
- For amenorrhea due to stress, tension or Liver qi stagnation, use with *Calm*.
- For amenorrhea due to Liver fire, use with *Gentiana Complex*.
- For hyperthyroidism, combine with *Thyrodex*.
- For severe blood stagnation, add *Circulation (SJ)*.

NUTRITION

- Avoid raw or cold foods such as sushi, salad, cucumber, tomatoes, ice cream, and refrigerated or iced drinks. Excessive intake of fruits also may cause coldness. Refrain from eating sour fruits, such as grapefruit and oranges.
- Eat cooked food and drink warm or room temperature beverages.
- Foods that are warm, such as lamb, beef, chives, cinnamon and pepper are recommended. Nuts and seafood such as oyster, lobster and shrimp should be included, as they tonify the Kidney. Alcohol can be consumed in small amounts (1 oz.) daily, as it invigorates the blood and warms the body.
- Ensure there is an adequate intake of vitamin B complex and vitamin E, which are important for production of sex hormones. Deficiency in zinc may also contribute to irregular menstruation.

LIFESTYLE INSTRUCTIONS

- Avoid sports that may expose the body to cold environment, such as skiing or cold-water sports.
- Stress can sometimes lead to irregular or absence of menstruation. Avoid stressful situations, or engage in stress-reduction activities, whenever possible.
- A regular and healthy lifestyle with adequate rest and relaxation is the basic requirement for a normal menstrual cycle.
- Hot compresses on the abdomen increase blood circulation, relax abdominal muscles, and relieve pain.

CLINICAL NOTES

- *Balance (Cold)* is usually used first in patients presenting with general menstrual disorders of cold and deficiency. When the condition is shown to be complicated by blood stagnation, Kidney yang deficiency, and cold, *Menotrol* should then be prescribed.
- Patients can also massage the lower abdomen to increase blood circulation and warm the womb. Instruct the patient to fold her hands together [overlapping *Laogong* (PC 8)] and place her palm on her lower abdomen (at *Guanyuan* (CV 4)) and massage in a circular motion, moving clockwise 36 times and counterclockwise 36 times. Practice twice daily, once when waking in the morning and once before going to bed at night. Ideally, a male practitioner (yang energy) should massage the patient's abdomen (influencing yin). During massage of the abdomen, the patient should feel the pressure, but not pain or discomfort.
- Herbs may not be effective in cases where there has been injury or surgical removal of the reproductive organs.
- Patients with a long history of back pain may need additional diagnostic workups to rule out structural damage to the vertebrae causing amenorrhea, infertility or irregular menstruation.
- Patients with infertility should check to see if chlamydia is the cause. Scarring and inflammation of the tubes may be a cause of blockage leading to infertility.
- Patients experiencing infertility should monitor basal body temperature to track ovulation. If there is no change in the temperature profile after the patient has been taking herbs for two months, the doctor should re-evaluate and consider modifying or changing the formula to properly address the patient's condition. If the patient does

become pregnant, herbs should be stopped immediately as there are blood-invigorating herbs that may be too strong for the patient. Please refer to B*lossom (Phase 1-4)* for additional information on female infertility.

☙ Patients with infertility should not go on strict diets or exercise excessively. They should also be advised not to use a douche.

CAUTIONS

☙ This formula is contraindicated during pregnancy and nursing.

☙ This formula is contraindicated in cases of heat and deficiency heat, and in cases of infection or inflammation.

☙ Patients who are on anticoagulant or antiplatelet therapies, such as Coumadin (Warfarin), should use this formula with caution, as there may be a slightly higher risk of bleeding and bruising.

☙ Patients who wear a pacemaker, or individuals who take anti-arrhythmic drugs or cardiac glycosides such as Lanoxin (Digoxin), should not take this formula. *Fu Zi* (Radix Aconiti Lateralis Praeparata) may interact with these drugs by affecting the rhythm and potentiating the contractile strength of the heart.

ACUPUNCTURE POINTS

Traditional Points:

☙ Needle *Sanyinjiao* (SP 6), *Geshu* (BL 17) and *Xuehai* (SP 10). Apply moxa to *Zusanli* (ST 36).

☙ *Qihai* (CV 6), *Shenque* (CV 8), *Xiawan* (CV 10), *Zhongwan* (CV 12), *Neiguan* (PC 6), *Gongsun* (SP 4), *Mingmen* (GV 4), *Sanyinjiao* (SP 6), *Dahe* (KI 12), and *Zhongji* (CV 3).

Balance Method by Dr. Richard Tan:

☙ Left side: *Yinlingquan* (SP 9), *Diji* (SP 8), *Sanyinjiao* (SP 6), *Hegu* (LI 4), and *Lingku*.

☙ Right side: *Zusanli* (ST 36) or *ah shi* points nearby, *Chize* (LU 5), *Kongzui* (LU 6) or *ah shi* points nearby, and *Diwuhui* (GB 42).

☙ Left and right side can be alternated from treatment to treatment.

☙ Note: *Lingku* is one of Master Tong's points on both hands. *Lingku* is located in the depression just distal to the junction of the first and second metacarpal bones, approximately 0.5 *cun* proximal to *Hegu* (LI 4), on the *yangming* line.

☙ For additional information on the Balance Method, please refer to *Twelve and Twelve in Acupuncture* and *Twenty-Four More in Acupuncture* by Dr. Richard Tan.

Ear Points:

☙ Uterus, Ovaries, Pituitary Gland, and Hypothalamus.

☙ Embed steel balls or needles. Switch ear every five days.

Auricular Acupuncture by Dr. Li-Chun Huang:

☙ Menstrual disorder (menoxenia): Uterus, Kidney, Liver, Pituitary, Ovary, and Endocrine.

☙ Amenorrhea and hypomenorrhea: Uterus, Ovary, Gonadotropin, Exciting Point, Pituitary Point, Endocrine, Kidney, Liver, and Sympathetic.

☙ Dysmenorrhea: Uterus, Pelvic, Liver, Sympathetic, Kidney, Ovary, Endocrine, Pituitary, and Lower *Jiao*.

☙ For additional information on the location and explanation of these points, please refer to *Auricular Treatment Formula and Prescriptions* by Dr. Li-Chun Huang.

MODERN RESEARCH

Amenorrhea is defined as the absence or abnormal stoppage of the menses.[1] Other than prepuberty, pregnancy, early lactation, and after menopause, amenorrhea is considered a pathologic condition and must be addressed.[2] Etiologies of amenorrhea include anatomical obstruction (such as stagnant accumulation of menstrual blood) and physiological abnormality (such as hormonal imbalance).[3] Therefore, optimal treatment must address both of these causes.

The excessive accumulation of menstrual blood leading to obstruction and pain is one of the most common presentations of amenorrhea. To address this condition, herbs are prescribed to eliminate the accumulated blood, improve blood circulation, and relieve pain. To eliminate accumulation of blood and clots, herbs with antiplatelet, anticoagulant, and thrombolytic functions are prescribed. Herbs with such functions include *Chi Shao* (Radix Paeoniae Rubrae), *Tao Ren* (Semen Persicae) and *Hong Hua* (Flos Carthami).[4,5,6] In fact, in one study, researchers found that herbs that activate blood circulation and eliminate blood stasis proved effective in inhibiting formation of clots in 73.4% of the test cases.[7] Lastly, to improve circulation, *Chuan Xiong* (Rhizoma Ligustici Chuanxiong) is added. *Chuan Xiong* (Rhizoma Ligustici Chuanxiong) is one of the most effective herbs to improve the circulation of blood to the body's periphery.[8]

Because the accumulation of blood often leads to severe abdominal pain, herbs are prescribed to alleviate pain and discomfort. There are many herbs with marked analgesic effects, including (but not limited to) *Fu Zi* (Radix Aconiti Lateralis Praeparata), *Chuan Niu Xi* (Radix Cyathulae), *Dang Gui* (Radicis Angelicae Sinensis), *Bai Shao* (Radix Paeoniae Alba), *Gan Cao* (Radix Glycyrrhizae), and *Yan Hu Suo* (Rhizoma Corydalis), which have shown excellent *in vitro* and *in vivo* effects. [9,10,11,12,13] Of all these herbs, *Yan Hu Suo* (Rhizoma Corydalis) is especially effective against visceral pain, and its analgesic effect has been compared with that of morphine. Though morphine is still more potent and has a faster onset of action, *Yan Hu Suo* (Rhizoma Corydalis) has far fewer side effects, slower development of tolerance, and has shown no evidence of creating dependence.[14] Furthermore, it has synergistic effects in combination with electro-acupuncture.[15] Overall, these herbs offer safe, effective, and reliable pain relief.

Hormonal imbalance is another common cause of amenorrhea. Chronic anovulation may be caused by polycystic ovarian disease where there is an acyclic production of estrogen, or it may be due to hypogonadism where there is a low or absent production of estrogen. In either case, proper balance and regulation of the endocrine system is necessary to restore normal menstruation. Herbs in this formula have a two-directional effect on the endocrine system. They balance and regulate the endocrine system to restore equilibrium. *Sheng Di Huang* (Radix Rehmanniae), *Ren Shen* (Radix Ginseng) and *Gan Cao* (Radix Glycyrrhizae) have all shown marked regulatory influence on the endocrine system. *Sheng Di Huang* (Radix Rehmanniae) and *Gan Cao* (Radix Glycyrrhizae) are more specific to the adrenal glands,[16,17] while *Ren Shen* (Radix Ginseng) has a more general influence on the entire endocrine system.[18] Specifically, administration of these herbs has been shown to regulate and balance the endocrine system by directly affecting the hypothalamus and the pituitary glands.[19]

PHARMACEUTICAL DRUGS & CHINESE MEDICINE: A COMPARATIVE ANALYSIS

Western Medical Approach: Amenorrhea and dysmenorrhea are conditions that almost all women suffer on occasional basis. As common as the conditions are, there are few drug treatments available. On one hand, hormone drugs, such as birth control pills and patches, are prescribed to regulate menstrual cycles. Though they are more effective, they often cause serious side effects, such as weight gain, hyperkalemia, clotting disorders, retinal thrombosis, cancer, liver damage, hypertriglyceridemia, hypertension, bleeding, and fertility impairment. On the other hand, those with dysmenorrhea may take non-steroidal anti-inflammatory agents (NSAID) to relieve pain and reduce inflammation and swelling. Though effective, they cause such serious side effects as gastric ulcer, duodenal ulcer, gastrointestinal bleeding, tinnitus, blurred vision, dizziness and headache. In short, drug treatment options are very limited between those that treat only symptoms and do not work well, and those that work well but may have significant side effects.

Traditional Chinese Medicine Approach: Herbal therapy is extremely effective to regulate menstruation and treat amenorrhea and dysmenorrhea. These herbs have analgesic effect to relieve pain, anti-inflammatory effect to reduce

FORMULAS

swelling and inflammation, and antispasmodic effect to relieve cramping. Furthermore, many herbs have been shown to have marked effect to regulate hormones to promote normal menstruation. However, this effect requires continuous use of herbs for at least one to two cycles. In short, herbal therapy is extremely beneficial for treatment of menstrual disorder as it treats both the symptoms and the cause of PMS and dysmenorrhea.

Summation: Drug offers limited options for treatment of amenorrhea and dysmenorrhea. Birth controls are effective, but these drugs carry significant short- and long-term side effects. NSAIDs relieve pain, but should be used as needed for only a short period of time. Herbs, on the other hand, are extremely effective for both immediate and prolonged benefits. Furthermore, they are very safe and are associated with few or no side effects. Individuals with such menstrual disorders should definitely explore these non-drug treatment options.

CASE STUDIES

A 41-year-old female presented with infertility and depression. Her practitioner diagnosed her as Kidney deficiency and Liver qi deficiency. Poor egg quality was a secondary explanation to her infertility. The patient's treatment consisted of acupuncture once a week and *Menotrol* (4 capsules three times daily). Shortly after the treatment started, the patient's cold symptoms abated and her menstrual cycle became regular (from 32 days to 28 days). She became pregnant after only two months of treatment.

L.M., San Diego, California

A 15-year-old female student presented with irregular periods for almost two years. Her period interval was noted to be 8 days every 4 months. Tongue body appeared enlarged and purple with the sides slightly more pale. She also had a thick, white tongue coating and a "rolling" pulse. Her condition was diagnosed as damp stagnation with underlying deficiency. After being treated with *Menotrol* for two months, the patient started having her menses. Her period interval has changed from 8 days every 4 months to 5 or 7 days every 1 to 1½ months.

T.G., Albuquerque, New Mexico

M.C., a 33-year-old female, presented with irregular menstruation for the past five years (about two to three times a year each time lasting four to five days). She complained of cramping pain, fatigue, lower back pain, bloating, poor circulation, dry skin and lips, and brittle nails. Her blood pressure was 139/90 mmHg and her heart rate was 92 beats per minute. Her tongue was slightly dusky, pale to pink in color, moist with a thin white coat. Her pulse was slippery. Her diagnosis was amenorrhea with blood deficiency, blood stagnation, and Spleen qi deficiency with phlegm and damp accumulation. *Menotrol* was prescribed. The patient's last period was in early January. After starting *Menotrol*, she menstruated again the second week of February, which was an exciting and positive sign because she usually menstruates once every five to six months. She will continue taking *Menotrol* until her cycle becomes regular. She also received weekly acupuncture treatments and began walking three to four times a week.

J.C., Whittier, California

J.W., a 44-year-old patient, presented with infertility and a history of miscarriage. She experienced high stress which she "bottles up" inside. Her hands and feet were cold. She also had back pain, low energy, severe menstrual cramps and premenstrual syndrome (PMS). Her tongue was pale and purplish, swollen with teeth marks. The tip was red. Pulses were wiry on both sides and slippery on the right. Her blood pressure was 125/86 mmHg and heart rate was 83 beats per minute. Lab report showed she had low FSH levels. The diagnosis was Spleen and Kidney yang deficiencies with Liver qi and blood stagnation. *Menotrol* was prescribed. After one month on *Menotrol*, the patient reported her menstrual cramping "miraculously disappeared" and her estrogen levels increased dramatically. She was afraid the herbs would interfere with her *in vitro* fertilization (IVF) procedure so she stopped taking them for six weeks. After the IVF was not successful and her tongue color became very purple in the center, the practitioner suggested she take the formula *Calm*. She was open to it. Within a week, her stress level decreased and her energy

FORMULAS

MENOTROL ™

level increased. Her tongue color changed from purple to pink and slightly dusky. She is presently continuing to take *Calm* and is actively trying to conceive naturally.

J.C.O., Whittier, California

[1] *Dorland's Illustrated Medical Dictionary 28th Edition*. W.B. Saunders Company 1994.
[2] Berkow, R. *The Merck Manual of Diagnosis and Therapy 16th Edition*. 1992.
[3] Fauci, A. et al. *Harrison's Principles of Internal Medicine 14th Edition*. McGraw-Hill Health Professions Division. 1998.
[4] *Zhong Xi Yi Jie He Za Zhi* (Journal of Integrated Chinese and Western Medicine), 1984; 4(12):745
[5] *Zhong Xi Yi Jie He Za Zhi* (Journal of Integrated Chinese and Western Medicine), 1983; 2:109
[6] *Hua Xi Yi Xue Za Zhi* (Huaxi Medical Journal), 1993; 8(3):170
[7] *Zhong Cao Yao* (Chinese Herbal Medicine), 1983; 14(7):27
[8] *Zhong Yao Xue* (Chinese Herbology), 1989; 535:539
[9] *Zhong Guo Zhong Yao Za Zhi* (People's Republic of China Journal of Chinese Herbology), 1992; 17(2):104
[10] *Zhong Yao Tong Bao* (Journal of Chinese Herbology), 1988; 13(7):43
[11] *Xin Yi Yao Xue Za Zhi* (New Journal of Medicine and Herbology), 1975; (6):34
[12] *Yao Xue Za Zhi* (Journal of Medicinals), 1971; (91):1098
[13] *Hu Nan Zhong Yi* (Hunan Journal of Traditional Chinese Medicine), 1989; 2:7
[14] *Zhong Yao Yao Li Yu Ying Yong* (Pharmacology and Applications of Chinese Herbs), 1983; 447
[15] *Chen Tzu Yen Chiu* (Acupuncture Research), 1994; 19(1):55-8
[16] *Zhong Yao Xue* (Chinese Herbology), 1998; 156:158
[17] *Zhong Hua Yi Xue Za Zhi* (Chinese Journal of Medicine), 1975; 10:718
[18] *Bai Qiu En Yi Ke Da Xue Xue Bao* (Journal of Baiqiuen University of Medicine), 1980; 6(2):32
[19] *Zhong Cheng Yao* (Study of Chinese Patent Medicine), 1989; 11(9):30

FORMULAS

MENSE-EASE ™

CLINICAL APPLICATIONS

- ☯ Dysmenorrhea with bloating, cramping, pain, or blood clots
- ☯ Endometriosis with severe menstrual cramping and pain
- ☯ Postpartum pain
- ☯ Pain in various gynecological disorders

WESTERN THERAPEUTIC ACTIONS

- ☯ Analgesic function to relieve pain [1,2,4,5]
- ☯ Antispasmodic effect to relieve cramping [4,5]
- ☯ Anti-inflammatory action to reduce swelling and inflammation [4,5]

CHINESE THERAPEUTIC ACTIONS

- ☯ Relieves cramping and pain
- ☯ Invigorates blood circulation
- ☯ Disperses blood stagnation
- ☯ Activates qi circulation

DOSAGE

Take 3 to 4 capsules on an empty stomach three times daily with warm water. Dosage may be increased to 5 to 6 capsules every four hours as needed to relieve pain. For best results, combine *Calm* with *Mense-Ease* and begin herbal treatment three days before the first day of menstruation.

INGREDIENTS

Ai Ye (Folium Artemisiae Argyi)
Chi Shao (Radix Paeoniae Rubrae)
Chuan Xiong (Rhizoma Ligustici Chuanxiong)
Dang Gui (Radicis Angelicae Sinensis)
Gui Zhi (Ramulus Cinnamomi)
Hong Hua (Flos Carthami)
Huai Niu Xi (Radix Achyranthis Bidentatae)

Mu Dan Pi (Cortex Moutan)
Pu Huang (Pollen Typhae)
Tao Ren (Semen Persicae)
Wu Yao (Radix Linderae)
Xiang Fu (Rhizoma Cyperi)
Yan Hu Suo (Rhizoma Corydalis)

FORMULA EXPLANATION

Mense-Ease is formulated specifically to treat women's disorders, such as dysmenorrhea, endometriosis, and other gynecological disorders. Such women's disorders are considered as qi and blood stagnation in the lower *jiao*. *Mense-Ease* contains herbs that activate qi and blood circulation, remove qi and blood stagnation, and relieve pain and cramps.

Pu Huang (Pollen Typhae) has an excitatory action on the uterus and works to invigorate the blood circulation and relieve pain by eliminating blood stasis. *Ai Ye* (Folium Artemisiae Argyi) and *Chi Shao* (Radix Paeoniae Rubrae) have antispasmodic effects on the smooth muscles to relieve pain. *Yan Hu Suo* (Rhizoma Corydalis), *Chuan Xiong* (Rhizoma Ligustici Chuanxiong), *Mu Dan Pi* (Cortex Moutan), *Gui Zhi* (Ramulus Cinnamomi), *Tao Ren* (Semen Persicae), *Dang Gui* (Radicis Angelicae Sinensis), *Huai Niu Xi* (Radix Achyranthis Bidentatae), and *Hong Hua*

FORMULAS

MENSE-EASE ™

(Flos Carthami) activate blood circulation, remove blood stasis, and relieve pain. *Wu Yao* (Radix Linderae) and *Xiang Fu* (Rhizoma Cyperi) are qi regulators that help to relieve abdominal bloating and distention.

SUPPLEMENTARY FORMULAS

- To enhance the effect to relieve pain, add ***Herbal Analgesic***.
- For premenstrual syndrome (PMS), irritability, stress, or emotional disorders, add ***Calm***.
- For irritability, stress, or emotional disorders with insomnia in patients with deficiency, add ***Calm ZZZ***.
- For dull pain and a cold sensation during the non-menstrual period, use ***Balance (Cold)***.
- For cystitis, urinary tract or lower *jiao* infections, use ***V-Statin*** with ***Herbal ABX***.
- For fever and fire signs, add ***Gardenia Complex***.
- For cysts in the uterus and ovaries, fibroids or endometriosis, use ***Resolve (Lower)***.
- For back pain, use ***Back Support (Chronic)***.
- For menses with blood clots, add ***Resolve (Lower)***.
- For severe blood stagnation, add ***Circulation (SJ)***.
- For infertility, use ***Blossom (Phase 1-4)***.
- To stop bleeding, add ***Notoginseng 9***.
- For headache associated with PMS, add ***Migratrol***.
- For gynecological pain due to scar tissue causing excessive qi and blood stagnation, add ***Mense-Ease*** and ***Resolve (Lower)***.

NUTRITION

- Foods and fruits that are cold or sour in nature should be avoided, especially one week prior to or during menstruation. Cold and sour foods create more stagnation, and may worsen the pain.
- Decrease the consumption of salt, red meats, processed foods, junk foods, and foods with high sodium content. Caffeine should be avoided as it acts as a stimulant to excite the central nervous system and as a diuretic to deplete many important nutrients.
- Increase the consumption of whole-grain foods, and broiled chicken, turkey and fish.
- Drink a large quantity of distilled water daily before, during, and after the menstruation.
- Menstrual cramps due to calcium deficiency should be treated with ingestion of foods rich in calcium, such as green vegetables, legumes, and seaweeds.
- Ensure there is an adequate intake of vitamin B complex and vitamin E, which are important for production of sex hormones. Deficiency of zinc may also contribute to irregular menstruation.
- A folk remedy for menstrual pain uses a stalk of ginger (sliced) with 3 pieces of green onion, 30 grams of brown sugar and 3 cups of water. Bring the mixture to a boil and cook for five minutes. Add a teaspoon of white pepper and serve.

LIFESTYLE INSTRUCTIONS

- Avoid sports that may expose the body to cold environments, such as snow skiing or cold water sports.
- Hot baths or hot showers aimed at the abdomen help to relieve menstrual pain and cramps.
- Hot compresses on the abdomen increase blood circulation, relax abdominal muscles, and relieve pain.
- Stress can sometimes lead to irregular or no menstruation. Avoid stressful situations, or engage in stress-reduction activities.
- A regular and healthy lifestyle with adequate rest and relaxation is the basic requirement for a normal menstrual cycle.
- Wear cloth that fully covers the body and do not expose the belly or the abdomen to the cold environment. Avoid wearing tight pants.

FORMULAS

MENSE-EASE ™

CLINICAL NOTES

- *Resolve (Lower)* and *Calm* can be used one week prior to each menstrual cycle at 2 to 4 capsules each twice daily to help move qi and blood in the uterus and prepare for smooth shedding of the uterine wall during menstruation. Unless the patient is extremely deficient in qi or blood, this principle can be applied to all patients, especially those with blood stagnation.

- *Imperial Tonic* is an excellent postpartum tonic. Women lose a tremendous amount of *jing* (essence) and blood after labor. The concept of replenishing the Kidney *jing* (essence) is not prevalent in the West. As a result, many women age faster and suffer from low back pain or symptoms of Kidney yin or *jing* (essence) deficiency later in their lives. This is a great formula to start one or two weeks after delivery. It helps replenish qi, blood, yin and yang that may have been lost during labor. Also, it is beneficial to nursing mothers, as more nutrients will be passed down to the baby. However, before tonifying the patient with *Imperial Tonic*, *Sheng Hua Tang* (Generation and Transformation Decoction) should be used for one week to clear out residual blood stagnation and to relieve pain. This will prevent future gynecological complications due to blood stagnation in the pelvis.

- For individuals who had cesarean-section, *Traumanex* can be used to relieve pain and facilitate recovery.

- For most patients, heat pads or moxa will always relieve pain. Be sure moxa treatment exceed 30 minutes, for maximum effect.

CAUTIONS

- This formula is contraindicated during pregnancy and nursing.

- Patients who are on anticoagulant or antiplatelet therapies, such as Coumadin (Warfarin), should use this formula with caution, as there may be a slightly higher risk of bleeding and bruising.

ACUPUNCTURE POINTS

Traditional Points:
- *Sanyinjiao* (SP 6), *Guilai* (ST 29), *Zhongji* (CV 3), *Zusanli* (ST 36), *Xuehai* (SP 10), *Qihai* (CV 6), *Geshu* (BL 17), *Diji* (SP 8), *Taichong* (LR 3), and *Xingjian* (LR 2).
- Needle *Yinlingquan* (SP 9), *Lougu* (SP 7), and *Sanyinjiao* (SP 6). Massage local tender points around *Sanyinjiao* (SP 6).

Balance Method by Dr. Richard Tan:
- Left side: *Yinlingquan* (SP 9), *Diji* (SP 8), *Sanyinjiao* (SP 6), *Hegu* (LI 4), and *Lingku*.
- Right side: *Zusanli* (ST 36) or *ah shi* points nearby, *Chize* (LU 5), *Kongzui* (LU 6), *Lieque* (LU 7) or *ah shi* points nearby, *Diwuhui* (GB 42), *Zulinqi* (GB 41).
- Left and right side can be alternated from treatment to treatment.
- Note: *Lingku* is one of Master Tong's points on both hands. *Lingku* is located in the depression just distal to the junction of the first and second metacarpal bones, approximately 0.5 *cun* proximal to *Hegu* (LI 4), on the *yangming* line.
- For additional information on the Balance Method, please refer to *Twelve and Twelve in Acupuncture* and *Twenty-Four More in Acupuncture* by Dr. Richard Tan.

Ear Points:
- Ear seeds are very effective for relieving menstrual pain. The primary points to select are: *Shenmen*, Sympathetic, Uterus, Endocrine, Brain Stem and Ovary. Adjunct points can be used on other affected areas such as the Back for back pain, Spleen for diarrhea and so on.
- Ear seeds can be placed one week before each menstrual cycle. The patient should massage the points for five minutes three times each day or as frequently as possible. To prevent the seeds from falling out, advise the

FORMULAS

MENSE-EASE ™

patient not to wash that ear during showers and not to rub the ear too hard with a towel while the ear is still wet. Each course of treatment is four months. Alternate ear each month.

Auricular Acupuncture by Dr. Li-Chun Huang:

❧ Menstrual disorder (menoxenia): Uterus, Kidney, Liver, Pituitary, Ovary, and Endocrine.
❧ Amenorrhea and hypomenorrhea: Uterus, Ovary, Gonadotropin, Exciting Point, Pituitary Point, Endocrine, Kidney, Liver, and Sympathetic.
❧ Dysmenorrhea: Uterus, Pelvic, Liver, Sympathetic, Kidney, Ovary, Endocrine, Pituitary, and Lower *Jiao*.
❧ Endometritis: Uterus, Cervix, Kidney, Liver, Ovary, Pituitary, Thalamus, Endocrine, Gonadotropin, *San Jiao*.
❧ For additional information on the location and explanation of these points, please refer to *Auricular Treatment Formula and Prescriptions* by Dr. Li-Chun Huang.

MODERN RESEARCH

Mense-Ease is formulated specifically to treat various gynecological disorders, such as dysmenorrhea, endometriosis, postpartum pain, and pain in various gynecological disorders. Independent research has confirmed that the ingredients of *Mense-Ease* exert strong analgesic, antispasmodic and anti-inflammatory effects.

Yan Hu Suo (Rhizoma Corydalis), containing corydaline, exerts a strong anti-inflammatory activity and is effective in both the acute and chronic phases of inflammation.[1] It also possesses strong analgesic activities that act directly on the central nervous system.[2] Because of this, *Yan Hu Suo* (Rhizoma Corydalis) works synergistically with acupuncture to relieve pain. According to a recent study, the analgesic effects of electro-acupuncture, when combined with *Yan Hu Suo* (Rhizoma Corydalis), are significantly greater than that of the control group that received electro-acupuncture only.[3]

Chi Shao (Radix Paeoniae Rubrae), containing daisein and paeoniflorin, has a strong antispasmodic effect to alleviate muscle spasms and cramping.[4] *Wu Yao* (Radix Linderae) has antispasmodic and muscle relaxant effects. [5]

Xiang Fu (Rhizoma Cyperi) inhibits the contraction of the uterus and relieves spasms. It also has an analgesic effect to relieve pain as well as an anti-inflammatory effect to reduce swelling.[5] It has been demonstrated in a research study that the use of *Xiang Fu* (Rhizoma Cyperi) greatly increases the pain threshold in mice. [4]

Mu Dan Pi (Cortex Moutan) has analgesic and anti-inflammatory effects and is commonly used for general aches and pains. It works directly on the central nervous system and has analgesic, tranquilizing and hypnotic effects. [4,5]

PHARMACEUTICAL DRUGS & CHINESE MEDICINE: A COMPARATIVE ANALYSIS

Western Medical Approach: Premenstrual syndrome (PMS) and dysmenorrhea are conditions that almost all women suffer on occasional basis. As common as these conditions are, there are few drug treatments available. On one hand, there are over-the-counter (OTC) drugs such as Midol and Motrin (Ibuprofen) that reduce swelling and inflammation. These drugs treat the symptoms, and do not regulate menstruation or change the long-term prognosis of the condition. Those who have PMS or dysmenorrhea are likely to have the same conditions on a monthly basis when treated with only these OTC drugs. On the other hand, there are prescription drugs such as birth control pills or patches that regulate menstrual cycles. Though they are more effective, they often cause serious side effects, such as weight gain, hyperkalemia, clotting disorders, retinal thrombosis, cancer, liver damage, hypertriglyceridemia, hypertension, bleeding, and fertility impairment. In short, drug treatment options are very limited between those that treat only symptoms and do not work well, and those that work well but may have significant side effects.

MENSE-EASE ™

Traditional Chinese Medicine Approach: Herbal therapy is extremely effective to regulate menstruation and relieve PMS and dysmenorrhea. These herbs have analgesic effect to relieve pain, anti-inflammatory effect to reduce swelling and inflammation, and antispasmodic effect to relieve cramping. Furthermore, many herbs have been shown to have marked effect to regulate hormones to promote normal menstruation. However, this effect requires continuous use of herbs for at least one to two cycles. In short, herbal therapy is extremely beneficial for treatment of menstrual disorders, as it treats both the symptoms and the cause of PMS and dysmenorrhea.

Summation: Drug offers limited options for treatment of PMS and dysmenorrhea. OTC drugs are ineffective and do not have lasting effects. Birth controls are effective, but these drugs carry significant short- and long-term side effects. Herbs, on the other hand, are extremely effective for both immediate and prolonged benefits. Furthermore, they are very safe and are associated with few or no side effects. Individuals with such menstrual disorders should definitely explore these non-drug treatment options.

CASE STUDIES

A 27-year-old female office worker presented with pain in her lower abdomen. The pain was more prominent before and during menses. She also had occasional bloody stools. The patient had a history of chronic yeast infections and endometriosis, which were resolved by surgeries. The practitioner diagnosed the condition as blood and qi stagnation with damp-heat in the lower *jiao*. After taking *Mense-Ease* and *Resolve (Lower)*, menstrual pain reduced and rectal bleeding abated.

N.H., Boulder, Colorado

A 51-year-old female postal worker noticed an irregularity in her menstrual cycle. For the past 3 years, she had noticed an increase in her menstrual irregularity. The patient noted moderate pain and heavy bleeding 8 days out of her whole cycle. Computerized Electrodermal Screening (EAV) detected higher than average readings, which was indicative of stress or irritation to her glands. The practitioner diagnosed this as peri-menopausal dysmenorrhea/menorrhagia due to qi and blood stagnation in lower *jiao*. After 2 months of taking *Mense-Ease* (2 capsules with each meal), the patient's menstrual discomfort improved 75% and her excessive bleeding was completely resolved.

D.H., Fort Myers, Florida

L.L., a 27-year-old female, presented with severe menstrual cramps, numerous dark blood clots, headache, acne breakouts with periods, extreme fatigue which forced her to lie in bed all day on the first day of the period. She stated that she must fast the first day otherwise she has nausea and vomiting. The blood pressure was 110/72 mmHg and the heart rate was 76 beats per minute. Her teethmarked tongue appeared dark purple with red dots on the tip and sides. Tongue coating was thin and white. The pulse was slippery and thin. The diagnosis was Liver blood stagnation with Spleen qi deficiency and Liver qi stagnation. *Mense-Ease* was prescribed. After taking it for two weeks, the patient's next period was much less debilitating. She reported fewer blood clots, no more headaches, normal body temperature, and less intense cramping. After two months, the symptoms have decreased by 50%. She was able to function and eat on day one of her period, whereas before, she was bed-ridden.

J.C.O., Whittier, California

A 28-year-old female dental hygienist presented with a palpable lump on her lower abdomen near acupuncture point *Zigongxue* (Uterus). She had severe premenstrual syndrome (PMS) affecting her emotionally, as well as large dark clots in her menstrual discharge. She had 1 week of constant dull pain on her left lower abdomen especially after her period. She described the pain as a grabbing, shooting type of pain as though someone was tightening a rope around her belly. She had a history of candida. She sought to get pregnant, and therefore discontinued taking her birth control pills. Laparoscopy was done in 1995 to remove her right ovary and in 1999 to remove endometriosis. Scar tissue was present in her left lower abdomen from a hernia operation when she was a youngster. Cysts were also

FORMULAS

MENSE-EASE ™

present on her left ovary. Lastly, the patient also had a history of hypothyroidism and hay fever. Her tongue color was unremarkable and her tongue coating appeared moist. Her tongue root coating would alternate from white to yellow. Her sublingual region was also unremarkable. The patient's pulse was constantly deep, thready and soft. The practitioner diagnosed this clinical picture as damp-heat in the lower *jiao* and Spleen qi deficiency leading to the accumulation of dampness. The practitioner prescribed *Mense-Ease* to regulate her menstruation, and *Resolve (Lower)* to treat endometriosis. The patient was instructed to take 3 to 5 capsules of each formula three times daily, starting 3 days before her period and to continue the dose throughout her menstrual flow and for 1 week afterwards. After taking the herbs, she became less emotional. She noted fewer episodes of cramps the first month and no pain during the second month of her herbal therapy. Although her lower abdominal pain lingered, the intensity lessened, the frequency reduced, and the affected area dwindled. The patient also finally discontinued her caffeine intake, which she also attributed to her pain. After 3 months of herbal treatment, surgery was done to remove 2 inches of tissue. Ultrasound confirmed the complete absence of ovarian cysts after 3 months of herbal therapy. Doppler ultrasound showed a favorable pulsatility index for uterine blood flow. There were no blockages present in her reproductive system. The practitioner concluded that *Mense-Ease* was quite effective in treating other patients with similar conditions. The efficacy of *Resolve (Lower)* was also proven clinically with ultrasound results.

T.K., Denver, Colorado

S.M. presented with dysmenorrhea, cramping with dark blood clots and fatigue. The tongue was purplish pale and the pulse was slippery and slow. She also had a pale complexion. The doctor diagnosed her with qi and blood stagnation and *Mense-Ease* was prescribed. After taking the formula, the patient reported relief of lower abdominal pain and reduction in blood clots.

B.F., Newport Beach, California

[1] Kubo, M. et al. *Biol Pharm Bull*. February 1994
[2] Zhu, XZ. Development of natural products as drugs acting on central nervous system. *Memorias do Instituto Oswaldo Cruz*. 86 2:173-5, 1991.
[3] Hu, J. et al. Effect of some drugs on electro-acupuncture analgesia and cytosolic free Ca^{++} concentration of mice brain. *Chen Tzu Yen Chiu*; 19(1):55-8. 1994
[4] Bensky, D. et al. *Chinese Herbal Medicine Materia Medica*. Eastland Press. 1993
[5] Yeung, HC. *Handbook of Chinese Herbs*. Institute of Chinese Medicine. 1996

FORMULAS

MIGRATROL ™

CLINICAL APPLICATIONS

- Migraine headache: acute and chronic
- Tension headache: acute and chronic
- Cluster headache: acute and chronic

WESTERN THERAPEUTIC ACTIONS

- Analgesic action to relieve pain [1,2,3,4,7,8,9]
- Anti-inflammatory influence to reduce inflammation [1,2,3,5,9]
- Treats various types of headaches [5,6,9,10,12,13]

CHINESE THERAPEUTIC ACTIONS

- Relieves pain
- Subdues hyperactive yang qi
- Tonifies blood and yin
- Extinguishes Liver wind
- Relieves qi and blood stagnation

DOSAGE

Take 3 to 4 capsules three times daily. For severe pain, the dosage may be increased to 6 to 8 capsules every 4 to 6 hours as necessary. For maximum effectiveness, take the herbs on an empty stomach with warm water.

INGREDIENTS

Bai Shao (Radix Paeoniae Alba)
Bai Zhi (Radix Angelicae Dahuricae)
Chuan Xiong (Rhizoma Ligustici Chuanxiong)
Dang Gui (Radicis Angelicae Sinensis)
Ge Gen (Radix Puerariae)
Ju Hua (Flos Chrysanthemi)

Long Gu (Os Draconis)
Man Jing Zi (Fructus Viticis)
Sang Ji Sheng (Herba Taxilli)
Shu Di Huang (Radix Rehmanniae Preparata)
Tian Ma (Rhizoma Gastrodiae)
Yu Jin (Radix Curcumae)

FORMULA EXPLANATION

Migratrol is an empirical formula based on the classic Chinese herbal formula *Si Wu Tang* (Tangkuei Four Combination) for tonifying Liver blood and yin. It is designed specifically to relieve the most common forms of migraine and tension headaches. The focus of this formula is directed at the *jueyin* and *shaoyang* meridians, the ones most commonly affected in migraine and tension headache syndromes. *Migratrol* contains herbs that tonify Liver blood and yin, subdue hyperactive yang qi, extinguish Liver wind, regulate Liver qi and blood, and relieve pain.

The four main herbs in *Migratrol* are in the classic herbal formula *Si Wu Tang* (Tangkuei Four Combination). *Shu Di Huang* (Radix Rehmanniae Preparata), *Dang Gui* (Radicis Angelicae Sinensis), *Bai Shao* (Radix Paeoniae Alba) and *Chuan Xiong* (Rhizoma Ligustici Chuanxiong) are combined to tonify Liver blood and yin. In addition, *Chuan Xiong* (Rhizoma Ligustici Chuanxiong) regulates and invigorates the blood, and is one of the primary herbs in the Chinese pharmacopoeia to treat headache. *Yu Jin* (Radix Curcumae) regulates wood element qi (Gallbladder/*shaoyang*), and relieves blood stasis. In combination with *Chuan Xiong* (Rhizoma Ligustici Chuanxiong), *Yu Jin* (Radix Curcumae) serves to invigorate and harmonize yin and yang, and Liver blood and qi. *Ju*

FORMULAS

MIGRATROL ™

Hua (Flos Chrysanthemi) tonifies Liver yin, clears Liver heat, and subdues hyperactive Liver yang. *Man Jing Zi* (Fructus Viticis), *Bai Zhi* (Radix Angelicae Dahuricae) and *Ge Gen* (Radix Puerariae) are combined for their benefits in relieving pain, relaxing muscle tension and relieving spasms by increasing peripheral blood circulation. *Tian Ma* (Rhizoma Gastrodiae) and *Long Gu* (Os Draconis) are added to extinguish Liver wind and subdue and anchor hyperactive Liver yang. *Sang Ji Sheng* (Herba Taxilli) is added to tonify Liver yin.

In summary, *Migratrol* contains herbs that address both acute and chronic aspects of headaches by treating excess and deficiency. It contains herbs to relieve pain by activating qi and blood circulation, calming hyperactive yang qi, and extinguishing Liver wind. Furthermore, it treats the underlying cause of headache by tonifying the blood and yin to remedy deficiencies in those areas.

SUPPLEMENTARY FORMULAS

- For acute headache with severe pain, add *Corydalin*.
- For headache from wind-heat, add *Lonicera Complex*.
- For headache from excess and heat conditions, add *Gardenia Complex*.
- For headache associated with infection, add *Herbal ABX*.
- For headache associated with infection of ear, nose and throat, add *Herbal ENT*.
- For headache caused by stress and tension, add *Calm*, *Calm (ES)*, or *Calm ZZZ*.
- For headache related to sinus congestion, add *Pueraria Clear Sinus* or *Magnolia Clear Sinus*.
- For headache with neck and shoulder stiffness, add *Neck & Shoulder (Acute)*.
- For migraine headache with Liver wind rising, combine with *Gastrodia Complex* or *Gentiana Complex*.
- If headache is caused by recent traumatic or musculo-skeletal injury, add *Traumanex*.
- For headache due to old trauma or injury or blood stagnation, add *Circulation (SJ)*.
- For Kidney yin deficiency, add *Nourish* or *Kidney Tonic (Yin)*.

NUTRITION

- Avoid intake of cold drinks, cold foods, and sour fruits: cold and sour substances constrict vessels, channels and collaterals.
- If headaches are food related, the diet must be regulated and controlled to reduce or eliminate triggers.
- Consume adequate amounts of fruits, vegetables, grains and raw nuts and seeds.
- One of the most common causes of headache is caffeine. Gradually decrease and stop consumption of caffeine-containing drinks, such as coffee, tea, cola, and specialty beverages with caffeine.
- Avoid foods containing tyramine, which can trigger headaches, such as alcohol, chocolate, bananas, citrus, avocado, cabbage, and potatoes. Also avoid cakes, dairy products (except yogurt), processed or packaged foods (because of colorants, preservatives and other additives), tobacco and junk food.
- Monosodium glutamate (MSG) should be avoided by individuals sensitive to it. MSG is generally found in canned soups, TV dinners, some meats, many pre-prepared frozen dishes and restaurant foods.

The Tao of Nutrition by Ni and McNease
- Headache
  - Recommendations: chrysanthemum flowers, mint, green onions, oyster shells, pearl barley, carrots, prunes, buckwheat, peach kernels, and green tea.
  - Avoid spicy food, lack of sleep, alcohol, smoking, excess stimulation, eye strain, and stress.
- For more information, please refer to *The Tao of Nutrition* by Dr. Maoshing Ni and Cathy McNease.

MIGRATROL ™

LIFESTYLE INSTRUCTIONS

- Avoid allergens as much as possible, as allergens may trigger headache.
- Installation of an air purifier will minimize the presence of allergens in the air and reduce the risk of allergy and headache.
- Avoid stressful situations and environments whenever possible. Ease tension with massage, warm baths, and an exercise program.
- Avoid direct exposure to air conditioning, fans, drafts or wind blowing on the head and neck region.
- Tension headaches can be relieved by gentle massage of the neck and shoulders to relax the muscles. A hot epsom salt bath or soaking the feet is also helpful.
- Headache due to poor circulation will respond to a vigorous scalp massage.
- Regular exercise, adequate rest, and normal sleeping habits are essential for optimal health.

CLINICAL NOTES

- The late Dr. John H.F. Shen created this formula. The formula explanation was provided by Ray Rubio, L.Ac..
- *Migratrol* is a great formula for both acute and chronic headache, especially if the headache is due in part to blood deficiency. It can be taken on a long-term basis to minimize recurrences and the severity of pain. The maintainance dose is 2 capsules twice daily.
- *Corydalin* is best for acute headaches with severe pain, and is most effective for symptomatic relief. *Migratrol* is most effective when taken on a long-term basis to control and prevent the recurrence of headaches.
- For headache in which herbs cannot achieve maximum relief, the cervical vertebrae (C1 to C3) should be checked for any abnormality. Check for specific trigger points in the neck or any uneven tension of cervical muscles bilaterally. If one side is stiffer than the other, this may be an indication of a cervical disorder. In cases where the neck and shoulder are also stiff due to misalignment resulting in headaches, *Neck & Shoulder (Acute)* can be added.
- For women who suffer from periodic headaches, especially preceding menstrual cycles, it is important to treat blood stagnation. The headaches usually subside with passage of blood clots. The recommended formulas include *Mense-Ease* and *Resolve (Lower)*.

CAUTIONS

- Patients with persistent pain not relieved by *Migratrol* or *Corydalin* should seek further examination to rule out structural or functional abnormalities.
- Patients who are on anticoagulant or antiplatelet therapies, such as Coumadin (Warfarin), should use this formula with caution, as there may be a slightly higher risk of bleeding and bruising.
- Should prominent signs of diminishing vision and vomiting occur in addition to the headache, refer the patient to a medical doctor immediately for a CT scan or MRI to rule out intracranial pressure due to a tumor, aneurysm, or cerebral stenosis.

ACUPUNCTURE POINTS

Traditional Points:
- *Renzhong* (GV 26), *Lieque* (LU 7), *Zusanli* (ST 36), *Xingjian* (LR 2), *Taichong* (LR 3), *Geshu* (BL 17), *Baihui* (GV 20), and *Xuehai* (SP 10).

Balance Method by Dr. Richard Tan:
- Migraine: On the same side of the migraine, needle *Fengshi* (GB 31), *Diwuhui* (GB 42), and *Shaofu* (HT 8).
- On the opposite side, needle *Taichong* (LR 3), *Xiguan* (LR 7), *Waiguan* (TH 5), and *Tianjing* (TH 10).

MIGRATROL ™

- ✆ For additional information on the Balance Method, please refer to *Dr. Tan's Strategy of Twelve Magical Points* and *Acupuncture 1, 2, 3* by Dr. Richard Tan.

Ear Points:
- ✆ Adrenal Gland, Hypothalamus, and Temporal Lobe.
- ✆ Use metal ear balls. Alternate ears every three days. Five sessions equals one treatment course.

Auricular Acupuncture by Dr. Li-Chun Huang:
- ✆ Migraine: Temple, Sympathetic, External Sympathetic, Nervous Subcortex, and Coronary Vascular Subcortex. Bleed Ear Apex
- ✆ Frontal headache: External Sympathetic, Forehead, Nervous Subcortex
  - ▪ For headache due to sinus or rhinitis, add Internal Nose
  - ▪ For headache due to ametropia: add Vision II
- ✆ Occipital headache: Occiput, Lesser Occipital Nerve, and Nervous Subcortex. Bleed Ear Apex.
  - ▪ For occiput headache due to cervical vertebral C3 to C4 degeneration, add Cervical Vertebral C3 and C4 (frontal and back of ear)
- ✆ Temporal headache: Temple, Sympathetic, External Sympathetic, Nervous Subcortex, and Coronary Vascular Subcortex. Bleed Ear Apex.
- ✆ Vertex headache: Vertex, External Sympathetic, and Nervous Subcortex. Bleed Ear Apex.
- ✆ For additional information on the location and explanation of these points, please refer to *Auricular Treatment Formula and Prescriptions* by Dr. Li-Chun Huang.

MODERN RESEARCH

Migratrol contains many herbs commonly used to treat a variety of headaches, including but not limited to migraine, tension and cluster headaches. The mechanism of action of the herbs includes analgesic effect to relieve pain, anti-inflammatory action to reduce inflammation, and specific constituents to target and treat headache.

Dang Gui (Radicis Angelicae Sinensis) is a commonly used herb in Chinese medicine and has pronounced strength to relieve various types of pain, including but not limited to migraine, pain of the low back and legs, and menstrual cramps.[1,2] Pharmacologically, it has shown analgesic and anti-inflammatory actions.[3] In comparison to aspirin, the anti-inflammatory action of *Dang Gui* (Radicis Angelicae Sinensis) is approximately 1.1 times stronger and its analgesic effect is approximately 1.7 times stronger.[4] More specifically, a preparation of *Dang Gui* (Radicis Angelicae Sinensis) was found to have an 82.9% effective rate in treating 35 patients with migraine headache.[5]

In addition to *Dang Gui* (Radicis Angelicae Sinensis), many herbs in this formula have also been used to treat headaches with good results. In one clinical study, 50 patients with headache were treated with herbal formulas with great success using such ingredients as *Dang Gui* (Radicis Angelicae Sinensis), *Chuan Xiong* (Rhizoma Ligustici Chuanxiong), *Bai Zhi* (Radix Angelicae Dahuricae), and *Ju Hua* (Flos Chrysanthemi).[6] All these herbs are ingredients of *Migratrol*.

Bai Shao (Radix Paeoniae Alba) is commonly used for its analgesic and antispasmodic effects.[7] Common applications include pain, spasms and cramps, and trigeminal pain.[8] Clinically, *Bai Shao* (Radix Paeoniae Alba) helps relieve pain and stiffness of neck and shoulder muscles associated with headache.

Bai Zhi (Radix Angelicae Dahuricae) has definite analgesic and anti-inflammatory activity, and is frequently used for a variety of headaches.[9] In addition to historical data, there have been various clinical studies proving *Bai Zhi* (Radix Angelicae Dahuricae) effectively treats headache. In one clinical study, patients with occipital headache were treated twice daily with *Bai Zhi* (Radix Angelicae Dahuricae). Out of 73 patients, 69 showed significant improvements, 3 showed slight improvement, and 1 showed no effect.[10] In another study, 54 out of 62 patients with chronic headache showed significant improvement using a 5% solution of *Bai Zhi* (Radix Angelicae Dahuricae) for 10 to 15 days per course of treatment, for 1 to 2 courses total.[11] In short, *Bai Zhi* (Radix Angelicae Dahuricae) is an extremely useful and effective herb for headache treatment.

In addition to the herbs listed above, *Ge Gen* (Radix Puerariae) and *Tian Ma* (Rhizoma Gastrodiae) in **Migratrol** show clear clinical effectiveness in treating headaches. In a clinical study of migraine headache, a *Ge Gen* (Radix Puerariae) preparation containing 100 mg of puerarin was reported 83% effective when used three times daily for 2 to 22 days.[12] Gastrodin, one of the ingredients of *Tian Ma* (Rhizoma Gastrodiae), showed good results in treating 156 patients with neurasthenic headache and 72 patients with vascular headache.[13]

In summary, **Migratrol** contains herbs that have shown through historical applications and clinical trials to be effective in treating a variety of headaches, including but not limited to migraine, tension and cluster headaches.

PHARMACEUTICAL DRUGS & CHINESE MEDICINE: A COMPARATIVE ANALYSIS

Western Medical Approach: Pain is a basic bodily sensation induced by a noxious stimulus that causes physical discomfort (as pricking, throbbing, or aching). Pain may be of acute or chronic state, and may be of nociceptive, neuropathic, or psychogenic type. For migraine, three classes of drugs commonly used to treat pain include non-steroidal anti-inflammatory agents (NSAID), opioid analgesics, and serotonin agonists. NSAID's [such as Motrin (Ibuprofen) and Voltaren (Diclofenac)] are generally used for mild to moderate pain, and are most effective to reduce inflammation and swelling. Though effective, they may cause such serious side effects as gastric ulcer, duodenal ulcer, gastrointestinal bleeding, tinnitus, blurred vision, dizziness and headache. Opioid analgesics [such as Vicodin (APAP/Hydrocodone) and morphine] are usually used for severe to excruciating pain. While they may be the most potent agents for pain, they also have the most serious risks and side effects, including but not limited to dizziness, lightheadedness, drowsiness, upset stomach, vomiting, constipation, stomach pain, rash, difficult urination, and respiratory depression resulting in difficult breathing. Furthermore, long-term use of these drugs leads to tolerance and addiction. Lastly, serotonin agonists, such as Imitrex (Sumatriptan), are specifically used for migraine. Common side effects of this drug include flushing, tingling feeling, feeling of warmth or heaviness, drowsiness, dizziness, upset stomach, diarrhea, vomiting, irritation of the nose, and muscle cramps. Though effective, these drugs do not change the course of illness, and do not reduce the frequency or severity of recurrent migraine attacks. In brief, it is important to remember that while drugs offer reliable and potent pain relief, they only treat symptoms and not the cause. They should be used only if and when needed. Frequent use and abuse leads to unnecessary side effects and complications.

Traditional Chinese Medicine Approach: Treatment of migraine is a sophisticated balance of art and science. Proper treatment of pain requires a careful evaluation of the type of disharmony (excess or deficiency, cold or heat, exterior or interior), characteristics (qi and/or blood stagnations), and locations (upper body, lower body, extremities, or internal organs). Furthermore, optimal treatment requires integrative use of herbs, acupuncture and *Tui-Na* therapies. All these therapies work together to tonify underlying deficiencies, strengthen the body, and facilitate recovery from chronic pain. TCM pain management targets both symptoms and the causes of pain, and as such, often achieves immediate and long-term success. Furthermore, TCM pain management is often associated with few or no side effects.

Summation: For treatment of mild to severe pain due to various causes, TCM pain management offers similar treatment effects with significantly fewer side effects. However, as is true of any therapeutic modality, it is important to recognize the limitations of TCM pain management. In some cases, such as acute, excruciating migraine, drugs are superior to herbs, as they are more immediately potent and have a more rapid onset of action (especially if given via injection). Therefore, optimal treatment may require the integration of western medicine to

MIGRATROL ™

treat acute pain, and herbal medicine to provide long-term healing of underlying causes and prevent recurrence of migraines.

CASE STUDY

M.L., a 13-year-old female, presented with migraine headache with no other significant complaints. She was diagnosed with qi and blood stagnation. *Migratrol* was prescribed at 6 grams daily. In the first two weeks, the patient reported the headache occurred approximately four times a week. During the third and fourth week of herbal treatment, the headache reduced to twice a week. During the fifth week, the headache was completely gone and the patient felt she had more energy. She also received acupuncture throughout the five weeks.

W.F., Bloomfield, New Jersey

[1] *Xin Zhong Yi* (New Chinese Medicine), 1980; 2:34
[2] *Lan Zhou Yi Xue Yuan Xue Bao* (Journal of Lanzhou University of Medicine), 1988; 1:36
[3] *Xin Yi Yao Xue Za Zhi* (New Journal of Medicine and Herbology), 1975; (6):34
[4] *Yao Xue Za Zhi* (Journal of Medicinals), 1971; (91):1098
[5] *Bei Jing Yi Xue* (Beijing Medicine), 1988; 2:95
[6] *Shan Xi Zhong Yi Za Zhi* (Shanxi Journal Chinese Medicine), 1985; 10:447
[7] *Shang Hai Zhong Yi Yao Za Zhi* (Shanghai Journal of Chinese Medicine and Herbology), 1983; 4:14
[8] *Zhong Yi Za Zhi* (Journal of Chinese Medicine), 1983; 11:9
[9] *Zhong Guo Zhong Yao Za Zhi* (People's Republic of China Journal of Chinese Herbology), 1991; 16(9):560
[10] *Xin Yi Xue* (New Medicine), 1976; 1:8
[11] *Xin Yi Yao Xue Za Zhi* (New Journal of Medicine and Herbology), 1976; 8:35
[12] *Zhong Hua Nei Ke Za Zhi* (Chinese Journal of Internal Medicine), 1977; 6:326
[13] *Zhong Guo Shen Jing Jing Shen Ke Za Zhi* (Chinese Journal of Psychiatric Disorders), 1986; 5:265

NECK & SHOULDER (Acute) ™

CLINICAL APPLICATIONS

☙ Neck and shoulder pain, possibly with redness, swelling, and inflammation
☙ Limited movement of the neck and shoulders, due to pain and stiffness
☙ Whiplash, muscle tightness and spasms
☙ Frozen shoulders with neck pain
☙ Pain associated with a slipped or bulging disk of the neck
☙ Acute neck and shoulder pain due to sports injuries, car accidents, prolonged body posture in a fixed position (such as working in front of a computer or sleeping in a poor position)
☙ Pain in the shoulder and scapula regions

WESTERN THERAPEUTIC ACTIONS

☙ Analgesic effect to relieve pain [1,2,3]
☙ Anti-inflammatory function to reduce inflammation and swelling [2,3]
☙ Muscle-relaxant action to alleviate muscle spasms and cramps [1,5]

CHINESE THERAPEUTIC ACTIONS

☙ Invigorates qi and blood circulation, eliminates qi and blood stagnation
☙ Opens channels and collaterals and relieves pain
☙ Reduces swelling and inflammation

DOSAGE

Take 4 capsules three times daily for moderate pain, or 7 to 8 capsules three times daily for severe pain. For maximum effectiveness, take the herbs with 6 to 8 ounces of warm water.

INGREDIENTS

Bai Shao (Radix Paeoniae Alba)
Chuan Xiong (Rhizoma Ligustici Chuanxiong)
Dang Gui Wei (Extremitas Radicis Angelicae Sinensis)
Gan Cao (Radix Glycyrrhizae)
Ge Gen (Radix Puerariae)

Hong Hua (Flos Carthami)
Qiang Huo (Rhizoma et Radix Notopterygii)
Wei Ling Xian (Radix Clematidis)
Yan Hu Suo (Rhizoma Corydalis)

FORMULA EXPLANATION

As the name implies, *Neck & Shoulder (Acute)* is designed to treat acute neck and shoulder pain. Acute neck and shoulder problems are often caused by accidents, such as car accidents, whiplash injuries, and prolonged body posture in a fixed position. In addition to pain, there is sometimes redness, swelling and inflammation.

Bai Shao (Radix Paeoniae Alba) and *Ge Gen* (Radix Puerariae) have strong antispasmodic effects to alleviate muscle spasms, cramps and pain. *Yan Hu Suo* (Rhizoma Corydalis) is a strong analgesic and is used in this formula to invigorate blood, activate qi and alleviate pain. To invigorate blood circulation and alleviate pain, *Hong Hua* (Flos Carthami), *Dang Gui Wei* (Extremitas Radicis Angelicae Sinensis) and *Chuan Xiong* (Rhizoma Ligustici Chuanxiong) are added. *Wei Ling Xian* (Radix Clematidis) is used to alleviate pain, promote qi stagnation and unblock stagnation in the channels due to external wind obstruction. With its warm and aromatic properties, *Qiang*

NECK & SHOULDER (Acute) ™

Huo (Rhizoma et Radix Notopterygii) opens the channels and alleviates pain in the upper body. Finally, *Gan Cao* (Radix Glycyrrhizae) harmonizes the formula and alleviates pain and spasms with an anti-inflammatory effect.

SUPPLEMENTARY FORMULAS

- To enhance the effect to relieve pain, add *Herbal Analgesic*.
- For recent trauma or bone fractures, combine with *Traumanex* initially, followed by *Osteo 8*.
- For old injury or stubborn pain due to chronic blood stagnation, use *Neck & Shoulder (Chronic)* or add *Circulation (SJ)*.
- With bone spurs or calcification, add *Flex (Spur)*.
- For shooting pain radiating down the arms, add *Arm Support*.
- For lower back, sciatic, or nerve pain, combine with *Back Support (Acute)* or *Back Support (Chronic)*.
- For joint pain or arthritis that worsens during cold and rainy weather, combine with *Flex (CD)*.
- For joint inflammation with redness, swelling, and burning pain, combine with *Flex (Heat)*.
- For severe spasms, combine with *Flex (SC)*.
- With hypertension, combine with *Gastrodia Complex*.
- With headache, add *Corydalin*.
- With migraine, add *Migratrol*.
- For stress-related neck pain, add *Calm*.
- For stress-related neck pain with insomnia, add *Calm ZZZ*.
- For osteoporosis, add *Osteo 8*.
- For herniated disk, add *Back Support (HD)*.
- For degeneration of muscles, tendons, ligaments and cartilage, add *Flex (MLT)*.

NUTRITION

- Eat plenty of whole grains, seafood, dark green vegetables, and nuts. These foods are rich in vitamin B complex and magnesium, which are essential for nerve health and relaxation of tense muscles.
- Adequate intake of minerals, such as calcium and potassium, are essential for pain management. Deficiency of these minerals will lead to spasms, cramps, and tense muscles.

LIFESTYLE INSTRUCTIONS

- Patients should avoid exposing affected areas to cold or drafts. Scarves, turtlenecks or similar clothing should be worn to protect the neck and avoid exposing the shoulders.
- Patients with frozen shoulders should be encouraged to exercise their shoulders as much as possible.
- Patients should also be advised to check their pillow to make sure it is not too high or too low. Mattresses should also be assessed for firmness.
- Hot bath with Epsom salts help to relax tense muscles and withdraw toxins from the tissues. Rest and relax in the bath for about 30 minutes.

CLINICAL NOTES

- Dr. Alex Chen, a master of traditional Chinese medicine with over 30 years of clinical experience, formulated *Neck & Shoulder (Acute)* specifically to relieve pain, reduce inflammation and stop muscle cramps. Herbs in this formula are routinely used in the trauma department of hospitals in China.
- Common causes of neck and shoulder injuries include traumas such as car accidents, sports injuries and/or repetitive stress syndrome of the neck and shoulder (i.e., from prolonged sitting in an upright position and/or staring at a computer monitor).

FORMULAS

NECK & SHOULDER (Acute) ™

✓ To consolidate the treatment effect, use *Flex (MLT)* or *Neck & Shoulder (Chronic)* for one week before discharging the patient.

Pulse Diagnosis by Dr. Jimmy Wei-Yen Chang:

✓ Thick and forceful pulse proximal to the right *chi* indicates pain on the upper *jiao* This pulse feels like a toothpick underneath the skin. The more forceful the pulse, the more severe the inflammation and pain are.

✓ Note: Dr. Chang takes the pulse in slightly different positions. He places his index finger directly over the wrist crease, and his middle and ring fingers alongside to locate *cun*, *guan* and *chi* positions. For additional information and explanation, please refer to *Pulsynergy* by Dr. Jimmy Wei-Yen Chang and Marcus Brinkman.

CAUTIONS

✓ Acute neck and shoulder pain, such as in whiplash, may be accompanied by spinal or anatomical injuries. The patient should be checked for structural and anatomical abnormalities if the overall condition does not improve after taking this herbal formula for 1 to 2 weeks.

✓ This formula is contraindicated during pregnancy and nursing, as it contains strong qi and blood activating herbs.

✓ Patients who are on anticoagulant or antiplatelet therapies, such as Coumadin (Warfarin), should use this formula with caution, as there may be a slightly higher risk of bleeding and bruising.

ACUPUNCTURE POINTS

Traditional Points:

✓ *Houxi* (SI 3) and *Shugu* (BL 65). Leave needles in for 15 minutes.

✓ *Hegu* (LI 4), *Shousanli* (LI 10), *Jianliao* (TH 14), *Chize* (LU 5), *Waiguan* (TH 5), *Quchi* (LI 11), *Fengchi* (GB 20), and *Dazhui* (GV 14).

Balance Method by Dr. Richard Tan:

✓ Needle the following points on the side opposite the pain: *Lingdao* (HT 4), *Tongli* (HT 5), *Shenmen* (HT 7), *Xuanzhong* (GB 39), and *Shugu* (BL 65).

✓ Needle the following points on the same side as the pain: *Houxi* (SI 3), *Zhongzhu* (TH 3), and *Sanyinjiao* (SP 6) or *ah shi* points nearby.

✓ After the needles are inserted, the patient should move his or her neck to loosen up the joint and the muscles.

✓ For additional information on the Balance Method, please refer to *Dr. Tan's Strategy of Twelve Magical Points* and *Acupuncture 1, 2, 3* by Dr. Richard Tan.

Ear Points:

✓ Neck pain: Cervical Vertebrae, Neck, Shoulder, Shoulder Blades, and Kidney. Embed ear seeds and instruct the patient to massage the points three to four times daily for two minutes each time. Switch ears every five days. Five treatments equal one course.

✓ Frozen shoulder: Shoulder, Shoulder Joint, Adrenal Gland or Shoulder, Clavicle, Adrenal Gland, Liver, Spleen, Subcortex.

✓ Fallen pillow syndrome/torticollis: Neck, Cervical Vertebrae and all the tender points around the area. Strong stimulation for 60 minutes. Needle once a day. Most patients will experience relief once the needles are inserted. If the pain is along the Liver and Gallbladder channels, needle Liver and Gallbladder as well. Similarly, if the pain is on the *taiyang* Urinary Bladder or Small intestine channel, needle the corresponding points accordingly.

NECK & SHOULDER (Acute) ™

Auricular Acupuncture by Dr. Li-Chun Huang:
- ☯ Torticollis (strained neck): Triangle Area of Cervical Vertebrae.
  - Occiput, Lesser Occiput Nerve, Large Auricular Nerve
- ☯ Periarthritis of shoulder: Shoulder, Shoulder Joint, Clavicle, and Large Auricular Nerve.
  - For pain of the shoulder upon abduction, use Clavicle, Shoulder Point (front and back of ear)
  - For anterior shoulder pain, use Shoulder Joint (front of ear), add Coronary Vascular Subcortex
  - For posterior shoulder pain, use Shoulder Joint (back of ear)
- ☯ For additional information on the location and explanation of these points, please refer to *Auricular Treatment Formula and Prescriptions* by Dr. Li-Chun Huang.

MODERN RESEARCH

Neck & Shoulder (Acute) contains herbs that have strong analgesic, anti-inflammatory and antispasmodic functions as confirmed by independent research.

Yan Hu Suo (Rhizoma Corydalis), containing corydaline, exerts strong anti-inflammatory activities and is effective in both the acute and chronic phases of inflammation.[2] It also possesses strong analgesic components that act directly on the central nervous system.[3] Because of its action on the central nervous system, *Yan Hu Suo* (Rhizoma Corydalis) works synergistically with acupuncture to relieve pain. It was demonstrated in one study that when combined with *Yan Hu Suo* (Rhizoma Corydalis), the analgesic effect of electro-acupuncture increased significantly when compared with the control group, which received electro-acupuncture only.[4] In addition, *Bai Shao* (Radix Paeoniae Alba) and *Ge Gen* (Radix Puerariae) contain daisein and paenoniflorin, which have strong antispasmodic effects to alleviate muscle spasms and cramps.[1,5] Finally, there are many herbs in this formula that increase blood circulation to expedite recovery.

PHARMACEUTICAL DRUGS & CHINESE MEDICINE: A COMPARATIVE ANALYSIS

Western Medical Approach: Pain is a basic bodily sensation induced by a noxious stimulus that causes physical discomfort (as pricking, throbbing, or aching). Pain may be of acute or chronic states. For acute neck and shoulder pain, two classes of drugs commonly used for treatment include non-steroidal anti-inflammatory agents (NSAID) and opioid analgesics. NSAID's [such as Motrin (Ibuprofen) and Voltaren (Diclofenac)] are generally used for mild to moderate pain, and are most effective to reduce inflammation and swelling. Though effective, they may cause such serious side effects as gastric ulcer, duodenal ulcer, gastrointestinal bleeding, tinnitus, blurred vision, dizziness and headache. Furthermore, the newer NSAID's, also known as Cox-2 inhibitors [such as Celebrex (Celecoxib)], are associated with significantly higher risk of cardiovascular events, including heart attack and stroke. Opioid analgesics [such as Vicodin (APAP/Hydrocodone) and morphine] are usually used for severe to excruciating pain. While they may be the most potent agents for pain, they also have the most serious risks and side effects, including but not limited to dizziness, lightheadedness, drowsiness, upset stomach, vomiting, constipation, stomach pain, rash, difficult urination, and respiratory depression resulting in difficult breathing. Furthermore, long-term use of these drugs leads to tolerance and addiction. In brief, it is important to remember that while drugs offer reliable and potent symptomatic pain relief, they should be used only if and when needed. Frequent use and abuse leads to unnecessary side effects and complications.

Traditional Chinese Medicine Approach: Treatment of pain is a sophisticated balance of art and science. Proper treatment of pain requires a careful evaluation of the type of disharmony (excess or deficiency, cold or heat, exterior or interior), characteristics (qi and/or blood stagnations), and locations (upper body, lower body, extremities, or internal organs). Furthermore, optimal treatment requires integrative use of herbs, acupuncture and *Tui-Na* therapies. All these therapies work together to tonify underlying deficiencies, strengthen the body, and facilitate recovery from chronic pain. TCM pain management targets both symptoms and the causes of pain, and as such, often achieves immediate and long-term success. Furthermore, TCM pain management is often associated with few or no side effects.

Summation: For treatment of mild to severe pain due to various causes, TCM pain management offers similar treatment effects with significantly fewer side effects.

CASE STUDIES

L.P., a 77-year-old female, presented with severe pain in the left wrist and right rib cage after a fall. She had numbness of the wrist and palm where she landed on the cement. The patient showed bruises on the right eye. The right wrist was painful to light movement and palpation. There were tender points on the right subclavicular area. There were no visible contusions on the right rib cage. The diagnoses were qi and blood stagnation with soft tissue damage. *Traumanex*, *Neck & Shoulder (Acute)* and *Flex (SC)* were prescribed at 2 capsules of each formula three times daily. The patient reported daily lowering of pain levels. Numbness was reduced to a light tingling after 2 days. She reported continuous and steady improvement each day. She was instructed to reduce the dosage to 2 capsules of each formula twice a day when the pain subsided. After the swelling was reduced, the patient was referred to a chiropractor for cervical and occipital adjustments.

M. H., West Palm Beach, Florida

A male presented with pain and decreased range of motion in the right shoulder. There was pain upon palpation on the Large Intestine and Small Intestine channels. The practitioner diagnosed the condition as *bi zheng* (painful obstruction syndrome) due to stagnation of qi and blood. The patient was instructed to take *Neck & Shoulder (Acute)*. Acupuncture treatments using Dr. Tan's Balance Method and *Tui Na* massage using Dr. Alex Chen's techniques were also applied. After six acupuncture and herbal treatments, he regained full shoulder range of motion without pain. After the pain was completely resolved, the practitioner switched the prescription to *Neck & Shoulder (Chronic)* at 3 capsules per day for maintenance care. Upon recurrence of pain, the patient was instructed to increase the dosage, which in turn resolved the pain sensations.

K.S., Encinitas, California

A 44-year-old female police officer presented with chronic headaches located in the occipital/temporal regions. She stated that stress aggravated the problem. There was acute tenderness at the *Fengchi* (GB 20) area as well as in the cervical spine. She also experienced pain on her zygoma. The practitioner diagnosed the condition as qi and blood stagnation in the Gallbladder, Urinary Bladder, and Small Intestine channels in addition to myofascial syndrome, which was stress-induced because of the nature of her job. She was treated with *Corydalin*, *Neck & Shoulder (Acute)* and *Calm (ES)*, which were all quite effective that they subsequently replaced her medication, Imitrex (Sumatriptan). The practitioner concluded that a critical aspect in the treatment was to assist patient in coping with their stress, which in turn made the herbal treatment more effective.

S.C., La Crescenta., CA

A 43-year-old female teacher presented with severe shoulder and neck muscle pain of two months duration. She attributed her musculoskeletal pain to stress from her job. She had a red-purple tongue and a deep rolling pulse. The practitioner diagnosed her condition as qi and blood stagnation. Within a week of taking *Neck & Shoulder (Acute)*, her pain reduced to about 50 to 60%. As an adjunct to the herbal treatment, acupuncture, massage and yoga were also added. After three weeks on the treatment plan, the patient's pain was almost completely resolved.

T.G., Albuquerque, New Mexico

FORMULAS

NECK & SHOULDER (Acute) ™

A 45-year-old female was involved in a car accident in August 1997. She was rear-ended by another vehicle, resulting in a whiplash. She had severe pain and inflammation on the back of her head and very limited movement of her neck. She could only move her head bilaterally 10 to 15 degrees. X-ray showed no structural damages. She started receiving *Tui-Na* treatments and taking *Neck & Shoulder (Acute)* at 7 capsules three times daily. After 2 days, pain and inflammation were reduced significantly. After 10 days, there was no inflammation and no pain at rest. She could now move her neck up to 40 degrees to the left, and 45 degrees to the right. She was able to return to work and drive safely on her own.

J.C., Diamond Bar, California

A 55-year-old horse trainer presented with a torn rotator cuff following a horse training accident. The pain in her left shoulder was so severe she was unable to sleep. NSAID's were taken without any relief. The patient took *Neck & Shoulder (Acute)*. At the close of 4 days of herbs, 60% of her pain was relieved. After 2½ weeks, she had no difficulty sleeping and the pain was no longer present.

J.H., Fort Myers, Florida

An 18-year-old male chef presented with neck and shoulder pain from a skateboard fall. X-rays revealed a diminished cervical curvature as well as a hypokyphotic curve at T2 to T3. The practitioner diagnosed the condition as a cervical sprain/strain. The patient was treated with *Neck & Shoulder (Acute)* and *Traumanex*, which produced a reduction in pain. The patient found it necessary to take the herbs with food to avoid stomach discomfort.

M.H., Jupiter, Florida

J.M., a 36-year-old female massage therapist presented with pain from a recent automobile accident (second accident in 6 months). She exhibited neck, back, arm, and leg pain. Airbags bent her right thumb. Her blood pressure was 120/70 mmHg and her heart rate was 72 beats per minute. X-rays showed herniation and soft tissue damage. She also complained of muscle spasms, hot sensation on trigger points, inability to move the right thumb, and the range of motion for the neck and trunk were both decreased. *Traumanex*, *Neck & Shoulder (Acute)* and *Back Support (Acute)* were all prescribed at 2 capsules each three times daily. J.M. responded quickly to these formulas and acupuncture treatments. Pain levels were reduced by half in a short period of time.

M.H., West Palm Beach, Florida

A 47-year-old female office manager complained of neck pain and low back pain that were aggravated by prolonged sitting. She has a past history of two whiplash injuries that can also have attributed to causing her neck pain. Upon examination, the practitioner found extreme spasms of the erector muscles, bilateral weakness of her sternocleidomastoid muscles and a lack of muscle tone in her lower back. With these symptoms, the patient was diagnosed with right-sided sciatica, arthralgia of the spine and stress-induced muscle spasms. The TCM diagnosis was concluded to be Liver qi stagnation. The treatment included acupuncture, moxa, and infrared heat. *Back Support (Acute)* and *Neck & Shoulder (Acute)* were prescribed for this patient. The results were as follows:

    3/29/01: stress: 8; pain: 9-10 (on a scale of 1 to 10; 10 rating = worse condition)
    5/05/01: 50% improvement
    5/19/01: 70% improvement
    8/16/01: No more pain. However, slight intermittent flaring of her condition was noted.

The practitioner and the patient both concluded that the *Back Support (Acute)* and *Neck & Shoulder (Acute)* have really helped.

T.W., Santa Monica, California

NECK & SHOULDER (Acute) ™

An 85-year-old retired female presented with excruciating pain in the neck and shoulder that caused difficulty sleeping. Objective findings included limited range of motion of the neck. The tongue had a dirty yellow coat and a red tip. The western diagnosis included psoriatic arthritis, arthritis, fibromyalgia, hiatal hernia, hypertension, depression, chronic constipation, leaky gut syndrome, sciatica and insomnia. The patient was instructed to take *Neck & Shoulder (Acute)* and *Corydalin*, 3 capsules of each three times daily in between meals. *Calm (ES)* was given at night to help sleep. The patient responded that the formulas were effective in reducing the acute pain in the neck and shoulder region. After the acute phase two weeks later, the patient was switched to *Gan Mai Da Zao Tang* (Licorice, Wheat, and Jujube Decoction) and *Shao Yao Gan Cao Tang* (Peony and Licorice Decoction), a combination recommended by Dr. Richard Tan that consistently helps patients with fibromyalgia.

J.B., Camarillo, California

[1] Bensky, D. et al. *Chinese Herbal Medicine Materia Medica*. Eastland Press. 1993
[2] Kubo, M. et al. Anti-Inflammatory activities of methanolic extract and alkaloidal components from corydalis tuber. *Biol Pharm Bull*. 17(2):262-5, February 1994
[3] Zhu, XZ. Development of natural products as drugs acting on central nervous system. *Memorias do Instituto Oswaldo Cruz*. 86 2:173-5, 1991.
[4] Hu, J, et al. Effect of some drugs on electro-acupuncture analgesia and cytosolic free Ca++ concentration of mice brain. *Chen Tzu Yen Chiu*; 19(1):55-8. 1994
[5] Yeung, HC. *Handbook of Chinese Herbs*. Institute of Chinese Medicine. 1996

FORMULAS

NECK & SHOULDER (Chronic) ™

CLINICAL APPLICATIONS

- Chronic pain of the neck and shoulders, including numbness and discomfort
- Limited movement of the neck and shoulders due to pain and stiffness
- Long-term neck and shoulder injuries with a slow recovery or continuing deterioration
- Injuries of the neck and shoulder muscles commonly caused by over-exertion
- Repetitive stress syndrome of the neck and shoulders (i.e., prolonged upright sitting position, or working in front of a computer)
- Arthritis of the neck

WESTERN THERAPEUTIC ACTIONS

- Anti-inflammatory effect to reduce inflammation and swelling [1]
- Analgesic action to alleviate muscle pain [2]
- Muscle-relaxant effect to relieve muscle cramps and spasms [4]
- Nourishes the muscles and the tendons to speed up recovery [5]

CHINESE THERAPEUTIC ACTIONS

- Disperses painful obstruction, strengthens sinews and tendons
- Disperses residual qi and blood stagnation in the channels and collaterals
- Relieves pain and muscle spasms due to chronic *bi zheng* (painful obstruction syndrome) of the neck and shoulders

DOSAGE

For moderate pain, take 4 capsules three times daily; for severe pain, take 7 to 8 capsules every six hours as needed. For maximum effectiveness, take the herbs with 6 to 8 ounces of warm water on an empty stomach.

INGREDIENTS

Bai Shao (Radix Paeoniae Alba)
Chuan Niu Xi (Radix Cyathulae)
Chuan Xiong (Rhizoma Ligustici Chuanxiong)
Dang Gui Wei (Extremitas Radicis Angelicae Sinensis)
Di Gu Pi (Cortex Lycii)
Gan Cao (Radix Glycyrrhizae)
Ge Gen (Radix Puerariae)
Hong Hua (Flos Carthami)
Mo Yao (Myrrha)
Mu Gua (Fructus Chaenomelis)

Qiang Huo (Rhizoma et Radix Notopterygii)
Qin Jiao (Radix Gentianae Macrophyllae)
Ru Xiang (Gummi Olibanum)
Sang Ji Sheng (Herba Taxilli)
Sheng Di Huang (Radix Rehmanniae)
Tao Ren (Semen Persicae)
Wu Jia Pi (Cortex Acanthopanacis)
Xu Duan (Radix Dipsaci)
Yan Hu Suo (Rhizoma Corydalis)

FORMULA EXPLANATION

As the name implies, ***Neck & Shoulder (Chronic)*** is designed to treat chronic neck and shoulder pain. Chronic neck and shoulder problems are characterized by pain, numbness, stiffness, discomfort, limited mobility, slow recovery or continuing deterioration. Effective treatment must focus on activating qi and blood circulation, opening the channels and collaterals, and nourishing the muscles and tendons.

NECK & SHOULDER (Chronic) ™

Qiang Huo (Rhizoma et Radix Notopterygii) treats soreness, pain and numbness in the neck, upper back and shoulders due to wind-damp obstruction. *Sang Ji Sheng* (Herba Taxilli), *Chuan Niu Xi* (Radix Cyathulae), *Sheng Di Huang* (Radix Rehmanniae) and *Xu Duan* (Radix Dipsaci) are used together to tonify the Kidney and the Liver, strengthen the tendons, and alleviate pain, stiffness and soreness of the muscles. *Mu Gua* (Fructus Chaenomelis) and *Qin Jiao* (Radix Gentianae Macrophyllae) dispel painful obstruction and cramping, relax the sinews and unblock the channels. *Wu Jia Pi* (Cortex Acanthopanacis) treats painful obstruction due to Liver and Kidney yin deficiencies. *Yan Hu Suo* (Rhizoma Corydalis) invigorates blood, activates qi and alleviates pain. *Tao Ren* (Semen Persicae), *Hong Hua* (Flos Carthami), *Ru Xiang* (Gummi Olibanum), *Mo Yao* (Myrrha), *Chuan Xiong* (Rhizoma Ligustici Chuanxiong), and *Dang Gui Wei* (Extremitas Radicis Angelicae Sinensis) invigorate blood and remove residual stasis in the channels and collaterals. *Bai Shao* (Radix Paeoniae Alba) and *Ge Gen* (Radix Puerariae) contain daisein and paeoniflorin and have strong antispasmodic effects to alleviate muscle spasm, cramps and pain. Aside from its anti-inflammatory effects, *Gan Cao* (Radix Glycyrrhizae) harmonizes the formula and alleviates muscle pain and spasms. *Sheng Di Huang* (Radix Rehmanniae) and *Di Gu Pi* (Cortex Lycii) tonify yin, clear deficient heat and keep the temperature of this formula cool.

SUPPLEMENTARY FORMULAS

- ☯ With bone spurs or calcification, add *Flex (Spur)*.
- ☯ For joint pain or arthritis that worsens during cold and rainy weather, combine with *Flex (CD)*.
- ☯ For joint inflammation with redness, swelling, and burning pain, combine with *Flex (Heat)*.
- ☯ With severe spasms, combine with *Flex (SC)*.
- ☯ To strengthen the soft tissues (muscles, tendons, ligaments), add *Flex (MLT)*.
- ☯ For bone fractures, combine with *Traumanex*.
- ☯ To improve blood circulation, add *Flex (NP)*.
- ☯ For lower back, sciatic, or nerve pain, combine with *Back Support (Acute)* or *Back Support (Chronic)*.
- ☯ With headache, add *Corydalin*.
- ☯ With migraine, add *Migratrol*.
- ☯ For osteoporosis, add *Osteo 8*.
- ☯ To enhance the effect to relieve pain, add *Herbal Analgesic*.
- ☯ For herniated disk, add *Back Support (HD)*.
- ☯ For old injury or stubborn pain due to chronic blood stagnation, add *Circulation (SJ)*.
- ☯ For shooting pain radiating down the arms, add *Arm Support*.
- ☯ For stress-related neck pain with insomnia, add *Calm ZZZ*.

CLINICAL NOTES

- ☯ Dr. Alex Chen, a master of traditional Chinese medicine with over 30 years of clinical experience, formulated *Neck & Shoulder (Chronic)* specifically to relieve pain, reduce inflammation and stop muscle cramps. Herbs in this formula are routinely used in the trauma department of hospitals in China.

Pulse Diagnosis by Dr. Jimmy Wei-Yen Chang:
- ☯ Thick and forceful pulse proximal to the right *chi* indicates pain on the upper *jiao*. This pulse feels like a toothpick underneath the skin. If there is soft tissue damage, the pulse proximal to the right *chi* will feel like a "turtle shell."
- ☯ Note: Dr. Chang takes the pulse in slightly different positions. He places his index finger directly over the wrist crease, and his middle and ring fingers alongside to locate *cun*, *guan* and *chi* positions. For additional information and explanation, please refer to *Pulsynergy* by Dr. Jimmy Wei-Yen Chang and Marcus Brinkman.

FORMULAS

NECK & SHOULDER (Chronic) ™

NUTRITION

☙ Eat plenty of whole grains, seafoods, dark green vegetables, and nuts. These foods are rich in vitamin B complex and magnesium, which are essential for nerve health and relaxation of tense muscles.

☙ Adequate intake of minerals, such as calcium and potassium, are essential for pain management. Deficiency of these minerals will lead to spasms, cramps, and tense muscles.

LIFESTYLE INSTRUCTIONS

☙ Patients should avoid exposing affected areas to cold temperatures or drafts. Adequate clothing such as turtlenecks should be worn to cover the neck and shoulder areas.

☙ Patients with frozen shoulders should be encouraged to exercise the shoulders as much as possible. Increase the range of motion for the shoulder will help to prevent adhesions of the tendons and ligaments.

☙ Patients should also be advised to check their pillow height to make sure it is not too high or too low. Mattresses should also be assessed for firmness.

☙ Hot baths with Epsom salts help to relax tense muscles and withdraw toxins from the tissues. Rest and relax in the bath for about 30 minutes.

CAUTIONS

☙ Chronic neck and shoulder pain may be accompanied by spinal or anatomical injuries. The patient should be checked for structural and anatomical abnormalities, especially if the overall condition does not improve after two to three weeks of herbal treatment.

☙ Patients who are on anticoagulant or antiplatelet therapies, such as Coumadin (Warfarin), should use this formula with caution as there may be a slightly higher risk of bleeding and bruising.

ACUPUNCTURE POINTS

Traditional Points:
☙ *Ah shi* points.
☙ *Shousanli* (LI 10), *Geshu* (BL 17), *Hegu* (LI 4), *Xuehai* (SP 10), and *Jianliao* (TH 14).

Balance Method by Dr. Richard Tan:
☙ Needle the following points on the side opposite the pain: *Lingdao* (HT 4), *Tongli* (HT 5), *Shenmen* (HT 7), *Xuanzhong* (GB 39), and *Shugu* (BL 65).
☙ Needle the following points on the same side as the pain: *Houxi* (SI 3), *Zhongzhu* (TH 3), and *Sanyinjiao* (SP 6) or *ah shi* points nearby.
☙ After the needles are inserted, the patient should move his or her neck to loosen up the joint and the muscles.
☙ For additional information on the Balance Method, please refer to *Acupuncture 1, 2, 3* by Dr. Richard Tan.

Ear Points:
☙ Neck pain: Cervical Vertebrae, Neck, Shoulder, Shoulder Blades, Kidney. Embed ear seeds and instruct the patient to massage the points three to four times daily for two minutes each time. Switch ears every five days. Five treatments equals one course.
☙ Frozen shoulder: Shoulder, Shoulder Joint, Adrenal Gland, Shoulder, Clavicle, Liver, Spleen, and Subcortex.

Auricular Acupuncture by Dr. Li-Chun Huang:
☙ Torticollis (strained neck): Triangle Area of Cervical Vertebrae.
  ▪ Occiput, Lesser Occiput Nerve, Large Auricular Nerve

NECK & SHOULDER (Chronic) ™

    ☙ Periarthritis of shoulder: Shoulder, Shoulder Joint, Clavicle, and Large Auricular Nerve.
- For pain of the shoulder upon abduction, use Clavicle, Shoulder Point (front and back of ear)
- For anterior shoulder pain, use Shoulder Joint (front of ear), add Coronary Vascular Subcortex
- For posterior shoulder pain, use Shoulder Joint (back of ear)

    ☙ For additional information on the location and explanation of these points, please refer to *Auricular Treatment Formula and Prescriptions* by Dr. Li-Chun Huang.

MODERN RESEARCH

Neck & Shoulder (Chronic) contains herbs with strong analgesic, anti-inflammatory and muscle-relaxant functions.

Yan Hu Suo (Rhizoma Corydalis), containing corydaline, exerts strong anti-inflammatory activity and is effective in both the acute and chronic phases of inflammation.[1] It also possesses strong analgesic components that act directly on the central nervous system.[2] Because of this action, *Yan Hu Suo* (Rhizoma Corydalis) works synergistically with acupuncture to relieve pain. It was demonstrated in one study that when combined with *Yan Hu Suo* (Rhizoma Corydalis), the analgesic effect of electro-acupuncture increased significantly when compared with the control group, that received electro-acupuncture only.[3]

In addition, *Bai Shao* (Radix Paeoniae Alba) and *Ge Gen* (Radix Puerariae) contain daisein and paenoniflorin, which have strong antispasmodic effects to alleviate muscle spasms and cramps.[4] Lastly, to specifically address the chronic nature of neck and shoulder injuries, many herbs are added in this formula to strengthen the muscles and tendons and speed up the overall recovery process.[5]

PHARMACEUTICAL DRUGS & CHINESE MEDICINE: A COMPARATIVE ANALYSIS

Western Medical Approach: Pain is a basic bodily sensation induced by a noxious stimulus that causes physical discomfort (as pricking, throbbing, or aching). Pain may be of acute or chronic state, and may be of nociceptive, neuropathic, or psychogenic type. For acute pain, use of non-steroidal anti-inflammatory agents (NSAID) and opioid analgesics offer immediate and reliable effects to relieve pain. Though these drugs have serious side effects, short-term use can be justified because the benefits often outweigh the risks. For chronic pain, on the other hand, use of NSAID's and opioid analgesics are usually not the desired treatment options, as they symptomatically relieve pain, but do not change the underlying course of illness. Unfortunately, the convenience of these drugs contributes to the vicious cycle of pain, followed by continuous and repetitive use of drugs to symptomatically relieve pain. When the effect of the drugs dissipates, patients are often left with nothing but more pain and more complications from side effects. Therefore, it is important to understand that while these drugs may be beneficial for acute pain, they do not adequately address most cases of chronic pain. Additional treatment modalities must be incorporated to ensure effective and complete recovery from chronic pain conditions. [Note: Common side effects of NSAID's include gastric ulcer, duodenal ulcer, gastrointestinal bleeding, tinnitus, blurred vision, dizziness and headache. Serious side effects of newer NSAID's, also known as Cox-2 inhibitors [such as Celebrex (Celecoxib)], include significantly higher risk of cardiovascular events, including heart attack and stroke. Side effects of opioid analgesics [such as Vicodin (APAP/Hydrocodone) and morphine] include dizziness, lightheadedness, drowsiness, upset stomach, vomiting, constipation, stomach pain, rash, difficult urination, and respiratory depression resulting in difficult breathing. Furthermore, long-term use of these drugs leads to tolerance and addiction.]

Traditional Chinese Medicine Approach: Treatment of chronic pain is a sophisticated balance of art and science. Proper treatment of pain requires a careful evaluation of the type of disharmony (excess or deficiency, cold or heat, exterior or interior), characteristics (qi and/or blood stagnations), and locations (upper body, lower body, extremities, or internal organs). Furthermore, optimal treatment requires integrative use of herbs, acupuncture and *Tui-Na* therapies. All these therapies work together to tonify underlying deficiencies, strengthen the body, and facilitate recovery from chronic pain. TCM pain management targets both the symptoms and causes of pain, and as

FORMULAS

such, often achieves immediate and long-term success. Furthermore, TCM pain management is often associated with few or no side effects.

Summation: For treatment of mild to severe pain due to various causes, TCM pain management offers similar treatment effects with significantly fewer side effects. Though TCM therapies may not be as potent as drugs for acute pain management, they are often superior [better effects with fewer side effects] for chronic pain management.

CASE STUDIES

A 46-year-old female presented with left sided pain which originated at the C2 to C7 cervical region followed by a tingling sensation on the lateral side of the left forearm and hand. The practitioner had treated the patient for several years for the same condition. Initially, the pain was only isolated around the neck region with slight radiation towards the middle and lower trapezium. The patient was subsequently diagnosed with hypothyroidism accompanied by intermittent pain, which appeared usually after a couple of days. Administration of the *Neck & Shoulder (Chronic)* formula had provided the patient with great relief as well as making the recurrence less severe and not as abrupt. Consequently, she was able to discontinue taking Motrin (Ibuprofen). The practitioner concluded that *Neck & Shoulder (Chronic)* was an excellent formula for degenerative disc disease.

C.H., San Jose, California

A 44-year-old female, who works as an accountant's assistant, presented with tightness to her neck and shoulders. She also complained of stress, depression and had a history of multiple surgeries. Her western diagnosis was spinal stenosis. Her TCM practitioner diagnosed her condition as *bi zheng* (painful obstruction syndrome) of the neck and shoulders. Prior to taking *Neck & Shoulder (Chronic)*, the practitioner prescribed *Ge Gen* (Radix Puerariae) with little result. *Neck & Shoulder (Chronic)* was the only herbal formula to which the patient responded to favorably.

D.M., Raton, New Mexico

A 22-year-old female presented with pain, tightness and tension in her neck, shoulders and upper back regions. The patient had been living with the condition for about the last 6 years. Initially her problems were due to stress; however, a severe car accident about 2½ years ago made the pain worse and constant. Symptoms exacerbated if under stress or when sick (sinus and head congestion). The pain on the right side of her back and neck was worse than her left. In particular, a point in her upper back where energy had been blocked since the car accident appeared quite weak. She had sought treatments from various physicians, chiropractors, physical therapists and massage therapists, which included *shiatsu*. Some of the treatments provided temporary relief but none had long-lasting effects. The patient was also taking birth control pills, zinc, echinacea, vitamin C, and Claritin (Loratadin). Additionally, she was given antibiotics for her sinus infection, Prevacid (Lansoprazole) for acid reflux, and a nasal spray prescription for her allergies. Her history and clinical picture directed the practitioner to diagnose the condition as qi and blood stagnation with *bi zheng* (painful obstruction syndrome) due to damp-cold. She was treated with acupuncture and began taking *Neck & Shoulder (Chronic)*. The patient's neck muscles gradually became unconstrained over a period of 3 ½ months.

J.M., Baltimore, Maryland

A 40-year-old female presented with neck tension and pain. There was decreased range of motion in her cervical spine but all reflexes and DTR's were within normal limits bilaterally. Upon taking *Neck & Shoulder (Chronic),* the patient immediately noticed a diminished stiffness in her trapezius region.

G.P., Lawndale, California

NECK & SHOULDER (Chronic)™

A 47-year-old female presented with localized pinpoint pain situated 3 *cun* lateral to *Shendao* (GV 11) within the region of *Shentang* (BL 44). The patient also complained of insomnia, poor night vision, dry, itchy and flaky skin patches, ridged nails and clumps of falling hair. Her menstruation was regular at 28-days with no clots. Her tongue had teeth marks, a crack in the middle *jiao* and a white tongue coat. Her pulse was thin, wiry and rapid but slippery in the Spleen position. The western diagnosis of her condition was reflex sympathetic dystrophy syndrome. The TCM diagnosis was qi and blood stagnation, Liver blood deficiency, and Kidney/Liver yin deficiency. After taking *Neck & Shoulder (Chronic),* her qi and blood stagnation subsided and her pain intensity decreased, as evident upon deep palpation. Her tongue cracks in the Spleen area also dwindled in size. Additionally, the patient reported improvement in sleep patterns because of pain relief.

M.D.P., Estes Park, Colorado

A male presented with pain and decreased range of motion in the right shoulder. There was pain upon palpation of the Large Intestine and Small Intestine channels. The practitioner diagnosed the condition as *bi zheng* (painful obstruction syndrome) due to stagnation of qi and blood. The patient was instructed to take *Neck & Shoulder (Acute)*. Acupuncture treatments using Dr. Tan's Balance Method and *Tui Na* massage using Dr. Alex Chen's techniques were also applied. After six acupuncture and herbal treatments, he regained full shoulder range of motion and no pain. After the pain was completely resolved, the practitioner switched the prescription to *Neck & Shoulder (Chronic)* at 3 capsules per day intended for maintenance care. Upon recurrence of pain, the patient was instructed to increase the dosage, which in turn resolved the pain sensation.

K.S., Encinitas, California

A 50-year-old retired male presented with severe neck and shoulder pain and stiffness, which is worse at night and disturbs sleep. The western diagnosis included degenerative disk disease at C5 to C7. The diagnosis was blood stagnation, *bi zheng* (painful obstruction syndrome), and deficiencies of Spleen yang and Kidney *jing* (essence). The patient was instructed to take *Neck & Shoulder (Chronic)* (6 capsules three times daily) and *Osteo 8* (2 capsules three times daily). Upon return, the patient commented that *Neck & Shoulder (Chronic)* was effective for relieving pain. In fact, it was the only treatment that clearly helped. The patient remained under the care of an acupuncturist and a chiropractor, and continued to take the herbs.

J.B., Camarillo, California

A 41-year-old female housewife presented with neck and shoulder pain and occipital headaches. Severe muscle spasms bilateral to C4 to C7 were found as well as neck and shoulder tightness. The patient also reported anxiety and insomnia due to pain and depression. Her pulse was wiry and her tongue was purple. Past histories include eight surgeries to correct her condition. The practitioner diagnosed the presentation as blood and qi stagnation. After taking *Neck & Shoulder (Chronic)*, a reduction in the severity of her neck and shoulder pain was noted. The patient also came to the realization that she was now less affected by damp and cold weather conditions. The practitioner also observed an improvement in the patient's neck range of motion.

Anonymous

[1] Kubo, M. et al. *Biol Pharm Bull.* February 1994
[2] Zhu, XZ. Development of natural products as drugs acting on central nervous system. *Memorias do Instituto Oswaldo Cruz.* 86 2:173-5, 1991.
[3] Hu, J. et al. Effect of some drugs on electro-acupuncture analgesia and cytosolic free Ca^{++} concentration of mice brain. *Chen Tzu Yen Chiu*; 19(1):55-8. 1994
[4] Bensky, D. et al. *Chinese Herbal Medicine Materia Medica.* Eastland Press. 1993
[5] Yeung, HC. *Handbook of Chinese Herbs.* Institute of Chinese Medicine. May 1996

NEURO PLUS ™

CLINICAL APPLICATIONS

- Alzheimer's disease or dementia with decreased mental and cognitive functions
- Parkinson's disease with decreased mental and physical functions
- Sequelae of stroke, such as poor speech, muscle paralysis, urinary and bowel incontinence, and constipation.
- Disorders associated with degeneration of the nervous system and characterized by impaired mental and/or physical functions
- A generalized decrease in mental functions, including forgetfulness, poor memory, difficulty concentrating, reduced comprehension, and possibly increased anxiety.
- Decreased physical functions, such as slurred speech, muscle rigidity, poor balance, difficulty walking, involuntary salivation, frequent urination, constipation, difficulty swallowing, or visual problems.
- Multiple sclerosis (MS)

WESTERN THERAPEUTIC ACTIONS

- Stimulates the nervous system to improve mental and physical functions [1,2,3,4]
- Increases blood circulation to the brain to improve mental functions [1,2,3,4]
- Increases blood circulation to the peripheral parts of the body to improve physical functions [3,9]

CHINESE THERAPEUTIC ACTIONS

- Tonifies the Kidney yin, yang and *jing* (essence)
- Regulates qi and blood circulation and removes blood stagnation
- Opens the sensory orifices to promote awareness and alertness

DOSAGE

Take 2 to 3 capsules three times daily on an empty stomach with warm water during the first week of herbal treatment. After the first week, increase the dosage to 4 capsules three times daily. *Neuro Plus* should be taken continuously for at least one to two months prior to making an evaluation and prognosis.

INGREDIENTS

Ba Ji Tian (Radix Morindae Officinalis)
Bai Zhi (Radix Angelicae Dahuricae)
Bai Zhu (Rhizoma Atractylodis Macrocephalae)
Bi Xie (Rhizoma Dioscoreae Hypoglaucae)
Dan Shen (Radix Salviae Miltiorrhizae)
Dong Chong Xia Cao (Cordyceps)
Du Zhong (Cortex Eucommiae)
Fu Ling (Poria)
Gou Qi Zi (Fructus Lycii)
Gui Ban (Plastrum Testudinis)
He Shou Wu (Radix Polygoni Multiflori)
Hong Hua (Flos Carthami)
Huang Qi (Radix Astragali)
Lu Jiao Shuang (Cornu Cervi Degelatinatium)
Meng Chong (Tabanus)
Qian Cheng Ta (Herba Lycopodii Serrati)

Ren Shen (Radix Ginseng)
San Qi (Radix Notoginseng)
Shan Yao (Rhizoma Dioscoreae)
Shan Zha (Fructus Crataegi)
Shan Zhu Yu (Fructus Corni)
Sheng Di Huang (Radix Rehmanniae)
Shi Chang Pu (Rhizoma Acori)
Shu Di Huang (Radix Rehmanniae Preparata)
Shui Zhi (Hirudo)
Tian Ma (Rhizoma Gastrodiae)
Tu Si Zi (Semen Cuscutae)
Wu Gong (Scolopendra)
Xi Yang Shen (Radix Panacis Quinquefolii)
Yi Zhi Ren (Fructus Alpiniae Oxyphyllae)
Yin Guo Ye (Folium Ginkgo)
Yuan Zhi (Radix Polygalae)

NEURO PLUS ™

FORMULA EXPLANATION

Neurodegenerative disorders are complex and pernicious diseases whose onset is insidious and is followed by progressive deterioration. The clinical manifestations are determined by the location and the seriousness of the disorder. The pathogenesis of neurodegenerative disorders is a mixture of deficient and excess conditions, represented by Kidney *jing* (essence) deficiency (a deficient condition), or blockage of the brain channel by blood stasis (an excess condition), or both.

Though it is the brain that shows the symptoms of neurodegenerative disorders, the cause lies in the Kidney. From the point of view of traditional Chinese medicine's disease differentiation through viscera and their inter-relations, the root of the disease is due to the deficiency of the Kidney and the bone marrow, whereas blood stasis and phlegm accumulation are considered symptoms, not the cause. Therefore, the keys to treating neurodegenerative disorders are to tonify the Kidney, eliminate phlegm, remove blood stasis, restore cognition, and promote perception.

Dong Chong Xia Cao (Cordyceps), *Ba Ji Tian* (Radix Morindae Officinalis), *Shu Di Huang* (Radix Rehmanniae Preparata), *Du Zhong* (Cortex Eucommiae), *Gou Qi Zi* (Fructus Lycii), *He Shou Wu* (Radix Polygoni Multiflori), *Yi Zhi Ren* (Fructus Alpiniae Oxyphyllae), *Tu Si Zi* (Semen Cuscutae), and *Shan Zhu Yu* (Fructus Corni) are used in this formula to nourish both Kidney yin and yang. Hence, the production of *jing* (essence) and the marrow are increased. *Ren Shen* (Radix Ginseng), *Shan Yao* (Rhizoma Dioscoreae), *Huang Qi* (Radix Astragali), *Xi Yang Shen* (Radix Panacis Quinquefolii), *Bai Zhu* (Rhizoma Atractylodis Macrocephalae), and *Fu Ling* (Poria) are used to reinforce the *yuan* (source) *qi*, calm the *shen* (spirit), and increase mental functions. *San Qi* (Radix Notoginseng), *Shan Zha* (Fructus Crataegi), *Shui Zhi* (Hirudo), *Dan Shen* (Radix Salviae Miltiorrhizae), *Hong Hua* (Flos Carthami), *Meng Chong* (Tabanus), *Tian Ma* (Rhizoma Gastrodiae), *Sheng Di Huang* (Radix Rehmanniae) and *Wu Gong* (Scolopendra) open the channels and collaterals, invigorate blood circulation and remove blood stasis. *Yuan Zhi* (Radix Polygalae), *Shi Chang Pu* (Rhizoma Acori) and *Bai Zhi* (Radix Angelicae Dahuricae) are used to open up the sensory orifices, eliminate phlegm and calm *shen* (spirit). *Gui Ban* (Plastrum Testudinis) and *Lu Jiao Shuang* (Cornu Cervi Degelatinatium) tonify the true yin and yang of the Kidney and generate qi and blood flow. *Yin Guo Ye* (Folium Ginkgo) and *Qian Cheng Ta* (Herba Lycopodii Serrati) are used to improve memory functions in patients with dementia or Alzheimer's disease.

SUPPLEMENTARY FORMULAS

- For post-stroke patients with deviation of the eyes and mouth, add **Symmetry**.
- To relieve constipation, combine with **Gentle Lax (Excess)** or **Gentle Lax (Deficient)**.
- For high cholesterol or triglycerides, combine with **Cholisma** or **Cholisma (ES)**.
- To minimize the risk of stroke in patients with hypertension, combine with **Gastrodia Complex** or **Gentiana Complex**.
- For cardiovascular disorders, combine with **Circulation**.
- For severe blood stagnation, add **Circulation (SJ)**.
- For high blood pressure and fast heart rate due to excess fire, add **Gardenia Complex**.
- For general forgetfulness not associated with Alzheimer's disease, use **Enhance Memory** instead.
- For heavy metal poisoning, add **Herbal DTX**.
- For adrenal insufficiency, add **Adrenoplex**.
- To enhance the effect to strengthen the constitution of the body, add **Cordyceps 3**.
- For compromised kidney functions, add **Kidney DTX**.
- With osteoporosis, add **Osteo 8**.
- With Kidney yang deficiency, add **Kidney Tonic (Yang)**.
- With Kidney yin deficiency, add **Kidney Tonic (Yin)**.

NEURO PLUS ™

NUTRITION

❧ Small frequent meals are recommended, instead of a few large meals. Avoid overeating, and stop when approximately 80% fullness is achieved.

❧ They should lose weight if obese. Cholesterol levels should be reduced if elevated.

❧ Encourage more "white meat" and less "red meat."

❧ Consume adequate amounts of vegetables for vitamins A, B1, B2, C and E.

❧ Avoid fried, smoked or barbecued foods.

❧ Stop smoking and avoid drinking alcohol.

❧ Avoid contact and exposure to aluminum, which may be found in antacids, cookware, aluminum foil, and certain foods. Drinking steam-distilled water has a chelating effect in the blood to remove unwanted aluminum from the body.

❧ Encourage a diet with a diverse source of all nutrients, including raw fruits, vegetables, whole grains, nuts, and seeds. B vitamins are important to maintain nerve health.

LIFESTYLE INSTRUCTIONS

❧ Exercise daily and maintain a positive, hopeful outlook toward the future.

❧ Regular workout and deep breathing exercises are excellent ways to oxygenate the blood and improve circulation to all parts of the body to facilitate recovery.

❧ When recuperating from a stroke, engage in regular and mild exercises, such as walking and swimming. However, make sure the activities are supervised as the risk of another accident (i.e. slip and fall) is high during the earlier period of recovery.

CLINICAL NOTES

❧ Since neurodegenerative disorders are characterized by the chronic and deteriorating nature of the illness, herbal treatment is considered effective if there is: 1) improvement in the signs and symptoms, or 2) lack of deterioration or stabilization of the overall condition.

❧ It has been noted by many practitioners that *Neuro Plus* is effective in treating patients with multiple sclerosis. The general consensus is approximately one out of four patients will have a marked improvement, while the others showed only minimal changes.

❧ To prevent deterioration of cognitive function, take 1 to 2 capsule of *Neuro Plus* twice daily.

CAUTIONS

❧ Stroke due to hemorrhage should *not* be treated with this herbal formula until the condition stabilizes.

❧ *Neuro Plus* contains herbs that invigorate blood circulation, remove blood stasis, and prevent clotting. Patients taking anticoagulant or antiplatelet drugs should *not* take this formula without first consulting a licensed health care practitioner. Concurrent use of both herbs and drugs requires close supervision.

❧ This formula is contraindicated during pregnancy and nursing.

❧ A slight increase in blood pressure has been observed in approximately 3 to 5% of patients, due in part to the warm herbs in the formula. Should this happen, reduce the dosage of the herbs. Increase in blood pressure associated with the herbs is self-limiting.

ACUPUNCTURE POINTS

Traditional Points:
1. **Main Points:** *Neiguan* (PC 6), *Renzhong* (GV 26) and *Sanyinjiao* (SP 6).

Neiguan (PC 6) nourishes the heart, calms the *shen* (spirit), and promotes smooth circulation of qi and blood. *Renzhong* (GV 26) opens up sensory orifices, stimulates the brain and awakens the *shen* (spirit). The combination of *Neiguan* (PC 6) and *Renzhong* (GV 26) has been found to increase the contractile strength of the heart and the cardiac output of blood circulation to the brain. *Sanyinjiao* (SP 6) is the meeting point of the three *yin* channels of foot. *Sanyinjiao* (SP 6) nourishes the Kidney, tonifies the *jing* (essence) and the marrow to improve the function of the brain.

2. **Local Points:** *Jiquan* (HT 1), *Chize* (LU 5), *Weizhong* (BL 40), and *Hegu* (LI 4) are local points that open up the channels and collaterals and improve the circulation of qi and blood. *Jiquan* (HT 1), *Chize* (LU 5), and *Hegu* (LI 4) are used for paralysis and tremor of the arms and the hands; and *Weizhong* (BL 40) is used for paralysis of the legs. *Fengchi* (GB 20), *Yifeng* (TH 17), *Wangu* (GB 12) and *Tianzhu* (BL 10) are four excellent points that help patients who have speech impairment or frequent aspiration of food particles, leading to respiratory infections.

    Shanshangdien (upper thunder point) and *Xiashangdien* (lower thunder point) are two extraordinary points that were discovered through clinical trial and experience. These two acupuncture points are very potent and should be reserved for those patients who have partial to complete paralysis.

    Shanshangdien (upper thunder point) is located on the lateral side of the neck, on the same level with Adam's apple, and between the sternal head and clavicular head of m. sternocleidomastoideus. It is three *cun* posterior to the Adam's apple and one *cun* posterior-inferior. It is located slightly inferior to *Futu* (LI 18). Its indications include frozen shoulder, shoulder pain, paralysis of the arm, stiff and rigid muscle of the arm, and tremor of the hand.

    Xiashangdien (lower thunder point) is located in the buttock region. *Xiashangdien* (lower thunder point) is the posterior tip of an equilateral triangle with greater trochanter and the iliac crest as the anterior two points. It is located slightly superior to *Huantiao* (GB 30). Its indications include pain in the lower back and hip region, muscular atrophy, sciatica, pain, weakness and muscular atrophy of the lower extremities, and hemiplegia.

3. **Needling Technique:** Stroke is an excess condition and sedation is warranted. This is because stroke is characterized by the *shen* (spirit) trapped inside the head with complete or partial closure of the sensory orifices. Therefore, the overall treatment focus should be to open up the sensory orifices, release *shen* (spirit), and awaken the brain.

    To achieve the maximum benefit from acupuncture, the location for some of the acupuncture points and their corresponding needling techniques are slightly different. *Neiguan* (PC 6) should be needled bilaterally first. Insert the needle 1 to 1.5 *cun*, then stimulate the point for at least one minute by slightly turning the needle and moving it up and down. The healthy side should be tonified while the diseased side should be sedated.

    Next, needle *Renzhong* (GV 26). Aim slightly upwards toward the top of the head and stimulate strongly until the patient shows tears in his or her eyes. Stimulation should be done with quick rapid movements, a motion similar to a woodpecker drilling trees.

    The third point is *Sanyinjiao* (SP 6). The point of insertion for *Sanyinjiao* (SP 6) should be moved 0.5 *cun* toward the dorsal side of the body (or towards Kidney channel) for greater stimulation. Tonify *Sanyinjiao* (SP 6) by moving the needle up and down until the patient shows a "jerking motion" of the lower leg three times.

    Jiquan (HT 1) should be needled with the patient raising his or her arm upward in the air. The point of insertion is moved 0.5 *cun* toward the fingers and away from the body. *Jiquan* (HT 1) should be sedated by moving the needle up and down until the patient shows "jerking motion" of the arm three times.

    Weizhong (BL 40) may be needled with the patient lying on the back or on the stomach. Point of insertion should be moved 0.5 *cun* higher toward the buttocks along the Urinary Bladder channel. The needle should be inserted 1 to 1.5 *cun* deep, and the point should be sedated until the leg shows a "jerking motion" three times.

    Hegu (LI 4) should be needled obliquely with the tip of the needle pointing toward *Sanjian* (LI 3). This point should be sedated until the index finger jerks three times.

    Shanshangdien (upper thunder point) should be needled perpendicularly 1 *cun* deep, and stimulated until there is an "electric sensation" that runs through the entire length of the arm. The needle is then withdrawn at

FORMULAS

NEURO PLUS ™

that time. *Shanshangdien* (upper thunder point) should never be needled downward toward the lung as it may puncture the lung and cause pneumothorax.

Lastly, *Xiashangdien* (lower thunder point) should be needled perpendicularly 1.5 to 3.0 *cun* deep, and stimulated until there is an "electric sensation" that runs through the entire length of the leg. The needle is then withdrawn at that time.

For maximum effect, acupuncture treatment should be conducted daily for 7 days during the first course of treatment, every other day for 3 weeks for the second course of treatment, and 2 to 3 times per week for the next 2 months of treatment. Three days of resting period is given between each course of treatment. Evaluations are made 1 month and 3 months after the initiation of treatment.

Balance Method by Dr. Richard Tan:
☯ Alzheimer's disease and dementia:
  - Left side: *Yongquan* (KI 1), *Dazhong* (KI 4), *Shangyang* (LI 1), and *Hegu* (LI 4).
  - Right side: *Shaoshang* (LU 11), *Jingqu* (LU 8), *Zhiyin* (BL 67), and *Jinggu* (BL 64).
  - Left and right side can be alternated from treatment to treatment.
☯ For additional information on the Balance Method, please refer to *Twelve and Twelve in Acupuncture, Twenty-Four More in Acupuncture*, and *Dr. Tan's Strategy of Twelve Magical Points* by Dr. Richard Tan.

MODERN RESEARCH

Neuro Plus consists of herbs that exert positive action in the treatment of neurodegenerative disorders, as confirmed by clinical and laboratory research.

Yin Guo Ye (Folium Ginkgo) has been used in China and Europe for treatment of dementia. In a placebo-controlled, double blind, randomized clinical trial with 309 patients over 52 weeks, *Yin Guo Ye* (Folium Ginkgo) was concluded to be "safe" and capable of "improving the cognitive performance and the social functioning of demented patients for 6 months to 1 year." The study was published by JAMA in October 1997.[1]

Ingredients isolated from the herb *Qian Cheng Ta* (Herba Lycopodii Serrati) exhibited promising effects in treating Alzheimer's disease. The mechanism of action of *Qian Cheng Ta* (Herba Lycopodii Serrati) is similar to that of Cognex (Tacrine), the first drug approved in the United States for Alzheimer's. According to the researchers, however, the herb may be more effective and cause fewer side effects than the pharmaceuticals. This herb has been used to treat approximately 100,000 patients with dementia in China, and clinical trials are in the planning stages in the United States.[2]

Shi Chang Pu (Rhizoma Acori) has demonstrated effectiveness in treating seizures and convulsions, especially those caused by primary or cerebral trauma.[3]

One of the main etiologies of neurodegenerative disorders is the lack of blood perfusion to the brain, which deprives it of essential nutrients and leads to deterioration in mental and physical functions. *Dan Shen* (Radix Salviae Miltiorrhizae) improves microcirculation and is commonly used to increase blood perfusion to the brain.[3,4] Two studies showed *Dan Shen* (Radix Salviae Miltiorrhizae) to have a protective effect against cerebral ischemia by increasing cerebral perfusion and reducing ultra-structural abnormalities.[5,6] Other studies demonstrated that with an increase in cerebral perfusion, *Dan Shen* (Radix Salviae Miltiorrhizae) reduced neurological deficits and repairs cellular damage.[7,8]

San Qi (Radix Notoginseng) has cardiotonic functions, which increase blood flow to the heart, decrease oxygen consumption of the cardiac muscle, lower blood pressure and the heart rate. Clinically, *San Qi* (Radix Notoginseng)

NEURO PLUS ™

and *Dan Shen* (Radix Salviae Miltiorrhizae) are commonly combined to treat circulatory problems, including but not limited to angina pectoris and atherosclerosis.[3,9]

Dan Shen (Radix Salviae Miltiorrhizae), *Shui Zhi* (Hirudo) and *Hong Hua* (Flos Carthami) inhibit coagulation, activate fibrinolysis, and are especially effective in treating and/or preventing stroke caused by blood clots blocking the blood vessels in the brain.[3,9]

Wu Gong (Scolopendra) has an excellent effect in stopping muscle spasms and cramps. It is commonly used clinically to treat seizures, convulsions, diphtheria and other conditions that exhibit muscle stiffness and spasm. Though mechanisms of actions differ, *Tian Ma* (Rhizoma Gastrodiae) also has anticonvulsive and muscle-relaxant effects. These two herbs are used together in this herbal formula to address muscle spasms, tremors, muscle rigidity and general musculoskeletal problems. [3,9]

PHARMACEUTICAL DRUGS & CHINESE MEDICINE: A COMPARATIVE ANALYSIS

Western Medical Approach: Neurological disorders are complicated illnesses that encompass many different diseases, including but not limited to Alzheimer's disease, Parkinson's disease and sequelae of stroke. From western medicine perspectives, these diseases are well defined, accurately diagnosed, but not successfully treated. Alzheimer's disease may be managed with Cognex (Tacrine) and Namenda (Memantine), which temporarily improves thinking but does not cure the disease nor alter its prognosis. However, Cognex (Tacrine) may cause clumsiness, unsteadiness, diarrhea, loss of appetite, nausea, vomiting, and liver damage, and Namenda (Memantine) may lead to extreme tiredness, dizziness, confusion, headache, sleepiness, constipation, vomiting, pain anywhere in the body, shortness of breath, and hallucination. Parkinson's disease may be managed with drugs that control symptoms, such as Sinemet (Levodopa and Carbidopa). However, these drugs only control symptoms, and do not cure the disease nor alter its prognosis. Common side effects include agitation, anxiety, nervousness, difficulty concentrating, dizziness or lightheadedness, headache, irritability, loss of appetite, nausea, blotchy spots on skin, insomnia and nightmares. Sequelae of stroke are only treated symptomatically with supportive care. Though there are drugs for treatment and prevention of stroke, there are none for management of stroke sequelae, such as poor speech, muscle paralysis, urinary and bowel incontinence, and constipation. In brief, drug treatment for these neurological disorders focus on treating symptoms, as there are no drugs that cure or alter the progression of these diseases.

Traditional Chinese Medicine Approach: TCM offers many options for treatment of these neurological disorders. This formula has been used in major hospitals in Tianjing, China with great success for treatment of Alzheimer's disease, Parkinson's disease and stroke sequelae. Alzheimer's and Parkinson's diseases are chronic illnesses that develop over a long period of time, and therefore, require long-term use of herbs to slowly stabilize and stop deterioration of the illness. Stroke, on the other hand, is an acute, sudden illness that causes immediate and dramatic changes. Similarly, use of TCM treatments (acupuncture and herbs) is likely to have immediate and significant results. In fact, near-complete recovery from stroke sequelae is sometimes possible, especially if treatments are initiated early, frequently, and aggressively.

Summation: Alzheimer's and Parkinson's diseases are two challenging conditions to both western and traditional Chinese medicine. Drugs and herbs may suppress symptoms, but they do not reverse the course of these illnesses. Furthermore, sequelae of stroke is poorly managed by western medicine but effectively treated with traditional Chinese medicine. Therefore, for post stroke patients, both acupuncture and herbal treatments must be initiated early, frequently, and aggressively to achieve maximum benefit and near-complete recovery.

NEURO PLUS ™

CASE STUDIES

A.H., a 61-year-old male, presented with foggy, unclear mind, difficulty concentrating on more than one task, poor memory, forgetfulness, decline of comprehension ability. Patient had also suffered from hypothyroidism for 12 years. The TCM diagnosis was Kidney qi deficiency. *Neuro Plus* was prescribed at 3 capsules twice daily. In two days, the patient showed remarkable improvement. His memory was extremely clear. He was able to recall information without looking at hand-written notes. His energy level increased and he was very alert. Best of all, he was able to multi-task three things at once (something that was totally impossible before). The patient also noticed an increase in libido. The patient had so much energy that his dosage was reduced to 2 capsules twice daily. The medical doctor reported she was very impressed with the results of this amazing formula.

M.H., West Palm Beach, Florida

A 78-year-old female with a past history of stroke presented with memory loss, insomnia, nightmares, and easily frightened. She frequently woke up in the middle of the night because of her dreams, which disturbed the entire nursing home. Her western medical diagnosis was dementia. The TCM diagnosis included qi and blood stagnation, Liver and Kidney yin deficiency, and Heart fire. She was given *Calm (ES)* and *Neuro Plus*. After taking the herbs for approximately one month, the patient was able to recall the practitioner's name for the very first time! In addition, her sleep, mood, complexion, and energy level improved greatly. The patient was much calmer and less irritable. Despite the fact that she still did not know the name of her town or the correct month, there were many improvements in all other areas. The practitioner concluded that the combination of *Calm (ES)* and *Neuro Plus* has enhanced the patient's quality of life.

P.R., Encinitas, California

A 52-year-old male presented with mania and anxiety due to working long hours and worrying too much about his finances. He had difficulty unwinding and sleeping at the end of the day. The patient also displayed unexpected bouts of hostility along with impulsive and belligerent outbursts of conversations. He had a family history of Alzheimer's disease. After taking low doses of *Neuro Plus*, the patient appeared to have returned to normal. He reverted back to his easy-going personality, both in relation to his work and his general lifestyle. Though the long-term success of *Neuro Plus* was still inconclusive, the improvement towards the well being of this patient was encouraging up to this moment.

L.C., Santa Monica, California

R.V. is a 91-year-old female who suffers from poor memory and Sundowner's syndrome. She has no short-term memory and is agitated and uncooperative at dusk. The only other symptom is loose stool. MRI shows no brain atrophy. The practitioner diagnosed her with Alzheimer's with Kidney yin and yang deficiencies. *Neuro Plus* was taken for 3 years at 1 capsule twice a day. The practitioner reported that *Neuro Plus* appears to have slowed down the progression of Alzheimer's. The patient experiences no more agitation at dusk and the periods of agitation that she does experience is dramatically reduced.

D.V., Newark, California

J.D. is an 83-year-old female who had a stroke 2 years ago. On the first visit, the patient shuffled into the clinic, sat down, and promptly fell asleep. She was unresponsive to questions. Clinical observation showed an extremely deficient and deep pulse. The tongue was pink and slightly dusky with greasy yellow-green tongue coat that was much thicker on her left side. J.D. started taking *Neuro Plus* daily (4 capsules three times daily) and received acupuncture treatment twice weekly. The points used were *Neiguan* (PC 6), *Sanyinjiao* (SP 6), *Yinlingquan* (SP 9), *Hegu* (LI 4) and *Taichong* (LR 3). The patient showed marked improvement. She can lift her feet, smile, and respond somewhat and stay awake throughout the entire treatment. The patient improved rapidly at two treatments per week. Her progress slowed when she had to reduce the treatment to once per week due to financial reasons.

However, she continued to improve. Her tongue coat became granular and brownish, changing over the course of treatment to a slightly-thick, more even white, or slightly yellow coat. After 4 months of treatments she has able to converse more normally. Her friends are happy because she can now talk with them on the phone. Treatment continues.

S.K., Toluca Lake, California

A 62-year-old female diagnosed with Alzheimer's disease presented with memory loss, disorientation and repetitive nonsensical speech patterns. The practitioner diagnosed the condition as qi and blood stagnation and Kidney qi deficiency. After taking *Neuro Plus*, the patient's speech and thoughts were more coherent, as well as a reduction of memory loss.

V.G., Carlsbad, California

A 45-year-old female presented with right-sided dyskinesis, lethargy, headaches and contractures. She was diagnosed with Parkinson's disease. After taking *Neuro Plus*, the patient displayed improvements in energy level, thinking and movement, which in turn enhanced her ability to function in activities of daily living. The patient was continually prescribed *Neuro Plus* at 8 grams per day.

G.P., Brea, California

K.L. is a 64-year-old retired male. The date of his first visit was January 29, 1995. Clinical manifestations included the following signs and symptoms: poor attention span, hand tremor, stiff tongue and inability to hold a rice bowl or chop sticks, poor balance and required help when walking. He also had partial urinary and fecal incontinence with frequent urination. A CT scan taken on December 22, 1995 confirmed cerebral atrophy. The patient's condition dramatically improved after taking *Neuro Plus* for only 5 days. On the sixth day, the patient's hand tremors stopped. He was much more energetic. His frequency of urination decreased, and did not require assistance to walk. He commented that *Neuro Plus* was like a "magic bullet" - and he said it without stuttering.

Anonymous

C.B. was a 56-year-old female who suffered from weight gain, right-side sciatic pain, insomnia, hot flashes and night sweats. She exhibited rapid, thin and thready pulse with peeled and cracked tongue. The practitioner diagnosed her with Kidney yin and blood deficiency with deficiency heat and blood stagnation. *Neuro Plus* and *Balance (Heat)* were prescribed. The patient reported the sciatic pain went away completely. Night sweats and hot flashes were reduced, therefore insomnia was no longer an issue.

S.C., Santa Monica, California

R.L., a 79-year-old female, presented post-stroke symptoms of paralysis on the right side (leg, arm and face). Her blood pressure was 140/80 mmHg and the heart rate was 90 beats per minute. She also had high cholesterol. She was diagnosed with wind-stroke with blood stagnation. *Neuro Plus* and *Cholisma* were prescribed at 4.5 grams and 1.5 grams each day, respectively. This patient also received acupuncture. After 10 weeks of treatment, the patient regained movement of her leg and partial movement of her arm and almost full movement of her face and mouth. *Neuro Plus* also helped the patient regain strength. These were very quick results. In addition, the cholesterol level dropped from 250 to 180 mg/dL.

W.F., Bloomfield, New Jersey

FORMULAS

---

[1] Le Bars, P. et al. A placebo-controlled, double-blind, randomized trial of an extract of ginkgo biloba for dementia. *JAMA* (Journal of American Medical Association);278:1327-1332. October 22, 1997

NEURO PLUS ™

[2] Skolnick, A. Old Chinese herbal medicine used for fever yields possible new Alzheimer's disease therapy. *JAMA* (Journal of American Medical Association); 227:776. March 12, 1997

[3] Yeung, HC. *Handbook of Chinese Herbs.* Institute of Chinese Medicine. 1996

[4] Nagai, M. et al. Vasodilator effects of des(alpha-carboxy-3'4-dihydroxyphenethyl)lithospermic acid (8-epiblechnic acid)' a derivative of lithospermic acids in salviae miltiorrhizae radix. *Biol Pharm Bull*, 19(2):228-32 Feb. 1996

[5] Wu, W. et al. The effect of radix saliva miltiorrhizae on the changes of ultrastructure in rat brain after cerebral ischemia. *J. Tradit Chin Med*, 12(3):183-6 Sept. 1992

[6] Kuang, PG. et al. The effect of radix saliva miltiorrhizae on vasoactive intestinal peptide in cerebral ischemia: an animal experiment. *J Tradit Chin Med*, 9(3):203-6 Sept. 1989

[7] Kuang, P. et al. Effect of radix saliva miltiorrhizae on nitric oxide in cerebral ischemia-reperfusion injury. *J Tradit Chin Med*, 16(3):224-7 Sept. 1996

[8] Protective effect of radix saliva miltiorrhizae on nitric oxide in cerebral ischemia-reperfusion injury. *J Tradit Chin Med*, 15(2):135-40. Jun. 1995

[9] Bensky, D. et al. *Chinese Herbal Medicine Materia Medica.* Eastland Press. 1993

NOTOGINSENG 9 ™

CLINICAL APPLICATIONS

- Bleeding
- Internal bleeding (upper gastrointestinal bleeding, stomach bleeding, duodenal bleeding, hemoptysis, hematuria, epistaxis, and excessive or irregular menstrual bleeding)
- External bleeding (from external and traumatic injuries)

WESTERN THERAPEUTIC ACTIONS

- Hemostatic effect to stop bleeding

CHINESE THERAPEUTIC ACTIONS

- Cools the blood
- Disperses blood stasis
- Stops bleeding

DOSAGE

Take 6 to 8 capsules to stop bleeding. If necessary, the herbs may be repeated three to four times daily until the bleeding stops.

INGREDIENTS

Ai Ye (Folium Artemisiae Argyi), charred
Ce Bai Ye (Cacumen Platycladi), charred
Di Yu (Radix Sanguisorbae), charred
He Zi (Fructus Chebulae)
Jing Jie (Herba Schizonepetae), charred

Qian Cao (Radix Rubiae)
San Qi (Radix Notoginseng)
Wu Bei Zi (Galla Chinensis)
Xian He Cao (Herba Agrimoniae)

FORMULA EXPLANATION

Notoginseng 9 is designed specifically to symptomatically stop bleeding. It contains herbs to cool the blood, disperse blood stasis, and stop bleeding in the upper, middle and lower *jiao*s.

San Qi (Radix Notoginseng) is one of the most important herbs to stop bleeding. It has the dual function to activate blood circulation and stop bleeding, therefore preventing the risk of blood stasis. Charred *Ce Bai Ye* (Cacumen Platycladi) cools the blood and stops respiratory bleeding. *Qian Cao* (Radix Rubiae) moves blood and stops irregular and excessive menstrual bleeding. Charred *Di Yu* (Radix Sanguisorbae) clears heat, cools the blood to stop bleeding in the gastrointestinal tract. Charred *Ai Ye* (Folium Artemisiae Argyi) warms the channels and collaterals, relieves pain and treats a variety of bleeding disorders. *Xian He Cao* (Herba Agrimoniae) has a good restraining function and is commonly used to treat various bleeding disorders. Charred *Jing Jie* (Herba Schizonepetae) also has an excellent hemostatic effect. *Wu Bei Zi* (Galla Chinensis) and *He Zi* (Fructus Chebulae) are astringent herbs to help stabilize and consolidate the effect.

In summary, *Notoginseng 9* is an excellent formula to stop bleeding due to various causes in the upper, middle and lower *jiao*s.

NOTOGINSENG 9 ™

SUPPLEMENTARY FORMULAS

- For gastric or duodenal ulcer bleeding, combine with *GI Care*.
- For colitis or intestinal bleeding with burning diarrhea, combine with *GI Care II*.
- For bleeding from Crohn's disease or irritable bowel syndrome (IBS), combine with *GI Harmony*.
- For bleeding due to ulcerative colitis, add *GI Care (UC)*.
- For external bleeding from injuries and trauma, stop the bleeding first and then use *Traumanex*.
- For cough with blood-streaked sputum, add *Respitrol (CF)*.
- For hemorrhoids, add *GI Care (HMR)*.
- For urinary tract infection, cystitis or abnormal uterine bleeding due to heat, add *V-Statin*.
- For menstrual pain, add *Mense-Ease*.
- For uterine fibroids or cysts, add *Resolve (Lower)*.
- For bleeding with high fever and excess heat, add *Gardenia Complex*.
- For blood stagnation, add *Circulation (SJ)*.
- For dryness and thirst, add *Nourish (Fluids)*.

NUTRITION

- Consume an adequate amount of calcium and magnesium, which are important for blood clotting.
- Consume an adequate amount of multivitamin, especially vitamin K, as they are essential for blood clotting. Foods rich in vitamin K include alfalfa, broccoli, cauliflower, egg yolks, kale, spinach, and all green leafy vegetables.

LIFESTYLE INSTRUCTIONS

- Avoid drinking alcohol, as it irritates the stomach and may cause ulcer and bleeding.
- Patients should find out the cause of bleeding and avoid it accordingly.

CAUTIONS

- This formula is used primarily to stop the "symptom," not the "cause," of bleeding. It is not to be taken long-term. Once bleeding stops, proper measures should be taken to identify and treat the cause of bleeding. *See* Supplementary Formulas section for appropriate formulas to use once the cause is determined.
- This formula should *not* be used in patients who are on anticoagulant or antiplatelet drugs, such as Coumadin (Warfarin) and Plavix (Clopidogrel), as it may counter the effectiveness of these drugs.
- Some drugs cause bleeding and prolong bleeding, and should be avoided. These drugs include aspirin and non-steroidal anti-inflammatory drugs, such as Motrin (Ibuprofen), Naprosyn (Naproxen), and others.
- Patients with profuse bleeding from serious injuries (such as acute trauma or accidents) should be sent to the emergency room immediately.

ACUPUNCTURE POINTS

Traditional Points:
- Blood in the urine: *Zhongji* (CV 3), *Xingjian* (LR 2), *Pangguangshu* (BL 28), *Yinlingquan* (SP 9), *Sanyinjiao* (SP 6), *Xuehai* (SP 10), *Shenshu* (BL 23), *Daling* (PC 7), and *Shenmen* (HT 7).
- Cough with blood: *Xingjian* (LR 2), *Yuji* (LU 10), *Laogong* (PC 8), *Feishu* (BL 13), *Quze* (PC 3), *Kongzui* (LU 6), *Yuji* (LU 10), *Rangu* (KI 2), and *Taixi* (KI 3).
- Nosebleed: *Shangxing* (GV 23), *Hegu* (LI 4), *Shaoshang* (LU 11), *Fengfu* (GV 16), and *Tianfu* (LU 3).
- Vomiting of blood: *Shangxing* (GV 23), *Erjian*, *Zhongwan* (CV 12), and *Yinbai* (SP 1).

NOTOGINSENG 9 ™

- Bleeding from Spleen deficiency: Needle and moxa *Zhongwan* (CV 12), *Zusanli* (ST 36), *Shenshu* (BL 23), *Yinbai* (SP 1), *Guanyuan* (CV 4), and *Taibai* (SP 3).
- Blood in the stool: *Dachangshu* (BL 25), *Changqiang* (GV 1), *Pishu* (BL 20), *Xiajuxu* (ST 39), and *Chengshan* (BL 57).

Balance Method by Dr. Richard Tan:
- Left side: *Hegu* (LI 4), *Yinlingquan* (SP 9)
- Right side: *Shaofu* (HT 8), *Laogong* (PC 8), *Zusanli* (ST 36)
- Alternate sides between treatments
- For additional information on the Balance Method, please refer to *Dr. Tan's Strategy of Twelve Magical Points* by Dr. Richard Tan.

Ear Acupuncture:
- Needle the area or organ area corresponding to bleeding, in addition to Adrenal and Subcortex.

Auricular Acupuncture by Dr. Li-Chun Huang:
- Epistaxis: Internal Nose, Diaphragm, Spleen, Pituitary, Lung, and Adrenal Gland.
- For additional information on the location and explanation of these points, please refer to *Auricular Treatment Formula and Prescriptions* by Dr. Li-Chun Huang.

MODERN RESEARCH

Notoginseng 9 is one of the most effective formulas to stop bleeding, as it contains many herbs with a fast onset of hemostatic effect. This formula has been used to treat various types of bleeding disorders, including internal and external bleeding.

San Qi (Radix Notoginseng) is one of the most useful and unique herbs to stop bleeding, as it has an excellent effect to stop bleeding with minimal effect of creating blood clots. Pharmacologically, it has shown marked hemostatic effect to decrease prothrombin time and stop bleeding.[1] Furthermore, the saponins of *San Qi* (Radix Notoginseng) have been shown to inhibit the aggregation of platelets, thereby minimizing the risks of clotting disorder.[2] Clinically, *San Qi* (Radix Notoginseng) has been used to treat various bleeding disorders, including but not limited to, upper gastrointestinal bleeding,[3] stomach bleeding,[4] hemoptysis due to bronchiectasis, pulmonary tuberculosis or pulmonary abscess,[5] and hematuria.[6]

In addition to *San Qi* (Radix Notoginseng), *Xian He Cao* (Herba Agrimoniae) has also demonstrated remarkable hemostatic effect, with mechanism of action attributed to an increase in platelets and a reduction in bleeding time.[7] Clinical research has confirmed its effect to treat upper gastrointestinal bleeding and menstrual bleeding.[8,9] *Di Yu* (Radix Sanguisorbae) also has good hemostatic effect,[10] and is most effective for upper gastrointestinal bleeding and profuse menstrual bleeding.[11,12] *Ce Bai Ye* (Cacumen Platycladi) has demonstrated marked influence to shorten bleeding time,[13] and has been used effectively to treat bleeding ulcers in 100 patients and bleeding hemorrhoids in 8 patients.[14,15] Administration of *Qian Cao* (Radix Rubiae) showed marked effectiveness in reducing bleeding time.[16] According to one study, it effectively stopped profuse bleeding after tooth extraction in 41 patients within 1 to 2 minutes.[17] Lastly, two other herbs with hemostatic effect include *Jing Jie* (Herba Schizonepetae) and *Ai Ye* (Folium Artemisiae Argyi), demonstrated efficacy using both fresh and charred forms.[18,19]

In summary, *Notoginseng 9* is an excellent formula to stop bleeding as it contains many herbs with remarkable hemostatic effects. It may be used to treat all types of bleeding, including but not limited to upper gastrointestinal bleeding, stomach bleeding, duodenal bleeding, hemoptysis, hematuria, menstrual bleeding, and bleeding due to various external and traumatic injuries.

FORMULAS

NOTOGINSENG 9 ™

PHARMACEUTICAL DRUGS & CHINESE MEDICINE: A COMPARATIVE ANALYSIS

Western Medical Approach: Bleeding is a very common condition that may be caused by external or internal injuries. Because of the wide variety of etiology, each condition is managed differently. For example, according to western medicine, treatments are different for uterine bleeding, gastrointestinal bleeding, bleeding from trauma, and bleeding from overdose of Coumadin (Warfarin).

Traditional Chinese Medicine Approach: TCM identifies the causes of bleeding and treat them differently. However, in addition to specific treatments (which requires time to diagnose and prepare treatment), general treatment is also available to immediately stop bleeding. *Notoginseng 9* is a formula that is designed to symptomatically stop bleeding. Once bleeding stops, it is then necessary to identify the cause and treat accordingly.

---

[1] *Zhong Cao Yao* (Chinese Herbal Medicine), 1986; 17(6):34
[2] *Xian Dai Zhong Yao Yao Li Xue* (Contemporary Pharmacology of Chinese Herbs), 1997; 282-283, 1997; 807:824
[3] *Shang Hai Zhong Yi Yao Za Zhi* (Shanghai Journal of Chinese Medicine and Herbology), 1983; 9:15
[4] *Yun Nan Zhong Yi Za Zhi* (Yunan Journal of Chinese Medicine), 1985; 1:28
[5] *Zhong Yi Za Zhi* (Journal of Chinese Medicine), 1965; 11:29
[6] *Ha Yi Da Xue Bao* (Journal of Ha Medical University), 1974; 7(2):51
[7] *Zhong Yao Yao Li Yu Ying Yong* (Pharmacology and Applications of Chinese Herbs), 1983:323
[8] *Shang Hai Zhong Yi Yao Za Zhi* (Shanghai Journal of Chinese Medicine and Herbology), 1979; 4:28
[9] *Shan Xi Zhong Yi* (Shanxi Chinese Medicine), 1985; 6(7):323
[10] *Zhong Yao Yao Li Yu Ying Yong* (Pharmacology and Applications of Chinese Herbs), 1983; 406
[11] *Zhe Jiang Zhong Yi Xue Yuan Xue Bao* (Journal of Zhejiang University of Chinese Medicine), 1985; 9(4):26
[12] *Zhe Jiang Zhong Yi Za Zhi* (Zhejiang Journal of Chinese Medicine), 1965; 8(3):4
[13] *Zhong Yi Yao Yan Jiu Zi Liao* (Research and Resource of Chinese Medicine and Herbology), 1965; (3):48
[14] *Zhong Hua Nei Ke Xue Za Zhi* (Journal of Chinese Internal Medicine), 1960; 8(3):249
[15] *Zhong Guo Gang Chang Bing Za Zhi* (Chinese Journal of Proctology), 1985; 4:5
[16] *Zhong Yi Yao Yan Jiu* (Research of Chinese Medicine and Herbology), 1991; (3):54
[17] *Yi Xue Wei Sheng Tong Xun* (Journal of Medicine and Sanitation), 1974; 1:54
[18] *Zhong Yao Cai* (Study of Chinese Herbal Material), 1989; 12(6):37
[19] *Zhong Yao Cai* (Study of Chinese Herbal Material), 1992; 15(2):22

FORMULAS

NOURISH ™

CLINICAL APPLICATIONS

❧ Tinnitus, blurred vision, dry eyes, dizziness, night sweats, visual disturbances and other symptoms of yin-deficient heat
❧ Hot flashes with night sweats, fluctuation of body temperature, and warm sensations
❧ Prevention of frequent genital herpes recurrence
❧ Chronic and recurrent infections of the genito-urinary regions, i.e., urinary tract infection, cystitis, pelvic inflammatory disease, inflammation of the genitourinary tract, and related discomforts.

WESTERN THERAPEUTIC ACTIONS

❧ Restores homeostasis to treat tinnitus, dizziness, hot flashes, and similar symptoms. [1,3,5]
❧ Analgesic and anti-inflammatory effects to reduce pain and inflammation [3,4]
❧ Antibiotic property to prevent or treat recurrent genitourinary infections [3,4]

CHINESE THERAPEUTIC ACTIONS

❧ Nourishes Liver and Kidney yin
❧ Controls flare-ups of yin-deficient heat

DOSAGE

Take 3 to 4 capsules three times daily on an empty stomach with warm water. For prevention of chronic and recurrent infections in the genito-urinary region, take 2 to 3 capsules three times daily.

INGREDIENTS

Fu Ling (Poria)
Gou Qi Zi (Fructus Lycii)
Huang Bai (Cortex Phellodendri)
Ju Hua (Flos Chrysanthemi)
Mu Dan Pi (Cortex Moutan)

Shan Yao (Rhizoma Dioscoreae)
Shan Zhu Yu (Fructus Corni)
Shu Di Huang (Radix Rehmanniae Preparata)
Ze Xie (Rhizoma Alismatis)
Zhi Mu (Radix Anemarrhenae)

FORMULA EXPLANATION

Nourish is formulated to treat Kidney yin deficiency with deficiency heat. Clinically, these patients will show such symptoms as tinnitus, blurred vision, dry eyes, dizziness, hot flashes, fluctuation of body temperature, and night sweats. Furthermore, chronic bacterial or viral infections, such as urinary tract infections or genital herpes, will also show Kidney yin deficiency with deficiency heat. Last, aging is a sign of Kidney yin deficiency, manifesting in signs such as soreness and weakness of the lower back and knees, tinnitus, vertigo, blurry vision, diminished hearing, heat sensations, thirst, dryness of mucous membranes, and so on.

Shu Di Huang (Radix Rehmanniae Preparata), *Shan Zhu Yu* (Fructus Corni), *Shan Yao* (Rhizoma Dioscoreae), *Ze Xie* (Rhizoma Alismatis), *Mu Dan Pi* (Cortex Moutan), and *Fu Ling* (Poria) compose the classic Kidney yin tonic formula *Liu Wei Di Huang Wan* (Six-Ingredient Pill with Rehmannia), one of the most famous herbal tonics. *Shu Di Huang* (Radix Rehmanniae Preparata) tonifies the Kidney yin and the Kidney *jing* (essence). *Shan Zhu Yu* (Fructus Corni) nourishes the Liver and prevents the leakage of Kidney *jing* (essence). *Shan Yao* (Rhizoma Dioscoreae) tonifies the Spleen and stabilizes the Kidney *jing* (essence). *Ze Xie* (Rhizoma Alismatis) clears deficiency fire from the Kidney. *Mu Dan Pi* (Cortex Moutan) sedates Liver fire. *Fu Ling* (Poria)

NOURISH ™

dissolves dampness from the Spleen. These six herbs are formulated with careful checks and balances to maximize the therapeutic effects and minimized unwanted effects.

In addition to nourishing Kidney and Liver yin, *Zhi Mu* (Radix Anemarrhenae) and *Huang Bai* (Cortex Phellodendri) are added to sedate deficiency fire. *Gou Qi Zi* (Fructus Lycii) and *Ju Hua* (Flos Chrysanthemi) benefit the eyes and treat dry and blurry vision by nourishing the Liver and Kidney yin.

SUPPLEMENTARY FORMULAS

- ❧ For menopause with deficiency heat symptoms (hot flashes and irritability), use with *Balance (Heat)*.
- ❧ For Kidney yin deficiency without deficiency fire, use *Kidney Tonic (Yin)* instead.
- ❧ For irritability, stress, or anxiety, combine with *Calm*.
- ❧ For menopause with stress or anxiety with insomnia and underlying deficiency, add *Calm ZZZ*.
- ❧ For osteoporosis, add *Osteo 8*.
- ❧ For low libido in women, add *Vitality*.
- ❧ For excess fire with severe hot flashes, add *Gardenia Complex*.
- ❧ As a constitutional tonic, combine with *Imperial Tonic*.
- ❧ For back pain, add *Back Support (Chronic)*.
- ❧ For hair loss, combine with *Polygonum 14*.
- ❧ For general deterioration in both mental and physical functions, use *Neuro Plus*.
- ❧ For hypertension, combine with *Gastrodia Complex*.
- ❧ For dysmenorrhea, use *Mense-Ease*.
- ❧ For irregular menstrual bleeding, add *Notoginseng 9*.
- ❧ To relieve side effects from chemotherapy and/or radiation treatments, use *C/R Support*.
- ❧ For acute attacks of herpes or urinary tract infection, use *Gentiana Complex*.
- ❧ For forgetfulness and to improve memory, add *Enhance Memory*.
- ❧ For adrenal insufficiency, add *Adrenoplex*.
- ❧ For impotence, lack of sexual interest, incomplete erection, and other sexual dysfunction, add *Vitality*.
- ❧ To tonify the individual to remedy the underlying constitutional deficiency, add *Cordyceps 3*.

NUTRITION

- ❧ Encourage a diet with a high content of raw foods, fruits and vegetables to stabilize blood sugar. Discourage dairy products and red meats, as they promote hot flashes.
- ❧ Avoid heat, over-exertion, stress, spicy or greasy foods, or anything else that may trigger a recurrent bacterial or viral attack.

The Tao of Nutrition by Ni and McNease

- ❧ Tinnitus
  - ▪ Recommendations: black sesame seeds, black beans, walnuts, grapes, celery, oyster shells, pearl barley, azuki beans, Chinese black dates, yams, lotus seeds, chestnuts, and chrysanthemum. Get plenty of sleep, massage the neck and head area, and try to live in a quiet and peaceful place, if possible.
  - ▪ Avoid loud noise, stress, tension, stimulating foods, spicy foods, smoking, alcohol, and coffee.
- ❧ Cataract
  - ▪ Recommendations: chrysanthemum, cilantro, spinach, cloves, water chestnuts, yams, lycium berries, black beans. Exercise the eyes regularly and get plenty of oxygen into the bloodstream. Steam the eyes over boiling spinach.
  - ▪ Avoid any type of spices, salt, garlic, eyestrain, constipation.

NOURISH ™

- ☙ Menopause
  - ▪ Recommendations: black beans, sesame seeds, soybeans, walnuts, lycium berries, mulberries, yams, licorice, lotus seeds, and chrysanthemum flowers.
  - ▪ Avoid stress, tension, and all stimulants.
- ☙ For more information, please refer to *The Tao of Nutrition* by Dr. Maoshing Ni and Cathy McNease.

LIFESTYLE INSTRUCTIONS

- ☙ Avoid stress, tension and anxiety as much as possible.
- ☙ Avoid cigarette smoking or exposure to second-hand smoke as it may dry up yin and body fluids.

CLINICAL NOTES

- ☙ Most patients with chronic or debilitating illness have an underlying Kidney yin deficiency. *Nourish* can be used to change the fundamental constitution of these patients so they respond better to the overall treatment.
- ☙ This formula can also be used to treat cataracts by nourishing the Kidney yin and the eyes. If the cataract is secondary to other disorders such as diabetes, hypertension or arteriosclerosis, additional herbal formulas should also be prescribed (See Supplementary Formulas).

CAUTION

- ☙ This formula should not be used for yang deficiency with such symptoms as intolerance of cold with cold hands and feet.

ACUPUNCTURE POINTS

Traditional Points:
- ☙ *Ququan* (LR 8), *Taixi* (KI 3), and *Sanyinjiao* (SP 6).
- ☙ *Jingming* (BL 1), *Taichong* (LR 3), *Xingjian* (LR 2), *Taiyang* (Extra 2), *Hegu* (LI 4), and *Xiaxi* (GB 43).

Balance Method by Dr. Richard Tan:
- ☙ Left side: *Hegu* (LI 4) and *Tongli* (HT 5).
- ☙ Right side: *Zusanli* (ST 36), *Taixi* (KI 3), *Guanyuan* (CV 4), *Shimen* (CV 5), and *Qihai* (CV 6).
- ☙ Left and right side can be alternated from treatment to treatment.
- ☙ For additional information on the Balance Method, please refer to *Dr. Tan's Strategy of Twelve Magical Points* by Dr. Richard Tan.

Ear Points:
- ☙ Menopause: Uterus, Ovary, Endocrine, *Shenmen*, Sympathetic, and Subcortex.
  - ▪ For emotional disturbance, add *Shenmen* and Heart.
  - ▪ For palpitation and irregular heart beat, add Heart and Small Intestine.
  - ▪ For hypertension, add depression point on the back of the ear.
  - ▪ For flushed cheeks, and excess perspiration, add Sympathetic, Cheeks and Lung.
- ☙ High pitched tinnitus: Inner Ear, Temporal Lobe, Pons, Adrenal Gland, and Pituitary Gland.
- ☙ Low pitched tinnitus: Middle Ear, Ear Drum, Eustachian Tube, Adrenal Gland, and Pituitary Gland.

FORMULAS

NOURISH ™

MODERN RESEARCH

Nourish is formulated based on *Liu Wei Di Huang Wan* (Six-Ingredient Pill with Rehmannia), a classic Chinese herbal formula which has a wide range of indications. Modern clinical applications of *Nourish* include tinnitus, spermatorrhea, gingivitis, diabetes, chronic nephritis, chronic genital herpes, and chronic urinary tract infection.[1,2]

Mu Dan Pi (Cortex Moutan) has analgesic and anti-inflammatory effects and is commonly used for general aches and pains. It works directly on the central nervous system and has analgesic, tranquilizing and hypnotic effects.[3,4]

It was demonstrated in one research study that many herbs in *Nourish* treat tinnitus. Out of 32 patients, 11 patients (34%) showed absence of tinnitus, 16 (50%) improved, and 5 (16%) showed no effect.[5] *Huang Bai* (Cortex Phellodendri) has a wide spectrum of antibiotic activities as it enhances phagocytosis of micro-organisms by white blood cells. The antibiotic activities of *Huang Bai* (Cortex Phellodendri) are ideal for preventing or treating recurrent genito-urinary infections. [3,4]

PHARMACEUTICAL DRUGS & CHINESE MEDICINE: A COMPARATIVE ANALYSIS

Western Medical Approach: As life expectancy continues to increase, women are expected to spend more and more of their life in post-menopause years. Therefore, it is becoming increasingly important to ensure a smooth transition during the menopause years. Western medicine used to consider hormone replacement therapy (HRT) as the standard treatment for menopause and related conditions. However, there is no longer a consensus as to when or how to use these drugs. While these drugs may alleviate hot flashes, they significantly increase risk of breast cancer, ovarian cancer, uterine cancer, and have a number of significant side effects. For most physicians and patients, the risks are simply far greater than the potential benefits. The bottom line is – synthetic hormone can never replace endogenous hormone. Therefore, no matter when or how they are prescribed, the potential for adverse reactions is always present.

Traditional Chinese Medicine Approach: TCM offers a gentle yet effective way to address menopause and its related conditions. Chinese herbs have demonstrated via numerous *in vivo* and *in vitro* studies to have marked effect to alleviate hot flashes, vasomotor instability, loss of bone mass, and other conditions associated with menopause. Most importantly, they are much gentler and safer on the body. In conclusion, menopause is simply a transition in the journey of life. It is not a disease, and therefore, should not be treated with synthetic drugs that pose significantly higher risks of cancer and other side effects. Herbs should be considered the primary option, and not the secondary alternative, as they are safe and natural, and more than sufficient to address almost all cases of menopause.

CASE STUDIES

A 27-year-old female health care provider presented with genital herpes. The affected area in the genital region was itchy, red and swollen with thick white discharge. The patient also felt menstrual pain. Her pulse was slippery, deep and strong. Her tongue body was pale purple with a red tip, and the sides were swollen with scalloped edges. The practitioner diagnosed the condition as damp-heat in the Liver and Liver qi stagnation. After taking *Nourish* and *Gentiana Complex*, a decrease in symptoms was noted. Symptoms flared up when the patient stopped using the formulas.

B.H., Pearl City, Hawaii

NOURISH ™

A 50-year-old male presented with hearing loss, ringing in the ear and diminished hearing. The TCM diagnosis was Kidney yin deficiency. The patient was prescribed *Nourish* with good results. The practitioner commented that *Nourish* works the best for such conditions.

R.C., MD, Ph.D., New York, NY

D.S., a 45-year-old female, presented with insomnia, mood swings, cramps and fatigue. The tongue was slightly purplish pale with teeth marks. The coating was thin and white. The pulse was deep and wiry. She was diagnosed with Spleen qi deficiency and blood deficiency. *Nourish, Calm, Schisandra ZZZ* were prescribed. The patient reported her sleep pattern improved, her moods balanced and her energy level increased. She was very happy with the herbs.

B.F., Newport Beach, California

A 53-year-old female patient presented with anxiety, depression and pale complexion. Her pulse was thin, weak and deep in all positions. She had cyclical bouts of rage, fatigue, sleeplessness, anxiety and severe depression. Periods were irregular. Her tongue was puffy and pale. The TCM diagnosis was blood and yin deficiencies with Liver qi stagnation, Kidney yin and yang deficiencies. *Shine* and *Nourish*, along with an iron supplement were prescribed. The patient noticed a change within the first 10 days and more so around her cycle. She felt as if a cloud had been lifted from above. She found herself smiling more. Restlessness was still bothering her but her sleep was much better. This patient has suffered from depression for a long time and is very deficient.

N.V., Muir Beach, California

---

[1] Yeung, HC. *Handbook of Chinese Herbal Formulas*. Institute of Chinese Medicine. 1995
[2] Bensky, D. et al. *Chinese Herbal Medicine Formulas and Strategies*. Eastland Press. 1990
[3] Yeung, HC. *Handbook of Chinese Herbs*. Institute of Chinese Medicine. 1986
[4] Bensky, D. et al. *Chinese Herbal Medicine Materia Medica*. Eastland Press. 1993
[5] Yang, DJ. Tinnitus treated with combined traditional Chinese medicine and western medicine. *Journal of Modern Developments in Traditional Medicine*. 9(5):270-1, 259-60, May. 1989

FORMULAS

NOURISH (Fluids) ™

CLINICAL APPLICATIONS

- Thirst and dryness
- Chronic consumptive disorders with dryness and yin and body fluids deficiency
- Lung disorders with chronic consumptive characteristics: post-infective cough, chronic bronchitis, laryngitis, bronchiectasis, tuberculosis, non-specific pneumonia, and smoking-related complications
- Stomach disorders with chronic consumptive characteristics: oral lesions, thirst, dryness of the mouth, nausea, vomiting, stomach and duodenal ulcers, gastritis, constipation and dry stools
- Cancer: dryness and thirst associated with chemotherapy and radiation
- Antibiotic-related side effects, such as dryness, thirst, and weakness
- Sjogren's syndrome

WESTERN THERAPEUTIC ACTIONS

- General tonic effect to improve the overall health
- Antitussive and expectorant effect to benefit the respiratory tract
- Anti-ulcer effect to benefit the gastrointestinal tract
- General hepatoprotective and detoxification effects
- Regulatory effect on the endocrine system to balance the hormones

CHINESE THERAPEUTIC ACTIONS

- Nourishes Lung and Stomach yin
- Replenishes body fluids
- Harmonizes the middle *jiao*

DOSAGE

Take 3 to 4 capsules three times daily. For maximum effect, take the herbs on an empty stomach with one tall glass of warm water and honey.

INGREDIENTS

Bai He (Bulbus Lilii)
Bei Sha Shen (Radix Glehniae)
Da Zao (Fructus Jujubae)
Geng Mi (Semen Oryzae)
Mai Men Dong (Radix Ophiopogonis)

Nan Sha Shen (Radix Adenophorae)
Tian Men Dong (Radix Asparagi)
Xi Yang Shen (Radix Panacis Quinquefolii)
Zhi Gan Cao (Radix Glycyrrhizae Preparata)

FORMULA EXPLANATION

Nourish (Fluids) is designed to treat various disorders originating from yin and/or body fluid deficiencies. Such deficiencies often occur as a result of over-work, over-exhaustion, chronic illness, dietary imbalances and chronic exposure to environmental toxins. The purpose of this formula is to strengthen the body, tonify yin, replenish body fluids, and restore the body to its optimal health.

Mai Men Dong (Radix Ophiopogonis) and *Tian Men Dong* (Radix Asparagi) are the chief herbs that enter the Lung and the Stomach to quickly replenish yin, relieve thirst and moisten dryness. *Bei Sha Shen* (Radix Glehniae), *Nan Sha Shen* (Radix Adenophorae) and *Bai He* (Bulbus Lilii) assist the chief herbs to nourish the yin and replenish the body fluids to relieve dryness. *Xi Yang Shen* (Radix Panacis Quinquefolii) nourishes both yin and qi to relieve fatigue or weakness that may be associated with yin deficiency. It is also slightly cool in property to clear the

FORMULAS

deficiency heat symptoms associated with yin deficiency. *Geng Mi* (Semen Oryzae), *Da Zao* (Fructus Jujubae), and *Zhi Gan Cao* (Radix Glycyrrhizae Preparata) harmonize the formula and tonify the middle *jiao*.

In summary, this is an excellent formula to tonify yin and replenish body fluids. It is most beneficial in individuals who have chronic consumptive disorders, or ones with such deficiencies caused by over-work or over-exhaustion.

SUPPLEMENTARY FORMULAS

- For chronic respiratory disorder, add **Respitrol (Deficient)**.
- For stomach or duodenal ulcer, add **GI Care**.
- For chronic constipation or constipation due to dryness, add **Gentle Lax (Deficient)**.
- For nausea, vomiting and fatigue after chemotherapy and radiation therapy, add **C/R Support**.
- For diabetes, add **Equilibrium**.
- For hepatitis, add **Liver DTX**.
- For hair loss, add **Polygonum 14**.
- For terminal stage cancer, add **CA Support**.
- For qi, blood, yin and yang deficiencies, add **Imperial Tonic**.
- For cough, add **Respitrol (CF)**.
- For excess fire or fever, add **Gardenia Complex**.
- For thirst unrelieved by yin tonics, add **Circulation (SJ)**.
- For Sjogren's syndrome with swollen glands, add **Herbal ENT** and **Resolve (AI)**.
- For menopause with yin-deficient heat, add **Balance (Heat)**.
- For Kidney yin deficiency, add **Nourish**.

NUTRITION

- Avoid eating spicy food, drinking alcohol or smoking cigarettes or cigars.
- Drink an adequate amount of water and fluids daily, especially on hot summer days.
- Honey, rice and all types of beans should be consumed regularly.

LIFESTYLE INSTRUCTIONS

- Patients with chronic consumptive diseases (such as cancer and chronic disorders of lung or stomach) should receive concurrent treatments to eliminate the cause and replenish the fluids.
- Engage in regular exercise.
- Avoid stress whenever possible.

CLINICAL NOTE

- In addition to the clinical applications listed above, this is also an excellent formula to use in diseases characterized by yin and/or body fluid deficiency, such as bronchitis, bronchial asthma, pneumonia, laryngopharyngitis, hoarse voice, whooping cough, tuberculosis, diabetes mellitus, hypertension, and arteriosclerosis.

CAUTIONS

- This formula should **not** be taken when there is an active infection or inflammation.
- This formula is contraindicated in cases of excess heat or dampness.

FORMULAS

NOURISH (Fluids) ™

ACUPUNCTURE POINTS

Traditional Points:
- *Fuliu* (KI 7), *Taixi* (KI 3), and *Chize* (LU 5).
- *Feishu* (BL 13), *Pishu* (BL 20), and *Lianquan* (CV 23).

Balance Method by Dr. Richard Tan:
- Left side: *Lingku*, *Hegu* (LI 4), *Rangu* (KI 2), *Dazhong* (KI 4), and *Fuliu* (KI 7).
- Right side: *Neiguan* (PC 6), *Zusanli* (ST 36), and *Feiyang* (BL 58).
- Alternate sides in between treatments.
- Note: *Lingku* is one of Master Tong's points on both hands. *Lingku* is located in the depression just distal to the junction of the first and second metacarpal bones, approximately 0.5 *cun* proximal to *Hegu* (LI 4), on the *yangming* line.
- For additional information on the Balance Method, please refer to *Dr. Tan's Strategy of Twelve Magical Points* by Dr. Richard Tan.

MODERN RESEARCH

Nourish (Fluids) is a unique formula as it is composed of herbs that have general protective and restorative effects on various systems in the body. Administration of herbs in this formula has been found to be very beneficial in individuals who are recovering from chronic consumptive disorders, or diseases characterized by dryness and deficiency of yin and body fluids. Clinically, this is an excellent formula to treat chronic and consumptive illnesses characterized by compromised functions of the respiratory, gastrointestinal, hepatic, and endocrine systems.

Nourish (Fluids) contains herbs with general effect that improve the overall health and facilitate recovery from chronic illnesses. For example, use of *Zhi Gan Cao* (Radix Glycyrrhizae Preparata) is associated with effects to increase body weight, muscle strength, and physical endurance.[1] *Xi Yang Shen* (Radix Panacis Quinquefolii) and *Bai He* (Bulbus Lilii) have an adaptogenic effect that improves both mental and physical health and performance.[2,3] Lastly, use of *Mai Men Dong* (Radix Ophiopogonis) daily in 100 geriatric patients was associated with a significant improvement in their overall health.[4]

Chronic and consumptive disorders are often related in part to the dysfunction of the endocrine system and the related glands. According to one study, 8 out of 9 patients with declining pituitary function were treated successfully by taking an herbal combination that contains *Zhi Gan Cao* (Radix Glycyrrhizae Preparata) as the main ingredient for 2 to 3 months.[5] Specifically, *Zhi Gan Cao* (Radix Glycyrrhizae Preparata) has been shown to have potent effect to stimulate the production of the adrenocortical hormones, such as glucocorticoids and mineralocorticoids. Administration of glycyrrhizin and glycyrrhetinic, two ingredients of *Gan Cao* (Radix Glycyrrhizae), clearly prolonged the therapeutic effect of cortisone as demonstrated by various laboratory studies. The same components also increase the mineralocorticoid effect to balance the water and electrolyte levels in the body.[6]

Nourish (Fluids) also uses many herbs with marked influences on the respiratory system. For example, *Bai He* (Bulbus Lilii) and *Zhi Gan Cao* (Radix Glycyrrhizae Preparata) both have marked antitussive and expectorant effects.[7] Clinically, these herbs have shown beneficial effects to treat chronic consumptive lung diseases, such as chronic bronchitis, bronchiectasis, tuberculosis, non-specific pneumonia, pulmonary tuberculosis, and complications of smoking.[8]

Nourish (Fluids) uses many herbs that influence and improve the overall gastrointestinal functions. Individuals with chronic illnesses often have dysfunction of the gastrointestinal system, where nutrients from foods cannot be properly digested and absorbed. For example, *Zhi Gan Cao* (Radix Glycyrrhizae Preparata) has a marked effect on the gastrointestinal tract to prevent and treat peptic ulcers, with mechanisms such as inhibition of gastric acid secretion, binding and deactivation of gastric acid, and promotion of recovery from ulceration.[9] Clinically, many

NOURISH (Fluids) ™

herbs in this formula may be used to treat gastrointestinal disorders, such as *Bai He* (Bulbus Lilii) for treatment of atrophic gastritis,[10] and *Zhi Gan Cao* (Radix Glycyrrhizae Preparata) for treatment of peptic ulcer and intestinal spasms.[11,12]

Individuals with chronic liver disorders often have underlying weakness and deficiency of the hepatic system. This formula uses herbs with hepatoprotective effects specifically to address such disorders. For example, the use of *Zhi Gan Cao* (Radix Glycyrrhizae Preparata) is associated with increased amount of cytochrome p-450 in the liver, which is responsible for the protective effect of the herb on the liver against chemicals or tetrachloride-induced liver damage and liver cancer.[13] In addition, use of glycyrrhizin, an active component in *Zhi Gan Cao* (Radix Glycyrrhizae Preparata), is associated with 77% rate of effectiveness in treating 30 patients with hepatitis B. The mechanism of this effect has been attributed to the action of the herb to reduce the damage to and death of liver cells, decrease inflammatory reaction, promote regeneration of liver cells, and lower the risk of liver cirrhosis and necrosis.[14]

Nourish (Fluids) contains many herbs that are beneficial for patients with cancer. Cancer is often diagnosed in traditional Chinese medicine as an excess condition (heat, phlegm and toxins) that consume yin and body fluids. Furthermore, cancer treatments, such as chemotherapy and radiation, further damage the body and cause more weakness and deficiency. To address these conditions, this formula uses herbs to support patients with cancer and alleviate general side effects associated with chemotherapy and radiation. For example, *Tian Men Dong* (Radix Asparagi) has been shown to be very effective in supporting/treating 42 patients with breast cancer and malignant lymphoma.[15,16] Furthermore, according to one clinical study, use of *Xi Yang Shen* (Radix Panacis Quinquefolii) was associated with a significant reduction of side-effects related to chemotherapy and radiation, such as dry mouth, nausea and vomiting.[17]

In summary, *Nourish (Fluids)* is an excellent adjunct formula for treatment of chronic and consumptive illnesses characterized by compromised functions of the respiratory, gastrointestinal, hepatic, and endocrine systems.

PHARMACEUTICAL DRUGS & CHINESE MEDICINE: A COMPARATIVE ANALYSIS

One striking difference between western and traditional Chinese medicine is that western medicine focuses and excels in crisis management, while traditional Chinese medicine emphasizes and shines in holistic and preventative treatments. Therefore, in emergencies, such as gun shot wounds or surgery, western medicine is generally the treatment of choice. However, for treatment of chronic idiopathic illness of unknown origins, where all lab tests are normal and a clear diagnosis cannot be made, traditional Chinese medicine is distinctly superior.

The general condition of "yin and body fluid deficiencies" may be present in many different scenarios, such as in cases of chronic consumptive disorder, chronic lung and stomach disorder, and individuals who received antibiotic, chemotherapy and radiation treatments. All these conditions are characterized by symptoms such as thirst, dryness, and the general presence of lack of body fluids and insufficient hydration of body tissues. These are non-specific and non-diagnostic signs and symptoms. Therefore, western medicine struggles to identify a diagnosis and treatment. On the other hand, these are obvious presentation of "yin and body fluid deficiencies" in traditional Chinese medicine. The use of herbs that nourish yin and promote generation of body fluids is extremely beneficial to correct these imbalances and restore normal health and body functions. From the prognosis perspective, use of this formula facilitates and shorten the course of recovery from many chronic and consumptive diseases.

[1] *Guo Wai Yi Xue Zhong Yi Zhong Yao Fen Ce* (Monograph of Chinese Herbology from Foreign Medicine), 1985; 7(4):48
[2] *Zhong Yao Xue* (Chinese Herbology), 1998; 737:738
[3] *Zhong Yao Cai* (Study of Chinese Herbal Material), 1990; 13(6):31
[4] *Zhong Guo Zhong Yao Za Zhi* (People's Republic of China Journal of Chinese Herbology), 1992; 17(1):21
[5] *Zhong Hua Yi Xue Za Zhi* (Chinese Journal of Medicine), 1975; 10:718
[6] *Zhong Yao Zhi* (Chinese Herbology Journal), 1993; 358

FORMULAS

NOURISH (Fluids) ™

[7] *Pharmacology and Applications of Chinese Herbs*, 1983; 264
[8] *Jiang Xi Yi Yao* (Jiangxi Medicine and Herbology), 1965; 1:562
[9] *Zhong Yao Zhi* (Chinese Herbology Journal), 1993; 358
[10] *Liao Ning Zhong Yi Za Zhi* (Liaoning Journal of Chinese Medicine), 1988; 4:18
[11] *Zhong Hua Nei Ke Xue Za Zhi* (Journal of Chinese Internal Medicine), 1960; 3:226
[12] *Zhong Hua Nei Ke Za Zhi* (Chinese Journal of Internal Medicine), 1960; 4:354
[13] *Zhong Yao Tong Bao* (Journal of Chinese Herbology), 1986; 11(10):55
[14] *Zhong Yao Tong Bao* (Journal of Chinese Herbology), 1987; 9:60
[15] *Jiang Su Yi Yao* (Jiangsu Journal of Medicine and Herbology), 1976; 4:33
[16] *Xin Yi Xue* (New Medicine), 1975; 4:193
[17] *Shang Hai Zhong Yi Yao Za Zhi* (Shanghai Journal of Chinese Medicine and Herbology), 1979; 4:29

FORMULAS

OSTEO 8 ™

CLINICAL APPLICATIONS

- Osteoporosis, decreased bone density
- Bone fracture, broken bones
- Individuals with risk factors of osteoporosis, such as menopause, old age, and use of tobacco, alcohol, and drugs
- Soreness, weakness and pain in the bones, lower back and knees.
- Inability to stand for a prolonged period of time.
- Pain or soreness that is aggravated by weight-bearing activities.
- Other symptoms may include tinnitus, hair loss, dryness, blurred vision and degeneration of muscle.

WESTERN THERAPEUTIC ACTIONS

- Increases bone density
- Increases adsorption of calcium into bones
- Facilitate recovery of bone fracture

CHINESE THERAPEUTIC ACTIONS

- Replenishes Kidney *jing* (essence)
- Tonifies Kidney yang and yin
- Tonifies qi and blood

DOSAGE

Take 3 to 4 capsules three times daily on an empty stomach with warm water. For prevention in patients with higher risk of osteoporosis, take 2 capsules daily.

INGREDIENTS

Dang Gui (Radicis Angelicae Sinensis)
E Jiao (Colla Corii Asini)
Gou Qi Zi (Fructus Lycii)
Gu Sui Bu (Rhizoma Drynariae)

Gui Ban (Plastrum Testudinis)
Lu Jiao (Cornu Cervi)
Ren Shen (Radix Ginseng)
Xu Duan (Radix Dipsaci)

FORMULA EXPLANATION

Osteo 8 is a well-balanced formula designed for women and men of all ages who want to maintain healthy bones. It contains herbs that tonify qi, blood, yin and yang. The main function of the formula is to replenish the vital *jing* (essence) of the Kidney to strengthen bones, increase bone density, and promote healing.

Most herbs in *Osteo 8* enter the Kidney to revitalize the body and replenish *jing* (essence). Osteoporosis or weakness of sinews and bones are the result of Kidney and Liver deficiencies. According to traditional Chinese medicine, the Kidney stores the *jing* (essence) that is vital for strong bones, and the Liver stores blood and controls the sinews and tendons. If the Liver and Kidney are deficient, bone, sinews and joints become weak. Therefore, treatment of bone disorders requires tonification of the Liver and Kidney.

Lu Jiao (Cornu Cervi), one of the most effective and precious herbs, is the principle herb in *Osteo 8*. It tonifies Kidney yang, replenishes Kidney *jing* (essence), nourishes blood and strengthens sinews and bones. *Gu Sui Bu* (Rhizoma Drynariae) and *Xu Duan* (Radix Dipsaci) are two herbs that tonify Kidney yang. *Gu Sui Bu* (Rhizoma

OSTEO 8 ™

Drynariae) and *Xu Duan* (Radix Dipsaci) strengthen the bones and are often used together to promote mending of bones and relieve soreness, weakness and pain of the bones. They are the best pair used to heal fractured bones and other injuries such as contusions, sprains and ligament injuries due to trauma.

Gui Ban (Plastrum Testudinis), *Gou Qi Zi* (Fructus Lycii) and *E Jiao* (Colla Corii Asini) are used to tonify the Kidney yin and *jing* (essence). *Gui Ban* (Plastrum Testudinis) nourishes Kidney yin and strengthens the bones by filling the marrow with *jing* (essence). *Gou Qi Zi* (Fructus Lycii) tonifies the Liver and the Kidney yin to treat secondary symptoms such as dizziness, dryness, blurred vision, tinnitus, thirst and night sweats. Neutral in property, it has a unique function to effectively nourish the different parts of the body without creating any stagnation. *E Jiao* (Colla Corii Asini), one of the essential herbs used in most anti-aging formulas, tonifies blood and nourishes yin. Together, these three herbs replenish Kidney yin and *jing* (essence) to maintain healthy bones and treat weakness and soreness of the back, hips and knees.

Finally, to enhance the overall wellness of the body, *Ren Shen* (Radix Ginseng) and *Dang Gui* (Radicis Angelicae Sinensis) are added to tonify *yuan* (source) *qi* and blood.

SUPPLEMENTARY FORMULAS

- For soreness and pain of the low back and knees, use with ***Back Support (Chronic)***.
- For neck and shoulder pain, use with ***Neck & Shoulder (Chronic)***.
- For arm pain, add ***Arm Support***.
- For bone spurs, add ***Flex (Spur)***.
- For fatigue and overall deficiency, use with ***Imperial Tonic***.
- For menopause with hot flashes and night sweats, use with ***Balance (Heat)***.
- For menopause patients with dryness or yin deficiency, use with ***Nourish***
- For menopause patients with irritability and insomnia, use with ***Calm*** or ***Calm (ES)***.
- For hair loss or premature gray hair, use with ***Polygonum 14***.
- For blood deficiency, insomnia and excessive dreams, use with ***Schisandra ZZZ***.
- For arthritis due to heat with redness, swelling and burning of joints, use with ***Flex (Heat)***.
- For arthritis due to coldness, with pain that worsens during cold and rainy weather, use with ***Flex (CD)***.
- For gout, add ***Flex (GT)***.
- For Kidney yang deficiency, add ***Kidney Tonic (Yang)***.
- For Kidney yin deficiency, add ***Kidney Tonic (Yin)***.
- For bone fractures, use with ***Traumanex***.
- For recovery from bone fracture with soft tissue injuries, use with ***Flex (MLT)***.

NUTRITION

- Consume a sufficient amount of calcium, either from diet or supplements. Make sure the supplement is of good quality so it breaks down and absorbs in the body. Calcium supplementation is most effective if it is combined with vitamin D and other minerals.
- Consumption of foods rich in plant estrogen is also beneficial, such as soybeans and yam.
- Consumption of oxtail, ox neck or bone-based soup with tomato and ginger is highly recommended.

LIFESTYLE INSTRUCTIONS

- Patients are advised stop drinking alcohol, smoking tobacco, and limit sexual activities to prevent loss of *jing* (essence).

OSTEO 8 ™

- Patients with osteoporosis have higher risk of bone fractures. They should refrain from activities with high risk of injury, such as lifting heavy objects or over exertion from strenuous exercises.
- Walking, *Tai Chi Chuan*, and other mild exercises are recommended in order to strengthen the bones and joints without increased risk of injury. Weight-bearing exercise is especially effective to improve bone strength.

CAUTIONS

- This formula should be used with caution in patients with an excess condition or heat accumulation.
- This formula should be used with caution in patients with damp-heat in the lower *jiao*.
- Patients who are on anticoagulant or antiplatelet therapies, such as Coumadin (Warfarin), should use this formula with caution, as there may be a slightly higher risk of bleeding and bruising.

CLINICAL NOTES

- Osteoporosis is six times more common in women than in men because a tremendous amount of *jing* (essence) is lost during the process of pregnancy and delivery. Post-menopausal osteoporosis is most common and happens between 51 to 75 years of age. Women who have children may see signs and symptoms of osteoporosis earlier than those who have less or no children.
- Men lose *jing* (essence) with excessive sexual activities. While they may not experience osteoporosis with old age, other signs of Kidney deficiency may include hair loss, loose teeth, weakness and soreness of the back and knees.

ACUPUNCTURE POINTS

Traditional Points:
- *Mingmen* (GV 4), *Dashu* (BL 11), and *Shenshu* (BL 23).
- *Sanyinjiao* (SP 6), *Shenshu* (BL 23), *Guanyuan* (CV 4), and *Pishu* (BL 20).

Balance Method by Dr. Richard Tan:
- Left side: *Shenmai* (BL 62), *Weizhong* (BL 40), *Tongli* (HT 5), and *Shaohai* (HT 3).
- Right side: *Taixi* (KI 3), *Yingu* (KI 10), *Houxi* (SI 3), and *Xiaohai* (SI 8).
- Left and right side can be alternated from treatment to treatment.
- For additional information on the Balance Method, please refer to *Dr. Tan's Strategy of Twelve Magical Points* by Dr. Richard Tan.

Auricular Acupuncture by Dr. Li-Chun Huang:
- Osteoporosis and cervical vertebral degeneration: Corresponding points (to the area of degeneration), Triangle Area of Cervical Vertebral of Posterior, C6, 7, C3, 4; and Large Auricular Nerve.
  - For dizziness, add Dizziness Area.
  - For shoulder pain, add Shoulder Joint.
  - For finger numbness, add Finger, Coronary Subcortex, and Large Auricular Nerve.
  - For back headache, add Occiput and Lesser Auricular Nerve. Bleed Ear Apex.
- For additional information on the location and explanation of these points, please refer to *Auricular Treatment Formula and Prescriptions* by Dr. Li-Chun Huang.

MODERN RESEARCH

Osteoporosis is a disorder characterized by a reduction in of bone mass density, leading to fractures after minimal trauma.[1] Osteoporosis is becoming one of the more common disorders as the population continues to age and life

OSTEO 8 ™

expectancies continue to increase. Osteoporosis occurs mostly in individuals between 51 to 75 years of age, and is six times more common in women than men.[2] There are numerous risk factors, including but not limited to aging, dietary habits, lifestyles, and family history. Chronic use of drugs also increases the risk of osteoporosis, with such examples as thyroid supplements, corticosteroids, ethanol, tobacco, and heparin. Osteoporosis is often treated with estrogen replacement therapy (ERT). While ERT may be effective for osteoporosis, it also increases the risk of breast and uterine cancer, endometrial carcinoma, malignant neoplasm, gallbladder disease, thromboembolitic disease, and photosensitivity.[3] Therefore, many people choose not to take ERT because of the side effects, cautions, and contraindications.

Osteo 8 is an herbal formula specifically for osteoporosis and other bone-related disorders. It contains herbs that increase the utilization of calcium, strengthen the bones, prevent fractures, and promote healing.

Lu Jiao (Cornu Cervi) is an herb that has been used for centuries to regulate growth and maturation. It is used to stimulate growth in pediatrics, and to delay aging in geriatric patients.[4] In addition, it has great effect to promote and facilitate the healing of broken bones.[5] Maintaining the integrity of bones requires an adequate amount of calcium. *Lu Jiao* (Cornu Cervi) and *Gui Ban* (Plastrum Testudinis) are both rich in numerous minerals, including calcium and magnesium, which are essential for bone growth.[6]

Use of *Gu Sui Bu* (Rhizoma Drynariae) has a marked impact on the skeletal system. It has been shown that *Gu Sui Bu* (Rhizoma Drynariae) has a definite beneficial effect in patients with bone fractures as it increases the adsorption of calcium into bones. Therefore, it can be used short-term to treat bone fractures, and long-term to prevent osteoporosis.[7] Furthermore, administration of *Gu Sui Bu* (Rhizoma Drynariae) also showed beneficial effect in treating osteoarthritis, a joint disease characterized by degeneration of the cartilage and bones.[8]

In addition to *Gu Sui Bu* (Rhizoma Drynariae), there are many other herbs that can be prescribed to strengthen both the bones and the tendons, such as *Gui Ban* (Plastrum Testudinis), *Gou Qi Zi* (Fructus Lycii) and *Xu Duan* (Radix Dipsaci).[5] These herbs have an excellent synergistic effect for treatment of bone fractures and soft tissue damages. In one study, it was found that such herbs that tonify the Kidney have a positive effect in treating osteoporosis, with results better than that of calcium alone. The researchers in this study concluded that use of herbs that tonify the Kidney is an "optimal method for osteoporotic treatment."[9]

Overall, *Osteo 8* contains herbs that are rich in calcium, increase adsorption of calcium into bones, and promote the growth and healing of bones. It is an ideal formula for both the prevention and the treatment of decreased bone density, bone fractures, or other bone-related disorders.

PHARMACEUTICAL DRUGS & CHINESE MEDICINE: A COMPARATIVE ANALYSIS

Osteoporosis is a bone disorder that primarily affects elderly individuals as they gradually lose bone mass density. As a result of osteoporosis, their bones become weak and fragile, and they have much higher risk of bone fracture from minor injuries. Furthermore, individuals with osteoporosis often require an extended period of time for recovery, which is often complicated with infection.

Western Medical Approach: The drug of choice for treating osteoporosis is biphosphonates, a category of drugs that include Fosamax (Alendronate), Actonel (Risedronate), Didronel (Etidronate), Aredia (Pamidronate), and Skelid (Tiludronate). On average, these drugs may increase bone mass density by 3 to 5% after continuous use for three years. However, they cause numerous side effects, such as stomach irritation, and may increase the risk of cancer (thyroid adenoma and adrenal pheochromocytoma) and fertility impairment (inhibition of ovulation, and testicular and epididymal atrophy). Furthermore, there is evidence that use of these drugs do not decrease the incidence of bone fracture. Though these drugs increase bone mass density, the bones remain brittle and are susceptible to fracture. In women with menopause, hormone replacement therapy may be used to decrease the loss of bone mass density. These drugs, however, must be prescribed and monitored very carefully, as use of these hormone substances have been shown to significantly increase risk of cancer, such as breast cancer (by 20 to 30%), endometrial cancer (by 6-8 folds), and ovarian cancer (by 10 to 20%). In brief, treatment of osteoporosis requires careful evaluation of risks versus benefits by both practitioners and patients.

Traditional Chinese Medicine Approach: Herbs have been used with great success to nourish underlying deficiencies, and prevent and treat osteoporosis. In fact, according to one clinical study, use of herbs for one year was associated with an average increase of 3.4% in bone mass density among 28 women with menopause (average age of 48.8 years). Furthermore, few or no side effects were reported throughout the study.

Summation: Drugs and herbs are both effective for prevention and treatment of osteoporosis. However, herbs are safe and natural, and should be considered the treatment of choice. Furthermore, patients are encouraged to adopt dietary and lifestyle recommendations described above to maximize the overall efficacy of their treatment program.

CASE STUDIES

A 49-year-old female practitioner of Oriental medicine has family history of osteoporosis in maternal grandmother and mother. While her grandmother did not have any incidence of physical injury leading to bone fracture, the mother had an ankle fracture on the right side, and lost three inches in height. The patient sought treatment for prevention and treatment of osteoporosis. Upon evaluation, the diagnosis was blood deficiency without visible signs of bone loss. The patient started on *Osteo 8* at dosage of 3 to 6 capsules per day. In addition, she also took a supplement of calcium, magnesium, and potassium (2 to 4 capsules per day). She exercised aerobically with weights three times a week. She also lowered her intake of high-fat foods and avoided caffeine. No other changes were made with the lifestyle. Prior to treatment, her baseline bone mass density (BMD) was 0.448 (on 9/19/01). After four month of treatment, her bone mass density (BMD) increased to 0.7 (1/16/02). The patient improved from "low normal" to "low risk" for osteoporosis. The practitioner commented that the "increase in bone density was remarkable."

C.C., Middletown, Connecticut

B.D., a 68-year-old female, wanted a natural alternative to Evista (Raloxifene) for osteoporosis prevention. She appeared thin and pale. She had a history of osteoporosis in her mother's side of the family. The TCM diagnosis was Kidney qi, *jing* (essence), yin and yang deficiencies. *Osteo 8* was prescribed at 2 capsules a day. She had a bone mass density test done 2 years ago and it was slightly low, and was therefore placed on Evista (Raloxifene). After one year on *Osteo 8*, the bone density tested normal. She repeated the test 1 year again later and the density tested normal again. Her medical doctor was quite impressed. [Note: This patient had a sensitive stomach. She started with 4 capsules daily but had to be reduced to 2 caps because of gastrointestinal discomfort.]

M.H., West Palm Beach, Florida

C.M., a 48-year-old female, presented with joint pain (hands, feet, knees) that worsened in cold and rainy weather, reporting a family history of arthritis and osteoporosis. She also suffered from tendonitis of both forearms. She had decreased range of motion, with calcification of joints in fingers. Her western diagnosis was rheumatoid arthritis; the TCM diagnosis was cold and damp obstruction. *Osteo 8* and *Flex (CD)* were prescribed at four capsules each, twice daily. Within one day, the symptoms began improving. After one week, joints and tendons were not stiff, and almost pain free. During the winter (the season in which her condition usually deteriorated), the symptoms even improved. The patient reported later that if she stopped taking the herbs, the symptoms returned.

C.D., Phoenix, Oregon

FORMULAS

OSTEO 8 ™

[1]. *Dorland's Illustrated Medical Dictionary 28th Edition*, 1994.

[2]. Berkow, R et al. *The Merck Manual of Diagnosis and Therapy 16th Edition*, 1992.

[3] Estrogen Supplements. *Drug Facts and Comparison*, 1999.

[4]. Bensky, D. et al. *Chinese Herbal Medicine Materia Medica*. Eastland Press. 1993

[5]. *Zhong Yao Xue* (Chinese Herbology), 1998.

[6]. *Chang Yong Zhong Yao Cheng Fen Yu Yao Li Shou Ce* (A Handbook of the Composition and Pharmacology of Common Chinese Drugs), 1994

[7]. *Zhong Yao Xue* (Chinese Herbology), 1998; 802:803

[8]. *Zhong Yao Tong Bao* (Journal of Chinese Herbology), 1987; 12(10):41

[9] Liu HD, Li E, Tong XX. Effects of replenishing kidney herbs on estrogen and 1,25-dihydroxyvitamin D3 of dexamethasone-induced rats model with osteoporosis. *Chung Kuo Chung His Chieh Ho Tsa Chih* 1993 Sep; 13(9):544-5,518

POLYGONUM 14 ™

CLINICAL APPLICATIONS

☯ Hair loss
☯ Premature gray hair
☯ Brittle, unhealthy hair with split ends
☯ Dry scalp, skin and nails

WESTERN THERAPEUTIC ACTIONS

☯ Increases blood circulation to the scalp [2]
☯ Provides essential nutrients for hair growth [5]

CHINESE THERAPEUTIC ACTIONS

☯ Replenishes the vital essence of the Liver and the Kidney
☯ Nourishes blood and promotes circulation to the scalp

DOSAGE

Take 4 capsules three times daily on an empty stomach with warm water. **Polygonum 14** should be taken continuously for two months prior to making an evaluation. Most patients report changes in hair texture within two months, and changes in hair color in four to six months.

INGREDIENTS

Bai Shao (Radix Paeoniae Alba)
Chuan Xiong (Rhizoma Ligustici Chuanxiong)
Da Zao (Fructus Jujubae)
Dang Gui (Radicis Angelicae Sinensis)
Gan Cao (Radix Glycyrrhizae)
Ge Gen (Radix Puerariae)
Gui Zhi (Ramulus Cinnamomi)

Han Lian Cao (Herba Ecliptae)
He Shou Wu (Radix Polygoni Multiflori)
Hei Zhi Ma (Semen Sesami Nigrum)
Huang Qi (Radix Astragali)
Nu Zhen Zi (Fructus Ligustri Lucidi)
Sang Shen Zi (Fructus Mori)
Shu Di Huang (Radix Rehmanniae Preparata)

FORMULA EXPLANATION

Polygonum 14 is designed specifically to treat hair loss, premature gray hair, and brittleness with split ends, which are all signs of Kidney yin with Liver blood deficiency. **Polygonum 14** is formulated to nourish Kidney yin and Kidney *jing* (essence), tonify Liver blood, and increase blood circulation to the scalp.

He Shou Wu (Radix Polygoni Multiflori) is an indispensable herb for treating any hair disorder. It replenishes the vital essence of the Liver and Kidney and tonifies the blood. *Han Lian Cao* (Herba Ecliptae), *Sang Shen Zi* (Fructus Mori), and *Nu Zhen Zi* (Fructus Ligustri Lucidi) tonify the Liver and the Kidney yin to benefit the hair. *Shu Di Huang* (Radix Rehmanniae Preparata), *Hei Zhi Ma* (Semen Sesami Nigrum) and *Bai Shao* (Radix Paeoniae Alba) are selected to tonify Liver blood and nourish the hair. Proper blood circulation to the scalp is also an important factor for healthy hair. *Huang Qi* (Radix Astragali), *Ge Gen* (Radix Puerariae) and *Gui Zhi* (Ramulus Cinnamomi) have ascending properties that carry the therapeutic functions of this formula to the scalp. *Chuan Xiong* (Rhizoma Ligustici Chuanxiong) and *Dang Gui* (Radicis Angelicae Sinensis) improve microcirculation and nourish the blood. *Da Zao* (Fructus Jujubae) and *Gan Cao* (Radix Glycyrrhizae) are used to harmonize the formula.

FORMULAS

POLYGONUM 14 ™

SUPPLEMENTARY FORMULAS

- For hair loss due to chemotherapy and radiation, combine with *C/R Support* to minimize side effects.
- For hair loss due to stress, add *Calm*.
- For post-partum hair loss, add *Schisandra ZZZ* or *Imperial Tonic*.
- For low libido, add *Vitality*.
- For prevention of osteoporosis, add *Osteo 8*.
- For forgetfulness, add *Enhance Memory*.
- To control appetite for weight loss, add *Herbalite*.
- To improve the shape and increase the size of the breasts, add *Venus*.
- To tonify blood, combine with *Schisandra ZZZ*.
- For depression, use *Shine*.
- For constipation, use *Gentle Lax (Deficient)*.
- For blurry vision or tinnitus, combine with *Nourish*.
- To tonify Kidney yang, add *Kidney Tonic (Yang)*.
- To tonify Kidney yin, add *Kidney Tonic (Yin)*.
- With blood stagnation, add *Circulation (SJ)*.

NUTRITION

- Biotin, found in green peas, oats, soybeans, sunflower seeds and walnuts, is essential for healthy hair and skin. Kelp and seaweed are also excellent choices to include in the daily diet.
- Protein is the essential make-up of hair. Therefore, the intake of food high in protein such as milk, fish, egg, and beans are recommended.
- Foods that are high in collagen will improve the elasticity and shine of hair, such as wild yam, taro, lotus root and tendons.
- Intake of vitamins A and B are also recommended, as they can improve circulation to the scalp and promote hair growth.
- Increase intake of water, vegetables, fruits, seeds and nuts for patients with dry skin.
- Those with dandruff can increase the intake of vitamin B6 and B12.
- Consume adequate amounts of vegetables for vitamins, as they improve circulation to the scalp and promote hair growth.

LIFESTYLE INSTRUCTIONS

- Avoid cigarette smoking and second-hand smoke, sugar, alcohol, caffeine and junk food.
- Stay out of the sun as it can dry and damage skin and hair.
- Stress can impair the delivery of nutrients to the scalp as it causes stagnation. Patient should be advised to stay away from stressful situations.
- Natural bristle brushes are recommended. Brushes with sharp tips should not be used as they might scrape the scalp. To invigorate circulation to the scalp, brush hair 100 times from the back of the head towards the front with the head down at least twice a day.
- Untangle hair with a brush before shampooing. Mild shampoo should also be selected to avoid over stimulation to the scalp. Water temperature should not be too hot to avoid further hair loss. The scalp can be massaged while shampooing. Be sure to rinse completely, leaving no shampoo or conditioning residues to clog up the hair pores. Hair should be dried by gently padding on the towel instead of rubbing back and forth.
- Blow drying and use of hair products such as gel, mousse, hairspray are not recommended. Chemical treatments, perms, and color should also be avoided.

FORMULAS

POLYGONUM 14 ™

- Avoid swimming as much as possible as chlorine does much damage to the hair. If one cannot avoid swimming, it is recommended that the patient wear a cap or rub some baby oil into the hair.
- Get regular exercise and establish a normal pattern of sleep.

CLINICAL NOTES

- *He Shou Wu* (Radix Polygoni Multiflori) has been known as a popular anti-aging herb since the Ming dynasty (14th Century) in China. It is often used by the sages and Taoist monks to enhance longevity.
- *Polygonum 14* is an herbal formula originally developed for Empress *Chi-Xi*, the last empress in the history of China. It was developed in the 19th century by a private doctor in the Forbidden City who used a relatively large amount of *He Shou Wu* (Radix Polygoni Multiflori) to enhance hair color and texture. Empress *Chi-Xi* took *Polygonum 14* throughout her life and it became the secret to her shiny, black hair even when she was in her eighties.
- *Polygonum 14* is a constitutional tonic that changes the fundamental color and texture of hair. Change in hair texture requires approximately one to two months, and change in hair color requires four to six months of continuous herbal treatment. Therefore, individuals who take *Polygonum 14* must be patient, as changes will not occur immediately.

CAUTIONS

- Some patients may experience loose stool after taking *Polygonum 14*, which can be alleviated by lowering the dosage, or taking it with food.
- Patients who are on anticoagulant or antiplatelet therapies, such as Coumadin (Warfarin), should use this formula with caution as there may be a slightly higher risk of bleeding and bruising.
- *Polygonum 14* is contraindicated in individuals with exterior or excess conditions.
- *Polygonum 14* should be taken continuously for at least two to three months for improvement.

ACUPUNCTURE POINTS

Traditional Points:
- *Shangxing* (GV 23), *Baihui* (GV 20), *Yinlingquan* (SP 9), *Sanyinjiao* (SP 6), and *Taixi* (KI 3).
- *Baihui* (GV 20). Apply moxa to *Zusanli* (ST 36) and *Sanyinjiao* (SP 6).

Auricular Acupuncture by Dr. Li-Chun Huang:
- Alopecia: Sympathetic, Kidney, Liver, Gallbladder, Spleen, Lung, Endocrine, Pituitary, and Coronary Vascular Subcortex.
- For additional information on the location and explanation of these points, please refer to *Auricular Treatment Formula and Prescriptions* by Dr. Li-Chun Huang.

MODERN RESEARCH

Polygonum 14 is designed specifically to treat hair loss, premature gray, and brittleness with split ends. The main ingredient, *He Shou Wu* (Radix Polygoni Multiflori), is commonly used to tonify the vital *jing* (essence) of the Liver and the Kidney, nourish the blood, and treat various hair disorders. To evaluate the effectiveness of herbs in treating gray hair, 36 patients were selected in a clinical trial. Out of 36 patients, 20 had partial white discoloration of hair and 16 had complete white discoloration of hair. The herbs selected were *He Shou Wu* (Radix Polygoni Multiflori), *Dang Gui* (Radicis Angelicae Sinensis) and *Shu Di Huang* (Radix Rehmanniae Preparata). The patients were advised to take the herbs once to twice daily continuously until there were significant changes, which could vary from one year to ten years. After ten years of clinical trial, it was concluded that the use of these herbs were 88.89%

effective, with 24 out of 36 patients showing significant improvement, and 8 patients showing moderate improvement. [1]

In addition to its function of nourishing hair, *He Shou Wu* (Radix Polygoni Multiflori) reduces absorption of cholesterol from the intestines, decreases the level of cholesterol in the blood, and regulates glucose metabolism.[2] Modern indications also include the treatment of cancer and constipation.[3] Other sources have reported *He Shou Wu* (Radix Polygoni Multiflori) to possess antiprogestational, antipyretic and sedative effects.[4]

Chuan Xiong (Rhizoma Ligustici Chuanxiong) increases peripheral blood circulation by reducing the agglutination and the peripheral activities of platelets. It is a channel guiding herb which directs the effectiveness of the formula to the scalp.[5]

PHARMACEUTICAL DRUGS & CHINESE MEDICINE: A COMPARATIVE ANALYSIS

One striking difference between western and traditional Chinese medicine is that western medicine focuses and excels in crisis management, while traditional Chinese medicine emphasizes and shines in holistic and preventative treatments. Therefore, in emergencies, such as gun shot wounds or surgery, western medicine is generally the treatment of choice. However, for treatment of chronic idiopathic illness of unknown origins, where all lab tests are normal and a clear diagnosis cannot be made, traditional Chinese medicine is distinctly superior.

In regards to premature aging of the hair characterized by hair loss, premature gray hair, and unhealthy hair, there is essentially no drug treatment available in western medicine. Rogaine (Minoxidil) is one of very limited options available, and its effect is often disappointing. Limited hair growth may occur only after continuous use for several months. Furthermore, hair loss occurs after drug use is discontinued. In short, drug treatment is only marginally beneficial and is only effective for a short period of time.

On the other hand, traditional Chinese medicine is significantly superior to western medicine to restore normal appearance and texture of hair. Furthermore, when used continuously for four to six months, it also helps to promote lasting hair growth. In addition to improving texture and volume of hair, this formula also has anti-aging effect to improve overall well being. Lastly, it is very safe and can be used for prolonged period of time.

CASE STUDIES

Two females, ages 54- and 55-years-old, presented with hair loss. The practitioner attributed their hair loss to blood deficiency with some underlying Liver yin and Spleen qi deficiencies. They were both treated with the *Polygonum 14* formula. The patients reported new hair growth as well as normalization of bowel movements. The practitioner concluded *Polygonum 14* to be quite effective in treating hair loss due to aging.

D.N., Pacific Palisades, California

C.W., a 40-year-old male, presented with tiredness, poor sleep, constipation, grey hair, over-work, and high cholesterol. His blood pressure was 130/80 mmHg and his heart rate was 80 beats per minute. There was no western diagnosis and the TCM diagnosis was found to be Liver blood deficiency. *Polygonum 14* was prescribed at 2 grams three times daily. This patient also received acupuncture as the overall treatment regime. The patient reported the quality of sleep improved after taking the herbs. Energy level increased and the constipation was relieved. Additionally, his cholesterol level dropped from 223 to 190 mg/dL.

W.F., Bloomfield, New Jersey

FORMULAS

POLYGONUM 14 ™

A 22-year-old male college student presented with dry skin and hair loss on the scalp, as noted by a patch near the vertex. He admitted to drug use and smoking, along with depression. His pulse was rapid and full while his tongue was crimson. The patient appeared restless. The practitioner diagnosed the condition as yin deficiency and fluid consumption, possibly from an overuse of stimulants. After taking *Polygonum 14* for less than 1 month, the patient observed that his hair felt less brittle and that he had not seen any hair strands on his pillow unlike in the past. The patch of lost hair was less noticeable and he detected new hair growth after 1½ months. The patient also reported an increased energy level, as well as a more cheerful disposition. He also appeared less restless. Additionally, he had refrained from drugs and smoking, from which he fortunately did not develop any withdrawal signs or cravings. Interestingly, with the use of *Polygonum 14*, the patient's hair not only felt healthier but also became darker, although his hair was naturally dark blonde.

F.V., Orlando, Florida

A 35-year-old female singer presented with hair loss, fatigue and low energy. She had a pale tongue, soft pulse and cold feet. The practitioner diagnosed her condition as Kidney yang deficiency. The patient was instructed to take *Polygonum 14*. The patient reported excellent results. The practitioner concluded that *Polygonum 14* had been quite effective in treatment of a variety of conditions, including Kidney yin deficiency and Spleen qi deficiency, but especially with hair loss symptoms.

L.T., Chicago, Illinois

---

[1] Zhao, HB. Treatment of white hair with polygonum (he shou wu) tincture. *Shangdong Journal of Traditional Chinese Medicine*. 4:41. 1983.
[2] Bensky, D. et al. *Chinese Herbal Medicine Materia Medica*. Eastland Press. 1993
[3] Tyler, VE. *The New Honest Herbal*. Philadelphia, PA: G.F. Stickley Co., 1987
[4] Duke, JA. *Handbook of Medicinal Herbs*. Boca Raton, FL: CRC Press, 1985
[5] Yeung, HC. *Handbook of Chinese Herbs*. Institute of Chinese Medicine. 1996

FORMULAS

PORIA XPT ™

(Expectorant)

CLINICAL APPLICATIONS

- ❧ Respiratory tract infection with profuse yellow or green sputum, and post-nasal drip
- ❧ Pneumonia or bronchitis with cough and dyspnea
- ❧ Common cold or influenza with chest congestion and fullness

WESTERN THERAPEUTIC ACTIONS

- ❧ Antitussive function to relieve cough
- ❧ Expectorant effect to expel phlegm and sputum from the upper respiratory tract
- ❧ Herbal antibiotic effect to inhibit the growth of harmful bacteria and viruses

CHINESE THERAPEUTIC ACTIONS

- ❧ Clears Lung heat
- ❧ Regulates Lung qi
- ❧ Lowers the adverse rising qi and relieves cough
- ❧ Transforms phlegm

DOSAGE

Take 4 to 6 capsules three times daily on an empty stomach with warm water.

INGREDIENTS

Bai Jie Zi (Semen Sinapis)
Chen Pi (Pericarpium Citri Reticulatae)
Da Zao (Fructus Jujubae)
Dan Nan Xing (Arisaema cum Bile)
Dong Gua Zi (Semen Benincasae)
Fu Ling (Poria)
Huang Qin (Radix Scutellariae)

Jie Geng (Radix Platycodonis)
Ting Li Zi (Semen Descurainiae seu Lepidii)
Xing Ren (Semen Armeniacae Amarum)
Yi Yi Ren (Semen Coicis)
Zhi Shi (Fructus Aurantii Immaturus)
Zhu Ru (Caulis Bambusae in Taenia)

FORMULA EXPLANATION

Poria XPT addresses the secondary stage of lung infection in which the superficial symptoms are no longer present. Instead there is an internal stagnation of phlegm and fire, which interferes with the descending function of Lung qi. Therefore, cough and profuse yellow or green sputum are the predominant symptoms.

Dan Nan Xing (Arisaema cum Bile) has a strong effect to treat blockage due to fire and phlegm. *Huang Qin* (Radix Scutellariae), *Ting Li Zi* (Semen Descurainiae seu Lepidii) and *Jie Geng* (Radix Platycodonis) work together to drain Lung fire while transforming phlegm. *Bai Jie Zi* (Semen Sinapis) and *Xing Ren* (Semen Armeniacae Amarum) eliminate phlegm, reverse rebellious Lung qi, and relieve cough. *Chen Pi* (Pericarpium Citri Reticulatae) and *Zhi Shi* (Fructus Aurantii Immaturus) regulate Lung qi and relieve chest congestion and fullness. *Zhu Ru* (Caulis Bambusae in Taenia) clears phlegm-heat to expel sputum and relieve the stifling sensation in the chest. *Fu Ling* (Poria), *Yi Yi Ren* (Semen Coicis) and *Dong Gua Zi* (Semen Benincasae) strengthen the Spleen and dispel phlegm through urination. *Da Zao* (Fructus Jujubae) is used to harmonize the stomach and moderate the strong properties of *Dan Nan Xing* (Arisaema cum Bile) and *Ting Li Zi* (Semen Descurainiae seu Lepidii).

PORIA XPT ™

(Expectorant)

SUPPLEMENTARY FORMULAS

- For infection with fever, chest congestion and dyspnea characterized by Lung heat, add *Respitrol (Heat)*.
- For cough, add *Respitrol (CF)*.
- For high fever, add *Gardenia Complex*.
- To enhance the overall antibiotic effect, add *Herbal ABX*.
- To treat infection of ear, nose and throat, add *Herbal ENT*.
- For sinus infection with yellow nasal discharge, add *Pueraria Clear Sinus*.
- For tonsillitis with swollen throat, add *Resolve (AI)* and *Herbal ENT*.
- For wind-heat, add *Lonicera Complex*.
- *Immune +* can be taken on a daily basis to build-up the immune system and prevent bacterial or viral infections. Start taking *Immune +* after symptoms of cold/flu have subsided.
- For plum-pit syndrome, add *Calm*.

NUTRITION

- Avoid foods that are greasy or spicy in nature as they create more dampness and heat.
- To avoid infection, a diet high in garlic, onions, and water is recommended.
- Adequate intake of vitamin C is important as it is greatly consumed by white blood cells when fighting infections.
- Avoid smoking and exposure to second-hand smoke, alcohol, seafood, and phlegm-producing foods such as sweets, dairy products, heavy or greasy foods.
- Eat plenty of foods that contain vitamin A and C, which strengthen the lung tissue and improve resistance to infection, respectively.

LIFESTYLE INSTRUCTIONS

- Patients are encouraged to expel sputum out so that the airway can be cleared to facilitate normal respiration and relieve chest congestion.
- Installation of an air purifier at home is recommended for recurrent respiratory disorders.
- A humidifier will increase moisture in the air, hydrate the mucous membranes of the nose and the lung, and hence increase resistance to infection.

CAUTIONS

- *Poria XPT* is designed for respiratory infections characterized by chest congestion with profuse yellow phlegm. It is not suitable for the initial stage of wind-heat or wind-cold.
- Some patients may experience stomach discomfort as a result of taking this formula. Should this occur, reduce the dosage or take the herbs with food.
- This formula is contraindicated during pregnancy and nursing.
- This formula is not recommended for long-term use. It should be discontinued when the desired effects are achieved.

ACUPUNCTURE POINTS

Traditional Points:
1. *Feishu* (BL 13), *Shanzhong* (CV 17), *Dazhui* (GV 14), and *Zusanli* (ST 36).
2. *Shanzhong* (CV 17), *Feishu* (BL 13), and *Yuji* (LU 10).

PORIA XPT ™

(Expectorant)

Balance Method by Dr. Richard Tan:
- Left side: *Ligou* (LR 5), *Zhubin* (KI 9), *Sanyinjiao* (SP 6), *Hegu* (LI 4), and *Quchi* (LI 11).
- Right side: *Yuji* (LU 10), *Taiyuan* (LU 9), *Fenglong* (ST 40), and *Chengshan* (BL 57).
- Left and right side can be alternated from treatment to treatment.
- To read more about Dr. Tan's acupuncture strategy, see his book *Dr. Tan's Strategy of Twelve Magic Points*.

MODERN RESEARCH

Poria XPT is designed to treat various types of respiratory tract infections, such as common cold, influenza, pneumonia or bronchitis. In addition to the infection, additional signs and symptoms include profuse yellow or green sputum, post-nasal drip, chest congestion and fullness, cough, and dyspnea. To treat both the cause and the symptoms, *Poria XPT* is formulated with herbs that have antibiotic, expectorant, antitussive and antipyretic effects.

Many herbs in this formula have marked antibiotic effects to treat respiratory tract infections. For example, *Huang Qin* (Radix Scutellariae) has broad antimicrobial effects against *Staphylococcus*, *Pseudomonas*, *Streptococcus*, and *Neisseria*.[1,2] *Huang Qin* (Radix Scutellariae) has antiviral activities and suppresses the replication of influenza A and B viruses.[3] It also has fungistatic activities against *Candida albicans* and *Cryptococcus neoformans*.[4] *Zhu Ru* (Caulis Bambusae in Taenia) also has an inhibitory effect against many pathogens, such as *Staphylococcus albus*, *Bacillus subtilis*, *E. coli*, and *Salmonella typhi*.[5]

Many herbs in this formula have an expectorant effect to eliminate sputum and phlegm, and an antitussive effect to suppress cough. *Dan Nan Xing* (Arisaema cum Bile) has expectorant properties and increases secretion of mucus in the respiratory tract. *Jie Geng* (Radix Platycodonis) has marked antitussive and expectorant effects to suppress and relieve cough.[6] *Bai Jie Zi* (Semen Sinapis) also has an expectorant effect.[7] Most importantly, *Xing Ren* (Semen Armeniacae Amarum) has a remarkable antitussive effect, with its mechanism attributed to inhibition of the respiratory reflex in the brain.[8]

Because infection is often accompanied by fever, *Huang Qin* (Radix Scutellariae) is used in this formula for its antipyretic effect to reduce body temperature.[9]

In summary, *Poria XPT* is an excellent formula to treat respiratory tract infections as it contains herbs that address both the cause and the symptoms of the illness.

PHARMACEUTICAL DRUGS & CHINESE MEDICINE: A COMPARATIVE ANALYSIS

Respiratory tract disorders (such as cough, dyspnea, and lung infection) are often complicated with presence of phlegm, and swelling and inflammation of the lung. Because the presence of phlegm in the lung creates discomfort and delays recovery, it is often necessary to expectorate the phlegm.

Western Medical Approach: There is only one approved expectorant available for treatment of phlegm – guaifenesin. This drug is mixed with other drug combinations, such as Robitussin and Triaminic, to treat the overall cold and flu complex of cough, nasal obstruction, chest congestion, and runny nose. Guaifenesin is relatively safe and free from side effects, but its potency is also limited.

Traditional Chinese Medicine Approach: Many herbs are extremely effective to stop the production, loosen the viscosity, and facilitate the elimination, of phlegm. Similar to western medicine, these herbs are often combined with others to treat other accompanying symptoms of illness, such as cough, nasal obstruction, and chest congestion.

Summation: Expectorants are effective to assist the elimination of phlegm in the chest, and are most effective when used with other medicinal substances to enhance the overall effect to treat various symptoms of respiratory tract

PORIA XPT ™

(Expectorant)

disorders. Guaifenesin is the only drug option available, and it is rather mild in potency. On the other hand, there are many herbs available to stop the production of phlegm and facilitate its elimination.

CASE STUDIES

A 59-year-old female presented with copious congestion, chest tightness and yellow-greenish phlegm. The patient's condition was diagnosed as heat in the Lung with phlegm congestion. The practitioner prescribed *Poria XPT*. Subsequently, the patient's phlegm resolved as well as her chest tightness and pain.

V.G., Carlsbad, California

A 59-year-old male physician presented with extreme fever (over 104°F), extreme difficulty breathing, pain in the chest, shortness of breath aggravated by exertion, unsteady walk, dizziness, and inability to speak more than one word per breath. His tongue was pale with red tip and body, and his was rapid and superficial. The diagnosis was phlegm heat in the Lung. The patient was treated with *Poria XPT* (6 capsules four times daily) and *Immune* + (6 capsules four times daily), along with other homeopathics and drugs [Combivent (Albuterol/Ipratropium) and aspirin]. The patient had a definite response to the herbs. The respiration became much easier, energy level and sense of vitality enhanced, and cough was no longer productive. The practitioner commented that "While all protocols employed resulted in benefit – it is without question that the herbal formulas generated imminent benefit and long term recuperation."

I.B.J., Miami, Florida.

D.C., a 50-year-old female, presented common cold symptoms of cough, chest congestion and difficult to expectorate phlegm. She had a slight fever. The tongue was red with yellow coating. The pulse was rapid and slippery. The doctor diagnosed her with Lung heat. The two formulas prescribed were *Respitrol (Heat)* and *Poria XPT*. In three days, the heat was relieved and the phlegm was cleared.

B.F., Newport Beach, California

[1] *Zhong Yao Xue* (Chinese Herbology), 1988; 137:140
[2] *J Pharm Pharmacol* 2000 Mar; 52(3):361-6
[3] Nagai et al. antiviral activity of plant flavonoid, 5,7,4'-trihydroxy-8-methoxyflavone, from scutellaria baicalensis against influenza A (H3N2) and B viruses. *Biol Pharm Bull*; 18(2):295-9. Feb. 1995
[4] Yang, D. et al. Antifungal activity in vitro of Scutellaria baicalensis. *Ann Pharm Fr*; 53(3):138-41. 1995
[5] *Zhong Yao Xue* (Chinese Herbology), 1998; 623:625
[6] *Zhong Yao Yao Li Yu Ying Yong* (Pharmacology and Applications of Chinese Herbs), 1983; 866
[7] *Zhong Yao Xue* (Chinese Herbology), 1998; 608:610
[8] *Life Sci*, 1980; 27(8):659
[9] *Zhong Hua Yi Xue Za Zhi* (Chinese Journal of Medicine), 1956; 42(10):964

P-Statin ™

CLINICAL APPLICATIONS

- Benign prostatic hypertrophy (BPH)
- Prostate enlargement with urinary frequency, urgency and nocturia. Feeling of incomplete emptying, terminal dribbling, and pain with urination.
- Varicocele
- *Lin zheng* (dysuria syndrome) with urinary urgency, painful urination, difficult urination with inflammation

WESTERN THERAPEUTIC ACTIONS

- Reduces the size of the prostate gland [3]
- Relieves pain and reduces inflammation associated with prostatic hypertrophy [4,5,6,7,8]
- Promotes normal urination [9,10]

CHINESE THERAPEUTIC ACTIONS

- Clears damp-heat
- Promotes normal urination
- Tonifies qi, blood and *jing* (essence)

DOSAGE

Take 3 to 4 capsules three times daily, with warm water, on an empty stomach. Dosage may be increased up to 8 to 10 capsules three times daily in acute conditions until symptoms subside, but for no more than four days. After relief of symptoms, dosage can then be reduced to 3 to 4 capsules daily. For prevention or maintenance, take 2 capsules twice daily.

INGREDIENTS

Chi Shao (Radix Paeoniae Rubrae)
Fu Ling (Poria)
Hu Po (Succinum)
Hua Shi (Talcum)
Huang Bai (Cortex Phellodendri)
Huang Qi (Radix Astragali)
Mo Yao (Myrrha)

Pu Gong Ying (Herba Taraxaci)
Ru Xiang (Gummi Olibanum)
Tao Ren (Semen Persicae)
Tong Cao (Medulla Tetrapanacis)
Wang Bu Liu Xing (Semen Vaccariae)
Yi Yi Ren (Semen Coicis)

FORMULA EXPLANATION

In traditional Chinese medicine, benign prostatic hyperplasia in geriatric men is a condition due to both excess and deficiency. Excess refers to the enlargement of the gland leading to stagnation of qi and blood and accumulation of damp-heat. Deficiency refers to the gradual depletion of qi, blood and Kidney *jing* (essence) accompanying aging. Therefore, optimal treatment must use herbs that tonify the underlying deficiency, clear damp-heat, and promote normal urination.

In this formula, many herbs are used to break up and resolve the enlargement and disperse stagnation. *Ru Xiang* (Gummi Olibanum) and *Mo Yao* (Myrrha) have excellent functions to activate blood circulation and disperse blood stagnation. This pair is commonly used to disperse masses throughout the entire body – not just the prostate. *Chi Shao* (Radix Paeoniae Rubrae) and *Tao Ren* (Semen Persicae) are used to enhance the effect of softening the

P-Statin ™

hardness and promoting normal urination. *Hu Po* (Succinum) is used to break up blood stagnation and open the orifices. Furthermore, *Tong Cao* (Medulla Tetrapanacis) and *Wang Bu Liu Xing* (Semen Vaccariae) are added to disperse and reduce swelling and inflammation. They also have excellent penetrating qualities to help restore healthy, continuous urinary flow. This combination exerts an excellent effect to resolve enlargement and disperse stagnation. In addition, *Huang Qi* (Radix Astragali) and *Fu Ling* (Poria) are markedly effective at tonifying qi and regulating water circulation. *Fu Ling* (Poria), *Hua Shi* (Talcum), *Tong Cao* (Medulla Tetrapanacis) and *Yi Yi Ren* (Semen Coicis) are diuretic herbs used to promote normal urination and relieve various discomforts associated with dampness and swelling. Bitter and cold, *Huang Bai* (Cortex Phellodendri) and *Pu Gong Ying* (Herba Taraxaci) clear damp-heat and toxic heat from the lower *jiao*.

In conclusion, *P-Statin* addresses both the cause and the symptoms of benign prostatic hyperplasia. It treats the cause by resolving enlargement of the prostate gland. It treats the symptoms by clearing damp-heat and promoting normal urination, alleviating discomfort and resolving or preventing inflammation. By targeting both the cause and the symptoms simultaneously, it offers both immediate and long-term support for these patients.

SUPPLEMENTARY FORMULAS

- For varicocele, add **Resolve (Lower)**. The dosages of **P-Statin** and **Resolve (Lower)** should be at a 3:1 ratio, respectively.
- For damp-heat accumulation with turbid, painful urination, use **Gentiana Complex**.
- For bacterial prostatitis, use with **V-Statin** or **Herbal ABX**.
- For kidney stones, add **Dissolve (KS)**.
- For Kidney yang deficiency with coldness or impotence, add **Kidney Tonic (Yang)**.
- For Kidney yin deficiency, add **Kidney Tonic (Yin)**.
- For edema and water accumulation, add **Herbal DRX**.
- For blood stagnation, add **Circulation (SJ)**.

NUTRITION

- Encourage the patient to eat foods rich in zinc, such as raw pumpkin seeds or pumpkin seed oil, and sunflower seeds. Studies have shown zinc deficiency to be linked to prostate disorders.[1]
- Foods with phytoestrogens, such as soy and yams, have a beneficial effect for prostate health.
- Increase the consumption of the following foods beneficial for general prostate health: organic, fresh, leafy vegetables, whole grains and raw wheat germ, carrots, citrus fruits, and natural enzymes. It is also recommended to eat cooked vegetables instead of raw ones.
- Avoid fruits such as watermelon and citrus that are cold or sour in nature.
- Avoid tobacco smoking, alcoholic beverages, junk food, tomatoes, tomato products, and spicy food. Reduce salt intake.

The Tao of Nutrition by Ni and McNease

- Recommendations: pumpkin seeds, anise tangerines, cherries, figs, litchis, sunflower seeds, mangos, and seaweeds.
- Avoid dairy products, rich foods, fatty foods, all stimulants such as alcohol, caffeine, and smoking; stress, tension, sex, and eating meat late in the day.
- For more information, please refer to *The Tao of Nutrition* by Dr. Maoshing Ni and Cathy McNease.

P-Statin ™

LIFESTYLE INSTRUCTIONS

❧ Take steps to reduce blood cholesterol levels if necessary. Studies have shown high cholesterol to be linked to prostate disorders.[1]

❧ Relaxation exercises help to relieve tension and facilitate bladder emptying.

❧ Abstain from sexual intercourse as much as possible until the condition is resolved, and then observe moderation.

CLINICAL NOTES

❧ Benign prostatic hyperplasia is a condition that becomes progressively more common and severe with aging. While the incidence of benign prostatic hyperplasia is 40 to 50% in men aged 51 to 60 years, the incidence is 80% in men older than 80 years of age. Therefore, BPH should be treated as early as possible to prevent the occurrence and deterioration of the condition.

❧ *P-Statin* is an excellent formula for prevention and/or maintenance, at 2 capsules twice daily.

❧ *P-Statin* and *Saw Palmetto Complex* both address benign prostatic hypertrophy (BPH). Both can be used for geriatric men who are beginning to develop enlarged prostates associated with aging and hormonal changes. *P-Statin* treats BPH by draining damp-heat and tonifying qi and *jing* (essence). *Saw Palmetto Complex* treats BPH by draining damp-heat and reducing swelling.

CAUTIONS

❧ *P-Statin* is designed to treat mild to moderate prostate enlargement. While it may help to promote normal urination, it is not suitable for treatment of prostate cancer, although it may be a helpful adjunct to other more specific treatment modalities for prostate cancer. Additional workup is necessary to confirm or rule out diagnosis of prostate cancer.

❧ This formula is not designed for long-term use. It should be discontinued when the desired effects are achieved.

❧ If use of this formula is necessary for extended maintainance, use only a reduced dosage.

ACUPUNCTURE POINTS

Traditional Points:

❧ *Hegu* (LI 4), *Sanyinjiao* (SP 6), *Guanyuan* (CV 4), *Zhongji* (CV 3), *Yanglingquan* (GB 34), *Qugu* (CV 2), and *Huiyin* (CV 1).

❧ Needle *Ciliao* (BL 32). Apply moxa to *Guanyuan* (CV 4) and *Zusanli* (ST 36).

Balance Method by Dr. Richard Tan:

❧ Left side: *Dazhong* (KI 4), *Zhaohai* (KI 6), *Zhongfeng* (LR 4), *Yangxi* (LI 5), *Yangchi* (TH 4), and Prostate point on the ear.

❧ Right side: *Jiexi* (ST 41), *Shenmai* (BL 62), *Lieque* (LU 7), and *Daling* (PC 7).

❧ Left and right side can be alternated from treatment to treatment.

❧ For additional information on the Balance Method, please refer to *Dr. Tan's Strategy of Twelve Magical Points* by Dr. Richard Tan.

Auricular Acupuncture by Dr. Li-Chun Huang:

❧ Prostatitis: Prostate, Urethra, Pelvic, Kidney, Lower Jiao, Liver, Spleen, *San Jiao*, and Endocrine.

❧ Hypertrophy of prostate: Prostate, Urethra, Pelvic, Kidney, Liver, Lower Jiao, Pituitary, Endocrine, *San Jiao*, and Gonadotropin.

FORMULAS

P-Statin ™

- Orchitis and epididymitis: Testis, Endocrine, Adrenal Gland, Kidney, Liver, Prostate, Pelvic, Internal Genital, and External Genital. Bleed Ear Apex.
- For additional information on the location and explanation of these points, please refer to *Auricular Treatment Formula and Prescriptions* by Dr. Li-Chun Huang.

MODERN RESEARCH

According to western medicine, benign prostatic hyperplasia is defined as enlargement of the prostate gland causing varying degrees of bladder outlet obstruction.[2] The exact etiology is unknown, but it is presumed to be linked to hormonal changes associated with aging. Clinically, patients often present with symptoms such as progressive urinary frequency, urgency and nocturia. Furthermore, many will experience a feeling of incomplete emptying, terminal dribbling, and pain with urination. Decreased size and force of the urinary stream is also commonly reported. Therefore, proper therapy requires treatment of both the cause and the symptoms.

P-Statin contains many herbs that have been used with marked success for treatment of benign prostatic hyperplasia and its associated symptoms. Studies have shown that *P-Statin* contains herbs to effectively reduce the size of the prostate, promote normal urination, relieve pain and reduce inflammation.

Huang Qi (Radix Astragali), *Hua Shi* (Talcum) and *Hu Po* (Succinum) are commonly used for treatment of prostatic hypertrophy. In one clinical study, patients with prostatic hypertrophy were treated on an empty stomach with a decoction of these three ingredients, with very positive results. That study reported that 38 of 52 patients reported complete remission of symptoms, 13 reported improvement in flow rate and reduction in prostate size, and 1 reported no improvement.[3]

As benign prostatic hyperplasia is often accompanied by inflammation of the prostate gland and painful urination, herbs are added to alleviate these conditions. *Ru Xiang* (Gummi Olibanum) and *Mo Yao* (Myrrha) have excellent analgesic effect, and are commonly used to treat various types of pain.[4,5] *Tao Ren* (Semen Persicae), *Tong Cao* (Medulla Tetrapanacis) and *Hu Po* (Succinum) show marked anti-inflammatory properties, and are used to reduce swelling and enlargement of the prostate gland.[6,7,8]

Altered patterns and distinct characteristics of urination are some of the most common symptoms of benign prostatic hyperplasia that must be addressed. Herbs with diuretic effect are often quite successful in reducing frequency and urgency of urination, improving the force of the urinary stream, and relieving dribbling and incontinence. Herbs with diuretic action that promote normal urination and increase urinary output include *Fu Ling* (Poria) and *Tong Cao* (Medulla Tetrapanacis).[9,10]

In summary, *P-Statin* is carefully crafted to address both the cause and the symptoms of benign prostatic hyperplasia. *P-Statin* contains herbs that treat the cause by reducing the size of the prostate gland, and herbs that treat the symptoms by promoting normal urination, relieving pain and reducing inflammation.

PHARMACEUTICAL DRUGS & CHINESE MEDICINE: A COMPARATIVE ANALYSIS

Western Medical Approach: Benign prostate hypertrophy (BPH) is a disorder that affects most men as they age. In western medicine, BPH may be treated with drugs that relax the bladder muscle to improve urination [such as Minipress (Prazosin)], or drugs that shrink the prostate [such as Proscar (Finasteride)]. However, Minipress (Prazosin) is an alpha-adrenergic drug originally used to treat hypertension, and may cause side effects such as hypotension, dizziness, lightheadedness, orthostatism, syncope, and if/when the drug is discontinued, rebound hypertension. Proscar (Finasteride) is effective, but requires three months or more to take effect, and may cause sexual dysfunction with side effects such as impotence, decreased libido, and decreased volume of ejaculate. Lastly,

FORMULAS

P-Statin ™

in severe cases of prostate hypertrophy, a catheter is inserted through the penis into the bladder to drain urine. Finally, western medicine considers surgical removal of the prostate to be the best option.

Traditional Chinese Medicine Approach: Many herbs can be used to effectively treat BPH. The main therapeutic benefits of this formula include analgesic effect to relieve pain, anti-inflammatory effect to reduce swelling and inflammation, and diuretic effect to promote normal urination. Though this formula does not cure BPH, it is quite effective to reduce the size of the prostate gland and relieve the symptoms.

Summation: Both western and traditional Chinese medicines are effective to treat BPH. Drug therapy is usually unsatisfactory, as its effectiveness is limited, and is associated with significant side effects. Herbal therapy, on the other hand, is both safe and effective, and has short- and long-term benefits. However, in serious cases of prostate cancer, patients should be referred to western medicine, as use of herbs as a sole treatment modality is not recommended.

[1] Balch, J. and Balch, P. *Prescriptions for Nutritional Healing.* Avery Publishing Group. 1997
[2] Beers, M. and Berkow, R. *The Merck Manual of Diagnosis and Therapy 17th Edition.* 1999.
[3] *Xin Zhong Yi* (New Chinese Medicine), 1987; 10:54
[4] *Zhong Yao Xue* (Chinese Herbology), 1998; 539:540
[5] *Zhong Yao Xue* (Chinese Herbology), 1998; 541:542
[6] *Zhong Yao Tong Bao* (Journal of Chinese Herbology), 1986; 11(11):37
[7] *Chang Yong Zhong Yao Cheng Fen Yu Yao Li Shou Ce* (A Handbook of the Composition and Pharmacology of Common Chinese Drugs), 1994; 1459:1462
[8] *Shang Hai Zhong Yi Yao Za Zhi* (Shanghai Journal of Chinese Medicine and Herbology), 1958; 11:33
[9] *Chang Yong Zhong Yao Cheng Fen Yu Yao Li Shou Ce* (A Handbook of the Composition and Pharmacology of Common Chinese Drugs), 1994; 1383:1391
[10] *Zhong Yao Cai* (Study of Chinese Herbal Material), 1991; 14(9):40

FORMULAS

PUERARIA CLEAR SINUS ™

CLINICAL APPLICATIONS

- ☯ Allergy, sinusitis or rhinitis with purulent yellow discharge
- ☯ Sinus infection with headache, pain, and nasal obstruction
- ☯ General nasal problems including stuffy nose, sneezing, loss of smell, yellow watery nasal discharge, etc.

WESTERN THERAPEUTIC ACTIONS

- ☯ Constricts blood vessels in the nasal mucosa to treat sinusitis and rhinitis [1]
- ☯ Reduces nasal mucous secretions [1]
- ☯ Antibiotic activities to treat sinus infection [1,2]
- ☯ Analgesic effect to relieve sinus headache and pain [1,2]

CHINESE THERAPEUTIC ACTIONS

- ☯ Dispels damp-heat accumulation
- ☯ Removes fluid congestion
- ☯ Unblocks nasal obstruction
- ☯ Clears heat and dispels purulent infection
- ☯ Alleviates sinus pain

DOSAGE

For treatment of sinusitis, rhinitis or sinus infection, take 4 to 6 capsules three times daily with warm water on an empty stomach one hour before or two hours after meals. For maintenance or prevention, take 3 capsules twice times daily.

INGREDIENTS

Bai Shao (Radix Paeoniae Alba)
Bai Zhi (Radix Angelicae Dahuricae)
Cang Er Zi (Fructus Xanthii)
Chuan Xiong (Rhizoma Ligustici Chuanxiong)
Da Huang (Radix et Rhizoma Rhei)
Da Zao (Fructus Jujubae)
Gan Cao (Radix Glycyrrhizae)

Ge Gen (Radix Puerariae)
Gui Zhi (Ramulus Cinnamomi)
Huang Qin (Radix Scutellariae)
Jie Geng (Radix Platycodonis)
Sheng Jiang (Rhizoma Zingiberis Recens)
Shi Gao (Gypsum Fibrosum)
Xin Yi Hua (Flos Magnoliae)

FORMULA EXPLANATION

Pueraria Clear Sinus is formulated to treat allergies, sinusitis or rhinitis due to damp-heat and fluid congestion. Clinically, common signs and symptoms include stuffy nose, sticky yellow discharge, loss of ability to smell, and sinus headache.

Xin Yi Hua (Flos Magnoliae) and *Cang Er Zi* (Fructus Xanthii) are the chief herbs in this formula. They have acrid, dispersing, and decongestant properties to unblock the nasal passages. *Huang Qin* (Radix Scutellariae), *Shi Gao* (Gypsum Fibrosum) and *Da Huang* (Radix et Rhizoma Rhei) clear heat, reduce inflammation and neutralize the warming properties of the chief herbs. *Gui Zhi* (Ramulus Cinnamomi) and *Bai Shao* (Radix Paeoniae Alba) harmonize the *wei* (defense) and *ying* (nutritive) levels to dispel external pathogenic influences. *Ge Gen* (Radix Puerariae) dispels wind-heat and alleviates pain. *Chuan Xiong* (Rhizoma Ligustici Chuanxiong) relieves sinus

FORMULAS

PUERARIA CLEAR SINUS ™

headache. *Jie Geng* (Radix Platycodonis) and *Bai Zhi* (Radix Angelicae Dahuricae) eliminate pus and resolve nasal discharge and post-nasal drip associated with the sinus infection. *Da Zao* (Fructus Jujubae), *Sheng Jiang* (Rhizoma Zingiberis Recens), and *Gan Cao* (Radix Glycyrrhizae) harmonize the formula and protect the middle *jiao*.

SUPPLEMENTARY FORMULAS

- For infection of the ear, nose and throat, add *Herbal ENT*.
- For nasal obstruction due to sinus infection, add *Herbal ABX*.
- For profuse yellow phlegm, post-nasal drip, dyspnea, or chest congestion, use *Poria XPT*.
- For wind-heat at the exterior, add *Lonicera Complex*.
- For Lung heat with cough, dyspnea and fever, add *Respitrol (Heat)*.
- For headache, add *Corydalin*.
- For migraine due to deficiency, add *Migratrol*.
- For nasal symptoms associated with environmental or toxic poisoning, add *Herbal DTX*.
- For excess heat, add *Gardenia Complex*.
- To strengthen the constitution of the body, use *Imperial Tonic*.
- To enhance immunity against allergies, take *Immune +* at a low dose (1 to 2 capsules a day) during non-allergy seasons.

NUTRITION

- Reduce or eliminate intake of dairy products, as they increase mucus production.
- Drink plenty of distilled water throughout the day to help drainage.
- Make sure the diet contains an adequate amount of vitamin A and C. Vitamin A is essential for healthy mucous lining of the respiratory tract. Vitamin C is well recognized for its effect to prevent and treat infection.

The Tao of Nutrition by Ni and McNease
- Allergy
  - Drink beet top tea as a water source.
  - Avoid wheat, citrus fruits, chocolate, shellfish, dairy products, eggs, potatoes, polluted meats, and polluted air.
- Chronic sinusitis
  - Recommendations: ginger, green onions, magnolia flower, bananas, garlic, black mushrooms, chrysanthemum flowers, mulberry leaves, and apricot kernel.
  - Avoid extremes of exposure to weather elements, coffee, smoking, stress, picking the nose, polluted air and smog.
- For more information, please refer to *The Tao of Nutrition* by Dr. Maoshing Ni and Cathy McNease.

LIFESTYLE INSTRUCTIONS

- Avoid allergens that may trigger sinusitis and rhinitis.
- Application of saline solution to the nose three to four times daily helps to reduce nasal congestion.
- Strengthen the immune system by increasing exercise, reducing worry and stress, and developing a normal sleep habit.
- Steam inhalation is helpful to drain sinus infections. Rinsing the nostrils with cold saline water is helpful to desensitize the nose to temperature and common allergens. Repeatedly suck in and blow out the cold saline water for 1 to 2 minutes every morning.

PUERARIA CLEAR SINUS ™

CLINICAL NOTES

❧ Approximately 25% of all sinusitis are related to food allergies. Therefore, it is extremely important to identify and avoid the allergen. Common allergens include milk, wheat, eggs, citrus fruits, corn and peanuts.

❧ Some patients may experience mild stomach discomfort while taking this herbal formula. If such a reaction occurs, ask the patient to reduce the dosage and increase the frequency of administration (instead of taking 4 capsules three times daily, take 2 capsules six times a day). Taking the herbs with food may prevent stomach discomfort.

❧ *Pueraria Clear Sinus* is more effective for sinus infections. *Magnolia Clear Sinus* is most effective for sinusitis and rhinitis due to seasonal allergies.

CAUTIONS

❧ This formula is contraindicated during pregnancy and nursing.

❧ This formula is designed for sinusitis or rhinitis due to damp-heat with yellow and sticky discharge. Sinusitis or rhinitis due to wind-cold with clear watery discharge should be treated with *Magnolia Clear Sinus*.

ACUPUNCTURE POINTS

Traditional Points:
❧ *Feishu* (BL 13), *Hegu* (LI 4), *Quchi* (LI 11), *Shangyang* (LI 1), and *Lingtai* (GV 10).
❧ *Shaoshang* (LU 11), *Quchi* (LI 11), and *Yingxiang* (LI 20).

Balance Method by Dr. Richard Tan:
❧ Left side: *Zusanli* (ST 36), *Gongsun* (SP 4), *Yinlingquan* (SP 9), *Sanjian* (LI 3), and *Quchi* (LI 11), *Yingxiang* (LI 20), *Zanzhu* (BL 2).
❧ Right side: *Jiexi* (ST 41), *Chize* (LU 5), and *Taiyuan* (LU 9), *Yingxiang* (LI 20), *Zanzhu* (BL 2).
❧ Left and right side can be alternated from treatment to treatment.
❧ For additional information on the Balance Method, please refer to *Dr. Tan's Strategy of Twelve Magical Points* and *Acupuncture 1, 2, 3* by Dr. Richard Tan.

MODERN RESEARCH

Pueraria Clear Sinus is formulated specifically to treat allergies, sinusitis or rhinitis. *Pueraria Clear Sinus* contains herbs that have such effects as vasoconstriction, antibiotic properties, and analgesic effect.

Xin Yi Hua (Flos Magnoliae) constricts the blood vessels of the nasal mucosa and is used to treat stuffy nose, rhinitis and nasosinusitis.[1] It also reduces nasal secretions and treats runny nose and nasal discharge.[2] It is commonly used in herbal formulas to relieve disorders of the nose.

Huang Qin (Radix Scutellariae) has a broad spectrum of antibiotic functions and treats sinus infection.[2] *Chuan Xiong* (Rhizoma Ligustici Chuanxiong) and *Bai Zhi* (Radix Angelicae Dahuricae) are commonly used to treat sinus headache.[1,2]

Huang Qin (Radix Scutellariae) has a wide range of therapeutic actions. It has a broad antimicrobial effect against *Staphylococcus, Pseudomonas, Streptococcus* and *Neisseria*.[2] It has also shown clear antifungal activities, especially against *Candida albicans, Cryptococcus neoformans* and *Pityrosporum ovale*.[3] Furthermore, it can be used to treat viral infections. One study shows that *Huang Qin* (Radix Scutellariae) starts to suppress the replication of influenza viruses within 6 to 12 hours.[4] Another study shows that *Huang Qin* (Radix Scutellariae) starts to reduce replication

FORMULAS

PUERARIA CLEAR SINUS ™

of influenza viruses within 4 to 12 hours in a dose-dependent manner.[5] In addition to its broad antibiotic effects, *Huang Qin* (Radix Scutellariae) also has excellent anti-inflammatory activities. One study concluded that the effectiveness of *Huang Qin* (Radix Scutellariae) is comparable to indomethacin, one of the strongest non-steroidal anti-inflammatory drugs.

PHARMACEUTICAL DRUGS & CHINESE MEDICINE: A COMPARATIVE ANALYSIS

Western Medical Approach: Sinusitis and rhinitis are two common nasal disorders. In western medicine, these two conditions are primarily treated with vasoconstrictive drugs that promote drainage, such as pseudoephedrine. Though effective, it is a strong stimulant and may cause many side effects, such as nervousness, restlessness, dizziness, difficulty sleeping, upset stomach, difficulty breathing, fast or irregular heartbeat, muscle weakness, palpitations, tremors, and hallucinations. In addition to vasoconstrictive drugs, antibiotic drug may be used to address infectious sinusitis and rhinitis. The main advantage of these two medications is that they are relatively effective, and reasonably safe, so long as they are prescribed correctly and monitored carefully.

Traditional Chinese Medicine Approach: Sinusitis and rhinitis are effectively treated with herbs that drain the sinus cavity, reduce nasal mucous secretions, and treat infection. These herbs may be given to treat acute, chronic infectious sinusitis and rhinitis. These herbs are very effective, and do not have the stimulating side effects that drugs have. Furthermore, antibiotic herbs are much safer and gentler than antibiotic drugs, and are able to treat infection without causing significant side effects or secondary infections. However, it is important to keep in mind that this formula is primarily a formula that treats sinusitis and rhinitis. Though it does have antibiotic effect, its potency is only moderate, and may not be suitable in cases of severe sinus or respiratory tract infections.

Summation: Both drugs and herbs are effective to treat sinusitis and rhinitis. In most cases, use of herbs is more than sufficient, as they effectively treat both conditions with little risk of side effects and adverse reactions. In cases of severe and stubborn sinus infection, additional therapies may be needed, such as antibiotic drugs or another antibiotic herbal formula.

CASE STUDIES

A robustly healthy female presented with flu symptoms. She had a sore throat and yellow mucus. The practitioner diagnosed her condition as wind-heat. In conjunction with acupuncture treatment, the practitioner also had the patient utilize a vaporizer for steaming her face. *Lonicera Complex* and *Pueraria Clear Sinus* worked quite effectively after taking them for 3 to 4 days at larger dosages. The practitioner also noted that *Pu Ji Xiao Du Yin* (Universal Benefit Decoction to Eliminate Toxin) could be used if the condition were more severe and had presence of heat and toxins.

S.C., La Crescenta, California

A 28-year-old male presented with dizziness, sinus drainage, ringing in the ears, bitter taste in the mouth, and night sweating for about five weeks. His tongue was dry with a red tip and a greasy yellow coating. His pulse was at 80 beats per minute, fast and superficial with Kidney, Spleen/Stomach deficient. His medical doctor diagnosed his condition to be caused by fluid in the ears. The practitioner diagnosed the condition as nasal obstruction due to heat. A combination herbal treatment of *Pueraria Clear Sinus* and *Zhi Bai Di Huang Wan* (Anemarrhena, Phellodendron, and Rehmannia Pills) was administered. Dizziness was resolved within two days of the treatment. The patient noted that the herbal formulas worked much better for his condition than the antihistamines.

S.T., San Jose, California

A 42-year-old midwife presented with sinus infection (for 10 days) with yellow green discharge, increased pressure and pain in the sinus cavity and the ears, and severe pain. Upon examination, it was found that there was also lymph

---

PUERARIA CLEAR SINUS ™

node swelling and pain. The TCM diagnosis was phlegm heat in the Lung and toxic heat in the throat. The patient was instructed to take **Pueraria Clear Sinus** (4 capsules three times daily) and **Herbal ABX** (4 capsules three times daily). Within one day, the patient responded that there was a lot less pain and marked decrease in swelling. She continued to improve with each dose and stated that she felt "all better" by the third day. The practitioner commented the formulas were "very amazing and powerful."

M.N., Knoxville, Tennessee

A 33-year-old male presented with frontal headaches with yellow nasal discharge. No body aches or fever were reported. His pulse was rapid. The practitioner diagnosed the condition as phlegm heat and wind-heat. The patient took **Pueraria Clear Sinus** for 10 days (6 capsules three times daily). Subsequently, his phlegm and headaches resolved.

M.K., Sherman Oaks, California

[1] Yeung, HC. *Handbook of Chinese Herbs*. Institute of Chinese Medicine. 1996
[2] Bensky, D. et al. *Chinese Herbal Medicine Materia Medica*. Eastland Press. 1993
[3] Yang, D. et al. Anti-fungal activity in vitro of scutellaria baicalensis. *Ann Pharm Fr*; 53(3):138-41. 1995
[4] Nagai, T. et al. Antiviral activity of plant flavonoid, 5,7,4-trihydroxy-8-methoxyflavone, from scutellaria baicalensis against influenza A (H3N2) and B viruses. *Biol Pharm Bull*; 18(2):195-9. Feb 1995
[5] Nagai, T. et al. Mode of action of the anti-influenza virus activity of plant flavonoid, 5,7,4-trihydroxy-8-methoxyflavone, from the roots of scutellaria baicalensis. *Antiviral Res*; 26(1):11-25. Jan 1995

FORMULAS

RESOLVE (AI)™

(Anti-Inflammatory)

CLINICAL APPLICATIONS

- Infection and inflammation with swelling: goiter, lymphedema, hemorrhoids, intestinal polyps, tonsillitis, appendicitis, infected lesions, dermatological swellings, mastitis, sinusitis, osteomyelitis, cellulitis, and thrombophlebitis
- Formation of hardness and nodules: any type of swelling, mass, enlargement, hardness, nodule, scrofula, boil, carbuncle, goiter, sore, lump, furuncle, abscess, polyp, hordeolum or hard-seated lesion in the body that may or may not have accompanying pus, pain or heat sensations
- Lymphatic blockage: this formula drains the lymphatic system to clear stagnation
- Pfeiffer's disease

WESTERN THERAPEUTIC ACTIONS

- Antibiotic properties to treat infection [1,2,3,4,5]
- Anti-inflammatory action to reduce swelling and inflammation [6,7,9,10,12]
- Antipyretic influence to reduce fever [8]
- Analgesic effect to relieve pain [10,11]

CHINESE THERAPEUTIC ACTIONS

- Clears heat and detoxifies
- Reduces swelling and promotes discharge of pus
- Invigorates blood circulation and relieves pain

DOSAGE

Take 3 to 4 capsules three times daily on an empty stomach. For maximum effectiveness, take up to 6 to 8 capsules three times daily with two tall glasses of warm water. Herbs may be taken with meals if they cause upset on an empty stomach.

INGREDIENTS

Bai Zhi (Radix Angelicae Dahuricae)
Chen Pi (Pericarpium Citri Reticulatae)
Chi Shao (Radix Paeoniae Rubrae)
Dang Gui (Radicis Angelicae Sinensis)
Fang Feng (Radix Saposhnikoviae)
Gan Cao (Radix Glycyrrhizae)
Jin Yin Hua (Flos Lonicerae)
Kun Bu (Thallus Laminariae seu Eckloniae)

Mo Yao (Myrrha)
Ru Xiang (Gummi Olibanum)
Tong Cao (Medulla Tetrapanacis)
Xia Ku Cao (Spica Prunellae)
Zao Jiao (Fructus Gleditsiae)
Zao Jiao Ci (Spina Gleditsiae)
Zhe Bei Mu (Bulbus Fritillariae Thunbergii)

FORMULA EXPLANATION

Resolve (AI) is an excellent formula to clear heat, eliminate toxins, reduce swelling, and invigorate blood circulation. Clinically, it can be used as a primary formula or as an adjunct formula to treat various conditions due to infection and inflammation characterized by the formation of hardness, nodules and swelling.

Jin Yin Hua (Flos Lonicerae) is an indispensable anti-inflammatory herb when it comes to treating toxic heat accumulation in the body. *Zhe Bei Mu* (Bulbus Fritillariae Thunbergii), *Xia Ku Cao* (Spica Prunellae), and *Kun Bu*

RESOLVE (AI) ™

(Anti-Inflammatory)

(Thallus Laminariae seu Eckloniae) are used in *Resolve (AI)* to penetrate the channels, soften hardness and expel phlegm accumulation. *Zao Jiao* (Fructus Gleditsiae), *Zao Jiao Ci* (Spina Gleditsiae), and *Bai Zhi* (Radix Angelicae Dahuricae) drain pus. Blood invigorating herbs such as *Ru Xiang* (Gummi Olibanum), *Mo Yao* (Myrrha), *Dang Gui* (Radicis Angelicae Sinensis), and *Chi Shao* (Radix Paeoniae Rubrae) are used to disperse stagnation, relieve pain and help with the regeneration or healing process. *Chen Pi* (Pericarpium Citri Reticulatae) regulates qi, dispels phlegm and has a synergistic effect with the blood invigorating herbs to soften hardness and relieve pain. *Fang Feng* (Radix Saposhnikoviae) dispels lingering wind that may reside in the channels and reduce superficial swelling. *Tong Cao* (Medulla Tetrapanacis) drains and expels dampness through urination. *Gan Cao* (Radix Glycyrrhizae) further helps with detoxification and also harmonizes the formula.

SUPPLEMENTARY FORMULAS

- To enhance the antibiotic effect of the herbs to treat infection, add *Herbal ABX*.
- For tonsillitis, add *Herbal ENT*.
- For high blood pressure and fast heart rate due to excess fire, add *Gardenia Complex*.
- For nasal polyps or sinusitis, add *Magnolia Clear Sinus* or *Pueraria Clear Sinus*.
- For mastitis, add *Resolve (Upper)*.
- For goiter, add *Thyrodex*.
- For constipation, add *Gentle Lax (Excess)*.
- For endometriosis, add *Resolve (Lower)*.
- For prostate enlargement, add *P-Statin*.
- For lymphatic drainage, add *Circulation (SJ)*.
- For herpes or shingles, add *Gentiana Complex* or *Dermatrol (HZ)*.
- For joint enlargement due to inflammation, add *Flex (Heat)*.
- For gout, add *Flex (GT)*.
- For cellulitis, add *Herbal ABX*.
- For water retention, add *Herbal DRX*.
- For chronic stubborn swelling with blood stagnation, add *Circulation (SJ)*.

NUTRITION

- Refrain from eating spicy, greasy, fried foods, BBQ, canned foods, fermentated or dairy products, seafood, alcohol, duck or the internal organs of any creature during the course of treatment.
- Drink plenty of water throughout the day.
- For tonsillitis, gargle with salt water for one minute, twice daily.

LIFESTYLE INSTRUCTIONS

- Mild exercise is recommended as it will help with qi and blood circulation in the body. However, individuals with dermatological swellings should avoid heavy exercise that induces sweating, as it may delay healing of sores on the skin.
- Do not scratch the lesions to avoid contraction of infection and formation of scars. When boils or cysts break and are draining, keep the local area clean to prevent infection to the other parts of the body. After handling a boil, hands should be washed thoroughly to avoid transferring bacterial infection to other areas.

RESOLVE (AI)™

(Anti-Inflammatory)

CLINICAL NOTES

- In western terminology, *-itis* means inflammation. Since **Resolve (AI)** is used to treat numerous conditions characterized by infection and inflammation, many of the clinical applications will end with *–itis,* such as mastitis, bronchitis, cholecystitis, thrombophlebitis, and tonsillitis.
- Inflammation of the lymphatic system will often cause subcutaneous formation of hardness and nodules. Such conditions can be effectively treated with **Resolve (AI)**.
- The primary effect of **Resolve (AI)** is to reduce inflammation and swelling to soften hardness and nodules. Though it contains herbs with an antibiotic effect, use of this formula alone may not be sufficient in treating acute infection with inflammation, such as in tonsillitis or sinusitis. Instead, another formula with heat-clearing, antibiotic actions should be added to potentiate the effect.

CAUTIONS

- This formula is contraindicated in cases of yin-type (deep-rooted) furuncles or carbuncles where the appearance is grayish dark and shows no signs of redness or pain.
- This formula is contraindicated during pregnancy and nursing.
- Use with caution in cases of Spleen qi deficiency or yang deficiency with coldness of the extremities.
- Though this formula has herbs with marked antibiotic and anti-inflammatory effects, certain conditions, such as acute appendicitis, are still better treated with surgery to avoid rupture of the appendix.
- Patients who are on anticoagulant or antiplatelet therapies, such as Coumadin (Warfarin), should use this formula with caution, as there may be a slightly higher risk of bleeding and bruising.
- This formula is not designed for long-term use. It should be discontinued when the desired effects are achieved.

ACUPUNCTURE POINTS

Traditional Points:
- *Weizhong* (BL 40), *Quchi* (LI 11), *Xuehai* (SP 10), *Shenzhu* (GV 12), *Lingtai* (GV 10), *Hegu* (LI 4), and *ah shi* points.
- Bleed veins around *Weizhong* (BL 40). Needle *xi* (cleft) points of the channel in which there is swelling.

Balance Method by Dr. Richard Tan:
- Bleed *Shaoze* (SI 1) and *Dadun* (LR 1).
- Depending on the case, select additional 'balance' points.
- For additional information on the Balance Method, please refer to *Dr. Tan's Strategy of Twelve Magical Points* and *Acupuncture 1, 2, 3* by Dr. Richard Tan.

Ear Points:
- Acute tonsillitis: Bleed the protruding vein in the back of the ear and apex of the tragus once a day. Needle and strongly stimulate the Throat, Pharynx and Tonsils.

Auricular Acupuncture by Dr. Li-Chun Huang:
- Simple goiter: Thyroid, Endocrine, Pituitary, Thalamus, *San Jiao*, Kidney, and Liver.
- Appendicitis: Appendix, Abdomen, and Sympathetic.
  - Endocrine, *Shenmen*, and Occiput.
- For additional information on the location and explanation of these points, please refer to *Auricular Treatment Formula and Prescriptions* by Dr. Li-Chun Huang.

FORMULAS

RESOLVE (AI) ™

(Anti-Inflammatory)

MODERN RESEARCH

Resolve (AI) is formulated specifically to treat infection and inflammation. The herbs in this formula have demonstrated pronounced antibiotic and anti-inflammatory activities. *Resolve (AI)* is most effective in treatment of swelling and inflammation due to infection, with the formation of abscesses, hardness and nodules.

Resolve (AI) contains many herbs with marked antibacterial, antiviral and antifungal activities. *Jin Yin Hua* (Flos Lonicerae) has demonstrated a broad spectrum of inhibitory actions against *Staphylococcus aureus, beta-hemolytic streptococcus, E. coli, Bacillus dysenteriae, Vibrio cholerae, Salmonella typhi, Diplococcus pneumoniae, Diplococcus meningitidis, Pseudomonas aeruginosa,* and *Mycobacterium tuberculosis.*[1,2] Decoction of *Bai Zhi* (Radix Angelicae Dahuricae) has an inhibitory effect against *E. coli, Bacillus dysenteriae, Bacillus proteus, Salmonella typhi, Pseudomonas aeruginosa, Vibrio cholerae, Mycobacterium tuberculosis hominis,* and species of *Shigella.*[3] *Fang Feng* (Radix Saposhnikoviae) has an antibacterial effect against *Shigella spp., Pseudomonas aeruginosa,* and *Staphylococcus aureus,* and an antiviral effect against influenza viruses.[4] *Xia Ku Cao* (Spica Prunellae) has demonstrated inhibitory action against *Shigella spp., Salmonella typhi, E. coli, Pseudomonas aeruginosa, Mycobacterium tuberculosis, Streptococcus,* and *dermatophytes.*[5] All together, herbs in *Resolve (AI)* provide a potent and wide spectrum antibiotic effect to ensure complete and effective treatment of infection.

Many herbs in *Resolve (AI)* have with marked anti-inflammatory, antipyretic and analgesic effects. This well-rounded action is necessary, as infection and inflammation are often accompanied by fever and pain. In this formula, *Bai Zhi* (Radix Angelicae Dahuricae) has potent anti-inflammatory effects.[6,7] *Jin Yin Hua* (Flos Lonicerae) has both anti-inflammatory and antipyretic properties.[8] *Chen Pi* (Pericarpium Citri Reticulatae) also exhibits anti-inflammatory activity to decrease the permeability of blood vessels, a symptom associated with inflammation or allergy.[9] *Dang Gui* (Radicis Angelicae Sinensis), on the other hand, has anti-inflammatory and analgesic influence, and is commonly used to treat both pain and inflammation.[10] It has been shown that *Dang Gui* (Radicis Angelicae Sinensis) is approximately 1.1 times stronger than aspirin to reduce inflammation, and 1.7 times stronger to relieve pain.[11] Lastly, *Gan Cao* (Radix Glycyrrhizae) is regarded by many as one of the most potent herbs to reduce inflammation. Contrary to most herbs, *Gan Cao* (Radix Glycyrrhizae) exerts an anti-inflammatory effect by stimulating the production of glucocorticoids and slows down the rate of breakdown of the same substances. *Gan Cao* (Radix Glycyrrhizae) has been used successfully for treatment of inflammation, edema, granuloma formation, edematous arthritis, and others. The anti-inflammatory influence of glycyrrhizin and glycyrrhetinic, two active components of *Gan Cao* (Radix Glycyrrhizae), is approximately 1/10th in comparison with cortisone.[12]

Resolve (AI) contains herbs that have a wide variety of clinical applications. In one report, 56 patients with appendicitis were treated for 7 days with an overall effectiveness of 92.8%.[13] Reported cases of mastitis were also treated with great success. Out of 35 patients, 31 recovered within 1 to 3 doses, 3 recovered after 4 to 6 doses, and 1 had no effect.[14] For treatment of peptic ulcer, use of herbs was also very successful. Out of 53 cases (14 had gastric ulcers, 33 had duodenal ulcers, and 6 had both), 35 experienced recovery within 30 days, 15 had significant improvement, and 3 had no response, after 30 days of treatment.[15] For thrombophlebitis, 111 patients were treated with complete recovery in 77 cases, significant improvement in 31 cases, and no improvement in 3 cases.[16] For chronic sinusitis, 68 patients were treated, with complete recovery in 66 cases and improvement in 2 cases.[17] Other conditions that have been treated with good success include acute appendicitis,[18] acute mastitis,[19,20] chronic bronchitis,[21,22] cholelithiasis,[23] nephritis,[24] hepatitis,[25] and tonsillitis.[26]

In summary, *Resolve (AI)* is comprised of herbs that are well documented for their antibiotic and anti-inflammatory effects. The clinical applications include swelling and inflammation due to infection, with such presentation as fever, abscess, nodules, hardness, discharge, and related symptoms.

RESOLVE (AI) ™

(Anti-Inflammatory)

PHARMACEUTICAL DRUGS & CHINESE MEDICINE: A COMPARATIVE ANALYSIS

Nodule is a general term that is used to describe many different types of goiter, lymphedema, swelling, mass, enlargement, hardness, scrofula, boil, carbuncle, sore, lump, furuncle, abscess, polyp, hordeolum or hard-seated lesion in the body. Though these conditions may have different etiology, they are all characterized by swelling, inflammation and possible infection.

Western Medical Approach: Many of these conditions have no treatment available. When infection is involved, antibiotics may be used orally or topically. When there is pain and inflammation, analgesic or anti-inflammation drugs may be used for symptomatic treatment. Lastly, surgery may be performed to remove the nodule or hardened tissues.

Traditional Chinese Medicine Approach: These nodules are considered to be stagnation of qi, blood, and phlegm. From pharmacological perspective, these herbs have antibiotic effect to treat infection, and anti-inflammatory effect to reduce swelling and inflammation. Furthermore, these herbs are also effective for hardness and nodules where there are no signs of infection and inflammation. For this application, however, herbs must be taken continuously for a few months to slowly dissolve and disperse these nodules and hardened tissues.

Summation: Nodules and hardened tissues encompass a wide variety of clinical conditions. When the cause is unknown, western medicine struggles to identify a diagnosis and a treatment. Traditional Chinese medicine, however, is quite effective as it offers a wide range of therapeutic substances to treat infection, reduce swelling and inflammation, and dissolve and disperse nodules and hardened tissues.

CASE STUDIES

D.C., a 45-year-old woman, presented with right-sided elbow pain that began after she received a cortisone injection. She also suffered from depression after having recently moved to a new location. The right elbow appeared swollen and slightly warm to the touch. Her hands and feet were always cold. TCM diagnosis was *bi zheng* (painful obstruction syndrome) with Liver qi stagnation. After taking *Resolve (AI)* and *Si Ni San* (Frigid Extremities Powder), her elbow pain was 75% better and no longer hurt steadily. It worsened with work but was bearable. The patient also received acupuncture and homeopathic therapy.

M.C., Sarasota, Florida

M.S., a 41-year-old female, presented with an allergic reaction: both eyes were itchy and weeping thick yellow fluids. This worsened with exposure to dust or chemicals. The TCM diagnosis was yin deficiency with damp-heat accumulation. After taking *Resolve (AI)* with *Ming Mu Di Huang Wan* (Improve Vision Pill with Rehmannia), the patient was 95% better. She continued to take the herbs and noticed that the symptoms would return when she stopped the herbs. This patient did not receive any acupuncture treatment.

M.C., Sarasota, Florida

[1] *Xin Yi Xue* (New Medicine), 1975; 6(3):155
[2] *Jiang Xi Xin Yi Yao* (Jiangxi New Medicine and Herbology); 1960; (1):34
[3] *Zhong Yao Yao Li Yu Ying Yong* (Pharmacology and Applications of Chinese Herbs), 1983; 796
[4] *Zhong Yao Tong Bao* (Journal of Chinese Herbology), 1988; 13(6):364
[5] *Zhong Yi Xue* (Chinese Herbal Medicine), 1989; 20(6):22
[6] *Chang Yong Zhong Yao Cheng Fen Yu Yao Li Shou Ce* (A Handbook of the Composition and Pharmacology of Common Chinese Drugs), 1994; 1459:1462
[7] *Zhong Guo Zhong Yao Za Zhi* (People's Republic of China Journal of Chinese Herbology), 1991; 16(9):560
[8] *Shan Xi Yi Kan* (Shanxi Journal of Medicine), 1960; (10):22
[9] *Zhong Yao Yao Li Yu Ying Yong* (Pharmacology and Applications of Chinese Herbs), 1983; 567

RESOLVE (AI) ™

(Anti-Inflammatory)

[10] *Xin Yi Yao Xue Za Zhi* (New Journal of Medicine and Herbology), 1975; (6):34
[11] *Yao Xue Za Zhi* (Journal of Medicinals), 1971; (91):1098
[12] *Zhong Cao Yao* (Chinese Herbal Medicine), 1991; 22(10):452
[13] *Yun Nan Zhong Yi Za Zhi* (Yunan Journal of Chinese Medicine), 1989; 10)5):14
[14] *Hu Bei Zhong Yi Za Zhi* (Hubei Journal of Chinese Medicine), 1989; 5:8
[15] *Si Chuan Zhong Yi* (Sichuan Chinese Medicine), 1990; 8(8):22
[16] *Liao Ning Zhong Yi Za Zhi* (Liaoning Journal of Chinese Medicine), 1991; 18(5):34
[17] *Shan Dong Zhong Yi Za Zhi* (Shandong Journal of Chinese Medicine), 1991; 10(2):36
[18] *He Bei Yi Yao* (Hebei Medicine and Herbology), 1984; 3:168
[19] *He Bei Zhong Yi Za Zhi* (Hebei Journal of Chinese Medicine), 1965; 10:47
[20] *Zhong Hua Wai Ke Za Zhi* (Chinese Journal of External Medicine), 1959; 4:362
[21] *Zhe Jiang Zhong Yi Za Zhi* (Zhejiang Journal of Chinese Medicine), 1985; 1:18
[22] *Zhe Jiang Zhong Yi Za Zhi* (Zhejiang Journal of Chinese Medicine), 1977; 2:31
[23] *Zhong Xi Yi Jie He Za Zhi* (Journal of Integrated Chinese and Western Medicine), 1985; 10:591
[24] *Xin Yi Xue* (New Medicine), 1976; 6:294
[25] *Jiang Su Zhong Yi* (Jiangsu Chinese Medicine), 1962; 3:39
[26] *Zhong Hua Er Bi Hou Ke Za Zhi* (Chinese Journal of ENT), 1959; 2:159

FORMULAS

RESOLVE (Lower) ™

CLINICAL APPLICATIONS

- ❧ Fibrocystic disorders in the lower half of the body, such as fibroids and cysts in the uterus and ovaries
- ❧ Palpable masses and benign tumors of the female reproductive organs
- ❧ Endometriosis
- ❧ Female infertility due to obstruction in the lower abdominal region (i.e. tubal obstruction)
- ❧ Pelvic pain due to obstruction in the lower abdominal region
- ❧ Scarring or blood stagnation in the pelvic cavity from surgery
- ❧ Varicocele in men causing infertility

WESTERN THERAPEUTIC ACTIONS

- ❧ Resolves fibroids in the uterus and ovaries [1,2,4]
- ❧ Treats female infertility due to fibroids in the uterus and ovaries [1,2]
- ❧ Antitumor effects to treat benign tumors of the female reproductive organs [1,2]
- ❧ Analgesic and anti-inflammatory action to relieve pain and swelling [3,5,6]
- ❧ Relieves pain associated with gynecological disorders [3,5,6]

CHINESE THERAPEUTIC ACTIONS

- ❧ Invigorates the blood circulation
- ❧ Dispels blood stasis and disperses nodules and masses
- ❧ Warms the abdomen and alleviates pain

DOSAGE

Take 3 to 4 capsules three times daily on an empty stomach with warm water. In cases of large fibroids, the dosage may be increased up to 8 to 10 capsules twice or three times daily. *Resolve (Lower)* should be taken continuously for one to two months prior to making a progress evaluation.

INGREDIENTS

Bie Jia (Carapax Trionycis)
Chi Shao (Radix Paeoniae Rubrae)
Chuan Xiong (Rhizoma Ligustici Chuanxiong)
Dang Gui (Radicis Angelicae Sinensis)
E Zhu (Rhizoma Curcumae)
Fu Ling (Poria)
Gui Zhi (Ramulus Cinnamomi)
Hong Hua (Flos Carthami)

Mu Dan Pi (Cortex Moutan)
Mu Li (Concha Ostreae)
Pu Huang (Pollen Typhae)
San Leng (Rhizoma Sparganii)
San Qi (Radix Notoginseng)
Tao Ren (Semen Persicae)
Yan Hu Suo (Rhizoma Corydalis)
Zhe Bei Mu (Bulbus Fritillariae Thunbergii)

FORMULA EXPLANATION

According to traditional Chinese medicine, a palpable mass in the lower abdominal region is often diagnosed as a stagnation of blood and phlegm. Fibrocystic disorders, such as endometriosis, fibroids and cysts in the uterus and ovaries, are examples of blood and phlegm stagnation in the lower *jiao*. *Resolve (Lower)* contains herbs that activate blood circulation, remove blood and phlegm stagnation, warm the abdomen and relieve pain.

RESOLVE (Lower) ™

Gui Zhi (Ramulus Cinnamomi), *Tao Ren* (Semen Persicae), *Hong Hua* (Flos Carthami) and *Chi Shao* (Radix Paeoniae Rubrae) unblock the blood vessels and remove blood stasis by promoting circulation. *Chuan Xiong* (Rhizoma Ligustici Chuanxiong), *Dang Gui* (Radicis Angelicae Sinensis), and *Mu Dan Pi* (Cortex Moutan) activate circulation, remove blood stasis and relieve pain. *Pu Huang* (Pollen Typhae) has an excitatory action on the uterus and works to invigorate the blood and relieve pain by eliminating blood stasis. *Yan Hu Suo* (Rhizoma Corydalis) is a strong analgesic and produces effects similar to morphine and codeine to relieve pain. *San Leng* (Rhizoma Sparganii) and *E Zhu* (Rhizoma Curcumae) have strong blood invigorating functions to dispel masses and alleviate pain. *Zhe Bei Mu* (Bulbus Fritillariae Thunbergii), *Mu Li* (Concha Ostreae) and *Bie Jia* (Carapax Trionycis) eliminate phlegm, soften abdominal masses, and dissipate nodules. *Fu Ling* (Poria) further helps to dispel phlegm and prevent the formation of dampness by strengthening the Spleen. *San Qi* (Radix Notoginseng) invigorates blood circulation and stops bleeding to prevent hypermenorrhea.

SUPPLEMENTARY FORMULAS

- For benign breast disorders, use with ***Resolve (Upper)***.
- For premenstrual syndrome (PMS) or irritability, use with ***Calm***.
- For stress and insomnia in patients with deficiency, add ***Calm ZZZ***.
- For dysmenorrhea, use ***Mense-Ease***.
- To treat infertility, use ***Blossom (Phase 1-4)***.
- To clear hot flashes in menopausal patients, combine with ***Balance (Heat)***.
- For infection in the genital area, add ***V-Statin***.
- For presence of hardness and nodules in the chest area, combine with ***Resolve (AI)***.
- To improve blood circulation throughout the body and in severe cases of varicocele or varicose veins, add ***Circulation (SJ)***.
- With edema, water retention or swelling of the legs, add ***Herbal DRX***.
- For patients with cancer who have extreme weakness and deficiency and cannot tolerate chemotherapy or radiation treatment, use ***CA Support***.
- To minimize the side effects of chemotherapy and radiation treatment in patients with cancer, combine with ***C/R Support***.

NUTRITION

- Avoid red meat, tap water, processed foods, junk foods, alcohol, dairy products (except for un-sweetened low-fat yogurt), iron supplements and those fruits and vegetables sprayed with pesticides.
- Avoid eating meats that have been treated with hormones, which may stimulate the growth of fibroids.
- Eliminate coffee from the diet as it may contribute to the growth of fibroids.
- Avoid cold and raw foods, such as watermelon, citrus, and sushi. Also refrain from drinking cold beverages, such as ice water.

LIFESTYLE INSTRUCTIONS

- Avoid all exposure to radiations, such as from microwave, television and computer monitor.
- Relaxation, maintaining a positive outlook on life and regular exercise are important to the recovery of cancer and to the progress in resolving fibroids and cysts, and for preventing recurrences.

RESOLVE (Lower) ™

CLINICAL NOTES

❧ *Resolve (Lower)* should be taken every day of the month except during menstruation to avoid profuse bleeding.

❧ If pain is present during the period, *Mense-Ease* should be administered starting the first day of menstruation. If pain is present before the onset of each cycle, both formulas can be taken together to invigorate blood and relieve pain.

❧ *Resolve (Lower)* should be taken for three months prior to making an evaluation on the progress of the treatment. If the cysts, fibroids or mass are reduced in size, continue giving the formula until the conditions are completely resolved. On the other hand, if the size remains constant, increase the dosage by 30 to 50% and continue for another three months prior to making the final evaluation. If the conditions remain the same, surgery should be considered.

Pulse Diagnosis by Dr. Jimmy Wei-Yen Chang:
❧ Thin, wiry and forceful on the left *chi* position.
❧ Note: Dr. Chang takes the pulse in slightly different positions. He places his index finger directly over the wrist crease, and his middle and ring fingers alongside to locate *cun*, *guan* and *chi* positions. For additional information and explanation, please refer to *Pulsynergy* by Dr. Jimmy Wei-Yen Chang and Marcus Brinkman.

CAUTIONS

❧ This formula contains herbs that have strong blood-invigorating functions and should be used with caution in patients with deficiencies. Patients with underlying deficiencies should be treated concurrently with *C/R Support*, *Imperial Tonic*, *Schisandra ZZZ*, or *Immune +*.

❧ This formula contains herbs that have strong blood-invigorating and stasis-removing functions. It is contraindicated for patients during pregnancy and nursing. It should be used with caution during menstruation, as bleeding may be increased.

❧ This formula should not be the only course of therapy. Consider surgical intervention if multiple masses exist, if the cyst is large, or if the fibroids do not respond to herbal therapy.

❧ Patients who are on anticoagulant or antiplatelet therapies, such as Coumadin (Warfarin), should use this formula with caution as there may be a slightly higher risk of bleeding and bruising.

ACUPUNCTURE POINTS

Traditional Points:
❧ *Neiguan* (PC 6), *Zhaohai* (KI 6), *Qimen* (LR 14), *Ganshu* (BL 18), *Taichong* (LR 3), *Xingjian* (LR 2), *Xuehai* (SP 10), and *Geshu* (BL 17).

Balance Method by Dr. Richard Tan:
❧ Left side: *Taichong* (LR 3), *Gongsun* (SP 4), *Zhaohai* (KI 6), *Waiguan* (TH 5), and *Lingku*.
❧ Right side: *Tongli* (HT 5), *Neiguan* (PC 6), *Xiajuxu* (ST 39), and *Fenglong* (ST 40).
❧ Left and right side can be alternated from treatment to treatment.
❧ Note: *Lingku* is one of Master Tong's points on both hands. *Lingku* is located in the depression just distal to the junction of the first and second metacarpal bones, approximately 0.5 *cun* proximal to *Hegu* (LI 4), on the *yangming* line.
❧ For additional information on the Balance Method, please refer to *Twelve and Twelve in Acupuncture* and *Twenty-Four More in Acupuncture* by Dr. Richard Tan.

FORMULAS

RESOLVE (Lower) ™

Auricular Acupuncture by Dr. Li-Chun Huang:

❧ Endometritis: Uterus, Cervix, Kidney, Liver, Ovary, Pituitary, Thalamus, Endocrine, Gonadotropin, and *San Jiao*.

❧ For additional information on the location and explanation of these points, please refer to *Auricular Treatment Formula and Prescriptions* by Dr. Li-Chun Huang.

MODERN RESEARCH

Resolve (Lower) consists of herbs that have been demonstrated in independent studies to resolve fibroids, treat cancer, and relieve pain.

E Zhu (Rhizoma Curcumae) has anticancer activities. It destroys tumor cells by degeneration, necrosis, shedding and diminution. In addition, it improves microcirculation and prevents the formation of fibrin clots. In a clinical study of 80 patients, *E Zhu* (Rhizoma Curcumae) was demonstrated to be effective for cervical cancer at various stages.[1] The antitumor activity of *E Zhu* (Rhizoma Curcumae) has also been demonstrated *in vitro* and *in vivo* through the induction of apoptosis.[2]

Chi Shao (Radix Paeoniae Rubrae) has inhibitory functions on the uterus at high concentrations. It also has anti-inflammatory and analgesic functions to relieve pain and swelling.[3] In addition, *Chi Shao* (Radix Paeoniae Rubrae) contains paenoniflorin, which has strong antispasmodic effects, to alleviate muscle spasms and cramps. [1]

Pu Huang (Pollen Typhae) is commonly used for various gynecological disorders. The most common clinical applications include postpartum abdominal pain, acute colicky pain in the lower abdomen, severe pain in the middle abdomen, and endometriosis. [4]

Chuan Xiong (Rhizoma Ligustici Chuanxiong) increases peripheral blood circulation by reducing the agglutination and the peripheral activities of platelets. It is a guiding herb that directs the ingredients of the formula to the affected area. [3]

Yan Hu Suo (Rhizoma Corydalis), containing corydaline, exerts strong anti-inflammatory functions and is effective in both the acute and chronic phases of inflammation.[5] *Yan Hu Suo* (Rhizoma Corydalis) also possesses strong analgesic properties that act directly on the central nervous system.[6] Because of this action, it works synergistically with acupuncture to relieve pain. It was demonstrated in one study that when combined with *Yan Hu Suo* (Rhizoma Corydalis), the analgesic effect of electro-acupuncture increased significantly when compared with the control group that received electro-acupuncture only.[7]

PHARMACEUTICAL DRUGS & CHINESE MEDICINE: A COMPARATIVE ANALYSIS

Fibrocystic disorders in the lower abdomen, such as fibroids, cysts and endometriosis, are very common among women. These disorders may cause irregular menstruation, severe pain, and infertility.

Western Medical Approach: These conditions are usually treated with hormonal drugs that suppress growth of these tissues, such as combination oral contraceptives, progestins and danazol. Unfortunately, these drugs have limited benefits but serious side effects, including breast tenderness, swelling, bleeding, thrombosis, embolism, depression, weight gain, elevated cholesterol and triglycerides, and many others. In many cases, an invasive procedure such as surgery is recommended to remove fibroids, cysts, and endometrial tissues.

Traditional Chinese Medicine Approach: These fibrocystic conditions are diagnosed as qi, blood and phlegm stagnation. Use of these herbs has been shown to be extremely effective to dissolve, disperse and disintegrate these tissues. These herbs have a potent and consistent effect, and generally show marked effect after three months of

FORMULAS

RESOLVE (Lower) ™

therapy. However, the length of treatment may be longer depending on the size of the masses and severity of the condition.

Summation: The best treatment for these fibrocystic conditions is the integration of western and traditional Chinese medicine. Since drug benefits are often less than satisfactory and have significant side effects, herbs should be used as the first line of therapy. In most cases, improvements are noted within three months. If so, herbal therapy should be continued until the condition is resolved. If herbs do not work, then surgery may be employed as the last alternative.

CASE STUDIES

A 36-year-old female presented with extreme headaches and lower abdominal cramping 1 week before her period. She also had heavy bleeding. The practitioner diagnosed the condition as blood stagnation in the lower *jiao* and in the *chong* (thoroughfare) and *ren* (conception) channels. Her gynecologist confirmed the presence of fibroids and endometriosis. Laproscopy was done on fibroid tumors, which were found in both ovaries. After taking *Resolve (Lower)*, 4 capsules three times daily, for four cycles along with acupuncture treatments one to two times a week for five months, the patient's headaches and abdominal cramping abated. Her periods were no longer painful. The practitioner concluded that regular prescriptions of *Resolve (Lower)* were quite effective for his patients with endometriosis and fibroids, especially those patients with underlying blood stagnation.

M.K., Sherman Oaks, California

A 42-year-old female medical doctor presented with uterine fibroids and painful menses. Upon further inquiry, the irritable patient also noted dark clots. Her pulse was wiry and her tongue was light purple. The practitioner diagnosed the condition as blood and phlegm stagnation. After taking *Resolve (Lower)*, the patient's menstrual pain and excessive bleeding lessened. The clots were smaller and the patient felt that the fibroids were dwindling in size. She was recommended for an MRI for confirmation.

D.M., Raton, New Mexico

A 36-year-old female patient presented with premenstrual abdominal pain, and pain and blood clots during her periods. The Western diagnosis was endometriosis; the TCM diagnosis was qi and blood stagnation. *Resolve (EM)* and *Dang Gui* (Radicis Angelicae Sinensis) were prescribed for use before and during periods. After the second month, the patient reported much less pain. *Resolve (Lower)* was prescribed for maintenance, two capsules, twice daily.

D.L., Doylestown, Pennsylvania

A 27-year-old female office worker presented with pain in her lower abdomen. The pain was more prominent before and during menses. She also had occasional bloody stools. The patient had a history of chronic yeast infections and endometriosis, which were resolved by surgeries. The practitioner diagnosed the condition as blood and qi stagnation with damp-heat in the lower *jiao*. After taking *Mense-Ease* and *Resolve (Lower)*, menstrual pain reduced and rectal bleeding abated.

N.H., Boulder, Colorado

A 28-year-old female dental hygienist presented with a palpable lump on her lower abdomen near acupuncture point *Zigongxue* (Uterus). She had severe premenstrual syndrome (PMS) affecting her emotionally as well as large dark clots in her menstrual discharge. She had 1 week of constant dull pain on her left lower abdomen especially after her period. She described the pain as a grabbing, shooting type of pain as though someone was tightening a rope around her belly. She had a history of candida. She sought to get pregnant, and therefore discontinued taking her birth

---

RESOLVE (Lower) ™

control pills. Laparoscopy was done in 1995 to remove her right ovary and in 1999 to remove endometriosis. Scar tissue was present in her left lower abdomen from a hernia operation when she was a youngster. Cysts were also present on her left ovary. Lastly, the patient also had a history of hypothyroidism and hay fever. Her tongue color was unremarkable and her tongue coating appeared moist. Her tongue root coating would alternate from white to yellow. Her sublingual region was also unremarkable. The patient's pulse was constantly deep, thready and soft. The practitioner diagnosed this clinical picture as damp-heat in the lower *jiao* and Spleen qi deficiency leading to the accumulation of dampness. The practitioner prescribed *Mense-Ease* to regulate her menstruation, and *Resolve (Lower)* to treat endometriosis. The patient was instructed to take 3 to 5 capsules of each formula three times daily, starting 3 days before her period and continue the dose throughout her menstrual flow and for 1 week afterwards. After taking the herbs, she became less emotional. She noted fewer episodes of cramps the 1st month and no pain during the 2nd month of her herbal therapy. Although her lower abdominal pain lingered, the intensity lessened, the frequency reduced, and the affected area dwindled. The patient also finally discontinued her caffeine intake, which she also attributed to her pain. After 3 months of herbal treatment, surgery was done to remove 2 inches of tissue. Ultrasound confirmed the complete absence of ovarian cysts after 3 months of herbal therapy. Doppler ultrasound showed a favorable pulsatility index for uterine blood flow. There were no blockages present in her reproductive system. The practitioner concluded that *Mense-Ease* was quite effective in treating other patients with similar conditions. The efficacy of *Resolve (Lower)* was also proven clinically with ultrasound results.

T.K., Denver, Colorado

[1] Bensky, D. et al. *Chinese Herbal Medicine Materia Medica*. Eastland Press. 1993

[2] Yang, H. et al. The antitumor activity of elemene is associated with apoptosis. *Chung Hua Chung Liu Tsa Chih*; 18(3):169-72. May 1996

[3] Yeung, HC. *Handbook of Chinese Herbs*. Institute of Chinese Medicine. 1996

[4] Bensky, D. et al. *Chinese Herbal Medicine Formulas and Strategies*. Eastland Press. 1990

[5] Kubo, M. et al. *Biol Pharm Bull*. February 1994

[6] Zhu, XZ. Development of natural products as drugs acting on central nervous system. *Memorias do Instituto Oswaldo Cruz*. 86 2:173-5, 1991.

[7] Hu, J, et al. Effect of some drugs on electro-acupuncture analgesia and cytosolic free Ca^{++} concentration of mice brain. *Chen Tzu Yen Chiu*; 19(1):55-8. 1994

FORMULAS

RESOLVE (Upper)™

CLINICAL APPLICATIONS

☯ Fibrocystic disorders in the upper body such as palpable masses or benign tumors of the breast and cysts
☯ Breast cancer or breast distention
☯ Lymphadenopathy or mastitis characterized by swollen and enlarged lymph nodes with nodules or fibroids

WESTERN THERAPEUTIC ACTIONS

☯ Anticancer activities which cause degeneration and necrosis of tumor cells [1,4]
☯ Antibiotic and anti-inflammatory functions to treat infection and inflammation [2,3]

CHINESE THERAPEUTIC ACTIONS

☯ Dispels blood, qi and phlegm stasis
☯ Disperses nodules and masses
☯ Unblocks the stagnant Liver qi
☯ Clears heat and detoxifies

DOSAGE

Take 3 to 4 capsules three times daily on an empty stomach with warm water. Take **Resolve (Upper)** continuously for one to two months prior to making an evaluation of progress.

INGREDIENTS

Bai Hua She She Cao (Herba Oldenlandia)
Chai Hu (Radix Bupleuri)
Dang Gui Wei (Extremitas Radicis Angelicae Sinensis)
Hou Po (Cortex Magnoliae Officinalis)
Lou Lu (Radix Rhapontici)
Lu Feng Fang (Nidus Vespae)
Niu Bang Zi (Fructus Arctii)

Pu Gong Ying (Herba Taraxaci)
Qing Pi (Pericarpium Citri Reticulatae Viride)
Tu Fu Ling (Rhizoma Smilacis Glabrae)
Wang Bu Liu Xing (Semen Vaccariae)
Zao Jiao Ci (Spina Gleditsiae)
Zhe Bei Mu (Bulbus Fritillariae Thunbergii)
Zhi Zi (Fructus Gardeniae)

FORMULA EXPLANATION

In traditional Chinese medicine, a palpable mass is diagnosed as a stagnation of blood and phlegm. Fibrocystic disorders in the upper half of the body, such as breast cancer or inflammation of the mammary glands, are often characterized by prolonged Liver qi stagnation with blood and phlegm obstruction.

Chai Hu (Radix Bupleuri), *Qing Pi* (Pericarpium Citri Reticulatae Viride) and *Hou Po* (Cortex Magnoliae Officinalis) unblock the stagnant Liver qi, relieve distention, and alleviate pain. All of the above herbs enter the Liver meridian, which passes through the breast. *Zao Jiao Ci* (Spina Gleditsiae) dissolves phlegm and invigorates qi circulation in the chest. *Bai Hua She She Cao* (Herba Oldenlandia) has an excellent antitumor effect. It increases white blood cells and inhibits the mitosis of tumor cells, causing the degeneration and necrosis of tumor cells. *Lu Feng Fang* (Nidus Vespae) relieves toxicity and has been used for mastitis to relieve inflammation of the mammary glands. *Lou Lu* (Radix Rhapontici) and *Zhe Bei Mu* (Bulbus Fritillariae Thunbergii) soften nodules to facilitate dissipation. *Tu Fu Ling* (Rhizoma Smilacis Glabrae) and *Pu Gong Ying* (Herba Taraxaci) clear toxic heat lodging in the nodules. *Wang Bu Liu Xing* (Semen Vaccariae) and *Dang Gui Wei* (Extremitas Radicis Angelicae Sinensis) have strong blood invigorating effects to dissolve stagnation and alleviate pain. *Niu Bang Zi* (Fructus Arctii) and *Zhi Zi* (Fructus Gardeniae) relieve toxic heat accumulation.

SUPPLEMENTARY FORMULAS

- Side effects of chemotherapy or radiation can be reduced by using *C/R Support*.
- For cancer patients those who are too weak to receive chemotherapy or radiation, use *CA Support* instead.
- For fatigue and immune enhancement, use *Immune +* or *Cordyceps 3*.
- For premenstrual syndrome (PMS), irritability, or anxiety, combine with *Calm*.
- For stress with insomnia in patients with deficiency, add *Calm ZZZ*.
- For an excess condition with stress, irritability, anxiety and restlessness, add *Calm ES*.
- For fatigue, dizziness, insomnia, excessive worrying or anemia, combine with *Schisandra ZZZ*.
- For dysmenorrhea, use *Mense-Ease*.
- For amenorrhea, use *Menotrol* after fibrocystic condition has resolved.
- For presence of hardness and nodules else where in the chest area, or swelling of the lymphatic system, combine with *Resolve (AI)*.
- To improve blood circulation throughout the body, add *Circulation (SJ)*.
- For infection or mastitis, add *Herbal ABX*.
- For signs and symptoms of excess heat, add *Gardenia Complex*.
- For patients with cancer who have extreme weakness and deficiency and cannot tolerate chemotherapy or radiation treatment, use *CA Support*.
- To minimize the side effects of chemotherapy and radiation treatment in patients with cancer, combine with *C/R Support*.

NUTRITION

- A diet based on organic fresh fruits and vegetables is highly recommended. The following foods are very beneficial to breast cancer patients: all mushrooms (shiitake especially), whole grains, broccoli, brussels sprouts, cabbage, cauliflower, yellow/orange vegetables (carrots, pumpkins, squash, sweet potatoes), garlic, onions, fresh berries, apples, cherries, grapes, and plums.
- Advise the patient to avoid red meat, tap water, processed foods, junk foods, alcohol, caffeine, dairy products (except for un-sweetened low-fat yogurt), iron supplements and those fruits and vegetables sprayed with pesticides.
- Avoid eating meats that have been treated with hormones, which stimulate the growth of fibroids.
- Eliminate coffee from the diet, as it may contribute to the growth of fibroids.

The Tao of Nutrition by Ni and McNease
- Mastitis
  - Recommendations: cooling foods, cabbage, cucumber, dandelion, lettuce, malt, reed root, lotus root, and honeysuckle.
  - Avoid spicy, stimulating foods, coffee, smoking, alcohol, dairy products, and breast feeding.
- For more information, please refer to *The Tao of Nutrition* by Dr. Maoshing Ni and Cathy McNease.

LIFESTYLE INSTRUCTIONS

- Avoid all exposure to radiations, such as from microwave, television and computer monitor.
- Relaxation, maintaining a positive outlook on life and regular exercise are important to the recovery of cancer patients and to the progress in resolving fibroids and cysts, and preventing recurrences.

FORMULAS

RESOLVE (Upper) ™

CLINICAL NOTES

- Upon resolution of the cysts or fibroids, *Resolve (Upper)* should be taken for another two weeks to consolidate the effects.
- Patients with deficiencies or weak constitutions should be treated concurrently with *C/R Support* or *Immune +* to ensure maximum effectiveness.
- *Resolve (Upper)* is a strong formula and is best used at the beginning stages of the disease.
- Patients who are under constant stress and anxiety are at higher risk of developing Liver qi stagnation. Prolonged Liver qi stagnation prevents recovery and contributes to continued deterioration in the overall condition. If at all possible, they need to remove stress from their lives to achieve maximum clinical effect.

CAUTIONS

- *Resolve (Upper)* is formulated for patients in the initial or early stages of masses in the breasts or lymphadenopathy. Patients with breast lump or large cyst should seek medical treatment to rule out tumor.
- Patients with deficiencies or a weak constitution should be treated concurrently with *Immune +* or *C/R Support*.
- *Resolve (Upper)* is contraindicated during pregnancy and nursing.
- *Resolve (Upper)* should be used with caution during menstruation as it may cause excessive bleeding.
- Patients who are on anticoagulant or antiplatelet therapies, such as Coumadin (Warfarin), should use this formula with caution, as there may be a slightly higher risk of bleeding and bruising.
- This formula is not designed for long-term use. It should be discontinued once the desired effects are achieved.
- *Resolve (Upper)* should be taken with food in individuals with a sensitive stomach.

ACUPUNCTURE POINTS

Traditional Points:
- *Jianjing* (GB 21), *Rugen* (ST 18), *Qimen* (LR 14), *Houxi* (SI 3), *Neiguan* (PC 6), *Ganshu* (BL 18), *Chize* (LU 5), and *Zusanli* (ST 36).
- *Shanzhong* (CV 17) and *Yingchuang* (ST 16).

Balance Method by Dr. Richard Tan:
- On the same side of the fibroid: needle *Neiguan* (PC 6), *Jianshi* (PC 5), *Ximen* (PC 4), *Lieque* (LU 7), *Tongli* (HT 5) and *Xiajuxu* (ST39), *Fenglong* (ST 40).
- On the opposite side of the fibroid: needle *Sanjian* (LI 3), *Sanyinjiao* (SP 6), *Lougu* (SP 7), and *Diji* (SP 8) or *ah shi* points nearby.
- For additional information on the Balance Method, please refer to *Dr. Tan's Strategy of Twelve Magical Points* by Dr. Richard Tan.

Ear Points:
- Mammary Gland, *Shenmen*, and Endocrine.
- Needle both ears and leave needles in for two to three hours. Ten treatments equal one course.

Auricular Acupuncture by Dr. Li-Chun Huang:
- Lobular breast hyperplasia: Breast, Chest, Pituitary, Ovary, Endocrine, *San Jiao*, and Liver.
- Mastitis: Breast, Chest, Liver, Occiput, Allergic Area, Endocrine, and Adrenal Gland. Bleed Ear Apex.
- Lymphadenitis: Corresponding point (to the area affected), *San Jiao*, Allergic Area, Adrenal Gland, Liver, Spleen, and Endocrine. Bleed Ear Apex.

FORMULAS

RESOLVE (Upper) ™

☙ For additional information on the location and explanation of these points, please refer to *Auricular Treatment Formula and Prescriptions* by Dr. Li-Chun Huang.

MODERN RESEARCH

The ingredients of *Resolve (Upper)* are carefully selected from a list of Chinese herbs that have demonstrated strong antitumor, antibacterial and antiviral effects. *Resolve (Upper)* is composed of herbs whose antitumor activities stop the proliferation of cancer cells at different stages for maximum synergistic functions.

Lu Feng Fang (Nidus Vespae) and *Pu Gong Ying* (Herba Taraxaci) are commonly used together to treat a variety of tumors as both have demonstrated anticancer activities.[1] The specific applications of *Lu Feng Fang* (Nidus Vespae) include breast lumps and mastitis. It was demonstrated in one study that *Lu Feng Fang* (Nidus Vespae) effectively treated 4 patients with acute mastitis.[2] In a follow-up study of 26 patients with mastitis treated with *Lu Feng Fang* (Nidus Vespae), 23 patients showed dramatic improvement, 1 showed moderate improvement, and 2 experienced no effectiveness.[3]

Bai Hua She She Cao (Herba Oldenlandia) inhibits the mitosis of tumor cells and causes degeneration and necrosis of tumor tissues. Modern applications of *Bai Hua She She Cao* (Herba Oldenlandia) include inflammation, ulceration and cancer.[4]

PHARMACEUTICAL DRUGS & CHINESE MEDICINE: A COMPARATIVE ANALYSIS

Western Medical Approach: Fibrocystic disorders in the chest region, such as palpable masses and mastitis, are very common among women. These disorders may cause pain and discomfort, and must be addressed immediately and carefully. In western medicine, antibiotic drugs are usually used to treat mastitis. Palpable masses are generally removed surgically.

Traditional Chinese Medicine Approach: These fibrocystic conditions are diagnosed as qi, blood and phlegm stagnation. Use of these herbs has been shown to be extremely effective to dissolve, disperse and disintegrate these tissues. These herbs have a potent and consistent effect, and generally show marked effect after three months of therapy. However, the length of treatment may be longer depending on the size of the masses and severity of the condition.

Summation: the best treatment for these fibrocystic conditions is the integration of western and traditional Chinese medicine. Herbs should be used as the first line of therapy, as they effectively address both infection and inflammation. For palpable masses, improvements will be noted within three months. If so, herbal therapy should be continued until the condition is resolved. If herbs do not work, then surgery may be employed as the last alternative.

CASE STUDY

J.S., a 34-year-female, presented with a non-cancerous fibrocystic breast lump on the right side. She had it for eight months and it felt achy and tender before her period. She also felt tired from overworking. The TCM diagnosis was Spleen yang deficiency with phlegm accumulation. *Resolve (Upper)* at one capsule three times daily, and *Immune +* at three capsules, three times daily were prescribed. Two weeks later, the patient reported the breast felt much better and her energy level was great. One month later, patient experienced only slight tenderness in the breast. She went back to her medical doctor for an examination and found that the lump had diminished in size. The patient was also advised to not wear underwire bras, to avoid further local qi stagnation.

M.C., Sarasota, Florida

FORMULAS

RESOLVE (Upper) ™

[1] Bensky, D. et al. *Chinese Herbal Medicine Materia Medica*. Eastland Press. 1993
[2] Lin, ZC. Miraculous effect of hornet nest (lu feng fang) in treating mastitis. *Journal of Traditional Chinese Medicine*.:5:40. 1959
[3] Yang, ZX. et al. Effectiveness of hornet nest (lu feng fang) in treating mastitis: a case report of 26 patients. *Journal of Traditional Chinese Medicine*; 11:407. 1963
[4] Yeung, HC. *Handbook of Chinese Herbs*. Institute of Chinese Medicine. 1996

RESPITROL (CF) ™

(Cough)

CLINICAL APPLICATIONS

☯ Cough
☯ Cough with associated symptoms such as sputum, chest congestion, wheezing and dyspnea
☯ Cough from acute conditions, such as common cold, influenza and lung infection
☯ Chronic cough induced by various conditions, such as infection, drugs, smoking and others
☯ Cough in tuberculosis or cancer of the lung

WESTERN THERAPEUTIC ACTIONS

☯ Antitussive effect to suppress cough
☯ Expectorant effect to eliminate phlegm and reduce congestion
☯ Bronchodilating effect to relieve wheezing and dyspnea
☯ Antibiotic effect to treat cough with infection

CHINESE THERAPEUTIC ACTIONS

☯ Releases wind from the exterior
☯ Eliminates phlegm
☯ Nourishes yin
☯ Descends Lung qi

DOSAGE

The standard dosage for adults is 4 to 6 capsules three times daily. The dosage should be carefully adjusted accordingly for pediatric and geriatric patients, based on age or body weight.

INGREDIENTS

Bai Jie Zi (Semen Sinapis)
Gan Cao (Radix Glycyrrhizae)
Mai Men Dong (Radix Ophiopogonis)
Sheng Jiang (Rhizoma Zingiberis Recens)
Su Zi (Fructus Perillae)

Tian Zhu Zi (Fructus Nandina)
Wu Mei (Fructus Mume)
Xing Ren (Semen Armeniacae Amarum)
Zi Su Ye (Folium Perillae)

FORMULA EXPLANATION

Respitrol (CF) is an empirical formula designed to treat cough due to various causes, including but not limited to external (wind-cold or wind-heat), or internal causes (heat, phlegm, or yin deficiency). This formula contains herbs that release wind from the exterior, eliminate phlegm, nourish yin, and descend Lung qi.

In this formula, *Zi Su Ye* (Folium Perillae) and *Sheng Jiang* (Rhizoma Zingiberis Recens) release wind-cold from the exterior, eliminate phlegm, and stop coughing. *Bai Jie Zi* (Semen Sinapis) eliminates phlegm and opens the airways. *Tian Zhu Zi* (Fructus Nandina) and *Xing Ren* (Semen Armeniacae Amarum) have marked effect to suppress cough, as they cause Lung qi to descend. *Mai Men Dong* (Radix Ophiopogonis) nourishes yin and relieves chronic cough due to Lung deficiency. *Su Zi* (Fructus Perillae) eliminates phlegm and descends Lung qi to relieve cough. Lastly, *Wu Mei* (Fructus Mume) astringes Lung qi and relieves cough. The use of *Mai Men Dong* (Radix Ophiopogonis) and *Wu Mei* (Fructus Mume) also help to control the warm, dispersing and drying nature of the formula from consuming yin and fluids. *Gan Cao* (Radix Glycyrrhizae) harmonizes the formula.

FORMULAS

RESPITROL (CF) ™

(Cough)

In short, **Respitrol (CF)** is an excellent empirical formula to symptomatically treat cough. However, if the cause can be identified, the overall treatment will be more effective if another formula is used to address the cause.

SUPPLEMENTARY FORMULAS

- For cough due to common cold or influenza, use with **Lonicera Complex**.
- For cough due to lung infection (such as in bronchitis or pneumonia), use with **Herbal ABX**.
- For cough with wheezing and dyspnea due to Lung heat, use with **Respitrol (Heat)**.
- For cough with wheezing and dyspnea due to Lung cold, use with **Respitrol (Cold)**.
- For sore throat from a respiratory infection, add **Herbal ENT**.
- For chronic cough with wheezing and dyspnea due to Lung deficiency, use with **Respitrol (Deficient)** or **Cordyceps 3**.
- For cough with chest congestion and profuse phlegm, use with **Poria XPT**.
- For yin deficiency with thirst and dryness, add **Nourish (Fluids)**.
- For high fever, add **Gardenia Complex**.
- For cough due to stress, add **Calm**.
- For immune deficiency, add **Cordyceps 3**.

NUTRITION

- Avoid drinking cold beverages, as they may cause constriction and induce cough.
- Individuals with poor swallowing reflex should consume food and beverages slowly. Aspiration of these contents into the lung increases the risk of cough and lung infection.
- Pear, loquat, lemon with honey, pineapples, lotus nodes and white radish are excellent foods to help reduce frequency and severity of cough.
- White radish is an excellent food to relieve cough. Take 1 white radish, approximately the size of a fist and cut it into thin slices. Mix it with 1 tablespoon of maltose and 1 cup of water and cook for 20 minutes. Serve the radish and the juice when they cool to room temperature. Another easier method is to mix the slices of white radish with honey. Wait for 30 minutes and drink the fluids that are secreted from the radish.

LIFESTYLE INSTRUCTION

- Airway irritation (smoke, dust and fumes) is a very common cause of cough. Try to avoid exposure to these environments as much as possible. If necessary, install an air filter to clean the air.

CLINICAL NOTES

- **Respitrol (CF)** is most effective when:
  - The cause of the cough is not known or a specific treatment is not possible.
  - The cough performs no useful function, or causes significant discomfort.
  - If the cause if known, then this formula may be used as an useful adjunct to suppress cough.
- Certain drugs, such as angiotensin-converting enzyme (ACE) inhibitors like Capoten (Captopril), Zestril (Lisinopril) and Vasotec (Enalapril), may cause non-productive cough in up to 20% of patients. This drug-induced cough may begin as soon as 1 week after starting that therapy, but may be delayed by as much as 6 months.[1]

CAUTIONS

- Cough is a symptom that has many causes, such as infection (bronchitis or pneumonia), pre-existing diseases (tuberculosis or emphysema), airway irritation (smoke, dust and fumes), and aspiration (upper airway secretion

RESPITROL (CF) ™

(Cough)

or gastric contents). It is very important to identify and treat the underlying cause, in addition to treating the symptom.

❧ In cases of lung infection, cough is a beneficial protective mechanism for clearing respiratory secretions and foreign materials. Optimal treatment in these situations requires use of medicines to treat the infection and the cough (if necessary) concurrently. Suppressing the symptom without treating the cause may delay the overall recovery. Though this formula contains herbs with antibiotic effect, it may be necessary to combine with additional formulas to reinforce the overall effect to treat infection.

❧ Do *not* use an excessive amount of this formula, as gross overdose of any medicinal substances will inevitably contribute to unwanted reactions. In this case, *Xing Ren* (Semen Armeniacae Amarum) and *Tian Zhu Zi* (Fructus Nandina) have excellent functions to stop coughing by suppressing respiratory reflex in the brain. Hence, gross overdose of these two herbs may suppress respiration and cause difficulty breathing.[2,3] Other potential side effects associated with gross overdose include dizziness, weakness, nausea, vomiting, abdominal pain, burning sensations in the upper abdominal region, increased blood pressure, and increased respiration.[4]

❧ Because this is a rather potent formula, it is *not* recommended for pediatric or geriatric patients, and it is contraindicated during pregnancy and nursing.

ACUPUNCTURE POINTS

Traditional Points:
❧ *Lieque* (LU 7), *Hegu* (LI 4), *Feishu* (BL 13), *Chize* (LU 5), *Feishu* (BL 13), *Taiyuan* (LU 9), *Taibai* (SP 3), *Fenglong* (ST 40), *Yuji* (LU 10), and *Xingjian* (LR 2).

Balance Method by Dr. Richard Tan:
❧ Left side: Needle *Jingqu* (LU 8), *Taiyuan* (LU 9), *Neiguan* (PC 6), *Xiajuxu* (ST 39), *Fenglong* (ST 40), and *Jiexi* (ST 41).
❧ Right side: Needle *Hegu* (LI 4), *Yangxi* (LI 5), *Sanyinjiao* (SP 6), and *Jiaoxin* (KI 8).
❧ Alternate sides with each treatment.
❧ For additional information on the Balance Method, please refer to *Dr. Tan's Strategy of Twelve Magical Points* by Dr. Richard Tan.

Ear Acupuncture:
❧ Lung, Trachea, *Shenmen*, and Liver.

Auricular Acupuncture by Dr. Li-Chun Huang:
❧ Cough from common cold: Lung, Internal Nose, Throat (Larynx, Pharynx), Trachea, Bronchus, and Stop Asthma.
❧ For additional information on the location and explanation of these points, please refer to *Auricular Treatment Formula and Prescriptions* by Dr. Li-Chun Huang.

MODERN RESEARCH

Respitrol (CF) is an empirical therapy for symptomatic relief of cough. It contains many herbs with antitussive effect to suppress cough, expectorant effect to eliminate phlegm and reduce congestion, bronchodilating effect to relieve wheezing and dyspnea, and antibiotic effect to treat cough from infection.

Many herbs in *Respitrol (CF)* have excellent antitussive effects to suppress cough, such as *Xing Ren* (Semen Armeniacae Amarum), *Tian Zhu Zi* (Fructus Nandina) and *Gan Cao* (Radix Glycyrrhizae). *Xing Ren* (Semen Armeniacae Amarum) suppresses cough via an inhibitory effect on the respiratory center in the brain, thereby exerting its antitussive effect.[5] *Tian Zhu Zi* (Fructus Nandina) has been used to treat various types of cough, including but not limited to acute bronchitis, whooping cough, and cough in children.[6] *Gan Cao* (Radix

FORMULAS

Glycyrrhizae) has marked antitussive and expectorant effects, and the mechanism of action has been attributed to its effect on the central nervous system.[7]

In addition to suppressing cough, *Respitrol (CF)* also uses herbs to relieve wheezing and dyspnea. For example, *Zi Su Ye* (Folium Perillae) has been shown to promote bronchodilation and relieve bronchospasm. It also reduces secretions from the bronchioli.[8] This formula also contains many herbs with expectorant effects to eliminate phlegm and reduce congestion, such as *Bai Jie Zi* (Semen Sinapis) and *Gan Cao* (Radix Glycyrrhizae).[9] Furthermore, *Gan Cao* (Radix Glycyrrhizae) also has an anti-inflammatory effect to reduce swelling and relieve chest congestion.[10] The mechanism of this action is attributed in part to the effect of *Gan Cao* (Radix Glycyrrhizae) to stimulate the production of glucocorticoid by the adrenal glands and to delay the metabolism by the liver.[11]

Furthermore, because cough is often a symptom of respiratory tract infection, many herbs with antibiotic effects are used in this formula. *Zi Su Ye* (Folium Perillae) has been shown to inhibit the activity of *Staphylococcus aureus*, with minimum inhibitory concentration (MIC) of 200 to 1,600 mg/ml.[12] *Sheng Jiang* (Rhizoma Zingiberis Recens) has been shown to have an inhibitory effect on *Salmonella typhi*, *Vibrio cholerae* and *Trichomonas vaginalis*.[13] *Mai Men Dong* (Radix Ophiopogonis) has an inhibiting influence on *Staphylococcus albus*, *Bacillus subtilis*, *E. coli* and *Salmonella typhi*.[14] *Wu Mei* (Fructus Mume) has demonstrated an inhibitory effect against *Staphylococcus aureus*, *Salmonella typhi*, *Bacillus subtilis*, *Bacillus dysenteriae*, *E. coli*, *Mycobacterium tuberculosis* and some dermatophytes.[15] Lastly, *Bai Jie Zi* (Semen Sinapis) has an inhibitory influence against some pathogenic fungi and dermatophytes.[16]

In summary, *Respitrol (CF)* is an empirical formula that treats cough and its associated conditions. It is formulated with herbs that suppress cough, eliminate phlegm, reduce chest congestion, relieve wheezing and dyspnea, and treat the infection.

PHARMACEUTICAL DRUGS & CHINESE MEDICINE: A COMPARATIVE ANALYSIS

Cough is a symptom that has many causes, such as infection, pre-existing diseases, airway irritation, and aspiration. Because cough is a natural reaction to eliminate foreign or harmful substance from the lungs, mild to moderate coughing is generally not treated. However, in cases where severe or constant cough interferes with resting and recovery, drugs and herbs should be used together to treat the symptom (cough) and the cause (numerous).

Western Medical Approach: Cough is usually treated with opioids, such as dextromethorphan and narcotic antitussives (such as codeine). These drugs have respiratory depressant effect to suppress cough. Though these drugs are effective, they may cause side effects such as hypersensitivity, tachycardia or bradycardia, syncope, respiratory depression, circulatory depression, nausea, vomiting, constipation, urinary retention, and in severe cases, tolerance and dependence.

Traditional Chinese Medicine Approach: Cough is usually treated with herbs that eliminate sputum, relieve chest congestion, and regulate the flow of Lung qi. In other words, herbs do not just suppress cough, but rather, to open up the airway and unblock chest congestion to relieve cough. Nonetheless, some herbs that relieve cough may have side effects, such as described above under Cautions.

Summation: It is generally not necessary to treat cough, as it is a natural defensive and desirable reaction. However, if treatment is deemed necessary, both the symptom and the cause must be addressed at the same time. In this case, both drugs and herbs are effective to treat cough. Drugs tend to "suppress" cough by depressing the respiratory tract. Herbs tend to "relieve" cough by opening the airway and unblocking obstruction. Both medicines have side effects, and must be carefully evaluated in choosing the most suitable therapy for the patient.

RESPITROL (CF) ™

(Cough)

[1] Fauci, Braunwald, Isselbacher, et al. Harrison's Principles of Internal Medicine 14th Edition. McGraw-Hill, 1998.
[2] *Zhong Yao Bu Liang Fan Ying Yu Zhi Liao* (Adverse Reactions and Treatment of Chinese Herbal Medicine), 1996; 218:220, 1996; 213:217
[3] Kariyone. T. *Atlas of Medicinal Plants.*
[4] *Zhong Yao Bu Liang Fan Ying Yu Zhi Liao* (Adverse Reactions and Treatment of Chinese Herbal Medicine), 1996; 218:220, 1996; 213:217
[5] *Life Sci*, 1980; 27(8):659
[6] Kariyone. T. *Atlas of Medicinal Plants.*
[7] *Zhong Yao Yao Li Yu Ying Yong* (Pharmacology and Applications of Chinese Herbs), 1983; 264
[8] *Zhong Yao Xue* (Chinese Herbology), 1998; 67:68
[9] *Zhong Yao Xue* (Chinese Herbology), 1998; 608:610
[10] *Zhong Cao Yao* (Chinese Herbal Medicine), 1991; 22(10):452
[11] *Zhong Yao Zhi* (Chinese Herbology Journal), 1993; 358
[12] *Zhong Guo Zhong Yao Za Zhi* (People's Republic of China Journal of Chinese Herbology), 1990; 25(2):31
[13] *Zhong Yao Xue* (Chinese Herbology), 1998; 69:72
[14] *Zhong Yao Xue* (Chinese Herbology), 1998; 845:848
[15] *Zhong Yi Za Zhi* (Journal of Chinese Medicine), 1984; 262
[16] *Chang Yong Zhong Yao Xian Dai Yan Jiu Yu Lin Chuan* (Recent Study & Clinical Application of Common Traditional Chinese Medicine), 1995; 439:441

FORMULAS

RESPITROL (Cold) ™

CLINICAL APPLICATIONS

- ☯ Common colds, head cold, influenza or respiratory disorders with sinus congestion, watery or white nasal discharge, sneezing and watery eyes
- ☯ Wheezing and/or dyspnea with intolerance to cold (temperature, food or drinks), grayish and cyanotic complexion of the face and body, chills, and absence of perspiration
- ☯ Cold-type lung disorders such as asthma, bronchitis, emphysema or lung infections with white sputum
- ☯ Used as immediate relief for sneezing, clear nasal discharge in people who are exposed to cold weather or water such as divers or swimmers.

WESTERN THERAPEUTIC ACTIONS

- ☯ Bronchodilating effect to relax the bronchial smooth muscle and relieve spasms
- ☯ Antitussive and expectorant properties to stop cough and eliminate phlegm
- ☯ Herbal antibiotic action to treat bacterial and viral infections
- ☯ Stimulating effect to increase bodily temperature and metabolic rate

CHINESE THERAPEUTIC ACTIONS

- ☯ Dispels cold, warms the interior
- ☯ Eliminates phlegm
- ☯ Regulates qi circulation to relieve wheezing and dyspnea

DOSAGE

Take 4 to 6 capsules three times a day with warm water on an empty stomach. For maximum effectiveness, start taking *Respitrol (Cold)* with the first sign of respiratory discomfort.

INGREDIENTS

Bai Jie Zi (Semen Sinapis)
Bai Shao (Radix Paeoniae Alba)
Cang Er Zi (Fructus Xanthii)
Gan Jiang (Rhizoma Zingiberis)
Gui Zhi (Ramulus Cinnamomi)
Hou Po (Cortex Magnoliae Officinalis)

Pi Pa Ye (Folium Eriobotryae)
Su Zi (Fructus Perillae)
Wu Wei Zi (Fructus Schisandrae Chinensis)
Xing Ren (Semen Armeniacae Amarum)
Zhi Gan Cao (Radix Glycyrrhizae Preparata)
Zi Wan (Radix Asteris)

FORMULA EXPLANATION

Respitrol (Cold) is formulated to treat cold-type respiratory disorders, including but not limited to, common cold, influenza, asthma, bronchitis, and infections of the respiratory tract. Diagnostic signs and symptoms of cold include chills, clear watery nasal discharge, sneezing, intolerance to cold, absence of fever, and grayish and cyanotic complexion of the face and body. *Respitrol (Cold)* contains herbs with functions to dispel cold, warm the interior, eliminate phlegm, and regulate qi circulation.

In this formula, *Xing Ren* (Semen Armeniacae Amarum) and *Hou Po* (Cortex Magnoliae Officinalis) eliminate phlegm, transform congested fluids and reduce wheezing. *Zi Wan* (Radix Asteris) expels wind and relieves dyspnea, chest discomfort, and wheezing. *Gui Zhi* (Ramulus Cinnamomi) works synergistically with *Bai Shao* (Radix Paeoniae Alba) to tonify and harmonize the qi in the *wei* (defense) and *ying* (nutritive) levels. Due to cold, water

FORMULAS

RESPITROL (Cold) ™

metabolism of the Lung may be impaired leading to a sudden blockage of fluids in the upper *jiao*. *Gan Jiang* (Rhizoma Zingiberis), *Bai Jie Zi* (Semen Sinapis), *Su Zi* (Fructus Perillae) and *Cang Er Zi* (Fructus Xanthii) warm the Lung, dispel the cold factor, arrest wheezing, and move water by regulating the qi flow of the Lung. *Wu Wei Zi* (Fructus Schisandrae Chinensis) is used to protect the Lung by preventing the leakage of qi. *Zhi Gan Cao* (Radix Glycyrrhizae Preparata) and *Bai Shao* (Radix Paeoniae Alba) relieve bronchial spasms, alleviate pain and harmonize the formula.

SUPPLEMENTARY FORMULAS

- For allergies, sinus headache, nasal obstruction, and white watery nasal discharge, combine with *Magnolia Clear Sinus*.
- For allergies, sinus headache, nasal obstruction, and sticky yellow nasal discharge, combine with *Pueraria Clear Sinus*.
- For coughing, add *Respitrol (CF)*.
- For infection of ear, nose and throat, add *Herbal ENT*.
- For thirst, dry mouth and throat, add *Nourish (Fluids)*.
- *Immune* + can be used as a maintenance formula for patients with underlying Lung deficiency manifesting in a weak immune system, recurrent colds and flu triggering asthma attacks.
- To tonify the overall constitution of the body, take *Imperial Tonic* on a daily basis.
- For maintenance and prevention of asthma attack, use *Cordyceps 3* and *Respitrol (Deficient)*.

NUTRITION

- Eliminate all cold and raw foods and beverages from the diet as they constrict the bronchial tubes causing spasms.
- Since asthma may be allergy related, eliminate foods from the diet that commonly cause allergy, such as milk, eggs, shellfish, fish, and nuts. Sulphites, used commonly in restaurants to preserve salads, french fries and avocado dips, are also linked to asthma attacks.
- White radish is an excellent food to relieve cough. Take 1 white radish, approximately the size of a fist and cut it into thin slices. Mix it with 1 tablespoon of maltose and 1 cup of water and cook for 20 minutes. Serve the radish and the juice when they cool to room temperature. Another easier method is to mix the slices of white radish with honey. Wait for 30 minutes and drink the fluids that are secreted from the radish.
- Lemon juice with honey is also very effective to relieve cough.
- A diet low in spicy, raw, greasy and sweet foods is also recommended.

The Tao of Nutrition by Ni and McNease
- Asthma
  - Recommendations: apricot kernels, almonds, walnuts, basil, carrots, pumpkins, winter melon, sunflower seeds, loofah, squash, figs, and daikon.
  - Avoid mucus-producing foods, cold foods, fruits, salads, all shellfish, dairy products, watermelon, bananas, mung beans, salty foods, cold weather, and especially ice cream.
- Common cold (wind-cold)
  - Recommendations: ginger, garlic, mustard greens and seeds, grapefruit peel, cilantro, parsnip, scallions, cinnamon, basil, soupy rice porridge, and eat as little as possible so as not to burden the system with a lot of digestion.
  - Avoid shellfish, heavy proteins and fats, meats, and all vinegars.
- For more information, please refer to *The Tao of Nutrition* by Dr. Maoshing Ni and Cathy McNease.

FORMULAS

RESPITROL (Cold) ™

LIFESTYLE INSTRUCTIONS

- Avoid exposure to pollen, dust, and drastic changes in temperature. Regular exercise with herbal therapy is the key to complete recovery.
- For asthma patients, vacuum and central heating filters should be changed frequently to keep dust, mold and dust mites to a minimum. Installation of an air purifier is recommended for patients who have family members with infectious respiratory disorders. It is recommended to replace carpets with hard surface floors to prevent dust, molds and other allergens from being trapped in the carpet. Bleach such as Clorox can be used to clear mold and fungus. Animal dander is also a major factor in causing allergies in patients. All contact (direct and indirect) with allergens should be avoided if possible to prevent allergic reactions.
- Some asthmatic patients may be allergic to aspirin. In those cases, acetaminophen products should be used instead.
- Patients should be advised to stop smoking, and stay away from second hand smoke.
- Patients should strengthen their immune system and body resistance in between asthma attacks. A balance of exercise and rest is important. Alternation of hot and cold water in the shower is also effective to desensitize the body to changes in temperature. Herbs that enhance the immune system, such as *Cordyceps 3* or *Immune +,* should also be taken on a regular basis.
- Patients are strongly encouraged to use hypo-allergenic products, and avoid those that contain artificial or chemical additives.

CLINICAL NOTES

- *Respitrol (Heat)* or *Respitrol (Cold)* should be taken for respiratory disorders with wheezing, dyspnea and shortness of breath. When the condition stabilizes, use *Respitrol (Deficient)* and *Cordyceps 3* during the remission stage of chronic respiratory disorders to strengthen the underlying constitution of the patient. *Respitrol (Deficient)* should not be taken during the acute stage of any respiratory disorder. Furthermore, *Cordyceps 3* is also very beneficial to strengthen the Lung and the Kidney, the two organs that are responsible to control respiration. Therefore, it is extremely important to ensure that the patient is compliant with taking *Respitrol (Deficient)* and/or *Cordyceps 3* to reduce the frequency and severity of asthma attacks.
- *Respitrol (Cold)* is suitable for common cold or influenza due to wind-cold. However, if the wind-cold transforms into wind-heat or Lung heat, *Lonicera Complex* or *Respitrol (Heat)* should be used, respectively.
- In cases where the patient is having an acute attack and the medication or inhaler is not readily available, two cups of coffee, hot cocoa and chocolate bars are good alternatives to help alleviate symptoms of wheezing or dyspnea. Caffeine has similar effect as the popular asthma drug theophylline.

CAUTIONS

- Patients with heat- or deficient-type respiratory disorders should use *Respitrol (Heat)* or *Respitrol (Deficient)*, respectively. See Supplementary Formulas for maintenance treatment of respiratory disorders.
- Patients with severe or acute asthma attacks may need additional herbal or drug treatment.
- This formula is contraindicated during pregnancy and nursing.
- This formula is contraindicated for long-term use. It should be discontinued when the desired effects are achieved. For long-term treatment, consider using *Respitrol (Deficient)* or *Cordyceps 3*.

ACUPUNCTURE POINTS

Traditional Points:
- *Fengfu* (GV 16), *Fengchi* (GB 20), *Hegu* (LI 4), *Geshu* (BL 17), *Lieque* (LU 7), *Qihu* (ST 13), *Zhongfu* (LU 1).
- Apply moxa to *Dingchuan* (Extra 6), *Gaohuang*, and *Feishu* (BL 13).

RESPITROL (Cold) ™

Balance Method by Dr. Richard Tan:
- Left side: *Shugu* (BL 65), *Jiexi* (ST 41), *Zusanli* (ST 36), and *Jingqu* (LU 8).
- Right side: *Gongsun* (SP 4), *Sanyinjiao* (SP 6), and *Hegu* (LI 4).
- Left and right side can be alternated from treatment to treatment.
- For additional information on the Balance Method, please refer to *Dr. Tan's Strategy of Twelve Magical Points* by Dr. Richard Tan.

Ear Points:
- Bronchi, Lung, Adrenal Gland, and Prostate Gland on both ears using ear seeds.

Auricular Acupuncture by Dr. Li-Chun Huang:
- Bronchial asthma: Bronchus, Trachea, Lung, Chest, Stop Asthma, Sympathetic, Adrenal Gland, Allergic Area, and Endocrine. Bleed Ear Apex.
- Common cold: Lung, Internal Nose, and Throat (Larynx, Pharynx).
  - For fever, bleed Ear Apex and Helix 1 to 6.
  - For dizziness, add Dizziness Area.
  - For pain and soreness all over the body, add Liver and Spleen. Bleed Helix 4.
  - For cough, add Trachea, Bronchus, and Stop Asthma.
- Bronchitis: Bronchus, Trachea, Lung (Lower), Spleen, Stop Asthma, and Sympathetic. Bleed Ear Apex.
- Bronchiectasis: Bronchus, Lung, Chest, Stop Asthma, Allergic Area, Sympathetic, Adrenal Gland, and Spleen.
- Emphysema: Sympathetic, Allergic Area, Chest, Lung, Bronchus, Stop Asthma, Spleen, Kidney, and Endocrine.
- For additional information on the location and explanation of these points, please refer to *Auricular Treatment Formula and Prescriptions* by Dr. Li-Chun Huang.

MODERN RESEARCH

Respitrol (Cold) is composed of herbs that have an antibiotic effect to treat the infection, bronchodilating effect to relieve wheezing and dyspnea, and antitussive and expectorant effects to relieve the associated symptoms.

Respitrol (Cold) contains several herbs with antibiotic effects against various types of pathogens. *Hou Po* (Cortex Magnoliae Officinalis) has an inhibitory effect against *Streptococcus matuans*, *Staphylococcus aureus*, *Bacillus subtilis*, *Diplococcus pneumoniae*, and *Bacillus dysenteriae*.[1,2,3] *Wu Wei Zi* (Fructus Schisandrae Chinensis) has an inhibitory effect *in vitro* against *Staphylococcus aureus*, *Bacillus anthracis*, *Salmonella typhi*, *Bacillus dysenteriae*, *Diplococcus pneumoniae*, *Vibrio cholerae*, and *Pseudomonas aeruginosa*.[4] *Zi Wan* (Radix Asteris) has an inhibitory influence against *E. coli*, *Bacillus dysenteriae*, *Bacillus proteus*, *Salmonella typhi*, *Bacillus paratyphosus*, *Pseudomonas aeruginosa*, *Vibrio cholerae*, and some dermatophytes and influenza viruses.[5] *Bai Jie Zi* (Semen Sinapis) has an inhibitory influence against some pathogenic fungi and dermatophytes, and has been used successfully to treat both tracheitis and pneumonia.[6,7,8] Lastly, *Pi Pa Ye* (Folium Eriobotryae) has an inhibitory effect *in vitro* against *Staphylococcus aureus*, and is effective in treating chronic tracheitis.[9,10]

Respitrol (Cold) has a marked effect to treat asthma, wheezing and dyspnea because many herbs in this formula have marked anti-asthmatic and bronchodilating effects. For example, *Xing Ren* (Semen Armeniacae Amarum) has an inhibitory effect on the respiratory center in the brain, thereby exerting its anti-asthmatic effects.[11] *Hou Po* (Cortex Magnoliae Officinalis) has a stimulating effect on the respiratory system to relieve wheezing and dyspnea.[12] Most importantly, *Gan Cao* (Radix Glycyrrhizae) has a remarkable anti-inflammatory effect to reduce the swelling and inflammation in the lung. In fact, the anti-inflammatory influence of glycyrrhizin and glycyrrhetinic acid, two compounds of *Gan Cao* (Radix Glycyrrhizae), is approximately 1/10th that of cortisone.[13]

RESPITROL (Cold) ™

Lastly, many herbs in **Respitrol (Cold)** treat the symptoms associated with these types of respiratory disorders. *Zi Wan* (Radix Asteris), *Bai Jie Zi* (Semen Sinapis), and *Gan Cao* (Radix Glycyrrhizae) have an expectorant effect to eliminate sputum and phlegm, and relieve chest congestion.[14,15,16] *Su Zi* (Fructus Perillae), *Xing Ren* (Semen Armeniacae Amarum), *Pi Pa Ye* (Folium Eriobotryae) and *Gan Cao* (Radix Glycyrrhizae) have an antitussive effect to relieve cough and dyspnea.[17,18,19,20]

In summary, **Respitrol (Cold)** is an excellent formula to treat respiratory disorders with cold manifestations. Not only does it have good antibiotic effect to treat respiratory tract infection, it also contains many herbs to relieve the associated symptoms.

PHARMACEUTICAL DRUGS & CHINESE MEDICINE: A COMPARATIVE ANALYSIS

Western Medical Approach: Treatment of asthma is generally divided into acute and chronic management. In western medicine, acute asthma is treated by bronchodilators that open the airway and reverse obstruction. Chronic asthma is managed by use of several categories of drugs, including bronchodilators, corticosteroids, theophylline, and cromolyn. Western medicine is extremely effective in treating acute asthma attacks, as use of bronchodilators [such as Proventil or Ventolin (Albuterol) inhalers] generally reverses airway obstruction within minutes. However, western medicine is not as successful in long-term management and prevention of asthma. These drugs do not change the underlying condition of the disease, nor do they improve the constitution of the patient. Therefore, long-term prognosis is often characterized by successful suppression of acute asthma attack, but no change in the frequency or severity of recurrent asthma attacks.

Traditional Chinese Medicine Approach: Asthma is treated based on the urgency of the current disease manifestation and the underlying condition of the patients. Urgency refers to the acute or chronic nature of the disease, while underlying condition refers to the fundamental constitution of the patients. By addressing both the disease and the fundamental constitution, use of herbs achieves both immediate and prolonged effects.

Summation: Both drugs and herbs are effective for treatment of asthma. Generally speaking, drugs are more effective for acute asthma, as they are more potent, and can be delivered via inhalation or intravenous injection to achieve faster onset of relief. However, long-term treatment of asthma with drugs is often less than optimal, as these drugs tend to create tolerance and dependence. Furthermore, they do not change the course of illness, and do not reduce the frequency and severity of recurrent asthma attacks. On the other hand, herbs are better for long-term prevention and management of asthma. Herbs strengthen the body and enhance its own ability to manage asthma. However, use of herbs may not be appropriate for acute asthma because they are less immediately potent than some pharmaceuticals, and have a slower onset of action. In conclusion, optimal treatment of asthma does not require choosing between drugs and herbs, but can be achieved by embracing the benefits of both, by using drugs for acute treatment and herbs for long-term healing and prevention.

CASE STUDY

B.F., a 55-year-old male, presented with cough, thick nasal discharge, headache and fatigue. The tongue was pale, flabby and slightly purple. The pulse was slow. He was diagnosed with common cold and wind-cold invasion. **Magnolia Clear Sinus**, **Respitrol (Cold)** and **Herbal ABX** were prescribed. The patient reported that the sinus cleared in three days.

B.F., Newport Beach, California

---

[1] *Planta med*, 1982; 44(2):100
[2] *Yao Jian Gong Zuo Tong Xun* (Journal of Herbal Preparations), 1980; 10(4):209
[3] *Xin Hua Ben Cao Gang Mu* (New Chinese Materia Medica), 1988; 58
[4] *Zhong Yao Xue* (Chinese Herbology), 1998; 878:881

FORMULAS

RESPITROL (Cold)™

[5] *Chang Yong Zhong Yao Cheng Fen Yu Yao Li Shou Ce* (A Handbook of the Composition and Pharmacology of Common Chinese Drugs), 1994; 1678:1681

[6] *Chang Yong Zhong Yao Xian Dai Yan Jiu Yu Lin Chuan* (Recent Study & Clinical Application of Common Traditional Chinese Medicine), 1995; 439:441

[7] *Hei Long Jiang Zhong Yi Yao* (Heilongjiang Chinese Medicine and Herbology), 1988; 1:29

[8] *Zhong Xi Yi Jie He Za Zhi* (Journal of Integrated Chinese and Western Medicine), 1986; 2:124

[9] *Chang Yong Zhong Yao Cheng Fen Yu Yao Li Shou Ce* (A Handbook of the Composition and Pharmacology of Common Chinese Drugs), 1994; 1970: 10

[10] *Yi Yao Wei Sheng* (Medicine, Medicinals, and Sanitation), 1972; 3:29

[11] *Life Sci*, 1980; 27(8):659

[12] *Zhong Yao Xue* (Chinese Herbology), 1998; 320:323

[13] *Zhong Cao Yao* (Chinese Herbal Medicine), 1991; 22(10):452

[14] *Chang Yong Zhong Yao Cheng Fen Yu Yao Li Shou Ce* (A Handbook of the Composition and Pharmacology of Common Chinese Drugs), 1994; 1678:1681

[15] *Zhong Yao Xue* (Chinese Herbology), 1998; 608:610

[16] *Zhong Yao Yao Li Yu Ying Yong* (Pharmacology and Applications of Chinese Herbs), 1983; 264

[17] *Zhong Yao Tong Bao* (Journal of Chinese Herbology), 1986; 8:56

[18] *Life Sci*, 1980; 27(8):659

[19] *Zhong Yao Xue* (Chinese Herbology), 1998; 651:653

[20] *Zhong Yao Yao Li Yu Ying Yong* (Pharmacology and Applications of Chinese Herbs), 1983; 264

FORMULAS

RESPITROL (Deficient) ™

CLINICAL APPLICATIONS

❧ Chronic respiratory disorders characterized by a weak or deficient body constitution
❧ Chronic breathing problems such as chronic asthma, bronchitis, and pulmonary emphysema
❧ General symptoms and signs of deficiency including shortness of breath characterized by difficulty in inhalation but normal exhalation, wheezing and shortness of breath that becomes worse with physical exertion, snoring sounds in the throat due to phlegm accumulation, low-pitched rhonchi, audible wheezes, frail cough with sputum, dry throat, aversion to wind, spontaneous sweating, red cheeks, red tongue with scanty coating, and a thready-rapid pulse.

WESTERN THERAPEUTIC ACTIONS

❧ Anti-asthmatic effect that treats asthma and relieves wheezing and dyspnea [1,10,11]
❧ Antitussive and expectorant functions which stop cough and eliminate sputum and phlegm [11,12]

CHINESE THERAPEUTIC ACTIONS

❧ Relieves wheezing, arrests cough
❧ Eliminates phlegm
❧ Tonifies the Lung and the Kidney
❧ Tonifies the Kidney to grasp the qi downward

DOSAGE

Take 3 to 4 capsules three times daily on an empty stomach with warm water. This formula may be taken continuously on a long-term basis for the maintenance and prevention of asthma.

INGREDIENTS

Bai Jie Zi (Semen Sinapis)
Chai Hu (Radix Bupleuri)
Chen Pi (Pericarpium Citri Reticulatae)
Dang Gui (Radicis Angelicae Sinensis)
Dong Chong Xia Cao (Cordyceps)
Hou Po (Cortex Magnoliae Officinalis)
Lai Fu Zi (Semen Raphani)
Rou Gui (Cortex Cinnamomi)

Su Zi (Fructus Perillae)
Ting Li Zi (Semen Descurainiae seu Lepidii)
Wu Wei Zi (Fructus Schisandrae Chinensis)
Xing Ren (Semen Armeniacae Amarum)
Zao Jiao Ci (Spina Gleditsiae)
Zhi Gan Cao (Radix Glycyrrhizae Preparata)
Zi Su Ye (Folium Perillae)
Zi Wan (Radix Asteris)

FORMULA EXPLANATION

Respitrol (Deficient) is formulated to treat deficient-type of respiratory disorders, including but not limited to, asthma, bronchitis, emphysema, and other chronic and debilitating respiratory disorders. Diagnostic signs and symptoms of deficiency include dyspnea, shortness of breath, wheezing, difficulty with inhalation, fatigue with dyspnea on mild physical exertion, and weak and chronic nature of respiratory illnesses. ***Respitrol (Deficient)*** contains herbs with functions to tonify the Kidney, regulate qi circulation, and eliminate phlegm.

Xing Ren (Semen Armeniacae Amarum), *Su Zi* (Fructus Perillae), *Zi Wan* (Radix Asteris), *Bai Jie Zi* (Semen Sinapis) and *Ting Li Zi* (Semen Descurainiae seu Lepidii) reverse rebellious Lung qi, eliminate phlegm, and relieve coughing and wheezing. *Wu Wei Zi* (Fructus Schisandrae Chinensis) is an astringent herb that prevents the leakage

RESPITROL (Deficient) ™

of Lung qi. *Lai Fu Zi* (Semen Raphani) tonifies the Spleen and reduces the production of phlegm. *Chen Pi* (Pericarpium Citri Reticulatae) and *Zao Jiao Ci* (Spina Gleditsiae) are expectorants. To prolong inhalation, *Rou Gui* (Cortex Cinnamomi) and *Dong Chong Xia Cao* (Cordyceps) warm the Kidney yang and restore its ability to grasp qi downward. *Hou Po* (Cortex Magnoliae Officinalis) and *Chai Hu* (Radix Bupleuri) regulate qi and relieve chest congestion. *Dang Gui* (Radicis Angelicae Sinensis) nourishes the blood. *Zi Su Ye* (Folium Perillae) disperses coldness and dilates the Lung. *Zhi Gan Cao* (Radix Glycyrrhizae Preparata) harmonizes the formula.

SUPPLEMENTARY FORMULAS

- For maintenance and prevention of asthma attack, use *Cordyceps 3* and *Respitrol (Deficient)* together.
- For coughing, add *Respitrol (CF)*.
- For infection of ear, nose and throat, add *Herbal ENT*.
- For thirst, dry mouth and throat, add *Nourish (Fluids)*.
- Take with *Immune +* to enhance immunity.
- For actual respiratory infection with sore throat, fever, headache, use *Lonicera Complex* or *Respitrol (Heat)* instead.
- To treat cold-type respiratory disorders with chills, clear nasal discharge, sneezing, nasal congestion, use *Respitrol (Cold)*.
- To treat allergies, use *Magnolia Clear Sinus* or *Pueraria Clear Sinus*.
- For deficiency of qi, blood, yin or yang, combine *Imperial Tonic* with *Respitrol (Deficient)* as a preventative treatment for asthma during remission periods.
- For Kidney yang deficiency, combine *Kidney Tonic (Yang)* with *Respitrol (Deficient)* as a preventative treatment for asthma during remission periods.

NUTRITION

- Eliminate all cold and raw foods and beverages from the diet as they constrict the bronchial tubes causing spasms.
- Since asthma may be allergy related, eliminate foods from diet that commonly cause allergy, such as milk, eggs, shellfish, fish, and nuts. Sulphites, used commonly in restaurants to preserve salads, french fries and avocado dips, are also linked to asthma attacks.
- White radish is an excellent food to relieve cough. Take 1 white radish, approximately the size of a fist and cut it into thin slices. Mix it with 1 tablespoon of maltose and 1 cup of water and cook for 20 minutes. Serve the radish and the juice when they cool to room temperature. Another easier method is to mix the slices of white radish with honey. Wait for 30 minutes and drink the fluids that is secreted from the radish.
- Lemon juice with honey is also very effective to relieve cough.
- Avoid mucus-producing foods such as sugar, fried or greasy foods, dairy products including cheese, food additives (MSG, metabisulfite), white flour products and junk food. Increase onions and garlic in the diet. A diet low in spicy, raw, greasy and sweet foods is also recommended.

The Tao of Nutrition by Ni and McNease
- Asthma
  - Recommendations: apricot kernels, almonds, walnuts, basil, carrots, pumpkins, winter melon, sunflower seeds, loofah, squash, figs, and daikon.
  - Avoid mucus-producing foods, cold foods, fruits, salads, all shellfish, dairy products, watermelon, bananas, mung beans, salty foods, cold weather, and especially ice cream.

RESPITROL (Deficient) ™

- Chronic bronchitis
  - Recommendations: carrots, apricot kernels, persimmons, white fungus, pears, honey jellyfish, ginger, water chestnuts, yams, sweet potatoes, daikon radish, walnuts, papaya, peach kernels, lotus roots, seaweed, and winter melon seeds. Always try to stay warm.
  - Avoid overworking, being chilled, stimulating foods, spicy foods, smoking, alcohol, caffeine, and cold drinks.
- For more information, please refer to *The Tao of Nutrition* by Dr. Maoshing Ni and Cathy McNease.

LIFESTYLE INSTRUCTIONS

- Patients with emphysema should avoid cigarettes and second-hand smoke. Avoid air pollution, dust, mold, fur, animal dander, chemicals, or artificial fragrances.
- It is helpful to maintain a stable temperature environment, avoiding sudden extremes of heat, cold, humidity, or dryness whenever possible.
- Some asthmatic patients may be allergic to aspirin. In those cases, acetaminophen products should be used instead.
- Patients should strengthen their immune system and body resistance in between asthma attacks. A balance of exercise and rest is important. Alternation of hot and cold water in the shower is also effective to desensitize the body to changes in temperature. Herbs that enhance the immune system, such as *Cordyceps 3* or *Immune +,* should also be taken on a regular basis.
- Avoid exposure to pollen, dust, and drastic changes in temperature. Regular exercise with herbal therapy is the key to complete recovery.
- For asthma patients, vacuum and central heating filters should be changed frequently to keep dust, mold and dust mites to a minimum. Installation of an air purifier is recommended for patients who have family members with infectious respiratory disorders. It is recommended to replace carpets with hard surface floors to prevent dust, molds and other allergens from being trapped in the carpet. Bleach such as Clorox can be used to clear mold and fungus. Animal dander is also a major factor in causing allergies in patients. All contact (direct and indirect) with allergens should be avoided if possible to prevent allergic reactions.

CLINICAL NOTES

- *Respitrol (Heat)* and *Respitrol (Cold)* should be taken for respiratory disorders with wheezing, dyspnea and shortness of breath. When the condition stabilizes, take *Respitrol (Deficient)* and *Cordyceps 3* during the remission stage of chronic respiratory disorders to strengthen the underlying constitution of the patient. *Respitrol (Deficient)* should not be taken during the acute stage of any respiratory disorder. Furthermore, *Cordyceps 3* is also very beneficial to strengthen the Lung and the Kidney, the two organs that are responsible to control respiration. Therefore, it is extremely important to ensure that the patient is compliant with taking *Respitrol (Deficient)* and/or *Cordyceps 3* to reduce the frequency and severity of asthma attacks.
- In cases where the patient is having an acute attack and the medication or inhaler is not readily available, two cups of coffee, hot cocoa and chocolate bars are good alternatives to help alleviate symptoms of wheezing or dyspnea. Caffeine has similar effect as the popular asthma drug theophylline.[6]

CAUTIONS

- Patients with heat- or cold-type respiratory disorders should use *Respitrol (Heat)* or *Respitrol (Cold)*, respectively. Please refer to Supplementary Formulas for maintenance treatment of respiratory disorders.
- Patients with severe or acute asthma attacks may need additional herbal or drug treatment.
- This formula is contraindicated during pregnancy and nursing.

RESPITROL (Deficient) ™

❧ Patients who are on anticoagulant or antiplatelet therapies, such as Coumadin (Warfarin), should use this formula with caution, as there may be a slightly higher risk of bleeding and bruising.

ACUPUNCTURE POINTS

Traditional Points:
❧ *Zusanli* (ST 36), *Fenglong* (ST 40), *Feishu* (BL 13), *Dashu* (BL 11), *Shanzhong* (CV 17), *Shenshu* (BL 23), *Chize* (LU 5), *Kongzui* (LU 6), *Taixi* (KI 3), and *Qihai* (CV 6).
❧ Apply moxa to *Guanyuan* (CV 4), *Mingmen* (GV 4), and *Dingchuan* (Extra 6).

Balance Method by Dr. Richard Tan:
❧ Left side: *Neiguan* (PC 6), *Kongzui* (LU 6), *Lingdao* (HT 4), *Fenglong* (ST 40), and *Zusanli* (ST 36).
❧ Right side: *Sanjian* (LI 3), *Piani* (LI 6), *Jiaoxin* (KI 8) *Sanyinjiao* (SP 6), and *Zhongfeng* (LR 4).
❧ Left and right side can be alternated from treatment to treatment.
❧ For additional information on the Balance Method, please refer to *Dr. Tan's Strategy of Twelve Magical Points* by Dr. Richard Tan.

Ear Points:
❧ Bronchi, Lung, Adrenal Gland, Prostate Gland on both ears using ear seeds.

Auricular Acupuncture by Dr. Li-Chun Huang:
❧ Bronchial asthma: Bronchus, Trachea, Lung, Chest, Stop Asthma, Sympathetic, Adrenal Gland, Allergic Area, and Endocrine. Bleed Ear Apex.
❧ Common cold: Lung, Internal Nose, and Throat (Larynx, Pharynx).
  ▪ For fever, bleed Ear Apex and Helix 1 to 6.
  ▪ For dizziness, add Dizziness Area.
  ▪ For pain and soreness all over the body, add Liver and Spleen. Bleed Helix 4.
  ▪ For cough, add Trachea, Bronchus, and Stop Asthma.
❧ Bronchitis: Bronchus, Trachea, Lung (Lower), Spleen, Stop Asthma, and Sympathetic. Bleed Ear Apex.
❧ Bronchiectasis: Bronchus, Lung, Chest, Stop Asthma, Allergic Area, Sympathetic, Adrenal Gland, and Spleen.
❧ Emphysema: Sympathetic, Allergic Area, Chest, Lung, Bronchus, Stop Asthma, Spleen, Kidney, and Endocrine.
❧ For additional information on the location and explanation of these points, please refer to *Auricular Treatment Formula and Prescriptions* by Dr. Li-Chun Huang.

MODERN RESEARCH

Respitrol (Deficient) is comprised of herbs with an anti-asthmatic effect to relieve wheezing and dyspnea, antitussive effects to stop coughing, and expectorant effect to eliminate phlegm and sputum. Clinical applications of *Respitrol (Deficient)* include asthma, bronchitis, emphysema, and other chronic and debilitating respiratory disorders.

Respitrol (Deficient) has marked effect to treat asthma, wheezing and dyspnea because many herbs in this formula have marked anti-asthmatic and bronchodilating effects. For example, *Xing Ren* (Semen Armeniacae Amarum) has an inhibitory effect on the respiratory center in the brain, thereby exerting its anti-asthmatic effects.[1] *Hou Po* (Cortex Magnoliae Officinalis) has a stimulating effect on the respiratory system to relieve wheezing and dyspnea.[2] Most importantly, *Gan Cao* (Radix Glycyrrhizae) has a remarkable anti-inflammatory effect to reduce the swelling and inflammation in the lung. In fact, the anti-inflammatory influence of glycyrrhizin and glycyrrhetinic acid, two compounds of *Gan Cao* (Radix Glycyrrhizae), is approximately 1/10th that of cortisone.[3]

RESPITROL (Deficient) ™

Furthermore, many herbs have bronchodilating effects to dilate the bronchi and reverse airway obstruction. *Dong Chong Xia Cao* (Cordyceps) has demonstrated bronchodilating effect, and has been used to treat chronic respiratory tract disorders with good success.[4] *Xing Ren* (Semen Armeniacae Amarum) has strong antitussive and anti-asthmatic functions, and is commonly used for treating cough, asthma, and acute or chronic bronchitis. *Zi Su Ye* (Folium Perillae) has been shown to promote bronchodilation and relieve bronchospasm.[5] *Chen Pi* (Pericarpium Citri Reticulatae) has been shown to dilate the bronchi, and may be used to treat chronic bronchitis characterized by severe coughing.[6,7] Lastly, *Dang Gui* (Radicis Angelicae Sinensis) has demonstrated a beneficial effect in treating wheezing and dyspnea caused by bronchospasm, with initial onset of action within 2 to 3 hours, and a duration of 8 to 24 hours.[8,9]

Hou Po (Cortex Magnoliae Officinalis) helps in the treatment of respiratory disorders caused by bacterial or viral infections. It also has both antibacterial and antiviral activities and is most effective against *Streptococcus*, *Staphylococcus* and *Shigella* species.[10]

Su Zi (Fructus Perillae), *Bai Jie Zi* (Semen Sinapis) and *Lai Fu Zi* (Semen Raphani) are three herbs commonly used together to treat various respiratory tract disorders, including but not limited to bronchitis, bronchial asthma, emphysema, pediatric asthma, and spasms of the diaphragm.[11] *Su Zi* (Fructus Perillae) has antitussive, expectorant and anti-asthmatic effects. *Bai Jie Zi* (Semen Sinapis) resolves phlegm, and *Lai Fu Zi* (Semen Raphani) has expectorant activities.[12]

In summary, **Respitrol (Deficient)** is an excellent formula to treat chronic respiratory disorders, as it contains herbs to dilate the bronchi, reverse airway obstruction, and relieve related symptoms.

PHARMACEUTICAL DRUGS & CHINESE MEDICINE: A COMPARATIVE ANALYSIS

Western Medical Approach: Treatment of asthma is generally divided into acute and chronic management. In western medicine, acute asthma is treated by bronchodilators that open the airway and reverse obstruction. Chronic asthma is managed by use of several categories of drugs, including bronchodilators, corticosteroids, theophylline, and cromolyn. Western medicine is extremely effective in treating acute asthma attacks, as use of bronchodilators [such as Proventil or Ventolin (Albuterol) inhalers] generally reverses airway obstruction within minutes. However, western medicine is not as successful in long-term management and prevention of asthma. These drugs do not change the underlying condition of the disease, nor do they improve the constitution of the patient. Therefore, long-term prognosis is often characterized by successful suppression of acute asthma attack, but no change in frequency or severity of recurrent asthma attacks.

Traditional Chinese Medicine Approach: Asthma is treated based on the urgency of the disease and the underlying condition of the patients. Urgency refers to the acute or chronic nature of the disease, while underlying condition refers to the fundamental constitution of the patients. By addressing both the disease and the fundamental constitution, use of herbs achieves both immediate and prolonged effects.

Summation: Both drugs and herbs are effective for treatment of asthma. Generally speaking, drugs are more effective for acute asthma, as they are more potent, and can be delivered via inhalation or intravenous injection to achieve faster onset of relief. However, long-term treatment of asthma with drugs is often less than optimal, as these drugs tend to create tolerance and dependence. Furthermore, they do not change the course of illness, and do not reduce frequency and severity of recurrent asthma attacks. On the other hand, herbs are better for long-term prevention and management of asthma. Herbs strengthen the body and enhance its own ability to manage asthma. However, use of herbs may not be appropriate for acute asthma because they are less immediately potent than some pharmaceuticals, and have a slower onset of action. In conclusion, optimal treatment of asthma does not require choosing between drugs or herbs, but embracing the benefits of both, by using drugs for acute treatment and herbs for long-term prevention.

RESPITROL (Deficient) ™

CASE STUDY

A 17-year-old male student presented with wheezing, shortness of breath and a dry, non-productive cough. It was worse with exertion and exposure to cold. He was extremely thin and unable to gain weight. The practitioner diagnosed the patient's condition as rebellious Lung qi with deficient Kidney not grasping Lung qi. The western diagnosis was chronic asthma. After taking *Respitrol (Deficient),* he was able to restrain his wheezing and keep it under control. Utilization of his inhaler was reduced from three to four times a day to once or twice a week. While on *Respitrol (Deficient)*, the patient also received acupuncture treatments twice a week for two weeks followed by once a week for two weeks.

Anonymous

[1] *Life Sci*, 1980; 27(8):659
[2] *Zhong Yao Xue* (Chinese Herbology), 1998; 320:323
[3] *Zhong Cao Yao* (Chinese Herbal Medicine), 1991; 22(10):452
[4] *Zhong Cao Yao* (Chinese Herbal Medicine), 1983; 14(5):32
[5] *Zhong Yao Xue* (Chinese Herbology), 1998; 67:68
[6] *Shang Hai Yi Yao Za Zhi* (Shanghai Journal of Medicine and Herbology), 1957; (3):148
[7] *Zhe Jiang Zhong Yi Za Zhi* (Zhejiang Journal of Chinese Medicine), 1985; 1:18
[8] *Zhong Cao Yao* (Chinese Herbal Medicine), 1983; 14(8):45
[9] *Tian Jing Zhong Yi* (Tianjing Chinese Medicine), 1986; 1:4
[10] Bensky, D. et al. *Chinese Herbal Medicine Materia Medica*. Eastland Press. 1986
[11] Bensky, D. et al. *Chinese Herbal Medicine Formulas and Strategies*. Eastland Press. 1990
[12] Yeung, HC. *Handbook of Chinese Herbs. Institute of Chinese Medicine*. 1996

FORMULAS

RESPITROL (Heat) ™

CLINICAL APPLICATIONS

- ☙ Respiratory disorders with heat manifestations
- ☙ Common cold or flu with fever, thick yellow nasal discharge, and/or cough
- ☙ Wheezing and dyspnea with a choking sensation, coughing with chest distention, fever, irritability, flushed face, and yellow sputum
- ☙ Pneumonia, pertussis, or respiratory tract infections with heat manifestations, such as cough, chest distention, fever and yellow sputum

WESTERN THERAPEUTIC ACTIONS

- ☙ Bronchodilating effect that relaxes the bronchial muscles and relieves spasms [1]
- ☙ Antitussive and expectorant function to stop cough and eliminate sputum and phlegm
- ☙ Antipyretic action to reduce fever and body temperature [14]

CHINESE THERAPEUTIC ACTIONS

- ☙ Clears Lung heat
- ☙ Dissolves phlegm
- ☙ Regulates qi circulation to relieve wheezing and dyspnea

DOSAGE

Take 4 to 6 capsules three times a day with warm water on an empty stomach. Patients should begin taking *Respitrol (Heat)* with the first sign of respiratory discomfort for maximum effectiveness.

INGREDIENTS

Da Zao (Fructus Jujubae)
Di Gu Pi (Cortex Lycii)
Gan Cao (Radix Glycyrrhizae)
Hou Po (Cortex Magnoliae Officinalis)
Jie Geng (Radix Platycodonis)
Lian Qiao (Fructus Forsythiae)
Pi Pa Ye (Folium Eriobotryae)

Sang Bai Pi (Cortex Mori)
She Gan (Rhizoma Belamcandae)
Shi Gao (Gypsum Fibrosum)
Ting Li Zi (Semen Descurainiae seu Lepidii)
Wu Wei Zi (Fructus Schisandrae Chinensis)
Xing Ren (Semen Armeniacae Amarum)

FORMULA EXPLANATION

Respitrol (Heat) is formulated to treat heat-type respiratory disorders, including but not limited to common cold, flu, asthma, bronchitis, and infections of the respiratory tract. Diagnostic signs and symptoms of heat include fever, cough, asthma, flushed face, perspiration, and yellow sputum. *Respitrol (Heat)* contains herbs with functions to clear Lung heat, dissolve phlegm, and regulate qi circulation.

Shi Gao (Gypsum Fibrosum) clears Lung heat, reduces fever, and relieves coughing. *Xing Ren* (Semen Armeniacae Amarum) stops coughing and calms wheezing. *Sang Bai Pi* (Cortex Mori) and *Di Gu Pi* (Cortex Lycii) clear Lung heat and stop coughing and wheezing. *Jie Geng* (Radix Platycodonis) clears Lung heat, expands the chest, and dissolves the phlegm. *Hou Po* (Cortex Magnoliae Officinalis) helps *Jie Geng* (Radix Platycodonis) expand the chest and relieve congestion. *She Gan* (Rhizoma Belamcandae) and *Pi Pa Ye* (Folium Eriobotryae) clear heat, relieve toxicity, and eliminate sputum and phlegm from the upper respiratory tract. *Ting Li Zi* (Semen Descurainiae seu

RESPITROL (Heat) ™

Lepidii) drains the Lung, eliminates phlegm and reduces wheezing. *Da Zao* (Fructus Jujubae) minimizes the harsh effect of *Ting Li Zi* (Semen Descurainiae seu Lepidii) to prevent damage to the Lung. *Lian Qiao* (Fructus Forsythiae) clears Lung heat and detoxifies. A small amount of *Wu Wei Zi* (Fructus Schisandrae Chinensis) is used to inhibit the leakage of Lung qi to prevent qi loss. *Gan Cao* (Radix Glycyrrhizae) relieves spasms, supplements qi and harmonizes all the herbs in this formula.

SUPPLEMENTARY FORMULAS

- For sinus infections with yellow nasal discharge, combine with *Pueraria Clear Sinus*.
- For profuse, thick, yellow phlegm with chest congestion, combine with *Poria XPT*.
- For wheezing and dyspnea with infection, add *Herbal ABX*.
- For coughing, add *Respitrol (CF)*.
- For infection of ear, nose and throat, add *Herbal ENT*.
- For thirst, dry mouth and throat, add *Nourish (Fluids)*.
- For excess heat or fire, add *Gardenia Complex*.
- As a constitutional tonic for asthma during remission, take *Cordyceps 3*.
- To boost the immune system, take *Immune +* after cold/flu symptoms subside.
- For dyspnea or chest tightness due to environmental or toxic poisoning, add *Herbal DTX*.
- For maintenance and prevention of asthma attack, use *Cordyceps 3* and *Respitrol (Deficient)*.

NUTRITION

- Eliminate all spicy, cold and raw foods and beverages from the diet as they constrict the bronchial tubes causing spasms.
- A diet low in spicy, raw, greasy and sweet foods is also recommended.
- To avoid infection, a diet high in garlic, onions, and water is recommended. Stay away from cigarette smoke, alcohol, seafood, food additives (MSG, metabisulfite), and phlegm-producing foods such as sweets, dairy products, and heavy or greasy foods.
- Supplying the body with vitamin C is important, as it is greatly consumed by white blood cells when fighting infections.
- Drink plenty of fluids throughout the day to facilitate the elimination of heat, phlegm and sputum.
- Since asthma may be allergy related, eliminate foods from diet that commonly cause allergies, such as milk, eggs, shellfish, fish, and nuts. Sulphites, used commonly in restaurants to preserve salads, french fries and avocado dips, are also linked to asthma attacks.
- White radish is an excellent food to relieve cough. Take 1 white radish, approximately the size of a fist and cut it into thin slices. Mix it with 1 tablespoon of maltose and 1 cup of water and cook for 20 minutes. Serve the radish and the juice when they cool to room temperature. Another easier method is to mix the slices of white radish with honey. Wait for 30 minutes and drink the fluids that are secreted from the radish.
- Lemon juice with honey is also very effective to relieve cough.

The Tao of Nutrition by Ni and McNease
- Asthma
  - Recommendations: apricot kernels, almonds, walnuts, basil, carrots, pumpkins, winter melon, sunflower seeds, loofah, squash, figs, and daikon.
  - Avoid mucus-producing foods, cold foods, fruits, salads, all shellfish, dairy products, watermelon, bananas, mung beans, salty foods, cold weather, and especially ice cream.
- Common cold (heat type)
  - Recommendations: mint, cabbage, chrysanthemum flowers, burdock root, cilantro, dandelion, apples, appears, and bitter melon. Drink plenty of fluids and get lots of rest

RESPITROL (Heat) ™

- Avoid shellfish, meats, vinegar, drafts, and hot foods.
- Chronic bronchitis
  - Recommendations: carrots, apricot kernels, persimmons, white fungus, pears, honey jellyfish, ginger, water chestnuts, yams, sweet potatoes, daikon radish, walnuts, papaya, peach kernels, lotus roots, seaweed, and winter melon seeds. Always try to stay warm.
  - Avoid overworking, being chilled, stimulating foods, spicy foods, smoking, alcohol, caffeine, and cold drinks.
- For more information, please refer to *The Tao of Nutrition* by Dr. Maoshing Ni and Cathy McNease.

LIFESTYLE INSTRUCTIONS

- Avoid exposure to pollen, dust, and drastic changes in temperature. Regular exercise with herbal therapy is the key to complete recovery.
- For asthma patients, vacuum and central heating filters should be changed frequently to keep dust, mold and dust mites to a minimum. Installation of an air purifier is recommended for patients who have family members with infectious respiratory disorders. It is recommended to replace carpets with hard surface floors to prevent dust, molds and other allergens from being trapped in the carpet. Bleach such as Clorox can be used to clear mold and fungus. Animal dander is also a major factor in causing allergies in patients. All contact (direct and indirect) with allergens should be avoided if possible to prevent allergic reactions.
- Some asthmatic patients may be allergic to aspirin. In those cases, acetaminophen products should be used instead.
- Patients should be advised to stop smoking, and stay away from second hand smoke.
- Patients should strengthen their immune system and body resistance in between asthma attacks. A balance of exercise and rest is important. Alternation of hot and cold water in the shower is also effective to desensitize the body to changes in temperature. Herbs that enhance the immune system, such as *Cordyceps 3* or *Immune +*, should also be taken on a regular basis.

CLINICAL NOTES

- *Respitrol (Heat)* or *Respitrol (Cold)* should be taken for respiratory disorders with wheezing, dyspnea and shortness of breath. When the condition stabilizes, use *Respitrol (Deficient)* and *Cordyceps 3* during the remission stage of chronic respiratory disorders to strengthen the underlying constitution of the patient. *Respitrol (Deficient)* should not be taken during the acute stage of any respiratory disorder. Furthermore, *Cordyceps 3* is also very beneficial to strengthen the Lung and the Kidney, the two organs that are responsible to control respiration. Therefore, it is extremely important to ensure that the patient is compliant with taking *Respitrol (Deficient)* and/or *Cordyceps 3* to reduce the frequency and severity of asthma attacks.
- Most cough during the day is due to heat or dryness. Cough at night is mostly due to Kidney deficiency, Spleen deficiency or dampness.
- In cases where the patient is having an acute attack and the medication or inhaler is not readily available, two cups of coffee, hot cocoa and chocolate bars are good alternatives to help alleviate symptoms of wheezing or dyspnea. Caffeine has similar effect as the popular asthma drug theophylline.[5]

CAUTIONS

- Patients with cold or deficient respiratory disorders should use *Respitrol (Cold)* or *Respitrol (Deficient)*, respectively. See Supplementary Formulas for maintenance treatment of respiratory disorders.
- Patients with severe or acute asthma attacks may need additional herbal or drug treatment.
- This formula is contraindicated during pregnancy and nursing.

RESPITROL (Heat) ™

☙ This formula is contraindicated for long-term use. It should be discontinued when the desired effects are achieved. For long-term treatment, consider using **Respitrol (Deficient)** or **Cordyceps 3**.

ACUPUNCTURE POINTS

Traditional Points:
☙ *Feishu* (BL 13), *Lieque* (LU 7), *Hegu* (LI 4), *Taiyuan* (LU 9), *Taibai* (SP 3), *Fenglong* (ST 40), and *Chize* (LU 5).
☙ *Ciliao* (BL 32), *Dazhui* (GV 14), *Feishu* (BL 13), and *Kongzui* (LU 6).

Balance Method by Dr. Richard Tan:
☙ Left side: *Sanjian* (LI 3), *Quchi* (LI 11), *Sanyinjiao* (SP 6), and *Yinlingquan* (SP 9).
☙ Right side: *Chize* (LU 5), *Jingqu* (LU 8), *Zusanli* (ST 36), and *Fenglong* (ST 40).
☙ Left and right side can be alternated from treatment to treatment.
☙ For additional information on the Balance Method, please refer to *Dr. Tan's Strategy of Twelve Magical Points* by Dr. Richard Tan.

Ear Points:
☙ Bronchi, Lung, Adrenal Gland, Prostate Gland on both ears using ear seeds.

Auricular Acupuncture by Dr. Li-Chun Huang:
☙ Bronchial asthma: Bronchus, Trachea, Lung, Chest, Stop Asthma, Sympathetic, Adrenal Gland, Allergic Area, and Endocrine. Bleed Ear Apex.
☙ Common cold: Lung, Internal Nose, and Throat (Larynx, Pharynx).
  ▪ For fever, bleed Ear Apex and Helix 1 to 6.
  ▪ For dizziness, add Dizziness Area.
  ▪ For pain and soreness all over the body, add Liver and Spleen. Bleed Helix 4.
  ▪ For cough, add Trachea, Bronchus, and Stop Asthma.
☙ Bronchitis: Bronchus, Trachea, Lung (Lower), Spleen, Stop Asthma, and Sympathetic. Bleed Ear Apex.
☙ Bronchiectasis: Bronchus, Lung, Chest, Stop Asthma, Allergic Area, Sympathetic, Adrenal Gland, and Spleen.
☙ Emphysema: Sympathetic, Allergic Area, Chest, Lung, Bronchus, Stop Asthma, Spleen, Kidney, and Endocrine.
☙ For additional information on the location and explanation of these points, please refer to *Auricular Treatment Formula and Prescriptions* by Dr. Li-Chun Huang.

MODERN RESEARCH

Respitrol (Heat) is formulated specifically to treat respiratory disorders with heat manifestations. From the traditional Chinese medicine perspective, "heat" in the respiratory tract is characterized by conditions such as wheezing, dyspnea, asthma, bronchitis, pneumonia, common cold, influenza, cough, chest distention, etc. Therefore, **Respitrol (Heat)** contains herbs to address both the cause and the symptoms of this disorder. The herbs in this formula have antibiotic effects to treat the infection, bronchodilating effect to relieve wheezing and dyspnea, and antitussive and expectorant effects to relieve the associated symptoms.

Several herbs in this formula have antibiotic effects against various types of pathogens. *Hou Po* (Cortex Magnoliae Officinalis) has an inhibitory effect against *Streptococcus matuans*, *Staphylococcus aureus*, *Bacillus subtilis*, *Diplococcus pneumoniae*, and *Bacillus dysenteriae*.[1,2,3] *Sang Bai Pi* (Cortex Mori) has an inhibitory effect against *Staphylococcus aureus*, *Salmonella typhi*, and *Bacillus dysenteriae*.[4] *Di Gu Pi* (Cortex Lycii) inhibits the activity of typhoid, paratyphoid and shigella.[5] *Wu Wei Zi* (Fructus Schisandrae Chinensis) has an inhibitory effect *in vitro*

RESPITROL (Heat) ™

against *Staphylococcus aureus, Bacillus anthracis, Salmonella typhi, Bacillus dysenteriae, Diplococcus pneumoniae, Vibrio cholerae,* and *Pseudomonas aeruginosa.*[6] Lastly, *Lian Qiao* (Fructus Forsythiae) has demonstrated a broad spectrum of inhibitory effects against *Staphylococcus aureus, Diplococcus pneumoniae, Bacillus dysenteriae,* alpha-hemolytic streptococcus, beta-hemolytic streptococcus, *Neisseria catarrhalis, Salmonella typhi, E. coli, Mycobacterium tuberculosis, Bacillus proteus, Bordetella pertussis, Corynebacterium diphtheriae,* leptospira, and some dermatophytes and influenza viruses.[7]

Respitrol (Heat) has marked effect to treat asthma, wheezing and dyspnea because many herbs in this formula have marked anti-asthmatic and bronchodilating effects. For example, *Xing Ren* (Semen Armeniacae Amarum) has an inhibitory effect on the respiratory center in the brain, thereby exerting its anti-asthmatic effects.[8] *Hou Po* (Cortex Magnoliae Officinalis) has a stimulating effect on the respiratory system to relieve wheezing and dyspnea.[9] Most importantly, *Gan Cao* (Radix Glycyrrhizae) has a remarkable anti-inflammatory effect to reduce the swelling and inflammation in the lung. In fact, the anti-inflammatory influence of glycyrrhizin and glycyrrhetinic acid, two compounds of *Gan Cao* (Radix Glycyrrhizae), is approximately 1/10th that of cortisone.[10]

In addition to treating the cause, *Respitrol (Heat)* is also formulated with herbs that treat the associated symptoms. For example, *Pi Pa Ye* (Folium Eriobotryae), *Gan Cao* (Radix Glycyrrhizae) and *Jie Geng* (Radix Platycodonis) all have antitussive and expectorant effects to relieve coughing and chest congestion.[11,12,13] Furthermore, *Shi Gao* (Gypsum Fibrosum) and *Di Gu Pi* (Cortex Lycii) have antipyretic effect to treat fever by lowering the body temperature.[14,15]

In summary, *Respitrol (Heat)* is an excellent formula to treat respiratory disorders with heat manifestations. Not only does it have good antibiotic effect to treat respiratory tract infection, it also contains many herbs to relieve the associated symptoms.

PHARMACEUTICAL DRUGS & CHINESE MEDICINE: A COMPARATIVE ANALYSIS

Western Medical Approach: Treatment of asthma is generally divided into acute and chronic management. In western medicine, acute asthma is treated by bronchodilators that open the airway and reverse obstruction. Chronic asthma is managed by use of several categories of drugs, including bronchodilators, corticosteroids, theophylline, and cromolyn. Western medicine is extremely effective in treating acute asthma attacks, as use of bronchodilators [such as Proventil or Ventolin (Albuterol) inhalers] generally reverses airway obstruction within minutes. However, western medicine is not as successful in long-term management and prevention of asthma. These drugs do not change the underlying condition of the disease, nor do they improve the constitution of the patient. Therefore, long-term prognosis is often characterized by successful suppression of acute asthma attack, but no change in frequency or severity of recurrent asthma attacks.

Traditional Chinese Medicine Approach: Asthma is treated based on the urgency of the disease presentation and the underlying condition of the patients. Urgency refers to the acute or chronic nature of the disease, while underlying condition refers to the fundamental constitution of the patients. By addressing both the disease and the fundamental constitution, use of herbs achieves both immediate and prolonged effects.

Summation: Both drugs and herbs are effective for treatment of asthma. Generally speaking, drugs are more effective for acute asthma, as they are more potent, and can be delivered via inhalation or intravenous injection to achieve faster onset of relief. However, long-term treatment of asthma with drugs is often less than optimal, as these drugs tend to create tolerance and dependence. Furthermore, they do not change the course of illness, and do not reduce frequency and severity of recurrent asthma attacks. On the other hand, herbs are better for long-term prevention and management of asthma. Herbs strengthen the body and enhance its own ability to manage asthma. However, use of herbs may not be appropriate for acute asthma because they are less immediately potent than some pharmaceuticals, and have a slower onset of action. In conclusion, optimal treatment of asthma does not require

RESPITROL (Heat) ™

choosing between drugs or herbs, but may be gained by embracing the benefits of both, by using drugs for acute treatment and herbs for long-term healing and prevention.

CASE STUDIES

A 36-year-old female computer technician presented with chills and fever, dry mouth and throat, body aches, and thirst. The chills and fever only lasted for one day. Tongue body was red with a thin, white tongue coating. Her pulse was superficial. Although warm to the touch, the patient complained of cold sensations. The practitioner diagnosed her condition as wind-heat invasion. The practitioner prescribed a full dose of *Respitrol (Heat)* for the first three days until the patient's symptoms subsided. The dose was subsequently reduced until all indications of the patient's condition were resolved.

T.G., Albuquerque, New Mexico

D.C., a 50-year-old female, presented common cold symptoms of cough, chest congestion and difficult to expectorate phlegm. She had a slight fever. The tongue was red with yellow coating. The pulse was rapid and slippery. The doctor diagnosed her with Lung heat. The two formulas prescribed were *Respitrol (Heat)* and *Poria XPT*. In three days, the heat was relieved and the phlegm was cleared.

B.F., Newport Beach, California

---

[1] *Planta med*, 1982; 44(2):100
[2] *Yao Jian Gong Zuo Tong Xun* (Journal of Herbal Preparations), 1980; 10(4):209
[3] *Xin Hua Ben Cao Gang Mu* (New Chinese Materia Medica), 1988; 58
[4] *Zhong Yao Xue* (Chinese Herbology), 1998; 648:650
[5] *Zhong Yao Xue* (Chinese Herbology), 1998; 244:245
[6] *Zhong Yao Xue* (Chinese Herbology), 1998; 878:881
[7] *Shan Xi Xin Yi Yao* (New Medicine and Herbology of Shanxi), 1980; 9(11):51
[8] *Life Sci*, 1980; 27(8):659
[9] *Zhong Yao Xue* (Chinese Herbology), 1998; 320:323
[10] *Zhong Cao Yao* (Chinese Herbal Medicine), 1991; 22(10):452
[11] *Zhong Yao Xue* (Chinese Herbology), 1998; 651:653
[12] *Zhong Yao Yao Li Yu Ying Yong* (Pharmacology and Applications of Chinese Herbs), 1983; 264
[13] *Zhong Yao Yao Li Yu Ying Yong* (Pharmacology and Applications of Chinese Herbs), 1983; 866
[14] Hsu, HY. et al. *Oriental Materia Medica, A Concise Guide*. Oriental Healing Arts Institute. 1986
[5] Gottlieb, W. *The Doctor's Book of Home Remedies*, 1990; p31-32
[15] *Yi Xue Zhong Yang Za Zhi* (Central Journal of Medicine), 1967; 223:664

FORMULAS

SAW PALMETTO COMPLEX ™

CLINICAL APPLICATIONS

☯ Enlargement of the prostate gland (benign prostatic hypertrophy)
☯ Urinary urgency with burning, painful urination and possible inflammation

WESTERN THERAPEUTIC ACTIONS

☯ Treats enlarged prostate through anti-androgenic properties [2,3,4]
☯ Reduces pain and dysuria associated with prostatic enlargement [5]

CHINESE THERAPEUTIC ACTIONS

☯ Reduces swelling
☯ Clears turbidity and damp-heat in the lower *jiao*
☯ Promotes urination

DOSAGE

Take 4 capsules three times daily on an empty stomach with warm water. For severe cases, the dosage can be increased up to 6 to 7 capsules three times daily.

INGREDIENTS

Ban Zhi Lian (Herba Scutellariae Barbatae)
Che Qian Zi (Semen Plantaginis)
Chen Pi (Pericarpium Citri Reticulatae)
Dang Gui (Radicis Angelicae Sinensis)
Fang Feng (Radix Saposhnikoviae)
Gan Cao (Radix Glycyrrhizae)
Huang Bai (Cortex Phellodendri)

Jin Yin Hua (Flos Lonicerae)
Mo Yao (Myrrha)
Ru Xiang (Gummi Olibanum)
Saw Palmetto Berries (Fructus Serenoa Repens)
Zao Jiao Ci (Spina Gleditsiae)
Zhe Bei Mu (Bulbus Fritillariae Thunbergii)

FORMULA EXPLANATION

Saw Palmetto Complex is specifically designed to treat benign prostatic hypertrophy (BPH), which is generally considered to be an accumulation of damp-heat in the lower *jiao*. *Saw Palmetto Complex* is formulated to eliminate damp-heat, reduce swelling, and promote normal urination.

Saw Palmetto Berries (Fructus Serenoa Repens) treats benign prostatic hypertrophy (BPH) and improves such symptoms as nocturia, dysuria, flow rate and post-micturition residue.[3] *Che Qian Zi* (Semen Plantaginis) works as a diuretic and has anti-inflammatory functions. *Huang Bai* (Cortex Phellodendri) and *Jin Yin Hua* (Flos Lonicerae) have antibacterial effects to treat possible infections. *Zhe Bei Mu* (Bulbus Fritillariae Thunbergii) disperses lumps and is used here to reduce the enlarged prostate. *Zao Jiao Ci* (Spina Gleditsiae) and *Ban Zhi Lian* (Herba Scutellariae Barbatae) decrease inflammation and dispel pus. *Ru Xiang* (Gummi Olibanum), *Mo Yao* (Myrrha) and *Dang Gui* (Radicis Angelicae Sinensis) invigorate blood, reduce pain and swelling, and break up stagnation. *Fang Feng* (Radix Saposhnikoviae) enters the Urinary Bladder channel and has antibacterial, antifungal and antipyretic functions. *Chen Pi* (Pericarpium Citri Reticulatae) regulates the qi flow and *Gan Cao* (Radix Glycyrrhizae) harmonizes the formula.

SAW PALMETTO COMPLEX ™

NUTRITION

❧ Encourage the patient to eat foods rich in zinc, such as raw pumpkin seeds or pumpkin seed oil. Studies have shown zinc deficiency to be linked to prostate disorders.[1]

❧ Advise the patient to eliminate tobacco smoking, alcoholic beverages, caffeine, and junk foods. Avoid spicy foods and decrease salt intake.

❧ Foods with phytoestrogen, such as soy and yams, have beneficial effect for prostate health.

❧ Increase the consumption of the following foods that are beneficial for prostate health: organic, fresh, leafy vegetables, whole grains and raw wheat germ, carrots, citrus fruits, and natural enzymes.

The Tao of Nutrition by Ni and McNease

❧ Prostate enlargement
  ▪ Recommendations: pumpkin seeds, anise tangerines, cherries, figs, litchis, sunflower seeds, mangos, and seaweeds.
  ▪ Avoid dairy products, rich foods, fatty foods, all stimulants such as alcohol, caffeine, and smoking; stress, tension, sex, and eating meat late in the day.

❧ For more information, please refer to *The Tao of Nutrition* by Dr. Maoshing Ni and Cathy McNease.

LIFESTYLE INSTRUCTIONS

❧ Advise the patient to reduce blood cholesterol levels. Studies have shown high cholesterol to be linked to prostate disorders.[1]

❧ Relaxation exercises help to relieve tension and facilitate bladder emptying.

SUPPLEMENTARY FORMULAS

❧ For Kidney yang deficiency with such signs and symptoms as coldness and weakness of the lower back and knees, urinary incontinence, terminal dripping, polyuria, combine with *Kidney Tonic (Yang)*.

❧ For bacterial prostatitis, use with *V-Statin* or *Herbal ABX*.

❧ For kidney stones, add *Dissolve (KS)*.

❧ For Kidney yin deficiency, add *Kidney Tonic (Yin)*.

❧ For edema and water accumulation, add *Herbal DRX*.

❧ For damp-heat accumulation with turbid, painful urination, use *Gentiana Complex*.

❧ For patients who do not respond to *Saw Palmetto Complex*, use *P-Statin* instead.

❧ For signs and symptoms of excess fire, add *Gardenia Complex*.

❧ For blood stagnation, add *Circulation (SJ)*.

CLINICAL NOTE

❧ *P-Statin* and *Saw Palmetto Complex* are both formulas for benign prostatic hypertrophy (BPH). Both formulas can be used for geriatric men who are beginning to develop enlarged prostate associated with aging and accompanying hormonal changes.
  ▪ *P-Statin* treats BPH by draining damp-heat and tonifying qi and *jing* (essence).
  ▪ *Saw Palmetto Complex* treats BPH by draining damp-heat and reducing swelling.

CAUTIONS

❧ *Saw Palmetto Complex* is designed to treat mild to moderate prostate enlargement. While it may help to promote normal urination, it is not suitable for treatment of prostate cancer, although it may be a helpful adjunct

FORMULAS

SAW PALMETTO COMPLEX ™

to other more specific treatment modalities for prostate cancer. Additional workup is necessary to confirm or rule out diagnosis of prostate cancer.

 ✿ Patients who are on anticoagulant or antiplatelet therapies, such as Coumadin (Warfarin), should use this formula with caution, as there may be a slightly higher risk of bleeding and bruising.

ACUPUNCTURE POINTS

Traditional Points:
✿ *Hegu* (LI 4), *Sanyinjiao* (SP 6), *Guanyuan* (CV 4), *Zhongji* (CV 3), *Yanglingquan* (GB 34), *Qugu* (CV 2), *Huiyin* (CV 1), and *Ciliao* (BL 32).
✿ Apply moxa to *Guanyuan* (CV 4) and *Zusanli* (ST 36).

Balance Method by Dr. Richard Tan:
✿ Left side: *Dazhong* (KI 4), *Zhaohai* (KI 6), *Zhongfeng* (LR 4), *Yangxi* (LI 5), *Yangchi* (TH 4), and Prostate point on the ear.
✿ Right side: *Jiexi* (ST 41), *Shenmai* (BL 62), *Lieque* (LU 7), and *Daling* (PC 7).
✿ Left and right side can be alternated from treatment to treatment.
✿ For additional information on the Balance Method, please refer to *Dr. Tan's Strategy of Twelve Magical Points* by Dr. Richard Tan.

Auricular Acupuncture by Dr. Li-Chun Huang:
✿ Prostatitis: Prostate, Urethra, Pelvic, Kidney, Lower Jiao, Liver, Spleen, *San Jiao*, and Endocrine.
✿ Hypertrophy of prostate: Prostate, Urethra, Pelvic, Kidney, Liver, Lower Jiao, Pituitary, Endocrine, *San Jiao*, and Gonadotropin.
✿ Orchitis and epididymitis: Testis, Endocrine, Adrenal Gland, Kidney, Liver, Prostate, Pelvic, Internal Genital, and External Genital. Bleed Ear Apex.
✿ For additional information on the location and explanation of these points, please refer to *Auricular Treatment Formula and Prescriptions* by Dr. Li-Chun Huang.

MODERN RESEARCH

Saw Palmetto Complex is formulated with ingredients that have been shown to treat benign prostatic hypertrophy (BPH).[2,3,4]

A number of recent studies have shown Saw Palmetto Berries (Fructus Serenoa Repens) to be effective in the treatment of benign prostatic hypertrophy (BPH). It treats BPH through its anti-androgenic properties. Namely, it prevents the conversion of testosterone to dihydrotestosterone (DHT) and inhibits DHT binding to cellular and nuclear receptor sites.[4] In a double-blind, placebo-controlled study of 110 patients, use of Saw Palmetto Berries (Fructus Serenoa Repens) was found to significantly improve symptoms associated with BPH such as nocturia, dysuria, flow rate and post-micturition residue. Clinically, the effectiveness of Saw Palmetto Berries (Fructus Serenoa Repens) was found to be comparable to Minipress (Prazosin) in a 12-week study, as measured by flowmeter and subjective assessments of irritation.[2]

Many of the herbs in *Saw Palmetto Complex* have diuretic properties to promote regular and painless urination. *Huang Bai* (Cortex Phellodendri) increases the muscle contraction of the bladder to increase the force of urination. *Che Qian Zi* (Semen Plantaginis) has diuretic functions that increase the output of urine, and *Zao Jiao Ci* (Spina Gleditsiae) reduces inflammation and dispels pus.[5]

FORMULAS

SAW PALMETTO COMPLEX ™

PHARMACEUTICAL DRUGS & CHINESE MEDICINE: A COMPARATIVE ANALYSIS

Western Medical Approach: Benign prostate hypertrophy (BPH) is a disorder that affects most men as they age. In western medicine, BPH may be treated with drugs that relax the bladder muscle to improve urination [such as Minipress (Prazosin)], or drugs that shrink the prostate [such as Proscar (Finasteride)]. However, Minipress (Prazosin) is an alpha-adrenergic drug originally used to treat hypertension, and may cause side effects such as hypotension, dizziness, lightheadedness, orthostasis, syncope, and if/when the drug is discontinued, rebound hypertension. Proscar (Finasteride) is effective, but requires three months or more to take effect, and may cause sexual dysfunction with side effects such as impotence, decreased libido, and decreased volume of ejaculate. Lastly, in severe cases of prostate hypertrophy, a catheter is inserted through the penis into the bladder to drain urine. Finally, western medicine considers surgical removal of the prostate to be the best option.

Traditional Chinese Medicine Approach: The treatment in TCM plan is to address both symptoms and cause of BPH. To alleviate the symptoms, herbs promote normal urination, relieve pain, and reduce edema. Furthermore, herbs reduce prostate hypertrophy by blocking the conversion of testosterone to dihydrotestosterone (DHT) and its binding to cellular and nuclear receptor sites. In short, by targeting both cause and symptoms, herbal therapy achieve both short- and long-term success.

Summation: Both western and traditional Chinese medicines are effective to treat BPH. Drug therapy is usually unsatisfactory, as its effectiveness is limited, and it is associated with significant side effects. Herbal therapy, on the other hand, is both safe and effective, and has short- and long-term benefits. However, in serious cases of prostate cancer, patients should be referred to western medicine as use of herbs as a sole treatment modality is not recommended.

CASE STUDIES

A 73-year-old retired man with a history of chronic prostatitis complained of difficulty urinating and incontinence. In addition, he also presented with pain in the prostate and rectal area. He had a history of chronic prostate hypertrophy and chronic infection. Pulse indicated Kidney yin deficiency. Tongue was red with bald patches, which the patient noted for many years. The patient was diagnosed with chronic prostatitis due to Kidney yin deficiency, and was treated with *Saw Palmetto Complex* (4 capsules three times daily). After taking *Saw Palmetto Complex* sporadically for 2 ½ months, the patient reported a decrease of symptoms and improved urinary functions. When refraining from taking the herbs, he noticed a return of his symptoms. Once the patient reinstated his herbal treatment, he felt his overall condition progressed and that his urinary dysfunction diminished.

V.W., Kilauea, Hawaii

A.W. is a 42-year-old male who presented with prostatitis, frequent urination and pain while sitting for a long period of time. All the above symptoms worsened with stress. Western diagnosis was benign prostatic hypertrophy with normal PSA level. The diagnosis was stagnation and damp-heat in the lower *jiao*. He was prescribed *Saw Palmetto Complex* at 6 grams a day. This patient did not receive acupuncture. After eight weeks of treatment, the patient reported the pain while sitting got much better and the urination did not hurt and was not as frequent. He was able to sleep through the night. The patient is now on a maintenance dosage of 3 grams a day.

W.F., Bloomfield, New Jersey

---

[1] Balch, J. and Balch, P. *Prescriptions for Nutritional Healing*. Avery Publishing Group. 1997
[2] Semino, M. et al. Symptomatic treatment of benign hypertrophy of the prostate. comparative study of prazosin and Serenoa repens. *Arch Esp Urol*; 45:211. 1992

FORMULAS

SAW PALMETTO COMPLEX ™

[3] Champault, G. et al. A double-blind trial of an extract of the plant Serenoa repens in benign prostatic hyperplasia. *Br. J. Clin Pharmacol*; 18:461. 1984

[4] Sultan, C. et al. Inhibition of androgen metabolism and binding by a liposterolic extract of Serenoa repens b in human foreskin fibroblasts. *J Steroid Biochem*; 20:5151984

[5] Yeung, HC. *Handbook of Chinese Herbs*. Institute of Chinese Herbs. 1996

FORMULAS

SCHISANDRA ZZZ ™

CLINICAL APPLICATIONS

- Insomnia with difficulty falling and staying asleep
- Disturbed sleep with excessive dreams and worries; "worrywarts"
- Poor memory with dizziness, weakness, fatigue, and anemia
- Fragile mental state with excessive worries, insomnia, disturbed sleep, dizziness, constant fatigue and weakness
- Postpartum depression with weakness and anemia

WESTERN THERAPEUTIC ACTIONS

- Mild sedative effect to facilitate falling and staying asleep [4,5,6,7,8]
- Adaptogenic effect to help the patient cope with stress, anxiety and excessive worries [9,10]
- Muscle-relaxant property to relieve muscle tension and tightness [7]
- Improves overall quality of sleep [4,5,6]

CHINESE THERAPEUTIC ACTIONS

- Nourishes the Spleen and the Heart
- Tonifies qi and blood
- Tranquilizes the *shen* (spirit)

DOSAGE

Take 4 capsules three times daily with warm water on an empty stomach. For treatment of insomnia and disturbed sleep, take 8 capsules 30 to 60 minutes before bedtime.

INGREDIENTS

Bai Zhu (Rhizoma Atractylodis Macrocephalae)
Da Zao (Fructus Jujubae)
Dang Gui (Radicis Angelicae Sinensis)
Fu Ling (Poria)
Huang Qi (Radix Astragali)
Long Yan Rou (Arillus Longan)
Mu Xiang (Radix Aucklandiae)
Ren Shen (Radix Ginseng)

Sheng Jiang (Rhizoma Zingiberis Recens)
Suan Zao Ren (Semen Zizyphi Spinosae)
Wu Wei Zi (Fructus Schisandrae Chinensis)
Xie Cao (Radix et Rhizoma Valerianae)
Yuan Zhi (Radix Polygalae)
Zhi Gan Cao (Radix Glycyrrhizae Preparata)

FORMULA EXPLANATION

Schisandra ZZZ is formulated to nourish the Spleen and the Heart, tranquilize the *shen* (spirit), and tonify qi and blood. Clinical applications of *Schisandra ZZZ* include insomnia, difficulty falling asleep and staying asleep, poor memory, dizziness, weakness, constant fatigue, postpartum depression due to anemia, etc.

Wu Wei Zi (Fructus Schisandrae Chinensis) replenishes the vital energy and has a regulatory effect on the central nervous system (CNS). *Ren Shen* (Radix Ginseng), *Huang Qi* (Radix Astragali), *Bai Zhu* (Rhizoma Atractylodis Macrocephalae) and *Fu Ling* (Poria) tonify the Spleen qi and enable it to generate blood to nourish the *shen* (spirit) of the Heart. *Dang Gui* (Radicis Angelicae Sinensis) and *Long Yan Rou* (Arillus Longan) tonify blood and calm the *shen* (spirit). *Suan Zao Ren* (Semen Zizyphi Spinosae) and *Yuan Zhi* (Radix Polygalae) are tranquilizing herbs with sedative and hypnotic effects. *Xie Cao* (Radix et Rhizoma Valerianae) is an herb that has tranquilizing and calming

FORMULAS

SCHISANDRA ZZZ ™

effects. *Zhi Gan Cao* (Radix Glycyrrhizae Preparata), *Sheng Jiang* (Rhizoma Zingiberis Recens) and *Da Zao* (Fructus Jujubae) improve the appetite, harmonize, and strengthen the gastrointestinal tract. *Mu Xiang* (Radix Aucklandiae) revives the Spleen and dispels stagnation.

SUPPLEMENTARY FORMULAS

- ❧ For depression, combine with *Shine*.
- ❧ For Spleen qi deficiency with loose stool and poor appetite, add *GI Tonic*.
- ❧ For Liver qi stagnation manifesting in irritability, restlessness, or PMS, combine with *Calm*.
- ❧ For severe insomnia with disturbed *shen* (spirit) in excess patients, use *Calm (ES)*.
- ❧ For insomnia due to stress in patients with deficiency, add *Calm ZZZ*.
- ❧ For menopausal symptoms, combine with *Balance (Heat)*.
- ❧ For dysmenorrhea, combine with *Mense-Ease*.
- ❧ For hair loss, dry or brittle hair, combine with *Polygonum 14*.
- ❧ To tonify the overall bodily constitution, combine with *Imperial Tonic*.
- ❧ For forgetfulness, add *Enhance Memory*.
- ❧ For coldness of the extremities, add *Balance (Cold)*.
- ❧ For Kidney yang deficiency, add *Kidney Tonic (Yang)*.
- ❧ For Kidney yin deficiency, add *Kidney Tonic (Yin)*.

NUTRITION

- ❧ Increase consumption of foods that contain high levels of tryptophan such as turkey, bananas, figs, dates, yogurt, milk, tuna, and whole grain crackers as they help promote sleep.
- ❧ Avoid foods that contain tyramine near bedtime. Tyramine increases the release of the brain stimulant norepinephrine. Foods with high content of tyramine include bacon, cheese, chocolate, eggplant, ham, potatoes, sugar, sausage, spinach, and tomatoes.
- ❧ A glass of warm milk with honey is helpful for mild insomnia.

LIFESTYLE INSTRUCTIONS

- ❧ Especially at night, patients with insomnia should avoid alcohol, caffeine, and tobacco.
- ❧ If insomnia is due to overwork, do not to work in the bedroom and remove anything that may be a reminder of the office or work. A warm bath or light snack before bedtime may also be helpful.
- ❧ Patient should be counseled to not worry about things they cannot control or change.

CLINICAL NOTE

- ❧ *Schisandra ZZZ* is excellent to take for a week after each menstrual cycle. It replenishes the blood and qi lost during each period.

CAUTIONS

- ❧ Patients who are on anticoagulant or antiplatelet therapies, such as Coumadin (Warfarin), should use this formula with caution, as there may be a slightly higher risk of bleeding and bruising.
- ❧ This herbal formula may cause drowsiness in individuals who are sensitive to herbs. Patients are advised not to drive or operate heavy machinery while taking this herbal formula. Similarly, alcohol is not recommended as it may intensify the effect.

SCHISANDRA *ZZZ* ™

ACUPUNCTURE POINTS

Traditional Points:
- ❧ *Shenmen* (HT 7), *Sanyinjiao* (SP 6), *Xinshu* (BL 15), *Pishu* (BL 20), *Taixi* (KI 3), *Weishu* (BL 21), and *Zusanli* (ST 36).
- ❧ Extra point *Anmian*, *Shenmen* (HT 7) and *Baihui* (GV 20).

Balance Method by Dr. Richard Tan:
- ❧ Left side: *Yinlingquan* (SP 9), *Xuehai* (SP 10), *Sanyinjiao* (SP 6), *Rangu* (KI 2), *Dazhong* (KI 4), *Fuliu* (KI 7), *Hegu* (LI 4), *Zhongzhu* (TH 3), *Zhizheng* (SI 7), and Ear S*henmen*.
- ❧ Right side: *Zusanli* (ST 36), *Jiexi* (ST 41), *Shaofu* (HT 8), and *Tongli* (HT 5), *Shaohai* (HT 3).
- ❧ Left and right side can be alternated from treatment to treatment.
- ❧ To read more about Dr. Tan's acupuncture strategy, see his book *Dr. Tan's Strategy of Twelve Magic Points*.

Ear Points:
- ❧ Insomnia: Heart, Kidney, and Parietal Lobe. Place magnetic ear balls or embed ear needles on one or both ears every evening and remove in them morning. Five days equal one course of treatment.
- ❧ Frequent dreams: Heart, Kidney, and Frontal Lobe. Embed needles and switch ear every three days. Patient should be instructed to massage those points at least three to four times each day for one to two minutes.
- ❧ Anemia: Bone Marrow, Kidney, Spleen, Ovaries or Testis, and Adrenal Gland.
- ❧ Excessive worry or neurasthenia:
  - o Main points: *Shenmen*, Heart, Subcortex, and Brain Stem.
  - o Adjunct points: Kidney, Spleen, Liver, Endocrine, and Stomach.

Auricular Acupuncture by Dr. Li-Chun Huang:
- ❧ Dream-disturbed sleep: Dream-Disturbed Sleep Area, Shenmen, Occiput, Heart, Neurasthenia Area, Neurasthenia Point, and Nervous Subcortex. Bleed Ear Apex.
  - ▪ For dream-disturbed sleep due to disharmony between the Heart and Kidney, add Kidney.
  - ▪ For dream-disturbed sleep due to deficiency of both Heart and Spleen, add Spleen.
  - ▪ For dream-disturbed sleep due to stagnancy of Liver qi, add Liver.
  - ▪ For nightmares, add Gallbladder.
- ❧ For additional information on the location and explanation of these points, please refer to *Auricular Treatment Formula and Prescriptions* by Dr. Li-Chun Huang.

MODERN RESEARCH

Schisandra ZZZ contains herbs having a wide range of clinical functions, including adaptogenic, muscle-relaxant, sedative, tranquilizing, and anti-aging properties.

Wu Wei Zi (Fructus Schisandrae Chinensis) has many functions and clinical applications. In addition to its use as a liver protectant, it has such uses as a general tonic, a nervous system regulator, gastrointestinal therapy, an adaptogen and others. *Wu Wei Zi* (Fructus Schisandrae Chinensis) possesses pronounced liver-protectant effect by protecting the hepatocyte plasma membrane and preventing the entry of toxic substances.[1] Furthermore, it repairs liver damage by increasing blood flow to the liver and increasing regeneration of liver cells.[2] In addition to its liver-protectant effect, *Wu Wei Zi* (Fructus Schisandrae Chinensis) stimulates the nervous system to increase reflex responses and improve mental alertness and treat memory loss, helps the body to adapt to stress by balancing body fluids, and improves failing senses.[3]

FORMULAS

SCHISANDRA ZZZ ™

Xie Cao (Radix et Rhizoma Valerianae) also has a wide range of functions, including but not limited to antispasmodic and sedative/hypnotic properties.[4,5] In a double-blind crossover study of 128 participants, it was found that those who took *Xie Cao* (Radix et Rhizoma Valerianae) had a significant improvement in sleep quality with less awakenings and less somnolence the next morning.[6] The clinical effects of *Xie Cao* (Radix et Rhizoma Valerianae) are thought to be similar to those of short-acting benzodiazepines.[7]

Chinese herbs that promote sleep include *Fu Ling* (Poria), *Suan Zao Ren* (Semen Zizyphi Spinosae), *Long Yan Rou* (Arillus Longan), and *Yuan Zhi* (Radix Polygalae). *Fu Ling* (Poria) has sedating and tranquilizing effects. *Suan Zao Ren* (Semen Zizyphi Spinosae) and *Yuan Zhi* (Radix Polygalae) have sedative and hypnotic effects. *Long Yan Rou* (Arillus Longan) has sedative effects.[8] They are commonly used to reduce the time necessary to fall asleep, reduce the number of awakenings at night, and improve the overall quality of sleep.

Common applications of *Ren Shen* (Radix Ginseng) include a general strengthening effect, adaptogenic effect against stress, and enhancement in mental and physical performance.[9] The general strengthening and adaptogenic effects include a non-specific increase in resistance to the noxious effects of physical, chemical or biological stress.[10]

PHARMACEUTICAL DRUGS & CHINESE MEDICINE: A COMPARATIVE ANALYSIS

Western Medical Approach: Insomnia is defined as difficulty falling and/or staying asleep. While there are many potential causes of insomnia, pharmaceutical treatment focuses primarily on using sedatives and hypnotics for symptomatic treatment. The sleeping pills most frequently used include benzodiazepines such as Halcion (triazolam), Restoril (temazepam), and Dalmane (flurazepam). The main advantages of these drugs are they are extremely potent, and generally induce sedation within 30 to 60 minutes. However, their effect generally lasts for a long period of time, resulting in drowsiness the following morning. Furthermore, if used for a long period of time, they cause tolerance and dependence, making it increasingly difficult to restore normal sleeping patterns. Finally, these drugs are also likely to cause other side effects, such as blurred vision, changes in sex drive or ability, shuffling walk, persistent, fine tremor or inability to sit still, difficulty breathing or swallowing, severe skin rash, yellowing of the skin or eyes, irregular heartbeat, and addiction. Therefore, these drugs should only be used when necessary for short-term treatment of insomnia, and not be relied upon on a long-term basis.

Traditional Chinese Medicine Approach: Insomnia [inability to fall and/or stay asleep] is the direct result of *shen* (spirit) disturbance. Therefore, the main focus of this formula is to use herbs that calm the *shen* (spirit) to treat insomnia. Furthermore, lack of sleep over a long period of time contributes to deficiency. Therefore, many tonic herbs are also used to supplement such weakness and deficiencies. It is important to remember that herbs do not "sedate" the patient to treat insomnia. Rather, they calm the *shen* (spirit) and nourish the deficiency to restore normal waking / sleeping cycles. Therefore, herbs should be taken continuously for at least one week to restore normal waking / sleeping cycles, as they do not work on an "as needed" basis like sleeping pills.

Summation: It is important to re-evaluate the patients periodically. Individuals who continue to have insomnia should be examined for secondary causes, such as pain, anxiety, stress, depression, and withdrawal from drug or alcohol. While drugs and herbs are both effective, insomnia can only be treated successfully on a long-term basis when these secondary causes are removed.

CASE STUDIES

E.E. is a 30-year-old postpartum female who presented difficulty falling and staying asleep, restlessness, overactive mind, difficulty concentrating, fearfulness and anxiousness. The pulse was thin, weak and rapid. The tongue was very red with peeled edges and quivering at the same time. The face, ear and neck were red and flushed. The practitioner diagnosed her with postpartum depression with Heart fire and Spleen and Heart qi and blood deficiencies. *Schisandra ZZZ* was prescribed at 3 capsules three times daily. Within the first week, the patient noticed reduced anxiety. She was able to fall asleep and the mind was calmer.

S.S., Topanga, California

A tired and exhausted patient presented with general aches and pain in the neck and low back. There was also a history of poor sleep and digestion with no constipation. The practitioner felt the patient had over-worked herself throughout the years and that the condition was due to "wear and tear." The diagnosis was qi and blood deficiencies with underlying yin and yang deficiencies. *Imperial Tonic, Schisandra ZZZ* and *Bu Zhong Yi Qi Tang* (Tonify the Middle and Augment the Qi Decoction) were given along with acupuncture and massage therapy. The treatment was concluded to be quite effective.

S.C., La Crescenta, California

An 18-year-old patient presented with life-long insomnia. She often needed one hour to fall asleep. Her sleep quality was quite poor, and she remained sluggish throughout the day. The practitioner diagnosed the case as qi and blood deficiency. The patient took 6 capsules of *Schisandra ZZZ* 30 minutes before bedtime. After 3 weeks of treatment, the patient was able to fall asleep within 15 minutes and awaken with more energy.

M.K., Sherman Oaks, California

D.S., a 45-year-old female, presented with insomnia, mood swings, cramps and fatigue. The tongue was slightly purplish pale with teeth marks. The coating was thin and white. The pulse was deep and wiry. She was diagnosed with Spleen qi deficiency and blood deficiency. *Nourish, Calm, Schisandra ZZZ* were prescribed. The patient reported her sleep pattern improved, her moods balanced and her energy level increased. She was very happy with the herbs.

B.F., Newport Beach, California

L.A., a 37-year-old female patient presented with insomnia, with difficulty falling and staying asleep. Other symptoms included neck and shoulder stiffness, TMJ pain, heavy menstrual flow, and cramping with blood clots. She complained of marital problems and held the stress and sadness within. She was also seeing a psychotherapist. The blood pressure was 123/86 mmHg and her heart rate was 88 beats per minute. The tongue appeared to be salmon pink in color, moist with numerous fissures from the center to the tip. The tongue was swollen and the tip was red. The pulse was slippery and thin. The TCM diagnosis was Spleen qi and Heart blood deficiencies with Liver qi stagnation. *Calm* was prescribed. *Calm* alone eased her tension, but did not help much with her energy. Her sleep improved slightly. The TMJ resolved after eight acupuncture treatments. After two months, *Schisandra ZZZ* was added. The patient then slept through the night much more soundly. However, she still complained about the neck and shoulder pain.

J.C.O., Whittier, California

H.G., a 55-year-old female, presented with agitation, anxiety, depression, and insomnia, and stated that she was easily angered. Her tongue was purple, with a thin white coating; her pulse was soft and wiry. The Western diagnosis was depressive-anxiety disorder; the TCM diagnosis was Liver fire rising with Liver qi stagnation. *Calm ES* was prescribed at three capsules, three times daily. Upon follow-up one week later, the patient reported a decrease of anxiety and agitation, but continuing insomnia. *Schisandra ZZZ* was added to her herbal regimen. One week later, the patient reported the insomnia completely resolved; but said that she experienced somnolence in the morning. She was told to reduce *Schisandra ZZZ* from three times daily to twice daily, eliminating the morning dose. After the dosage adjustment, the patient reported calm, uninterrupted sleep, and waking feeling energized, without lethargy or grogginess. She continues to take *Schisandra ZZZ* on an as-needed basis.

C.L., Chino Hills, California

FORMULAS

SCHISANDRA ZZZ ™

A 53-year-old male miner presented with insomnia, depression, stress, anxiety and fatigue. He had difficulty falling asleep, which was aggravated by relentless worrying. Other symptoms included palpitations and occasional dizziness. A choppy pulse and a pale tongue were present, along with a pale complexion. The practitioner diagnosed the condition as Heart and Spleen blood deficiency. After the initial treatment, his sleep improved from 2 to 3 hours per night to 5 to 6 hours per night. The patient was no longer fatigued and felt much calmer. Because of his occupation and the nature of his condition, he was unable to take the western medication since drowsiness was one side effect. The combination of *Schisandra ZZZ* and *Calm (ES)* made it possible to manage his condition with no known side effects. The practitioner recommended continuous application of the herbal combination of *Schisandra ZZZ* and *Calm (ES)* for his medical condition.

D.M., Raton, New Mexico

M.P., a 74-year-old female, presented with insomnia. She was prescribed Ambien (Zolpidem) by her medical doctor but could not take it because of an allergy to the medication where her tongue would swell and burn. She was then put on Zyprexa (Olanzapine) and Paxil (Paroxetine). The patient reported she also had an allergic reaction (tongue swelling) to Zyprexa (Olanzapine). The patient, described by the practitioner, was a very anxious, nervous type of person who would hyperventilate when stressed. Her husband also has multiple medical problems and she stated she was worried about him. Her blood pressure was 120/70 mmHg and her heart rate was 70 beats per minute. The TCM diagnosis was Spleen and Heart disharmony with qi and blood deficiencies. *Schisandra ZZZ* was prescribed at 4 to 6 capsules at night. The patient reported that taking 4 capsules allowed her to sleep for four hours and then she was awake. Dosage was then increased to 6 capsules at night and she reported she was able to sleep five to six hours. The patient is still currently under care and the practitioner is adjusting the dose slowly.

M.H., West Palm Beach, Florida

A 42-year-old female presented with insomnia due to family-related stress. She reported having difficulty falling asleep due to excessive thoughts, thus creating morning fatigue that "feels like a hangover." The TCM diagnosis was insomnia due to Spleen and Heart qi deficiencies with *shen* (spirit) disturbance. After she began taking three capsules of *Schisandra ZZZ* at bedtime, the patient reported much improved sleep without difficulty falling or staying asleep.

C.L., Chino Hills, California

E.P., a 32-year-old female, presented with a 2½-year history of vertigo, associated with insomnia, palpitations, anxiety and nausea. She also suffered from irritable bowel syndrome with alternating diarrhea and constipation. She had an unsteady gait and was unable to drive. For the Western diagnosis of anxiety disorder, the TCM diagnosis was Liver fire. Initially, *Calm* and *Gentiana Complex* were prescribed at two capsules each, three times daily, but then the dosage was increased to three capsules of each, three times daily. After three weeks, the signs and symptoms of irritable bowel syndrome were resolved, and *Gentiana Complex* was discontinued. On the sixth treatment, the patient reported all symptoms improved. However, work-related stress anxiety remained. On the 15th visit, *Calm* was changed to *Schisandra ZZZ* to help with her insomnia. After taking this formula for nine days, the patient reported much improvement in her sleeping patterns, from 5 to 6 hours of interrupted sleep to 6 to 7 hours of uninterrupted sleep. The patient was treated with acupuncture five times throughout the course of herbal treatment.

C.L., Chino Hills, California

A 50-year-old female public information specialist who was emotionally labile presented with pain in the shoulder, neck, thoracic, lumbar and foot. Her lumbar discs at L4 and L5 were herniated. In addition to migraines and bouts of constipation, she also complained of anxiety, depression and insomnia, all of which may be attributed to some side effects of taking multiple pharmaceuticals. The practitioner diagnosed her condition as qi and blood stagnation as well as Liver depression. *Corydalin* and *Schisandra ZZZ* were given. *Corydalin* significantly reduced her pain. She was able to lessen the use of oxycontin and Duragesic (Fentanyl) patches significantly. In fact, the dosages of

FORMULAS

SCHISANDRA ZZZ ™

oxycontin and Duragesic (Fentanyl) patches were reduced by as much as 75%. Furthermore, the practitioner observed that *Corydalin* was also effective to maintain other patients who suffered from occasional pain. The majority of patients (about 90%) who took *Corydalin* responded favorably, especially since most were experiencing digestive side effects with ibuprofen.

F.G., Sykesville, Maryland

[1] Nagai, H. et al. *Planta Medica*. 55(1):13-17. 1989.

[2] Takeda, S. et al. *Nippon Yakurigaku Zasshi*. 88(4):321-30. 1986

[3] Chevallier, A. *Encyclopedia of Medicinal Plants*. New York, NY: DK Publishing. 1996

[4] Hazelhoff, B. et al. Antispasmodic effects of valeriana compounds: an in-vivo and in-vitro study on the guinea pig ileum. *Arch Int Pharmacodyn*; 257:274. 1982

[5] Hendriks, H. et al. central nervous depressant activity of valerenic acid in the mouse. *Planta Med*; Feb 28. 1985

[6] Leathwood, PD. et al. Aqueous extract of valerian root (Valeriana officinalis l.) improves sleep quality in man. *Pharmacol Biochem Behav*; 17:65. 1982

[7] Von Eickstedt, KW. *Arzneimittelforschung*; 19:995. 1969

[8] Yeung, HC. Handbook of Chinese Herbs. *Institute of Chinese Medicine*. 1996

[9] Olin, B, et al. Ginseng. *The Lawrence Review of Natural Products by Facts and Comparison*. Sep 1990

[10] Brekhman II, *Dardymov IV*, Lloydia 32:46, 1969

FORMULAS

SHINE ™

CLINICAL APPLICATIONS

☙ Depression [1,3,4,5,6,7]

☙ Depression with low energy, prolonged sadness or irritability, and lack of interest in daily activities

WESTERN THERAPEUTIC ACTIONS

☙ Antidepressant effect to elevate mood and energy [1,3,4,5,6,7]

☙ Promotes the digestion and utilization of energy

CHINESE THERAPEUTIC ACTIONS

☙ Relieves food, qi, blood, and phlegm stagnation

☙ Promotes movement of qi

☙ Releases constraint

DOSAGE

Take 4 capsules three times daily with warm water on an empty stomach. Dosage may be increased up to 5 to 7 capsules if the condition is severe.

INGREDIENTS

Chai Hu (Radix Bupleuri)
Chuan Xiong (Rhizoma Ligustici Chuanxiong)
Da Zao (Fructus Jujubae)
Gan Cao (Radix Glycyrrhizae)
Guan Ye Lian Qiao (Herba Hypericum)
He Huan Pi (Cortex Albiziae)
Long Gu (Os Draconis)
Lu Cha (Folium Camellia Sinensis)

Mu Li (Concha Ostreae)
Shen Qu (Massa Fermentata)
Shi Chang Pu (Rhizoma Acori)
Xiang Fu (Rhizoma Cyperi)
Yu Jin (Radix Curcumae)
Yuan Zhi (Radix Polygalae)
Zhi Zi (Fructus Gardeniae)

FORMULA EXPLANATION

Shine is formulated specifically to treat depression, which according to traditional Chinese medicine is a disease caused by prolonged stagnation of qi, blood, dampness, or food. The treatment protocol is to break up all stagnation and moisten the internal organs.

Xiang Fu (Rhizoma Cyperi) and *Chai Hu* (Radix Bupleuri) promote the flow of Liver qi and reduce hypochondriac distention. *Yu Jin* (Radix Curcumae) and *Chuan Xiong* (Rhizoma Ligustici Chuanxiong) relieve stagnation by invigorating blood flow. *Shen Qu* (Massa Fermentata) helps digestion by removing food stagnation. *Gan Cao* (Radix Glycyrrhizae) and *Da Zao* (Fructus Jujubae) nourish the Heart and moisten internal dryness. *Yuan Zhi* (Radix Polygalae) and *He Huan Pi* (Cortex Albiziae) calm the *shen* (spirit) and relieve depression. *Lu Cha* (Folium Camellia Sinensis) lifts the mood. *Zhi Zi* (Fructus Gardeniae) sedates heat in the Heart and relieves irritability. *Shi Chang Pu* (Rhizoma Acori) opens the orifices, eliminates phlegm to increase alertness, and calms the *shen* (spirit). *Long Gu* (Os Draconis) and *Mu Li* (Concha Ostreae) have tranquilizing functions to alleviate insomnia and dream-disturbed sleep. Finally, *Guan Ye Lian Qiao* (Herba Hypericum), also known as St. John's Wort, was clinically found to be effective against depression, and enhances the overall effectiveness of this formula.

SHINE ™

SUPPLEMENTARY FORMULAS

- For vegetative depression with withdrawal, no desire to speak, poor appetite, and insomnia, combine with *Schisandra ZZZ*.
- For depression with stress, anxiety, restlessness (manic-depressives), add *Calm (ES)*.
- For a quick boost of energy and vitality, combine with *Vibrant*.
- For constant fatigue and lack of energy, combine with *Imperial Tonic*.
- To strengthen the constitutional weakness and deficiency, use with *Cordyceps 3*.
- For loss of sexual desire, combine with *Vitality*.
- For over-weight or excessive weight gain, combine with *Herbalite*.
- For patients who are "burnt out" with adrenal insufficiency, use with *Adrenoplex*.
- For difficulty with concentration, poor memory or forgetfulness, use with *Enhance Memory*.
- With insomnia in patients who worry excessively or have anemia, *Schisandra ZZZ*.
- For insomnia with stress in patients with deficiency, add *Calm ZZZ*.
- With headache, add *Corydalin*.
- For heat sensations, irritability or nightmares due to excess fire, add *Gardenia Complex*.
- For chronic depressive patients who do not respond to any of the above treatment or show little result, add *Circulation (SJ)*.

NUTRITION

- Avoid greasy and fried foods. A diet high in saturated fat may cause sluggishness, fatigue and slow thinking.
- Depression may be due in part to nutritional deficiency. Foods such as white bread, flour, saturated animal fats, hydrogenated vegetable oils, sweets, soft drinks, and canned goods deprive the body of vitamin B and increase the probability of depression.
- Avoid a diet too low in complex carbohydrates as it may cause serotonin depletion and depression.
- Stay away from wheat products, sugar, alcohol, caffeine, dairy products and processed foods.
- Eat plenty of fresh fruits, vegetables, and whole grains.

LIFESTYLE INSTRUCTIONS

- Exercise outdoors and under the sun will help to lift depression. It has been found that exercise helps people who are depressed by making them more energetic and stress-tolerant.
- A balanced lifestyle of work, rest and exercise is extremely important to achieve better mental and physical health.
- Massaging the nerves along the spine will help to relieve tension associated with depression.

CAUTIONS

- This formula is contraindicated during pregnancy and nursing.
- Use of *Guan Ye Lian Qiao* (Herba Hypericum) is sometimes associated with rash and photosensitivity. Patients should avoid exposure to sunlight or wear protective clothing.
- The concurrent use of *Guan Ye Lian Qiao* (Herba Hypericum) and antidepressant drugs should be avoided, as the combination may lead to serotonin syndrome. *Guan Ye Lian Qiao* (Herba Hypericum) has been shown to inhibit the uptake of serotonin, norepinephrine, and dopamine *in vitro* at high concentrations. The antidepressant drugs include monoamine oxidase inhibitors (MAOI), tricyclic antidepressants (TCA), and selective serotonin reuptake inhibitors (SSRI).
- Use of *Guan Ye Lian Qiao* (Herba Hypericum) may induce cytochrome P-450 system of the liver, leading to increased metabolism and decreased plasma concentration of certain drugs, such as cyclosporine

FORMULAS

SHINE ™

(Sandimmune/Neoral), ethinyloestradiol and desogestrel (combined oral contraceptive), theophylline (Theo-Dur), digoxin (Lanoxin), and indinavir (Crixivan).[2]

ACUPUNCTURE POINTS

Traditional Points:
- *Qimen* (LR 14), *Taichong* (LR 3), *Xingjian* (LR 2), *Guanyuan* (CV 4), *Shanzhong* (CV 17), and *Ganshu* (BL 18).
- *Taichong* (LR 3), *Shuaigu* (GB 8), and *Neiguan* (PC 6).

Balance Method by Dr. Richard Tan:
- Left side: *Qiuxu* (GB 40), *Yanglingquan* (GB 34), *Shenmen* (HT 7), *Tongli* (HT 5), *Shaohai* (HT 3).
- Right side: *Taichong* (LR 3), *Ligou* (LR 5), *Zhongzhu* (TH 3), *Waiguan* (TH 5), and *Tianjing* (TH 10).
- Bilateral Ear *Shenmen*.
- Alternate sides with each treatment.
- For additional information on the Balance Method, please refer to *Dr. Tan's Strategy of Twelve Magical Points* by Dr. Richard Tan.

Auricular Acupuncture by Dr. Li-Chun Huang:
- Depression, anxiety, stress, and nervousness: *Shenmen*, Liver, Heart, Occiput, Nervous Subcortex, Anxious Point, and Be Happy Point. Bleed Ear Apex
- For additional information on the location and explanation of these points, please refer to *Auricular Treatment Formula and Prescriptions* by Dr. Li-Chun Huang.

MODERN RESEARCH

Shine is comprised of herbs with demonstrated effectiveness to relieve depression, elevate mood and energy, promote digestion, and improve the utilization of energy.

Guan Ye Lian Qiao (Herba Hypericum), also known as St. John's Wort, is an herb used in both China and European countries dating back to the Middle Ages. It was used historically in treatment of inflammation, gastritis and insomnia; more recently, however, its use centers almost exclusively on the treatment of depression.[1] *Guan Ye Lian Qiao* (Herba Hypericum) is thought to work primarily by increasing the level of serotonin and secondarily by inhibiting the enzyme monoamine oxidase (MAO).[3,4] The effectiveness of this herb in treating depression has been demonstrated in many studies. Recently, one study using the Hamilton Depression Scale found *Guan Ye Lian Qiao* (Herba Hypericum) to be clinically effective in the treatment of depression with ratings close to 70% treatment response.[5,6,7,8] In another study including 1757 mild-to-moderate depressed patients, *Guan Ye Lian Qiao* (Herba Hypericum) was found to be significantly superior to placebo and "similarly effective" to antidepressant drugs.[9] Side effects of *Guan Ye Lian Qiao* (Herba Hypericum) are rare, with rash and photosensitivity being the most common.[10]

Lu Cha (Folium Camellia Sinensis) has a wide range of functions and is commonly used with different clinical applications. *Lu Cha* (Folium Camellia Sinensis) is an effective central nervous system stimulant and can increase body metabolism and boost energy levels.[11] *Lu Cha* (Folium Camellia Sinensis) has cancer protective functions as it inhibits the formation of cancer-inducing compounds and suppresses the mutation of bone marrow cells.[12,13] In addition to its cancer protective effect, *Lu Cha* (Folium Camellia Sinensis) also reduces cholesterol levels. Overall, *Lu Cha* (Folium Camellia Sinensis) prolongs life span, contributes to longevity, and protects against severe fatal diseases.[14,15]

FORMULAS

SHINE ™

In addition to *Guan Ye Lian Qiao* (Herba Hypericum) and *Lu Cha* (Folium Camellia Sinensis), many Chinese herbs are included to elevate mood and energy, promote digestion, and improve the utilization of energy.

PHARMACEUTICAL DRUGS & CHINESE MEDICINE: A COMPARATIVE ANALYSIS

Western Medical Approach: Depression is an emotional disorder that affects millions of people worldwide. In western medicine, the biomedical understanding of depression is relatively new, as antidepressant drugs were mostly developed only in the last two decades. Though there are several categories of drugs for depression, the most commonly used are the serotonin specific reuptake inhibitors (SSRI), such as Prozac (Fluoxetine), Zoloft (Sertraline), and Paxil (Paroxetine). As the name implies, these drugs have specific effect to increase serotonin activities in the brain to lift depression. However, despite their specific mechanism, they often require 4 to 6 months before they exert their effect to lift depression. Furthermore, they are associated with a great number of side effects, including but not limited to nausea, vomiting, weight loss, sexual dysfunction, and increased risk of suicide. Therefore, these drugs must be prescribed and monitored carefully to avoid such adverse reactions.

Traditional Chinese Medicine Approach: Depression is characterized by stagnation of qi, blood, food, and phlegm. Therefore, optimal treatment requires use of herbs to relieve such stagnation. These same herbs have also been found to have excellent effect to increase energy levels and lift depression. Generally speaking, most patients begin to benefit within approximately two weeks. Most importantly, these herbs are safe and natural, and are associated with few or no side effects.

Summation: Depression is a emotional disorder that should be addressed cautiously. Though use of drugs is effective, one must carefully evaluate the potential benefits versus risks. Once decision is made to start drug therapy, the patient must be monitored carefully to ensure that the drugs do not cause serious side effects. In comparison, herbs are also effective, and definitely much safer. It provides an additional option that definitely should be explored. Furthermore, in addition to drug or herbal therapies, counseling and behavior therapy should be initiated as they are extremely helpful toward long-term improvement. Lastly, exercise is also helpful as this increases one's inherent ability to deal with stress and depression.

CASE STUDIES

A 26-year-old female presented with chronic depression, which may have been due to not working for a few years. She was diagnosed with bipolar. Signs of depression manifested as constant somnolence and a lack of interest in any activity. According to traditional Chinese medicine, she was diagnosed with phlegm stagnation, evidenced by a "puffy" tongue body with a thick white tongue coating and a "rolling" pulse. Within a month of taking *Shine*, her somnolence subsided and she became more active during the day, which in turn made her less depressed.

T.G., Albuquerque, New Mexico

A woman presented with depression and irritability. Her anxiety was enhanced upon hearing that her western doctor was to discontinue her Vicodin (APAP/Hydrocodone) prescription, and the consequence of withdrawal. Hence, she was quite angry with her doctor. Her diagnosis included hepatitis C, fibromyalgia and Liver qi stagnation. The patient began taking *Shine*. In a separate event, a serious altercation with her spouse exacerbated her condition to a point where she considered suicide. After immediate administration of *Shine*, she began feeling much calmer. A half hour after ingesting the herbs, she said that thoughts of suicide were dismissed. The practitioner concluded that *Shine* was quite effective in treating patients with similar conditions.

M.H., Jupiter, Florida

FORMULAS

SHINE ™

J.M., a 36-year-old female, presented with depression. She was a single mother with two children and a pending divorce. Her psychologist wanted her on medication. She had poor appetite for food but increased cravings for candy and carbohydrates and alcohol. She was crying, unfocused and said she felt scattered emotionally and deflated energetically. Her blood pressure was 118/72 mmHg and her heart rate was 78 beats per minute. The diagnosis was qi and blood stagnation with Liver and Spleen disharmony. *Shine* was prescribed at 4 capsules three times daily. Results were apparent within 24 hours. J.M.'s depression began lifting the next day. She reported that she felt more solid, grounded and focused again. She was also more interested in moving physically and felt emotionally more stable. As the symptoms resolved, the dosage was reduced to 4 capsules twice daily and finally at once daily. The practitioner reported that the patient had previously been seeing another acupuncturist, and was on an herbal formula from another company. She reported that with the other formula, she felt stuck and was unable to move forward. With *Shine*, she felt the difference dramatically.

M.H., West Palm Beach, Florida

A 58-year-old male teacher presented with palpitations, which began one year ago following the death of his significant other. Stress or jogging appeared to exacerbate his condition. His symptoms were indicative of mitral valve prolapse. The diagnosis was Liver oppressing the Heart and Liver yang rising. The tongue was pink with a red tip and the pulse was wiry and pounding. Along with acupuncture treatment, the patient was given 4 capsules of *Shine* three times daily for about six months. The patient displayed a 75% (subjective) improvement within two weeks. The palpitations became less frequent. Feelings of stress reduced significantly along with a milder pounding sensation in the chest. After six weeks, the pulse was still full but had lost some of its wiry quality. The diagnosis was changed to Heart qi and blood deficiency. Within ten weeks, the pulse became slow and leisurely. Palpitations were also rare after seven months of treatment. Herbs were eventually discontinued with acupuncture maintenance every three to four weeks. The practitioner concluded that *Shine* was quite effective in reducing the stress level as well as the palpitations of the patient in a prompt and efficient manner.

C.C., Cromwell, Connecticut

A 42-year-old female finance administrator presented with "plum-pit" syndrome, belching, constipation, and irritability especially when angered. Her tongue was pale and her pulse was wiry. The patient's demeanor was always uptight or tense and short-tempered. In addition, the patient reported constant burping. The practitioner diagnosed the condition as follows: (1) Liver qi stagnation with dampness in the middle *jiao* and lower *jiao*, in turn, attacking the Stomach leading to continuous belching; (2) stagnation causing phlegm to congeal and stick, resulting in a "plum-pit" syndrome; and (3) stagnation of the Large Intestines causing constipation. The patient was instructed to take *Shine*. As a result of taking one bottle of *Shine* during the course of the treatment, significant improvements in the elimination of "plum-pit" qi and constipation were noted. Belching was also relieved by 90%. Upon taking the second bottle of *Shine*, the patient felt queasy and edgy and decided to stop taking the herbs. The patient however noted a positive change in mood and a more uplifted spirit. The practitioner concluded that the side effects might have been due to the fact that the patient had a deficient constitution.

P.L, San Diego, California

H.E., a 20-year-old female, presented with depression, difficulty with concentration, difficulty falling asleep, very active mind and short-temper. She startles easily. Her tongue was dry with white coating. Pulse was wiry. The diagnosis was Liver qi stagnation and Gallbladder/Heart disharmony. *Wen Dan Tang* (Warm the Gallbladder Decoction) and *Shine* were prescribed at 2 capsules each three times daily. Patient reported much improvement in symptoms after using herbs. She also reported that symptoms came back after stopping the herbs.

S.F., Greenbrae, California

SHINE ™

A 53-year-old female patient presented with anxiety, depression and pale complexion. Her pulse was thin, weak and deep in all positions. She had cyclical bouts of rage, fatigue, sleeplessness, anxiety and severe depression. Periods were irregular. Her tongue was puffy and pale. The TCM diagnosis was blood and yin deficiencies with Liver qi stagnation, Kidney yin and yang deficiencies. *Shine* and *Nourish*, along with an iron supplement were prescribed. The patient noticed a change within the first 10 days and more so around her cycle. She felt as if a cloud had been lifted from above. She found herself smiling more. Restlessness was still bothering her but her sleep was much better. This patient has suffered from depression for a long time and is very deficient.

N.V., Muir Beach, California

L.W., a 22-year-old male, presented with septic facial acne. Very depressed, he did not want to be seen in public. The TCM diagnosis was damp-heat with Liver qi stagnation. After one week of taking *Dermatrol PS* and *Shine*, the acne was 80% resolved and the depression improving. After washing his face with a mild soap, the patient applied a topical skin wash (Yin Care) diluted with tea tree oil. The acne was gone in 28 days. The patient now socializes happily with family and friends.

H.C., Stephens City, Virginia

[1] Olin, B. et al. *Facts and Comparisons The Review of Natural Products*. St. John's Wort, March 1994
[2] *PDR for Nutritional Supplements 1st Edition*, Medical Economics, 2001
[3] Bombardelli, E. et al. *Fitoterapia*; 66(1):43-68. 1995
[4] Suzuki, O. et al. *Planta Med*; 2:272. 1984
[5] Ernst, E. *Fortschr Med*; 113(25): 354-55. 1995
[6] Mueller, W. et al. *Deutsche Apotheker Zeitung*; 136:17-22,24. Mar 28, 1996
[7] DeSmet, P. et al. *Br. Med J*; 313:241-42. Aug 3, 1996
[8] Harrer, G. et al. *Phytomedicine*; 1:3-8. 1994
[9] Linde, K. et al. *Br Med J*; 313(7052):253-58. 1996
[10] Muldner, VH. and Zoller, M. *Arzneimittelforschung*; 34:918. 1984
[11] Olin, R. et al. *The Lawrence Review of Natural Products by Facts and Comparison*. Green Tea. May 1993
[12] Wang, H. and Wu, Y. Inhibitory effect of Chinese tea on N-nitrosation in vitro and in vivo. *IARC Sci Publ*;105:546. 1991
[13] Imanishi, H. et al. Tea tannin components modify the induction of sister-chromatid exchanges and chromosome aberrations in mutagen-treated cultured mammalian cells and mice. *Mutat Res*;259(1):79. 1991
[14] Uchida, S. et al. Radioprotective effects of (-)-epigallocatechin 3-0-gallate (green tea tannin) in mice. *Life Sci*;50(2):147. 1992
[15] Sadakata, S. et al. Mortality among female practitioners of Chanoyu (Japanese "tea-ceremony"). *Tohoku J Exp Med*; 166(4):475. 1992

FORMULAS

SILEREX ™

CLINICAL APPLICATIONS

- Various skin disorders such as rash, itching, dermatitis, and eczema
- Skin allergies induced by drugs, chemicals or foods

WESTERN THERAPEUTIC ACTIONS

- Antihistaminic effect to neutralize allergic reactions [3]
- Anti-inflammatory effect to relieve swelling and inflammation [1,2]
- Antibiotic properties to treat skin infections [1,2]

CHINESE THERAPEUTIC ACTIONS

- Disperses the wind to relieve itching
- Clears heat, cools the blood
- Drains dampness

DOSAGE

Take 5 to 6 capsules with warm water on an empty stomach every six hours as needed. Using **Silerex** prior to exposure to the allergen may prevent or reduce the risk of developing an allergy.

INGREDIENTS

Bai Ji Li (Fructus Tribuli)
Bai Xian Pi (Cortex Dictamni)
Che Qian Zi (Semen Plantaginis)
Dang Gui (Radicis Angelicae Sinensis)
Di Fu Zi (Fructus Kochiae)
Fang Feng (Radix Saposhnikoviae)
Jing Jie (Herba Schizonepetae)

Ku Shen Gen (Radix Sophorae Flavescentis)
Lian Qiao (Fructus Forsythiae)
Mu Dan Pi (Cortex Moutan)
Niu Bang Zi (Fructus Arctii)
Sheng Di Huang (Radix Rehmanniae)
Zhi Zi (Fructus Gardeniae)

FORMULA EXPLANATION

Silerex is formulated to treat various dermatological disorders, including rash, itching, eczema, dermatitis, and skin allergies to drugs, chemicals or foods. **Silerex** is comprised of herbs that disperse wind, clear heat, cool blood and drain damp.

Jing Jie (Herba Schizonepetae), *Bai Ji Li* (Fructus Tribuli) and *Fang Feng* (Radix Saposhnikoviae) relieve exterior wind, which is commonly regarded as the cause of itching. *Zhi Zi* (Fructus Gardeniae) clears heat to reduce redness and inflammation of the affected areas. *Mu Dan Pi* (Cortex Moutan), *Niu Bang Zi* (Fructus Arctii) and *Lian Qiao* (Fructus Forsythiae) cool and detoxify the blood to relieve itching. *Ku Shen Gen* (Radix Sophorae Flavescentis), *Che Qian Zi* (Semen Plantaginis), and *Di Fu Zi* (Fructus Kochiae) drain dampness through urination and treat weepy lesions. *Bai Xian Pi* (Cortex Dictamni) has antifungal effects to relieve fire toxicity. Finally, *Dang Gui* (Radicis Angelicae Sinensis) and *Sheng Di Huang* (Radix Rehmanniae) tonify and move the blood to extinguish wind, to relieve rash and itching.

FORMULAS

SILEREX ™

SUPPLEMENTARY FORMULAS

- For signs and symptoms of excess fire, add *Gardenia Complex*.
- For severe itching, add *Dermatrol (PS)*.
- For heavy metal poisoning, chemical allergy or any other unknown allergy, combine with *Herbal DTX*.
- To enhance the overall antibiotic effect, use *Herbal ABX*.
- For pus or swelling on the lesions, add *Resolve (AI)*.
- For respiratory discomfort associated with allergies, add *Respitrol (Heat)* or *Respitrol (Cold)*.
- For headache, add *Corydalin* or *Migratrol*.
- To clear heat and detoxify, use *Herbal ABX* or *Liver DTX*.
- If the allergy is due to ingestion of food, cleanse the colon with *Gentle Lax (Excess)*.
- For itching that worsens with stress, add *Calm* or *Calm (ES)*.
- With yin deficiency and heat, add *Nourish*.

NUTRITION

- Avoid seafoods, sushi, duck, goose, onions, garlic, sugar, alcohol, and foods that are raw, spicy, fried and greasy. Many meats and dairy products increase skin irritation by increasing the acidity of body tissue.
- Increase the consumption of flax seed oil, which helps to reduce inflammation in the body.

The Tao of Nutrition by Ni and McNease
- Eczema
    - Recommendations: potatoes, broccoli, dandelion, mung bean, seaweed, pearl barley, corn-silk, water chestnut, winter melon, and watermelon.
- Hives
    - Recommendations: wintermelon rind, chrysanthemum, vinegar, papaya, ginger, dried prunes, black sesame, black beans, and pearl barley.
    - Avoid shellfish and allergic foods.
- Allergy
    - Drink beet top tea as a water source.
    - Avoid wheat, citrus fruits, chocolate, shellfish, dairy products, eggs, potatoes, polluted meats, and polluted air.
- For more information, please refer to *The Tao of Nutrition* by Dr. Maoshing Ni and Cathy McNease.

LIFESTYLE INSTRUCTIONS

- The best long-term treatment is to identify and avoid the allergen. In addition, balancing and strengthening one's health and immunity will also reduce the frequency of allergic reactions while strengthening the patient's immunological balance.
- Cotton or silk clothing is recommended over synthetic fibers for better ventilation.

CLINICAL NOTES

- For itching of the genital region, use *Gentiana Complex* both internally and externally. For external treatment, wash the affected area with mild soap first. Then mix 5 grams each of *Ku Shen Gen* (Radix Sophorae Flavescentis), *She Chuang Zi* (Fructus Cnidii Monnieri), and *Gentiana Complex*, with 2 cups of warm water. Soak the affected area in the herbal solution for 5 minutes before rinsing off with water. Repeat the process once daily until itching is relieved.

SILEREX ™

- The optimal approach to address allergies is prevention, not treatment. Empirical wisdom suggests isolating the allergen and minimizing the patient's exposure to said allergen as much as possible.

CAUTIONS

- The optimal treatment of allergies is to avoid the allergens. *Silerex* relieves the symptoms, but does not cure the allergy. Therefore, it is not recommended to take this formula for a long time simply to suppress the symptoms. Every effort should be made to identify and avoid the allergen.
- If the condition does not improve after using *Silerex* for 2 to 3 weeks, consider modifying the herbal formula.
- Patients who are on anticoagulant or antiplatelet therapies, such as Coumadin (Warfarin), should use this formula with caution, as there may be a slightly higher risk of bleeding and bruising.

ACUPUNCTURE POINTS

Traditional Points:
- *Xuehai* (SP 10), *Geshu* (BL 17), *Fengchi* (GB 20) and *Chize* (LU 5).
- *Quchi* (LI 11) and *Xuehai* (SP 10).

Balance Method by Dr. Richard Tan:
- Left side: *Sanjian* (LI 3), *Quchi* (LI 11), *Gongsun* (SP 4), *Yinlingquan* (SP 9) and *Taichong* (LR 3).
- Right side: *Fenglong* (ST 40), *Jiexi* (ST 41), *Diwuhui* (GB 42), *Taiyuan* (LU 9) and *Chize* (LU 5).
- Left and right side can be alternated from treatment to treatment.
- To read more about Dr. Tan's acupuncture strategy, see his book *Dr. Tan's Strategy of Twelve Magic Points*.

Ear Points:
- Lung, Large Intestine, Adrenal Gland, and corresponding point of the affected area(s).
  - Pruritus: *Shenmen*, Lung, Subcortex, Adrenal Gland, and Urticaria Point. Adjunct points: Liver, Spleen, Heart, Endocrine, Pancreas, Gallbladder, Ovary, Testicles. Select three to five points and needle both ears every other day. Five to ten days is one treatment course. Rest for 1 week in between treatment courses.
  - Urticaria: Lung, Urticaria, Adrenal Gland, *Pingchuan*, and Liver. Needle one to two points each time every other day. Ten treatments equal one course.

Auricular Acupuncture by Dr. Li-Chun Huang:
- Contact dermatitis: Allergic Area, Sympathetic, Adrenal Gland, Liver, Spleen, Lung, Endocrine and Corresponding points (to the area affected). Bleed Ear Apex.
  - For dermatitis with severe pain, add *Shenmen*, Occiput
- Eczema: Allergic Area, Lung, Sympathetic, Spleen, *Shenmen*, Endocrine, Occiput, Diaphragm, and Corresponding points (to the area affected). Bleed Ear Apex.
- For additional information on the location and explanation of these points, please refer to *Auricular Treatment Formula and Prescriptions* by Dr. Li-Chun Huang.

MODERN RESEARCH

The herbs in *Silerex* have demonstrated clinical efficacy in treating various skin disorders, including but not limited to redness, swelling, carbuncles, erythema, mumps, rashes, eczema and dermatitis.[1, 2]

Fang Feng (Radix Saposhnikoviae) neutralizes toxins associated with herbs and/or chemicals. It is used for contact dermatitis or allergic dermatitis.[1,2] *Jing Jie* (Herba Schizonepetae) has antipyretic properties and is commonly used to treat skin disorders such as measles and urticaria.[1,2] *Ku Shen Gen* (Radix Sophorae Flavescentis) and *Bai Ji Li*

FORMULAS

SILEREX ™

(Fructus Tribuli) have antihistamine-like activities and may relieve general itching and pruritis.[1,2] *Niu Bang Zi* (Fructus Arctii) and *Zhi Zi* (Fructus Gardeniae) have excellent antibiotic effects and are especially useful if the wounds on the skin eruptions are open and infected. *Che Qian Zi* (Semen Plantaginis) has anti-inflammatory activities to reduce swelling and inflammation. *Di Fu Zi* (Fructus Kochiae) is most commonly used for eczema, pruritis and urticaria.

In a research study analyzing the effectiveness of Chinese herbs in treating itching associated with measles, 30 patients were given an herbal formula containing *Niu Bang Zi* (Fructus Arctii) as the main ingredient. Out of the 30 patients, 7 patients experienced significant improvement, 15 experienced moderate improvement, and 5 experienced slight improvement.[3]

PHARMACEUTICAL DRUGS & CHINESE MEDICINE: A COMPARATIVE ANALYSIS

Western Medical Approach: Skin disorders such as rash, itching, dermatitis, and eczema commonly occur as a result of oral ingestion of or direct physical contact with a incompatible substance. As a result, allergic and hypersensitive reactions occur either in localized areas or throughout the entire body. In western medicine, these skin disorders are treated with drugs that symptomatically relieve itching and irritation. Commonly used drugs include antihistamines [such as Benadryl (Diphenhydramine)] and corticosteroids [such as hydrocortisone]. In most cases, these drugs are used topically for a short period of time, and are therefore associated with limited side effects. However, oral use of these drugs is likely to cause more side effects. Furthermore, it is important to remember that the best way to avoid allergic skin reactions is to avoid the allergens whenever possible.

Traditional Chinese Medicine Approach: Skin disorders such as rash and eczema are characterized by wind-heat. Certain herbs that treat wind-heat have been shown to have marked antihistamine effect, and are excellent to alleviate skin itching and discomfort. Furthermore, many herbs also have anti-inflammatory effect to reduce swelling and inflammation. In short, oral ingestion of herbs is very effective to alleviate signs and symptoms of general skin disorders such as rash, eczema and dermatitis.

Summation: Drugs and herbs are both effective for treating skin disorders such as rash, dermatitis, and eczema. Though neither therapies "cure" allergy, they both effectively alleviate symptoms. Topical use of drugs alleviates symptoms safely and effectively, but oral use of the drugs tends to cause more side effects. On the other hand, herbs can be used safely and effectively via both oral and topical administrations.

---

[1] Bensky, D. et al. *Chinese Herbal Medicine Materia Medica*. Eastland Press. 1993
[2] Yeung, HC. *Handbook of Chinese Herbs*. Institute of Chinese Medicine. 1996
[3] Jiangxu Research Clinic of Dermatological Disorders. Observation of Tuimingwan in the treatment of measles, a case report of 30 patients. *Clinical Research Journal of Dermatological Disorders*; 3:215. 1972

FORMULAS

SYMMETRY ™

CLINICAL APPLICATIONS

- Bell's palsy
- Facial paralysis
- TMJ (temporo-mandibular joint) pain
- Trigeminal neuralgia
- Migraine headache due to wind, phlegm and blood stagnation
- Convulsions, epilepsy, seizures and twitching of muscles

WESTERN THERAPEUTIC ACTIONS

- Analgesic effect to relieve pain
- Anti-inflammatory effect to reduce swelling and inflammation
- Antiseizure and anti-epileptic effects to treat post-stroke sequelae and relieve nerve-related pain

CHINESE THERAPEUTIC ACTIONS

- Releases exterior wind
- Opens the channels and collaterals
- Activates qi and blood circulation

DOSAGE

Take 4 to 6 capsules three times daily. This herbal therapy should begin immediately on notice of the first warning signs. If necessary, the dosage may be increased to 8 capsules three times daily on day one of herbal therapy to achieve faster onset of action. If the herbs are irritating to the stomach where the patient reports nausea or epigastric discomfort, take the herbs after meals.

INGREDIENTS

Bai Fu Zi (Rhizoma Typhonii)
Bai Zhi (Radix Angelicae Dahuricae)
Chuan Xiong (Rhizoma Ligustici Chuanxiong)
Dang Gui (Radicis Angelicae Sinensis)
Fang Feng (Radix Saposhnikoviae)
Jiang Can (Bombyx Batryticatus)

Jing Jie (Herba Schizonepetae)
Quan Xie (Scorpio)
Si Gua Luo (Retinervus Luffae Fructus)
Wu Gong (Scolopendra)
Yan Hu Suo (Rhizoma Corydalis)

FORMULA EXPLANATION

According to traditional Chinese medicine, trigeminal neuralgia and facial paralysis are two conditions characterized by wind attacking the channels and collaterals in the facial regions, leading to blocked circulation of qi and blood. As a result, there is often severe pain, numbness, loss of muscle tone, and paralysis of the muscles. Optimal treatment of this condition requires use of herbs to release exterior wind, open the channels and collaterals, and activate qi and blood circulation.

Symmetry is formulated based on *Qian Zheng San* (Lead to Symmetry Powder), a classic formula that treats deviation of the eyes and mouth by restoring symmetry of the face. Following this general principle, *Symmetry* uses *Fang Feng* (Radix Saposhnikoviae), *Bai Zhi* (Radix Angelicae Dahuricae) and *Jing Jie* (Herba Schizonepetae) to release exterior wind, and *Quan Xie* (Scorpio) and *Wu Gong* (Scolopendra) to dispel interior Liver wind. In addition, *Bai Fu Zi* (Rhizoma Typhonii) and *Jiang Can* (Bombyx Batryticatus) dispel wind and eliminate phlegm obstruction. *Dang Gui* (Radicis Angelicae Sinensis) tonifies blood in the channels and collaterals, and treats the underlying deficiency. *Yan Hu Suo* (Rhizoma Corydalis) and *Chuan Xiong* (Rhizoma Ligustici Chuanxiong) activate qi and blood circulation and relieve pain. *Si Gua Luo* (Retinervus Luffae Fructus) opens the peripheral channels and collaterals.

Overall, **Symmetry** is a strong formula to treat various disorders of the face, including but not limited to trigeminal neuralgia, facial paralysis, TMJ, and migraine headache.

SUPPLEMENTARY FORMULAS

- For post-stroke patients with mental and physical deterioration, combine with **Neuro Plus**.
- For severe nerve pain, combine with **Flex (NP)**.
- For severe and acute migraine headache, combine with **Corydalin**.
- For chronic and moderate migraine headache due to blood deficiency, combine with **Migratrol**.
- With neck and shoulder pain, add **Neck & Shoulder (Acute)**.
- With excessive stress, add **Calm** or **Calm (ES)**.
- For postpartum Bell's palsy with qi and blood deficiency, add **Imperial Tonic**.
- With high blood pressure or prevention of stroke, add **Gastrodia Complex** or **Gentiana Complex**.

NUTRITION

- Consume adequate amounts of vegetables for vitamins A, B_1, B_2, C and E.
- Encourage a diet with a diverse source of all nutrients, including raw fruits, vegetables, whole grains, nuts, and seeds. B vitamins are important to maintain nerve health.
- Avoid cold, icy food and beverages, fried, smoked or barbecued foods. Stop smoking and avoid drinking alcohol.
- Advise patients to avoid all aluminum, which may be found in antacids, cookware, aluminum foil, and certain foods. Drinking steam-distilled water has a chelating effect in the blood to remove unwanted aluminum from the body.

LIFESTYLE INSTRUCTIONS

- Advise the patients to exercise daily and maintain a positive, hopeful outlook toward the future.
- Regular workout and deep breathing exercises are excellent ways to oxygenate the blood and improve circulation to all parts of the body to facilitate recovery.
- When recovering from a stroke or Bell's palsy, engage in regular and mild exercises, such as walking and *Tai Chi*. However, it is important to advise the patient to avoid exposure to wind and cold. In addition, biking, direct exposure to the fan or air conditioning are all strictly prohibited.

CLINICAL NOTES

- For deviation of the eyes and mouth, topical application of herbs is also beneficial. The topical preparation may be prepared by mixing extract powder of *Bai Jie Zi* (Semen Sinapis) with concentrated green tea. This herbal paste is to be applied topically to the affected area at night, and removed in the morning (the affected side in Bell's palsy can be determined by the side of the eye that cannot close). This process may be repeated daily, or every other day.
- Early and frequent treatment of Bell's palsy will ensure proper recovery. Acupuncture and moxa are extremely effective to treat this condition. In acute cases, patients are recommended to receive acupuncture treatment three times a week. Moxa on the local area for at least 20 minutes each day will also enhance recovery.

FORMULAS

SYMMETRY ™

- Stress or Liver qi stagnation may be triggering factors for many women who suffer from Bell's palsy. In such cases, maintenance and prevention formulas such as **Calm** or **Calm (ES)** should be taken regularly to prevent repeated attacks in the future.
- Bell's palsy is the prodromal sign of a future stroke in some patients. After successfully treating the symptoms, patients should be put on another formula to nourish yin or lower Liver wind to prevent future attacks. See Supplementary Formulas for details.
- For trigeminal neuralgia, use of herbs topically is also very beneficial. One topical preparation that has been used with great success contains *Ma Qian Zi* (Semen Strychni) 30g, *Chuan Wu* (Radix Aconiti Preparata) 15g, *Cao Wu* (Radix Aconiti Kusnezoffii) 15g, *Ru Xiang* (Gummi Olibanum) 15g, and *Mo Yao* (Myrrha) 15g. This topical preparation is made by grinding all the ingredients into a fine powder and then mixing it with oil to form an herbal paste. A small amount of herbal paste is to be applied topically to acupuncture points around the affected area, such as *Taiyang*, *Xiaguan* (ST 7), *Jiache* (ST 6), etc. [Note: These five herbs must be used only topically, and **not** internally, as internal ingestion of some of these herbs may be toxic.]
- This formula is an adjunct formula to acupuncture treatment. Optimal results will occur when acupuncture, electro-stimulation and herbs are all included in the treatment regime.

CAUTIONS

- This formula is relatively strong and potent, and it contains herbs that are considered slightly toxic in traditional Chinese medicine. Therefore, the dosage should be prescribed carefully according to the age, body weight and severity of the condition. See age-to-dose chart and weight-to-dose chart for details.
- This formula is contraindicated during pregnancy and nursing. It should be used with extreme caution in pediatric and geriatric patients, and only when the benefits outweigh the risks.
- *Dang Gui* (Radicis Angelicae Sinensis) may enhance the overall effectiveness of Coumadin (Warfarin), an anticoagulant drug. Patients who take anticoagulant or antiplatelet medications should **not** take this herbal formula without supervision by a licensed health care practitioner.

ACUPUNCTURE POINTS

Traditional Points:
- Facial paralysis:
  - Needle the affected side (the side with the eye that cannot close): *Jiache* (ST 6), *Dicang* (ST 4), *Xiaguan* (ST 7), *Sibai* (ST 2), *Yangbai* (GB 14), *Taiyang*, *Yingxiang* (LI 20), *Chengjiang* (CV 24), *Yifeng* (TH 17), *Fengchi* (GB 20), *Hegu* (LI 4), and *Zanzhu* (BL 2).
  - In more severe cases, treatment that is more aggressive is necessary. Thread the needle underneath the skin from *Dicang* (ST 4) towards *Jiache* (ST 6), *Yangbai* (GB 14) towards *Yuyao*, *Zanzhu* (BL 2) towards *Jingming* (BL 1), *Yingxiang* (LI 20) towards *Sibai* (ST 2), and *Renzhong* (GV 26) towards *Dicang* (ST 4). These points are needled subcutaneously at least 1 *cun* parallel to the skin. Once the needle is inserted, be careful to not have the tip of the needle penetrate out of the skin.
- Trigeminal neuralgia:
  - Strongly stimulate the following points: *Zanzhu* (BL 2), *Xiaguan* (ST 7), *Daying* (ST 5), *Yuyao*, *Sibai* (ST 2), *Chengjiang* (CV 24), *Yintang*, *Xiaguan* (ST 7), and *Tinggong* (SI 19).
  - Alternate points in Group 1 and 2 from treatment to treatment. Needle and bleed these points.
    - Group 1: *Shangxing* (GV 23), *Wuchu* (BL 5), *Chengguang* (BL 6), *Tongtian* (BL 7), and *Luoque* (BL 8).
    - Group 2: *Qianding* (GV 21), *Baihui* (GV 20), *Toulinqi* (GB 15), *Muchuang* (GB 16), *Zhengying* (GB 17), and *Chengling* (GB 18).
  - Select a few points and alternate between them. *Hegu* (LI 4), *Taiyang*, *Yangbai* (GB 14), *Zanzhu* (BL 2), *Tongziliao* (GB 1), *Xiaguan* (ST 7), *Juliao* (GB 29), *Jiache* (ST 6), *Daying* (ST 5), and *Tinghui* (GB 2).

SYMMETRY ™

Balance Method by Dr. Richard Tan:
- Left side: *Sanjian* (LI 3), *Zhongzhu* (TH 3), and *Ququan* (LR 8).
- Right side: *ah shi* points around *Chize* (LU 5) to *Kongzui* (LU 6), *Quze* (PC 3) to *Ximen* (PC 4), *Shaohai* (HT 3) to *Lingdao* (HT 4), *Zulinqi* (GB 41), and *Xiangu* (ST 43).
- Alternate sides from treatment to treatment. Patient should receive acupuncture treatment at least twice a week for optimal result.
- For additional information on the Balance Method, please refer to *Dr. Tan's Strategy of Twelve Magical Points* by Dr. Richard Tan.

Auricular Acupuncture by Dr. Li-Chun Huang:
- Trigeminal neuralgia: Auricular Temporal Nerve, Brain Stem, and *San Jiao*. Bleed Ear Apex.
  - For neuralgia of the first branch of the trigeminal nerve, add Forehead, Eye
  - For neuralgia of the maxilla nerve, add Upper Jaw, Upper Palate
  - For neuralgia of the mandibular nerve, add Lower Jaw, Lower Palate
- Facial paralysis: Cheek Area, Brain Stem, Sanjiao, Endocrine, Adrenal Gland, Mouth, Sympathetic, Liver, Spleen, and Coronary Vascular Subcortex. Bleed Ear Apex and Helix 5.
- For additional information on the location and explanation of these points, please refer to *Auricular Treatment Formula and Prescriptions* by Dr. Li-Chun Huang.

MODERN RESEARCH

Symmetry is designed specifically to treat disorders affecting the facial regions, such as facial paralysis or hemiplegia in stroke sequelae, Bell's palsy, TMJ (temporo-mandibular joint) pain and trigeminal neuralgia.

Bai Fu Zi (Rhizoma Typhonii), *Jiang Can* (Bombyx Batryticatus) and *Quan Xie* (Scorpio) are the three principle herbs in this formula. Together, these three herbs have shown remarkable effect via numerous clinical studies to treat facial paralysis and trigeminal neuralgia. According to one study, concurrent use of acupuncture and herbs [*Bai Fu Zi* (Rhizoma Typhonii), *Jiang Can* (Bombyx Batryticatus), *Quan Xie* (Scorpio) and others] were successful in treating 52 of 60 patients with facial paralysis.[1] According to another study, concurrent use of acupuncture and herbs [*Bai Fu Zi* (Rhizoma Typhonii), *Jiang Can* (Bombyx Batryticatus), *Quan Xie* (Scorpio) and others] for 2 days to 1 year was associated with 95% effective rate in 88 patients with facial paralysis.[2] For trigeminal neuralgia, one study reported 94.2% rate of effectiveness among 52 patients when treated with *Bai Fu Zi* (Rhizoma Typhonii), *Jiang Can* (Bombyx Batryticatus), *Quan Xie* (Scorpio) and others.[3]

Symmetry also contains many herbs with analgesic effect to relieve pain. *Yan Hu Suo* (Rhizoma Corydalis), *Bai Zhi* (Radix Angelicae Dahuricae) and *Dang Gui* (Radicis Angelicae Sinensis) all have excellent analgesic and anti-inflammatory effect. *Yan Hu Suo* (Rhizoma Corydalis) may be used to treat pain of various origins.[4,5] *Bai Zhi* (Radix Angelicae Dahuricae) is most effective for treating headache.[6,7] *Dang Gui* (Radicis Angelicae Sinensis) is excellent for migraine headache, with potency comparable to acetylsalicylic acid.[8,9] Lastly, *Bai Fu Zi* (Rhizoma Typhonii) in formulas has been shown to have good success to treat numbness of the facial nerves.[10]

Many herbs in *Symmetry* also have marked antiseizure and anti-epileptic effect, to prevent seizure and epilepsy, and to treat nerve-related pain. Herbs with such actions include *Jiang Can* (Bombyx Batryticatus),[11] *Quan Xie* (Scorpio),[12] and *Wu Gong* (Scolopendra).[13]

In summary, *Symmetry* restores symmetry to the face, and treats disorders such as facial paralysis, Bell's palsy, TMJ (temporo-mandibular joint) pain, trigeminal neuralgia and migraine headache.

FORMULAS

SYMMETRY ™

PHARMACEUTICAL DRUGS & CHINESE MEDICINE: A COMPARATIVE ANALYSIS

Western Medical Approach: Neurological disorders are complicated illnesses that encompass many different diseases, including but not limited to Bell's palsy, facial paralysis, TMJ (temporo-mandibular joint) pain, trigeminal neuralgia, and others. From western medicine perspectives, these diseases are well defined, accurately diagnosed, but not successfully treated. Though there are some drugs available for symptomatic treatment, such as use of antiseizure or tricyclic antidepressants for nerve pain, none are very effective and all have serious side effects. Furthermore, there are simply no effective pharmaceutical treatments for either the symptoms or the cause of conditions such as Bell's palsy and facial paralysis. As a result, these conditions continue to deteriorate, creating more debilitation and suffering.

Traditional Chinese Medicine Approach: TCM has long excelled in treatment of such neurological disorders with both acupuncture and herbs. There are numerous options available to stimulate the central and peripheral nervous systems, to help to relieve symptoms and restore normal functions. Generally speaking, prognosis is excellent if treatment begins within three months from the onset of illness, positive within one year, and hopeful if within three years. TCM treatments using both acupuncture and herbs should be explored and aggressively implemented as early and as much as possible to achieve maximum results. Time delay before treatment only decreases the overall success rate.

Summation: TCM treatments offer safe and effective options for treatment of these neurological disorders, and are clearly significantly superior to western medicine.

CASE STUDY

A 50-year-old female suffered from deviation of eye and mouth on the right side of the face. The patient had yellow tongue coating, and a wiry-fine-slippery-rapid pulse. Upon more inquiry, the condition was diagnosed as wind attacking the channels and collaterals, with underlying deficiencies. The patient was treated with both electro-acupuncture and modified *Symmetry*. In addition, the patient was instructed to apply herbs topically to the affected area at night, removing them in the morning (the topical preparation was made by mixing *Bai Jie Zi* (Semen Sinapis) with concentrated green tea). After three courses of treatment, the overall condition was greatly improved. The deviation was not noticeable at rest, and only slightly noticeable when laughing. The patient continued to be treated on a regular basis, and eventually reported complete recovery.

Anonymous

[1] *Nei Meng Gu Zhong Yi Yao* (Traditional Chinese Medicine and Medicinals of Inner Magnolia), 1990; 9(4):18
[2] *Shi Zhen Guo Yao Yan Jiu* (Research of Shizhen Herbs), 1996; 7(1):13
[3] *Si Chuan Zhong Yi* (Sichuan Chinese Medicine), 1998; 2:25
[4] *Zhong Yao Yao Li Yu Ying Yong* (Pharmacology and Applications of Chinese Herbs), 1983; 447
[5] *Biol Pharm Bull*, 1994:Feb; 17(2):262-5
[6] *Xin Yi Xue* (New Medicine), 1976; 1:8
[7] *Xin Yi Yao Xue Za Zhi* (New Journal of Medicine and Herbology), 1976; 8:35
[8] *Xin Yi Yao Xue Za Zhi* (New Journal of Medicine and Herbology), 1975; (6):34
[9] *Bei Jing Yi Xue* (Beijing Medicine), 1988; 2:95
[10] *Hu Bei Zhong Yi Za Zhi* (Hubei Journal of Chinese Medicine), 1982; 1:33
[11] *Jiang Su Yi Yao* (Jiangsu Journal of Medicine and Herbology), 1976; 2:33
[12] *Si Chuan Zhong Yi* (Sichuan Chinese Medicine), 1991; 9(11):12
[13] *Zhong Yao Xue* (Chinese Herbology), 1998; 704:706

THYRODEX ™

CLINICAL APPLICATIONS

- Hyperthyroidism
- Hyperthyroidism with low-grade fever, tachycardia (90 to 120 heartbeats per minute), tremors of the tongue and fingers, enlarged thyroid gland, unilateral or bilateral swollen and bulging eyes
- Hyperthyroidism with palpitations or tachycardia, fatigue, weight loss, fidgeting, irritability, bad temper, aversion to heat, perspiration, hunger and increased appetite, increased blood pressure, etc.
- Grave's disease

WESTERN THERAPEUTIC ACTIONS

- Lowers the level of thyroid hormone in the blood [2,3]
- Reduces enlargement of the thyroid gland [2,3,4]
- Treats the unwanted "sympathetic excess" signs and symptoms of hyperthyroidism [2,3,5]

CHINESE THERAPEUTIC ACTIONS

- Softens hardness, resolves nodules, and eliminates phlegm
- Clears toxic heat and drains Liver fire
- Tranquilizes the *shen* (spirit)
- Tonifies qi and yin

DOSAGE

Take 3 to 4 capsules three times daily. Patients with hyperthyroidism (other than thyrotoxicosis) should notice dramatic improvement within one to one-and-a-half months of herbal treatment.

INGREDIENTS

Bie Jia (Carapax Trionycis)
Chuan Niu Xi (Radix Cyathulae)
Fang Feng (Radix Saposhnikoviae)
Gan Cao (Radix Glycyrrhizae)
Huang Qi (Radix Astragali)
Mu Li (Concha Ostreae)
Xia Ku Cao (Spica Prunellae)

Xuan Shen (Radix Scrophulariae)
Yuan Zhi (Radix Polygalae)
Zhe Bei Mu (Bulbus Fritillariae Thunbergii)
Zhi Mu (Radix Anemarrhenae)
Zhi Zi (Fructus Gardeniae)

FORMULA EXPLANATION

According to traditional Chinese medicine, hyperthyroidism is a combination of qi and yin deficiencies, Liver fire rising, and phlegm stagnation. The fundamental causes are qi and yin deficiencies while the symptoms and signs show Liver fire and phlegm stagnation. Treatment, therefore, must address both the cause and the symptoms simultaneously.

Bie Jia (Carapax Trionycis) nourishes yin and resolves hard lumps. *Xuan Shen* (Radix Scrophulariae) and *Zhi Mu* (Radix Anemarrhenae) have three important functions: replenishing the *jing* (essence), clearing heat and resolving hard lumps in the body. *Zhi Zi* (Fructus Gardeniae) and *Xia Ku Cao* (Spica Prunellae) clear heat, and purge Liver fire. They reduce the "sympathetic excess" signs and symptoms commonly associated with hyperthyroidism, such as increased heart rate, increased blood pressure, tremor, etc. *Zhe Bei Mu* (Bulbus Fritillariae Thunbergii) resolves

FORMULAS

THYRODEX ™

phlegm and further assists *Xia Ku Cao* (Spica Prunellae) to disperse lumps and hardenings. Clinically, *Zhe Bei Mu* (Bulbus Fritillariae Thunbergii) and *Mu Li* (Concha Ostreae) are commonly used to treat goiter. *Chuan Niu Xi* (Radix Cyathulae) stimulates blood circulation and enhances the overall effectiveness of the formula. *Yuan Zhi* (Radix Polygalae) calms the *shen* (spirit) and relieves nervousness and anxiety. *Gan Cao* (Radix Glycyrrhizae) harmonizes all the herbs of the formula. *Fang Feng* (Radix Saposhnikoviae) and *Huang Qi* (Radix Astragali), two principle herbs in the formula *Yu Ping Feng San* (Jade Windscreen Powder), have excellent effects to strengthen *wei* (defensive) *qi* and stop perspiration.

SUPPLEMENTARY FORMULAS

- For high blood pressure and fast heart rate due to excess fire, add *Gardenia Complex*.
- For anxiety and nervousness, add *Calm (ES)*.
- For insomnia, add *Schisandra ZZZ* or *Calm ZZZ*.
- For hypertension, use *Gastrodia Complex* or *Gentiana Complex*.
- For enlarged thyroid, use with *Resolve (AI)*.
- For thirst with dry mouth and throat, add *Nourish (Fluids)*.
- With Kidney yin deficiency, add *Nourish* or *Kidney Tonic (Yin)*.
- With blood stagnation, add *Circulation (SJ)*.
- For dysmenorrhea, use *Mense-Ease*.

NUTRITION

- Consume plenty of the following foods: broccoli, brussels sprouts, cabbage, cauliflower, kale, mustard greens, peaches, pears, soybeans, spinach, and turnips. These foods may help to suppress thyroid hormone production.[1]
- Short-term consumption of foods rich in iodine will provide temporary relief of hyperthyroidism due to a negative feedback mechanism. Long-term consumption, however, is not recommended because foods rich in iodine will facilitate production of thyroid hormone. Foods rich in iodine include sea salt, iodized salt, kelp, and sargassum.

LIFESTYLE INSTRUCTIONS

- Eliminate all stimulants, such as cigarette smoking, second-hand smoke, and caffeine from tea, coffee or soft drinks.
- Avoid vigorous exercise, hot tubs and saunas.
- Advise the patients to engage in relaxing exercises, such as walking, *Qi Gong* or *Tai Chi Chuan*.

CLINICAL NOTES

- Patients with hyperthyroidism (other than thyrotoxicosis) should notice dramatic improvement within one to one-and-a-half months of herbal treatment. Most symptoms should completely subside within three to six months of treatment. Protrusion of the eye(s) may persist despite herbal treatment.
- Practitioners should suspect hyperthyroidism when the following manifestations are present:
  - Young adults (especially female) who have a bad temper, hunger with excessive appetite, palpitations and profuse perspiration.
  - Young adults (especially female) who are fidgety and irritable, have early menses with a light flow, amenorrhea, and significant weight loss.
  - Young adults with sudden onset of difficulty with physical movement, numbness of legs, or possible collapse of leg muscles while walking.

THYRODEX ™

CAUTIONS

- This formula is contraindicated during pregnancy and nursing.
- Patients with thyrotoxicosis or thyroid storm require emergency medical treatment. Warning signs and symptoms of thyroid storm or thyrotoxicosis include high fever, tachycardia, fidgeting, irritability, nausea, vomiting, obvious weight loss, profuse perspiration, delirium, and possible loss of unconsciousness.

ACUPUNCTURE POINTS

Traditional Points:
- *Huatoujiaji* points (Extra 15), *Jianshi* (PC 5), *Sanyinjiao* (SP 6), *Yinxi* (HT 6), *Fuliu* (KI 7), *Taixi* (KI 3), and *Neiguan* (PC 6).
- *Xingjian* (LR 2) and *Quchi* (LI 11).

Balance Method by Dr. Richard Tan:
- Left side: *Xuanzhong* (GB 39), *Yangfu* (GB 38), *Guangming* (GB 37), *Daling* (PC 7), and Thyroid point on the ear.
- Right side: *Xingjian* (LR 2), *Taichong* (LR 3), *Fuliu* (KI 7), and *Yangxi* (LI 5).
- Left and right side can be alternated from treatment to treatment.
- For additional information on the Balance Method, please refer to *Dr. Tan's Strategy of Twelve Magical Points* by Dr. Richard Tan.

Auricular Acupuncture by Dr. Li-Chun Huang:
- Hyperthyroidism: Thyroid, Pituitary, Endocrine, Thalamus, Nervous Subcortex, Kidney, Liver, and Heart. Bleed Ear Apex
  - For arrhythmia and tachycardia, add Reducing Heart Rate Point.
  - For nervousness, hot temper insomnia, and irritability, add Occiput, Anxious, and Neurasthenia Point.
  - For hunger to enhance satiety, add Hunger Point.
  - For fatigue, add Spleen.
  - For impotence with hyperthyroidism, add Internal Genital and Gonadotropin.
- For additional information on the location and explanation of these points, please refer to *Auricular Treatment Formula and Prescriptions* by Dr. Li-Chun Huang.

MODERN RESEARCH

Thyrodex is an herbal formula developed by Professor Xiao-Ping Zhang of Anhui Hospital of Traditional Chinese Medicine. It is an empirical formula designed to treat patients with hyperthyroidism. It has been used for over 30 years in China and has helped several thousand patients with hyperthyroidism. Hyperthyroidism is defined as an increase in the circulating thyroid hormone leading to many signs and symptoms similar to "sympathetic excess," such as increased blood pressure, tachycardia, weight loss, etc. Treatment should focus on reducing the amount of thyroid hormone, decreasing the enlargement of the thyroid gland and minimizing the signs and symptoms of hyperthyroidism.

Zhe Bei Mu (Bulbus Fritillariae Thunbergii), *Mu Li* (Concha Ostreae), *Xuan Shen* (Radix Scrophulariae), and *Zhi Mu* (Radix Anemarrhenae) are Chinese herbs historically prescribed to dissolve lumps and hardenings. Clinically, they have been used with great results for treating goiter and hyperthyroidism.[2,3]

In addition to reducing thyroid hormone and thyroid enlargement, *Zhi Zi* (Fructus Gardeniae) and *Xia Ku Cao* (Spica Prunellae) clear heat and purge Liver fire.[4] They reduce the "sympathetic excess" signs and symptoms commonly

FORMULAS

associated with hyperthyroidism, such as increased blood pressure, increased heart rate, tremor, etc. Furthermore, for patients with hyperactivity and insomnia, *Yuan Zhi* (Radix Polygalae) calms the *shen* (spirit) with its sedative and tranquilizing effects.[5]

PHARMACEUTICAL DRUGS & CHINESE MEDICINE: A COMPARATIVE ANALYSIS

Western Medical Approach: Hyperthyroidism is a common disorder that is well understood, but it only has limited treatment options: drugs or surgery. In most cases, patients prefer non-invasion drug therapy first. Unfortunately, these drugs [such as tapazole and propylthiouracil) are ineffective and cannot consistently control thyroid hormones within an optimal range. Fluctuation of thyroid hormone levels contributes to presentation of hyperthyroidism or hypothyroidism, depending on whether the drug is under or over dosed, respectively. Eventually, most patients receive either surgery or radioactive iodine treatments. These treatments are invasive and irreversible, as they literally destroy the thyroid gland. After these invasive treatments, many patients develop hypothyroidism, and must take synthetic thyroid hormone for the rest of their life.

Traditional Chinese Medicine Approach: Hyperthyroidism is a disorder characterized by Liver fire rising with underlying qi and yin deficiencies. Hyperthyroidism has been treated in China for thousands of years successfully by using herbs that suppress the sympathetic excess to control the symptoms, and herbs that nourish underlying deficiencies to regulate the endocrine system. By targeting both the symptoms and the cause, herbs exert immediate and long-term effectiveness for management of hyperthyroidism. However, herbal therapy in this case has certain limitations. Patients in thyroid storm crisis must be referred to western medicine for urgent treatment. Furthermore, use of herbs will not reverse protrusion of the eyes, no matter the dose or duration.

Summation: Hyperthyroidism can be treated with both western medicine and traditional Chinese medicine. Ideally, all options should be explored (including drugs, herbs and others), as many cases of mild to moderate hyperthyroidism respond well to such treatment. If these treatments are effective, they spare the patients emotional grief, financial burden, and unnecessary exposure to risks associated with surgery and radioactive iodine treatments. If all other options fail, then surgery or radioactive iodine treatments can be considered as last alternatives, as these treatments are invasive and irreversible. It is important that practitioners and patients are informed and educated to understand all available options; so they may decide together on the most appropriate therapy.

CASE STUDIES

M.D., a 52 year old female, presented with nodule on the left thyroid, palpitation, agitation, shortness of breath with chest pressure, nausea, frequent urination, restless sleep and soft bowel movement. Her blood pressure was 110/70 mmHg and her heart rate was from 90 to 120 beats per minute. The western diagnosis was hyperthyroidism. Her TCM diagnosis was Liver fire with Liver and Kidney yin deficiencies with phlegm stagnation. *Thyrodex* was prescribed. Within one week of acupuncture and herbs, the patients started to feel better. Attached is her lab report showing great improvement over a four-month period. All her symptoms continued to steadily and gradually improve. This is a great formula. Her medical doctor does not understand how her condition improved but had canceled her scheduled radiation treatment. She was very happy.

Date	T4	T3	TSH
January	1.73	H4.59	L0.02
April	1.03	2.82	0.04

M.N., Knoxville, Tennessee

THYRODEX ™

A 22-year-old female web design developer presented with a rapid strong heartbeat, lower abdominal gas and pain with erratic bowel movements. Other symptoms included hair and skin changes, chronic fatigue, irritability, poor memory, and lack of concentration. An earlier TSH level reading was 0.009 and free T3 levels were 4.9. She also displayed a fine tremor and reflexes at +3. The pulse was regular, strong and wiry while the tongue was red. The practitioner diagnosed the patient with hyperthyroidism. The diagnosis was Liver qi stagnation, Liver and Spleen disharmony and fire depleting Heart yin. The patient was treated with acupuncture as well as dietary modifications. She took 4 capsules of *Thyrodex* three times daily for 4 months, then 4 capsules two times daily for 2 months, finishing with 2 capsules two times daily for one month. In addition, Vitamins B and E were taken along with Lemon Balm Tincture. After the treatment regimen, most symptoms abated with only occasional palpitations and shakiness. Energy levels were considerately better. Improvements in digestion, bowel movement, and sleeping patterns were observed. The lab results were as follows:

Date	TSH	T3	T4
12/00	0.04	119	1.30
03/01	1.56		0.09
06/01	0.59	90	1.10

Anonymous

A 39-year-old female with hyperthyroidism had been diagnosed with Grave's disease. Subjective and objective signs and symptoms included goiter, exophthalmus, and insomnia. Objective laboratory analysis indicated elevation of thyroid hormone (T4) and decreased TSH. Conventional pharmaceutical and alternative medical treatments failed to improve her condition. When she sought Chinese medicine as a last measure prior to possible surgical intervention, she was instructed to take *Thyrodex* (4 capsules three times daily). After a short period of taking *Thyrodex*, she noticed significant improvements in sleep habits and energy levels. The patient felt less irritable and anxious. Her eye discomfort also resolved. Furthermore, there were no side effects from the herbs whatsoever. The practitioner concluded an overall positive outcome and diminishing signs and symptoms of Grave's disease using *Thyrodex*. Upon follow-ups visits, the lab results for thyroid hormones were within normal limits.

D. S., San Diego, California.

A 46-year-old female with hyperthyroidism presented with the following symptoms: feelings of warmth and thirst, perspiration, fast metabolism, difficulty sleeping, chronic sore throat (worse at night), migraines, poor appetite in the morning, and frequent diarrhea. The pulse was thin and deep on the left side, and full on the right side. The tongue was pale and scalloped with a slight thick white coat. The diagnosis was Kidney yin deficiency with Liver yang rising, accompanied by Spleen qi deficiency with dampness. The patient was instructed to take *Thyrodex* (4 capsules three times daily). After 6 months of treatment using *Thyrodex*, the lab results showed normal levels of T4 and TSH (T3 was not tested). The patient's attitude and overall demeanor was quite upbeat. She continued to take *Thyrodex* (2 capsules three times daily). Both the medical doctor and the acupuncturist closely monitored her condition.

R.H., Ft. Collins, Colorado

M.C., a 55-year-old female, presented with trouble sleeping. Lab results showed hyperthyroidism, goiter and hypertension. Her blood pressure was 166/98 mmHg and her heart rate was 90 beats per minute. The diagnosis was Liver fire rising. *Thyrodex* was prescribed at 4 capsules three times a day. Thyroid hormones dropped from 10.34 to 4.88 in two months. Swelling in the neck was also better.

W.F., Bloomfield, New Jersey

THYRODEX ™

D.E., a 49-year-old woman with a history of hyperthyroidism, presented with heart palpitations, sweating easily (especially at night), hunger, weight loss, and becoming easily agitated. Her blood pressure was 120/88 mmHg, with heart rate of 98 beats per minute. The Western diagnosis was hyperthyroidism; the TCM diagnosis was Stomach fire, Heart yin deficiency, and *wei* (defensive) *qi* deficiency. The patient was taking Tapazole at 2.5 to 5 mg per day. The practitioner prescribed *Thyrodex* at 3 to 4 capsules, three times daily, and acupuncture treatments. After commencing herbal treatment, the patient gradually reduced her Tapazole from 5.0 mg to 2.5 mg per day. In the course of two months of herbal treatment, the patient showed significant improvement with no more palpitations, sweating, or excessive hunger. Even with drug therapy reduced by 50%, TSH levels remained approximately the same, under herbal treatment. The patient continues to receive both herbal and acupuncture treatments.

D.L., Doylestown, Pennsylvania

A 39-year-old female presented with elevated blood pressure, palpitations, hot flashes, anxiety, and swelling in her neck, with a heart rate of 92 beats per minute. The Western diagnosis was hyperthyroidism; the TCM diagnosis was Liver and Kidney yin deficiencies. After she began taking *Thyrodex*, the patient experienced diminished hot flashes and anxiety. Her blood pressure remained unchanged but the goiter diminished in size. After *Gastrodia Complex* was added to the herbal treatment, the patient noticed improvement after just one bottle.

P.W., Paulet, Vermont

[1] Balch, JF and Balch, PA. *Prescriptions for Nutritional Healing*. Avery Publishing Group. 1997
[2] Yeung, HC. *Handbook of Chinese Herbs*. Institute of Chinese Medicine. 1993
[3] Zhang, XP. Treatment of Endocrine Disorders with Herbs. Presentation given by Professor Zhang at the Seminar hosted by California Association of Acupuncture and Oriental Medicine. July 1998
[4] Bensky, D. et al. *Chinese Herbal Medicine Materia Medica*. Eastland Press. 1993
[5] Ling, YK. et al. *Chinese Herbology*. Shanghai Scientific Press. 1984

FORMULAS

THYRO-*forte* ™

CLINICAL APPLICATIONS

- ❧ Hypothyroidism
- ❧ Hypothyroidism with fatigue, lack of energy, dull facial expression, hoarse voice, drooping eyelids, puffy and swollen eyes and face, weight gain, constipation, aversion to cold, dry hair and skin, low body temperature, decreased heart rate and blood pressure, muscle weakness or sluggishness, and other related symptoms.
- ❧ Chronic thyroiditis

WESTERN THERAPEUTIC ACTIONS

- ❧ Stimulates the production of thyroid hormones [1,2]
- ❧ Increases basal metabolism [3,4,5]
- ❧ Improves physiological functions [6,7,8,10,11,12,13]
- ❧ Enhances energy levels

CHINESE THERAPEUTIC ACTIONS

- ❧ Tonify Kidney, Heart and Spleen yang
- ❧ Nourish Kidney yin
- ❧ Tonify qi

DOSAGE

Take 4 capsules three times daily on an empty stomach. Depending on the severity of hypothyroidism, the dosage may need to be adjusted upwards or downwards.

INGREDIENTS

Fu Ling (Poria)
Fu Zi (Radix Aconiti Lateralis Praeparata)
Gou Qi Zi (Fructus Lycii)
Gui Ban (Plastrum Testudinis)
Hai Zao (Sargassum)
Kun Bu (Thallus Laminariae seu Eckloniae)
Lu Jiao (Cornu Cervi)

Mu Dan Pi (Cortex Moutan)
Ren Shen (Radix Ginseng)
Rou Gui (Cortex Cinnamomi)
Shan Yao (Rhizoma Dioscoreae)
Shan Zhu Yu (Fructus Corni)
Shu Di Huang (Radix Rehmanniae Preparata)
Ze Xie (Rhizoma Alismatis)

FORMULA EXPLANATION

According to traditional Chinese medicine, hypothyroidism is a condition characterized by yang deficiency. While the fundamental etiology is Kidney yang deficiency, complications may involve yin deficiency of the Kidney and yang deficiencies of the Spleen and Heart. Treatment, therefore, must address both yang and yin deficiencies of the organs involved.

Rou Gui (Cortex Cinnamomi) and *Fu Zi* (Radix Aconiti Lateralis Praeparata) are two of the strongest and most commonly used herbs to fortify the yang of Kidney, Heart and Spleen, three organs implicated in patients with hypothyroidism. In addition, *Rou Gui* (Cortex Cinnamomi) treats insufficient *ming men* (life gate) fire, a condition characterized by accelerated aging process. *Fu Zi* (Radix Aconiti Lateralis Praeparata) tonifies and restores depleted yang, a condition characterized by lower basal metabolism and compromised physiological functions. The combination of these two herbs has an excellent synergistic function to tonify yang and treat the underlying cause of

THYRO-*forte* ™

hypothyroidism. *Lu Jiao* (Cornu Cervi) and *Gui Ban* (Plastrum Testudinis) are excellent herbs to tonify Kidney yang, Kidney yin, and Kidney *jing* (essence), and they are safe and effective when used at a large dose or for a long period of time.

Hai Zao (Sargassum) and *Kun Bu* (Thallus Laminariae seu Eckloniae) dispel phlegm and soften nodules. In other words, they have great effect to reduce the hypertrophy and enlargement of the thyroid glands. In addition, these two herbs are rich in iodine and will stimulate the production of thyroid hormone, especially in cases of hypothyroidism due to lack of iodine in the diet.

Shu Di Huang (Radix Rehmanniae Preparata), *Shan Zhu Yu* (Fructus Corni), *Shan Yao* (Rhizoma Dioscoreae), *Ze Xie* (Rhizoma Alismatis), *Mu Dan Pi* (Cortex Moutan), and *Fu Ling* (Poria) compose the classic Kidney yin tonic formula *Liu Wei Di Huang Wan* (Six-Ingredient Pill with Rehmannia), one of the most famous herbal tonics. *Shu Di Huang* (Radix Rehmanniae Preparata) tonifies the Kidney yin and the Kidney *jing* (essence); *Shan Zhu Yu* (Fructus Corni) nourishes the Liver and prevents the leakage of Kidney *jing* (essence); and *Shan Yao* (Rhizoma Dioscoreae) tonifies the Spleen and stabilizes the Kidney *jing* (essence). *Ze Xie* (Rhizoma Alismatis) clears deficiency fire from the Kidney; *Mu Dan Pi* (Cortex Moutan) sedates Liver fire; and *Fu Ling* (Poria) dissolves dampness from the Spleen. These six herbs are formulated with careful checks and balances to maximize the therapeutic effects and minimize unwanted side effects. In addition, *Gou Qi Zi* (Fructus Lycii) is used to tonify Liver and Kidney yin. In addition to treating the underlying cause of the illness, *Ren Shen* (Radix Ginseng) tonifies qi and immediately raises the energy level of hypothyroid patients.

SUPPLEMENTARY FORMULAS

- For an immediate energy boost, add *Vibrant*.
- For edema and water accumulation, add *Herbal DRX*.
- To tonify Kidney yang, add *Kidney Tonic (Yang)*.
- To tonify Kidney yin, add *Kidney Tonic (Yin)*.
- For long-term increase in energy, add *Imperial Tonic*.
- For constipation, add *Gentle Lax (Deficient)*.
- For dry hair and skin, add *Polygonum 14*.
- For lack of libido in men or women, add *Vitality*.
- For adrenal insufficiency, use with *Adrenoplex*.
- To strengthen constitutional weakness and deficiency, add *Cordyceps 3*.
- For poor appetite or loose stool, add *GI Tonic*.

NUTRITION

- Avoid fluoride and chlorine (which are found in many toothpastes and in tap water), since these elements may block the iodine receptors in the thyroid glands, leading to reduced hormone production and eventually hypothyroidism. Drink steam-distilled water only.
- Minimize intake of foods that suppress the production of thyroid hormone, such as brussel sprouts, peaches, pears, spinach, turnips, cabbage, broccoli, kale and mustard greens.
- Encourage the consumption of foods (or supplements) rich in vitamin B complex to promote the proper generation and utilization of energy.
- Increase the intake of foods rich in iodine, such as seaweed. Iodine is the building block of thyroid hormone, and is essential for normal thyroid health.
- According to traditional Chinese medicine, vegetables are generally cold in nature and meats are usually warm in property. Since individuals with hypothyroidism often have yang deficiency and cold presentations, increased consumption of meats (especially lamb) will help warm up the body and dispel cold.

FORMULAS

THYRO-*forte* ™

LIFESTYLE INSTRUCTIONS

- Regular exercise helps to stimulate thyroid hormone secretion and increases the tissue sensitivity to the hormone. Exercise is also beneficial by raising the basal body metabolism.
- Induce perspiration by taking hot water baths, saunas, or steam baths.

CLINICAL NOTES

- Patients with hypothyroidism should notice improvement within one month, starting with increased energy and elevated body temperature. Stabilization and maximum effect may not be observed until the individual has been ingesting the herbs for one to two months.
- Progress of hypothyroid treatment can be monitored by checking the body temperature, heart rate, and blood pressure. It is best to check these parameters first thing in the morning to avoid fluctuations.
- *Thyro-forte* and thyroid supplement drugs may be taken concurrently without conflict.
- It is important to be aware that long-term use of thyroid supplements (such as levothyroxine) has been associated with loss of as much as 13% of bone mass. Therefore, patients who have been or are currently using thyroid supplements should take calcium supplements to replenish the loss of bone mass.

CAUTIONS

- This formula is contraindicated during pregnancy and nursing.
- Patients who wear a pacemaker, or individuals who take anti-arrhythmic drugs or cardiac glycosides such as Lanoxin (Digoxin), should not take this formula. *Fu Zi* (Radix Aconiti Lateralis Praeparata) may interact with these drugs by affecting the rhythm and potentiating the contractile strength of the heart.

ACUPUNCTURE POINTS

Traditional Points:
- *Pishu* (BL 20), *Shenshu* (BL 23), *Zusanli* (ST 36), *Guanyuan* (CV 4) and *Qihai* (CV 6).
- Apply moxa to *Shenshu* (BL 23), *Guanyuan* (CV 4) and *Zusanli* (ST 36).

Balance Method by Dr. Richard Tan:
- Left side: *Hegu* (LI 4), *Yangxi* (LI 5), *Fuliu* (KI 7), *Sanyinjiao* (SP 6), and Thyroid point on the ear.
- Right side: *Taiyuan* (LU 9), *Xuanzhong* (GB 39), *Yangfu* (GB 38), *Guangming* (GB 37), and *Zusanli* (ST 36).
- Left and right side can be alternated from treatment to treatment.
- For additional information on the Balance Method, please refer to *Dr. Tan's Strategy of Twelve Magical Points* by Dr. Richard Tan.

Auricular Acupuncture by Dr. Li-Chun Huang:
- Hypothyroidism: Thyroid, Pituitary, Exciting Point, Thalamus, Endocrine, Gonadotropin, Sanjiao, Kidney, Liver, and Sympathetic.
- For additional information on the location and explanation of these points, please refer to *Auricular Treatment Formula and Prescriptions* by Dr. Li-Chun Huang.

MODERN RESEARCH

Thyro-forte is an herbal formula developed specifically for patients with hypothyroidism. Herbs in this formula function to stimulate the production of thyroid hormone, increase basal metabolism, improve physiological functions, and enhance energy levels.

FORMULAS

THYRO-*forte* ™

Synthesis of thyroid hormone requires adequate quantities of iodine.[1] Without iodine as the raw material, the thyroid glands continually attempt to produce thyroid hormone without success. This eventually leads to hypertrophy and enlargement of the thyroid glands. Rich in iodine, *Hai Zao* (Sargassum) and *Kun Bu* (Thallus Laminariae seu Eckloniae) will stimulate the production of thyroid hormone, and effectively reduce the hypertrophy and enlargement of the thyroid glands (in cases of hypothyroidism due to lack of iodine in diet).[2]

In addition to supplying adequate quantities of iodine, it is imperative to ensure that the basal metabolism is increased and the physiological functions are improved. Basal metabolism may be increased with yang tonic herbs. Studies have shown that *Rou Gui* (Cortex Cinnamomi) and *Fu Zi* (Radix Aconiti Lateralis Praeparata) have stimulating effects on the body, leading to excitation of the cardiovascular,[3] gastrointestinal,[4] and immune systems.[5] Furthermore, physiological functions can be improved with yin tonic herbs. Numerous herbs in this formula have shown marked stimulating effects on the endocrine system to increase the production of various endogenous hormones. Examples include *Shu Di Huang* (Radix Rehmanniae Preparata),[6] *Shan Zhu Yu* (Fructus Corni),[7] and *Shan Yao* (Rhizoma Dioscoreae).[8] *Ze Xie* (Rhizoma Alismatis), *Mu Dan Pi* (Cortex Moutan) and *Fu Ling* (Poria) do not have direct effects on the production of thyroid hormone, they are added to balance the tonic herbs and minimize any unwanted effects. Altogether, these six herbs compose *Liu Wei Di Huang Wan* (Six-Ingredient Pill with Rehmannia), a Kidney yin tonic formula commonly used to treat various disorders characterized by aging and decline in physiological functions.

Lastly, *Ren Shen* (Radix Ginseng) is added here as it has numerous physiologic effects. In addition to improving energy, *Ren Shen* (Radix Ginseng) improves learning and memory,[9] stimulates the pituitary gland to increase the release of various endogenous hormones,[10,11] balances the cardiovascular system by restoring homeostasis,[12] and enhances the immune system.[13]

PHARMACEUTICAL DRUGS & CHINESE MEDICINE: A COMPARATIVE ANALYSIS

Western Medical Approach: Hypothyroidism is one of the most common disorders in developed countries. The disease is well understood, and treatment is simple and straightforward. In western medicine, hypothyroidism is the lack of thyroid hormone, and therefore, treatment is to use synthetic thyroid hormone to supplement the insufficiency. Synthroid (Levothyroxine) is generally considered to be the drug of choice, and when used carefully, it is generally safe and effective. Because Synthroid (Levothyroxine) is very potent, it must be monitored carefully, as inappropriate dosing contributes to hyper- or hypothyroid signs and symptoms. It has also been noted that Synthroid (Levothyroxine) may contribute to hypersensitivity problems, presumably because it is synthetic and may have compatibility issues. Lastly, it has been observed that long-term use of synthetic thyroid hormones is associated with increased loss of bone mass density. In short, synthetic thyroid hormone is the only drug treatment available for hypothyroidism patients. Furthermore, once synthetic thyroid hormone therapy begins, endogenous production slowly decreases and the body becomes more and more dependant on the exogenous source. Eventually, the patient will become dependent on thyroid drugs for life. In conclusion, though synthetic thyroid hormone is effective, it must be prescribed correctly, monitored carefully, and potential complications must be address with preventative measures (such as taking calcium supplements daily to avoid developing osteoporosis).

Traditional Chinese Medicine Approach: Many herbs effectively treat hypothyroidism. Because this condition is diagnosed as Kidney yang deficiency, it is treated with warm herbs that tonify Kidney yang. These herbs have been shown to have marked effect to increase body temperature, elevate body metabolism, and improve mood to alleviate many symptoms associated with hypothyroidism. Furthermore, these herbs also have marked effect to regulate endocrine system and stimulate thyroid glands to increase production of thyroid hormones. Because herbs are effective to treat both symptoms and cause, they often exert both immediate and long-lasting effects. However, there is one major limitation to herbal therapy. Because these herbs work primarily by stimulating the thyroid gland to produce thyroid hormone, those who cannot produce thyroid hormone (such as those who have had a complete

THYRO-*forte* ™

thyroidectomy) will not benefit from herbs. They must be treated with synthetic thyroid hormone to ensure proper regulation of growth and metabolism.

Summation: Both drugs and herbs treat hypothyroidism effectively. The main benefit of drug therapy is potency and consistency, and the main disadvantages are the potential adverse reactions and long-term dependence on the drugs. The main advantage of herbal therapy is its effectiveness to manage both symptoms and cause of hypothyroidism, and the main drawback is the absence of means to treat patients who can no longer produce thyroid hormone internally. Optimal treatment depends on complete understanding by informed and educated practitioner *and* patient of the pros and cons of both modalities of medicines, deciding together on the most appropriate therapy.

CASE STUDIES

A 47-year-old female presented with low energy and excess uterine bleeding. She had been diagnosed with hypothyroid and uterine fibroids. The patient stated she wanted to get off Synthroid (Levothyroxine). Her RBC, TSH and T4 levels were low. Her pulse was thready and her tongue was pale. The practitioner diagnosed the case as Kidney deficiency with Liver blood deficiency due to excess bleeding. A raw herbal formula was used to shrink the fibroids and control the uterine bleeding for 6 months. Once the bleeding and fibroids were under control, the patient was instructed to take *Thyro-forte*. Immediately, the patient experienced an increase in energy and overall health. The combination of 4 capsules three times daily of *Thyro-forte* accompanied with Synthroid (Levothyroxine) was too potent, so the dose was reduced to 3 capsules three times daily with positive results. Without the *Thyro-forte* treatment, the patient noticed a drop in energy level.

F.V., Orlando, Florida

A 30-year-old female diagnosed with hypothyroidism displayed signs and symptoms of low energy, diarrhea, depression, coldness, and a low body temperature of 96.9° F. She was given *Thyro-forte*. Shortly after administering *Thyro-forte*, she reported an enhanced energy level along with an increase of overall body warmth by over 50% (basal temperature was increased to 97.8° F). The patient's bouts with diarrhea and depression appeared to have resolved. She felt stronger, happier, and more energetic.

S. T., San Jose, California

L.D., a 31-year-old female, presented with fatigue, dizziness, low body temperature, coldness, and muscle weakness. Her blood pressure was 100/60 mmHg and her heart rate was 65 beats per minute. Her western diagnoses were hypotension and hypoglycemia. Laboratory results showed she had decreased thyroid activity and adrenal medullary insufficiency. The diagnosis was yang deficiency. She was prescribed *Thyro-forte* and *Adrenoplex* at 2.5 and 1.5 grams per day, respectively. She did not receive any acupuncture. After two months, she felt much more energized and the dizziness was gone. She no longer felt cold.

W.F., Bloomfield, New Jersey

T.M., a 53-year-old female, presented with constant fatigue, muscle aches and pain, dry skin and trouble with communication, with sensations of tightness in her throat. The western diagnoses were fibromyalgia and a low T4 level; the TCM diagnosis was Spleen qi and blood deficiencies. *Thyro-forte* was prescribed along with *Si Ni San* (Frigid Extremities Powder), *Gui Pi Tang* (Restore the Spleen Decoction) and *An Mian Pian* pills. After nine months of treatment with acupuncture and herbs, the patient was able to completely cease use of thyroid drugs.

M.C., Sarasota, Florida

THYRO-*forte* ™

E.B., a 75-year-old female, presented with hypothyroidism. It started a number of years ago and she took Thyroxin until recently when a new medical doctor switched her, against her will, to Levoxyl that contains no T3. Thyroxin contains T3. The client attributed this to the severe reduction in her energy and recent weight gain despite a program of aerobic exercise 5 days a week, weight lifting, and careful attention to her diet. After 12 noon everyday she lost any desire to do anything. The patient described herself as lethargic and discouraged. The patient weighed 151 pounds. Her blood pressure was 148/80 mmHg with a heart rate of 56 beats per minute. A year ago, before switching to the new thyroid drug, she weighed 133 pounds. No lab reports were available. She presented with excellent spirit but clearly distressed about her loss of energy and her weight gain. Her tongue was pale with a purplish cast. The Spleen pulse was large and empty. The TCM diagnosis was Spleen qi and yang deficiency with dampness. *Thyro-forte* was prescribed at 2 capsules three times daily. The patient reported increased energy levels to 8 out of 10 from the 2 out of 10 she rated herself before the herbal treatment. Her weight, however, did not change. About a year and a half after the herbal treatment, the patient persuaded her M.D. to put her back on Thyroxin and she then tapered off the *Thyro-forte* thereafter.

H.H., San Francisco, California

---

[1] Fauci, et al., *Harrison's Principles of Internal Medicine 14th Edition*, 1998; 2012:2019
[2] Yen, ZH, et al., *Chinese Herbology*, 1998; 629:631
[3] Zhou, YD, *Journal of Herbology*, 1983; 18(5):394
[4] Chen, Y, *Journal of Chinese Herbology*, 1981; 6(5):32
[5] Wang, YS, *Pharmacology and Applications of Chinese Herbs*, 1983; 443
[6] Yen, ZH, et al., *Chinese Herbology*, 1998; 156:158
[7] Jiang, Y, *Pharmacology and Clinical Applications of Chinese Herbs*, 1989; 5(1):36
[8] He, ZQ, *Journal of University of Chinese Herbology*, 1991; 22(3):158
[9] *Encyclopedia of Chinese Herbs*, 1994
[10] Song, R, *Journal of Baiqioen University of Medicine*, 1980; 6(2):32
[11] Shu, SK, *Study of Chinese Patent Medicine*, 1989; 11(9):30
[12] *CA*, 1992; 116:34223d
[13] Yen, ZH, et al., *Chinese Herbology*, 1998; 729:736

FORMULAS

TRAUMANEX ™

CLINICAL APPLICATIONS

- Sports injuries including external injuries, traumas, bruises, contusions, sprains, etc.
- Broken bones or fractures with severe pain, inflammation and swelling
- Post-surgical recovery

WESTERN THERAPEUTIC ACTIONS

- Antispasmodic function to relieve muscle spasms and cramps [1,2,3,5,7]
- Anti-inflammatory actions to reduce inflammation and swelling [2,3,9]
- Stops bleeding and traumatic hemorrhage [2,9]

CHINESE THERAPEUTIC ACTIONS

- Invigorates the blood
- Removes blood stagnation
- Relieves pain
- Helps to regenerate bones and soft tissues

DOSAGE

Take 5 to 6 capsules every six hours at the initial stage of injury. After the condition stabilizes, reduce the dosage to 3 to 4 capsules three times daily. For maximum effectiveness, take the herbs on an empty stomach with warm water. The herbs can be taken after meals if stomach discomfort should occur.

INGREDIENTS

Bai Shao (Radix Paeoniae Alba)
Da Huang (Radix et Rhizoma Rhei)
Dang Gui Wei (Extremitas Radicis Angelicae Sinensis)
Er Cha (Catechu)
Fu Ling (Poria)
Gan Cao (Radix Glycyrrhizae)
Hong Hua (Flos Carthami)

Mo Yao (Myrrha)
Mu Dan Pi (Cortex Moutan)
Mu Xiang (Radix Aucklandiae)
Ru Xiang (Gummi Olibanum)
Su Mu (Lignum Sappan)
Tao Ren (Semen Persicae)
Yan Hu Suo (Rhizoma Corydalis)

FORMULA EXPLANATION

Traumanex is formulated for both internal and external injuries, such as broken bones, bone fractures, sports injuries, bruises, contusions, sprains, etc. It can be used to enhance recovery and prevent scarring. This is an excellent formula to activate qi and blood circulation, remove qi and blood stagnation, relieve pain, and facilitate healing by regenerating bone and soft tissues.

Yan Hu Suo (Rhizoma Corydalis) and *Su Mu* (Lignum Sappan) dispel blood stasis and alleviate pain. *Er Cha* (Catechu) reduces swelling, drains dampness and absorbs seepage from sores or wounds. *Ru Xiang* (Gummi Olibanum), *Mo Yao* (Myrrha), *Mu Xiang* (Radix Aucklandiae), *Dang Gui Wei* (Extremitas Radicis Angelicae Sinensis), *Hong Hua* (Flos Carthami) and *Tao Ren* (Semen Persicae) promote the healing of wounds and relieve pain by invigorating blood circulation. *Da Huang* (Radix et Rhizoma Rhei) and *Mu Dan Pi* (Cortex Moutan) reduce inflammation by clearing heat. *Bai Shao* (Radix Paeoniae Alba) has strong analgesic, antispasmodic and anti-inflammatory effects. *Fu Ling* (Poria) tonifies the Spleen and indirectly promotes the regeneration of muscles. *Gan Cao* (Radix Glycyrrhizae) relaxes the tendons and muscles and harmonizes the formula.

SUPPLEMENTARY FORMULAS

- To stop bleeding, add *Notoginseng 9*.
- For severe pain, use with *Herbal Analgesic*.
- For headache, use with *Corydalin* or *Migratrol*.
- For neck and shoulder pain, add *Neck & Shoulder (Acute)* or *Neck & Shoulder (Chronic)*.
- For lower back pain, combine with *Back Support (Acute)* or *Back Support (Chronic)*.
- For upper back pain, combine with *Back Support (Upper)*.
- For pain in the arm (shoulder, elbow, wrist and hand), add *Arm Support*.
- For severe pain due to herniated disk, add *Back Support (HD)*.
- For pain due to knee injuries, add *Knee & Ankle (Acute)* or *Knee & Ankle (Chronic)*.
- For chronic pain due to damaged soft tissues (muscles, ligaments, tendons and cartilages), add *Flex (MLT)*.
- For muscle spasms and cramps, combine with *Flex (SC)*.
- For chronic arthritic pain that worsens during cold and rainy weather, combine with *Flex (CD)*.
- For inflammation of joints with redness and swelling, consider using *Flex (Heat)* instead.
- For bone spurs, use with *Flex (Spur)*.
- For external injury with open wound and/or infection, use with *Herbal ABX*.
- During the recovery phase of bone fractures or broken bones, use with *Osteo 8*.
- For post-surgical constipation, add *Gentle Lax (Deficient)*.
- For severe blood stagnation and bruising, add *Circulation (SJ)*.
- For signs and symptoms of excess fire, add *Gardenia Complex*.

NUTRITION

- Advise the patients to eat half of a fresh pineapple daily. Pineapple is rich in bromelain and will reduce swelling and inflammation.
- Patients with broken bones or fractures should consume an adequate amount of calcium during recovery.
- Patients with broken bones or fractures should avoid foods with preservatives because phosphorus in preservatives can lead to bone loss.
- Patients are advised to avoid cold food and drinks, as cold will cause more stagnation. They should also avoid spicy food to prevent aggravating the inflammatory condition.

LIFESTYLE INSTRUCTIONS

- Avoid exercise with high risk of injury, especially during the recovery phase.
- For external injury with open wounds, be sure to clean the affected area thoroughly to prevent infection.
- Vitamin E oil can be applied to the wounds to minimize scarring. However, vitamin E oil should be applied only after the open wounds have closed/healed.

CLINICAL NOTES

- *Traumanex* is an herbal formula originally used by *Kung-Fu* masters and monks in the *Shaolin* temple to treat various internal and external injuries. It has excellent functions to relieve pain, treat soft tissue injuries, facilitate healing of broken bones or bone fractures.

TRAUMANEX ™

- There are three excellent formulas for post-surgical recovery. *Traumanex* should be taken after the surgery for 5 to 10 days to facilitate the immediate healing of wounds. Continue herbal treatment with *Flex (MLT)* and *Osteo 8* for one month to facilitate healing and recovery of soft tissues and bones, respectively.
- The following is a folk remedy to treat acute back pain from sprain and strain. Crack open 2 crabs (ocean) with a wooden stick (do not use a knife or any metal instruments) and put then into a clay pot with enough vodka or whiskey to cover both crabs. Place the clay pot into another bigger pot with water and steam it for one hour. Serve the crab meat along with the soup.

CAUTIONS

- This formula is contraindicated during pregnancy and nursing.
- Do not use this formula if the patient has internal hemorrhage. *Traumanex* has many herbs that activate blood circulation and may delay coagulation.
- Patients who are on anticoagulant or antiplatelet therapies, such as Coumadin (Warfarin), should use this formula with caution as there may be a slightly higher risk of bleeding and bruising.
- This formula may cause mild gastrointestinal discomfort, which can be minimized by taking the herbs with food or decreasing the dosage.
- This formula is not designed for long-term use. It should be used only during the acute phases of injuries, and discontinued when the desired effects are achieved.

ACUPUNCTURE POINTS

Traditional Points:
- *Ah shi* points.

Balance Method by Dr. Richard Tan:
- The treatment protocol is different for each case, depending on the location and severity of injuries.
- For additional information on the Balance Method, please refer to *Twelve and Twelve in Acupuncture* and *Twenty-Four More in Acupuncture* by Dr. Richard Tan.

Ear Points:
- Knee injuries: Knees, Adrenal Gland, and Pituitary Gland.
- Post-operative pain: Needle the reflective location of the surgery, Subcortex, *Shenmen*, and Lung. Needle twice a day with strong stimulation and leave the needles in for one to two hours. These points are more effective to relieve sharp pain associated with surgery and not as well for distension and pain as the result of abdominal surgery.
- Post-operative flatulence: Select and needle the sensitive points along the Large Intestine and Small Intestine, Stomach, Sympathetic, and Spleen. Strongly stimulate for one to two hours to help alleviate distension and promote passage of gas.

Auricular Acupuncture by Dr. Li-Chun Huang:
- Acute sprain and contusion: Corresponding points (to the area of injury).
  - For pain, add Large Auricular Nerve, and Lesser Occipital Nerve. Bleed Ear Apex.
  - For tranquillizing the mind, add *Shenmen*.
- For additional information on the location and explanation of these points, please refer to *Auricular Treatment Formula and Prescriptions* by Dr. Li-Chun Huang.

FORMULAS

TRAUMANEX ™

MODERN RESEARCH

Traumanex is formulated specifically to treat both internal and external injuries, such as broken bones, bone fractures, sports injuries, bruises, contusions, sprains, etc. Pharmacologically, herbs in this formula have an antispasmodic function to relieve muscle spasms and cramps, anti-inflammatory action to reduce inflammation and swelling, and hemostatic effect to stop bleeding.

Bai Shao (Radix Paeoniae Alba) and *Gan Cao* (Radix Glycyrrhizae) are commonly combined to relieve muscle spasms and cramps. Clinically, they may be used for musculoskeletal spasms and leg cramps associated with external or sports injuries. They may also be used for smooth-muscle cramps, such as abdominal and intestinal cramps or dysmenorrhea.[1] *Bai Shao* (Radix Paeoniae Alba) and *Gan Cao* (Radix Glycyrrhizae) have strong antispasmodic and anti-inflammatory effects as confirmed by modern research. Furthermore, *Bai Shao* (Radix Paeoniae Alba) and *Gan Cao* (Radix Glycyrrhizae) are effective in treating both skeletal and smooth muscles. [2,3]

For treatment of musculoskeletal disorders using *Bai Shao* (Radix Paeoniae Alba) and *Gan Cao* (Radix Glycyrrhizae), 30 out of 42 patients reported relief of trigeminal pain;[4] 11 out of 11 patients experienced reduction of muscle spasm and twitching in the facial region;[5] and out of 33 elderly patients with pain in the lower back and legs, 12 patients reported significant improvement, 16 reported moderate improvement, 4 reported slight improvement and 1 reported no effect.[6]

For treatment of smooth muscle disorders, the combination of *Bai Shao* (Radix Paeoniae Alba) and *Gan Cao* (Radix Glycyrrhizae) relieved abdominal pain and cramps due to intestinal parasites in 11 out of 11 patients;[7] and in 185 patients with epigastric and abdominal pain, 139 patients reported significant improvement, 41 reported moderate improvement, and 5 reported no effect.[8] Lastly, *Bai Shao* (Radix Paeoniae Alba) has tranquilizing and analgesic effects to relieve pain.[9]

Tao Ren (Semen Persicae), *Hong Hua* (Flos Carthami) and *Dang Gui Wei* (Extremitas Radicis Angelicae Sinensis) have excellent functions to invigorate blood circulation and facilitate healing. It was demonstrated in a clinical study with 775 cases of swelling and subcutaneous hemorrhage due to acute sprains that *Hong Hua* (Flos Carthami) can effectively improve and/or cure the condition within 3 to 5 days.[2,9]

Su Mu (Lignum Sappan), *Ru Xiang* (Gummi Olibanum) and *Mo Yao* (Myrrha) are commonly used together to treat trauma-induced pain and swelling.[2,9]

Da Huang (Radix et Rhizoma Rhei) has a wide range of effects on the treatment of sports or traumatic injuries. Taken internally, it shortens coagulation time or stops bleeding. Used externally (as powder or paste), it treats traumatic hemorrhage with no adverse reactions or side effects. [2,9]

PHARMACEUTICAL DRUGS & CHINESE MEDICINE: A COMPARATIVE ANALYSIS

Western Medical Approach: Trauma injuries are generally treated with drugs that reduce inflammation and relieve pain. Two classes of drugs commonly used for treatment include non-steroidal anti-inflammatory agents (NSAID) and opioid analgesics. NSAID's [such as Motrin (Ibuprofen) and Voltaren (Diclofenac)] are generally used for mild to moderate pain, and are most effective to reduce inflammation and swelling. Though effective, they may cause such serious side effects as gastric ulcer, duodenal ulcer, gastrointestinal bleeding, tinnitus, blurred vision, dizziness and headache. Furthermore, newer NSAID's, also known as Cox-2 inhibitors [such as Celebrex (Celecoxib)], are associated with significantly higher risk of cardiovascular events, including heart attack and stroke. Opioid analgesics [such as Vicodin (APAP/Hydrocodone) and morphine] are usually used for severe to excruciating pain. While they may be the most potent agents for pain, they also have the most serious risks and side effects, including but not limited to dizziness, lightheadedness, drowsiness, upset stomach, vomiting, constipation, stomach pain, rash, difficult urination, and respiratory depression resulting in difficult breathing. Furthermore, long-term use of these drugs leads to tolerance and addiction. In brief, it is important to remember that while drugs offer reliable and potent symptomatic pain relief, they should be used only if and when needed. Frequent use and abuse leads to unnecessary side effects and complications.

Traditional Chinese Medicine Approach: Treatment of trauma injuries is focused on relieving acute symptoms and promoting long-term recovery. Symptoms of pain, inflammation and swelling are usually treated with herbs that activate qi and blood circulation, as these herbs have excellent analgesic and anti-inflammatory effects. Furthermore, herbs that activate qi and blood also promote blood circulation to the affected area to facilitate and speed up the recovery process. In other words, by relieving symptoms and promoting recovery, use of herbs achieves both immediate and prolonged benefits.

Summation: Both drugs and herbs are effective and play slightly different roles in trauma management. In mild to moderate cases, drugs and herbs are approximately equally effective. In severe cases, such as bone fractures or severe physical injuries, drugs have stronger analgesic effect. After the acute condition stabilizes, herbs should definitely be used as they facilitate and shorten the recovery process. In short, drugs and herbs have contrasting benefits, and may be utilize in different stages of trauma recovery for optimal care.

CASE STUDIES

C.K., a 12-year-old boy, presented with a painful and swollen elbow, with bruises due to a go-cart accident in which he was pinned under the roll bar. The patient was asked to take three capsules of *Traumanex*, four times a day, with food to avoid stomach upset. The accident happened on Thursday: the boy was able to return to school on Monday with 100% recovery, and experienced no stomach upset. A topical herbal tincture *Po Sum On*, along with acupuncture, massage and homeopathic remedies, were all part of the treatment regimen.

M.C., Sarasota, Florida

D.D., a 41-year-old nurse, presented with a work-related injury. She had severe back pain that was the result of a fall from lifting a patient. She said she heard a popping sound in her back when she fell. MRI confirmed her diagnosis of the herniated lumbar disc. She was 9 weeks post-injury and had scheduled for steroid epidurals. She refused injections and came to our clinic for 'safe and non-invasive care.' Her blood pressure was 140/80 mmHg and the heart rate was 80 beats per minute. TCM diagnoses included qi and blood stagnation and soft tissue damage. *Back Support (Acute)*, *Flex (SC)* and *Traumanex* were prescribed at 3 capsules each three times a day. After the herbs, the patient was able to reduce Vicodin (APAP/Hydrocodone) use from 2 to 0.5 tablets per day, and none at all on some days. She had increased blood pressure from stress over the injury, which was up to 170/110 mmHg. After the herbs and massage, the blood pressure came down to normal and is staying down. She had received no additional physical therapy. She did remarkably well in a short period of time.

M.H., West Palm Beach, Florida

An 18-year-old male chef presented with neck and shoulder pain from a skateboard fall. X-rays revealed a diminished cervical curvature as well as a hypokyphotic curve at T2 to T3. The practitioner diagnosed the condition as a cervical sprain/strain. The patient was treated with *Neck & Shoulder (Acute)* and *Traumanex*, which produced a reduction in pain. The patient found it necessary to take the herbs with food to avoid stomach discomfort.

M.H., Jupiter, Florida

FORMULAS

TRAUMANEX ™

J.M., a 36-year-old female massage therapist presented with pain from a recent automobile accident (second accident in 6 months). She exhibited neck, back, arm and leg pain. Airbags bent her right thumb. Her blood pressure was 120/70 mmHg and her heart rate was 72 beats per minute. X-rays showed herniation and soft tissue damage. She also complained of muscle spasms, hot sensation on trigger points, inability to move the right thumb and the range of motion for the neck and trunk were both decreased. *Traumanex*, *Neck & Shoulder (Acute)* and *Back Support (Acute)* were all prescribed at 2 capsules each three times daily. J.M. responded quickly to these formulas and acupuncture treatments. Pain levels were reduced by half in a short period of time.

M.H., West Palm Beach, Florida

L.P., a 77-year-old female, presented with severe pain in the left wrist and right rib cage after a fall. She had numbness of the wrist and palm where she landed on the cement. The patient showed bruises on the right eye. The right wrist was painful to light movement and palpation. There were tender points on the right subclavicular area. There were no visible contusions on the right rib cage. The diagnoses were qi and blood stagnation with soft tissue damage. *Traumanex*, *Neck & Shoulder (Acute)* and *Flex (SC)* were prescribed at 2 capsules of each formula three times daily. The patient reported daily lowering of pain levels. Numbness was reduced to a light tingling after two days. She reported continuous and steady improvement each day. She was instructed to reduce the dosage to 2 capsules of each formula twice a day when the pain subsided. After the swelling was reduced, the patient was referred to a chiropractor for cervical and occiput adjustments.

M. H., West Palm Beach, Florida

[1] Bensky, D. et al. *Chinese Herbal Medicine Formulas and Strategies*. Eastland Press. 1990
[2] Bensky, D. et al. *Chinese Herbal Medicine Materia Medica*. Eastland Press. 1993
[3] Tan, H. et al. Chemical components of decoction of radix paeoniae and radix glycyrrhizae. *China Journal of Chinese Materia Medica*. 20(9):550-1,576, Sept. 1995
[4] Huang, DD. *Journal of Traditional Chinese Medicine*. 11:9. 1983
[5] Luo, DP. *Hunan Journal of Traditional Chinese Medicine*. 2:7. 1989
[6] Chen, Hong. *Yunnan Journal of Traditional Chinese Medicine*. 4:15. 1990
[7] Zhang, RB. *Jiangxu Journal of Traditional Chinese Medicine*. 5:38-39. 1966
[8] You, JH. *Guanxi Journal of Chinese Herbology*. 5:5-6. 1987
[9] Yeung, HC. *Handbook of Chinese Herbs*. Institute of Chinese Medicine. 1996

FORMULAS

VENUS ™

CLINICAL APPLICATIONS

- Small or underdeveloped breasts
- Women who want to increase or maintain a healthy breast shape
- Enhances lactation in nursing women

WESTERN THERAPEUTIC ACTIONS

- Regulates the endocrine system to increase the production of sex hormones [1]
- Stimulates the growth and development of breasts [2,3,4,5]
- Improves blood circulation [6]
- Increases the generation of new tissue [7]

CHINESE THERAPEUTIC ACTIONS

- Tonifies Kidney yang and *jing* (essence)
- Opens channels in the breasts
- Invigorates blood circulation

DOSAGE

Take 2 to 4 capsules on an empty stomach three times daily to enhance healthy breasts. For maximum effectiveness, the exercises listed under Clinical Notes should be done twice daily. Dosage should be lowered to 1 to 2 capsules daily for women taking this formula to enhance lactation. Discontinue use if the baby has diarrhea.

INGREDIENTS

Bai Zhi (Radix Angelicae Dahuricae)
Chuan Mu Tong (Caulis Clematidis Armandii)
Dang Gui (Radicis Angelicae Sinensis)
Huang Qi (Radix Astragali)

Lu Rong (Cornu Cervi Pantotrichum)
Tong Cao (Medulla Tetrapanacis)
Wang Bu Liu Xing (Semen Vaccariae)
Yin Yang Huo (Herba Epimedii)

FORMULA EXPLANATION

Venus is designed for women with small and/or underdeveloped breasts due to various reasons such as degeneration, aging, over-developed pectoris muscles, malnutrition and sudden weight loss. Small breasts in women are usually due to heredity, interruption of growth during adolescence, and nutritional deficiencies.

Venus contains potent Kidney yang and *jing* (essence) tonics that will stimulate the growth of reproductive organs and increase libido. *Lu Rong* (Cornu Cervi Pantotrichum), the chief ingredient in *Venus*, is often medically used for developmental delays in children. It tonifies the *ming men* (life gate) fire, replenishes *jing* (essence) and blood. In medical terminology, it stimulates the pituitary gland to release growth hormones that will promote the growth of reproductive organs including the breasts. When Kidney yang is restored, sex drive also increases. *Yin Yang Huo* (Herba Epimedii) is also a well-known herb to tonify Kidney yang and enhance libido. The Spleen is the organ responsible for generating muscle and tissue, and *Huang Qi* (Radix Astragali) is used to tonify the Spleen and help with toning and firming the muscles around the breasts. *Dang Gui* (Radicis Angelicae Sinensis) is well known as an herb that treats all types of obstetric and gynecologic disorders. It tonifies blood, promotes blood circulation, and regulates menstruation. Its phyto-estrogenic effect stimulates the estrogenic receptors of the breasts and helps them grow to their fullest potential. *Chuan Mu Tong* (Caulis Clematidis Armandii), *Tong Cao* (Medulla Tetrapanacis) and

FORMULAS

VENUS ™

Wang Bu Liu Xing (Semen Vaccariae) invigorate blood circulation and promote lactation. Historically, they have been used on postpartum women to support mammary glands and promote lactation. In women who are not nursing, however, these herbs will simply enlarge the breast tissue. *Bai Zhi* (Radix Angelicae Dahuricae), an herb that enters the Stomach channel and passes through the breasts, is used as a channel-guiding herb to draw nutrients from the other tonic herbs to the breast area.

In conclusion, *Venus* contains many herbs that have remarkable influences on the hormones and development of the sex organs. In the past, these herbs were used mainly to promote lactation in nursing mothers. More recently, with the understanding of modern science, these herbs are known to have a great effect to increase breast size.

SUPPLEMENTARY FORMULAS

- For healthy, shiny hair, add *Polygonum 14*.
- Fro low libido, add *Vitality*.
- For weight loss and to control the appetite, add *Herbalite*.
- For fatigue and weakness or decrease in libido due to qi and blood deficiencies, add *Imperial Tonic*.
- For postpartum recovery, add *Imperial Tonic*.
- For anemia, dizziness or blood deficiency, add *Schisandra ZZZ*.
- For stress or decrease in libido due to Liver qi stagnation, add *Calm*.
- For women with a cold constitution, add *Balance (Cold)*.
- For menopause, add *Balance (Heat)* or *Nourish*.
- For adrenal burnout, add *Adrenoplex* .
- For osteoporosis, add *Osteo 8*.
- For Kidney yang deficiency, add *Kidney Tonic (Yang)*.
- For Kidney yin deficiency, add *Kidney Tonic (Yin)*.
- For infertility, add *Blossom (Phase 1-4)*.

NUTRITION

- Patients are advised to eat a nutritious diet and increase the consumption of lamb because it is an excellent Kidney tonic. Intake of protein (beans, eggs, etc.) and foods high in collagen such as tendons, chicken wings, and animal skin can be increased. Other recommendations include lotus seeds, sunflower seeds, peanuts, strawberries, dates, yam, papaya, taro, onions, celery, chives, spinach, oranges, carrots, milk and cheese.
- Fried, fatty food, sugar, dairy and caffeine should be avoided as much as possible.
- For low libido, intake of vitamin E can be increased. Foods high in vitamin E include wheat germ oil, almonds, sunflower seeds or oil, peanuts, soybeans, whole-wheat products and asparagus.

LIFESTYLE INSTRUCTIONS

- Tight bras are not recommended since the constriction impairs proper circulation to the breasts.
- It is helpful to use cold water to shower the breasts to achieve the firming and massaging effect. Avoid using water that is too hot on the breasts as that may loosen surrounding tissue.
- Proper posture is important to prevent breasts from sagging. Swimming is recommended. Exercises that involve excessive vertical (up and down) movement of the breasts are not recommended as they might cause stretching or lengthening of the surrounding tendons and ligaments that support the breasts.

VENUS ™

CLINICAL NOTES

Exercises for the Breasts: Several exercises can be done to help promote healthier breast size and firmness. They help strengthen the connective tissues around the breasts and promote the growth of new cells. These exercises should be done twice daily in addition to taking the herbs for maximum shaping, toning and lifting effect.

Breast Massage: There are two steps for this breast massage exercise.
- Step 1: The purpose of this massage is to maintain and achieve a healthy breast shape and firmness. This exercise prevents ligament laxity that causes drooping of the breast. Massage the breasts in a circular motion going outwards. Gradually increase the size of the circular motion to cover the neck and shoulder. Repeat for 3 to 5 minutes (Picture 1).
- Step 2: Stroke the bottom of one breast upward using right and left hands in alternating motion. Repeat 50 times for each breast and make sure to cover the entire bottom curve (Picture 2).

Praying Style Exercise: The purpose of this exercise is to strengthen the pectoral muscles to help bring circulation to the chest. First, stand up straight with palms together in a prayer position in front of chest. Make sure both elbows form a straight horizontal line across chest (Picture 3). Next, push palms together to feel muscles under the breasts contracting. While pushing palms together, raise arms up to forehead with elbows still in a straight line and hold for 2 to 3 seconds. After 2 to 3 seconds, release contraction and bring back to original position in middle of chest. Repeat this procedure 10 times (Picture 4).

Expand the Chest Exercise: The purpose of this exercise is to strengthen the upper chest muscles to enhance breast firmness to prevent drooping. First, clasp hands behind your back with palms facing down (Picture 5). Next, take a deep breath in, thrust chest outward and lift clasped hands behind your back. Tighten your lower back muscles and arch your whole body including your neck. Return to a relaxed position with hands clasped behind the back. Repeat this procedure 10 times (Picture 6).

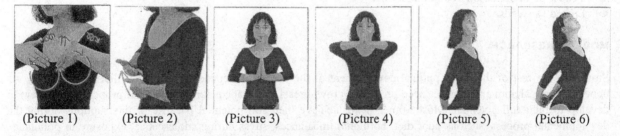

(Picture 1)   (Picture 2)   (Picture 3)   (Picture 4)   (Picture 5)   (Picture 6)

Some patients may notice breast tenderness after intake of these herbs. That is an indication of growth and the patient should not be worried. Along with the exercise, patients should notice a difference in tone after 4 to 6 weeks, while actual growth may be from 3 to 6 months. Full growth potential and desired results depend on body constitution, genetics, consistent intake of herbs, diet and exercise. As is the case in not achieving desired weight loss, the main reason for lack of response to the herbs is from lapses in taking the herbs or doing exercise. Finally, patients should be advised that this formula and exercise could only enhance breasts to their maximum genetic potential and not beyond. A small-breasted woman from a family of small-breasted women may see improvement in the tone and shape of her breasts, but should not expect to greatly exceed her genetic inheritance.

VENUS ™

CAUTIONS

- ☯ This formula is contraindicated in patients with acute infection or heat accumulation, fibrocystic disorders of the breast, hormone-dependent cancer, or have a personal or family history of breast cancer or cancer of any gynecological organs.
- ☯ Menopausal patients should take this formula with caution, as it may be too warming.
- ☯ This formula is contraindicated during pregnancy.
- ☯ Patients who are on anticoagulant or antiplatelet therapies, such as Coumadin (Warfarin), should use this formula with caution, as there may be a slightly higher risk of bleeding and bruising.
- ☯ This formula should not be taken for more than six months as it has warming properties.

ACUPUNCTURE POINTS

Traditional Points:
- ☯ Needle *Shanzhong* (CV 17).
- ☯ Apply moxa to *Zusanli* (ST 36).
- ☯ Massage *Qihai* (CV 6), *Geshu* (BL 17), *Shanzhong* (CV 17), *Sanyinjiao* (SP 6), *Qimen* (LR 14), *Rugen* (ST 18), and *Shaoze* (SI 1).

Balance Method by Dr. Richard Tan:
- ☯ Left side: *Yinlingquan* (SP 9), *Lougu* (SP 7), *Sanyinjiao* (SP 6), *Sanjian* (LI 3), *Waiguan* (TH 5), and the Breast point on the ear.
- ☯ Right side: *Lieque* (LU 7), *Zusanli* (ST 36), and *Xiajuxu* (ST 39).
- ☯ Left and right side can be alternated from treatment to treatment.

Ear Points:
- ☯ Tender point on the Chest and Endocrine.
- ☯ Embed ear seeds.

MODERN RESEARCH

Similar to the rest of the body, optimal development of the breasts is dependent on proper diet and nutrition. As bones require calcium and muscles need protein to grow, breasts need adequate nutrition and proper environment to develop to their full potential. Most women never achieve their full potential because of interruptions during the developmental process, such as poor diet, hormonal imbalances, stress during adolescence, exposure to pollutants, pesticides and chemicals, and lack of certain vitamins and minerals during puberty. In reality, such interruptions are common events in daily life that affect many, many women.

To achieve the desired shape and size of the breast, *Venus* uses herbs that act to fulfill the breasts' natural potential and stimulate additional growth. Herbs in *Venus* have been shown to have remarkable effects to regulate the endocrine system, increase the production of sex hormones and enhance the growth of the breasts.

To fulfill the natural growth potential of the breast, *Lu Rong* (Cornu Cervi Pantotrichum) is used to stimulate the endocrine system and increase hormone production. Historically, it was used with great success to treat children with slow growth and development. More recently, it has been documented through *in vitro* and *in vivo* studies that it increases the production of hormones responsible for developing the sex characteristics.[1] In addition, *Wang Bu Liu Xing* (Semen Vaccariae) and *Chuan Mu Tong* (Caulis Clematidis Armandii) are commonly used together to stimulate the growth of the sex organs.[2] In fact, it has been found that *Wang Bu Liu Xing* (Semen Vaccariae) given on a daily basis was effective in promoting the growth and metabolism of breast tissue.[3,4] Furthermore, *Dang Gui*

VENUS ™

(Radicis Angelicae Sinensis) is used in *Venus* to awaken the estrogen receptors in the breast to stimulate additional growth. One study found that *Dang Gui* (Radicis Angelicae Sinensis) has estrogen-like action and its use was associated with an increase in the sex organs.[5] In short, the use of these herbs restores natural growth potential and stimulates additional growth of the breasts.

In addition, many herbs are added to improve blood circulation and promote the generation of tissues. *Lu Rong* (Cornu Cervi Pantotrichum) and *Dang Gui* (Radicis Angelicae Sinensis) are used to improve blood circulation throughout the body.[6] *Huang Qi* (Radix Astragali) is used to stimulate the growth of new tissues.[7] These herbs provide the essential nutrients and the optimal environment for proper and optimal development of the breasts.

In summary, the size and shape of the breasts are not predetermined solely by genetics. Various factors affect the growth and development of the breasts, and numerous methods can be employed to achieve the natural potential and stimulate additional growth. *Venus* contains herbs that have been documented through research studies to regulate the endocrine system, increase the production of sex hormones, and enhance the growth of breasts.

PHARMACEUTICAL DRUGS & CHINESE MEDICINE: A COMPARATIVE ANALYSIS

Western Medical Approach: In western medicine, there is no drug treatment for insufficient lactation and breast enhancement.

Traditional Chinese Medicine Approach: This herbal formula has been used historically to address insufficiency lactation, and is currently used for breast enhancement. This formula nourishes the body and promotes blood circulation to breast tissues. Historically, it has been used with great success to relieve pain and resolve insufficient lactation. Today, it is most useful to nourish breast tissues and increase their size. This formula works within days when combined with dietary recommendations for insufficient lactation, but may require 3 to 6 month of continuous use for breast enhancement.

---

[1] *Chem Pharm Bull*, 1988; 36:2587:2593

[2] *Zhong Yao Xue* (Chinese Herbology), 1998; 582:584

[3] *Zhong Guo Zhong Yao Za Zhi* (People's Republic of China Journal of Chinese Herbology), 1990; 15(7): 52

[4] *Chi Jiao Yi Sheng Za Zhi* (Journal of Barefoot Doctors), 1975; (8): 26

[5] Liu, J. and Gong, H. Screening Some of the Estrogen-Like Herbs. The 5th Symposium on Research in Chinese

[6] *Report of Medicine*, 1991; 26(9): 714

[7] Xue, JX. et al. Effects of the combination of astragalus membranaceus (Fisch.) Bge. (AM), angelica sinensis (Oliv.) Diels (TAS), cyperus rotundus L. (CR), ligusticum chuanxiong Hort (LC) and paeonia veitchii lynch (PV) on the hemorrheological changes in "blood stagnating" rats. *Chung Kuo Chung Yao Tsa Chih*; 19(2): 108-10, 128. Feb 1994

VIBRANT ™

CLINICAL APPLICATIONS

☯ Tiredness, fatigue, lack of energy
☯ Chronic fatigue syndrome: constant fatigue, lethargy, lack of interest
☯ Sports formula: to increase mental and physical performance

WESTERN THERAPEUTIC ACTIONS

☯ Increases basal metabolism to increase energy levels and sense of well-being [8,17,18,21,22]
☯ Adaptogenic function help the patient adapt to stress, and improve mental and physical functions [17,18,20]

CHINESE THERAPEUTIC ACTIONS

☯ Tonifies the *yuan* (source) *qi*
☯ Awakens the *shen* (spirit)

DOSAGE

Take 3 to 4 capsules up to three times daily on an empty stomach with warm water.

INGREDIENTS

Ci Wu Jia (Radix et Caulis Acanthopanacis Senticosi) *Ji Xue Cao* (Herba Centellae)
Huang Qi (Radix Astragali) *Lu Cha* (Folium Camellia Sinensis)

FORMULA EXPLANATION

Vibrant is formulated to help people with demanding lifestyles cope with fatigue and lack of energy. *Vibrant* has herbs with excellent adaptogenic functions to improve both mental and physical performance. In terms of traditional Chinese medicine, these herbs tonify the *yuan* (source) *qi*, strengthen the Spleen, and awaken the *shen* (spirit).

Ci Wu Jia (Radix et Caulis Acanthopanacis Senticosi) is one of the most commonly used herbs in Asia, Europe and America. It is approved by the German Commission E as a tonic that has invigorating and fortifying effects to treat fatigue and debility. It also enhances capacity for work and improves concentration. Its indications include convalescence, prevention of colds and flu, and chronic fatigue syndrome. [1,2,3,4,5]

When used together, *Ci Wu Jia* (Radix et Caulis Acanthopanacis Senticosi) and *Huang Qi* (Radix Astragali) tonify the *yuan* (source) *qi* and have an excitatory effect on the central nervous system. They are both excellent herbs to promote well-being and health. *Huang Qi* (Radix Astragali) tonifies qi and ascends yang. It is especially helpful for patients who have shortness of breath, fatigue, and malaise.

Lu Cha (Folium Camellia Sinensis) is a beverage consumed in large quantities by people in Asian countries. It has shown to have excellent antibacterial, antiviral, immune-enhancing, and stimulating effects. [6,7] Consumption of *Lu Cha* (Folium Camellia Sinensis) provides an immediate boost of energy to enhance both mental and physical performance.

Ji Xue Cao (Herba Centellae), also known as gotu kola, has adaptogenic effects, and is commonly used to address both mental and physical conditions. Numerous studies have demonstrated its effectiveness to improve memory and to overcome stress, fatigue, mental confusion, and deterioration in mental function. [20,21,22]

VIBRANT ™

SUPPLEMENTARY FORMULAS

- As a long-term, overall constitutional tonic, use with *Imperial Tonic*.
- To enhance immunity, take with *Immune +* or *Cordyceps 3*.
- For stress and anxiety, combine with *Calm*.
- For anger and severe emotional disturbances, combine with *Calm (ES)*.
- For difficulties falling asleep or staying asleep, take *Schisandra ZZZ*.
- To enhance memory and concentration, add *Enhance Memory*.
- For Spleen qi deficiency, add *GI Tonic*.
- For adrenal deficiency, add *Adrenoplex*.
- For Kidney yang deficiency, add *Kidney Tonic (Yang)*.
- For Kidney yin deficiency, add *Kidney Tonic (Yin)*.
- For sluggishness due to blood stagnation, add *Circulation (SJ)*.

NUTRITION

- Advise the patient to eat a well-balanced diet with an adequate amount of raw foods, fruits and vegetables.
- Encourage the patients to drink at least 8 glasses of water daily.
- Eat more fish and fish oils, onions, garlic, olives, olive oil, herbs, spices, yogurt, fiber, tofu and other soy products.
- Sea vegetables, such as kelp and dulse, replenish the body with minerals like magnesium, potassium, calcium, iodine and iron.
- Decrease intake of red meat, alcohol, fats, caffeine, and highly processed foods. Avoid shellfish, fried foods, junk foods, and processed foods.
- Ensure adequate intake of vitamin B complex to process and utilize energy.
- Avoid the use of stimulants, such as coffee, caffeine, and high-sugar products.
- Food allergy or chemical hypersensitivity can drain energy and cause fatigue. Additional tests should be done to confirm or rule out allergy and/or hypersensitivity.

The Tao of Nutrition by Ni and McNease
- Chronic fatigue syndrome
  - Recommendations: winter melon, pumpkin, pumpkin seed, yam, sweet potato, lima bean, black bean, soy bean, strawberry, watermelon, pineapple, chestnut, papaya, figs, garlic, onions, and pearl barley.
  - Avoid dairy products, alcohol, coffee, sugar, fatty or fried foods, overly spicy foods, cold and raw foods, tomato, eggplant, bell pepper, and shellfish.
- For more information, please refer to *The Tao of Nutrition* by Dr. Maoshing Ni and Cathy McNease.

LIFESTYLE INSTRUCTIONS

- Daily exercise is advised to increase basal metabolic rate.
- Make sure the patient gets plenty of rest and goes to bed at a sensible hour.
- Get regular exercise and adequate rest.
- Take a bath for about 20 minutes prior to bedtime. Sea salt or epsom salts can be added to the bath water.
- Engage in activities such as *Tai Chi Chuan*, walking or meditation that allow calmness of mind without creating stagnation or excessive fatigue.
- Avoid exposure to heavy metals, such as lead, cadmium, aluminum, copper and arsenic, all of which can suppress the immune system and cause fatigue.

VIBRANT ™

CLINICAL NOTE

❧ *Vibrant* has a rapid onset of action and can be used on an as-needed basis in the early morning, late afternoon, before meetings, exams, or whenever there is fatigue or lack of energy.

CAUTIONS

❧ Avoid drinking coffee or other beverages containing caffeine while taking *Vibrant* to prevent over-stimulation of the central nervous system.

❧ Possible side effects of *Vibrant* include dry mouth and a slight increase in blood pressure or heart rate.

ACUPUNCTURE POINTS

Traditional Points:

❧ *Guanyuan* (CV 4), *Zhongwan* (CV 12), *Zhongji* (CV 3), *Guanyuan* (CV 4), and *Pishu* (BL 20).

❧ Apply moxa to *Guanyuan* (CV 4), *Shenshu* (BL 23), *Mingmen* (GV 4), and *Zhongji* (CV 3).

Balance Method by Dr. Richard Tan:

❧ Left side: *Hegu* (LI 4), *Yinlingquan* (SP 9), *Waiguan* (TH 5), and *Fuliu* (KI 7).

❧ Right side: *Lingdao* (HT 4), *Zusanli* (ST 36), and *Lieque* (LU 7).

❧ Left and right sides can be alternated from treatment to treatment.

❧ For additional information on the Balance Method, please refer to *Dr. Tan's Strategy of Twelve Magical Points* by Dr. Richard Tan.

Auricular Acupuncture by Dr. Li-Chun Huang:

❧ Fatigue: Sympathetic, Kidney, Liver, Spleen, Speed Recovered Fatigue, *San Jiao*, Anxious, Nervous Subcortex, and Thyroid. Bleed Ear Apex.

❧ For additional information on the location and explanation of these points, please refer to *Auricular Treatment Formula and Prescriptions* by Dr. Li-Chun Huang.

MODERN RESEARCH

Vibrant is formulated to help people with demanding lifestyles cope with fatigue and lack of energy. *Vibrant* has herbs which help the patient adapt to stress, increase basal metabolism, boost energy, and improve mental alertness and physical performance.

Lu Cha (Folium Camellia Sinensis) has a wide range of functions and is commonly used in different clinical applications. *Lu Cha* (Folium Camellia Sinensis) is an effective central nervous system stimulant that increases body metabolism and boosts energy levels.[8] *Lu Cha* (Folium Camellia Sinensis) has cancer-protective functions, as it inhibits the formation of cancer-inducing compounds and suppresses the mutation of bone marrow cells.[9,10] In addition to its cancer-protective effect, *Lu Cha* (Folium Camellia Sinensis) also reduces cholesterol levels. Overall, *Lu Cha* (Folium Camellia Sinensis) prolongs life span, contributes to longevity, and protects against life-threatening diseases.[11,12]

Huang Qi (Radix Astragali) is one of the most frequently used Chinese herbs and is historically used for its function to tonify the *wei* (defensive) *qi*. In terms of Western medicine, modern research has discovered repeatedly that *Huang Qi* (Radix Astragali) increases both specific and non-specific immunity.[13,14,15] In a clinical study of 115 leucopenic patients, it was found that the use of *Huang Qi* (Radix Astragali) is associated with an "obvious rise of the white blood cell (WBC) count" with a dose-dependent relationship.[16]

Ci Wu Jia (Radix et Caulis Acanthopanacis Senticosi) has been used for centuries in both Russia and China for its "adaptogenic" effect to normalize high or low blood pressure, to stimulate the immune system, and to increase work capacity. Clinical effects of *Ci Wu Jia* (Radix et Caulis Acanthopanacis Senticosi) include increased energy levels, protection against toxins and free radicals, and control of atherosclerosis.[17] One study showed *Ci Wu Jia* (Radix et Caulis Acanthopanacis Senticosi) effectively increased human physical working capacity.[18] The overall adaptogenic effect of *Ci Wu Jia* (Radix et Caulis Acanthopanacis Senticosi) is attributed to stimulation of the pituitary-adrenocortical system.[19]

Ji Xue Cao (Herba Centellae) has adaptogenic effects, and is commonly used to address both mental and physical conditions. Numerous studies have demonstrated its effectiveness to improve memory and to overcome stress, fatigue, mental confusion,[20] and deterioration in mental function.[21,22]

PHARMACEUTICAL DRUGS & CHINESE MEDICINE: A COMPARATIVE ANALYSIS

One striking difference between western and traditional Chinese medicine is that western medicine focuses and excels in crisis management, while traditional Chinese medicine emphasizes and shines in holistic and preventative treatments. Therefore, in emergencies, such as gun shot wounds or surgery, western medicine is generally the treatment of choice. However, for treatment of chronic idiopathic illness of unknown origins, where all lab tests are normal and a clear diagnosis cannot be made, traditional Chinese medicine is distinctly superior.

In cases of chronic energetic disorders, where all tests are normal but there are still general and non-diagnostic signs and symptoms, western medicine offers few treatment options since there is not a clear diagnosis. On the other hand, traditional Chinese medicine is beneficial as it excels in maintainance and preventative therapies. Herbs can be used to regulate imbalances and alleviate associated signs and symptoms. Therefore, herbal therapy should definitely be employed to prevent deterioration and to restore optimal health.

CASE STUDIES

A 35-year-old medical doctor complained of excessive stress and fatigue. He commented that he began to feel extremely tired around 11:00 AM, and again at 3 PM (lunch hour was from 12 to 1 PM). Because the fatigue caused lack of concentration, it made working quite difficult. He began to take *Vibrant*, 4 capsules in the morning and 4 capsules in the afternoon. He experienced an immediate increase in energy and concentration, which enabled him to work without any difficulty.

J.C., Diamond Bar, California

A 35-year-old female complained of bedwetting, fatigue, low back pain, abdominal pain, loss of appetite and depression. The doctor diagnosed her with Kidney *jing* (essence), yin and yang deficiencies. *Imperial Tonic* and *Vibrant* were prescribed. The patient reported that bedwetting, depression and pain went away and the energy level went from 2 to 10, on a scale of 1 to 10. As an added and unexpected joy for her, the patient stated she also lost 10 pounds even though she had been eating more.

S.C., Santa Monica, California

S.W. suffered from tiredness, restless sleep, and occasional, recurrent nasal congestion during allergy season. She was diagnosed with Kidney yin and yang deficiency and *wei* (defensive) *qi* deficiency. The practitioner prescribed *Immune* + to build the *wei* (defensive) *qi*, and *Vibrant* to sustain and build her Kidney yin and yang over time. The patient greatly commented on the positive results of *Vibrant* to increase her daily energy level and positive outlook.

J.P., Naples, Florida

FORMULAS

VIBRANT ™

[1] Blumenthal, M. et al. *German Commission E Monographs*: Therapeutic Monographs on Medicinal Plants for Human Use. Austin, TX: American Botanical Council. 1997

[2] Newall, CA. et al. *Herbal Medicines: A Guide for Health-care Professionals*. London: The Pharmaceutical Press. 1996

[3] Leung, AY. and Foster, S. *Encyclopedia of Common Natural Ingredients Used in Food, Drugs, and Cosmetics 2nd edition*. New York: John Wiley and Sons. 1996

[4] Bradley, P. (ed.). *British Herbal Compendium* Vol. 1. Dorset, England: British Herbal Medicine Association. 1992

[5] Brown, DJ. 1996 *Herbal Prescriptions for Better Health*. Rocklin, CA: Prima Publishing. 1996

[6] Gutman, RL. and Beung-Ho Ryu. Rediscovering Tea: An exploration of the scientific literature. *HerbalGram* 37. pp. 33-48. 1996

[7] Snow, JM. Monograph – Camellia sinensis (L.) Kuntze (Theaceae). *The Protocol Journal of Botanical Medicine* Vol. 1, No. 2.

[8] Olin, R. et al. *The Lawrence Review of Natural Products by Facts and Comparison*. Green Tea. May 1993

[9] Wang, H. and Wu, Y. Inhibitory effect of Chinese tea on N-nitrosation in vitro and in vivo. IARC Sci Publ;105:546. 1991

[10] Imanishi, H. et al. Tea tannin components modify the induction of sister-chromatid exchanges and chromosome aberrations in mutagen-treated cultured mammalian cells and mice. *Mutat Res*;259(1):79. 1991

[11] Uchida, S. et al. Radioprotective effects of (-)-epigallocatechin 3-0-gallate (green tea tannin) in mice. *Life Sci*;50(2):147. 1992

[12] Sadakata, S. et al. Mortality among female practitioners of Chanoyu (Japanese "tea-ceremony"). *Tohoku J Exp Med*; 166(4):475. 1992

[13] Chu, DT. et al. Immunotherapy with Chinese medicinal herbs. I. Immune restoration of local xenogenetic graft-versus-host reaction in cancer patients by fractionated astragalus membranaceus in vitro. *Journal Of Clinical & Laboratory Immunology*. 25(3):119-23, Mar. 1988

[14] Sun, Y. et al. Immune restoration and/or augmentation of local graft versus host reaction by traditional Chinese medicinal herbs. *Cancer*. 52(1):70-3, July 1. 1983

[15] Sun, Y. et al. Preliminary observations on the effects of the Chinese medicinal herbs astragalus membranaceus and Ganoderma lucidum on lymphocyte blastogenic responses. *Journal of Biological Response Modifiers*. 2(3):227-37, 1983

[16] Weng, XS. *Chung Juo Chung Hsia I Chieh Ho Tsa Chih*. August 1995

[17] Sprecher, E. Eleutherococcus Senticosus on the way to being a phytopharmacon. *Pharma Ztg*; 134:9. 1989

[18] Asano, K. et al. Effect of Eleutherococcus senticosus extract on human physical working capacity. *Planta Med*;48(3):175. 1986

[19] Filaretov, AA. et al. Effect on adaptogens on the activity of the pituitary-adrenocortical system in rats. *Bull Eksper Bio Med*;101(5):573. 1986

[20] Bartram, T. *Encyclopedia of Herbal Medicine 1st edition*. Dorest, England: Grace Publishers. 1995

[21] Kapoor, LD. *CRC Handbook of Ayruvedic Medicinal Plants*. Boca Raton, FL: CRC Press. 1990

[22] Murray, M. Centella asiatica (Gotu Kola) Monograph. *American Journal of Natural Medicine*. Volume 3, No. 6 Jul/Aug:22-26. 1996

FORMULAS

VITAL ESSENCE ™

CLINICAL APPLICATIONS

☯ Male infertility
☯ Male sexual and reproductive disorders, such as infertility, low sperm count, poor sperm motility, mobility and morphology, premature ejaculation, spermatorrhea, etc.

WESTERN THERAPEUTIC ACTIONS

☯ Regulates the sex organs and hormone production
☯ Balance hormone productions to treat sexual and reproductive disorders
☯ Anti-aging and adaptogenic effects to improve general health

CHINESE THERAPEUTIC ACTIONS

☯ Tonifies Kidney yin and Liver blood
☯ Replenishes Kidney *jing* (essence)
☯ Revitalizes Kidney yang and *ming men* (life-gate) fire

DOSAGE

Take 3 to 4 capsules three times daily. Dosage can be increased up to 6 to 8 capsules three times daily. For optimal results, this formula should be taken continuously for 2 to 3 months, or until successful pregnancy of partner.

INGREDIENTS

Che Qian Zi (Semen Plantaginis)
Chuan Xiong (Rhizoma Ligustici Chuanxiong)
Dang Gui (Radicis Angelicae Sinensis)
Fu Ling (Poria)
Fu Pen Zi (Fructus Rubi)
Gou Qi Zi (Fructus Lycii)
He Shou Wu (Radix Polygoni Multiflori)

Huang Qi (Radix Astragali)
Jiu Cai Zi (Semen Allii Tuberosi)
Shu Di Huang (Radix Rehmanniae Preparata)
Tu Si Zi (Semen Cuscutae)
Wu Wei Zi (Fructus Schisandrae Chinensis)
Xian Mao (Rhizoma Curculiginis)
Yin Yang Huo (Herba Epimedii)

FORMULA EXPLANATION

Vital Essence is mainly composed of herbs that tonify Kidney yin, yang and *jing* (essence). Tonifying Kidney yin will boost sperm count. Warming the Kidney yang will increase sperm mobility and motility. Replenishing Kidney *jing* (essence) will improve sperm morphology.

Gou Qi Zi (Fructus Lycii), *Shu Di Huang* (Radix Rehmanniae Preparata) and *Dang Gui* (Radicis Angelicae Sinensis) tonify Kidney yin and Liver blood. They replenish the foundation of the Kidney. *Jiu Cai Zi* (Semen Allii Tuberosi), *Tu Si Zi* (Semen Cuscutae), *Xian Mao* (Rhizoma Curculiginis) and *Yin Yang Huo* (Herba Epimedii) vitalize the Kidney yang, increase libido and improve sperm mobility and motility. *Fu Pen Zi* (Fructus Rubi) and *He Shou Wu* (Radix Polygoni Multiflori) are essential Kidney *jing* (essence) tonics for the treatment of male infertility. *Chuan Xiong* (Rhizoma Ligustici Chuanxiong) moves blood and prevents the tonic herbs from creating stagnation in the body. *Huang Qi* (Radix Astragali) tonifies the *zhong* (central) *qi* to enhance energy. *Fu Ling* (Poria) and *Che Qian Zi* (Semen Plantaginis) are dampness-eliminating herbs that offset the cloying properties of the yin and *jing* (essence) tonics. *Fu Ling* (Poria) also strengthens the Spleen to ensure maximum absorption of the Kidney tonics. *Che Qian Zi* (Semen Plantaginis) ensures the absence of blockage in the lower *jiao*. Finally, *Wu Wei Zi* (Fructus Schisandrae Chinensis), an astringent, is added to prevent further leakage of *jing* (essence).

FORMULAS

VITAL ESSENCE ™

SUPPLEMENTARY FORMULAS

- With impotence, erectile dysfunction or low libido, add *Vitality*.
- With prostatitis, add *Saw Palmetto Complex* or *P-Statin*.
- With difficulty in ejaculation, add *Wei Ling Xian* (Radix Clematidis) and *Shi Chang Pu* (Rhizoma Acori) with *Resolve (Lower)*.
- With thick or condensed semen due to deficiency fire of the Kidney, add *Nourish*.
- For varicocele, add *Resolve (Lower)* and *P-Statin*.
- For decreased sperm motility or mobility, add *Vitality*.
- For low sperm count, add *Polygonum 14*.
- With premature ejaculation or spermatorrhea, add *Vitality* and *Jin Suo Gu Jing Wan* (Metal Lock Pill to Stabilize the Essence).
- For stress and anxiety, add *Calm* or *Calm (ES)*.
- To improve the quality of sperm for *in vitro* fertilization (IVF), add *Polygonum 14*.

NUTRITION

- Patients should be advised to eat more clams, oysters, sea cucumbers and lamb.
- Excessive use of certain herbs such as echinacea, ginkgo biloba and St. John's Wort have been associated with infertility and should be avoided.
- Consume an adequate amount of selenium (200 to 400 mcg daily), as deficiency has been associated with reduced sperm count and sterility in men.
- Consume an adequate amount of vitamin C and bioflavonoids (2,000 to 6,000 daily), as they are important in sperm production.
- Consume an adequate amount of vitamin E (200 to 400 IU daily), which helps to balance hormone production.
- Adequate intake of zinc (80 mg daily) is important for normal functioning of the reproductive organs.
- Avoid alcohol, coffee and cigarette smoking.

LIFESTYLE INSTRUCTIONS

- Avoid excessive sexual intercourse or ejaculation. While taking herbs, sexual activity should be reduced to once a week until the sperm lab report shows normal.
- Certain artificial lubricants may prevent the sperm from reaching the cervix. Saliva may also have a negative effect on the spermatozoa.
- Avoid drinking alcohol, which reduces sperm count.
- Avoid smoking and exposure to second-hand cigarette smoking.
- Avoid stress as much as possible.

CLINICAL NOTES

- Semen analysis is extremely important, as sperm factors account for approximately 40% of all cases of infertility. Parameters evaluated include ejaculate volume, viscosity, appearance, pH balance, sperm count, motility and sperm morphology. Semen composition of fructose less than 120 mg/dL is indicative of ejaculatory duct obstruction or agenesis of seminal vesicles. Most patients may already have an analysis. They should be instructed to re-test and compare the results after taking herbs for two to three months.
- Hormonal analysis is also important. Testosterone level studies are indicated for patients displaying loss of libido and possible hypogonadotropic abnormality. Normal FSH at baseline analysis correlates with improvement in semen parameters.
- Testicular volume estimation for impaired spermatogenic function or oligospermia should be performed.

FORMULAS

VITAL ESSENCE ™

Pulse Diagnosis by Dr. Jimmy Wei-Yen Chang:
- Weak pulse on the left *chi* position.
- Note: Dr. Chang takes the pulse in slightly different positions. He places his index finger directly over the wrist crease, and his middle and ring fingers alongside to locate *cun*, *guan* and *chi* positions. For additional information and explanation, please refer to *Pulsynergy* by Dr. Jimmy Wei-Yen Chang and Marcus Brinkman.

CAUTIONS

- Certain medications, such as Zantac (Ranitidine) and Tagamet (Cimetidine), may decrease sperm count and even cause impotence.
- It is important to remember that this formula is designed to treat infertility. They do ***not*** offer any protection against sexually transmitted diseases.
- *Dang Gui* (Radicis Angelicae Sinensis) may enhance the overall effectiveness of Coumadin (Warfarin), an anticoagulant drug. Patients who take anticoagulant or antiplatelet medications should ***not*** take this herbal formula without supervision by a licensed health care practitioner.

ACUPUNCTURE POINTS

Traditional Points: .
- Needle and moxa *Dahe* (KI 12), *Qugu* (CV 2), *Sanyinjiao* (SP 6), *Guanyuan* (CV 4), and *Zhongji* (CV 3).
- Needle and moxa *Qugu* (CV 2), *Yinlian* (LR 11), *Dadu* (SP 2), and *Ciliao* (BL 32).
- Needle and moxa *Shenshu* (BL 23), *Guanyuan* (CV 4), *Rangu* (KI 2), *Fuliu* (KI 7), *Zusanli* (ST 36), and *Sanyinjiao* (SP 6).

Balance Method by Dr. Richard Tan:
- Left side: *Lingku*, *Lieque* (LU 7), *Shuiquan* (KI 5), and *Sanyinjiao* (SP 6).
- Right side: *Yangxi* (LI 5) and *Zusanli* (ST 36).
- Alternate sides from treatment to treatment
- Note: *Lingku* is one of Master Tong's points on both hands. *Lingku* is located in the depression just distal to the junction of the first and second metacarpal bones, approximately 0.5 *cun* proximal to *Hegu* (LI 4), on the *yangming* line.
- For additional information on the Balance Method, please refer to *Dr. Tan's Strategy of Twelve Magical Points* by Dr. Richard Tan.

MODERN RESEARCH

Male sperm disorders account for approximately 40% in failed pregnancies. Disorder of sperm production can evolve from an assortment of conditions that include, but are not limited to, spermatogenesis, azoospermia, varicocele, retrograde ejaculation, in addition to endocrine, genetic, social, pharmaceutical and psychological factors. As men age, the sperm density and testosterone levels appear to decrease while estradiol and estrone levels increase. This formula is designed with both general and specific effects to treat male infertility. It contains herbs that address the general health of individuals, such as ones with anti-aging and adaptogenic effects. More specifically, it incorporates herbs with marked influences to regulate the endocrine system, balance the hormones, and treat sexual and reproductive disorders.

In this formula, *He Shou Wu* (Radix Polygoni Multiflori) is well-known for its anti-aging effect as it demonstrated marked effect to improve general health and increase life expectancy.[1] *Tu Si Zi* (Semen Cuscutae) has an adaptogenic effect to improve both mental and physical health.[2] Though these two herbs do not treat male infertility directly, they address the underlying deficiency associated with many cases of infertility.

FORMULAS

VITAL ESSENCE ™

To address the many possible causes of male infertility, this formula uses herbs with various pharmacological effects to treat the entire person. *He Shou Wu* (Radix Polygoni Multiflori) has a broad influence on the endocrine system to regulate the secretion of hormones.[3] *Wu Wei Zi* (Fructus Schisandrae Chinensis) and *Xian Mao* (Rhizoma Curculiginis) have a specific effect to stimulate the reproductive organs and increase their weight.[4] *Fu Pen Zi* (Fructus Rubi) also stimulates the reproductive organs to increase the production of the sex hormones.[5,6] Administration of *Yin Yang Huo* (Herba Epimedii) increases sperm production, stimulates the sensory nerves, and increases sexual desire and activity. It also increases the secretion of endogenous hormones, such as corticosterone, cortisol, and testosterone.[7,8] Clinically, the herbs in this formula have been used with marked effect to treat many sexual and reproductive disorders. According to one clinical study, use of *Gou Qi Zi* (Fructus Lycii) in one formula was associated with marked success to treat male infertility with low sperm count and poor sperm motility. After treatment, 33 out of 42 patients had normal sperm counts and mobility, and they successfully conceived children.[9]

In conclusion, *Vital Essence* is one of the best formulas to treat male infertility. Not only does it treat the underlying sexual and reproductive disorders, it also restores the overall health and well-being of the patients.

PHARMACEUTICAL DRUGS & CHINESE MEDICINE: A COMPARATIVE ANALYSIS

One striking difference between western and traditional Chinese medicine is that western medicine focuses and excels in crisis management, while traditional Chinese medicine emphasizes and shines in holistic and preventative treatments. Therefore, in emergencies, such as gun shot wounds or surgery, western medicine is generally the treatment of choice. However, for treatment of chronic idiopathic illness of unknown origins, where all lab tests are normal and a clear diagnosis cannot be made, traditional Chinese medicine is distinctly superior.

Western Medical Approach: There is no drug treatment for male infertility. Those with sperm disorders (low sperm count, poor sperm motility, mobility and morphology) are usually treated with physical medicine, such as artificial insemination. However, there are no options available to increase sperm quantity and quality.

Traditional Chinese Medicine Approach: One main function of Kidney yang is regulation of sexual and reproductive functions. *Vital Essence* is a Kidney yang tonic formula that emphasizes more on maintaining reproductive functions and treating reproductive disorders, such as low sperm count, poor sperm motility, mobility and morphology. Though this formula is definitely effective, it does not have an instantaneous effect, but rather requires continuous use of two to three months for maximum effect.

Summation: Reproductive disorder is perhaps best treated with integration of western and traditional Chinese medicine. Herbal therapy has been found to be exceptionally effective for male infertility to increase sperm quantity and quality. In most cases, use of herbal therapy is sufficient for mild to moderate cases of male infertility. In severe cases where herbs improve the condition but the patient still cannot achieve fertilization, artificial insemination can also be employed to enhance the success rate.

[1] *Zhong Yao Yao Li Yu Lin Chuang* (Pharmacology and Clinical Applications of Chinese Herbs), 1989; 5(3):19
[2] *Chang Yong Zhong Yao Cheng Fen Yu Yao Li Shou Ce* (A Handbook of the Composition and Pharmacology of Common Chinese Drugs), 1994; 1563:1564
[3] *Zhong Yao Yao Li Yu Lin Chuang* (Pharmacology and Clinical Applications of Chinese Herbs), 1989; 5(3):19
[4] *Shang Hai Zhong Yi Yao Za Zhi* (Shanghai Journal of Chinese Medicine and Herbology), 1989; 2:43
[5] *Chang Yong Zhong Yao Xian Dai Yan Jiu Yu Lin Chuan* (Recent Study & Clinical Application of Common Traditional Chinese Medicine), 1995; 691:692
[6] *Zhong Yi Za Zhi* (Journal of Chinese Medicine), 1984; (7):63
[7] *Zhong Yao Da Ci Dian* (Dictionary of Chinese Herbs), 1977; 2251
[8] *Zhong Xi Yi Jie He Za Zhi* (Journal of Integrated Chinese and Western Medicine), 1989; 9(12):737-8,710
[9] *Xin Zhong Yi* (New Chinese Medicine), 1988; 2:20

FORMULAS

VITALITY ™

CLINICAL APPLICATIONS

- ☯ Enhancement of sexual function and performance
- ☯ Treatment of sexual and reproductive disorders
- ☯ Low libido in women and men
- ☯ Common uses: impotence, premature ejaculation, spermatorrhea, etc.

WESTERN THERAPEUTIC ACTIONS

- ☯ Increases the secretion of endogenous hormones [1,2,3]
- ☯ Increases the secretion of testosterone, corticosterone, and cortisol [1,2,3]

CHINESE THERAPEUTIC ACTIONS

- ☯ Warms Kidney yang
- ☯ Replenishes Kidney *jing* (essence)
- ☯ Increases sexual desire

DOSAGE

Take 3 to 4 capsules three times daily on an empty stomach with warm water. The last dosage after dinner or before bedtime can be served with grain-based liquor such as vodka to enhance the overall effect, as this formula was traditionally prepared as an herbal tincture.

INGREDIENTS

Ba Ji Tian (Radix Morindae Officinalis)
Dang Gui (Radicis Angelicae Sinensis)
Du Zhong (Cortex Eucommiae)
Fu Zi (Radix Aconiti Lateralis Praeparata)
Gou Qi Zi (Fructus Lycii)
Jiu Cai Zi (Semen Allii Tuberosi)
Ren Shen (Radix Ginseng)
Rou Gui (Cortex Cinnamomi)

Shan Yao (Rhizoma Dioscoreae)
Shan Zhu Yu (Fructus Corni)
She Chuang Zi (Fructus Cnidii)
Shu Di Huang (Radix Rehmanniae Preparata)
Suo Yang (Herba Cynomorii)
Tu Si Zi (Semen Cuscutae)
Yin Yang Huo (Herba Epimedii)

FORMULA EXPLANATION

Vitality is an excellent formula to tonify Kidney yang and Kidney *jing* (essence). Clinically, deficiencies of Kidney yang and Kidney *jing* (essence) are characterized by impotence, premature ejaculation, low sperm count, low libido, and general sexual disorders. In western terminology, these herbs increase the production of sex hormones; and in TCM terminology, these herbs tonify Kidney yang and Kidney *jing* (essence). This formula works to enhance libido in women as it boosts the testosterone levels and Kidney yang.

The direct translation of the chief herb *Yin Yang Huo* (Herba Epimedii) is "horny goat herb." It was originally discovered by a farmer who noticed the increase in proliferation in one of his herds of goats that were grazing on this herb. *Yin Yang Huo* (Herba Epimedii) increases sexual activity, increases sperm production, stimulates the sensory nerves and therefore increases sexual desire. Weakness of Kidney yang and depletion of Kidney *jing* (essence) contribute to symptoms of impotence, decreased libido, spermatorrhea, premature ejaculation and other sexual dysfunctions. The treatment protocol is to increase the Kidney yang and tonify the Kidney *jing* (essence). *Fu*

FORMULAS

Zi (Radix Aconiti Lateralis Praeparata), *Rou Gui* (Cortex Cinnamomi), *Jiu Cai Zi* (Semen Allii Tuberosi), *Du Zhong* (Cortex Eucommiae), *Tu Si Zi* (Semen Cuscutae), *Ba Ji Tian* (Radix Morindae Officinalis), *Suo Yang* (Herba Cynomorii), and *She Chuang Zi* (Fructus Cnidii) warm and tonify the Kidney yang. *Shan Zhu Yu* (Fructus Corni), *Shu Di Huang* (Radix Rehmanniae Preparata), *Gou Qi Zi* (Fructus Lycii), *Shan Yao* (Rhizoma Dioscoreae) and *Dang Gui* (Radicis Angelicae Sinensis) tonify the Kidney *jing* (essence) and blood. *Dang Gui* (Radicis Angelicae Sinensis) also moves blood and directs the effect to the lower abdomen. *Ren Shen* (Radix Ginseng) is used to replenish the vital energy and prolong stamina.

SUPPLEMENTARY FORMULAS

- To boost energy and vitality, use with *Vibrant* or *Imperial Tonic*.
- To strengthen constitutional weakness and deficiency, use with *Cordyceps 3*.
- For soreness and weakness of the lower back, combine with *Back Support (Chronic)*.
- For arthritic pain that worsens during cold and rainy weather, combine with *Flex (CD)*.
- For heat-type arthritis with redness, swelling and inflammation, combine with *Flex (Heat)*.
- For adrenal deficiency, add *Adrenoplex*.
- For poor memory and forgetfulness, add *Enhance Memory*.
- To treat male infertility, use *Vital Essence*.
- To treat female infertility, use *Blossom (Phase 1-4)*.
- To tonify Kidney yin, add *Kidney Tonic (Yin)*.
- To tonify Kidney yang, add *Kidney Tonic (Yang)*.

NUTRITION

- Eliminate alcohol from the diet as it decreases the body's ability to produce testosterone.
- Intake of vitamin E should be increased. Foods high in vitamin E include wheat germ oil, almonds, sunflower seed or oil, peanuts, soybeans, whole wheat products and asparagus. Kiwi and fresh oyster can also be taken together as an aphrodisiac.
- Shellfish, oyster, shrimps, cashews, beef and mushrooms are all foods that either contain high protein or zinc that may increase libido. However, these foods often are high in cholesterol and should not be over-consumed or otherwise will cause blockage and achieve the opposite effect.
- Impotence is sometimes caused by circulatory problems. In such cases, increase the consumption of foods rich in niacin (eggs, peanut butter, avocado, and fish) and vitamin E (raw wheat germ and vegetable oil).
- Zinc is also beneficial in preventing impotence and reduced sperm count. Zinc is found in such foods as pumpkin seeds, sunflower seeds, oysters, soy, and eggs. Avoid eating foods that deplete the body of zinc, such as alcohol and coffee.

The Tao of Nutrition by Ni and McNease
- Impotence
  - Recommendations: scallions, scallion seeds, lamb, sea cucumber, shrimps, rooster, bitter melon seeds, ginseng, black beans, kidney beans, yams, and lycium fruit. Maintaining a calm composure.
  - Avoid obscene visual stimulation, dairy products, sweets, masturbation, overwork, and too much sex.
- For more information, please refer to *The Tao of Nutrition* by Dr. Maoshing Ni and Cathy McNease.

LIFESTYLE INSTRUCTIONS

- Avoid cigarette smoking or exposure to second-hand smoke.
- Vigorous exercise, hot tubs, saunas and tight underwear lead to increased temperature in the testicles and reduced sperm count.

VITALITY ™

- Refrain from sexual activity when exhausted or under stress. Do not overindulge in sexual activity when any weakness in function or performance is present.
- Exercises for men with impotence and premature ejaculation:
  - Tip-toe and clench one's teeth while urinating. This simple posture will tighten and strengthen the muscles surrounding the groin to help condition the Kidney qi. This is also a good exercise to help with terminal dripping in elderly patients. Women can practice this exercise by squatting and tip-toeing over the toilet while urinating. This exercise for women will strengthen and tighten the muscles and ligaments surrounding the reproductive organs to help treat prolapse of the bladder and uterus or frequent urinary urges due to Kidney yang deficiency. It also tightens the muscles surrounding the vagina and can be recommended to the partners of those taking *Vitality* or those who have low libido to enhance pleasure. Results can be expected in a few months if practiced daily and consistently.
- Exercises for women with low libido:
  - Walking on the balls of the feet with the navel pulled towards the spine and the heels off the ground, taking care to breathe deeply. Engaging in the Kegel exercise (attempting to use vaginal muscles to stop and start the flow of urine rapidly and frequently at each time of urinating) while also clenching the teeth and breathing through the nose. Exercises such as the following may be helpful if practiced regularly.
- There are five conditions when sexual activity should be avoided: when one is hungry, full, drunk, emotionally unstable (angry, sad, fearful, hateful or worrying) or recovery from a chronic illness.

CLINICAL NOTES

- *Vitality* is an excellent male and female tonic to increase sexual prowess and strengthen sexual energy. It is important to keep in mind that *Vitality* nourishes the body from within to change the underlying constitution of the person. It does not provide an immediate boost of sexual power.
- The practitioner may be able to find in chiropractic or medical supply catalogs a small piece of furniture that fits around the toilet to provide a safe, stable platform to support the feet several inches off the floor, promoting a more natural 'squatting' posture for the individual seated on the toilet. This may assist in promoting complete evacuation of the bladder and bowels, enhancing the effort to strengthen normal function and organ position.

Pulse Diagnosis by Dr. Jimmy Wei-Yen Chang:
- Weak pulse on the left *chi* position.
- Note: Dr. Chang takes the pulse in slightly different positions. He places his index finger directly over the wrist crease, and his middle and ring fingers alongside to locate *cun*, *guan* and *chi* positions. For additional information and explanation, please refer to *Pulsynergy* by Dr. Jimmy Wei-Yen Chang and Marcus Brinkman.

CAUTIONS

- Patients who wear a pacemaker, or individuals who take anti-arrhythmic drugs or cardiac glycosides such as Lanoxin (Digoxin), should not take this formula. *Fu Zi* (Radix Aconiti Lateralis Praeparata) may interact with these drugs by affecting the rhythm and potentiating the contractile strength of the heart.
- Patients who are on anticoagulant or antiplatelet therapies, such as Coumadin (Warfarin), should use this formula with caution, as there may be a slightly higher risk of bleeding and bruising.
- *Vitality* should be used with caution in patients with pre-existing hypertension, since many herbs in this formula are warm or hot in nature and may raise the blood pressure.
- This formula is contraindicated in individuals with exterior or excess conditions, such as infections or inflammations.
- Because this formula is warm to hot in property, prolonged use may be associated with reactions such as thirst, dry mouth, warm sensations, constipation, flushed face, and nosebleeds. To avoid these reactions, decrease the dosage or temporarily discontinue the formula.

FORMULAS

VITALITY ™

ACUPUNCTURE POINTS

Traditional Points:
❧ *Shenshu* (BL 23), *Mingmen* (GV 4), *Guanyuan* (CV 4), *Rangu* (KI 2), and *Sanyinjiao* (SP 6).

Balance Method by Dr. Richard Tan:
❧ Left side: *Xuehai* (SP 10), *Taixi* (KI 3), *Zhongfeng* (LR 4), *Yangxi* (LI 5), and *Lingku*.
❧ Right side: *Lieque* (LU 7), *Daling* (PC 7), *Zusanli* (ST 36), *Shenmai* (BL 62), and *Yanglingquan* (GB 34).
❧ Left and right side can be alternated from treatment to treatment.
❧ Note: *Lingku* is one of Master Tong's points on both hands. *Lingku* is located in the depression just distal to the junction of the first and second metacarpal bones, approximately 0.5 *cun* proximal to *Hegu* (LI 4), on the *yangming* line.
❧ For additional information on the Balance Method, please refer to *Dr. Tan's Strategy of Twelve Magical Points* by Dr. Richard Tan.

Auricular Acupuncture by Dr. Li-Chun Huang:
❧ Impotence: Internal Genital, External Genital, Gonadotropin Point, Kidney, Liver, Libido, Exciting Point, Endocrine, and Pituitary.
❧ Emission: *Shenmen*, Kidney, Liver, Heart, Neurasthenia Point (front and back of ear), Neurasthenia Area (front and back of ear), Nervous, Subcortex, and Dream-Disturbed Sleep Area.
❧ For additional information on the location and explanation of these points, please refer to *Auricular Treatment Formula and Prescriptions* by Dr. Li-Chun Huang.

MODERN RESEARCH

Yang tonics have been used for thousands of years in traditional Chinese medicine to treat male sexual disorders. *Vitality* is formulated with yang-restoring Chinese herbs that are directly linked to the increased secretion of endogenous hormones, such as corticosterone, cortisol and testosterone. [1,2]

Rou Gui (Cortex Cinnamomi), *Suo Yang* (Herba Cynomorii), *Yin Yang Huo* (Herba Epimedii) and *Fu Zi* (Radix Aconiti Lateralis Praeparata) have been studied extensively and have demonstrated effects to enhance the production of corticosterone and testosterone. *Yin Yang Huo* (Herba Epimedii) significantly increased the level of corticosterone; and *Rou Gui* (Cortex Cinnamomi) and *Yin Yang Huo* (Herba Epimedii) significantly increased the level of testosterone. [1] The findings in this study were verified by another study in which *Rou Gui* (Cortex Cinnamomi), *Yin Yang Huo* (Herba Epimedii) and *Fu Zi* (Radix Aconiti Lateralis Praeparata) restored yang deficiency by increasing cortisol secretion. [2]

Yin Yang Huo (Herba Epimedii) has been studied extensively for its influence on the secretion of endogenous hormones. It has demonstrated effects to increase the levels of corticosterone, cortisol, and testosterone. [1,2] In addition, it has androgen-like effects as it stimulates sexual activity, increases sperm production, and heightens sexual desire. [3] In addition, other herbs such as *Ba Ji Tian* (Radix Morindae Officinalis), *Du Zhong* (Cortex Eucommiae), *Tu Si Zi* (Semen Cuscutae) and *Gou Qi Zi* (Fructus Lycii) have similar functions and are commonly used in treatment of male sexual disorders. Clinical applications of *Vitality* include, but not are limited to, impotence, spermatorrhea, frequent urination, and male infertility. [3]

PHARMACEUTICAL DRUGS & CHINESE MEDICINE: A COMPARATIVE ANALYSIS

One striking difference between western and traditional Chinese medicine is that western medicine focuses and excels in crisis management, while traditional Chinese medicine emphasizes and shines in holistic and preventative treatments. Therefore, in emergencies, such as gun shot wounds or surgery, western medicine is generally the treatment of choice. However, for treatment of chronic idiopathic illness of unknown origins, where all lab tests are normal and a clear diagnosis cannot be made, traditional Chinese medicine is distinctly superior.

Western Medical Approach: Sexual disorders such as erectile disorder, is treated with drugs such as Viagra (Sildenafil) and Cialis (Tadalafil). These drugs generally have a quick onset of effect, and they work primarily by increasing blood flow to the penis. However, these drugs may cause side effects such as headache, upset stomach, diarrhea, dizziness or lightheadedness, flushing, nasal congestion, blindness, breast enlargement, rash, painful erection, prolonged erection, fainting, chest pain, and itching or burning during urination. Furthermore, these drugs are only effective for men, and not for women.

Traditional Chinese Medicine Approach: One main function of Kidney yang is regulation of sexual and reproductive functions. *Vitality* is a Kidney yang tonic formula that emphasizes more to maintain sexual functions and treat sexual disorders, such as decreased libido in men and women, impotence, premature ejaculation, and spermatorrhea. Though this formula is very effective, it does not have an instantaneous effect, but rather requires continuous use of two to three months for maximum effect.

Summation: Both drugs and herbs are effective for treating sexual disorders. Drugs have quick onset of action, but they only have one specific indication, are effective only for men, and have numerous significant side effects. Herbs have a gradual onset of action, but may be used in both men and women to treat a wide variety of sexual disorders. Furthermore, herbs are safe and natural, and have few or no side effects. Finally, it is important to remember that neither drugs nor herbs prevent pregnancy nor do they protect either partner from sexually transmitted diseases and HIV.

CASE STUDIES

A 65-year-old male presented with generalized male sexual dysfunction, possibly due to old age and/or use of high blood pressure medications. The diagnosis was Kidney yang and qi deficiencies. The patient was instructed to take *Vitality* with good results noted within one week.

R.C., M.D., Ph.D., NY, New York

T.S. is female who presented with pain (especially of the joints of the limbs), coldness of the fingers and difficulty falling asleep. Objective findings revealed that her fingers were icy and cyanotic. Her leg muscles appeared to be abnormally tight. Her blood pressure was 110/80 mmHg and her heart rate was 78 beats per minute. She also received monthly rheumatoid arthritis shots. Western diagnosis for this patient was fibromyalgia. The TCM diagnosis was yang deficiency. *Vitality* was prescribed and the patient reported she felt the formula worked well in improving her condition and relieving the pain.

M.W., San Diego, California

[1] Kuang, AK. et al. Effects of Yang-restoring herb medicines on the levels of plasma corticosterone, testosterone and triiodothyronine. *Chung His I Chieh Ho Tsa Chih*, 9(12):737-8,710 Dec. 1989

[2] Chen, M. et al. Effect of monoamine neurotransmitters in the hypothalamus in a cortisol-induced rat model of Yang-deficiency. *Chung His I Chieh Ho Tsa Chih*, 10(5):292-4' 262 May 1990

[3] Bensky, D. et al. *Chinese Herbal Medicine Materia Medica*. Eastland Press. 1993

FORMULAS

V-Statin ™

CLINICAL APPLICATIONS

- ❧ Vaginitis
- ❧ Pelvic inflammatory disease (PID)
- ❧ Genito-urinary infections in women and men
- ❧ Genital itching, soreness or pain in men or women
- ❧ Yellow or green vaginal discharge with offensive odor and cottage cheese consistency
- ❧ Infection or eczema of the scrotum, male genital infection with itching
- ❧ Pyelonephritis, urinary tract infection (UTI), cystitis with dysuria, turbid, yellow urine
- ❧ Infertility in women due to inflammation and infection of the pelvis (ovaries, uterus, fallopian tubes)

WESTERN THERAPEUTIC ACTIONS

- ❧ Antibiotic effects to treat infection [2,3,4,5,6,7,8,9]
- ❧ Anti-inflammatory effects to reduce inflammation and swelling [10,11,12,13,14,15,16]
- ❧ Analgesic action to relieve pain [17,18,19,20]
- ❧ Diuretic action to promote normal urination [21,22,23,24,25]

CHINESE THERAPEUTIC ACTIONS

- ❧ Clears damp-heat in the lower *jiao*
- ❧ Clears damp-heat in the Liver, Gallbladder and Urinary Bladder channels
- ❧ Promotes diuresis
- ❧ Invigorates blood circulation in the lower *jiao*

DOSAGE

Take 3 to 4 capsules three times daily with warm water on an empty stomach. Dosage may be increased to 6 to 8 capsules three times daily, if necessary. This formula should be taken consistently for at least one to two weeks to ensure complete eradication of the pathogen(s) and to avoid stimulating possible bacterial and viral resistance. It is important to advise the patient not to discontinue the use of herbs prior to completion of the whole course of herbal treatment.

INGREDIENTS

Bian Xu (Herba Polygoni Avicularis)
Chai Hu (Radix Bupleuri)
Che Qian Zi (Semen Plantaginis)
Da Huang (Radix et Rhizoma Rhei)
Dang Gui (Radicis Angelicae Sinensis)
Deng Xin Cao (Medulla Junci)
Di Fu Zi (Fructus Kochiae)
Feng Wei Cao (Herba Pteris)
Gan Cao (Radix Glycyrrhizae)
Hong Hua (Flos Carthami)
Hua Shi (Talcum)
Huai Niu Xi (Radix Achyranthis Bidentatae)

Huang Qin (Radix Scutellariae)
Long Dan Cao (Radix Gentianae)
Pao Zai Cao (Herba Physalis Angulatae)
Qu Mai (Herba Dianthi)
Sheng Di Huang (Radix Rehmanniae)
Shui Ding Xiang (Herba Ludwigiae Prostratae)
Tao Ren (Semen Persicae)
Xian Feng Cao (Herba Bidentis)
Ya She Huang (Herba Lippiae)
Ze Xie (Rhizoma Alismatis)
Zhi Zi (Fructus Gardeniae)

V-Statin ™

FORMULA EXPLANATION

V-Statin addresses damp-heat in the lower *jiao* manifesting in vaginitis, cystitis, urinary tract infection, pelvic inflammatory disease, vaginal discharge, genital itching, male genital infection and pyelonephritis.

Long Dan Cao (Radix Gentianae) clears damp-heat from the Liver, a channel that travels through the genital region. *Zhi Zi* (Fructus Gardeniae), *Da Huang* (Radix et Rhizoma Rhei) and *Huang Qin* (Radix Scutellariae) all clear damp-heat and treat infection. They work synergistically to relieve symptoms such as foul yellow vaginal discharge, dysuria, genital itching and male genital infection. *Feng Wei Cao* (Herba Pteris), *Ya She Huang* (Herba Lippiae), and *Pao Zai Cao* (Herba Physalis Angulatae), indigenous herbs from Taiwan, are used to detoxify and reduce inflammation and infection of the genital organs. *Di Fu Zi* (Fructus Kochiae) clears heat and relieves genital itching.

Shui Ding Xiang (Herba Ludwigiae Prostratae) and *Xian Feng Cao* (Herba Bidentis) are very strong herbs used in Taiwan to treat infection of the urinary system such as cystitis, urinary tract infection, nephritis, pyelonephritis, dysuria, and turbid yellow urine. These herbs reduce inflammation, clear heat and promote diuresis.

Bian Xu (Herba Polygoni Avicularis), *Hua Shi* (Talcum), *Deng Xin Cao* (Medulla Junci), *Ze Xie* (Rhizoma Alismatis), *Che Qian Zi* (Semen Plantaginis), and *Qu Mai* (Herba Dianthi) dispel dampness in the lower *jiao* and promote urination. Together, they dispel water and treat *lin zheng* (dysuria syndrome). To prevent the diuretic herbs from draining too much fluid from the body, *Sheng Di Huang* (Radix Rehmanniae) and *Dang Gui* (Radicis Angelicae Sinensis) are added to nourish yin and blood.

Chai Hu (Radix Bupleuri) is a guiding herb to the Liver channel, which passes through the genital region. *Huai Niu Xi* (Radix Achyranthis Bidentatae), descending in nature, directs the overall effect of the formula downward to the lower *jiao*, and thus, to the genital region.

To enhance the overall efficacy of the formula, *Tao Ren* (Semen Persicae) and *Hong Hua* (Flos Carthami) are added to increase blood circulation to the lower *jiao*. Proper blood circulation increases delivery of herbs to the affected area and in exchange helps to flush out toxins in the blood. Finally, *Gan Cao* (Radix Glycyrrhizae) is used to harmonize the formula.

SUPPLEMENTARY FORMULAS

- To enhance the antibiotic effect to treat infection, use with **Herbal ABX**.
- For diabetes, use with **Equilibrium**.
- For chronic recurrent vaginitis, use with **Vitality**.
- For menopausal patients, use with **Balance (Heat)** or **Nourish**.
- For prostate disorders with burning urination, use with **Saw Palmetto Complex**.
- For patients who experience slight loose stools after taking **V-Statin,** combine with **GI Tonic**.
- To activate blood circulation throughout the entire body, add **Circulation (SJ)**.
- For signs and symptoms of excess fire, add **Gardenia Complex**.
- For bleeding, add **Notoginseng 9**.

NUTRITION

- Natural, plain yogurt with live culture helps to minimize yeast infection by establishing a normal environment in the genital tract.
- Eat plenty of fruits and vegetables, which provide the nutrients needed to resist infection and facilitate healing.
- Regular consumption of unsweetened cranberry juice will help to prevent and treat urinary tract infection.

FORMULAS

V-Statin ™

The Tao of Nutrition by Ni and McNease
- ❧ Candida yeast infection
  - Recommendations: dandelions, beet tops, carrot tops, barley, garlic, rice vinegar, mung beans, and citrus fruits.
  - Avoid sugar, excessive fruits, yeast-containing foods, processed foods, cheese, fermented foods, soy sauce, smoking, alcohol, and caffeine.
- ❧ Chronic bladder infections
  - Recommendations: watermelon, pears, carrots, celery, corn, mung beans, corn-silk, squash, wheat, water chestnuts, barley, red beans, millet, oranges, cantaloupe, grapes, strawberries, lotus roots, loquats, and plenty of water.
  - Avoid heavy proteins, meat, dairy products, onions, scallions, ginger, black pepper, and alcohol.
- ❧ For more information, please refer to *The Tao of Nutrition* by Dr. Maoshing Ni and Cathy McNease.

LIFESTYLE INSTRUCTIONS

- ❧ During the treatment period, avoid sexual intercourse to prevent further irritation or infection, and to prevent communicating the infection to one's partner.
- ❧ Substances that irritate the genital area should be avoided, such as spermicides, lubricants, condoms, diaphragms, cervical caps and contraceptive sponges. Select toilet tissue or feminine hygiene products that are not dyed, chlorine-bleached, or scented.
- ❧ Use hypo-allergenic or fragrance-free substances whenever possible, such as fabric softener, soap, laundry detergents, deodorant sprays, bathwater additives, shower gels, and related products.
- ❧ Candida cannot be killed with the normal washing and drying methods. Patients suffering from yeast infection can try to soak their underwear in bleach for 24 hours before washing them. Ironing may also be an alternative as candida is killed at high temperature.[30]
- ❧ Refrain from douching or the insertion of foreign objects in the vagina. In the case of severe itching, refrain from scratching or from *excessive* washing of the affected area.
- ❧ Wear loose clothing and refrain from wearing tight slacks, vinyl, or tight denim. Wear silk or cotton underwear for better ventilation. Avoid polyester, snug, nonporous or nonabsorbent underpants.
- ❧ Patients with urinary tract infections and cystitis should drink more water (more frequently) and urinate more often, to prevent pathogens from lingering in the urinary tract and bladder.

CLINICAL NOTES

- ❧ From a TCM perspective, *V-Statin* has a localized effect to treat damp-heat in the genital area. *Gentiana Complex* has a broader effect to treat damp-heat in the Liver and Gallbladder channel.
- ❧ The powder of *She Chuang Zi* (Fructus Cnidii) and *Ku Shen Gen* (Radix Sophorae Flavescentis) can be applied topically to relieve itching. Wash affected area thoroughly using a mild soap and apply 5 grams of each herb onto the external genitalia, leave for 3 to 5 minutes and rinse off. Repeat this procedure twice daily.
- ❧ Vaginitis tends to recur in women who have diabetes or have frequently taken antibiotics.
- ❧ When a woman has frequent recurrences of lower *jiao* infections, the male partner should also be checked for urethral discharge, penile lesions, other infections, past venereal disease or parasitic infection. It is best to simultaneously treat the male partner to prevent recurrences of vaginitis, urinary tract infection or cystitis.
- ❧ Patients who do not respond or improve after taking antibiotics or this formula consistently for two weeks usually have chronic vaginitis. They need to take *Kidney Tonic (Yang)* with *V-Statin* at a 1:2 or 1:3 ratio, respectively.
- ❧ Vaginitis is common in women during the menopausal phase, as hormonal changes may disturb the pH balance of the vagina, leading to infections.

FORMULAS

V-Statin ™

- ⚘ Women with vaginitis should be careful before, during and after menstruation as this is when they are most susceptible to infection. Patients should pay extra attention to personal hygiene.
- ⚘ Inflammation and infection of the reproductive organs may cause local swelling and obstruction, leading to infertility. This condition is similar to damp-heat in the lower *jiao* in traditional Chinese medicine.
- ⚘ Advise the patient to wipe from front to back after a bowel movement to avoid infection.
- ⚘ Patients should be advised to urinate after sexual intercourse to prevent bacteria from infecting the urethra to causing urinary tract infection.

Pulse Diagnosis by Dr. Jimmy Wei-Yen Chang:
- ⚘ Forceful, thick and long pulse on and proximal to the left *chi* position..
- ⚘ Note: Dr. Chang takes the pulse in slightly different positions. He places his index finger directly over the wrist crease, and his middle and ring fingers alongside to locate *cun*, *guan* and *chi* positions. For additional information and explanation, please refer to *Pulsynergy* by Dr. Jimmy Wei-Yen Chang and Marcus Brinkman.

CAUTIONS

- ⚘ This formula should be used with caution by patients with deficiency and cold of the Spleen and Stomach.
- ⚘ This formula is contraindicated during pregnancy and nursing.
- ⚘ Patients who are on anticoagulant or antiplatelet therapies, such as Coumadin (Warfarin), should use this formula with caution as there may be a slightly higher risk of bleeding and bruising.
- ⚘ This formula is contraindicated for long-term use. It should be discontinued when the desired effects are achieved.

ACUPUNCTURE POINTS

Traditional Points:
- ⚘ *Sanyinjiao* (SP 6), *Yinlingquan* (SP 9), *Qihaishu* (BL 24), *Shangliao* (BL 31), *Ciliao* (BL 32), *Zhongliao* (BL 33), *Xialiao* (BL 34), *Guanyuan* (CV 4), and *Sanjiaoshu* (BL 22).
- ⚘ *Zhongji* (CV 3), *Qugu* (CV 2), and *Sanyinjiao* (SP 6).

Balance Method by Dr. Richard Tan:
- ⚘ Left side: *Dadu* (SP 2), *Taibai* (SP 3), *Taixi* (KI 3), Dazhong (KI 4), *Taichong* (LR 3), *Hegu* (LI 4), and *Yangxi* (LI 5).
- ⚘ Right side: *Zhiyin* (BL 67), *Zuqiaoyin* (GB 44), *Daling* (PC 7), and *Lieque* (LU 7).
- ⚘ For additional information on the Balance Method, please refer to *Dr. Tan's Strategy of Twelve Magical Points* by Dr. Richard Tan.

MODERN RESEARCH

V-Statin is designed to treat infection and inflammation of the genito-urinary tract. Clinically, it addresses disorders such as vaginitis, pelvic inflammatory disease, urinary tract infection, cystitis, dysuria, pyelonephritis, and infertility in women due to inflammation and infection. Herbs in this formula have marked effectiveness to treat infection, reduce inflammation, promote normal urination, and alleviate related symptoms.

Many herbs in this formula have marked antibiotic properties, including both antibacterial and antiviral activities. This formula incorporates numerous herbs for two important reasons. First, the use of multiple herbs within an herbal formula has been shown to increase the antibiotic effect more than ten-folds. Second, isolated use of single ingredients is often ineffective and increases the risk of development of bacterial and viral resistance.[1] Given these two reasons, it is necessary to combine herbs with appropriate properties to ensure effectiveness in treating the

FORMULAS

V-Statin ™

infection and minimizing the potential risk of the micro-organisms developing resistance and/or mutation. Herbs with antibiotic properties include *Long Dan Cao* (Radix Gentianae), *Zhi Zi* (Fructus Gardeniae), *Da Huang* (Radix et Rhizoma Rhei), *Huang Qin* (Radix Scutellariae), *Bian Xu* (Herba Polygoni Avicularis), *Chai Hu* (Radix Bupleuri) and *Dang Gui* (Radicis Angelicae Sinensis).[2,3,4,5,6,7] In fact, some of these herbs have potent, wide-spectrum inhibitory effects against micro-organisms that are most often found to cause genito-urinary infections.[8] It has also been shown that in cases where standard antibiotics drugs are ineffective due to pathogenic resistance, the addition of *Huang Qin* (Radix Scutellariae) will restore the bacteriocidal and bacteriostatic activities of the antibiotic drugs.[9]

In addition to having antibiotic properties, many herbs have potent effects to reduce inflammation and relieve pain. The combination of these herbs significantly suppresses capillary permeability, reduces inflammation and swelling, and alleviates pain. Herbs with marked anti-inflammatory effects include *Huang Qin* (Radix Scutellariae), *Chai Hu* (Radix Bupleuri), *Huai Niu Xi* (Radix Achyranthis Bidentatae), *Tao Ren* (Semen Persicae), *Sheng Di Huang* (Radix Rehmanniae), *Dang Gui* (Radicis Angelicae Sinensis) and *Gan Cao* (Radix Glycyrrhizae).[10,11,12,13,14,15,16] Among the herbs having clearly-identified analgesic effects are *Dang Gui* (Radicis Angelicae Sinensis), *Da Huang* (Radix et Rhizoma Rhei), *Zhi Zi* (Fructus Gardeniae), and *Gan Cao* (Radix Glycyrrhizae).[17,18,19] In fact, it has been shown that Chinese herbs, such as *Dang Gui* (Radicis Angelicae Sinensis), are as potent as drugs in the relief of pain and reduction of inflammation. Research demonstrates that the anti-inflammatory effect of *Dang Gui* (Radicis Angelicae Sinensis) is approximately 1.1 times stronger than aspirin, and its analgesic properties are approximately 1.7 times stronger than aspirin.[20]

Many herbs in this formula promote normal urination to alleviate burning sensations and pain associated with infection and inflammation of the genito-urinary tract. Herbs with diuretic influence include *Long Dan Cao* (Radix Gentianae), *Bian Xu* (Herba Polygoni Avicularis), *Ze Xie* (Rhizoma Alismatis) and *Qu Mai* (Herba Dianthi).[21,22,23,24,25]

In addition to their general pharmacological effects, some herbs have specific influence against certain disorders. For example, the combination of *Hua Shi* (Talcum) and *Gan Cao* (Radix Glycyrrhizae) was effective in treating 10 patients with urinary tract infection, within three to four days.[26] In another study, 58 patients with dysuria were successfully treated with an herbal formula that contained *Long Dan Cao* (Radix Gentianae), *Dang Gui* (Radicis Angelicae Sinensis), *Chai Hu* (Radix Bupleuri), *Ze Xie* (Rhizoma Alismatis), *Zhi Zi* (Fructus Gardeniae), *Sheng Di Huang* (Radix Rehmanniae), and *Gan Cao* (Radix Glycyrrhizae).[27] For chronic nephritis, the daily administration of 60 grams of *Deng Xin Cao* (Medulla Junci) was associated with complete recovery within thirty days in 25 out of 30 patients.[28] Lastly, 33 patients with acute nephritis were treated by injection of a 20% *Dang Gui* (Radicis Angelicae Sinensis) solution to key acupuncture points once daily, with good results.[29]

PHARMACEUTICAL DRUGS & CHINESE MEDICINE: A COMPARATIVE ANALYSIS

Western Medical Approach: There are many disorders characterized by infection and inflammation of genital regions, including vaginitis, cystitis, pelvic inflammatory disease, urinary tract infection, and many others. In western medicine, these conditions are generally treated with antibiotic drugs, including antibacterial, antiviral and antifungal agents. As a category, these drugs are very effective to treat such infections and inflammations. However, these drugs are very potent, and may cause many side effects, such as secondary infection.

Traditional Chinese Medicine Approach: Herbal therapy is also very effective for treating these infections and inflammations. Many herbs have been shown to have marked antibacterial, antiviral and antifungal properties. Furthermore, some have analgesic effect to relieve pain, and others have diuretic effect to relieve dysuria. Lastly, though these herbs are generally safe, they should be discontinued once the desired effects are achieved, as extended use may consume and weaken the body.

FORMULAS

V-Statin ™

Summation: Drugs and herbs are both effective for treating infections and inflammations of genito-urinary systems. In general, drugs are more effective for bacterial and fungal infections, but their safety profiles vary depending on the exact antibiotic prescribed. Herbs are equally effective for bacterial, viral and fungal infections. For severe infections and inflammations, they are slightly less immediately potent than drugs, but are much safer and have significantly fewer side effects. Lastly, in both therapies, the chosen substance(s) should always be taken until the course of therapy is completed. Those who have weakness and deficiency from the infection and/or its treatment should take herbs to strengthen the body and facilitate recovery.

CASE STUDIES

A 27-year-old female clerk presented with bloating and inability to urinate. Pain and a burning sensation also followed upon urination. The color of her urine was yellow. She had a red tongue color with a dry tongue coating, which appeared yellow towards the base. Pulse analysis was rapid and rolling. A western diagnosis assessment of urinary tract infection (UTI) was concluded, with a TCM diagnosis of damp-heat in the lower *jiao*. The patient started urinating immediately after the treatment with *V-Statin*. Urinary tract infection was resolved within 10 days of continuous administration of *V-Statin*.

T.G., Albuquerque, New Mexico

J.H., an 83-year-old diabetic female, presented with a recent history of episodes of burning, painful, dribbling and frequent urination. The urgency and pressure woke her at night and she would have to get up to urinate several times between bedtime and morning. The patient reported that she has had bladder infections throughout her life but these were occuring more often than in the past. Her doctor was treating the infection with Cipro (Ciprofloxacin) and the client was tired of taking drugs and afraid of its side effects. Actual lab work was not available but the patient reported the urine analysis showed very high bacteria count in which the practitioner suspected *E coli*. Her blood pressure was 153/82 mmHg and heart rate was 80 beats per minute. The diagnosis was damp-heat in the lower *jiao*, specifically the Urinary Bladder. *V-Statin* was prescribed at 1 to 2 capsules twice daily. The patient began taking the herbs as soon as she finished the current prescription for Cipro (Ciprofloxacin). She was pleased to report that she had been symptom free and infection free for nearly 2 years of taking the prophylactic dose of the herbs. She stated that she certainly did not miss either the pain or the infection or the repeated rounds of antibiotics. The practitioner concluded that this is an excellent example of the successful use of an herbal formula as a preventative measure.

H.H., San Francisco, California

A 31-year-old female presented with a family history of chronic psoriasis, and outbreaks mainly on her elbows, knees and sacrum. She also suffered from vaginal itching and burning sensations. The TCM diagnosis was toxic damp-heat in the Liver. *V-Statin* and *Dermatrol (PS)* were prescribed. A topical wash, Yin Care, was prescribed for external application for the psoriasis and vaginally for local itching. The patient received acupuncture and herbal treatments for two years. She was advised to stop smoking, eat less spicy food, and refrain from alcohol intake, but was unable to change her lifestyle. Nonetheless, her condition continued to improve, and she noticed that if she did not take the herbs, the symptoms would return.

M.C., Sarasota, Florida

---

[1] *Zhong Yao Xue* (Chinese Herbology), 1988; 140:144
[2] *Zhong Yao Yao Li Yu Ying Yong* (Pharmacology and Applications of Chinese Herbs), 1983; 295
[3] *Zhong Yao Zhi* (Chinese Herbology Journal), 1984; 578
[4] *Zhong Yao Xue* (Chinese Herbology), 1988; 137:140
[5] *Yi Xue Xue Bao* (Report of Medicine), 1983; 18(9):700
[6] *Zhong Yao Xue* (Chinese Herbology), 1998; 103:106
[7] *Huo Xue Hua Yu Yan Jiu* (Research on Blood-Activating and Stasis-Eliminating Herbs), 1981; 335

FORMULAS

V-Statin ™

[8] *Zhong Yao Xue* (Chinese Herbology),1998; 251:256

[9] *J Pharm Pharmacol* 2000 Mar; 52(3):361-6

[10] *Chem Pharm Bull*, 1984; 32(7):2724

[11] *Zhong Yao Yao Li Yu Ying Yong* (Pharmacology and Applications of Chinese Herbs), 1983; 888

[12] *Zhong Yao Tong Bao* (Journal of Chinese Herbology), 1988; 13(7):43

[13] *Zhong Yao Tong Bao* (Journal of Chinese Herbology), 1986; 11(11):37

[14] *Zhong Yao Yao Li Yu Ying Yong* (Pharmacology and Applications of Chinese Herbs), 1983; 400

[15] *Xin Yi Yao Xue Za Zhi* (New Journal of Medicine and Herbology), 1975; (6):34

[16] *Zhong Cao Yao* (Chinese Herbal Medicine), 1991; 22(10):452

[17] *Si Chuan Zhong Yi* (Sichuan Chinese Medicine), 1988; 9:11

[18] *Shen Yang Yi Xue Yuan Xue Bao* (Journal of Shenyang University of Medicine), 1984; 1(3):214

[19] *Zhong Yao Xue* (Chinese Herbology),1998; 759:765

[20] *Yao Xue Za Zhi* (Journal of Medicinals), 1971; (91):1098

[21] *Zhong Yao Yao Li Yu Ying Yong* (Pharmacology and Applications of Chinese Herbs), 1983; 295

[22] *Chang Yong Zhong Yao Cheng Fen Yu Yao Li Shou Ce* (A Handbook of the Composition and Pharmacology of Common Chinese Drugs), 1994; 1665:1667

[23] *Sheng Yao Xue Za Zhi* (Journal of Raw Herbology), 1982; 36(2):150

[24] *Chang Yong Zhong Yao Xian Dai Yan Jiu Yu Lin Chuang* (Recent Study & Clinical Application of Common Traditional Chinese Medicine), 1995; 267:269

[25] *Zhong Yao Xue* (Chinese Herbology),1998; 353:354

[26] *Liao Ning Yi Yao* (Liaoning Medicine and Herbology), 1976; (2):69

[27] *Ji Lin Zhong Yi Yao* (Jilin Chinese Medicine and Herbology), 1991; (2):12

[28] *Fu Zhou Yi Yao* (Fuzhou Medicine and Medicinals), 1983; (3):30

[29] *Xin Yi Xue* (New Medicine), 1976; 6:294

[30] Gottlieb, W. *The Doctor's Book of Home Remedies*. 1990, p. 638

FORMULAS

Section 6

General Index

索引

GENERAL INDEX

Abdominal pain, 33
Abreva, 154
Abscess, 33, 487, 640
Absorption
  herb-drug interaction, 148
Abuse
  alcohol. *See* Addiction
  substance. *See* Addiction
Acamprosate, 160
Accolate, 154
Accupril, 154
Acetaminophen / Codeine, 185
Aches, 366. *See also* Pain
Acid reflux, 33, 430
Aciphex, 154
Acne, 33, 338
Acromioclavicular separation, 33
Actigall, 154
Actos, 154
Acutrim, 154
Acyclovir, 188
Adaptogenic effect
  Flex (MLT), 381
  Imperial Tonic, 505
  Kidney Tonic (Yang), 517
  Kidney Tonic (Yin), 521
  Schisandra ZZZ, 685
  Vibrant, 730
  Vital Essence, 735
ADD, 33, 283
Addiction, 34
  alcohol, 276
  detoxification, 535
  drug, 276
  smoking, 276
Addison's disease, 34
Adefovir, 170
ADHD, 33, 283
Adhesions, pelvic, 242
Adrenal insufficiency, 34, 196
Adrenoplex, 196
Advil, 154
Aging, 34
  premature, 92, 196
Agitation, 34
AIDS, 34
  immune, weakened, 498
Air pollution, 481
Albuterol, 180, 186
Alcohol

abuse. *See* Addiction
  hangover, 65
  liver cirrhosis, 535
Alefacept, 156
Alendronate, 169
Aleve, 155
Alfuzosin, 185
Allegra, 155
Allergy, 35
  nose, 635
  seasonal, 555
  skin, 698
Allopurinol, 188
Almotriptan, 158
Alopecia, 35
Alprazolam, 187
ALT, 38. *See also* SGPT, SGOT
Aluminum / Magnesium, 174, 176
Alupent, 155
Alzheimer's disease, 35, 592
Amantadine, 183
Ambien, 155
Amenorrhea, 35, 232, 311, 521, 560
Amevive, 156
Amitriptyline, 167
Amlodipine, 177
Amoxicillin, 156
Amoxicillin / Clavulanic Acid, 158
Amoxil, 156
Amphotericin B
  herb-drug interaction, 150
Ampicillin, 180
Analgesic effect
  Arm Support, 202
  Back Support (Acute), 207
  Back Support (HD), 222
  Back Support (Upper), 227
  Balance (Cold), 232
  Calm, 269
  Circulation (SJ), 311
  Corydalin, 325
  Dermatrol (HZ), 333
  Flex (CD), 366
  Flex (GT), 372
  Flex (Heat), 376
  Flex (MLT), 381
  Flex (NP), 385
  Flex (SC), 391
  Flex (Spur), 396
  Gardenia Complex, 401

GENERAL INDEX

GENERAL INDEX

GENERAL INDEX

GENERAL INDEX

GENERAL INDEX

GENERAL INDEX

GENERAL INDEX

GENERAL INDEX

Corticosterone, 739, 742
Cortisol, 739
Corydalin, 325
Cough, 50, 657, 674, 677
   chronic, 657
   frail, 668
   post-infective, 610
Coumadin
   herb-drug interaction, 149
Cramps, 50, 391
   menstrual, 82
Craving, 492
Crohn's disease, 50, 447, 459
Crying, 50
Cyclobenzaprine, 169
Cystitis, 51, 418, 744
   acute, 414
   chronic and recurrent, 605
Cysts, 50, 652
   lower body, 646
   upper body, 652
Dairy product intolerance, 51
Dalmane, 164
Damp, 138
Danazol, 164
Danocrine, 164
Darvocet, 164
Darvon, 164
Daypro, 164
Defense Level, 127
Defensive, Qi, Nutritive, Blood Differentiation, 127
Deficiency, 117
   blood, 119, 134
   heat, 116, 139
   qi, 118, 132
   yang, 118, 122
   yin, 117
Degeneration, 51
   knee, 530
   knee and ankle, 530
Degenerative disorder, 366, 508
Dehydration, 51
Delirium, 51
Demadex, 165
Dementia, 52, 356, 596
Denavir, 165
Dependence. *See* Addiction
Depression, 52, 692
   lupus, due to, 550
   postpartum, 685

Dermatitis, 52, 465, 698, 700
Dermatological disorder, 333, 338
Dermatrol (HZ), 333
Dermatrol (PS), 338
Desloratadine, 163
Detergents, 481
Detox, 52
Detoxification, 481. *See also* Detox
   alcohol, 535
   general, 481
   kidney, 511
   liver, 535
   smoking, 535
Dexedrine, 165
Dextroamphetamine, 165
Diabeta, 165
Diabetes, 53, 360, 517, 608
   neuropathy, 385
Diarrhea, 53, 436, 459, 517
   acute, 436
   blood, with, 447
   chronic, 447
   damp-heat, 436
   excess type, 436
   food poisoning, due to, 436
   infection, due to, 436
   mucus or blood, with, 436
   mucus, with, 447
   pus, with, 447
   traveler's, 105, 436
Diazepam, 185
Dicolfenac, 186
Didronel, 165
Diet, 53, 141
Diethylpropion, 183
Diflucan
   herb-drug interaction, 149
Diflunisal, 165
Digestive system, weak and deficient, 459
Dilantin, 165
   herb-drug interaction, 149
Diltiazem, 160
Dimetapp, 165
Diphenhydramine, 159, 182
Discharge, 54
   nasal, 555
   vaginal, 744
Disease
   Addison's, 34
   Alzheimer's, 35, 592

GENERAL INDEX

GENERAL INDEX

GENERAL INDEX

GENERAL INDEX

GENERAL INDEX

GENERAL INDEX

GENERAL INDEX

GENERAL INDEX

GENERAL INDEX

GENERAL INDEX

GENERAL INDEX

GENERAL INDEX

GENERAL INDEX

Respitrol (CF), 657
Respitrol (Cold), 662
Respitrol (Deficient), 668
Respitrol (Heat), 674
Restless leg syndrome, 95
Restlessness, 269, 283. *See also* Stress, ADD, ADHD
Restoril, 181
Retinitis, 418
Rheumatic heart disease, 311
Rheumatism. *See* Arthritis
Rheumatoid arthritis, 376. *See also* Arthritis
Rhinitis, 487, 555, 635. *See also* Sinusitis
   allergic, 320
   clear watery discharge, with, 555
   purulent yellow discharge, with, 635
Rhonchi, 668
Rib
   fracture, 227
   pain, 95, 227
Rifadin
   herb-drug interaction, 149
Rifampin
   herb-drug interaction, 149
Rifaximin, 187
Ringing of ears. *See* Tinnitus
Ritalin, 181
Robaxin, 182
Robitussin, 182
Rogaine, 182
Rosiglitazone, 158
Rotator cuff
   tendonitis/tear, 95
Runny nose. *See* Common cold
Sadness, 692. *See also* Depression
Saliva, drooling of, 55
Salivation, involuntary, 592
Salpingitis, 95
San Jiao Bian Zheng (Triple Burner Differentiation), 130
Satisfaction, lack of, 196
Saw Palmetto Complex, 680
Scabies, 96
Scalp, dry, 621
Scapular pain, 96, 227
Schisandra ZZZ, 685
Schizophrenia, 96, 276
Sciatica, 96, 215, 225, 517
   chronic, 366
   deficiency, with, 366
Scrofula, 96, 640

Scrotum, 96
   eczema, 744
   infection, 744
   itching, 744
Sedative effect
   Balance (Heat), 236
   Calm, 269
   Calm (ES), 276
   Calm ZZZ, 289
   Schisandra ZZZ, 685
Seizure, 96, 702
   children, in, 283
   hypertension, with, 408
Selegiline, 167
Semen. *See* Sexual dysfunction
Senna, 182
Senokot, 182
Sequelae, post-stroke, 702, 705
Sertraline, 188
Seven Emotions, 140
Sexual
   disorder, 517, 735, 739
   dysfunction, 96, 320, 521
   functions, diminished, 196
Sexually transmitted disease, 96
SGOT, 96
   elevated, 535
SGPT, 96
   elevated, 535
Shaoyang, 130
Shaoyin, 130
Shen (spirit), 144
Shi lin (stone dysuria), 349
Shin splints, 97
Shine, 692
Shingles, 97, 333
Shortness of breath. *See* Asthma, cough, dyspnea
Shoulder, 202
   acromioclavicular separation, 202
   bursitis, 202
   capsulitis, 45, 202
   frozen, 63, 202, 579
   inflammation and pain, 202, 579
   pain, 97
   pain, acute, 579
   pain, chronic, 586
   periarthritis, 202
   redness and swelling, with, 579
   rotator cuff tear, 202
   stiffness, 586

GENERAL INDEX

GENERAL INDEX

GENERAL INDEX

Section 7

Other Information

另外信息

Section 7

Other

Information

WWW.DrTanShow.COM

This website has the most current seminar schedule, books and Dr. Tan's forum.

Medical Board

- This forum is set up for people to discuss Chinese medical issues, especially for acupuncture and herbs related to Dr. Tan's balance method.

Wisdom Board

- For discussion of Chi Cultivation, Feng Shui and Ba Zi reading –
ancient Chinese fortune telling methods.

Open Topic

- This forum is posted for any other questions and issues that are not fall into the two main categories, such as: Chinese philosophy, playing bridge on Yahoo, etc.

QUOTES FROM DR. TAN'S STUDENTS

"He teaches people not only what to do but also how to think."

"Thank you Dr. Tan for the wonderful techniques you've shared. Your teaching continues to be a great source of inspiration for me in my practice."

"I think I speak for all acupuncturists when I say "thank you". You have enlightened us again and again with your knowledge and humor over the years."

"Sitting in his seminar feels like watching a fantastic show."

"His teaching completely changed my practice of Chinese medicine and changed my life a great deal."

"I love to visit Dr. Tan's website. The experience is like visiting a museum."

"Chi Initiation and Cultivation allowed me to discover within myself the treasure of daily self-healing."

"I never thought that the wisdom of a happier life could be so simple and practical."

"Being an acupuncturist you can not miss visiting the forum session on Dr. Tan's website (drtanshow.com)! It is so rich and valuable in terms of clinical experience and discussion!"

"Listening to his lecture in the retreat workshop makes us smile, laugh and cry. Everyone in my group felt tremendously inspired."

ORDER FORM (Books)

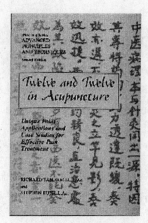

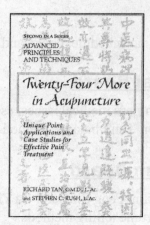

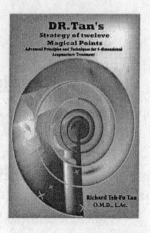

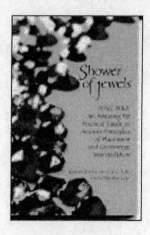

Twelve and Twelve in Acupuncture
by Richard Tan and Stephen Rush. The first of two books that describes the Balance Method of acupuncture.

Twenty-Four More in Acupuncture
by Richard Tan and Stephen Rush. The second of two books that describes the Balance Method of acupuncture.

Dr. Tan's Strategy of Twelve Magical Points
is a book on advanced principles and techniques in acupuncture. It is perfect for difficult disorders.

Shower of Jewels
by Richard Tan and Cheryl Warnke, helps to improve your environment and your life through *Feng Shui* - "the Art of Placement."

Qty	Title	Unit Price	Subtotal
	copies of *Twelve and Twelve in Acupuncture*	$ 25.00	
	copies of *Twenty Four More in Acupuncture*	$ 25.00	
	copies of *Dr. Tan's Strategy of Twelve Magic Points*	$ 24.00	
	copies of *Shower of Jewels*	$ 26.00	
	Sales Tax (8.25% for California Residents)		
	Shipping and Handling ($5.00 for up to 2 books)		
	Total Amount of Order		

Name _____

Address _____

City _____ State _____ Zip _____

Phone _____

Email Address: _____

[ ] Check Enclosed (payable to Dr. Richard Tan)

[ ] Charge my credit card (Visa or MasterCard only)

Card No. _____ Exp _____

Signature: _____

Please allow one to two weeks for delivery. Thank you for your order.

You May Purchase the Books By Phone, Fax, Mail, Or on Dr. Tan's website:

Dr. Richard Tan, D.O.M., L.Ac.
4550 Kearny Villa Rd., Ste 107
San Diego, CA 92123

Tel: (858) 277-1421
Fax: (858) 277-9037
www.drtanshow.com

ORDER FORM (Books)

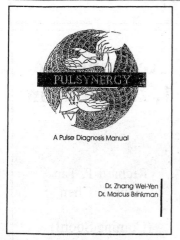

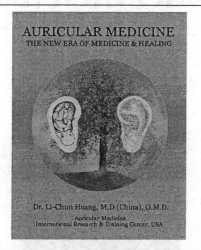

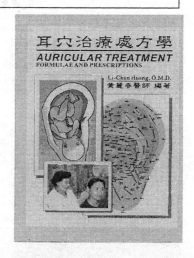

Pulsynergy

by Dr. Jimmy Wei-Yen Zhang (Chang) and Marcus Brinkman. This is a revolutionary book that enables practitioners to gain valuable insights on differential diagnosis based on pulse. Dr. Chang discusses in this text many unique pulse patterns associated with modern disorders that have never been discussed in the history of traditional Chinese medicine. It is one of the best books for both students and practitioners who wish to gain keen insight on pulse diagnosis.

Auricular Medicine,

Second Edition by Dr. Li-Chun Huang is by far the most complete textbook on Auricular Medicine. Dr. Huang revised the textbook from its first edition and added many new research results and new experiences. It covers all aspects of Auricular Medicine, including Auricular Diagnosis and Auricular Treatment. It is the best book for both study and reference of Auricular Medicine and also a very good reference book for acupuncturists.

Auricular Treatment

Formulas and Prescription by Dr. Li-Chun Huang. This book focuses on Auricular Treatment. It covers the theories and methods of Auricular Treatment. It includes many prescriptions for different diseases, which have been proved to be efficient by Dr. Li-Chun Huang through her 35 years of practice.

Qty	Title	Unit Price	Subtotal
	copies of *Pulsynergy*	$ 25.00	
	copies of *Auricular Medicine*	$ 115.00	
	copies of *Auricular Treatment*	$ 70.00	
	Sales Tax (8.25% for California Residents)		
	Shipping and Handling ($2.00 for the Clinical Manual set and $6 each for all other books)		
	Total Amount of Order		

Name _____   [ ] Check Enclosed (Payable to Lotus Institute)

Address _____   [ ] Charge my credit card (Visa or MasterCard only)

City _____ State ____ Zip _____   Card No. _____ Exp _____

Phone _____   Signature: _____

You May Purchase the Books By Phone, Fax, Mail, Website or E-Mail:

Lotus Institute of Integrative Medicine
PO Box 92493
City of Industry, CA 91715

Tel: (866) 90-Lotus; (626) 780-7182
Fax: (626) 609-2929
E-Mail: info@elotus.org
Website: www.elotus.org

ORDER FORM (Books)

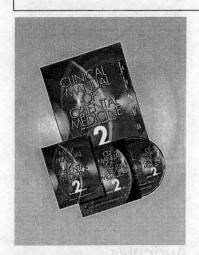

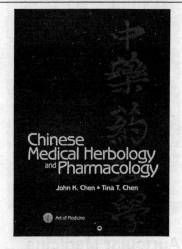

Acupuncture 1, 2, 3 for Pain

by

Richard T. Tan
Tina T. Chen

(Coming Soon!)

Clinical Manual of Oriental Medicine 2 –

Clinical Manual of Oriental Medicine, 2nd Ed.
Every feature complete in book format. More than 500 symptoms indexed, 350 drugs correlated and 99 herbal formulas discussed in-depth

CDManual of Oriental Med, V.2
Full electronic version for instant reference, search and/or printing ease.

MiniManual of Oriental Med, 2nd Ed.
Formula ingredients and functions and acupuncture points in a pocket manual.

Chinese Medical Herbology & Pharmacology

by Dr. John and Tina Chen is one of the most comprehensive and authoritative texts on Chinese Herbal Medicine. Contents include detailed descriptions
of Oriental medicine, western science, and safety data, It contains 670 in-depth herb monographs and 1150 illustrations (color and black-and-white photographs, classic line drawings, and chemical structure diagrams).

Acupuncture 1, 2, 3 for Pain

by Richard Tan and Tina Chen is a book that is focused on the treatment of pain. Full of illustration, this text makes acupuncture as easy as 1, 2, 3.

Qty	Title	Unit Price	Subtotal
	Sets of *Clinical, Mini and CD Manual of Oriental Medicine: Free when you attend any of our seminars*	$ 50.00	
	copies of *Chinese Medical Herbology and Pharmacology*	$ 89.95	
	copies of *Acupuncture 1,2,3 for Pain*	$ 25.00	
	Sales Tax (8.25% for California Residents)		
	Shipping and Handling ($2.00 for the Clinical Manual set and $6 each for all other books)		
	Total Amount of Order		

Name _____   [ ] Check Enclosed (Payable to Lotus Institute)

Address _____   [ ] Charge my credit card (Visa or MasterCard only)

City _____ State _____ Zip _____ Card No. _____ Exp _____

Phone _____   Signature: _____

You May Purchase the Books By Phone, Fax, Mail, Website or E-Mail:

Lotus Institute of Integrative Medicine
PO Box 92493
City of Industry, CA 91715

Tel: (866) 90-Lotus; (626) 780-7182
Fax: (626) 609-2929
E-Mail: info@elotus.org
Website: www.elotus.org